HANDBOOK OF
Religion and Health

Harold G. Koenig, M.D.
Michael E. McCullough, Ph.D.
David B. Larson, M.D.

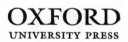

OXFORD
UNIVERSITY PRESS

2001

OXFORD
UNIVERSITY PRESS

Oxford   New York

Athens   Auckland   Bangkok   Bogotá   Buenos Aires   Calcutta
Cape Town   Chennai   Dar es Salaam   Delhi   Florence   Hong Kong   Istanbul
Karachi   Kuala Lumpur   Madrid   Melbourne   Mexico City   Mumbai
Nairobi   Paris   São Paulo   Shanghai   Singapore   Taipei   Tokyo   Toronto   Warsaw
and associated companies in
Berlin   Ibadan

Library of Congress Cataloging-in-Publication Data
Koenig, Harold George.
Handbook of religion and health
Harold G. Koenig, Michael E. McCullough, David B. Larson.
p. cm.
Includes bibliographical references and index.
ISBN 0-19-511866-9
1. Health—Religious aspects.   I. McCullough, Michael E.
II. Larson, David B., 1947– .   III. Title.
BL65.M4 K646   2000
291.1′78321—dc21   99-054710

1   3   5   7   9   8   6   4   2
Printed in the United States of America
on acid-free paper

SIR JOHN TEMPLETON

Foreword

THE PUBLICATION OF THE *Handbook of Religion and Health* is a signal achievement in the history of medicine. For the first time, in one place, empirical research findings that support the existence of a protective or preventive effect of religious involvement are comprehensively reviewed and critiqued. As those of us who have labored in this field for many years have long suspected, the relationship between religion and health, on average and at the population level, is overwhelmingly positive. Now we can say, finally, that we know this to be true.

The publication of the *Handbook of Religion and Health* is also personally gratifying to me. When I began conducting epidemiologic research and writing reviews in this area nearly two decades ago, my mentors and colleagues told me repeatedly that I was wasting my time. My idea of establishing the "epidemiology of religion" as a field of study, they assured me,

was misguided and, quite frankly, ridiculous. They implored me to find some other, more "acceptable" area of epidemiology, instead of wasting my time investigating the health effects of religiousness. I might have given up were it not for my joyous discovery of two other fellow researchers also foolish enough to be "wasting" their careers in the same pursuit.

Those brave and reckless souls were Drs. Harold Koenig and Dave Larson, two of the authors of this book. Somehow, serendipitously (or, perhaps, miraculously), the three of us had stumbled simultaneously onto this crazy notion that the spiritual lives of human beings might have something to say about their physical, mental, and emotional well-being. To our great surprise, we each discovered that scores and scores of studies had actually been published on this topic over the past several decades. Yet, hardly anyone seemed to notice, or care. It is not overdramatizing things in the least to note that there was a time about fifteen years ago when those of us actively investigating the linkages between religion and health could have fit around a single conference table. A very small one.

Today, the epidemiology of religion and the larger field of clinical research on religion and spirituality are well established in the scientific world and in the public consciousness. The U.S. National Institutes of Health has convened invited conferences, established expert working groups, and funded considerable empirical research in this area, beginning with a study of mine a decade ago. Prestigious scientific societies, including the American Academy for the Advancement of Science, the American Public Health Association, the American Psychological Association, and the Gerontological Society of America, have sponsored special symposia on religion and health. Private foundations, such as Templeton, RWJ (Robert Wood Johnson), and Fetzer, have generously funded research initiatives. Invited commentaries have appeared in mainstream medical journals such as *JAMA*. Cover stories have appeared in popular magazines like *Time* and *Macleans* as well as in feature stories on all the major broadcast networks and in other outlets ranging from National Public Radio to the Christian Broadcasting Network. What has caused this sudden explosion of attention?

As a working scientist, I would like to believe that this recent high visibility of the religion and health field is the result of the tireless efforts of the now many epidemiologists and social and behavioral scientists who are conducting research and publishing in this area. But that explanation does not suffice. That this field is now indeed a full-blown *field* is due in very large part to the herculean efforts of the authors of the *Handbook of Religion and Health*.

Dr. Koenig, a physician and a professor at Duke University, has devoted his career to advancing the understanding of the clinical correlates and applications of the spiritual lives of patients. He has published far more on this topic than anyone else in the entire religion and health field and is almost alone in considering religion as a resource for promoting recovery from illness, not just prevention of morbidity

and mortality. Dr. Larson, a physician and epidemiologist, gave up successful careers in both academic medicine and government service to establish the National Institute for Healthcare Research (NIHR), a Washington-based think tank dedicated to promoting research and education on the interconnections of religion and health. Currently, more than two-thirds of all U.S. medical schools include coursework or lectures on the topic of religion and spirituality. This incredible sea change in medical education is the result almost entirely of the vision and efforts of Dr. Larson. The third coauthor, Dr. Mike McCullough, a prolific young psychologist, is the director of research at NIHR and is quickly becoming the leading expert on the scope of published research in this field.

I can think of no other team of medical scientists more equipped to have written the *Handbook of Religion and Health*. Two features of this book particularly stand out: its mind-boggling comprehensiveness and its evenhandedness. Drs. Koenig, McCullough, and Larson are no mere evangelists. They are fair-minded in their presentation of existing findings; they let the data speak for themselves. The result, as this book shows, will give skeptics pause and debunkers fits. More important, this book provides an indispensable resource for medical care providers, health professions students, and researchers eager to explore this field but unsure where to begin.

The body-mind revolution in biomedical science several decades ago radically transformed the clinical practice of medicine and changed the direction of medical education and research. The *Handbook of Religion and Health* heralds the arrival of a newer and broader body-mind-spirit perspective that promises to transform medicine and medical research just as radically. At long last, the much awaited "new paradigm" has come, and the *Handbook of Religion and Health* is its definitive sourcebook.

Jeff Levin, Ph.D., M.P.H.

Dr. Levin is the author of *God, Faith, and Health*, editor of *Religion in Aging and Health*, and coeditor of *Essentials of Complementary and Alternative Medicine*.

Preface

IN THE *Handbook of Religion and Health* we review and discuss research that has examined the relationships between religion and a variety of mental and physical health conditions. This analysis is critical, comprehensive, and systematic; it includes more than 1,200 studies and 400 research reviews conducted during the twentieth century. We examine both the positive and the negative "effects" of religion on health across the life span from childhood to adolescence, from young adulthood to middle age, and from later life to end of life. On the basis of this research, we develop comprehensive theoretical models grounded on known behavioral, psychological, social, and physiological mechanisms to help explain how religion might influence health. We also review research that explores the association between religious involvement and use of health services and research that examines the role of religion in disease prevention and treatment compliance. We discuss the relevance of the findings to health and religious professionals and make recommendations for future research. We conclude with an overview of methods and measures for conducting such research.

As we enter the third millennium, the *Handbook of Religion and Health* lays a foundation for the emergence of a new way of practicing medicine that considers the body, mind, and spirit. According to Michael Novak, in a *New York Times* op-ed piece (May 24, 1998), the twenty-first century will be "the most religious century" in recent times. In that article, Novak quotes Norman Mailer as saying, "Religion, to me, is now the last frontier." Whether or not religion is the last frontier, the relationship between religion and health is certainly a new and sometimes puzzling frontier for medical researchers, health professionals, and religious professionals today. In the chapters ahead, we hope to put some of the pieces of this puzzle into place.

Durham, North Carolina   *H. G. K.*
March 2000

Contents

HANDBOOK OF RELIGION AND HEALTH

Introduction

ALTHOUGH CHAPTER 2 PRO-
vides a more detailed history of the
precarious and turbulent 8,000-year
relationship among religion, science,
and medicine, a brief overview will help set the
stage for this book. Over the years, the discussion of whether religion has negative, neutral,
or positive effects on health has been characterized by controversy. For centuries the religious
establishment regulated and controlled science,
medicine, and health care. This control was so
complete in the Middle Ages that the church
was the official body that issued medical licenses
to physicians, and many practitioners in those
days (particularly those who served the general
population) were monks or priests. Even the
nursing profession originally emerged from
religious orders devoted to caring for the
sick. Religious orders were also responsible
for building and staffing the first medical hospitals almost 1,700 years ago, and many of the

first hospitals that provided compassionate care
("moral treatment") to the mentally ill, particularly in the United States, were built and run
by religious groups such as the Quakers.

On the other hand, for thousands of years it
was believed that physical and mental disorders
resulted from demon possession or other spiritual forces and therefore must be dealt with in
spiritual terms. In recent history, such views
culminated in 1487 with the publication of *Malleus Maleficarum*, which officially sanctioned the
persecution and burning of witches, many of
whom had chronic mental illness or were suffering from acute psychosis caused by eating
moldy bread (ergotism). The Inquisition, as it
was called, lasted for more than 200 years; the
last "witch" was decapitated in 1782 (Zilboorg &
Henry, 1941).

Over the past 500 years the church's power
has declined and the influence of medical science has increased, allowing the latter to break

3

free from the church's control and domination. The schism between religion and medicine has continued to widen. Within the past few years, however, there has been a resurgence of interest in a new rapprochement between these healing traditions, and even discussion about the role that religion can play in improving health and the quality of health care.

REASONS FOR CURRENT INTEREST

Why such renewed interest by researchers and clinical practitioners in patients' religious beliefs and practices, areas that have traditionally been considered off limits because they were either too personal or irrelevant to health? There are several reasons. First is the role that religion continues to play in the lives of many people despite tremendous advances in education, psychology, and medicine. With such scientific progress, one might think that religious beliefs and practices should be declining and that the secularization of our society would be nearly complete by now. But this has not occurred.

In 1994, 96% of the population of the United States believed in God or a higher power, 90% believed in heaven, 79% believed in miracles, 73% believed in hell, and 65% believed in the devil (Princeton Religion Research Center, 1996). More than half of Americans (55%) believed that the Bible is the literal or inspired word of God. Not only are religious beliefs widespread, but also public and private religious practices remain the norm. In 1995, 43% of Americans reported that they had attended church or synagogue within the past seven days; 90% said they prayed, often several times per day; and 80% read the Bible. Many of these religious beliefs and practices relate to mental or physical health in one way or another and therefore have the potential to impact health, health beliefs, or health behaviors.

A second reason for the growing interest in religion's relationship to health comes from recent demographic and economic trends. An explosion of births after World War II (76 million babies born between 1945 and 1967), ad-

vances in medical science that have improved survival rates in both infancy and old age, and a declining birth rate in recent decades have resulted in a U.S. population that is rapidly aging. Social programs that provide health care (Medicare) and economic support (Social Security) for aging Americans are increasingly being threatened by rising costs. Between 1980 and 1998, the Medicare budget increased from $38 billion to more than $200 billion; by the year 2007, it will exceed $400 billion. Total health care expenditures in the United States are expected to rise to $2.1 trillion in 2007 from $1.1 trillion in 1998 (Smith, Freeland, et al. 1998). And this swelling of health care costs will have occurred before the United States experiences the greatest increase in the number of older persons (with attendant health problems) it has ever known: By the year 2040, almost 25% of Americans will be over age 65 (more than 70 million people—twice the number of older adults alive in 2000).

The United States is not alone in having a rapidly aging population and growing financial concerns about how to meet the economic and health care needs of its citizens. In the years ahead, many people around the world will slip through the ever-widening cracks in government-sponsored health programs, requiring that other resources be found to fill these gaps. Given their philosophy and their tradition of caring for downtrodden, needy, vulnerable members of society and their long history of involvement in health ministries, religious bodies may be of particular help in the growing health care crisis (Gatz & Smyer, 1992; Koenig, George, & Schneider, 1994; Schneider 1999). Even more exciting is the possibility that devout religious belief and practice might help prevent the development of health problems and/or speed their resolution, reducing or obviating the need for expensive health services. Anticipating future problems with health care financing, the United States Public Health Service has for the past decade focused on health promotion and disease prevention (*Healthy People 2000*, 1991).

A third reason for the renewed interest in religion and spirituality is the changing face of medicine, which has created disillusionment over the cost and the impersonal, routinized nature of modern health care; the number of medical mistakes and complications; and the side effects of drugs and other medical treatments. Medical education is heading toward a bimodal split between providing doctors with the high-technology/analytic/reductive skills required for diagnosing and treating physical diseases and the exact antithesis—training doctors to help persons to alter their lifestyles, to prevent disease, and to be sensitive to social, psychological, and spiritual factors in the lives of patients. The training necessary to deal with one type of problem seems the exact opposite of that needed for dealing with the other type of problem. Patients are caught in the middle, wishing to have their diseases diagnosed and treated competently and with the latest technology, yet having social, psychological, and spiritual needs that are being ignored because of an increasingly streamlined health care system that overemphasizes the physical over the spiritual.

Medical school selection processes and training create doctors who are likely to have difficulty handling nonreductive categories of social and spiritual disease. Consequently, many physicians are uncomfortable with the "humanness" of patients, whereas many patients are profoundly uncomfortable with the absence of a humane and/or spiritual aspect to their care. Scientific medicine has been magnificently successful but is challenged to figure out how the ancient and venerable tradition of "doctor as healer" fits in and how to connect practically at the bedside with the way most human beings deal psychologically with life-threatening disease, which is broadly spiritual/religious. This leaves a large vacuum to fill—a vacuum that has created a demand for psychosocial-spiritual care that is not being met by traditional sources, but has opened the door to a whole host of charlatans and alternative medicine practitioners (Eisenberg, Davis, et al. 1998; Relman, 1998; Angell & Kassirer, 1999).

The renewed focus by medical professionals on religion and health has also stimulated much public and media interest that has sensational-ized the topic. Associated Press articles have appeared in newspapers around the country with titles such as "Doctors Find Attending Church Good for the Body" (Associated Press, 1996). Popular magazines—including *Time, Reader's Digest, Prevention,* and *McCall's*—regularly run cover stories with the headlines such as "Faith and Healing" (Wallis, 1996), "Doctors Report: Faith *Can* Heal You" (McConnell, 1998), "Add Years to Your Life: Unlock the Secret Healer Within" (Michaud, 1998), "How Faith Keeps You Well" (Williams, 1998), and similar glamorous titles. Major television networks have produced special reports such as "Religion and the Power of Prayer to Heal the Sick" (Weymeyer, 1995) and NPR radio has aired programs such as "Religion and Health in the Elderly" (Schmelzer, 1994). While many of these articles and programs are inspiring and thought provoking, where does the serious academician or interested layperson turn if she or he wants to learn more about the research on which such claims are based? With few exceptions, most published research reviews of the religion-health relationship have focused on the positive findings and seldom mention the studies in which either no association or even a negative relationship was found.

From a scientific perspective, the question of religion's effects on health is an important one that has not yet been fully answered. Well-respected health professionals on both sides of the debate articulately and passionately plead their case. Do religious beliefs and activities really keep one mentally or physically healthier and reduce mortality, as some claim? If so, this finding has major implications for a struggling health care system. If these beliefs and behaviors have no effect on health, then this, too, is important information. On the other hand, if religious doctrines and practices have negative or adverse influences on mental or physical health (Watters, 1992), then perhaps religion should be considered neither a resource nor an ally. If religion is inimical to health, then government support of religious institutions (through tax breaks and other means) should be reconsidered for public health reasons, and perhaps religious beliefs and practices should be discouraged by health care providers, the media, and others.

IDENTIFYING THE RESEARCH

In this book, we review research conducted during the twentieth century that has examined associations between religion and a wide range of health outcomes and behaviors. To identify the research, we employed a combination of three strategies. First, we used computer literature searches (Medline, Current Contents, Psychlit, Soclit, HealthStar, Cancerlit, CINAHL, and others) to systematically identify quantitative studies that have examined the religion/spirituality-health relationship. These computer searches, however, go back only as far as the middle 1960s. Thus, after retrieving the articles identified by the computer searches, we consulted the footnotes and references in these papers to identify relevant studies that were not detected by the computer search; these studies were then retrieved and the process repeated until no new studies could be found. Finally, in order to identify studies not located by these methods, we examined articles and books that have reviewed research on the topic. In this manner, we located more than 1,600 studies and reviews that examine the religion-health relationship (see part VIII).

EVALUATING THE RESEARCH

After identifying the relevant research, we summarize and discuss the studies retrieved and then develop comprehensive conceptual models to illustrate the mechanisms by which religion can influence health, and vice versa. The approach used to evaluate studies focuses on research design, statistical analysis, and interpretation of results. Studies that identify subjects through systematic, random, or probability sampling provide the most generalizable results. Likewise, studies that use appropriate statistical tests that control for relevant confounders and take into account measurement error are given more weight. This does not mean, however, that studies that employ non-

random samples or that do not control for relevant covariates provide no useful information; it means only that results from the first group of studies are more reliable.

The most powerful data are those obtained from randomized clinical trials (first-level evidence); the next most powerful evidence is gathered from prospective cohort studies (second-level); the third level of evidence is obtained from cross-sectional studies; finally, data from a case series or a single case report provide the weakest, fourth-and-fifth-levels of evidence. Because of the newness of this field and the ethical issues involved in double-blinded controlled trials of religious interventions on health, studies that provide first-level evidence are relatively few. By far, most of the research in this area involves third-level evidence—data from cross-sectional studies. A number of well-designed prospective cohort studies also exist that provide second-level evidence. Although we review studies that provide all levels of evidence, special emphasis is given to results from prospective cohort studies and, to the extent that they are available, from clinical trials.

To give the reader a sense of the quality of studies reviewed, we assigned a quality score ranging from 0 to 10 to each study (see part VIII). A score of 0 indicates poor quality, and a score of 10 indicates high quality. The quality scores are based on a review of the methods and the results sections of each paper. When assigning scores, following a procedure described by Cooper (1984), we took into consideration the overall study design (e.g., clinical trial, prospective cohort, cross-sectional), the sampling method (random, systematic, or convenience), quality and number of religious measures, quality of outcome measure, inclusion of control variables, and interpretation of results.

To obtain a sense of how reliable we were in assigning these scores, we compared our scores on 76 studies with scores independently assigned to those studies by an outside reviewer (Andrew Futterman, Ph.D., associate professor of psychology at the College of the Holy Cross and a scientist who is both familiar with our scoring criteria and active in this field of research). The rating for one study (Byrd, 1988) was excluded from this analysis because of the controversial and somewhat unique nature of this report and the difficulty we had in coming to a consensus on the quality of the study's methodology. For the remaining 75 studies, scores assigned on a 0 to 10 scale by the authors and the blinded outside reviewer were compared. Continuous scores were moderately correlated with each other (Pearson $r = .57$).

Since we used scores to differentiate higher (7–10) from lower (0–6) quality studies, we also examined agreement with respect to this categorization. Scores were dichotomized into these two groups and compared. The kappa of agreement (κ) between the authors' and the outside reviewer's scores was 0.49 (where κs of 0.40 to 0.75 indicate good agreement, according to Landis & Koch, 1977). More specifically, there was 75% overall agreement in category assignments (56 of 75 studies).

GENERALIZABILITY OF RESEARCH RESULTS

Most of the studies reviewed here include subjects living in the United States, Europe, or Israel who are from traditional Christian or Jewish backgrounds. In order to determine whether results from this research generalize more broadly, we have made every effort to include studies that examine the religion-health intersection in Muslims, Hindus, and Buddhists and in members of other world religions. Unfortunately, research on health outcomes in these religious groups is relatively rare and can be difficult to access and, at times, hard to interpret, particularly when subjects are studied outside their natural environment and culture.

ORGANIZATION OF CHAPTERS

The results of this review are summarized and discussed in separate chapters for each health condition. Chapters typically begin with some background about the health topic, including information about definition or classification of the condition, impact on public health, and biological, psychological, social, and behavioral correlates. This is usually followed by a discus-

sion of why religion might relate to the health condition of interest and then by a brief description of each of the studies that have examined the relationship. We review as many of the studies as possible, including "positive studies" (religion positively related to health outcome), "no association studies" (religion unrelated to health outcome), and "negative association studies" (religion negatively related to health outcome). The better studies, however, are emphasized and their results given priority in the discussions. Each chapter ends with a summary of the findings and brief statement about conclusions. Although our review focuses primarily on published research, we also include unpublished or preliminary research findings when available.

OVERVIEW OF CONTENTS

The contents of this book are divided into seven major units. In part I, we define and distinguish the terms "religion" and "spirituality" and examine their many dimensions. We then present a detailed outline of the colorful history of religion, science, and medicine as they have evolved and interacted during the past 8,000 years. In part II, we first examine popular notions concerning the positive effects of religious involvement on health. Included here are references to religious scriptures, the writings of clergy, the claims of faith healers and popular writers, the opinions of religious health professionals, and the views of a few leaders in the fields of psychology and medicine who see religion/spirituality as having an influence on health. We then examine the skeptical side, exploring how religion may negatively affect health. Included here are the opinions of Freud, Ellis, Watters, and other distinguished health professionals, as well as reports of negative health outcome associated with religious belief. In the final chapter of this part, we reveal what patients with serious health problems say about the role that religion plays in helping them cope with illness. These largely subjective and superficial discussions set the stage for our more objective review of clinical and epidemiological literature in the chapters to follow.

In part III, we focus on research that examines religious involvement and mental health. Religion's associations with positive mental states (well-being, life satisfaction, happiness) and negative mental states (depression and suicide, anxiety, chronic psychosis, and substance abuse) are explored. We also review religion's relationships to delinquency and crime, marital stability and happiness, and personality traits relevant to health (anger and hostility, hope and optimism, locus of control). The review includes studies in the young, the old, the healthy, the sick, prisoners, African Americans, Mexican-Americans, mainline Protestants, Pentecostals, Catholics, Jews, Muslims, Hindus, and other populations. We discuss studies that use religious beliefs and behaviors in the therapy of patients with depression and anxiety disorders and review the effects of devout religious commitment on the speed of recovery from depression and other psychiatric disorders. On the basis of this research, we develop a hypothetical causal model to illustrate biological, psychological, and social pathways by which effects might be mediated.

The chapter on religion and well-being explores relationships between religious beliefs and practices and positive mental states such as happiness and life satisfaction. This chapter is different from the chapters to follow, which are concerned primarily with negative mental states. Here we examine whether devout religiousness and active participation in the religious community are associated with positive mood, joy, fulfillment, and living a full life.

In the chapter on depression, we review studies that explore whether religion prevents or speeds recovery from depression. This research includes both cross-sectional studies that focuses on associations between religious variables and depressive symptoms at one point in time and prospective cohort studies that examine religious involvement as a predictor of future depression (or absence thereof). We review studies that examine recovery from depression and thus how religiousness affects prognosis. We also compare the efficacy of religious and secular psychotherapy for depression. We devote an entire chapter to religious involvement and suicide, the most feared consequence of severe depression.

In the chapter on religion and anxiety, we review studies of religious involvement and symptoms of fear/anxiety, as well as associations with clinical conditions such as obsessive-compulsive disorder, panic disorder, generalized anxiety disorder, and posttraumatic stress disorder. Mental health professionals have long maintained that these conditions (the neuroses) are far more common among religious than nonreligious persons because of the former's lack of flexibility, closed-mindedness, and repression of normal sexual and aggressive drives. We review the results of large epidemiological studies that have now objectively examined the truth of this claim.

The chapter on religion and psychosis is an important one in which we explore relationships between religious beliefs and delusional disorder, schizophrenia, psychotic depression, and mania. Between 10% and 54% of psychotic disorders are accompanied by bizarre religious delusions and preoccupations—the manic individual who believes he is Jesus Christ, the delusionally depressed patient who is convinced that he or she has committed the unpardonable sin, the schizophrenic patient who insists that his or her roommate is the Devil. We examine whether religion causes or exacerbates such disorders, results from these disorders, or is turned to as a source of comfort or hope by sufferers.

In the chapter on substance abuse, we examine associations between religious involvement and the abuse of alcohol or recreational drugs. We study the relationships between alcohol abuse and frequency of church attendance, prayer, scripture reading, "born-again" status, and religious denomination and look at age differences as they affect these relationships. We also review studies on the influence of religious background and activity on use of marijuana, cocaine, and other illicit drugs by teenagers and younger adults. Finally, we examine the role of Alcoholics Anonymous, Al-Anon, and Narcotics Anonymous in the treatment and rehabilitation of persons with substance abuse problems, as well as the role that religion plays in these programs.

The chapters on juvenile delinquency, marital stability, and health-related personality traits (hostility, optimism/hope, sense of control) round out the section on mental health. Is religion really irrelevant to delinquent behavior in youth, as investigators in the 1970s maintained? Is there a link between religion and delinquency in adolescence? What is the relationship with adult criminal activities? Do religious beliefs, activities, and commitment deter such behaviors, and why might they do so (or not)?

Next, we examine whether religion fosters or hinders the development of stable, satisfying marriages. While religious beliefs can prevent separation or divorce, they may also promote unhappiness and dissatisfaction for persons who find themselves trapped in cold and sterile relationships. Do religious persons report that their marriages are happier than they really are in order to conform to social expectations? In the chapter on personality, we examine whether religious persons are less hostile, more optimistic, and more likely to experience a sense of control over their lives. While clergy make such pronouncements regularly from pulpits across the country, to what extent are these claims backed by objective research? In the final chapter of part III we describe how religion, through a web of complex mechanisms that extend from childhood to old age, is capable of influencing mental health.

In part IV, we focus on physical disorders, exploring relationships between religion and heart disease, hypertension, stroke, immune system dysfunction, cancer, mortality, physical disability, pain, somatic symptoms, and health behaviors (e.g., smoking, diet, weight control, exercise). At the conclusion of this section, we develop a causal model to help explain how religion might influence physical health.

In the chapter on religion and heart disease, we explore associations between coronary heart disease (CHD) and religious affiliation, religious orthodoxy, frequency of church attendance, dependence on religion for strength, and other indicators of religiousness. Included here are large epidemiological studies of thousands of persons followed for more than a quarter of a century, from midlife to old age. We also review the effects of social support and religious coping on physical functioning and survival following open-heart surgery (coronary artery bypass grafting, cardiac valve replacement, and heart transplantation). Finally, we examine psychosocial, behavioral, and spiritual interventions that are now being tested to see whether they can improve CHD prognosis and possibly even reverse coronary artery disease.

The chapter on religion and hypertension discusses the effects of religious beliefs and practices on systolic and diastolic blood pressures. Here we include results from a study, performed at Duke University, of almost 4,000 persons followed for six years, during which the investigators examined the cross-sectional associations and the longitudinal effects on blood pressure of attending church, praying, studying the Bible, and viewing religious TV. We also review the results from almost three dozen other studies that have examined this association and hypothesize reasons for the relationships observed.

The chapter on cerebrovascular disease and the brain examines how religious activity and stroke are related, investigates the possible influences of religion on the development of Alzheimer's disease, and discusses new research on the neurological basis for religious experience. Included here is a prospective study of stroke incidence involving thousands of older adults followed as part of the Established Populations for Epidemiologic Studies of the Elderly (EPESE) project at Yale. New research from the neurology laboratories at the University of California at San Diego claims that a "God module" may exist in the brain that could provide a neurobiological explanation for religious experience.

In the chapter on the immune system dysfunction, we explore whether religious beliefs and practices affect the level and activity of lymphocytes, antibodies, cytokines, and other substances that protect us from disease and outside invaders. We review results from a recent study at Duke University that examined the relationships between religious activity, the cytokine interleukin-6, and other immunological/inflammatory substances in blood. Cross-sectional and longitudinal data on immune function and religious activity were examined in more than 1,700 subjects. A study from the University of Iowa has replicated this finding, and other studies at Stanford University and the University of Miami show associations between religious activity, on one hand, and number of lymphocytes, lymphocyte activity, and antibody production, on the other. We also review studies that examine the effects of social support (like that provided by religious congregations) on immune function and on survival of patients with breast cancer and other malignancies.

In the chapter on religion and cancer, we take an in-depth look at how health behaviors and psychological factors affect the development and course of cancer. Members of certain religious groups experience death rates from cancer that are about half those of the general population. Studies of cancer in Mormons, Seventh-Day Adventists, Hutterites, Amish, Jews, liberal Protestants, conservative Protestants, Catholics, and other religious groups are examined. Diet, health behaviors, and religious influences are explored as possible explanations for the protective effects observed. We also examine the effects of religious beliefs and practices on the risk of developing cancer, ability to cope with cancer, and cancer prognosis.

In the chapter on religion and mortality we examine how membership in certain religious groups and level of religious involvement or commitment affects survival. Mormons, Seventh-Day Adventists, and members of other devout religious groups tend to live longer than people in the general population. This has been attributed largely to the avoidance of negative health habits that lead to cancer, cardiovascular disease, and other physical illness. Religious affiliation alone, however, tells us very little about the effects that religious belief, practice, and level of commitment have on survival. In this chapter we review studies that examine associations with church attendance, dependence on religion for strength and support, and other indicators of religious commitment that go far beyond simple affiliation.

Understanding the relationship between religion and functional disability is particularly important, given recent projections of large increases in the number of severely disabled persons over the next 30 to 40 years; while there were only about 3 million severely disabled elderly persons in the United States in 1990, by 2030 there will be almost four times that number. Studies have examined what effect being religious has on the perception of disability. Do more devoutly religious persons see themselves as less (or more) disabled than those who are less religious with the same amount of objective disease? Are more religiously active persons less likely to become physically disabled when followed over time? Do religious persons cope better with severe disability than those who are not religious? What effect does development of physical disability have on religious activity? These questions have now been examined in large epidemiologic studies of thousands of subjects.

In chapter 23, we explore relationships between religious involvement and pain and other somatic symptoms. Psychological and social factors strongly influence the experience of physical pain. Because of the close links between religion and psychological and social factors, religious beliefs and practices may similarly influence pain intensity. We discuss how different religious groups view pain and suffering and how these views affect their experience of pain. Studies that explore possible effects of religious involvement on the perception of pain by patients with terminal cancer, institutionalized older patients with arthritis, and persons with other chronic health problems are reviewed. The second half of the chapter examines associations between religion and nonpain somatic symptoms. Here we explore the relationship between frequency of physical health complaints and religious beliefs and practices. Because religious activities are often mobilized in response to pain or nonpain somatic symptoms, subjects must be studied over time in order to evaluate the ultimate effects of religion on symptom severity.

In the final chapter of this section, we explore associations between religion and health behaviors such as smoking, exercise, diet, weight control, sexual practices, and other activities likely to influence the development and prognosis of physical disease. Several studies have now documented a relationship between religious involvement and cigarette smoking. We discuss the results from a recent study at Duke University that examined the cross-sectional and longitudinal effects of public and private religious behaviors on the smoking habits of several thousand older adults. Using data from a national sample of almost 3,500 adults, researchers at Purdue University have documented a link among diet, weight, and religiosity that could impact physical and mental health in numerous ways. Religiousness may also affect sexual practices such as engaging in premarital sex or extramarital affairs and use of multiple sexual partners, all of which increase the risk of contracting sexually transmitted diseases, such as AIDS, syphilis, and other viral infections, that have long-term health and social consequences.

At the conclusion of part IV, we develop a conceptual model to help guide our understanding of how religion influences physical health. This model relies on recent findings in the fields of psychosomatic medicine and psychoneuroimmunology that have received increasing attention in the mainstream medical literature. The model also considers religious influences on health habits, health care–seeking behaviors, and adherence to medical treatment. Our goal is to shed light on the psychological, social, behavioral, and physiological pathways by which religious beliefs and practices might influence physical health and ultimately influence disease and mortality.

Part V addresses the relationships between religion and disease prevention, treatment compliance, and use of health services. The first chapter examines the effects of religious affiliation, belief, and practice on use of preventive health services and on compliance with medical treatments. Do the devoutly religious use fewer preventive services and comply less well with treatments because their faith lies in a power higher than the medical profession? Or do religious teachings that emphasize care for the physical body, respect for physicians, and social responsibility promote greater use of preventive services and better treatment compliance?

In the next chapter, we examine associations between religious involvement and use of health services. This includes general medical services such as care from primary-care physicians and visits by home health providers, as well as acute inpatient services and long-term care services, and mental health services such as care provided by mental health specialists, psychotropic medication, and inpatient psychiatric services. We examine and discuss religious influences on excess use, appropriate use, and underuse of these services. The increasing demand for health services and the decreasing availability of such services makes it imperative that we better understand how religious commitment and affiliation affect their use. Several studies have now examined this relationship, including a study of 542 high utilizers at Duke University Hospital that related religious affiliation, attendance, and intrinsic religiosity to use of acute inpatient services. We conclude this section by developing a theoretical model to help explain how religion might affect service use.

In part VI, we examine the implications of this research for health professionals and religious professionals. We describe how this knowledge can be applied to better meet people's needs. Primary care physicians working on the front lines encourage behaviors among patients that promote health and discourage those that endanger health and predispose to disease. Psychiatrists and psychologists help people with mental disorders and emotional difficulties who struggle to relate to other people and to cope with life's problems. Many of these mental conditions have both genetic and developmental origins that increase patients' vulnerability to stress. These people need resources to help them cope with the daily stresses that often precipitate mental crises. In the chapter on health professionals, we discuss whether primary care physicians and mental health professionals should address religious issues with their patients and how this can be done in a sensitive and appropriate manner. We also review the growing research on how physicians and patients feel about addressing religious issues in the context of the physician-patient relationship, how frequently discussion of these issues actually occurs, and how often physicians and patients would like it to occur.

Nurses deal even more closely with patients than do doctors. In the acute hospital and nursing home setting, nurses have considerable control over patients' daily routines. Hospital nurses control when patients eat, bathe, use the restroom, go to sleep, visit with loved ones, take medications, and engage in most other activities. They also control access to books, magazines, chaplain services, and other religious resources. Nurses are ideally positioned to bring comfort and hope to those who are dependent on them for care. Patients may be more likely to mention religious issues or spiritual needs to nurses because they feel more comfortable with them or don't want to bother the busy doctor about "things like that."

Social workers are in a position similar to that of nurses, and they may be even more likely to encounter religious issues and spiritual needs. Social workers must often arrange for and coordinate community services to help patients live outside the hospital. They do a great deal of counseling both with the patient and with his or her family. As health services become less and less available, social workers will be forced to look for alternative community resources for patients. Religious communities, if they are committed to promoting the mental and physical health of members, may help to ensure that people's needs are met outside the hospital.

In the chapter on religious professionals we discuss what research on religion and health means to chaplains, pastoral counselors, religious educators, community clergy, and religious congregations. The information presented here is particularly relevant to the work of chaplains, those specialists designated in our health care system to meet the religious and spiritual needs of patients. Chaplains are highly trained clergy who spend most of their time working in acute care hospitals, nursing homes, government institutions (e.g., prisons, armed forces), and other health care settings. Considerable space in this chapter is devoted to the pressures now being placed on chaplains by hospital administrators in response to imperatives from managed-care organizations to cut costs, underscoring the need

for research to demonstrate the cost effectiveness of chaplain services. We also examine the chaplain's role in the health care setting and discuss whether this role should be reduced or expanded.

Pastoral counselors (community clergy and licensed pastoral counselors) are responsible for a surprisingly large proportion of the psychotherapy that persons receive in the United States, and they are likely to provide even more services in the decades ahead. Many religious persons prefer pastoral counselors to secular therapists when they need help coping with emotional problems. The limits of both secular and religious interventions are discussed, as are indications for referral.

We also discuss the implications of this research for religious educators and for the content of curriculums taught in seminaries and divinity schools. Clergy in the twenty-first century will need substantially more education than they currently receive about the mental and physical health needs of members in their congregations. Churches will likely end up having to shoulder much of the responsibility for meeting the emotional and perhaps even the physical care needs of millions of baby boomers who would otherwise fall through the ever-widening cracks in government-funded health programs as financial resources dwindle during the twenty-first century.

Community clergy, in addition to acquiring the skills necessary to help members of their congregation meet their own health needs, must be prepared to develop health programs in their churches that promote healthy behaviors, facilitate early detection of disease, and ensure compliance with medical therapies. While this may seem like an unnecessary drain on already scarce church resources, it will ultimately be less time consuming and costly to prevent disease and promote health than to care for a congregation of sick people. In this chapter, we discuss the role of clergy as collaborators with health care professionals, social service agencies, and mental health organizations in helping to meet the health needs of church members and others in the community. We also discuss the responsibilities of members of congregations to care for one another and to participate in health programs, both as utilizers of these programs and as volunteer helpers and financial contributors.

In Part VII, we outline directions for future research on religion and health, review methods for conducting such research, and examine tools for measuring the religious variable. In the chapter on areas of research needing further study, we review what types of studies are needed to advance the field. This information will be useful for private and federal funding agencies that wish to sponsor research in this area but need help deciding which topics should receive priority. In the chapter on research methods, we present basic concepts for conducting research, such as identifying a hypothesis, choosing a study design, selecting a sample, attending to measurement issues, analyzing the data, and interpreting results. We also examine the peer review process, discuss how to evaluate different sources of scientific information, and address the issue of publication bias. In the final chapter, we review many of the instruments used to measure the religious variable, discussing their strengths and weaknesses and when to use them.

In the final section of the book, part VIII, we include a review and critique of more than 1,600 studies and reviews on the religion-health relationship. In a single line for each study, we note the first author and year of publication, the study design (e.g., cross-sectional, prospective), sampling method (e.g., random, convenience), number of subjects, type of subjects (e.g., adults, medical patients, adolescents), geographical location of study, number and type of religious variables, study findings, whether analyses were controlled, and overall rating of study quality. Studies are listed by health condition and, when possible, by order of chapters in the book. Part VIII is followed by a detailed index to help readers locate studies and topics of interest.

COMPREHENSIVENESS

Because of the extensive involvement of persons throughout the world in religious groups that promote beliefs and activities relating directly to health, health practices, or health care, the overall impact of religion on health could have enormous public health significance. This book is unique in its ambitious goals to (1) comprehensively and thoroughly review, critique, and integrate existing research on religion and health, (2) examine the clinical implications of this research, (3) make recommendations for future research, and (4) provide advice on how to design and conduct studies that avoid the flaws and weaknesses of previous work. While other publications have examined specific aspects of religion and health in different populations (e.g., the elderly, African Americans), no publication has yet addressed religion's potential impact on a broad range of mental and physical health problems in persons of different ages, religious backgrounds, and racial groups and developed unifying theoretical models to help bring together and make sense of the findings.

Studies on religion and health have been widely published in medical, nursing, sociological, psychological, social work, demographic, and religious journals. Because of the parochialism of our disciplines, professionals in one field often have no idea what is happening in another. This volume, with hundreds of references to research studies, clinical reports, and research reviews, provides a central resource to which professionals in a broad range of disciplines can turn in order to identify the research, learn about the meaning of the findings, and discover how the findings can be applied to their specific areas of interest.

PART I

HISTORICAL CONTEXT

1

Definitions

URING A RECENT SERIES OF
conferences in which 60 leading researchers and scientists in medicine,
psychology, substance abuse, and
the neurosciences met and discussed issues related to religion and health, it was difficult to
find definitions of religion and spirituality that
were acceptable to everyone (Larson, Swyers, &
McCullough, 1997). These scientists concluded
that both religion and spirituality have a "sacred
core" that consists of "feelings, thoughts, experiences, and behaviors that arise from a search
for the sacred. The term 'search' refers to attempts to identify, articulate, maintain, or transform. The term 'sacred' refers to a divine being
or Ultimate Reality or Ultimate Truth as perceived by the individual" (p. 21). Discussants
emphasized that the term "sacred" should not
be applied to things that are simply very important in life (such as our children, our job, or our
marriage); instead, the term "sacred" should

be used for concepts with "divine attributes"
because of their nature or because of their association with the divine.

"Religion" was distinguished from "spirituality" by the addition of two criteria. First, certain
forms of religion might involve a search for
nonsacred goals either in or outside a religious
setting. For example, *extrinsic* religiosity involves using religion—attending religious services, for example—as a means to nonsacred
goals such as increasing social contacts, improving status in the community, or attaining some
other benefit not associated with the divine.
Second, religion must involve rituals or prescribed behaviors (associated with the search
for the sacred) that have received validation and
support from a definable group of people (but
not necessarily validation from the culture,
since religious cults and sects typically reject
the dominant culture).

Because we need definitions of spirituality

17

and religion that can be operationalized for research purposes, it is necessary to define these terms in greater detail. For this reason, we turn to Webster's Dictionary (1980, pp. 1200, 1373).

Religion is defined as:

(a) belief in a divine or superhuman power or powers to be obeyed and worshiped as the creator(s) and ruler(s) of the universe, (b) the expression of such a belief in conduct and ritual. . . . [or] (a) any specific system of belief, worship, conduct, etc., often involving a code of ethics and a philosophy [e.g., the Christian *religion*, the Buddhist *religion*]; (b) any system of belief, practice, ethical values, etc., resembling, suggestive of, or likened to such system [humanism as a religion].

Spirituality is defined as:

1. spiritual character, quality, or nature
2. [often plural] the rights, jurisdictions, tithes, etc., belonging to the church or to the ecclesiastic
3. the fact or state of being incorporeal [without material body or substance].

Neither definition (particularly the one for spirituality) is satisfactory in terms of identifying specific components of religion and spirituality that might be objectively assessed and utilized to distinguish a spiritual person from a religious person. Thus, further elaboration on both definitions is needed.

In stepping back and examining what the terms "religion" and "spirituality" attempt to capture, we see that there are characteristics that are distinctive and may be useful in identifying and separating each concept for research purposes (Table 1.1). In summary, then, we de-fine and distinguish religion and spirituality as follows (see Figure 1.1):

Religion: Religion is an organized system of beliefs, practices, rituals, and symbols designed (a) to facilitate closeness to the sacred or transcendent (God, higher power, or ultimate truth/reality) and (b) to foster an understanding of one's relationship and responsibility to others in living together in a community.

Spirituality: Spirituality is the personal quest for understanding answers to ultimate questions about life, about meaning, and about relationship to the sacred or transcendent, which may (or may not) lead to or arise from the development of religious rituals and the formation of community.

RELIGIONS IN THE UNITED STATES AND WORLD

Table 1.2 presents various religious groups and the number of adherents of each in the United States and in the world. This information is important because much of the research on religion and health has been conducted in the United States.

SPIRITUALITY IN THE UNITED STATES

There are five types of spirituality (broadly defined) in the United States. By the word "moored" we mean *moored to an established religious tradition*. The vast majority of research in the United States has been conducted with subjects who would considered themselves type

TABLE 1.1 Characteristics distinguishing religion and spirituality

Religion	Spiritual
Community focused	Individualistic
Observable, measurable, objective	Less visible and measurable, more subjective
Formal, orthodox, organized	Less formal, less orthodox, less systematic
Behavior oriented, outward practices	Emotionally oriented, inward directed
Authoritarian in terms of behaviors	Not authoritarian, little accountability
Doctrine separating good from evil	Unifying, not doctrine oriented

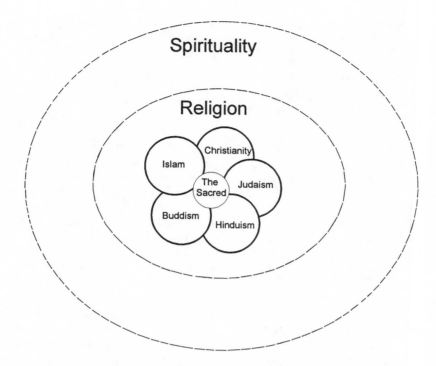

FIGURE 1.1 Schematic diagram of distinctions between religion and spirituality.

4 or type 5 moored spirituality. These divisions were provided to us by the American theologian Martin Marty, former editor of *Christian Century* and a professor at the University of Chicago.

1. *Humanistic spirituality* (about 7% of population)
   Focus on the human spirit
   Believe in human self-transcendence on own terms
   Have no transcendent reference (agnostic)
   Accept no tie or claim, no higher power
   Have a highly developed ethical system
   Albert Camus and Ernest Hemingway exemplify
2. *Unmoored spirituality* (about 7% of population)
   Belong to upper middle class; cultural elite
   Includes many educators and mental health professionals
   Are individualistic; not religious or institutional
   Believe in energy, connection, nature,
   crystals, healing touch, astrology, parapsychology
   Shirley MacLaine exemplifies
3. *Moored spirituality–Eastern type* (<3% of population)
   Comprises Buddhists, Taoists, Shintoists, Hindus
4. *Moored spirituality–Western type I* (about 25% of population)
   Includes evangelical, conservative Protestants, Catholics, Eastern Orthodox, Jews, Muslims
   Feel responsible to someone (Theocratic)
   Offer prayers that are very specific and directed
   Believe in faith healing, anointing with oil
   Focus on a God who intervenes
   John Wimber exemplifies
5. *Moored spirituality–Western type II* (about 60% of population)
   Includes mainline Protestants, Catholics, Eastern Orthodox, Jews, Muslims
   Believe all of our lives are under God
   Don't expect specifics; pray for God's will
   Are much less likely to discern God's will

TABLE 1.2 Major religious groups in the United States and world

Religion	No. of Adherents
United States[a]	
Christian	151,225,000
Jewish	3,137,000
Muslim	527,000
Buddhist	401,000
Hindu	227,000
World[b]	
Christian	1,927,953,000
Jewish	14,117,000
Muslim	1,099,634,000
Buddhist	323,894,000
Hindu	780,547,000

a. Bendell, 1997, pp. 252–258.

b. *World Almanac*, 1997, p. 646.

MAJOR DIMENSIONS OF RELIGION

Because of a pressing need to be specific in our descriptions (for research purposes), we discuss the major components or dimensions of religion here. Because there is controversy over these dimensions also, we are as comprehensive and as inclusive as possible. For illustration purposes, we focus on the Judeo-Christian religious tradition (with which we, the authors, are most familiar). Twelve dimensions have been identified from the work of Glock (1962), Allport and Ross (1967), King and Hunt (1972), Batson (1976), Paloutzian and Ellison (1982), and Pargament, Ensing, et al. (1990). They include the following.

1. *Religious belief.* This is the most basic level of religion. Does the individual believe or not believe in God? Is he or she agnostic (simply doesn't know whether God exists) or atheistic (believes that God does not exist)? Religious belief is often measured in terms of orthodoxy of belief. How closely do the individual's beliefs conform to the established doctrine of a religious body? For example, to what extent do the individual's beliefs conform to the Christian faith as established in the early ecumenical creeds and confessions of the church? Alternatively, how strictly does the individual observe the rites and traditions of Judaism?

2. *Religious affiliation or denomination.* Religious affiliation refers to identification with a particular religious group. This is not equivalent to membership in a religious group or adherence to the beliefs or practices of that group. For example, researchers often ask whether the subject is Protestant, Catholic, or Jewish; has another affiliation; or has no affiliation. Affiliation and "denomination" are often used interchangeably, although they are not the same. Denomination usually refers to the specific group within Protestant Christianity with which the person is affiliated. Examples of denominations are Baptists, Methodists, and Presbyterians. Responses to questions about religious affiliation or denomination usually provide little information about the level of religiousness of the person, since within any religious group or denomination there exists a range of individuals, from those who are only nominally affiliated to those who are active and involved.

3. *Organizational religiosity.* Organizational religiosity refers to participation in church, synagogue, or temple activities and is a measure of the social dimension of religion. Organizational religiosity is contrasted to nonorganizational religious activities such as personal prayer, scripture reading, or religious TV viewing, all of which can be done in private. The lowest level of organizational religiosity is church or synagogue membership. Membership, however, means different things in different religious groups. For example, being a member of a Baptist church means something quite different (active identification with and participation in church) from membership in the Catholic Church (where membership has less meaning attached to it).

Typically, organizational religiosity refers to attendance at religious services, either on the Sabbath or during the week. It can also refer to religious social activity such as attending church or synagogue dinners, socials, picnics, or other social meetings. Organizational religiosity means participation in Bible or scripture study groups, prayer groups, or home fellowship groups. Holding church offices, such as deacon or elder, is included in this category. Participating in communion or any of the other sacraments or rituals of the church, synagogue, or temple may be categorized under organizational religiosity, just as giving financial support to the church is (although religious giving or tithing may be seen as a consequence of religiousness; this is discussed later).

4. *Nonorganizational religiosity.* Private prayer (other than at mealtimes) is considered the primary religious activity that defines this category. According to the theologian Michael Novak (1999), "For Jews and Christians, prayer is a conversation with their Creator—'the love that moves the sun and all the stars,' Dante wrote—and a break from the humdrum of the everyday." Prayer may be divided into at least six different types, depending on the activity involved: petitionary prayer, intercessory prayer, prayer of adoration, prayer of confession, contemplative prayer, and meditative prayer. Petitionary prayer involves making specific, directed requests or petitions to God; a specific outcome is requested (e.g., please heal my painful knee). Intercessory prayer involves praying for another person or persons and is also usually (although not necessarily) directed to a specific divine being for a specific outcome. A prayer of adoration involves praising, thanksgiving, or displaying honor or love toward God or other divine being. A prayer of confession involves admitting to a particular sin or mistake and asking forgiveness from God; part of this prayer may also involve some type of penance or activity directed at correcting the mistake.

A contemplative prayer is usually nondirected and is without any specific goal attached to it. In the Christian tradition, it may simply involve listening to God, with or without reference to a specific topic. In other traditions, it may involve sitting quietly and clearing the mind of thoughts and is thus similar to meditative prayer. Meditation usually involves clearing the mind of thoughts and focusing, concentrating, or directing attention to a specific word or phrase. The most common example of meditative prayer is Buddhist meditation or transcendental meditation (TM) or mindfulness meditation. Meditation does not necessarily have to relate to to the transcendent; in fact, the Relaxation Response developed by Herbert Benson (1975) is simply a behavioral reflex that occurs when a person clears her mind of other thoughts and repeats a single word, phrase, or syllable over and over again.

Other nonorganizational religious activities include reading religious scriptures or inspirational literature, watching religious television, and listening to religious radio. Again, these activities can be done from the privacy of home and do not require interaction with others.

5. *Subjective religiosity.* Subjective religiosity taps that internal sense of religion's importance in the individual's life. How religious does the person consider himself to be? This is an entirely subjective dimension that relies upon self-report. While related, subjective religiosity is not the same as religious commitment or intrinsic religious orientation. A person may see herself as very religious and yet score relatively low on more objective measures of religious commitment or intrinsic motivation.

6. *Religious commitment/motivation.* Religious commitment is a term loosely used to reflect degree or level of religiosity. It attempts to capture how internally committed the person is to his religion. What real difference does religion make in the person's life? One of the best indicators of religious commitment, in our estimation, is intrinsic religious motivation, or intrinsic religiosity. Intrinsic religiosity is contrasted with extrinsic religiosity. The Harvard psychologist Gordon Allport developed the intrinsic-extrinsic concept in the 1950s while studying religious prejudice. His original intention was to identify the truly religious person who is internally committed to and motivated by religious beliefs. Allport describes the intrinsically religious person:

> Persons with this orientation find their master motive in religion. Other needs, strong as they may be, are regarded as of less ultimate significance, and they are, so far as possible, brought into harmony with the religious beliefs and prescriptions. Having embraced a creed, the individual endeavors to internalize it and follow it fully. It is in this sense that he lives his religion. (Allport and Ross 1967, p. 434).

In contrast, the extrinsically religious person is interested in religion only in order to achieve a different, nonreligious goal. Again, according to Allport,

Persons with this orientation [extrinsic religiosity] are disposed to use religion for their own ends. The term is borrowed from axiology to designate an interest that is held because it serves other, more ultimate interests. Extrinsic values are always instrumental and utilitarian. Persons with this orientation may find religion useful in a variety of ways—to provide security and solace, sociability and distraction, status and self-justification. The embraced creed is lightly held or else selectively shaped to fit more primary needs. In theological terms the extrinsic type turns to God, but without turning away from self. (Allport & Ross, 1967, p. 434)

Allport and Ross later added on a third class of individual because they found that some persons showed markedly strong agreement with both intrinsic and extrinsic statements and yet tended to make more prejudiced statements than did intrinsic believers. These persons have been called indiscriminantly pro-religious.

7. *Religious "quest."* Religion as quest is a religious orientation that is distinct and separate from either intrinsic or extrinsic religiosity. According to C. Daniel Batson,

These persons view religion as an endless process of probing and questioning generated by the tensions, contradictions, and tragedies in their own lives and in society. Not necessarily aligned with any formal religious institution or creed they are continually raising ultimate "whys," both about the existing social structure and about the structure of life itself. While it may seem strange to call such an individual religious, there is actually a long history of such a view. It goes at least as far back in Western thought as the Hebrew prophets and much farther back in Eastern religions. (Batson, 1976, p. 32)

In his studies of altruistic behavior, Batson claimed that persons with a strong Quest orientation were more responsive to the wishes of a person seeking aid than were those with an intrinsic orientation (who tended to persistently offer help even when the subject didn't want any) (Batson & Gray 1981; Batson & Flory, 1990).

8. *Religious experience.* Religious experience is that dimension of religion examined by the American psychologist William James (1902) in his classic book *Varieties of Religious Experience.* In that book, James focused on the dramatic, spectacular, and sometimes bizarre religious experiences of patients and famous people in history. Examples of religious experience that make up this dimension include religious conversion (gradual and sudden types), "born-again" experiences, mystical experiences, physical or emotional healing, and other experiences relating to God, the transcendent, or ultimate reality.

Religious conversion may involve a gradual turning to religion or transforming of nominal belief into something deeply personal and meaningful over a period of many years. Alternatively, religious conversion can be dramatically sudden and completely life changing, so much so that personality may even be altered. In conservative or evangelical Protestant Christianity, the term "born again" refers to a life-changing personal experience with Jesus Christ that "saves" the person experiencing it. The phrase comes from an interaction between Jesus and the pharisee Nicodemus in John 3:1 of the New Testament. In recent times, however, it has become more of a label than an indication of true religious conversion; Gallup polls indicate that nearly 40 percent of Americans say they are born again, and nearly 60 percent of persons in the southeastern United States make this claim.

Other religious experiences include mystical experiences that involve "becoming one" with the universe or with God, or related phenomena. While such experiences tend to be more common among those who perform Eastern religious practices, there is a mystical tradition in Christianity, in particular in Catholicism.

Physical or emotional healing initiated by a spiritual or religious activity can also be categorized as religious experience. Religious conversion may be accompanied by such physical or emotional healing, which people tend to remember long afterward and retell as their "testimony."

Religious experience can also include feelings of closeness to God or the transcendent, feelings of awe or wonder related to other spiritual experiences, or fear and terror related to negative religious experiences.

9. *Religious well-being*. Paloutzian and Ellison (1982) developed a dimension of religion called "spiritual well-being" (SWB). As they conceptualize it, SWB is composed of religious well-being and existential well-being (ten questions measure each of these two components). The existential well-being questions assess primarily general well-being and life satisfaction, whereas the religious well-being questions tap feelings of having a personally meaningful, satisfying, and fulfilling relationship with God. More will be said about Paloutzian and Ellison's SWB scale in chapter 33.

10. *Religious coping*. Religious coping involves religious behaviors or cognitions designed to help persons cope with or adapt to difficult life situations or stress. These coping activities may involve praying to God to change a situation or to give emotional strength (petitionary prayer), consciously deciding to trust or depend on God, consciously deciding to "turn a situation over" to God, reading inspirational scriptures for comfort or relief of anxiety, talking with a minister or chaplain to help work through a problem, or employing any other religious thoughts or behaviors that are used to relieve stress. Pargament has written a book titled *The Psychology of Religion and Coping* (1997) that explores this concept in great depth. Religious coping as described here is not a form of extrinsic religiosity, although the distinction is not entirely obvious without explanation.

11. *Religious knowledge*. Religious knowledge concerns the amount of information and knowledge that a person has about the major tenets or doctrines and history of her religious faith. For Christians, this knowledge is commonly measured by asking about familiarity with the Ten Commandments, the Sermon on the Mount, the two great commandments, the names of biblical prophets, and so forth. Questions about teachings in the Koran or the Torah can tap religious knowledge among Muslims or Jews, respectively.

12. *Religious consequences*. Devout religious belief and practice should also have practical consequences in the way people live. To what extent do the individual's actions and decisions conform to the basic tenets of his religious tradition? For Christians and members of other religious faiths, this may involve giving money to support the church, the poor, or the hungry (tithing and gifts), acts of altruism (helping a neighbor in need), volunteering (offering one's time and talent for a good cause), or helping out in the church (e.g., as part-time custodian, secretary, or deacon).

SUMMARY AND CONCLUSIONS

While there is much controversy and little agreement on definitions of religion and spirituality, we have presented definitions for these concepts that will help the reader better understand how these terms are used in this book. Definitions have also been crafted so that they may be operationalized and measured in research studies that explore relationships with and impact on health outcomes. We described 11 dimensions of religion based on the work of behavioral scientists who have studied this area for the past 50 years. We focused primarily on religion because most of the research that links spirituality and health has thus far operationalized spirituality in terms of religion (given the difficulty of measuring spirituality as a separate concept). We now turn to the colorful history that lies behind the tumultuous relationship among religion, science, and medicine.

2

A History of Religion, Science, and Medicine

Historical Timeline

THE TIMELINE PRESENTED here includes key events that have shaped the historical relationship among religion, science, and medicine. It includes, in chronological order, major incidents in the history of science, medicine, medical psychology, nursing, and the care of the sick, particularly as they relate to religion. It also includes here important religious events, related and unrelated to medicine, to provide a historical benchmark for comparison. Although we have tried to include events relevant to many of the world's great religions, we focus primarily on Western religious traditions and Christianity in particular; see Sullivan (1989) for a more thorough treatment of the history of medicine, science, and the Eastern religious traditions.

2,000,000–13,000 B.C.	Early Stone Age (paleolithic period), beginning when stone tools are first used by humanoid creatures and ending after the last ice age (Encarta Encyclopedia, 1999).

A special acknowledgement and thanks to Sam Thielman, Garry Crites, and Ann Bonner for their help in compiling and proofreading this historical timeline.

400,000–150,000 B.C.	Earliest true human beings (*Homo sapiens*) appear in Africa, China, and Europe.
13,000–8,000 B.C.	Middle Stone Age (mesolithic period).
8,000–3,000 B.C.	New Stone Age (neolithic period); agricultural villages arise during this period.
7,000 B.C.	Mesopotamian civilization develops in what is today known as Iraq.
6,000–5,000 B.C.	Artifacts from the predynastic period in Egypt indicate that mental illness and physical illness were not distinguished from each other, both being understood in religious terms (evil spirits, demon possession) (Zilboorg & Henry, 1941).
5000 B.C.	Egyptian civilization develops in the Nile Valley.
5000–1500 B.C.	In Pharaonic times there is little distinction between religion and magic (heka); both are regarded as controlling factors in daily life (Nunn, 1996, p. 96).
	The ancient healing art of laying on of hands is depicted in the hieroglyphics, pictographs, and cuneiform writings of Egyptian, Assyrian, and Persian civilizations (Krieger, 1975).
	Hypnotism is used by shamans of primitive tribes in northern Asia to influence the sick (Zilboorg & Henry, 1941).
4,500–3,000 B.C.	Beginning of Bronze Age (which lasts until iron-made tools appear—around 1200 B.C. in Greece).
3200–1025 B.C.	In Mesopotamian medicine, supernaturalistic and naturalistic paradigms are mixed; treatment is sometimes applied through magic and sometimes applied through natural methods (e.g., herbs, or mixtures made up of parts of animals, roots). Diseases are believed to be caused by unappeased ghosts who attack or possess humans, leaving the mark of illness upon them (Prioreschi, 1995, p. 424).
3100–2650 B.C.	As a means of maintaining health, Egyptians nurture their preoccupation with excrement and the bowels by treating themselves with enemas for three consecutive days every month; some use enemas once every day. At this time, fecal matter is believed to be the primary suspect in death and disease (Prioreschi, 1995, p. 333).
3000 B.C.	In the Ebers Papyrus, a section referred to as the "Treatise on the Heart" indicates that what we now know as the pulse is a key diagnostic tool used for distinguishing levels of disease (Prioreschi, 1995, p. 335).
2650–1800 B.C.	Traditionally, the first and greatest physician of ancient Egypt lives during the Old Kingdom and is named Imho-

tep, though in fact there is no historical evidence of his being a physician at all. Imhotep is later worshipped as a god (Prioreschi, 1995, p. 357).

Some forms of massage and physical medicine are practiced in ancient Egypt as a means of curing disease (Nunn, 1996, p. 136).

Drug therapy in ancient Egypt is mainly empirical and seeks to relieve symptoms rather than heal disease (Nunn, 1996, p. 136).

In the Middle Kingdom of ancient Egypt (2000–1800 B.C.), the priest exorcises evil spirits using the name of the central god, Horus. In the eyes of the central government, this is a favorable action by the exorcist and is seen as appeasing the gods (Prioreschi, 1995, p. 327).

Egyptian remedies for trauma rarely contain incantations, unlike the treatment used for medical conditions. Deities are such an accepted part of life that invoking their help is done as a first resort when treating medical conditions. Incantations are directly addressed to disease-demons, commanding them to leave the body (Nunn, 1996, p. 96).

2300–1500 B.C.	Hinduism emerges partly out of the Indus Valley civilization (2300–1700 B.C.), partly out of the Indo-Aryan Vedic civilization (1500 B.C. and later), and partly out of the undated hunting/collecting, nomadic, agricultural folk tradition of India.
	In the Indus Valley civilization, the priest performs rituals of dancing, recites incantations, and uses amulets to cure patients of a variety of ills. Herbs, water, and cow by-products are also often administered (Prioreschi, 1995, p. 235).
2000–500 B.C.	Early Chinese society believes that life is controlled by spirits and demons and that the ancestral spiritual world needs to be pacified in order to avoid disease and chaos in this life (Prioreschi, 1995, p. 119).
	Dissection of the body is not practiced in ancient China because it would violate the precepts of ancestor worship. Body parts are considered to be part of one's parents; thus, disease is treated by medication, not mutilation (Prioreschi, 1995, p. 139).
	Acupuncture is a critical method of treatment in China, tapping into many of the body's channels and anatomical connections to bring about healing (Prioreschi, 1995, p. 136).
2000–1900 B.C.	Abraham is called by God, and the monotheistic religious tradition of Judaism emerges (and, later, Islam and Christianity).

2000–63 B.C.	In Old Testament times, the sick are examined and kept under careful observation by the priest (Prioreschi, 1995, p. 486).
	"Biblical medicine is exclusively supernaturalistic; no other naturalistic medicine paradigm developed as seen in other ancient cultures. Moreover, this supernatural paradigm is entirely religious, separated from incantations and exorcisms" (Prioreschi, 1995, p. 482).
1900 B.C.	The Kahum papyrus, the most ancient document on gynecology known, is written around this period (Prioreschi, 1995, p. 343).
1700 B.C.	A simple theory of disease gradually develops in Ionian philosophy (Ionia is an area in the Peloponnesus section of Greece). The four elements (earth, air, fire, and water) are associated with the four humors (black bile, blood, yellow bile, and phlegm) in the four organs (spleen, heart, liver, and brain), and good health is seen as a result of a proper balance among these humors. Illness is treated by drugs to correct imbalances (Pollak, 1963, p. 50).
1550–332 B.C.	The concept of protection from the eye of Horus (the primary Egyptian god) comes into being. Egyptian medicine urges a supernaturalistic paradigm of medicine, combining the naturalistic approach of the physician, the non-scientific healing of the priest, and the magic of the sorcerer (Prioreschi, 1995, p. 330).
1500–1000 B.C.	In early Hebraic times, the Old Testament suggests that it is God who afflicts persons with "madness, blindness and confusion of mind" because of their sins (Deuteronomy 28:28, NIV).
	"I put to death and I bring to life, I have wounded and I will heal, and no one can deliver out of my hand" (Deuteronomy 32:39, NIV).
	"He said, 'If you listen carefully to the voice of the Lord your God and do what is right in his eyes, if you pay attention to his commands and keep all his decrees, I will not put on you any of the diseases I brought on the Egyptians, for I am the Lord, who heals you'" (Exodus 15:26, NIV).
	"I will bring health and healing to it [the city of Jerusalem]; I will heal my people and will let them enjoy abundant peace and security" (Jeremiah 33:6, NIV).
1000–500 B.C.	In the Homeric tradition of ancient Greece, mental illness is thought to originate in influences by the gods of mythology.
900 B.C.	A separation between priests and physicians appears in

biblical texts. While the physician has clear-cut duties, he has no responsibility for mental illnesses; demonic powers are believed responsible for any condition for which organic factors can not be identified, and these are handled by the priest (Alexander, 1966).

900–500 B.C.	As a part of Vedic healing, disease demons are transferred from a patient to his enemy. Astrology also plays a role in determining methods of treatment in India during this time (Prioreschi, 1995, p. 236).
600 B.C.	Hindus believe that meditation leads to true knowledge, which leads them to freedom from the cycle of death (disease) and rebirth and facilitates the reuniting with Brahman, the absolute existence (Prioreschi, 1995, p. 211).
600–300 B.C.	In Avestan times (old Persia), there are three healers: the physician, the surgeon, and the incantation priest. Naturalistic and supernaturalistic medicine are practiced side by side (Prioreschi, 1995, p. 461).
600–500 B.C.	Buddhism emerges out of northeastern India, as Sakyamuni, or Gautama Buddha, begins his teachings. The Buddha reportedly gives authorization to a Pirit service, a religious ritual used for the curing of the sick. Early Buddhism approves both religious beliefs/ritual (Pirit) and medicine as valid tools for healing (Kitagawa, 1989, p. 20).
	The Mahayana tradition of Buddhism places a greater emphasis on personal faith, whereas the Esoteric tradition stresses the magical power of Buddhist divinities. The folk Buddhist tradition, on the other hand, is associated with spirit cults and various cults of faith healing involving magical incantations. Buddhists rarely rely on faith healing alone, and most go to see doctors as well (Kitagawa, 1989, pp. 20–21).
600 B.C.–A.D. 600	In the Classical period a new medical paradigm develops that views disease as the result of natural causes and healing as the result of the inherent virtues of medicinal drugs (Prioreschi, 1995, p. 241).
500–300 B.C.	Hippocrates (460–357 B.C.), known as the "father of modern medicine," describes illness in terms of four bodily fluids (blood, phlegm, yellow bile, and black bile). He also describes a variety of mental disorders (e.g., psychosis, phobia, mania, melancholia, paranoia), which he ascribes to disease of the brain.
	Plato (429–347 B.C.) mixes science with mystical elements, emphasizing the need to treat the "soul" as well as the physical body (rather than being mystical, however, Plato may simply be expressing his belief that the physical is merely a reflection of ideas). His student Aristotle (384–

322 B.C.), reportedly "laid the foundation of the science of psychology" (Zilboorg & Henry, 1941, p. 54).

300 B.C.–0

In the Western world, physical and mental illnesses are believed to have natural causes, yet are affected by Divine forces. Because of heavy influences by the Greek Asclepian cult, treatment is administered primarily through astrology, magic, and herbs (Asclepius was Apollo's son—the god of medicine).

200–100 B.C.

Therapeutics of Chinese medicine rest upon five main principles: guidance toward Tao, diet, drugs, acupuncture, and moxibustian (a technique used to influence the movement of chi in the body's vessels). Sometimes massage and exercise are added (Prioreschi, 1995, p. 153).

50 B.C.–0

In order to control a famine, Caesar orders the banishment of all foreigners from Rome—80,000 men—but exempts physicians and teachers. From that time on (46 B.C.), all free foreigners who practice as physicians in Rome are entitled to the freedom of the city (Pollak, 1963, p. 63).

After he is cured of a rheumatic condition by his physician (10 B.C.), emperor Augustus grants all physicians exemption from taxes (Pollak, 1963, p. 63).

During this period of history, the mentally ill are kept in dark cells and dungeons, according to Cicero (106–43 B.C.) and Plutarch (A.D. 46–120).

0–300

Jesus focuses on the meaning of suffering and the healing of the whole person; little distinction is made between healing of the body, mind, and spirit. Emphasis is placed on the power of the *thought life* to affect health (Matthew 15:17–20). Early Christians believe that sickness, whether or not caused by sin, can be healed through prayer (James 5:14).

Physical healing does not become a dominant and widespread Christian practice until about the fourth or fifth century A.D. During the first three centuries, mainstream Christianity does not promise physical healing (as did the pagan healing cults) (Ferngren, 1992). "Caring for" rather than curing the sick is the chief ministry of the early Christian community.

According to Ferngren (1992, pp. 13–14), caring for the sick was Christianity's truly novel contribution to health care. At that time, pagans did not care for their sick in any organized fashion or on any widespread basis. The Jewish community provided care primarily to its own. The Christian Church, on the other hand, offered care not only to Christians but also to non-Christians.

100–300

In ancient Chinese literature there are many passages that identify physicians with sorcerers, connecting illness with demonic influence. An etymological lexicon written in 100 states "Sorcerer Pend was the first physician" (Pollak, 1963, p. 69).

According to Mahayana Buddhism, to exist is to suffer. To end suffering, one must end existence (Prioreschi, 1995, p. 218).

Chong Chueh teaches that, as a rule, illnesses are brought about by sinful conduct, and purification is achieved through public confession, giving healing and protection against diseases (Prioreschi, 1995, p. 123).

Rabbi Judah, president of the Sanhedrin, edits the *Mishnah*, one of the primary sources of discussion on medical matters in the ancient world.

Clement of Alexandria (150–215), one of the early church fathers who is well versed in Greek, argues that health by medicine has its origin in and its existence from God as well as resulting from human cooperation. He notes that the art of healing learned by human wisdom is from God. This view is reinforced by Origen (185–254), who notes that just as God allows trees to grow, so also does he give medical knowledge to humans.

While medicine and skills of physicians are seen as blessings from God, it is sinful to put one's entire faith in them since their efficacy depends primarily on God who can heal without them (Amundsen, 1982, p. 333).

Galen (130–200) is a Greek anatomist, physician, and writer whose theories form the basis of European medicine for the next 1,200 years (until the beginning of the Renaissance).

In the western world, during the reign of Emperor Alexander Severus (222–235), the training of physicians is regulated by the state. Practical bedside instruction is required by the state, but patients are not always edified by that practice. Some complain of being sicker after being pawed over by countless trainees (Pollak, 1963, p. 64).

As the persecution of Christians around the Roman Empire reaches its peak, the two Christian physicians, Cosmas and Damian, are beheaded, in 290. These two brothers are widely known as miracle healers, yet their cures are done out of piety and not for gain. Patients spend one or more nights in the church to receive either a saintly vision or advice from the saints in the morning. Both reportedly lead to cures. The healing specialties of these brothers are sicknesses of the glands, and the stomach and infectious diseases (Pollak, 1963, p. 73).

300–400

The Roman Emperor Constantine experiences a dramatic conversion to Christianity in 312; soon afterward, the Edict of Milan is issued, which ends the persecution of Christians. Constantine moves the traditional day of sabbath worship from Saturday to "the day of the sun" (Sunday).

Pagan practices start to be regulated during Constantine's lifetime and are outlawed by Constantine's son Constantius, who closes temples and restricts sacrifices in 356 and by Theodosius, who bans private pagan worship in 392.

An early draft of the Nicene Creed is agreed upon by bishops of the Christian Church at the council of Nicaea in 325. Later, at the Council of Constantinople (381), the Creed as we know it today is produced. The Theodosian Edict of 381 dictates that all Christianity must be Nicene. This official statement of faith outlines the basic nature of Jesus, God, and the Holy Spirit (doctrine of the Trinity) and is honored by most Christian denominations to this day.

The content of the New Testament (the "Canon") is established in the Eastern Church in 367 and in the Western Church in 382; at the Council of Carthage in 397, it becomes official for the entire Church (the first Christian Bible).

In the ancient world, medicine is generally practiced as a private trade; it is not available to members of the general population, who are cared for by their families. This all changes after the Emperor Constantine, in 337, the year of his deathbed baptism, makes Christianity the official religion of the Roman empire (Amundsen, 1998, p. 68).

According to the medical historian Roy Porter, "Charity was the supreme religious virtue. In the name of love, and with the conviction that every human was a soul to be saved, believers were enjoined to care for those in need: the destitute, the handicapped, the poor, the hungry, those without shelter, and perhaps above all, the sick" (Porter, 1993, p. 1452).

Until the Christian era (after 350), there is no evidence of buildings (i.e., hospitals) devoted to the care and treatment of sick persons in the general population (Granshaw, 1993, p. 1181).

Eastern Orthodox Christians, at the insistence of St. Basil, Bishop of Caesarea, establish the first great hospital in Asia Minor around 370. It is scattered among hotels, poorhouses, homes for the aged, buildings for diseases, and a special hospital for lepers. This is done to honor the biblical obligation, in Matthew 25:36, 40, to clothe the poor and to heal the sick (Pollak, 1963, p. 74).

400–1400

The period in Western European history from the fall of the West Roman Empire in the fifth century through the fifteenth century is known as the Middle Ages (or the Dark Ages, although many historians no longer use this term, since it suggests inaccurately that no classical learning went on).

Religion takes a firm hold on science, and, between 200 and 1700, almost all mental disorders are understood in terms of demonic possession, say Zilboorg and Henry (1941). The historians Alexander and Selesnick (1966) likewise emphasize that the psychiatry of the Middle Ages could scarcely be distinguished from prescientific demonology, and mental treatment was conducted largely through exorcisms (p. 52). This view of history, however, is controversial. The Inquisition is not even established until 1233, and then the focus is not so much on the persecution of witches and the demon possessed as it is on identifying and reforming heretics (Kroll, 1973). This is discussed further later.

Demonology during this period is not as closely connected with physical health as it is with mental health. For example, Soranus's *Gynecology* is well respected by the early Church fathers Tertullian (160–220) and Augustine (354–430). Many Christians in antiquity and in the medieval period also accept Galen's teachings (especially on the humors).

400–550

Augustine presents a perspective on secular medicine that is positive, and similar to that of many other Christian church leaders. He and others are vigorous in their efforts to encourage caring for the sick. The practice of medicine is seen as material evidence of God's love and compassion for human suffering (Amundsen, 1982, p. 349).

There is great respect for physicians among Jews. The Jewish Talmud prohibits Jews from living in a city in which there is no physician (Dorff, 1998, p. 14).

A hospital for the mentally ill is established in Jerusalem in 490 (Alexander, 1966).

The first permanent medical hospital in China is founded in 491 by Hsiao Tzu-Liang, a Buddhist prince (Prioreschi, 1995, p. 103).

In 534, St. Benedict of Nursia writes "The Rule of St. Benedict" for the monks of the monastery of Monte Cassino. In the eighth century, this work becomes the central monastic rule in the West. According to this rule, all monks and nuns are resolved to love and serve the sick (Pollak, 1963, p. 79).

550–700

Mohammed the Prophet is born in 570. Islamic religious tradition emerges as the Qur'an (basic scriptures of Islam) is revealed to Mohammed (610–632). A body of medical knowledge is universally attributed by Islamic religious authorities to the prophet Mohammed. Most of this is old Arab medicine (dating before Mohammed and based largely on tradition and experience). Nevertheless, some elite Muslims study at the Sasanian Medical School at Jundaysabur (Persia). Also, by the tenth century, some Muslim physicians, such as Ibn-Zakariyya Al-razi, are classically trained and rather sophisticated (Al-razi works on differentiating smallpox from measles, according to the historian Hodgson).

Although the Qur'an does not speak specifically of medical treatment, it sets a high value on health and on the restoration of health (Rahman, 1989, p. 154).

500–1200

The first period of medieval medicine is designated as "Monastic" or "Monastery" medicine, since it is practiced and taught under the direction of the Church (Pollak, 1963, p. 79).

Between 541 and 767, 16 waves of plague afflict Europe. Saints and relics are revered. Many sufferers seek pagan remedies for sickness, including sorcery (Amundsen, 1998, pp. 71–72).

Knowledge about and practice of medicine between the fifth and the tenth centuries is handed down from master to pupil. By the twelfth century, medicine is taught in medical schools and as part of the education of the clergy. Education is based upon the teachings of Hippocrates, Galen, and later physicians. Despite Zilboorg/Henry's and Alexander/Selesnick's commentaries on the subject, Kroll (1973) notes that "no major medical work taught at the universities prior to the fourteenth century pays attention to demonology" (p. 281).

In the sixth century, many mentally sick persons are cared for in monasteries run by the Church. The Church encourages humane treatment of mental patients, who from the twelfth century on are even brought into people's homes and included in family life (Gheel, Belgium) (Braceland & Stock, 1963).

John of Salibury, Archbishop of Lyons, Agobard, and Abelard are religious leaders of the day who speak out against the idea that the devil produces mental disease. The Franciscan monk Bartholomaeus, a professor of theology, writes the *Encyclopedia of Bartholomaeus* (1255–1230), which discusses mental illnesses in terms of natural rather than supernatural causes. Bartholomaeus tries to localize the cause of insanity to the regions of the brain around the lateral ventricles (Kroll, 1973).

Scientific medicine in the Middle Ages is largely folk medicine, which is strongly influenced by mythology and Christian teachings but does not focus on demonology. Persons felt to be demon possessed and those believed to have simple infections, receive largely the same treatment—with herbs and animal parts combined with ritual prayers.

In the Middle Ages, the physician has very little science upon which to base treatments. In these times, the only "scientific guide" is astrology. According to Sarton (1931), "Belief in astrology was universal. It would not have occurred to any good medieval physician to question these principles any more than to a modern one to doubt the indications of a good thermometer" (p. 790).

Between 500 and 1000, physicians are of two basic types: strictly secular practitioners and physician monks. The vast majority, trained in western Europe, are little more than craftsmen who acquire their skills by apprenticeship. A few wealthy persons see secular physicians for a fee. Most persons seek miraculous healing, rely upon folk remedies, or seek help from clergy with medical skills (Amundsen, 1998, p. 83).

Care for the poor and sick throughout this period is provided primarily by the Church (Amundsen, 1998, p. 83).

1000–1200

The Knights Hospitallers (equivalent to modern hospital physicians) are monks who operate hospitals in Jerusalem at the time of the crusades (Stevens, 1989). Clergy-operated monasteries continue as the primary institutions of healing. In medieval Europe, hospitals "were usually associated with a church or monastery, with religion defining life within them" (Granshaw, 1993, p. 1182).

Young Hindu physicians are taught that it is critical that "Thou shall renounce lust, anger, greed, ignorance, vanity, egotistic feelings, envy, harshness, falsehood, idleness, nay all acts that soil the good name of man." The Caraka Samhita teaches that physicians are not to attempt to treat cases that seem hopeless, since this may tarnish their reputation as physicians (Prioreschi, 1995, pp. 264–265).

The physician-rabbi Moses Maimonides (1135–1204) writes the Mishned Torah, which summarizes the Jewish law, especially with regard to health practices (e.g., diet, exercise, hygiene, sleep).

The summoning of a physician and the taking of medication that is dispensed are considered the duty of all with illnesses who are Christians in England during this time. Failure to make use of a physician and his medications is considered a grievous sin (Pollak, 1963, p. 92).

Although there is a tradition of lay physicians dating back to the sixth century, in the twelfth and thirteenth centuries the centers of medical training shift to monasteries and Church-supported universities or "cathedral schools"; interestingly, despite being led by prominent Churchmen, these schools of medicine do not focus on supernatural healing (Kroll, 1973).

Within the medieval universities, religious authorities confer licenses to practice medicine (Gelfand, 1993, p. 1122).

1200–1400

Until well into the Renaissance (the period between the Middle Ages and modern times), the doctor is generally also a priest. Because some clergy begin to spend more of their time treating sick persons than on ecclesiastical duties, the church proclaims edicts that strongly encourage clergy to focus on theological matters, not medicine or surgery, which are to be left to the laity. There is less pressure against practicing medicine than practicing surgery ("ecclesia abhorret a sanguine"). The Church does not condemn the practice of medicine or surgery but simply emphasizes that theological study is a more important activity for priests (Amundsen, 1978). As a result, the practice of medicine and surgery becomes separated further and further from religious influence.

The Fourth Lateran Council (1215) forbids the practice of surgery by clergy in major orders (subdeacons, deacons, priests, bishops) but permits surgery by clergy in minor orders (e.g., porters, acolytes, lectors) (Amundsen, 1998, p. 85).

As noted earlier, the Inquisition is established in 1233, primarily to identify and reform heretics. The persecution of witches and the demon possessed, however, becomes more common in the late 1400s and continues for another 200 years (Kroll, 1973).

Hospitals designed specifically to care for the mentally ill are established in Spain in the early 1400s under the guidance of priests. The care given to the insane in these early asylums is much better than that provided later in the large, state-sponsored asylums of the sixteenth and seventeenth centuries.

Toward the end of the twelfth century, the Alexian Brothers (or Beghards) begin to care for the poor and sick in Western Europe, an activity that has persisted to the present. During the plague epidemics of the twelfth–fifteenth centuries, these devoutly religious men risk their own lives nursing the sick, burying the dead, and caring for the mentally ill. They continue to nurse the sick in urban areas of Europe for centuries, despite disregard and lack of support by the Church at times until they are made a religious order in the mid-1400s (Kauffman, 1976, 1978).

There is an intellectual awakening: Institutions of higher learning are reopened (1200–1300) and are largely supported by the Church. The word "doctor" is first used to indicate a learned person skilled in a profession. Science and the Church, however, begin to butt heads. The Church condemns Aristotelian empiricism, which incorporates the Greek scientific tradition and becomes widely popular between 1200–1240 (Kroll, 1973).

The Theologian and philosopher Thomas Aquinas (1225–1274) synthesizes Christian faith and Aristotelian philosophy, which is finally accepted in the mid-fourteenth century (Kroll, 1973). Under Aquinas's influence, medieval scientists begin to see their work as uncovering God's plan. Aquinas writes about the importance of dreams and the workings of the unconscious (almost 700 years before Freud).

In fourteenth-century England, there is a rather clearly distinguished categorization of healers: surgeons, physicians, and "leche." The physician is university trained, with a B.M., or doctorate. The leche can be a physician but is usually a lay practitioner of lower status.

The later period of medieval medicine is known as "The Age of Scholastic Medicine." The relationship between religion and medicine undergoes a crucial shift that separates the two ever so slightly as doctors become certified by the state, rather than by the Church (Pollak, 1963, p. 91).

1400–1700

The Renaissance in Western Europe begins. Increasing numbers of mentally ill persons populate Europe from 1300 on. Many cases of mental illness during this period may be due to "ergotism," an acute psychosis that results from eating moldy bread (Packer, 1998).

People with mental illness are forced to live on the streets and are seen as a menace.

The Renaissance ushers in an age of obsession with demonology. A movement to exterminate witches (often the growing population of mentally ill) culminates with the publication of *Malleus Maleficarum* (1487), which provides details about the diagnosis and treatment of the demon possessed. The treatment is exorcism; if that fails, "A man also, or woman that hath a familiar spirit, or that is a wizard, shall surely be put to death; they shall stone them with stones: their blood shall be upon them" (Leviticus 20:27).

Thousands of persons are burned or decapitated over the next 200 years (Zilboorg & Henry, 1941). In America, the Salem witch trials in 1692 involve nearly 100 accused and result in 19 executions (Gamwell & Tomes, 1995).

Kroll and Bachrach (1984), after carefully reviewing the historical details, disagree with Zilboorg and Henry, Alexander and Selesnick, and other historians about the role of demon possession and sin in the etiology of mental illness in the Middle Ages. They conclude that these "generalizations are based upon a very selective use of materials often wrenched from context and buttressed by tortuous arguments to sustain the thesis of medieval superstition and backwardness" (p. 507). After reviewing 57 descriptions of mental illness from pre-Crusade chronicles and saints' lives, Kroll and Bachrach find that in only 16% is the cause of the mental illness attributed to sin or wrongdoing. Natural causes for mental illness, such as humoral imbalance, poor diet, excessive alcohol intake, overwork, and grief, are widely known and understood. According to Kroll and Bachrach, compassionate treatment consistent with Christian teachings is encouraged by many religious physicians/priests of the day.

1400–1550

The religious establishment during this period sinks to a new low. According to the historian Marvin O'Connell, the Church in the fifteenth and sixteenth centuries is characterized by "A venal, slothful, and ignorant clergy; a laity shot through with superstition; colossal financial chicanery from indulgence-hawkers to corrupt officials of the Roman curia who routinely sold benefices and dispositions; an administrative chaos which made it virtually impossible to fix responsibility for the abuses and hence to apply the practical means to root them out; popes who were hedonists and simoniacs . . . all these were commonplace in Christian Europe at the moment the Protestant Reformation began" (O'Connell, 1998, p. 111).

As the Christian Church's authority begins to be shaken, the practice of medicine becomes more a secular discipline, and the split between religion and science widens.

In 1517, Martin Luther (1483–1546) posts his Ninety-five Theses on the door of a large church in Wittenberg, initiating the Catholic-Protestant split.

In 1525, the Anabaptist tradition, later to develop into the Mennonite and Amish faith traditions, arises in Switzerland.

In 1534, King Henry VIII of England establishes the supremacy of the crown over the Church in England, renouncing the supremacy of the pope in Rome. The Anglican tradition begins (the Episcopal church is the American branch of the Anglican Communion).

In 1543, Copernicus publishes *De Revolutionibus*, which concludes that the earth revolves around the sun, conflicting with the dominant view in the religious world that the earth is the center of the universe. In that same year, Andreas Vesalius unifies the work and knowledge of anatomy in a text that historically establishes medical education and medical examination and increases the standing of the profession (Pollak, 1963, p. 75).

Paracelsus (1493–1541) is a devout Protestant who believes that the essence of religion is found in faith, personal experience, and spirituality. He is also a highly successful and renowned physician, who argues effectively against orthodox medicine's Galenic view of anatomy, humoral pathology, and botanical therapy (which he sees as largely materialistic and atheistic). Attacking humoral doctrine (which sees disease as an imbalance among blood, bile, water, and phlegm), Paracelsus instead replaces it with a chemically based theory and practice of medicine. Paracelsians, or chemical physicians, as they are called, are widespread in Northern Europe and England in the sixteenth century. Paracelsus argues that for medicine to be effective it has to recognize the interrelationship between the somatic and the spiritual (Gelfand, 1993, p. 1124; Porter, 1993, p. 1461).

1550–1600

John Calvin (1509–1564) begins a reform movement in Europe that eventually leads to the Presbyterian, United Church of Christ, Congregational, and Reformed churches. According to Calvinistic doctrines, deacons have a specific task in medicine as attendants to the sick, bringing them spiritual comfort as well as physical care for their diseases (Marland & Pelling, 1996, p. 130). Well-known Calvinists of more recent times include Anton Boisen, Karl Menninger, Norman Vincent Peale, and Seward Hiltner.

Calvin denies any direct miraculous power from the sacraments or the act of laying on of hands. "It was a more sure and notable proof of divine power to remove a grievous disease in a moment, and at a single touch. Though He could have done it with a nod alone, my interpretation is simply that Christ laid his hands on the sick to commend them to the Father, and to win them grace and deliverance from their diseases" (Marland & Pelling, 1996, p. 155).

At the Council of Trent, Catholic authorities meet between 1545 and 1563 to confront the Protestant reformation; Catholic doctrines and practices are revised in response to the cry for reform of abuses.

Founded in Solothurn, Switzerland, in 1572, the Brotherhood of Cosmas and Damian is regarded as the first medical professional society (Pollak, 1963, p. 73).

1600–1700

According to Zilboorg and Henry (1941), the word "psychologia" is used for the first time—the "science of man's behavior was being born and christened."

Francis Bacon (1561–1626), known as the great leader in the reformation of modern science, advocates experimentation, verification, and proof, helping to banish authority and dogmatism from scientific thought. He relegates theological questions to the region of faith, insisting that experience and observation are the only remedies against prejudice and error.

The philosopher Rene Descartes (1590–1650) studies chemistry and anatomy, dissecting animals to demonstrate that life in both man and animals can be explained by physiological processes. He accepts William Harvey's doctrine of the circulation of the blood and argues that the seat of the mind of man is the pineal gland in the brain. Natural theories begin to replace religious explanations as the followers of Descartes reduce the immortal soul to consciousness or thought.

Moliere (1622–1673) notes in jest that clinical medicine, at that time naturalistic and nonscientific, is nothing more than "clysterium donare, postea seignare, ensuita purgare"—"To give enemas, then to bleed, then to purge" (Prioreschi, 1995, p. 11).

The renowned Anglican literary scholar Robert Burton (1577–1640), author of the classic *The Anatomy of Melancholy*, at Oxford, and the astrological physician Richard Napier (1559–1634) support both organic and spiritual models of mental illness (Porter, 1993, p. 1460).

In 1633 Galileo (1564–1642) is rebuked by the Inquisition for supporting the Copernican view of the universe in his book, *Dialogue Concerning the Two Chief World Systems* (1632). He is forced to recant and arrested.

Baptist religious tradition emerges from seventeenth-century English Puritanism.

1650–1700

The Sisters of Charity of St. Vincent de Paul organize Catholic nuns to serve both religious and secular hospitals. By 1789, there are 426 hospitals run by the Sisters of Charity in France alone (Porter, 1993, p. 1543). Not until the 1830s do Protestants have anything similar, when a Lutheran pastor starts a nursing school in Kaiserwerth, Germany, to train women (called "deaconesses") for a life of service to the sick. Later, Florence Nightingale applies this concept to a secular setting to train the first "nurses" (Numbers & Amundsen, 1998, p. 2). For a more detailed history of the emergence of the nursing profession out of religious orders, see Nelson (1997).

John Locke (1632–1704), an English philosopher and founder of British empiricism, claims that all knowledge results from investigation of things by the bodily senses. A wall of separation between religion, on the one hand, and science and the practice of medicine, on the other, begins to rise more rapidly as the scientific revolution picks up speed.

"A sound mind in a sound body, is a short, but full description of a happy state in this World; he that has these two, has little more to wish for; and he that wants either of them, will be little the better for anything else" (John Locke, *Some Thoughts Concerning Education*, 1693).

The greatest of the natural philosophers, Sir Isaac Newton, composes his famous work *Philosophiae Naturalis Principia Mathematica* (1687), which sets up mathematical and mechanical systems of physiology and therapeutics to help guide a more scientific medicine. Newton argues that the entire universe can be explained in terms of physical laws. According to *Eerdman's Handbook to the History of Christianity*, Newton "believed that his scientific discoveries were communicated to him by the Holy Spirit, and regarded the understanding of Scripture as more important than his scientific work" (Dowley, 1982, p. 490).

The French scientist and religious philosopher Blaise Pascal (1623–1662) does experiments that help establish hydrodynamics, advancing the work of Galileo.

In the late 1600s, the Church holds the position that secular methods of cure (medical or surgical) are God given and work only through the exercise of God's power.

1700–1800

The Age of the Enlightenment begins in France. This is a time of challenge to traditional religious values. It is argued that reason is the essence of human nature and that science can explain the universe. The French and American revolutions take place.

The French Revolution (1792–1802) has an enormous effect on the practice of medicine. Nearly all of the old medical institutions and scientific academies are abolished, and medical practice is deregulated so completely that almost anyone can purchase a legal permit to practice medicine. As a consequence, government assumes much closer control of medicine. These reforms help to unify medicine and surgery, and the central "school of health" in Paris becomes the world center for medicine during the first half of the nineteenth century (Gelfand, 1989, p. 1131–1132).

Julien de La Mettrie (1709–1751) publishes *L'Homme machine* (1749), which argues that humans are wholly material beings, that modern anatomy and physiology can find no evidence of a soul or spirit. Soon afterward, Denis Diderot (1713–1784) publishes his *Rêve d'Alembert*, which argues that human consciousness is entirely organic in origin. These works characterize the Enlightment period (Porter, 1993, p. 1457).

Gamwell and Tomes (1995) note, "The rise of science in the eighteenth century slowly eroded the foundations of religion and ultimately led to the secular science of the modern world" (p. 19).

The Wesleyan-Methodist tradition begins in England (as an offshoot of the Anglican tradition) with the work of John and Charles Wesley. John Wesley (1703–1791) writes extensively on health topics, including volumes such as *Thoughts on Nervous Disorders* (1784), *The Duty and Advantage of Early Rising* (1789), and his most famous work on the subject, *Primitive Physick* (1747). *Primitive Physick* becomes one of the most popular medical manuals of the eighteenth century.

Franz Anton Mesmer (1734–1815) embraces astrology, believing that the stars have influences on human beings. He first claims that cures may be obtained by stroking magnets ("Theory of Magnetism") but later discards the magnets, becoming convinced that he can influence others by stroking them with only his hands.

In 1765, the first medical school in North America is established at the College of Philadelphia, which later (1791) merges with the medical school of the University of Pennsylvania.

In 1767, King's College organizes a medical faculty and becomes the second institution in the North American colonies to confer a doctor of medicine degree; it later becomes the College of Physicians and Surgeons, Columbia University.

In the early 1800s, there are only three medical hospitals in the United States: the New York Hospital, the Pennsylvania Hospital, and the Massachusetts Hospital. The first official nursing organization in the United States is initiated in Emmitsburg by the Catholic Sisters of Charity in 1803, following a French model. The sisters perform home nursing as well as offer institutional care (Nelson, 1997).

Treatment for mental illness is often harsh—mass confinement of the mentally ill, who are herded into insane asylums mainly to protect others from them. Blood-letting and purging enemas continue as the primary forms of medical treatment offered by Benjamin Rush (1745–1813) in America and by others of his day.

1780–1830	The Second Great Awakening, a Protestant revival, sweeps the United States. Calvinistic teachings on man's depraved nature are disputed, and some theologians shift from a doctrine of predestinarianism to the doctrine of free will. It is possible, through good works and community volunteerism, for humans to influence their own salvation. This movement has great social force in America and helps prepare the country for a new approach to the treatment of mental illness (Taubes, 1998).
1800–1850	William Tuke, a devout Quaker, starts the York retreat in England. He believes that a purely medical approach to mental illness will fail to produce cures, since insanity is a disruption of the mind and spirit and needs compassionate psychological and spiritual treatment. He discourages the use of frequent bleedings, purgings, and ice baths and instead institutes a regimen of exercise, work, and recreation, treating patients like normal adults who are expected to behave according to societal norms. Tuke's results are astonishing, and his "moral treatment" quickly spreads to America, where the "Friends Asylum" is established in Philadelphia in 1817 (the second oldest mental hospital in the United States).

Moral treatment is the first established form of psychiatric care in the United States. Rather than view mental illness as demonic possession or a form of debasement, the proponents of moral treatment see mental illness as a physical disease (Taubes, 1998).

Most insane asylums in America during the early 1800s are a mixture of science and religion (Gamwell & Tomes, 1995). Patients are often "rewarded" for self-control by being allowed to attend religious services. Referring to this trend, Amariah Brigham (coeditor of the *American*

Journal of Insanity and superintendent of the Hartford Retreat) writes: "No doubt that these services are beneficial to our patients. Permission to attend them is solicited by nearly all and many are induced to exercise their self-control in order to enjoy this privilege" (p. 24) (Seventeenth Annual Report, 1841).

The American social reformer Dorothea Dix (1802–1887), a former Methodist turned Unitarian who herself suffers from depression, begins in the 1840s to fight politically for the humane care of the insane poor (Gamwell & Tomes, 1995).

In 1844, Samuel Woodward founds the American Psychiatric Association, then known as the Association of Medical Superintendents of American Institutions for the Insane (AMSAII). The association's official publication is the *American Journal of Insanity* (later renamed the *American Journal of Psychiatry*).

The American Medical Association is established in 1847.

In 1830, the Church of Jesus Christ of Latter-Day Saints (the Mormon Church) is established in New York by Joseph Smith.

Two Christian doctors, Peter Parker and David Livingstone, ignite a medical-missionary movement (1840s) which progresses to involve nearly all major religious denominations and continues to this day (Numbers & Amundsen, 1988, p. 2).

1850–1875   Study of the brain and the nervous system replaces the "flow of bodily humors" as the key to mental health (1850–1870).

Strange "scientific" theories of personality and mental illness are proposed and flourish, including physiognomy (the study of facial features) and phrenology (the study of facial features and features of the skull that are believed to reflect the underlying brain). "Hydrotherapy," "electrotherapy," health foods, and tranquil natural settings are used to treat the mentally ill (Gamwell & Tomes, 1995).

Rudolph Virchow, a German pathologist and anthropologist, develops the cellular theory of pathology, leading to the foundation of pathological histology (*Die Cellularpathologie*, 1858).

Charles Darwin (1809–1882) introduces his theory that man descended long ago from marine animals, through amphibians, marsupials, and the ape species (*Origin of Species by Means of Natural Selection, or the Preservation of Fa-*

voured Races in the Struggle for Life, 1859), challenging the religious anthropocentric view of man.

In 1858, a vision reported by Bernadette Soubirous (1844–1879) results in Lourdes, France, becoming a prominent healing shrine (it is visited by 3 million people per year). While believers have claimed that thousands of miracles have occurred there, the Catholic church has authenticated only 64 (Porter, 1993, pp. 1456–1457).

The first General Conference of the Seventh-Day Adventists (SDAs), based on the teachings of William Miller, a Baptist farmer-preacher from upstate New York, is held in 1863. Strong emphasis is placed on health. Following the book *Philosophy of Health: Natural Principles of Health and Cure* (1848), SDAs emphasize fresh air, exercise, a meat-free diet, sexual purity, drug-free medicine, avoidance of stimulants, and sensible dress. Ellen White (1864), widely known and respected as an SDA prophetess, administers hydropathic treatments and supervises the founding of many sanitariums.

1875–1890

The English biologist and educator Thomas Huxley (1825–1895) writes extensively on natural science and becomes a prominent scientific opponent of religion. An agnostic, Huxley becomes a fierce proponent of Darwin's theory of evolution. It is in this period that modern medical science begins to openly oppose religious dogma and tradition.

Christian Science is born in 1866 as Mary Baker Eddy (1821–1910) spontaneously recovers from a serious injury. She emphasizes the mind-body relationship in *Science and Health with Key to the Scriptures* (1875), claiming that the mind through prayer is capable of physical healing. She practices both homeopathy and mesmerism before establishing the Christian Science Church. In 1908, she starts publishing the *Christian Science Monitor*. Unity School of Practical Christianity, Church of Religious Science, and Divine Science are related groups that spin off from the Christian Science tradition (Numbers & Amundsen, 1998, p. 2).

Evangelical Christianity, which had its origins in the preaching of John Wesley and George Whitefield in the mid-1700s, spreads rapidly in the late 1800s and early 1900s through revivals led by Charles Finney, Dwight Moody, and Billy Sunday.

The term "psychiatrist" is used for the first time in Germany in the 1880s. "Scientific" psychiatrists study the brain and nervous system and distinguish themselves from the old "asylum doctors." These new doctors want to distance themselves from religion as they fight to establish their identity as a respectable scientific discipline, modeling themselves after other medical specialties, such as surgery and the new, budding field of neurology.

With tremendous advances in medicine and the discovery of the germ theory of disease, researchers begin to seek organic causes for mental illness. With few exceptions (e.g., syphilis), however, organic causes for mental illness cannot be identified.

German psychiatrists such as Emile Kraeplin make detailed observations of the mentally ill, and in 1883 Kraeplin writes his *Compendium of Psychiatry* (revised in 1896), carefully describing illnesses including manic-depression and dementia praecox (later called schizophrenia by Eugene Bleuler).

As the spiritual aspects of treatment are reduced or eliminated, abuses in the care of mental patients in asylums become more prevalent.

Louis Pasteur (1822–1895) introduces the germ theory of disease in *Memoire sur les corpuscles organisés qui existent dans l'atmosphere* (1861). At the same time, there is a resurgence of faith healing during revivals, pilgrimages to shrines, and exposure to relics.

Robert Koch (1843–1910) describes the life history of the bacterium that causes anthrax (1876); he later isolates the bacterial causes of tuberculosis (1882) and of cholera (1884).

In 1879, a wealthy Pittsburgh businessman, Charles Russell, begins publishing *Zion's Watch Tower and Herald of Christ's Presence*, which becomes the major publication of the Jehovah's Witnesses.

The Baptist evangelist Charles Spurgeon (1834–1892) notes that "The greatest earthly blessing that God can give to any of us is health, with the exception of sickness. . . . A sick wife, a newly made grave, poverty, slander, sinking of spirit, might teach us lessons nowhere else to be learned so well" (Porter, 1993, p. 1465).

1885–1900

The Association of American Physicians is founded in 1886 and has a profound effect on the development of clinical research in the United States as it opens its membership not only to those who practice and teach internal medicine but also to basic scientists (pathologists, bacteriologists, physiologists).

Jean Charcot (1825–1893), the Paris physician and neurophysiologist known for his work on diseases of the nervous system, contributes important insights into the nature of hysteria. Charcot is reported to have said that science has reluctantly accepted the "faith-cure" (referring to the miracles at Lourdes). Nevertheless, he declares that faith-cures were "an ideal method, since they often attained their ends when all other means have failed" (Berdoe, 1893, p. 481).

The Johns Hopkins Medical School and Hospital begins accepting its first students in 1893; William Osler becomes its first professor of medicine and W. S. Halstead its first professor of surgery.

1890–1915

From the academic side, "psychology" begins to emerge as a subdiscipline of philosophy. As an outgrowth of naturalistic determinism (the belief that all things can be understood in terms of natural scientific principles and laws), American psychologists such as J. H. Leuba, E. D. Starbuck, and William James begin to study religion scientifically. While James and Starbuck are somewhat sympathetic toward religion, Leuba is not and argues that religious experience is both naive and illusory.

The first scientific research study on the psychology of religion is published in an academic journal (Leuba, 1896). Leuba (1912) later becomes a major figure in the academic world studying the psychology of religion.

The sociologist Emile Durkheim (1897) writes his classic volume *Le Suicide*, identifying religious organizations as important groups in society that act to enhance social cohesion, reduce anomie, and protect persons from self-destructive acts (a notion he later expands in a 1912 publication).

E. D. Starbuck (1899) writes the first academic textbook on the psychology of religion.

William James (1901) writes his *Varieties of Religious Experience*, a classic description of the more extreme forms of religious belief and experience.

In 1906, the Emmanuel Movement is begun in Boston by the Episcopal clergyman Elwood Worcester, who acknowledges the primacy of mind over body and believes that through prayer one can achieve physical healing by activating divine forces. This is one of the first examples in recent times of cooperation between clergy and physicians.

Sir William Osler, a professor of medicine at Johns Hopkins, writes "The Faith That Heals" in the *British Medical Journal* (Osler, 1910).

The birth of American Pentecostalism (including Assemblies of God and Churches of God) occurs between 1907 and 1911, with a heavy emphasis on faith healing and miracles (Azusa Street revival). Prominent leaders in this group later include Oral Roberts, Kenneth Copeland, and Jim Bakker.

The American Evangelical-Fundamentalist tradition advances with the publication of *The Fundamentals*, a 12-volume series published between 1910 and 1915. The term "fundamentalism" refers to the beliefs of those who subscribe to evangelical orthodoxy as outlined in the volumes named earlier. Neo-evangelicals who evolve from this tradition late in the twentieth century include Carl Henry, Billy Graham, James Dobson, C. Everett Koop, and Francis Schaeffer. Popular magazines that present the view of evangelical Christianity include *Christianity Today* (founded in 1956) and *Focus on the Family* (founded in the1980s).

1900–1940

Science, however, is moving another direction. The great hope of the new sciences of psychology and sociology is for a new solution to the old problems of mental and emotional diseases, but *sans réligion* (Lannert, 1991).

In 1905, John Strutt claims that the age of some rocks is at least 2 billion years, contradicting the assertion in Genesis that the universe was created around 4000 B.C. (although people have believed the earth to be millions of years old since the eighteenth century).

Sigmund Freud (1856–1939), a Viennese physician, initially seeks the neurophysiological origins of mental illness; failing in this endeavor, he develops the first comprehensive psychological theory for neurosis and a treatment ("the talking cure").

Freud eloquently describes the irrational and neurotic influences of religion on the human psyche in *Future of an Illusion* (1927) and in numerous other publications (1907, 1913, 1930, 1933a, 1933b, 1939). In 1930, at the age of 73, Freud writes that religion results in "depressing the value of life and distorting the picture of the real world in a delusional manner—which presupposes an intimidation of intelligence."

Carl Jung presents a different view of religion in *Modern Man in Search of Soul* (1933). He argues that "losing a religious outlook on life" can be the cause of much neurosis and mental disturbance.

Mental health professionals who administered the "talking cure" of Freud became known as psychotherapists, from the work "psyche," which means *soul*, and "therapist," which means *servant*; thus, the psychotherapist is "a servant of the soul" (Lannert, 1991).

Albert Einstein (1879–1955) develops his special theory of relativity ($e = mc^2$) in 1905 and his general theory of relativity in 1916, rejecting Newton's carefully ordered universe. Later, Einstein makes his famous remark, "Science without religion is lame. Religion without science is blind" (Einstein, 1941).

1930-1940

In the 1930s, a Baptist commission reviewing missionary activity of the church calls for less evangelism and more humanitarianism: "The use of medical or other professional service as a direct means of making converts, or public [religious] services in wards and dispensaries from which patients cannot escape, is subtly coercive, and improper" (Numbers & Amundsen, 1988, p. 3).

Psychology emerges as a discipline in its own right and distances itself from philosophy and religion, instead modeling itself after scientific disciplines like physics. Almost no research is devoted to the study of religion or its relationship to mental health. By 1935, the brief flourish of interest in the psychology of religion at the turn of the century has ended.

1940-1950

In 1948, George Gamow describes the "big bang" theory, which suggests that the universe began as an explosion approximately 14 billion years ago. This theory leaves open the possibility of an instantaneous creation by a Creator.

The National Institutes of Health is reorganized and expanded after World War II and begins giving out research grants to clinical departments.

1950-1980

Church-related hospitals, first established around the turn of the twentieth century, care for more than a quarter of all hospitalized patients in the United States (Numbers & Amundsen, 1998, p. 2). Porter notes that "in the mid 20th century, almost a thousand Catholic hospitals were handling some 16 million patients a year" (Porter, 1993, p. 1453).

The Harvard psychologist Gordon Allport (1950) writes *The Individual and His Religion*, in which he examines the nature of "mature" religion and begins to develop the notion of "intrinsic" versus "extrinsic" religiosity.

The U.C. Berkeley sociologists Charles Glock and Rodney Stark report on the dimensions of religiousness and relate them to different psychological attitudes (Glock & Stark, 1965, 1966; Stark & Glock, 1968). Only isolated studies of the relationship between religion and health appear during this time (e.g., those of Gordon Allport, David Moberg, Bernard Spilka, C. D. Batson, and Allen Bergin).

Studies of religion continue to be frowned on by mainstream scientists. Modern biological psychiatry emerges.

In 1962, the inaugural issue of the *Journal of Religion and Health* appears.

In 1962-1965, a series of meetings of Catholic leaders results in the Second Council of the Vatican (Vatican II). Sweeping changes occur in the Catholic Church.

The Johns Hopkins epidemiologist George Comstock publishes evidence in the *Journal of Chronic Disease* that frequent church attendees have lower mortality rates (Comstock & Partridge, 1972).

In 1978, Oral Roberts's City of Faith Medical and Research Center in Tulsa, Oklahoma, opens. The goal is to treat patients' medical, physiological, and spiritual problems.

1980–1990

Mormon and Adventist surgeons make remarkable technological advances with experiments involving artificial and baboon hearts (Numbers & Amundsen, 1998, p. 3).

As many as 100 million charismatic Christians around the world express beliefs in divine healing, and many millions make pilgrimage to Lourdes, France, in hope of healing.

Increasing research appears in mainstream medical, sociological, and psychological journals on religion and health (e.g., by William P. Wilson, David B. Larson, Jeffrey S. Levin, Ellen Idler, Harold G. Koenig, Kenneth Pargament, and Christopher Ellison).

The American Psychological Association's journal, *Psychotherapy* devotes an entire issue to "Psychotherapy and Religion" (Bradford & Spero, 1990), reflecting growing interest and acceptance of the link between the two.

1990–2000

During "the decade of the brain," psychiatrists focus on biological and neurological causes for mental illness and on pharmacological treatments.

Psychiatric Annals, a widely read journal for continuing psychiatric education, devotes one entire issue to the problem of evil (Haroun, 1997).

In 1992, Pope John Paul II apologizes for the Catholic Church's condemnation of Galileo. In 1996, he suggests that evolution may be a part of God's master plan.

Scientists say the universe is 13 billion years old and that Earth is only a speck in one of 50 billion galaxies spread across 12 billion light years of space (Will, 1998).

Forty percent of major scientists in the physical sciences say they believe in God (Larson & Witham, 1997); a subsequent survey by the same authors, however, reveals that only 7% of scientists admitted to the elite National Academy of Science profess a belief in God (most of those who believe are mathematicians).

Increasing numbers of studies are published in mainstream psychiatric and medical journals that examine the possible relationship between religion and health. By the end of the century, more than 60 medical schools (of the 126 schools in the United States) have courses on religion, spirituality, and medicine.

PART II

DEBATING RELIGION'S
EFFECTS ON HEALTH

3

Religion's Positive Effects

THE COMMON ASSUMPTION that religious faith is good for health has many sources. Religious scriptures, religious professionals, faith healers, popular writers, religious health professionals, and a few leading health professionals sympathetic to religion all make this claim. Not surprising, then, there have been movements, both in the past and, increasingly, in the present, to integrate religion into the clinical practice of medicine and psychology. We now examine these sources in greater detail.

RELIGIOUS SCRIPTURES

Religious scriptures, such as the Judeo-Christian Bible, indicate that devout religious practices are rewarded by good health. Take, for example, the following Scriptures:

These are the commands, decrees and laws the Lord your God directed me to teach you to observe in the land that you are crossing the Jordan to possess, so that you, your children and their children after them may fear the Lord your God as long as you live by keeping all his decrees and commands that I give you, and *so that you may enjoy long life* [italicized for emphasis]. (Deuteronomy 6:1–2, NIV)

"Because he loves me," says the Lord, "I will rescue him; I will protect him, for he acknowledges my name. He will call upon me, and I will answer him; I will be with him in trouble, I will deliver him and honor him. *With long life will I satisfy him* and show him my salvation." (Psalms 91:14–16, NIV)

Praise the Lord, O my soul; and forget not all his benefits—
who forgives all your sins and *heals all your diseases,*

who redeems your life from the pit and crowns
you with love and compassion,
who satisfies your desires with good things, so
that *your youth is renewed* like the eagle's. (Psalms
103:2–5, NIV)

Do not be wise in your own eyes: fear the Lord
and shun evil. This will bring *health to your body
and nourishment to your bones*. (Proverbs 3:8,
NIV)

My son, pay attention to what I say; listen
closely to my words. Do not let them out of
your sight, keep them within your heart; for
they are life to those who find them and *health
to a man's whole body*. (Proverbs 4:22, NIV)

If you obey my commands, you will remain in
my love, just as I have obeyed my Father's commands and remained in his love. I have told you
this so that my joy may be in you and that *your
joy may be complete*. (John 15:10–11, NIV)

But the fruit of the Spirit is love, *joy, peace*,
patience, kindness, goodness, faithfulness, gen-
tleness and *self-control*. (Galatians 5:22–23, NIV)

Dear friend, I pray that you may enjoy *good health*
and that all may go well with you, *even as your
soul is getting along well*. (3 John 1:2, NIV)

Descriptive terms like "long life," "health to
your body," "joy," and "peace" suggest that religion has both mental and physical health benefits. The faithful have for centuries taken these
pronouncements as truth based upon the highest authority.

Religious Professionals

Sermons by ministers and rabbis often encourage devout religious belief and practice to
achieve not only spiritual growth but also
greater well-being, happiness, purpose in life,
and fulfillment in marriage, family, job, and
relationships with others. Likewise, the liturgy
and hymns during religious services often include themes having to do with joy, peace, confidence, overcoming adversity, or other positive
health consequences of having triumphed over
evil forces. Note the selected stanzas taken from
a few common hymns:

When darkness seems to hide His face,
I rest upon His unchanging grace;
In every high and stormy gale,
My anchor holds within the vale.
His oath, His covenant, His blood
Support me in the whelming flood;
When all around my soul gives away,
He then is all my hope and stay.
                              —*The Solid Rock*
                       (by Mote & Bradbury)

A wonderful Savior is Jesus my Lord,
He taketh my burden away;
He holdeth me up, and I shall not to be moved,
He giveth me strength as my day.
                        —*He Hideth My Soul*
                    (by William J. Kirkpatrick)

Fear not, I am with thee; O be not dismayed,
For I am thy God, and will still give thee aid;
I'll strengthen thee, help thee, and cause thee
    to stand,
Upheld by my righteous, omnipotent hand.
When thro' fiery trials thy pathway shall lie,
My grace, all-sufficient, shall be thy supply;
The flame shall not hurt thee; I only design
Thy dross to consume, and thy gold to refine.
                    —*How Firm a Foundation*
                           (by John Rippon)

When peace like a river, attendeth my way,
When sorrows like the sea billows roll;
Whatever my lot, Thou hast taught me to say,
"It is well with my soul."
                   —*It Is Well with My Soul*
                         (by Philip P. Bliss)

You're my heart and my soul,
My joy and my strength.
You're my hope and my reason to live.
In Your presence there is peace and fullness
    of joy . . .
                      —*I Will Celebrate You*
                        (by Richard Garcia)

Thro' many dangers, toils, and snares
I have already come;
'Tis grace hath bro't me safe this far,
And grace will lead me home.
                          —*Amazing Grace*
                  (by John Newton & John Rees)

Indeed, not only are clergy some of the primary sources from which we hear the health
benefits of religion; they are also important

sources of mental health care in this country. There are nearly 500,000 churches, synagogues, and mosques in the United States, with more than 300,000 clergy. Since counseling activities by clergy take up 10 to 20% of their time, religious professionals provide nearly 150 million hours of mental health services per year (not including the activities of nearly 100,000 full-time nuns or chaplains for whom such data are not available) (Weaver, 1995).

While clergy have counseled members of their congregations for centuries, this service did not become organized or incorporate psychotherapeutic principles from the mental health sciences until the pastoral care movement began in the early 1900s. Two physicians (W. S. Keller, in Cincinnati, Ohio, and R. C. Cabot, in Boston) and a minister (Anton Boisen) began the pastoral care education movement in the 1920s and 1930s. Their efforts led to the formation of the Council for Clinical Training of Theological Students, which eventually split into the Council for Clinical Training, in New York City, and the Institute of Pastoral Care, in Boston (Wicks, Parsons, et al., 1985).

The pastoral care movement received much impetus through the writings of Seward Hiltner, Wayne Oates, and the Protestant theologian Albert Outler (author of *Psychotherapy and the Christian Message*, 1954). In 1964, the American Association of Pastoral Counselors was organized and began publishing a professional journal, the *Journal of Pastoral Care*. This organization now has a national board that provides certification and continuing education for pastoral counselors throughout the United States. The pastoral care movement has been closely affiliated with the inclusion of chaplains in medical and other settings and with the development of chaplaincy training programs (clinical pastoral education) in hospitals.

FAITH HEALING

Largely outside mainstream Protestant and Catholic Christianity, there have arisen charismatic groups that include televangelists and faith healers who, in dramatic fashion and with much showmanship, produce physical "heal-

ings" among eager and excited audiences. People in wheelchairs stand up and walk; the blind see; the deaf hear; participants faint, shake, and experience other unusual physical and emotional reactions. Tens of thousands of people flocked to hear Kathryn Kuhlman (1962) and Oral Roberts (1995), and many more come today to participate in faith healing meetings held by Benny Hinn (1997) and others. Often desperate and as a last resort, millions of hope-filled faithful over the years have made pilgrimages to holy places like Lourdes, France, in search of healing.

Positive Confession Movement

Similar to faith healers, the positive confession movement of Kenneth Hagin (1982) and Kenneth Copeland (1996) has had significant impact on the beliefs of many evangelical Christians. Hagin and Copeland teach that health and prosperity were provided by the death of Jesus Christ on the cross and that all a believer needs to do is claim a "promise" and speak it into existence by the word of the Christian's mouth. Similar is the teaching of Paul Yong-Gi Cho (1987), pastor of one of the largest evangelical churches in the world, in Seoul, Korea. These groups have been roundly criticized by mainstream religious groups, especially dispensationalist theologians.

Fundamentalism and Faith Healing

The term "fundamentalist" is a somewhat technical term that is used by the general public in a nontechnical way. The term is often used to refer to any Christian to the right of center, especially the far right. Many fundamentalists, however, would be vehemently opposed to faith healers or avoiding physicians. Historically, fundamentalist Christianity flourished in the early twentieth century as a response to Modernism. It held to traditional beliefs such as scriptural inerrancy, the virgin birth, and salvation through Christ's blood. It also avoided social action, seeing it as a liberal hallmark. The fundamentalists from dispensational backgrounds (many Southern Baptists, for example) believe that healing as a gift passed away at the end of the apostolic age.

Healing in Non-Christian Religions

Just as Lourdes does for Christians, places of healing exist for Hindus (Benares, along Ganges River), Jews (the old temple wall in Jerusalem), and Muslims (Mecca, in Western Saudia Arabia). In the United States, there are Jewish centers for healing and renewal (such as Elat Chayyim in Accord, New York, and the National Center for Jewish Healing, in New York City) and Buddhist healing centers (Medicine Buddha Healing Center in San Jose, California). In May 1998, the Dalai Lama visited New York City to spend a day at Beth Israel Medical Center with 20 physicians and research scientists from around the country to find common ground between modern Western medical technology and ancient Buddhist practices. The visit was organized by Beth Israel's Institute of Neurology and Neurosurgery, the Tibet House, and Columbia University's Center for Meditation and Healing, and several follow-up meetings have been planned to incorporate Buddhist ideas and practices into traditional medicine (Brozan, 1998).

POPULAR SECULAR AND CHRISTIAN WRITERS

A number of well-known and loved American writers such as Norman Vincent Peale and Dale Carnegie have included references to religious scriptures in their best-selling self-help books, *The Power of Positive Thinking* (1952) and *How to Win Friends and Influence People* (1936). Hence, the wisdom of health (Peale) and success (Carnegie) appears grounded in the sacred writings of the Judeo-Christian tradition.

Another group of popular writers who address health issues has emerged among evangelical Protestants as a result of the growing industry of Christian counseling. These Christian writers have produced many practical guidebooks and self-help manuals. They include Tim LaHaye (*How to Win over Depression*, 1974),

Bruce Larson (*Living on the Growing Edge*, 1968), David Seamands (*Healing for Damaged Emotions*, 1983), and Robert Schuller (*Tough Times Never Last, but Tough People Do!*, 1983). These Christian writers provide an interesting mix of cognitive behavioral psychotherapy, positive thinking, and practical suggestions based on the Bible, an approach that has become known as pop evangelical psychology. Their influence has been profound, both on the public and on the practices of many Christian counselors and other mental health professionals. Christian counseling has become professionalized with the rise of evangelical seminaries with established and credible schools of psychology (such as the Rosemead Graduate School of Professional Psychology at Biola University, in La Mirada, California, and the Fuller School of Psychology at the Fuller Theological Seminary, in Pasadena, California).

RELIGIOUS HEALTH PROFESSIONALS

Religious health professionals include medical physicians, psychiatrists, psychologists, and other health workers who have been trained in the secular tradition but who use religion in their clinical practices to complement (not replace) traditional therapies.

Medical Practice

Perhaps the first organization of religious health professionals was the Emmanual Movement. The Emmanual Movement had its beginnings in Boston, in the early 1900s (just prior to the advent of the pastoral care movement). In 1908, an Episcopal minister, Elwood Worcester, and a prominent physician at Tufts Medical School, Dr. I. Cariat, coauthored *Religion and Medicine*, a book that was later included in the Surgeon General's *Progress of Medicine during the Nineteenth Century* (Wicks, Parsons, et al., 1985).

In the early 1970s, Granger Westberg, clinical adjunct professor of preventive medicine at the University of Illinois at Chicago School of

Medicine, founded a number of Wholistic Health Centers in the Midwest (Westberg, 1984). As with the Emmanuel Movement, the attempt was to integrate religion and medical care by involving religious professionals and churches. While the concept of "parish nursing" began out of this movement (see chapter 29), the Emmanuel Movement and its offshoots did not gain momentum and had little influence in medical circles.

Psychiatric Practice

A psychiatrist and former dean of medical education at Duke University, Dan Blazer, reviews the history of recent attempts to integrate religion into the practice of psychiatry in his book *Freud vs. God* (1998). Before the rise of the "Christian psychiatry" movement in this country, the Swiss physician Paul Tournier made attempts to integrate religion into the mental health care of his patients. Tournier was primarily a clinician and was virtually unknown in the academic field of psychiatry. He wrote mostly for a Christian audience and, according to Blazer, was unique in that he did not attempt to "Christianianize psychiatry or psychologize Christianity." Tournier's book *The Meaning of Persons* (1957) received wide readership both in the United States and in Europe.

The Christian psychiatry movement in the United States (which grew out of the evangelical Protestant tradition) was started by William P. Wilson, at Duke University, and Mansell Pattison, at the University of Georgia, in the 1970s and early 1980s. Both individuals were prominent psychiatrists (Wilson was head of biological psychiatry at Duke, and Pattison was chairman of the department of psychiatry at Georgia) who made attempts to organize training programs for psychiatrists interested in practicing Christian psychiatry (a form of psychiatry that integrates Christian beliefs and practices into the psychotherapy and treatment of mental disorder).

Soon after the emergence of Christian psychiatry, a network of Christian psychiatry units in hospitals and independent treatment centers was started in the mid-1980s and early 1990s.

These centers are designed specifically to attract evangelical Christian clients. The Minirth-Meier New Life treatment centers, the Rapha mental health centers, and the Kairos mental health centers are the best known of these. Christian psychiatrists and mental health workers staff these centers. Frank Minirth and Paul Meier have written a number of popular self-help books related to this practice that have been hugely successful (Minirth et al., 1994).

Among popular psychologists, Gary Collins (*Christian Counseling: A Comprehensive Guide*, 1988) and James Dobson (*Dare to Discipline*, 1970) have acquired enormous followings during the past three decades, largely as a result of their many popular self-help books and family guides. In academic psychology, the Brigham Young University professor Allen Bergin has for 20 years led efforts in the field of psychology to integrate patients' religious beliefs and values into the practice of psychotherapy (or at least to see them as relevant). In 1980 he wrote an articulate piece on psychotherapy and religious values, in which he argued that, unless psychologists sincerely considered and conceptually integrated the religious belief systems of clients into their work, they would not be be fully effective professionals. In that article he hypothesized that "Religious communities that provide the combination of a viable beliefs structure and a network of loving, emotional support should manifest lower rates of emotional and social pathology and physical disease" (Bergin, 1980, p. 102). He went on to suggest that such a hypothesis could be tested empirically using the scientific method.

Similar attempts have been made to integrate religion and spirituality into the practice of medicine. Perhaps the best-known contemporary writers in this area are the Yale surgeon Bernie Siegel (*Love, Medicine and Miracles*, 1986), the Texas cardiologist Larry Dossey (*Healing Words*, 1995), and the Georgetown internist Dale Matthews (*The Faith Factor*, 1998). All argue that the religious or spiritual dimension of patients should be considered in medical care. Christian physicians and dentists in the United States for the past two decades have organized themselves into the rapidly growing

Christian Medical and Dental Society (CMDS), which in 2000 has more than 14,000 dues-paying members around the country, 95% of whom are physicians (in 1995 it had only 7,000 members).

The fact that a substantial number of health professionals are themselves religious, have made efforts to partner with religious professionals, and use patients' religious beliefs to speed healing contributes to the view that religion can have positive effects on health, particularly mental health.

LEADING HEALTH PROFESSIONALS SYMPATHETIC TO RELIGION

Another source of support for religion's health benefits comes from the lectures and writings of leading academic health professionals. These individuals, while sympathetic to the possible benefits of religion, would probably feel uncomfortable labeling themselves religious health professionals. Practitioners in this category include the eminent psychologists Carl Jung and Martin Seligman. A Swiss psychologist, Jung was a contemporary of Sigmund Freud. In his classic work *Modern Man in Search of Soul*, Jung wrote the following:

> During the past 30 years, people from all the civilized countries of the earth have consulted me. I have treated many hundreds of patients, the larger number being Protestants, a smaller number Jews, and not more than five or six believing Catholics. Among all my patients in the second half of life—that is to say, over thirty-five—there has not been one whose problem in the last resort was not that of finding a religious outlook on life. It is safe to say that every one of them fell ill because he had lost that which the living religions of every age have given to their followers, and none of them has been really healed who did not regain his religious outlook. (Jung, 1933, p. 229)

Likewise, Martin E. P. Seligman, president of the American Psychological Association in 1998, recently discussed, in a speech given to the John Templeton Foundation group, the current epi-demic of depression among younger persons in the United States. He noted:

> If you ask yourself, why didn't our grandparents become depressed at the same rate we do when they were thwarted—when the people they love rejected them and they didn't get the job they wanted, when their children died. Why did they have less of a rate? Well I think they had communal buffers. Larger buffers. They had their relationship to God. They had belief in a nation, patriotism. They had belief in a community, and they had large extended families. Now this is the spiritual furniture that our parents and grandparents sat in when they failed. This spiritual furniture, all of these things, belief in God, community, nation has become threadbare in our lifetime. (Seligman, 1998, p. 158)

A prominent medical professional who has emphasized the potential benefits of religion and spirituality on health is the Harvard professor Herbert Benson. Benson helped create the growing field of mind-body medicine during the past three decades, publishing extensively on the health effects of the Relaxation Response in top-tier medical and scientific journals such as the *New England Journal of Medicine, The Lancet*, and *Science* (Benson, 1975, 1977; Benson, Shapiro, et al., 1971) and writing many popular books in this area (Benson, 1975, 1984, 1996; Benson & Stuart, 1993). Since the mid-1990s he has directed a Harvard Medical School continuing medical education course entitled "Spirituality and Medicine" that has attracted worldwide attention. Over the past century, then, a number of highly regarded and respected mental health and medical professionals have spoken out in favor of the health benefits of religious belief and practice.

This position has even affected the training of medical doctors. In 1992, only four of 125 medical schools in the United States offered courses on religion and medicine. By 1999, more than 60 medical schools offered such courses. Among the medical schools that offer courses on religion/spirituality and medicine are Johns Hopkins University, Harvard University, the University of Pennsylvania, and Case

Western Reserve University (see chapter 29 for a list of other schools). Thus, some of the country's leading medical schools now offer students either elective or required courses that integrate religion and spirituality into medicine.

SUMMARY AND CONCLUSIONS

In this chapter, we have focused primarily on the Judeo-Christian tradition in the United States. Physical and emotional healing, however, play a vital role in the belief systems of Hindus, Buddhists, Muslims, and Jews, as well. Clearly, many people closely associate religion and health. Scriptures in both the Hebrew Bible and the New Testament emphasize the mental and physical health benefits of obedience to God. Likewise, Christian hymns speak of comfort, peace, and joy as part of the Christian religious experience. One of the primary tasks of the clergy in the United States is counseling, and religious professionals are a major source of mental health care for people in the United States. The field of pastoral care has grown into a recognized and respectable discipline.

In contrast, the often dramatic and always controversial activities of faith healers and miracle workers have attracted hundreds of thousands of people through television and radio, popular books, and conferences. Their work has often overshadowed the more mundane, less attention-seeking work of hundreds of thousands of religious professionals who have consistently labored to help members of their congregations overcome emotional and physical health problems.

Many health professionals are themselves religious and have made attempts to integrate religious beliefs and healing methods into their practices. Christian psychiatry and psychology have rapidly grown in America with the opening of specialized units and treatment centers that use Christian methods for treating mental disorders alongside traditional biological and psychosocial therapies. Perhaps one of the most credible sources of support for the health benefits of religious faith are nonreligious health professionals, academic leaders in psychology and medicine, who have written about and spoken on this topic. There is now considerable momentum among U.S. medical schools to educate young doctors about the religious beliefs and practices of patients and how they relate to health and illness.

Thus, it is clear that much of the general public and a growing number of health professionals believe that religion and good health are somehow related. Are there any dissenters in this regard? Chapter 4 examines the other side of the debate.

4

Religion's Negative Effects

IN CHAPTER 3 WE DISCUSSED THE positive effects of religion on health as suggested by religious scriptures, religious hymns, religious professionals, faith healers, popular writers, religious health professionals, and a number of nonreligious health professionals. In this chapter we examine what skeptics say about religion's health benefits. Indeed, there is a sizable group of reputable health professionals who argue that religious beliefs and practices have either no effect or adverse effects on mental health and, in some instances, on physical health.

CLARIFYING THE QUESTION

As we discuss the possible negative effects of religion on health, it is important to keep clear just what our question is: Do religious beliefs and practices cause negative changes in health?

Just because a religious person has mental or physical illness does not necessarily mean that the person's religious faith caused the health problems. This applies equally well to the devoutly religious person who has excellent mental and physical health; that is, we cannot assume that religiousness is responsible for the excellent health.

Indeed, health problems often affect the experience and expression of religious beliefs. For example, mentally ill persons may express bizarre religious beliefs and unusual religious preoccupations, just as they may express eccentric political beliefs or engage in strange eating behaviors. We would not conclude that someone's bizarre political ideas are the cause of his mental illness but would more likely decide that they occur as *a result of* the mental problems. The same probably applies to religion.

A second example is the very religious person with severe medical illness. Should we automatically conclude that the person's religious-ness caused the physical health problems? Or is it possible that the severely ill person, in attempting to cope with the illness, has turned to religion for comfort? In the second instance, religious beliefs and activities might be viewed as a consequence of the medical illness. Such "cause and effect" considerations are particularly relevant as we examine reports based on personal observation or clinical experience (which is always limited and difficult to generalize from).

We now examine the views of well-known and influential mental health professionals concerning the possible adverse effects of religion.

SIGMUND FREUD

When one thinks of the fathers of modern psychiatry, Freud tops the list. His works have had an enormous influence on psychiatric practice over the past 100 years. In fact, the notion that talking about problems might bring about emotional relief and resolution of internal conflict received widespread professional acceptance largely as a result of Freud's writings on the subject. Indeed, Freud was a masterful writer, brilliant thinker, and articulate speaker and teacher who was able to synthesize information from many sources into new ideas and then effectively communicate these ideas to others.

Just as he clearly and convincingly taught about the inner workings of the human mind, Freud presented his views on religion without ambiguity. These views were not favorable. One of his first papers on the topic, *Obsessive Acts and Religious Practices* (1907), compared religious practices such as prayer and religious rituals to the obsessive acts of the neurotic:

> I am certainly not the first to be struck by the resemblance between what are called obsessive acts in neurotics and those religious observances by means of which the faithful give expression to their piety. . . . It is easy to see wherein lies the resemblance between neurotic ceremonial and religious rites; it is in the fear of pangs of conscience after their omission, in the complete isolation of them from all other activities (the feeling that one must not be dis-

turbed), and in the conscientiousness with which the details are carried out. . . . The protestations of the pious that they know they are miserable sinners in their hearts correspond to the sense of guilt of the obsessional neurotic; while the highest observances (prayers, invocations, etc.) with which they begin every act of the day, and especially every unusual undertaking, seem to have the significance of defensive and protective measures. (Freud, 1907, pp. 25, 27, 31)

In 1913, Freud published *Totem and Taboo*; in 1919, he published *Psychoanalysis and Religious Origins*. In these works, he developed his psychoanalytic theory of religion, rooting it in the Oedipus complex:

> God the Father once walked upon earth in bodily form and exercised his sovereignty as chieftain of the primal human horde until his sons united to slay him. It emerges further that this crime of liberation and the reactions to it had as their result the appearance of the first social ties, the basic moral restrictions and the oldest form of religion, totemism. But the later religions too have the same content, and on the one hand they are concerned with obliterating the traces of that crime or with expiating it by bringing forward other solutions of the struggle between the father and son, while on the other hand they cannot avoid repeating once more the elimination of the father. (Freud, 1919, p. 96)

Freud's greatest and best-known work on religion is *Future of an Illusion* (1927), written by him at age 70. It is here that he brings together all of his previous writings on religion and predicts its future as human civilization advances and matures.

> Religion would thus be the universal obsessional neurosis of humanity; like the obsessional neurosis of children, it arose out of the Oedipus complex, out of the relation to the father. If this view is right, it is to be supposed that a turning-away from religion is bound to occur with the fatal inevitability of a process of growth, and that we find ourselves at this very juncture in the middle of that phase of development. Our behavior should therefore be modeled on that of a sensible teacher who does not

oppose an impending new development but seeks to ease its path and mitigate the violence of its eruption. Our analogy does not, to be sure, exhaust the essential nature of religion. If, on the one hand, religion brings with it obsessional restrictions, exactly as an individual obsessional neurosis does, on the other hand it comprises a system of wishful illusions together with a disavowal of reality, such as we find in an isolated form nowhere else but amentia, in a state of blissful hallucinatory confusion. . . . Our God, Logos [reason], will fulfill whichever of these wishes nature outside us allows, but will do it very gradually, only in the unforeseeable future, and for a new generation of man. He promises noncompensation for us, who suffer grievously from life. On the way to this distant goal your religious doctrines will have to be discarded, no matter whether the first attempts fail, or whether the first substitutes prove untenable. And you know why: in the long run nothing can withstand reason and experience, and the contradiction which religion offers to both is all too palpable. (Freud, 1927, pp. 43, 54)

Freud went on to write *Moses and Monotheism* (1939), a monograph that he completed in the final year of his life. It continued along the same theme as the others but was directed at Judaism. Thus, for more than 30 years, during the prime of his career, Freud relentlessly and systematically disassembled the religious beliefs and traditions of his day.

ALBERT ELLIS

The work of the psychologist Albert Ellis in the 1950s helped pave the way for the later development of cognitive-behavioral psychotherapy by Aaron Beck in the 1960s and 1970s. Ellis developed the psychotherapeutic technique called Rational Emotive Therapy (RET) and is the founder and president of the Rational Emotive Therapy Institute in New York City. Ellis has for years been a prominent and respected leader in the field of psychology, and his published research dates back to the 1940s.

In 1980, Ellis responded in the *Journal of Consulting and Clinical Psychology*, a leading journal of the American Psychological Association,

to an opinion piece on religious values and psychotherapy written by Allen Bergin. Ellis emphasizes his point in the following passage:

Devout, orthodox, or dogmatic religion (or what might be called religiosity) is significantly correlated with emotional disturbance. People largely disturb themselves by believing strongly in absolutistic shoulds, oughts, and musts, and most people who dogmatically believe in some religion believe in these health-sabotaging absolutes. The emotionally healthy individual is flexible, open, tolerant, and changing, and the devoutly religious person tends to be inflexible, closed, intolerant, and unchanging. Religiosity, therefore, is in many respects equivalent to irrational thinking and emotional disturbance. . . . The elegant therapeutic solution to emotional problems is to be quite unreligious and have no degree of dogmatic faith that is unfounded or unfoundable in fact. . . . The less religious they are, the more emotionally healthy they will tend to be. (Ellis, 1980, p. 637)

In a more recent article, published in *Free Inquiry* (1988), Ellis identifies 11 pathological characteristics of religiosity:

1. Religion discourages self-acceptance.
2. Religion discourages self-interest.
3. Religion discourages self-directedness.
4. Religion tends to make healthy human-to-human relationships difficult.
5. Religion encourages intolerance of others.
6. Religion encourages inflexibility.
7. Religious people have difficulty accepting and living in the real world.
8. Religious people have difficulty accepting ambiguity and uncertainty.
9. Religious people use scientific thinking only until it conflicts with their religious beliefs, after which they began thinking irrationally.
10. Religious people are prone to fanatical commitments, in contrast to emotionally healthy nonbelievers who commit passionately but not fanatically.
11. Emotionally stable people tend to be risk-takers in that they recognize what they want and take appropriate risks to achieve their goals; in contrast, religious people are too suffused with guilt to pursue their goals, because their worldview requires self-sacrifice.

WENDELL WATTERS

Wendell Watters, professor of psychiatry at Mc-Master University in Ontario, Canada, in his book *Deadly Doctrine* (1992), argues that Christian doctrine and teachings are incompatible with the development and maintenance of sound mental health and can even lead to physical health problems. He states that Christian beliefs have a negative effect on the development of self-esteem, in part because Christian teachings discourage pride and warn believers not to think too well of themselves. The Christian Church, he says, discourages its adherents from developing into self-reliant adults and instead encourages a type of infantile dependence on Church leaders. Watters also links Christian doctrine with the development of schizophrenia:

> Earlier in this volume I attempted to show that Christian doctrine and teachings are incompatible with many of the components of sound mental health, notably self-esteem, self-actualization and mastery, good communication skills, related individuation and the establishment of supportive human networks, and the development of healthy sexuality and reproductive responsibility. . . . Christian doctrine can contribute indirectly to the development of schizophrenia in a child born with limited capacity to adapt. . . . We have demonstrated that Christian teachings interfere with the process of "related individuation" and that a child who is under-individuated shows poor ego boundaries and runs the risk of remaining fused with or absorbed into the stronger organism, the parent. (Watters, 1992, pp. 140–141, 146)

Elsewhere, Watters establishes a connection between Christian doctrine and the development of major affective disorders.

> Kaplan and Sadock sum up the problem with these words: "It is widely believed that persons prone to depression are characterized by low self-esteem, strong superego, clinging and dependent interpersonal relations, and limited capacity for mature and enduring object relations." As we have demonstrated throughout this book, these characteristics are inevitable

products of the Christian belief system, one that preaches self-abasement as a means of ingratiating oneself with the deity, that discourages ego development and inner-directedness, and promotes superego growth and outer-directedness with its reliance on external authority. . . . Christian doctrine and liturgy have been shown to discourage the development of adult coping behaviors and the human-to-human relationship skills that enable people to cope in an adaptive way with the anxiety generated by stress. (Watters, 1992, pp. 148, 149)

Finally, Watters sums up the health implications of his arguments:

> Evidence that religion is irrelevant would not move me to write a book; there are already many excellent works on that topic. However, evidence that religion is not only irrelevant but actually harmful to human beings should be of interest, not only to other behavioral scientists, but to anyone who finds it difficult to live an unexamined life. Finally, the argument advanced in this volume should stir the political decision makers who complain about the high cost of health care even while continuing to subsidize that very institution that may be actually making the public "sick." (Watters, 1992, p. 12)

The federal government subsidizes religious institutions in the United States by allowing members to deduct donations to these organizations from their taxes. If Watters is right, perhaps the government should stop this practice.

Thus, prominent mental health professionals passionately argue that religious beliefs and practices, particularly those based in the Christian tradition, have negative effects on mental health—the exact opposite of what religious professionals, religious health professionals, and some non-religious health professionals claim (see chapter 3).

NEGATIVE HEALTH CONSEQUENCES OF RELIGION

Religious beliefs may adversely impact health, particularly physical health, in a number of ways.

Stopping Life-saving Medications

Of particular concern is the use of religion to *replace* traditional medical care. Members of some religious groups may decide to stop life-saving medications in order to prove their faith. Likewise, some aggressive faith healers encourage followers to stop medical treatments as a way to demonstrate the faith necessary for divine healing. Such recommendations are based on isolated biblical passages taken out of context that emphasize the need to depend entirely on God—not on human methods—for cure. Consequently, diabetics may discontinue their insulin, hypothyroid patients their thyroid hormone, asthmatics their bronchodilators, and epileptics their antiseizure medications, all in the name of faith, and often with disastrous consequences (Coakley & McKenna, 1986; Smith, 1986).

The British psychiatrist Louis Rose (1971) and the Minnesota surgeon William Nolen (1974) have authored popular books in which they claim to have followed up on hundreds of dramatic faith healing cures and found little to substantiate these claims. Even the Catholic Church recognizes only 64 "true healings" among the millions of people who have made pilgrimages to the shrine of St. Bernadette Soubirous in Lourdes, France, since 1858, when medical documentation began (Lourdes, 1999). Only seven of these healings were documented after 1950, none since 1970. Medical advances in the past half-century have uncovered scientific explanations for the cause and cure of many illnesses previously shrouded in mystery.

This brings up an interesting question. To what extent are religious experience, mysticism, faith healing, miracles, and the like related to such phenomena as hysteria, hypochondriasis, and hypnotizability? Hood has reported that scores on his Mysticism Scale are strongly correlated with the hypochondriasis and hysteria subscales of the MMPI (Hood, 1975). Recall that the famous Paris physician and neurophysiologist Jean Charcot (1825–1893) attributed miracles and religious ecstasy to simple hysteria (Porter, 1993). Also consider Levin, Wickramasekera, et al.'s (1998) report on the relationship between religiousness and hypnotizability. These investigators examined the association between "absorption" and religiosity in 83 adult survivors of cancer or other life-threatening disease. Subjects completed the Tellegen Absorption Scale and Religious Orientation Scale. Prior research had established that absorption and hypnotizability are highly correlated. Levin et al. discovered that intrinsically religious subjects had absorption scores at least 20% higher than did predominantly extrinsic, proreligious, or nonreligious subjects. Investigators interpreted these results in a positive way, suggesting that certain religious cognitions may generate an internally focused state that enhances health and attenuates disease through self-soothing psychophysiological mechanisms.

Failing to Seek Timely Medical Care

Believers have claimed miraculous cures from faith healing throughout modern history. Seeking help from faith healers or turning exclusively to religious activities (e.g., prayer) instead of seeking timely medical attention can delay necessary medical care and lead to adverse health outcomes. Religious persons may first seek help from religious sources for a number of reasons, including negative past experiences with the medical profession, inability to afford traditional care, social pressure from other members of their religious group, and attempts to adhere to religious doctrines taken out of context. This may delay diagnosis and necessary treatment, allowing serious or acute illnesses (e.g., cancer, infection) to advance quickly.

Lannin and colleagues (1998), at Eastern Carolina University in Greenville, North Carolina, reported in the *Journal of the American Medical Association* a study that examined the reasons that breast cancer mortality in the United States is so much higher in African American women than white women. Investigators studied 540 patients with newly diagnosed breast cancer and 414 control women matched by age, race, and area of residence. The outcome variable was breast cancer stage at diagnosis. Investigators found that "cultural beliefs" were a significant predictor of late stage (III or IV) at diagnosis. Among these cultural beliefs were "fundamentalist" religious beliefs such as "The devil can cause a person to get cancer" and "If a person prays about cancer, God will heal it without medical treatments" (see chapter 3 for a discussion of fundamentalist theology and faith healing). The researchers concluded that both socioeconomic and cultural beliefs accounted for the delay in diagnosis among African American women.

While Lannin et al. found that religious beliefs were related to late cancer stage at diagnosis in the uncontrolled analysis, they did not report on the independent effects of these beliefs on stage of diagnosis after race, education, and socioeconomic factors were taken into account. Religious beliefs were much more common among African Americans, the uneducated, and the poor, all potent risk factors for late stage at diagnosis. While cultural factors did independently predict late stage at diagnosis, religious beliefs were only two of 24 variables that were combined into a single category that the researchers labeled "cultural factors." Again, investigators did not examine the effect of religious belief *by itself* on stage of diagnosis when other variables were controlled. Furthermore, at least one qualitative study of breast symptom discovery and cancer diagnosis did not find that religious beliefs of African American women "constrained or prohibited the evaluation and treatment of breast symptoms" (Facione & Giancarlo, 1998).

In another study published in the *Journal of the American Medical Association*, Simpson (1989) examined the survival of devout Christian Scientists, who often abstain from cigarettes and alcohol but rarely consult doctors for health problems. This study examined the longevity of 2,630 male and 2,938 female Christian Scientists who received their college educations at Principia College, a four-year liberal arts college in Elsah, Illinois, between 1934 and 1982. The comparison group was 17,743 male and 12,105 female students who received their college educations in the College of Liberal Arts and Sciences at the University of Kansas, Lawrence. The life table method was used to compare

mortality separately in men and women, using five-year time blocks. Significantly higher death rates were found in male Christian Scientists ($p = .042$) and female Christian Scientists ($p = .003$). These results replicated the findings of Wilson (1965), who reported that the death rate of Christian Scientists from cancer was double the national average.

In a commentary written for the *New England Journal of Medicine*, the Christian Scientist leader Nathan Talbot (1983) indicated that Christian Scientists are "caring and responsible people who love their children and want only the best possible care for them" (p. 1641). Nevertheless, he noted that this "care" included treating sick children with prayer alone, even for serious conditions like leukemia, club feet, spinal meningitis, bone fracture, and diphtheria, all of which, Talbot claims, have been healed by prayer alone.

On the other hand, involvement in certain religious groups may actually speed time to breast cancer diagnosis. Zollinger and colleagues (1984) prospectively studied 282 Seventh-Day Adventist and 1675 non-Adventist breast cancer patients in California. Investigators found that the probability of not having died from breast cancer 10 years after diagnosis was 60.8% among Seventh-Day Adventists and 48.3% among non-Adventists. When stage at diagnosis was taken into account, however, the difference in survival disappeared. In other words, Seventh-Day Adventist women simply had their breast cancers diagnosed at an earlier stage than non-Adventist women. The close-knit family and social community of Seventh-Day Adventists, along with their focus on health, may have led to early diagnosis.

A more recent study directly compared the mortality rate of Christian Scientists with that of Seventh-Day Adventists (both groups abstain from smoking and alcohol). It found significantly greater death rates for Christian Scientists (Centers for Disease Control, 1991). Seventh-Day Adventists and Christian Scientists have similar ethical systems, but their theological beliefs are very different. While Seventh-Day Adventists readily seek medical treatment, Christian Scientists see sickness and poverty as illusory, as error that needs to be corrected by metaphysical study. Thus, religion may have different effects on health care–seeking behavior and physical health, depending on the particular religious group one is affiliated with.

The following case of AIDS and Religious Enthusiasm was reported to us by one of our colleagues. Jane (fictitious name) was a young woman in her twenties who had end-stage AIDS and was in and out of the hospital regularly. Jane was a member of a small religious group somewhere in the southeastern United States and had recently married a young man within her Church. Jane's doctors had recently discovered that she and her husband were having unprotected intercourse, even after her diagnosis. No amount of education or warning could convince her husband to take protective measures. When asked why he persisted in putting himself at risk, the husband replied that God had communicated to him that He would protect him from contracting the AIDS virus. We advised our colleague to try to get permission from Jane to contact her pastor and see if the pastor could reason with the husband. The use of religion to justify irresponsible behavior is an extrinsic use of religion that may indeed have negative health consequences.

Refusing Blood Transfusions

The refusing of blood transfusions is common practice among Jehovah's Witnesses and may lead to death. Jehovah's Witnesses believe that a person must not sustain his life with another creature's blood; there is no distinction between drinking blood through the mouth and taking it directly into the blood vessels. It is their religious conviction that God (Jehovah) will turn his back on anyone who receives blood transfusions. Consequently, Jehovah's Witnesses avoid blood transfusions for themselves and their children because they believe that the procedure bars the recipient from eternal salvation.

For adults, such refusals are typically accepted on the grounds that the transfusions represent an invasion of the right of privacy and a violation of the person's freedom of religious practice. Parents' refusal of blood transfusions

for children, on the other hand, has been more controversial (Swan, 1997). Jehovah's Witnesses have appeared before the U.S. Supreme Court more than 50 times to establish their religious freedoms; however, they have typically lost cases involving children's health.

Refusing Childhood Immunizations

At least five studies have reported harm resulting from religious belief against childhood immunizations. Rodgers et al. (1993) reported high attack and case fatality rates during a measles outbreak among children of religious groups refusing measles vaccination. Etkind et al. (1992) and Novotny et al. (1988) reported pertussis (whooping cough) outbreaks in children of groups that claimed exemptions on religious grounds to state requirements for pertussis vaccination. Likewise, outbreaks of rubella (German measles) have been reported among the Old Order Amish in Pennsylvania and elsewhere in the United States, largely in unvaccinated children and young adults (MMWR, 1991).

Most recently, Conyn-van Spaendonck et al. (1996) conducted a population-based study of a poliovirus epidemic in the Netherlands that occurred in 1992–1993. They surveyed 2,400 children ages 5–14 and 3,000 adults ages 40–64; a total of 3,182 persons responded. Investigators examined fecal samples for virus isolation and characterization. Crude excretion rate for wild polio virus type 3 in the general population was 2.5/1,000 persons (5.5 in children and 0.0 in adults) but 29.7 for members of the Reformed church (7/236) and 70.7 for members of the Orthodox Reformed church (7/99) (all children), compared with 1/201 for members of the traditional Dutch Reformed church. The proportion of children who were never vaccinated was 28.6% for Orthodox Reformed, 62.5% for Reformed, and 66.7% for Old Orthodox Reformed church members, compared with less than 5% for other religious groups. They concluded that the risk of poliomyelitis during the 1992–1993 outbreak was restricted to religious subpopulations that had rejected vaccination.

Refusing Prenatal Care and Physician-assisted Delivery

Spence and colleagues studied perinatal and maternal mortality in the religious group Faith Assembly (Kaunitz et al., 1984; Spence et al., 1984). Members of this religious group practice out-of-hospital, nonphysician-attended birthing without prenatal care. According to Hobart Freeman, founder of the Indiana-based Faith Assembly religious group, "Satan controls the visible, sensory realm of nature, and he works through the occult forces of medicine, science, and education" (Hughes, 1990, p. 108). Spence et al. compared maternal and perinatal mortality in Kosciusko and Elkhart counties (where members of Faith Assembly live) between 1975 and 1982 with that of other Indiana counties during the same period (26,618 vs. 681,497 deliveries, respectively). Compared to other Indiana women, Faith Assembly women were less likely to have at least one prenatal visit (0% vs. 99%).

The researchers found that perinatal mortality among Faith Assembly children was 48/1,000 live births, compared to 18/1,000 live births for the state ($p < .01$). The maternal mortality rate for Faith Assembly women was 872/100,000 live births, versus 9/100,000 live births in rest of the state ($p < .001$). Thus, perinatal mortality was three times higher and maternal mortality was nearly 100 times higher among Faith Assembly members than among the general population. This finding prompted the Indiana General Assembly to pass a law requiring doctors to report the withholding of medical care, even if parents object for religious reasons. A follow-up study after this law was passed compared perinatal and maternal mortality between 1975 and 1982 with the rates between 1983 and 1985, after the General Assembly passed the law. Perinatal mortality declined by nearly one-half, and maternal mortality was virtually eliminated (Spence & Danielson, 1987).

Fostering Child Abuse

Bottoms et al. (1995) note that religious beliefs can foster, encourage, and justify child abuse. These investigators examined cases of religion-related child abuse and described cases that involved withholding of medical care for religious reasons, abuse related to attempts to rid a child of evil, and abuse perpetrated by clergy. Most of the background information for this article consisted of case reports, not systematic studies. The core of the report, however, consisted of results from a national survey of 19,272 mental health professionals that was designed to gather information about reports of religion-related abuse. This included ritualistic child abuse (specifically, the torturing or killing of a child to rid him of evil), the withholding of medical care for religious reasons, and other forms of child abuse committed for religious reasons.

Their initial sampling frame consisted of 5,998 clinical psychologists (APA members), 7,381 psychiatrists (APA members), and 5,896 clinical social workers (NASW members). The study was conducted in two phases: a post-card survey to identify child abuse allegations involving ritualistic, ceremonial, supernatural, religious, or mystical practices, followed by a more in-depth questionnaire. A total of 6,939 postcards were returned (36% response rate) (2,722 clinical psychologists, 2,083 psychiatrists, 2,134 social workers). Among the respondents, 2,136 had encountered as least one religion-related abuse at some time in their careers. Detailed surveys were sent to all 2,136, of whom 797 returned surveys, of which 720 were deemed valid (34% response rate). These surveys provided details on a total of 1,652 ritualistic or religion-related child abuse cases self-reported by either adult survivors or child clients. Of those, 417 were religion-related cases, divided into (a) abuse involving withholding of medical care for religious reasons, (b) abuse related to attempt to rid a child of the devil or evil spirits, and (c) abuse perpetrated by clergy.

Note that these 417 alleged cases were reported by 720 mental health professionals (during their entire careers), who represented 34% of 2,136 reporting ritualistic or religion-related abuse, who made up 31% of 6,939 mental health professionals, who represented 36% of the original sampling frame of 19,272 potential informers. Corroborative evidence of abuse or harm was present in less than 50% of the 417 cases, and corroborative evidence of religion-related case elements was present in about two-thirds of these. In only 5% of cases involving medical neglect, 9% of cases involving ridding of evil, and 9% of clergy abuse cases was the evidence strong enough to lead to a court conviction (this included cases of religious abuse perpetrated by patients who were psychotic at the time). Of the 417 cases, 271 were considered "pure" (not mixtures of more than one type): 25 were pure cases of medical neglect; 69 involved reports of removing evil spirits from children; and 177 involved abuse by clergy. On the basis of the approximately 200 cases identified and corroborated in this study out of 19,272 respondents looking back over their entire careers, one might conclude from this study that religion-related child abuse is not very common.

Defending the Rights of Children to Receive Medical Care

Regardless of how frequently it occurs, child abuse—including the withholding of medical care from children—is a serious problem. Certain religious groups have obtained special exemptions from state child abuse and neglect reporting laws on the basis of the claim that they treat the child by religious methods, such as prayer (Skolnick, 1990). While the Supreme Court ruled in 1944 that "the right to practice religion freely does not include liberty to expose the community or child to communicable disease or the latter to ill health or death" (Bullis, 1991, p. 551), 46 of 50 states in 1990 included a religious exemption that protects parents from prosecution for the harm that results to children from religiously motivated medical neglect (Bullis, 1991). This prompted the American Academy of Pediatrics (1997) to issue a position statement in the journal *Pediatrics* in which it asserts that "the AAP advocates that all legal interventions apply equally whenever children are endangered or harmed, without exemptions based on parental religious beliefs" (p. 279).

Rita Swan, once a devout Christian Scientist, left that organization after her young son died from meningitis after treatment by a Chris-

tian Science practitioner. Swan now heads a private advocacy organization called Children's Health Care Is a Legal Duty (CHILD) and has published emotion-stirring pieces in major medical journals on the withholding of medical care from children by Christian Scientists, Jehovah's Witnesses, and other faith-healing groups (Swan, 1983, 1997; Asser & Swan, 1998). For more than 15 years she has advocated for the rights of children to receive medical care. During this time, her private organization has documented the deaths of many children due to the withholding of medical care on religious grounds.

Asser and Swan (1998) reported that 172 children died between 1975 and 1995 from what the researchers believed was parental withholding of medical care on religious grounds. Of the children who died, 113 did so after their neonatal period, and 59 died during the prenatal or perinatal period. Investigators reported graphic examples of children dying from food aspiration, childhood cancer, pneumonia, meningitis, diabetes, asthma, and other treatable childhood illnesses. Investigators reported that 140 of the deaths were from conditions whose survival rates with medical care exceed 90%.

The 172 cases were distributed across 23 denominations from 34 states. However, 83% of the total fatalities came from five religious groups: 50 from Indiana (primarily from Faith Assembly), 16 from Pennsylvania (primarily from Faith Tabernacle), 15 from Oklahoma and Colorado (primarily from Church of the First Born), 5 deaths from End Time Ministries in South Dakota, and 28 deaths from members of the Christian Science Church nationwide. Excluding cases from Faith Assembly (where child fatalities declined dramatically after several prosecutions and the death of the group's leader), 35% of the deaths occurred from 1988 to 1995, a span that constitutes 38% of the total time period under study. Asser and Swan concluded that child death due to neglect on religious grounds continues to proceed largely unchecked.

The methodology of this study makes it difficult to determine exactly how often withholding of medical care from children on religious grounds actually occurs. The authors them-

selves admit that "Calculations of overall incidence and mortality rates are not possible in
this study as the number of children in the
group sampled is not available and the cases
were collected in a *non-rigorous manner*" ([our
italics] p. 628). By "non-rigorous manner" the
authors refer to the fact that most of these cases
were collected over the past 15 years from news-
paper articles, public documents, trial records,
and personal communications, primarily from
the files of Swan's public advocacy group,
CHILD. Furthermore, prediction of whether or
not these children would have survived with
medical care was based on the clinical experience of only one pediatrician (the study's lead
author) and published statistics from the appropriate era (statistics that changed as medical
care improved). Thus, much of the science in
this study was subjective and could have been
heavily influenced by the bias of study investigators.

Condoning Other Forms of Religious Abuse

In spring 1999 the Haworth Press published
the first issue of a new journal, the *Journal of
Religion and Abuse*. That issue included titles
such as, "Power to Wound, Power to Mend:
Toward a Non-abusing Theology," "Investigating and Prosecuting Clergy Sexual Abuse," and
"The Problem with False Shepherds." Other,
more subtle forms of religious abuse exist in
addition to the more obvious ones that involve
religious cults or abuse of children.

While membership in close religious groups
may enhance social support for those who abide
by the prescriptions and proscriptions of the
group, individuals who deviate from accepted
standards may be judged negatively and consequently be marginalized. Sorenson and colleagues (1995) examined the association between religious involvement and depression
among unmarried adolescent mothers and
found higher rates of depression among those
subjects who were more religiously active. Investigators concluded that religion may foster feelings of guilt or shame, eroding feelings of competence, self-worth, and hopefulness, and
encourage the withdrawal of community support to those who do not conform to social
norms.

If a religious person becomes physically ill,
members of his religious group may pray for
his healing. If the person is healed, this reaf-
firms the religious beliefs of the group. If the
person is not healed, however, he may be
blamed for the illness, which may be viewed as
the sufferer's fault (it can't be God's fault, since
he wishes to heal people and has the power to
do so). Perhaps the person's faith isn't strong
enough, or there is unconfessed sin in his life.
This attitude may cause the physically ill person
to doubt his own faith and to feel as if he has
done something wrong. Such thoughts and feelings in turn may lead to discouragement and
worsen the ill person's depression as he becomes further victimized, now feeling additional guilt for not being healed. Such a sequence can greatly diminish the sick person's
ability to draw comfort and support from his
personal faith and from his religious community (see chapter 29 for a further discussion of
this issue).

Replacing Mental Health Care with Religion

Religious practices are sometimes used to replace (rather than complement) traditional
mental health care as well as physical care. This
is not surprising, since there is such a great
overlap between mental health and spiritual
health, which at times may be indistinguishable.
Some religious groups advocate complete
avoidance of contact with the mental health
system. Perhaps best known for its aggressive
posture toward psychiatry is the Church of Scientology, which has a Citizen's Commission on
Human Rights "dedicated to exposing and erad-
icating criminal acts and human rights abuses
by psychiatry." This group has been particularly
vocal in speaking out against the use of psychiatric drugs such as Prozac and frequently pickets
the American Psychiatric Association's annual
meetings.

Some popular Christian writers such as Martin and Diedre Bobgan have also advocated
avoiding mental health care, especially psychotherapy, referring to Thomas Szasz's *Myth of*

Psychotherapy (1978) for validation of their viewpoint. They are less opposed to the use of psychotropic medication for severe mental disorders such as schizophrenia, panic disorder, and major depression. The Bobgans have spoken out against secular and even Christian psychotherapy in books such as *Prophets of Psychoheresy*, volumes 1 and 2 (1989, 1990), which critique mental health professionals such as Gary Collins, James Dobson, Paul Meier, and Frank Minirth, who integrate secular techniques with a Christian perspective (see chapter 3). The Bobgans encourage people to choose either "the psychological way" or "the spiritual way" and recommend that they not combine the two (Bobgan & Bobgan, 1981). The popular Christian counselor and author Jay Adams has lent his support to the Bobgans' viewpoint (see Bobgan & Bobgan, 1989, pp. 105–106). While adverse mental health outcomes are less easy to document than physical health outcomes, such antagonistic attitudes toward the mental health professions can delay or prevent the provision of necessary psychiatric care.

UNHEALTHY AND HEALTHY BELIEF SYSTEMS

Simply having faith, any faith, may not be as important as *what* a person believes. There is some evidence that religious beliefs that portray God (or a higher power) as distant, uninterested, punishing, or vindictive have less salutary health effects than belief systems that present God as merciful, kind, forgiving, and understanding or as a collaborative partner (Pargament, 1997). In a cross-sectional study of 577 consecutively hospitalized patients age 55 or over, Koenig, Pargament, et al. (1998) found that appraisals of God as benevolent or as a collaborative partner were related to better mental health. Religious beliefs that viewed God as a punishing deity and demonic forces as responsible for health problems were associated with worse mental health. As always with cross-sectional studies, however, it is not possible to determine whether these beliefs were responsible for the poorer mental health or whether psychological distress was responsible for the beliefs.

Involvement in religious cults that indoctrinate, isolate, and alienate members from their families and from the general community often has negative effects on members' mental and physical health. Examples of religious cults whose members experienced negative health consequences from their cult activities include the People's Temple, led by the Rev. Jim Jones, whose more than 900 members ended their lives by ingesting cyanide in Jonestown, Guyana, on November 18, 1978; the Branch Davidians, led by David Koresh, whose 72 members died near Waco, Texas, on April 19, 1993, after seven weeks of siege by officers of the federal Bureau of Alcohol, Tobacco, and Firearms; the Solar Temple cult, whose 72 members committed suicide in four separate incidents between 1994 and 1997 in St. Casimir (Quebec), Grenoble (France), Switzerland, and Montreal. In another example, 39 members of the Heaven's Gate cult led by Marshall Applewhite ended their lives by suicide in Encinitas, California, on March 26, 1997, believing that aliens hiding behind the Hale-Bopp comet would take them to a better place. The content of one's faith, then, can influence health for better or worse.

OTHER REPORTS

A number of other reports have appeared concerning religious beliefs or practices that impact negatively on health. Opler (1936) described chronic nervous apprehension in an Apache couple who were completely dependent on ritual activities of an Apache shaman for their health maintenance. Jilek (1974) reported an exacerbation of depression among tribe members involved in certain religious ceremonies conducted by the Salish Indians of Canada. Prince (1964) reported that Yoruba possession cults in Nigeria encourage dissociation and multiple personality formation. Koos (1977), describing the Puerto Rican healing tradition known as Espirisimo, reported the negative psychological consequences experienced by persons undergoing long-term training to develop their "faculties" for communication with the spirit world. Snow (1978) describes how urban African American folk healers may worsen anxiety both in individual patients and in entire communities. In a study of American fundamentalists, Pattison, Lapins, et al. (1973) reported that the 20% of his sample who experienced faith healing also had chronic difficulty coping with stress. Ness (1980), studying a mainline Protestant Church in Canada, found that frequency of religious attendance and giving of "testimonials" were positively associated with physical symptoms on the Cornell Medical Index. Again, cause-effect relationships are difficult to prove in most of these studies.

RELIGIOUS EXPERIENCE AND MENTAL ILLNESS

Mental illnesses such as schizophrenia, acute mania, or psychotic depression can be accompanied by bizarre religious delusions. For example, the acute manic may believe that he or she is the reincarnated Jesus Christ, God, or some other divine being with special powers. The acutely psychotic schizophrenic may hear voices from God or from the devil telling him or her to do certain things. The person with psychotic depression may have the delusion that he or she has committed an unpardonable sin and is destined for eternal damnation. The obsessive-compulsive may pray or perform detailed, time-consuming religious rituals over and over again to relieve intolerable anxiety or guilt.

Even the textbook of psychiatric nomenclature and categorization, the Diagnostic and Statistical Manual of Mental Disorders (DSM), has for years used religious examples to illustrate cases of serious mental illness. Larson and colleagues (1993) found that of the 45 case examples in the DSM-III-R glossary that illustrated technical terms, including illogical thinking, incoherence, poverty of content and speech, poverty of affect, catatonic posturing, delusions of being controlled and other types of delusional thought, hallucinations, and magical thinking, 22.2% ($n = 10$) had substantial religious content. While such references have been removed from DSM-IV in an effort to be culturally sensitive, this underscores the point that religious beliefs and experiences often accompany mental illness. Many patients who suffer with mental illness, however, may also turn to religion as a source of comfort and strength to help them cope with their trials.

It is not surprising that mental health professionals have often concluded that religious beliefs and practices have a negative impact on mental health, particularly when so many of their patients express religious ideas (and so many of their colleagues do not; this point is discussed later in this chapter). Whether religious beliefs and practices actually *cause* mental illness, as many have assumed, or are a result of the mental illness remains a subject of debate.

REASONS FOR DIVERGENT VIEWS

It is difficult to understand how prominent and reputable mental health professionals can hold such divergent views about the effects of religion on health. On the one hand, as we saw in chapter 3, religious and many secular health professionals argue that religion has positive effects on mental health. On the other hand, there is also a relatively large group of well-known and respected health professionals who believe that religion has negative health effects. Why such a difference of opinion?

Personal Belief or Disbelief

The views of health professionals are to a large extent based on personal belief, opinion, and clinical experience working with mentally ill patients, rather than on systematic research. The views of religious professionals and religious health professionals are similarly based on personal experience and opinion, not on systematic research. While it is evident to many that bias plays a strong role in the views of religious professionals and religious health professionals, less easily recognized is the fact that bias also plays a strong role in the perspective of secular health professionals presented in this chapter. We now review some studies that have examined religious beliefs and backgrounds of health professionals that may influence their views about religion.

Mental Health Professionals. Marx and Spray (1969) asked the religious affiliation of 1,371 psychiatrists, 1,465 clinical psychologists, and 1,154 psychiatric social workers in Chicago, Los Angeles, and New York. They found that 21.3% were Protestant, 9.5% Catholic, 33.6% Jewish, 14.6% none, 10.6% agnostic, and 10.4% atheists. This distribution of affiliation was in marked contrast to that found in the general U.S. population, where about 60% are Protestant, 25% Catholic, 3% Jewish, and less than 10% unaffiliated, agnostic, or atheist. They concluded that Jews and unbelievers were markedly overrepresented in the mental health professions. Similarly, Ragan and colleagues (1980) conducted a survey of religious belief and practice among a random sample of 555 members of the American Psychological Association. They found that only 43% believed in God, 27% attended church twice a month or more, and 9% held leadership positions in their congregations.

Bergin and Jensen (1990) surveyed 425 therapists who represented 59% of a national sample of U.S. clinical psychologists, psychiatrists, clinical social workers, and marriage and family therapists. Like earlier researchers, they found the proportion who were unaffiliated or considered themselves atheist or agnostic (combined) to be 30% for psychologists, 24% for psychiatrists, 9% for social workers, and 13% for marriage and family therapists, compared with 9% of the general population. When asked to respond to the statement "My whole approach to life is based on my religion," the category "uncertain/disagree/strongly disagree" was chosen by 67% of psychologists, 61% of psychiatrists, 54% of social workers, and 38% of marriage and family therapists, compared with 28% of the general population. With regard to church attendance, the differences were less striking; 33% of psychologists, 32% of psychiatrists, 44% of social workers, and 50% of marriage and family therapists said they attended services regularly (compared to 40% of the general population).

Religious beliefs and practices of mental health professionals may differ depending on which areas of the country they practice in.

For example, Shafranske and Malony (1990b) surveyed 47 psychologists randomly selected from a roster of licensed psychologists in California. Only 26% of this sample believed in a personal God in the traditional sense, 5% indicated that they participated in an organized religious body as their primary source of spirituality, and 80% had very limited or no involvement in organized religion (51% had no religious affiliation).

What about the religious beliefs and behaviors of mental health professionals outside the United States? Neeleman and King (1993) surveyed 231 psychiatrists at general and psychiatric hospitals in London, England. Religious background and belief were each assessed by 16 questions. Almost three-quarters (73%) of psychiatrists reported no religious affiliation (vs. 38% of their patients), and 78% attended religious services less than once a month. Belief in God was more common among women than men psychiatrists (39% vs. 19%). Interestingly, 92% of these psychiatrists believed that religion and mental illness were connected and that religious issues should be addressed in treatment. Almost one-half (42%) of the psychiatrists believed that religiosity can lead to mental illness, and 58% never made referrals to clergy.

Such studies in the United States and Great Britain indicate that mental health professionals, particularly psychologists and psychiatrists, are significantly less religious in belief or activity than either persons in the general population or psychiatric patients. Such differences in belief may affect how mental health professionals view the influence of religion on the health of the mentally ill and on people in general.

Primary Care Physicians. To what extent might there be a bias against religion among primary care physicians and other health professionals who provide medical care to patients? Unfortunately, there is less information on the religious beliefs and practices of physicians and other medical providers than there is for mental health professionals.

Koenig, Bearon, and Dayringer (1989) surveyed a random sample of 160 family physicians and general practitioners in Illinois concerning the role of religion in the clinical care of elderly patients. Nearly 37% of physicians believed that in certain circumstances patients might wish their doctor to pray with them (the same percentage also reported having prayed with patients). In contrast, a parallel study that examined whether elderly patients would like their doctors in certain circumstances to pray with them found that 78% of 72 persons surveyed said they would (Koenig, Smiley, and Gonzales, 1988).

Next, Koenig, Hover, et al. (1991) surveyed 130 physicians, 38 nurses, 77 inpatients, and 60 family members of patients at Duke University Medical Center in Durham, North Carolina, in order to compare religious beliefs, activities, and religious coping among these four groups. Physicians were less likely to attend religious services weekly (35%) than were patients (62%), families (59%), or nurses (51%). Physicians were also less likely to use religion as their most important coping behavior when dealing with stress; only 9% of physicians did so, compared with 44% of patients, 56% of families, and 26% of nurses. Physicians were also less likely to be affiliated with conservative Protestant religious denominations (2% of physicians vs. 43% of patients and 49% of family members).

Oyama and Koenig (1998) more recently surveyed 380 family medicine outpatients and 31 family medicine physicians in North Carolina and Texas about their religious beliefs and practices. Compared with physicians, patients were significantly more likely to pray once a day (61% vs. 29%), more likely to hold intrinsic religious attitudes, and more likely to be affiliated with a religious tradition. Finally, a survey of 269 family physicians attending an annual meeting of the American Academy of Family Physicians found that 99% of physicians agreed that a patient's spiritual beliefs can contribute to healing (MacDonald, 1996). However, when a random national sample of 1,000 adults was surveyed by the ICR Research Group for *USA Weekend*, only 10% said that a doctor had talked to them about their spiritual faith as a factor in physical health (McNichol, 1996).

On the basis of the limited research cited, primary care physicians, like mental health professionals, appear to be less religious than pa-

tients and therefore may have difficulty recognizing the religious and spiritual needs and desires of those patients.

Personal Advantage

Divergent views between religious professionals and health care professionals may result when each professional sides with the dominant views of his respective subculture. For example, the job of religious professionals is to preach the benefits of religious faith and to encourage congregants to participate in religious activities. If religious professionals were to criticize religious beliefs and practices as unhealthy, they would be ostracized by those within their profession (and probably dismissed by their congregations). Similarly, religious mental health professionals emphasize the positive aspects of religious faith and deemphasize the negative aspects in order to appeal to religious clients. Finally, both religious professionals and religious health professionals likely interact with and receive support from those who believe as they do and consequently reinforce each other's belief systems in social, family, and work settings. Again, the benefits of religion are emphasized, while any negative aspects are minimized. In this way the religious subculture maintains itself.

The same phenomenon occurs among scientific health professionals. They may see religion as irrational, wishful thinking, or even delusional, greatly different from the careful logic and rational thinking that guide life within the scientific subculture. Some mental health professionals may see religion as a competing paradigm for viewing and understanding human behavior, as a challenge to their worldview, and possibly even as a threat to their source of livelihood. Medical physicians may see religion as a competing method of healing that causes patients to delay seeking health care or to fail to comply with medical treatments. These negative attitudes toward religion are reinforced in social and work settings, creating social pressure to believe as one's colleagues do or risk being seen as different and consequently marginalized. In these ways, either a negative or a positive view of religion is perpetuated and reinforced within the local subculture.

Lack of Reliance on Research Data

We have seen that opinions based on personal beliefs and limited clinical experience and reinforced within one's work and social settings can influence professionals' views of and feelings about religion. This is particularly true when there is a lack of research data to guide attitudes and practices, when such data are not widely known, or when the data are purposefully ignored.

On the one hand, religious professionals have relied primarily if not entirely upon tradition and "sacred stories" handed down through Church history and seldom questioned. Clergy have been reluctant to conduct scientific research to test the truth of their doctrines because such doctrines are believed because of faith, not facts. In addition, many of the clergy are skeptical about whether the tools of science are capable of examining "things of the spirit," and with good reason. Finally, the secular professions largely control access to and expertise in research, making it difficult for religious professionals to conduct research, even if they wanted to.

On the other hand, researchers in the medical and psychological sciences have made only half-hearted attempts to examine the health benefits or risks of religious beliefs and practices. When such studies have been done, the results have not been widely disseminated within the field or integrated into clinical practice. As noted earlier, scientists who have attempted to conduct such research have often been discouraged from pursuing this line of investigation and may even have had their academic careers shortened. In fact, conducting research on religion and health became known as an "antitenure factor." Finally, until recently research funding for such studies from the National Institutes of Health has been almost unobtainable. It is little wonder that, over the years, few researchers or research groups have been capable of sustaining a research focus on the religion-health relationship.

Investigators who did attempt to study this area frequently had to do the work on their own time, given the lack of funding. Consequently, many studies of religion and health have not been the best in terms of research design (see chapter 32). Subjects often ended up being those most readily available—students in psychology or sociology classes or psychiatric patients. Even some of Freud's psychosexual theories were criticized early on because his research was conducted on subjects that were outside the societal norms; the validity of extrapolating from a test group to a culture should be suspect if the test group is tainted in some way. If religious variables were included in well-designed, large-scale studies, they were typically one or two items (most often denomination) not capable of capturing the kind of detail necessary to adequately assess the impact of religious involvement on health.

In summary, the major reasons for the thriving debate and divergence of opinion concerning religion's health effects is (1) a lack of adequate research data and (2) a lack of easy access to research that has been done. We now review the research that shows a negative relationship between religious involvement and good health. The studies were identified from our comprehensive review of the literature (which includes more than 1,200 separate research studies; see part VIII).

RESEARCH THAT SHOWS NEGATIVE HEALTH EFFECTS OF RELIGION

Authoritarianism

Hassan and Khalique (1981), studying 360 Indian and Muslim college students from the subcontinent of India, found that religiosity was positively related to anxiety, intolerance of ambiguity, rigidity, and authoritarianism. Gregory (1957) reported that religious orthodoxy was associated with authoritarian personality traits in 596 California college students. Jones (1958) found that religion was associated with high scores on authoritarianism in 197 young American Naval cadets. Putney and Middleton (1961) indicated that highly orthodox religious beliefs correlated with authoritarianism in 1,126 American college students. Weima (1965) found a similar association between religiousness and authoritarianism in a sample of mostly Catholic college students in Utrecht, Holland. None of these studies, however, controlled for possible confounding variables, and most studies used measures of authoritarianism that were contaminated by items that tapped orthodox religious values.

While it has been claimed that authoritarianism is associated with negative mental health outcomes (e.g., drive for power, hostility, prejudice, sadomasochism, guilt), these may be more assertions than realities determined by careful scientific research, according to a researcher at the University of California at Berkeley, Rodney Stark (1971). Using a national probability sample of northern whites, Stark found no relationship between authoritarianism, measured by the traditional F scale, and religious orthodoxy or religious attendance; in fact, the relationship was negative among conservative Protestants and Catholics.

Prejudice

A number of studies have found a positive correlation between religiousness and prejudice. Blum and Mann (1960) reported that undergraduates who belonged to religious organizations were more prejudiced than those who did not belong to such groups. Eiseman and Cole (1964) reported a positive correlation between prejudice and conservative religious attitudes in denominational college students, a finding corroborated by others (Feagin, 1964; Maranell, 1967). Allport and Ross (1967), however, argued that only a certain type of religiousness (i.e., extrinsic religiosity) was related to greater prejudice, whereas the truly religious person (who scored high on intrinsic religiousness) was actually less prejudiced than the average person. Others have failed to demonstrate a relationship between prejudice and religiosity and emphasize more important determinants, such as social class (Rosenbloom, 1959).

Anxiety, Dependency, and Depression

In his book *The Open and Closed Mind*, Rokeach (1960) reported results from two samples of college students ($n = 202$ and $n = 207$) that showed religious individuals were more likely to be anxious than nonbelievers. Believers also complained more of working under tension, sleeping fitfully, and experiencing other symptoms. Dunn (1965), studying the personality traits of religious persons, likewise reported that these individuals were more perfectionistic, withdrawn, insecure, depressed, worried, and inept. Religious women were somewhat more likely to express masculine interests, whereas religious men tended to have somewhat feminine interests. In contrast, Strunk (1959) found that 60 male divinity students were more aggressive in social contacts than were 50 business administration students.

Dreger (1952) examined personality correlates of religious attitudes among college students using projective techniques. Religious subjects expressed more dependency feelings than did nonreligious subjects. Bateman and Jensen (1958) examined the effect of religious background on modes of handling anger and found that persons with extensive religious training were more likely to turn anger in on themselves than to direct it outward at the environment. Pyron (1961) examined the relationship between "openness to change" and religiousness among 128 persons (population not described) and found that those with higher religious scores were more opposed to change. Some investigators have noted that strongly held religious beliefs are "characteristic" of the premorbid schizophrenic (Dittes, 1971; Clark, 1981; Spero, 1983). Others have reported negative effects of religion on behavioral disturbances in children. For example, Sajwaj and Hedges (1973) discuss the negative consequences of forcing a six-year old retarded boy to pray at mealtimes.

With regard to personal adjustment and its relationship to religious attitude and certainty, Wright (1959) reported that those who appeared more liberal in their religious attitude or less certain of their religious responses tended to be better adjusted. Likewise, Cowen (1954) found a significant negative association between orthodox religious belief and self-esteem. Both Ellis (1962) and Branden (1994) described the negative effects of religion on mental health that result from beliefs in original sin and divine omnipotence, which, they reasoned, undermine self-esteem and feelings of personal mastery.

Strawbridge and colleagues (1998) reported that religiosity may buffer the effects of some stressors but may exacerbate others. Their cross-sectional study of 2,537 participants ages 50–102 in Alameda County found that religiosity (measured as organizational and nonorganizational religiosity) buffered the effects of financial and health problems but exacerbated depression among those facing family crises. These authors concluded that, "As an antidote for depression, . . . religiosity should be prescribed with great care; it might make the patient better, but it also just might make things worse" (p. S124). Investigators reasoned that because family cohesion is valued highly by the religious, when there are problems caused by unruly children, marital conflict, or difficulties caring for an older parent or other relative, greater religiousness may exacerbate the stress experienced. Religious coping resources may be most helpful for stressors perceived as resulting from outside the individual (e.g., like poor health or financial stress). For family problems thought to result from personal or spiritual defects or shortcomings, the authors speculated, religious resources may be less helpful.

Alcoholism

Walters (1957), studying the religious backgrounds of 50 alcoholics, reported that a larger proportion of alcoholics in the study group were church members than in a control group, and mothers of alcoholics were more involved in religious activities than were mothers of control group members. No statistics were used in this study, and the author admitted that religious alcoholics may have been more likely to seek treatment than nonreligious alcoholics, skewing the results. Peele (1990) reviewed several studies that show that religious-based alcohol rehabilitation programs (such as Alcoholics Anonymous) are less effective than traditional treatment programs.

Social and Community Integration

Thorndike (1939) examined 37 separate factors to determine what makes a city "good" to live in, such as low levels of infant mortality and a high percentage of young people enrolled in schools. He correlated this "goodness" score with the percentage of the population that reported being church members. In 295 cities, he found a negative correlation ($r = -.22$) between the goodness score of a sample and the percentage of the sample that claimed church membership (his analyses, however, were uncontrolled for socioeconomic factors). Likewise, Angell (1951) studied factors related to community social health and moral integration in 28 cities and found no association between social health and church membership. Pugh (1951) found that nonchurch members had higher "social values" than church members and African American Baptist ministers (social values were not defined but were taken from Allport-Vernon Study of Values scale).

Wright and Cox (1971) conducted two cross-sectional surveys of sixth graders in England, one in 1963 ($n = 2276$) and one in 1970 ($n = 1963$). Strong religious beliefs and practices among the children were inversely related to favorable attitudes toward gambling, drunkenness, smoking, lying, stealing, premarital sexual intercourse, and suicide in both studies. However, changes in attitude toward these behaviors (toward greater permissiveness) between 1963 and 1970 were about the same in highly religious subjects as in highly nonreligious subjects. In other words, there was a general shift among both the religious and the nonreligious toward greater permissiveness. The authors concluded that "changes towards a more permissive point of view are in no way delayed or impeded by [religious] commitment."

In a major review of the research on religion and mental health in the *American Journal of Psychiatry*, Victor Sanua, a professor in the Department of Social and Psychological Foundations at the City University of New York, concluded that "The contention that religion as an institution has been instrumental in fostering general well-being, creativity, honesty, liberalism, and other qualities is not supported by empirical data. Both Scott and Godin point out that *there are no scientific studies* [italics added] which show that religion is capable of serving mental health" (Sanua, 1969, p. 1203).

Physical Health

One research group from London, England, has reported two studies that found worse health outcomes six to nine months later among medical patients who scored high on a spiritual beliefs scale at baseline (King, Speck, & Thomas, 1994; King, Speck, & Thomas, 1999). These studies used a broad definition of spiritual beliefs (as distinct from traditional religious involvement and activity) and have serious methodological flaws, which we review in chapter 22. Nevertheless, their findings are noteworthy.

SUMMARY AND CONCLUSIONS

A number of highly respected health professionals view religion as having a negative influence on mental health, physical health, or both. There is little doubt that people with mental illness often present with bizarre and distorted religious ideas and that religious beliefs and practices are used in pathological ways. Devoutly religious persons may also have high expectations of themselves and of others. They may condemn themselves for having family problems or other difficulties that they think religious people shouldn't have. At other times, they may judge harshly and alienate those who do not believe or behave as they do. Such attitudes do not foster good mental health or build community.

We have also seen that certain religious beliefs can interfere with the timely seeking of medical care and may delay diagnosis and treatment, leading to worse health outcomes. Religious beliefs may prevent sufferers from complying with medical treatments by encouraging them to rely on faith rather than on traditional medical care; they may therefore refuse potentially life-saving blood transfusions, prenatal care, childhood vaccinations, or other standard treatments or prevention measures.

Nevertheless, the claims of religious abuse and negative effects of religion on health rest largely on isolated case reports and highly selected case series, rather than on population-based systematic research studies. There is no doubt that some systematic research does show either no relationship between religion and health or a negative relationship. Many of these reports, however, are older studies of college students and adolescents without mature religious faith, utilize samples that were brought together by convenience, involve cross-sectional study designs (making causal inferences impossible), or fail to control for other relevant variables in analyses.

What remains largely unknown (on the basis of the evidence presented in this chapter) is whether traditional religious beliefs and practices, as engaged in by the majority of adults in the United States and around the world cause negative health effects or result in abuse. If religion is capable of causing negative health effects, it is important to determine how often this actually occurs. For example, do most religious persons in the United States rely on religious healing instead of traditional medical care? Or do they tend to rely on *both* traditional medicine and religious healing methods, seldom seeking one in exclusion of the other? Likewise, do the majority of clergy in the United States sexually abuse children or dominate the lives of people in their congregations? Or do these behaviors occur relatively rarely? If religious beliefs and practices have negative health consequences, do the health benefits outweigh the negative effects? Indeed, these are testable research questions.

5

Religious Coping

The Patient's Experience

ELIGIOUS AND HEALTH PRO-
fessionals may debate the benefits or
risks to health that religion conveys,
but people with serious health prob-
lems, people fighting against life-threatening or
life-disabling diseases, tell us the most about
how religion relates to health. Even if no relationship existed, religion would be relevant to
health care if patients perceived that it improved their coping with health problems and
therefore wished health care providers to address spiritual issues as part of their medical or
psychiatric care.

How does one go about studying the role
that religion plays in helping people cope with
serious health problems? The investigator must
first systematically identify a group of people
with serious medical illness—cancer, heart failure, AIDS, end-stage renal disease, or chronically disabling conditions such as stroke or arthritis. The illnesses must be severe enough and
cause sufficient stress to require considerable

adaptation. For example, older persons who are
experiencing both losses related to aging and
multiple physical health problems are frequently under a great deal of stress and provide
an ideal group to study. Another stressed population is family caregivers of persons with dementia, end-stage cancer, AIDS, or other illness
that present heavy care demands.

Having identified a population to study, the
investigator must then assess subjects' use of
religion as a coping behavior. One way is to
simply ask an open-ended question about what
enables the respondents to cope with the fear,
helplessness, uncertainty, and physical discomfort that accompany their illnesses. The subjects
must then spontaneously choose, on the basis of
their history of personal experience, the single
most helpful coping strategy. This method probably underestimates religious coping, since some
people feel uncomfortable talking about religion
to health care professionals and researchers,
whom they perceive as unreceptive to it.

A second way of assessing patients' religious coping experiences is to provide a list of different coping strategies and then to ask subjects to choose those that have been most helpful. This provides subjects with a bit more information about what types of coping strategies the researcher is interested in and gives the subjects permission to check religious coping methods if they have been helpful.

A third way of acquiring information about the importance of religious coping is to directly ask patients whether they use religion to cope with health problems. This method is likely to overestimate religious coping; some people feel obligated to respond positively to such questions since a positive response is usually socially desirable (given the largely religious culture in which we live). Subjects may also wish to please the interviewer and therefore give the response they perceive the interviewer wants or expects.

Consequently, researchers find rates of religious coping that vary widely, depending on the method chosen to acquire this information. Open-ended questions have yielded rates of religious coping varying between 1% and 42% (depending on the population and on the part of the world in which the subjects live) (Cederblad et al., 1995; Koenig, 1998b). Questions that directly ask about the use of religious coping receive positive responses 80–90% of the time (Princeton Religion Research Center, 1982; Americana Healthcare Corporation, 1980–1981). We now review research that examines religious coping in different physical illnesses, age groups, and crisis situations. The studies reviewed were identified in our comprehensive literature search (see Introduction) and include both positive and negative studies. We discuss studies in order of year of publication, when applicable, whether the study was conducted in or outside the United States.

RELIGIOUS COPING IN SPECIFIC MEDICAL CONDITIONS

Kidney Disease

Greenberg, Spitz, et al. (1975) qualitatively examined the coping behaviors of seven chronic hemodialysis patients living in Connecticut and their families. Most patients and families were Catholic. The investigators concluded that factors related to adjustment were (1) the defense mechanisms used, especially denial; (2) the patient's ability to cope with the dependency demands of the dialysis procedure; and (3) the presence of responsible family members willing to emotionally support the patient. There was no mention of prayer or other religious behaviors, which were apparently not assessed directly.

Baldree et al. (1982) examined the coping behaviors of 35 dialysis patients (54% African American) who had been on hemodialysis for at least six months. Subjects ranged in age from 21 to 60 years and lived in Chicago. The investigators found that prayer was the third most common coping behavior on a checklist of 40 possible coping strategies (Jalowiec & Powers Coping Scale).

O'Brien (1982) conducted a three-year prospective study of 126 chronic hemodialysis patients in Washington, D.C. (75% African American and 69% Protestant). Perceptions of religion's usefulness in coping with end-stage renal disease and dialysis were assessed. More than half (52.4%) indicated that religion was "usually" or "always" associated with their adjustment to hemodialysis. Compared to Catholics and Protestants, Jews were more likely to indicate that religion was never related to adjustment (12% vs. 23% vs. 63%, respectively). Three years after the baseline interview, 63 subjects were reinterviewed. More than one-quarter (27%) indicated that religion's importance for adjusting to dialysis had increased during the previous three years. Only 1 of 63 subjects had experienced a decline in religion's importance. Overall, 40% (25/63) reported an increased use of religion in adjusting to illness, 44% reported no change, and 16% indicated a decrease. With regard to religious attendance, 33% had increased their frequency of attendance compared to baseline, 38% had stayed the same, and 29% had decreased (because of increased physical limitations in the majority of cases). The author concluded that religion as a coping behavior becomes increasingly important to hemodialysis patients over time. Note, however, that 50% of the sample was lost to follow-up.

Tix and Frazier (1997) conducted a nine-month prospective study of 239 subjects who received renal transplants at the University of Minnesota Hospital and 179 subjects classified as "significant others." Subjects were surveyed 3 months (T1) and 12 months (T2) after surgery. Of the T1 sample, 174 patients and 123 significant others participated in the T2 survey. At baseline 42% of patients were Protestant, 35% were Catholic, and 64% were men; the average age was 42. T1 measures included a 10-item scale assessing the overall degree to which religion was used to cope with transplant-related stresses. Psychological distress was measured at T1 and T2 by a 17-item composite measure of depression, anxiety, and hostility (subscales of Derogatis's Brief Symptom Inventory); life satisfaction was measured by Diener's five-item Satisfaction with Life Scale.

Regression analyses revealed that religious coping at T1 was related to greater life satisfaction at T1 and T2 for patients and significant others and to less psychological distress at T1 for significant others. Religious coping at T1 did not predict life satisfaction or distress at T2 when T1 life satisfaction/distress was controlled. When analyses were stratified by religious denomination, religious coping was associated with higher life satisfaction for Protestants but not for Catholics. Among Protestant patients, greater T1 religious coping significantly predicted greater T2 life satisfaction when T1 life satisfaction was controlled. Among significant others of Catholic patients, greater T1 religious coping predicted increased psychological distress at T2 (for unclear reasons) after controlling for T1 distress. The researchers concluded that religious coping, especially among Protestants, is associated with better adaptation to the stress of transplant surgery.

Cancer

See chapter 20 for a description of studies by Sodestrom and Martinson (1987), Johnson and Spilka (1991), Spilka, Zwartjes, et al. (1991), Raleigh (1992), Halstead and Fernsler (1994), and Roberts, Brown, et al. (1997) in the United States and by Kesselring, et al. (1986) and Ginsburg, et al. (1995) in other countries.

Cardiovascular Disease

Croog and Levine (1972) examined changes in religiousness among 324 men during a 12-month period following myocardial infarction (MI). Subjects were ages 30–60, had suffered their first MI, and had no serious prior health problems; 62% were Catholic, 23% Protestant, and 15% Jewish, and all were from Boston or Worcester, Massachusetts. Subjects were surveyed at 1 month (T2) and 12 months (T3) after the MI. They were asked at T2 about religious attitudes/behaviors immediately prior to the myocardial infarction (T1). By religious denomination, 73% of Catholics, 48% of Protestants, and 40% of Jews indicated that religion was important or very important at T1; likewise, 79%, 52%, and 42%, respectively, indicated that religion was important or very important at T2. At T3, 21% of Catholics, 21% of Protestants, and 26% of Jews reported an increase in religiousness, whereas 16%, 11%, and 23%, respectively, reported a decrease. For church attendance, 9% of Catholics, 11% of Protestants and 13% of Jews had an increase, whereas 14%, 29%, and 9%, respectively, had a decrease.

When questioned at T3, 13% of Catholics, 5% of Protestants, and 2% of Jews (9% average) experienced a change in their religious feelings or views toward religion, virtually all in a positive direction. Given the stability of religion over time in populations without health problems (and these men generally did not have multiple health problems), an increase in religiousness for nearly 10% of subjects during a nine-month period indicates considerable change. At T2, 11% (12%, 15%, and 2%, respectively) had seen or planned to see clergy for support (the second largest group sought for support). About 13% indicated that payment for sins was influential in causing heart attack (but this was ranked fifteenth out of 16 possible causes for MI).

Jalowiec and Powers (1981) surveyed 50 volunteer patients at a university clinic in Chicago, including 25 newly diagnosed hypertensives and 25 people who sought care at the emergency room for nonserious acute illnesses. A 40-item scale, developed by the authors, measured coping behaviors. Investigators reported that out of 40 possible coping behaviors, pray/trust in God was rated second among hypertensive patients and tenth among other patients.

Saudia et al. (1991) surveyed 100 patients one day before each underwent coronary artery bypass graft (CABG) surgery at the University of Alabama Medical Center in Birmingham. The sample was mostly Protestant (87%) and male (75%). Subjects were asked whether prayer was used to cope prior to surgery and whether it was helpful (on a scale from 0 to 15). Ninety-five percent reported using prayer, and 70% rated prayer "extremely helpful" (a score of 15) for coping with surgery. Only two subjects rated the helpfulness of prayer less than 10.

Sears and Greene (1994) examined religious coping in 79 consecutive candidates for heart transplantation at the University Medical Center in Jackson, Mississippi. The average age of the sample was 53, and most subjects were male (85%) and white (87%) and had diagnoses of either ischemic cardiomyopathy (37%) or congestive heart failure (30%). Investigators assessed religious interest and administered the short form of Pargament's Religious Problem-Solving Scales (categorized into self-directing, collaborative, and deferring strategies) (Pargament, Kennell, et al., 1988). Three groups of subjects were formed: the deferring/collaborator group, who had highest interest in religion ($n = 9$); the self-director group (coped without God's help), who had the least interest in religion ($n = 37$); and eclectics, whose religious coping depended on the type of stressor being experienced ($n = 24$). Eclectics scored higher on the Spielberger anxiety scale than self-directors (39.9 vs. 33.6, $p < .05$), and deferring/collaborators scored in the intermediate range (37.5).

Harris et al. (1995) examined the role of religion in heart transplant recipients' health and well-being in a prospective study of 40 adult heart transplant patients. Subjects were interviewed 2, 7, and 12 months after transplant at a Pennsylvania university medical center. Of the subjects, 80% were male, 80% were white, 55% were Protestant, and 40% were Catholic. More

than half (51%) indicated that prayer was used to cope at two months posttransplant, and there was no significant change over time in this proportion. Church attendance increased significantly from 18% two months after heart transplantation to 44% at one year ($p < .05$), although the influence of religious beliefs on life declined slightly from 46% to 37% ($p < .05$). Religious beliefs and practices at the baseline interview (two-month) predicted better physical functioning, lower anxiety, higher self-esteem, fewer health worries, and less difficulty with the transplant medical regimen and better compliance when assessed 10 months later.

Ai et al. (1998) examined the role of religiosity in the recovery of 151 patients following CABG. Subjects were on average 64.7 years old and lived in or around Ann Arbor, Michigan. Investigators cross-sectionally assessed religious variables and psychological distress one year following the procedure. Psychological distress was measured using Derogatis's SCL-90-R. During the 12-month period after surgery, 76% of patients said religion was "pretty important" or "very important"; 54% attended religious services on a regular basis; and 68% prayed. Using logistic regression, investigators found that prayer was more likely among subjects who experienced depression during the first month following CABG ($\beta = .70$, $p = .037$). However, after controlling for post-CABG depression, social support, and number of other illnesses using ANCOVA, investigators found that prayer was associated with less current psychosocial distress ($F = 8.4$, $p < .005$).

HIV-Infected Persons

Carson (1993) surveyed 100 volunteer subjects who were HIV-positive (70%) or had AIDS (30%). Kobasa's Personal Views Survey was used to determine "hardiness" (a construct related to longer survival in this population). A spirituality scale was constructed by summing responses to questions concerning frequency of prayer, meditation, use of imagery or visualization, reading religious literature, and attending spiritual retreats and church services. More than half of subjects rated their participation in prayer, meditation, and other spiritual activities with a mean score that indicated from some to a great deal of activity, with prayer receiving the highest score. Attendance at spiritual retreats, and at religious services and reading religious literature were rated by the majority of subjects with a mean score that indicated no to very little participation. Total Spiritual Scale score was related to greater hardiness ($r = 0.18$, $p = .04$), although only prayer ($r = 0.23$, $p = .01$) and meditation ($r = 0.26$, $p = .005$) were related to hardiness when individual items were examined (analyses uncontrolled).

Folkman, Chesney, Cooke, et al. (1994) examined spirituality and caregiver burden among 82 HIV-positive caregivers of patients with AIDS (caregivers were also partners of patients), 162 HIV-negative caregivers, and 61 HIV-positive partners of healthy men in the San Francisco Bay area. Subjects were administered a 10-item measure of religious and spiritual beliefs and activities developed by the investigators. HIV-positive caregivers had significantly higher religiosity/spirituality than HIV-negative caregivers; religiosity/spirituality of the 61 HIV-positive partners of healthy men was intermediate between the other two groups. Among HIV-positive caregivers, religiosity was inversely related to caregiver burden (after controlling for other variables in a regression model, $\beta = -.16$, $p = .03$) but was unrelated to caregiver burden in HIV-negative caregivers.

Jenkins (1995) examined religious coping style among 422 HIV-positive military personnel at three United States military medical centers. The sample was 93% male and 63% white and had a mean age of 33 years. Three styles of religious coping were examined: self-directed coping without God's help (40.5% of sample), and two styles based on collaboration between self and God (collaborative/self, which emphasized the role of self [18.0%], and collaborative/deferral, which emphasized the role of God [41.5%]). African Americans were much more likely than Caucasians to cope using the collaborative/deferral style and much less likely to use the self-directed coping style ($p < .001$). Religious coping was used more often by those with advanced health problems (a commonly observed pattern in many studies). Clinically depressed individuals reported significantly more religious discontent and pleading ($p < .001$), indicating an association between distress and negativistic, desperate religious approaches to coping. The author concluded that religious approaches may have particular value for programs that target coping and quality of life among HIV-positive African Americans.

Kaldjian et al. (1998) surveyed 90 HIV-positive patients on the HIV/AIDS floor of Yale-New Haven Hospital. Of the sample 90% were Christian and 3% were Muslim; 7% reported no affiliation. Investigators reported that 44% of patients felt guilty about their HIV infection, 32% expressed a fear of death, and 26% felt their disease was a form of punishment (17% said it was a punishment from God). Prior discussions about resuscitation status were more likely in the 81% of patients who believed in God's forgiveness ($p < .05$) and were less likely among those who perceived HIV infection as punishment ($p < .01$). A living will was more common in the 69% of patient who prayed daily and in those whose belief in God helped them when thinking about death. Fear of death was less likely among those who read the Bible frequently ($p = .01$) and attended church regularly ($p = .02$). Ninety-eight percent of the sample believed in a divine being called God whose love is unconditional (96%); 84% expressed a personal relationship with God; 82% said that their belief in God helped when thinking about death; and 63% believed in life after death. Fifty-six percent of patients could identify someone in their lives who served as a spiritual counselor, and half of the remaining 44% desired spiritual counseling (but only 30% of these patients had spoken with a hospital chaplain). Fifty-six percent of patients believed that it would be important to discuss spiritual needs with their physician, and 46% indicated that an opportunity to pray with their physician would be helpful.

Diabetes

In one of the few studies that have evaluated religious coping in diabetics, Zaldivar and Smolowitz (1994) surveyed 104 Hispanic diabetics who attended an outpatient medical clinic in New York City (47% from the Dominican Republic and 35% from Puerto Rico). Seventy-eight percent responded affirmatively to the statement "I have diabetes because it is God's will," 25% to the statement "I have diabetes because God is punishing me," 55% to the statement "My priest helps me control my diabetes," and 81% to the statement "Only God can control my diabetes." These results underscore the importance of involving clergy in the treatment of Hispanic diabetics in some inner-city populations.

Landis (1996) examined spiritual well-being and mental health among 94 diabetics in Galveston, Texas. Of the sample population, 65% were female, 33% were African American, 83% were Christian, and 70% were insulin-requiring diabetics; the mean age was 46. Spiritual well-being (SWB) was measured by Paloutzian and Ellison's SWB scale, psychological distress by the Psychosocial Adjustment to Illness Scale, and illness "uncertainty" by the Mishel Uncertainty in Illness Scale. SWB was inversely correlated with uncertainty ($r = -.49, p < .001$) and psychological distress ($r = -.47, p = .001$). More important, the religious well-being (RWB) subscale of the SWB scale was also inversely related to uncertainty ($r = -.26, p < .01$) and psychological distress ($r = -.34, p < .001$). Using hierarchical regression, Landis found that uncertainty and existential well-being (EWB) predicted psychosocial adjustment, but RWB did not (however, RWB may have had an indirect effect on psychosocial adjustment through EWB). When asked what most helped them to cope with diabetes, 34% said family and friends, 29% said their ability to manage the disease, and 18% named spiritual support such as belief in God, prayer, hope for a cure, and purpose.

Cystic Fibrosis

Evaluating the use of nonmedical treatments by cystic fibrosis patients, Stern et al. (1992) surveyed all 402 cystic fibrosis patients and their families seen on the inpatient and outpatient services of a pediatric hospital in Cleveland, Ohio. The median age of subjects was 18 years; mean education was 14 years; 96% were white, 56% were male, 58% were Protestant, and 36% were Catholic. The use of religion as a nonmedical treatment included visiting faith healers, making a religious pilgrimage, having a " healing article," or participating in a prayer group. Religious treatments were by far the most common type of alternative nonmedical therapy. Sixty-six percent of participants ($n = 264$) used at least one type of nonmedical therapy, and 57% ($n = 231$) used at least one religious treatment (48% group prayer, 14% faith healing, 4% religious pilgrimage, 12% healing article or religious object). Among those using group prayer, 92% believed it helped in maintaining health and conveying a sense of support; 70% of those visiting faith healers, 80% of those using religious objects, and 73% of those making religious pilgrimages reported a similar benefit. No patient or family member reported any adverse effect from these religious activities on well-being or self-esteem.

Use of religion as a nonmedical therapy in the United States is widespread regardless of specific medical illness, according to a report by Eisenberg, Kessler, et al. (1993) published in the *New England Journal of Medicine*. These investigators examined unconventional therapies for health problems in the United States by surveying a random national sample of 1539 adults. They found that 25% of subjects indicated use of prayer as an unconventional therapy, which was second only to exercise (26%) in frequency.

Elderly Medically Ill

Conway (1985) questioned 65 African American and white elderly women about how they had coped with stressful medical problems within the past year. Subjects, many with recent health problems, were recruited from low-income housing projects for the elderly in Kansas City. Responding to a checklist of religious and nonreligious coping behaviors, 91% reported that they used prayer as a coping mechanism. One of the two most common cognitive methods for coping with stressful medical illness was "thinking of God or your religious beliefs," endorsed by 86%. When asked who helped them when faced with stressful medical problems, the respondents most frequently named God (85%), a professional (78%), a friend (60%), a family member (57%), or a minister (28%).

African Americans, 58% of the sample, were more likely than whites to indicate that God was helpful (80% vs. 53%, $p < .05$) and that church members were helpful (26% vs. 6%, $p < .05$).

Koenig, Cohen, Blazer, et al. (1992) interviewed a consecutive sample of 850 older patients admitted to the medical and neurological services of the Veterans Administration hospital in Durham, North Carolina. Subjects were age 65 or older; 28% were African American, and 92% were Protestant; 25% had been admitted with cardiovascular disease and 22% with cancer. Twenty-one percent indicated that religion was the most important factor that enabled them to cope. When asked to rate on a 0–10 visual analog scale how much they used religion to cope, 56% indicated 7.5 or higher (a large extent or more). In that study, religious coping was inversely related to depression both cross-sectionally and longitudinally (see chapter 7).

Koenig (1998b) next examined religious coping among 338 men and women consecutively admitted to the Duke University Medical Center in Durham, North Carolina. All participants were over age 60, 52% were women, and 33% were African American. When asked to respond spontaneously to the open-ended question "What is the most important factor that enables you to cope?," 42% indicated that religion (e.g., prayer, God, faith, my church) was what helped the most. When asked to rate on a 0–10 visual analog scale the extent to which they used religion to help them cope, 67% indicated 7.5 or higher (a large extent or more). Factors that predicted greater reliance on religion included being female, being African American, having less education, and facing more stressful life events.

Terminally Ill

Carey (1974) surveyed 84 terminally ill patients (ages 13–82, 48% Protestant, 37% Catholic, and 14% non-Christian) at Lutheran General Hospital in Park Ridge, Illinois. Chaplains rated emotional adjustment using a six-item adjustment scale and a five-item physical discomfort scale. Six religious belief and religious orientation questions were also administered. Catholics scored higher than Protestants, who scored

higher than non-Christians on emotional adjustment (63% vs. 49% vs. 17% high adjustment, a relationship that persisted after controlling for sex and education). Among the 61 patients who provided information on religious beliefs, 87% believed in a personal God, 77% believed in Jesus as the son of God, 66% believed in an afterlife and place of permanent happiness, and 34% believed in a place of permanent unhappiness.

Of six religious belief items, Carey found that only belief in Jesus was related to adjustment (66% of believers had high emotional adjustment vs. 29% of nonbelievers). Intrinsic religiosity was also related to better adjustment (80% showed high levels of adjustment, vs. 63% for indiscriminately proreligious, 50% for extrinsically religious, and 53% for indiscriminately nonreligious). Regression analysis revealed that the six most powerful predictors of good adjustment were (1) less physical discomfort, (2) feeling of concern by next of kin, (3) previous discussion of death with dying person, (4) extrinsic religious orientation ($\beta = -.30$), (5) higher education level, and (6) feeling of concern from one's local clergy ($\beta = .25$). Thus, extrinsic religiosity (use of religion as a means to another end, rather than as an end in itself) was associated with poorer adjustment.

Gibbs and Achterberg-Lawlis (1978) surveyed 16 cancer patients in a rehabilitation program at the University of Texas Health Center in Dallas. Members of the research team chose patients who were closest to death—those with life expectancies measured in weeks—to participate in the study. Of the sample, 50% were African American, 50% were white, 56% were female, and 75% were Baptist or Church of Christ; mean age was 49. Investigators asked questions about strength of religious beliefs, religious orientation, and seven other aspects of religious belief and practice. Strength of religious beliefs was significantly related to low ratings of conscious fear ($F = 28.0$, $p < .001$) and positive ratings of death imagery ($F = 5.2$, $p < .05$). Patients who indicated that their church was a major source of emotional support experienced less sleep difficulty and displayed less denial of their impending death. Thus, religious patients had fewer fears of death. Interestingly, anxiety level as assessed by Templer's Death Anxiety Scale was lower for the terminally ill population than for a control group of healthy eye clinic patients.

Smith, Nehemkis, et al. (1983–1984) interviewed 20 patients with terminal illness in a medical oncology section and nursing home care unit of a large veterans hospital in Long Beach, California (19 patients had metastatic cancer). Religiousness was measured using a two-item scale: importance of religion, rated from 1 to 9, and church attendance, rated from 1 to 5. Death anxiety was assessed by four scales: (1) conscious fear of death, measured by a single item; (2) the Collett-Lester Fear of Death subscale; (3) fantasy level, measured by 16 images developed by Feifel and Nagy; and (4) Spilka et al.'s Death Perspective Scale (DPS). Church attendance was inversely related to all four fear-of-death measures but was significantly related only to the Feifel and Nagy images scale ($r = -.51, p < .05$). Church attendance was also positively related to an "afterlife-of-reward" subscale of the DPS ($r = .46, p < .05$). Importance of religion was positively related to the afterlife-of-reward and courage subscales of the DPS ($r = .80, p < .01$ and $r = .55, p < .05$) and negatively related to an indifference subscale ($r = -.71, p < .01$) but was unrelated to any fear of death measures.

In one of the only studies of medically ill adolescents on this topic, Silber and Reilly (1985) surveyed 114 newly hospitalized young persons, ages 11–19, at Children's Hospital National Medical Center in Washington, D.C. Of the participants, 66% were female, 51% were African American, and 81% attended public school. The sample was divided among patients with severe and likely fatal disease ($n = 24$), severe but likely not fatal disease ($n = 53$), and moderately severe disease ($n = 37$). The investigators administered a nine-item Spiritual and Religious Concerns Questionnaire (SRQ). Most subjects believed in God, and about half were actively practicing their religion. Severity of medical illness was significantly related to level of spiritual and religious concern, with more severely ill patients scoring higher on the SRQ (regardless of sex or race). In particular, nearly half of the adolescents with severe, possibly fatal illness reported that they had experienced a marked change in their religious and spiritual concerns as a result of their illness.

Reed (1986) compared 57 terminally ill and 57 healthy persons from the southeastern United States on religiousness and sense of well-being. Terminally ill patients had Stage III or IV cancer; the healthy control group consisted of volunteers recruited from community organizations and neighborhood groups. Terminally ill and healthy groups were matched on age, gender, education, and religious affiliation. A 13-item Religious Perspective Scale (a revision of King and Hunt scales) and Campbell's 9-item Index of Well-Being were administered to all participants. Terminally ill patients scored significantly higher than healthy subjects on religiousness ($p < .001$). Interestingly, there was no significant difference in well-being between terminally ill and healthy groups (10.10 vs. 10.03, $p = $ ns). There was a significant correlation between religiousness and well-being in the healthy group ($r = .43, p < .001$), although this association did not reach statistical significance in the terminal group ($r = .14, p = $ ns).

Reed (1987) expanded the above study to include 300 subjects divided into three groups: 100 terminally ill patients with incurable cancer hospitalized an average of six days (Group 1); 100 nonterminally ill patients hospitalized an average of five days (Group 2); and 100 healthy nonhospitalized persons free of any serious illnesses (Group 3). The three groups were matched as in the 1986 study. Group 1 patients (terminal) had significantly greater religiousness than Groups 2 or 3 ($p = .02$), and there was no difference in overall well-being among the three groups. Each group was asked about changes in their spiritual views recently. Such changes were reported by 44% of terminal patients (89% toward greater spirituality), 42% of nonterminal hospitalized patients (55% toward greater spirituality), and 28% of healthy subjects (57% toward greater spirituality). Only 11% of terminal patients whose spiritual beliefs had changed indicated that they had eschewed specific religious teachings and rituals of childhood or expressed more questions and doubts about their spiritual beliefs. Moving from Group 3 to Group 1 (healthy to severely ill), there was a diminishing incidence of reference to loss of faith or disregard of childhood religious beliefs and an increasing percentage of statements about strengthened spirituality ($p < .01$).

Psychiatric Patients

There are very few studies that examine the use of religious beliefs and behaviors by psychiatric patients to cope with stress or that explore the spiritual needs of such patients. Fitchett et al. (1997) examined 51 adult psychiatric inpatient and 50 adult general medical/surgical inpatients (matched by gender and age) at a Chicago hospital. Diagnoses among psychiatric patients were major depression (39%), bipolar disorder (28%), minor mood disorder (14%), schizoaffective disorder (14%), and paranoia, substance abuse, panic disorder, or adjustment disorder (14%). More than two-thirds (68%) of psychiatric inpatients responded "a great deal" to a question that asked to what extent religion was a source of comfort and support (vs. 72% for medical-surgical patients). The vast majority of the psychiatric patients in this study (88%) reported experiencing three or more religious needs during hospitalization (vs. 76% for medical-surgical patients). Only 24% of the psychiatric patients, however, had talked with a member of the clergy about the current hospitalization (vs. 81% of medical-surgical patients). We return to the issue of meeting psychiatric patients' spiritual needs in chapter 29.

These studies indicate that religious coping in the setting of medical or psychiatric illness is very common, especially among older adults and African Americans. Most of these studies find that use of religion increases with increasing severity of medical illness or life stress, suggesting that persons turn to religion as stress level increases or death approaches.

RELIGIOUS COPING AMONG HEALTHY ADULTS

High rates of religious coping among persons with health problems, then, particularly those with acute or life-threatening illness, may be due to a transient turning to religion during a time of crisis. The old saying "There are no atheists in foxholes" may explain the near ubiquitous use of religion in these settings, particularly among acutely hospitalized patients. In order to avoid this "foxhole effect," we examine how persons living in the community cope with stress.

In the 1980s, a Gallup poll asked a national random sample of 1,485 adults to indicate whether the following statement was true for them: "I receive a great deal of comfort and support from my religious beliefs" (Princeton Religion Research Center, 1982). Possible responses were "completely true" (38%), "mostly true" (40%), "mostly untrue" (11%), and "completely untrue" (7%). This suggests that almost 80% of the U.S. population receives comfort and support from religious beliefs. Despite the forces of secularization, the importance of religion to Americans has not changed much since 1982. Recent Gallup polls indicate that religious belief and practice in the United States (as measured by importance placed on religion, church membership and attendance, confidence in organized religion, percentage with a religious preference, proportion who say religion can answer problems, belief in God, and belief in the honesty and ethical standards of the clergy) are actually more common today than in 1982 (Princeton Religion Research Center, 1999).

Manfredi and Pickett (1987) interviewed 51 persons age 60 or over who were living in a senior citizen housing complex in Rhode Island. They administered the Lazarus Ways of Coping Checklist after identifying a stressful event experienced by each subject in the past month. Out of 66 possible coping strategies, prayer was the coping behavior most frequently used.

Koenig, George, and Siegler (1988) examined the use of religion and other emotion-regulating coping strategies by 100 community-dwelling older adults who were participating in the Duke Longitudinal II Study of Aging. Respondents were asked how they coped with the worst event or situation (1) in their whole lives, (2) in the past 10 years, and (3) in their lives currently. The questions were asked in an open-ended way, allowing subjects to spontaneously report whatever they felt was most helpful. Forty-nine percent of stressful events were health-related, and 29% were family-related. Investigators found that 17% of 556 coping strategies were religious (the most common category of response). Women mentioned religious coping more frequently than did men (58% vs. 32%). The most common religious responses were placing trust and faith in God, praying, and finding help and strength from God (74% of all religious coping behaviors).

Mattlin et al. (1990) examined coping strategies used by 977 white married couples (n = 1,556) living in Detroit, Michigan. Subjects were asked how they had coped with the most stressful event or situation during the past year. A checklist of coping responses was offered. More than half of the sample (55%) indicated that religion was used "some" or "a lot" for dealing with stressors. Religious coping was used more often when subjects were dealing with illness and death (more serious stressors) than when they were dealing with practical or interpersonal problems.

Pargament, Ensing, et al. (1990) examined religious coping activities as predictors of outcome to significant negative life events in 586 adult members of mainline churches in the Midwestern United States (66% were female, 96% white, 39% college educated). Subjects were drawn systematically and proportionally from active and inactive members of 10 churches. They were asked whether they had used religion to cope with a serious life event in the previous year. Seventy-eight percent indicated that they had used religion in coping, from a slight amount to a great deal (similar to the findings of the 1982 Gallup poll findings mentioned earlier). Mental health, assessed using the General Health Questionnaire, was positively related to spiritually based religious coping activities (β = .25), intrinsic religiosity (β = .11), and religious experience (β = .18). Religious coping activities added significant additional variance to mental health (incremental r-square = .03, $p < .001$) after nonreligious coping variables and control variables were added to the model.

Ellison and Taylor (1996) surveyed a random sample of 1,344 community-dwelling adults who participated in the National Survey of Black Americans. Investigators identified those in the sample who were having major life crises that caused great mental distress or personal problems that were too great to handle alone. Among the questions asked was, "Did you pray or get someone to pray for you?" Almost 80% turned to prayer as a coping resource. This practice was again more likely among persons who were dealing with health problems or bereavement, persons with low general personal mastery, and women (multiple covariates controlled).

RELIGIOUS COPING AMONG CAREGIVERS

Does religion help family caregivers cope with the stress of caring for a sick loved one? Caregiving can be particularly stressful when one is caring for a family member with terminal cancer or dementia or for a child with chronic health problems. Studies have found high rates of depression and anxiety among caregivers, who are also at increased risk for developing physical health problems (Esterling, Kiecolt-Glaser, Bodnar, et al., 1994; Esterling, Kiecolt-Glaser, & Glaser, 1996; Kiecolt-Glaser & Glaser, 1994; Kiecolt-Glaser, Glaser, et al., 1996a; Kiecolt-Glaser, Marucha, et al., 1996).

Caregivers of Alzheimer's Patients

Baines (1984) was one of the first investigators to ask caregivers about the importance of religious activities in helping them cope with stress. Nearly three-quarters (74%) of caregivers in Baines's study reported that prayer was their primary method of coping.

Wright, Pratt, et al. (1985) examined the relationship between spiritual support and caregiver burden in a sample of 240 caregivers of loved ones with Alzheimer's disease. A single item assessed spiritual support. Caregiver burden scores were inversely related to spiritual support ($-.25$, $p < .01$, uncontrolled). Spiritual support was more strongly related to caregiver burden than was support from extended family, support from friends and neighbors, or support from community services.

Using an open-ended format, Segall and Wykle (1988–1989) asked 59 African American family caregivers how they coped with stress. Subjects spontaneously discussed factors that helped them deal with the stress of caregiving. Almost two-thirds (65%) mentioned religious beliefs and practices as essential for coping. Subjects were later asked to rate on a 1–5 scale how much they used prayer and how much they used faith; average scores were 4.3 and 4.0, respectively (out of a maximum possible score of 5.0).

Wood and Parham (1990) surveyed 85 rural African American ($n = 36$) and white ($n = 49$) caregivers in Virginia of relatives with Alzheimer's disease. Coping strategies were measured using Conway's (1985) scale. The investigators found that religious coping was common among both African Americans and whites, although, as Conway had discovered, African Americans were considerably more likely than whites to pray, think about religion, and report that they had received support from their ministers and from God.

Robinson and Kaye (1994) examined 17 caregiver wives of Alzheimer's patients and 23 noncaregiver wives of healthy adults to explore the relationship among spiritual perspective, social support, and depression in these groups. Reed's Spiritual Perspective Scale (SPS), the CES-D depression scale, and three scales of social support were administered to both groups. Unlike previous studies, this study revealed no association among SPS, CES-D, and social support in either caregivers or noncaregivers. The small sample size, however, probably limited the study's power to detect significant relationships.

Burgener (1994) surveyed coping behaviors among 84 caregivers of Alzheimer's patients in northern New York. The cases, identified through the Alzheimer's Association, were 44% male and 82% white; mean age of caregivers was 71. Cases were compared to 81 home-dwelling age-matched elderly controls who were participating in meal programs and senior centers (14% male, 72% white). An eight-item religiosity scale measured organizational and nonorganizational religious activity, and a variety of questions assessed religious support. Caregiver stress was measured by the Relatives' Stress Scale, well-being by a single item, and six domains of physical and mental health by the Medical Outcomes Study SF-20. Among caregivers, general well-being was associated with religious attendance ($r = .34$, $p < .01$), participation in organized religious activities ($r = .43$, $p < .01$), having the need for contact with the religious community met ($r = .38$, $p < .01$), and having spiritual needs met ($r = .46$, $p < .001$). Religious attendance was also correlated with social functioning ($r = .30$, $p < .01$). After controlling for other variables using multiple regression, religious attendance and "degree of spiritual needs met" predicted lower caregiver stress ($p < .01$), and religious attendance predicted higher social functioning ($\beta = .34$, $p < .01$). Researchers concluded that caregivers who worship regularly and who report that their spiritual needs are being met cope better with stress than caregivers who don't.

Caregivers of Cancer Patients

Kirschling and Pittman (1989) studied spiritual well-being and coping among 70 family members (mean age 62) who were caring for terminally ill relatives admitted to hospice programs in two northwestern states. The Paloutzian-Ellison Spiritual Well-being (SWB) scale and Bradburn's Affect Balance Scale were administered. Several persons ($n = 6$) did not complete the SWB scales because they were not religious or didn't believe in God. The SWB scale and subscales were all related to positive and negative affect in the expected directions, but none of the associations were significant except between existential well-being and negative affect ($-.38$, $p < .001$). The elimination of nonreligious caregivers may have reduced sample variability, making it more difficult to obtain significant associations.

Rabins, Fitting, Eastham, and Zabora (1990), at Johns Hopkins University, prospectively followed 62 caregivers of persons with either Alzheimer's disease or recurrent metastatic cancer to determine predictors of emotional adaptation during a two-year period. Multiple regression was used to examine the effects of a variety of baseline predictors on mood and well-being (measured by Bradburn's Affect-Balance Scale). About 30% of the variance in positive mood and well-being (i.e., adaptation) was explained by number of social contacts; strength of religious faith, however explained an additional 13% of the variance in positive mood and well-being ($F = 15.4$, $p < .0001$). Thus, a strong religious faith and frequent social contacts were the two major predictors of adaptation in this group. Keilman and Given (1990) also found an inverse correlation between spiritual/philosophical scores on the Coping Resources Inventory and depressive symptoms on the CES-D in a sample of 100 caregivers of cancer patients ($r = -.24$, $p < .001$, uncontrolled).

Caregivers of Elderly, Children, and HIV Patients

Salts et al. (1991) interviewed 30 married elderly couples from a southern U.S. community, examining the interaction between religiousness and caregiver status. Couples were categorized into four groups: active couples (neither couple disabled), short-term caregivers (one spouse disabled from an illness expected to improve), long-term caregivers (one spouse disabled from an illness not expected to improve), and survival couples (both members of the couple disabled and needing care). Three categories based on religious activity were formed: *no religion* (1 of 11 active couples, 0 of 5 short-term caregivers, 2 of 8 long-term caregivers, 1 of 5 survival couples); religious activities only (church activities serving as a major source of social interaction outside the home) (7 of 11 active couples, 0 of 5 short-term caregivers, 1 of 8 long-term caregivers, 3 of 5 survival couples); and religion used as an important coping resource (3 of 11 active couples, 5 of 5 short-term caregivers, 5 of 8 long-term caregivers, 1 of 5 survival couples). One couple was classified as a live-in caregiver couple, and they coped through religion. Researchers concluded that "Not only were religious activities and beliefs found to play a vital role in the lives of virtually all the couples, but the role of religion appeared to vary systematically in relation to the various health-related patterns observed" (p. 51).

Rutledge, Levin, et al. (1995) cross-sectionally surveyed 102 parents of children with chronic illness to determine the change over time in religious coping among parents who were caring for a chronically ill child (average age 7 years). The sample was recruited from outpatient clinics and support groups in Virginia. Of the sample, 69% were women, 90% were white, 58% were Protestant, 24% were Catholic, and 16% were Jewish. Four questions examined change in religious coping; responses were summed and dichotomized into "stable" versus "change." Nonreligious coping was measured with five items, which were similarly summed and dichotomized into stable versus change. The investigators found little change in the use of religious resources as a result of caring for a chronically ill child. Parents with "stable" religious coping were more likely to experience stable use of financial, familial, and social coping (e.g., nonreligious coping resources).

Folkman (1997) conducted in-depth interviews with caregivers and partners of persons dying of AIDS to determine the factors related to the caregivers' adjustment. Interviews were conducted every two months before and after the patient's death over a two-year period ($n = 156$). Nonbereaved caregivers and partners of AIDS patients ($n = 117$) were also studied. Religious and spiritual beliefs and activities were measured using a nine-item scale developed by Folkman, Chesney, Pollack, et al. (1992). The spiritual scale included the following items:

1. Meditation/prayer helps me find solutions to my problems.
2. Believing in a higher self/God gives meaning to my life.
3. Meditation/prayer makes me feel better.
4. Events in my life reflect an overall purpose and plan.
5. I attend religious or spiritual services.
6. I do personal meditation.
7. I read spiritual or metaphysical literature.
8. I talk to others about my spiritual concerns.
9. I consult a spiritual or religious leader.

Scores on spiritual beliefs and activities, other coping behaviors, and mental health outcomes were averaged over a two-year period and correlated (this was not a prospective analysis). At baseline in the combined sample of bereaved and nonbereaved caregivers, spiritual beliefs and activities were significantly related to positive affect ($r = .15$, $p = < .05$), planful problem solving ($r = .20$, $p < = .001$), and positive reappraisal ($r = .27$, $p = < .01$). When analyses were stratified by bereavement status, spirituality scores significantly correlated with positive appraisals in bereaved caregivers ($\beta = 0.47$, $p < .0001$), and positive appraisals were significantly related to positive affect and well-being ($\beta = 0.28$, $p < .0001$); however, there was no direct relationship between positive affect and spiritual beliefs and activities ($\beta = .04$, ns). The same pattern was observed in nonbereaved caregivers. On the basis of these quantitative and qualitative findings, Folkman concluded that "spiritual beliefs and experiences may be especially helpful in supporting adaptive coping during the days and weeks surrounding the partner's death" (p. 1214).

In summary, religious or spiritual beliefs and behaviors are commonly used to cope with the stress of caring for a sick family member or loved one. These behaviors are generally associated with greater meaning and purpose, more positive appraisals, greater well-being, and faster adaptation to the caregiving role.

RELIGIOUS COPING DURING NATURAL DISASTERS OR LIFE CRISES

Because religious behaviors may help persons to maintain emotional and psychological stability during situations associated with severe, uncontrollable stress, they are commonly used to deal with natural disasters and other major non-health-related life crises.

Nuclear Waste Spill

Cleary and Houts (1984) examined the psychological impact of the Three Mile Island (TMI) incident on persons who were living in the local area (Harrisburg, Pennsylvania). Four hundred and three persons living within five miles of TMI were surveyed by telephone on two occasions separated by six months. The investigators reported that neither baseline church attendance nor social support predicted lower than expected distress on the follow-up evaluation; number of friends, however, was related to better outcomes.

Hurricanes

Weinrich, Hardin, et al. (1990) studied the effects of stress caused by Hurricane Hugo, which hit the southeastern United States in 1989. They examined the experiences of 61 nursing students who provided care to hurricane victims in South Carolina three weeks after the event. Student nurses were asked about their perceptions of victims' disaster stress reactions, coping skills, and strategies. The most frequently observed coping strategies were talking about their experiences (95%), humor (82%), religion (74%), and altruism (47%).

Likewise, Sattler et al. (1994) interviewed 322 survivors seven weeks after Hurricane Iniki hit Hawaii. Investigators found that women were more likely to use religion to cope during and after the hurricane, and religious coping—measured using a four-item religious coping scale—was positively related to greater psychological stress ($r = .22$). As have others, these researchers found that religious coping was positively related to emotional distress during the period surrounding the acute stressor, as persons turned to religion for comfort in times of severe need. This was also seen in the Ai et al. (1998) study of patients experiencing the stress of open-heart surgery, where the association reversed over time as religious coping eventually led to improved adaptation. Studies of prayer in persons with chronic pain demonstrate this same pattern (see chapter 23).

War

Zeidner and Hammer (1992) surveyed 261 Jewish northern Israelis who experienced missile attacks during the Gulf War. The sample was 55% female and 48% single persons; the mean age was 29 years. Coping activities were measured using Carver's COPE scales, which include a question about "increased engagement in religious activities." Investigators measured "spiritual/philosophical" resources using a subscale of the Coping Resources Inventory. Again, high levels of religious activities and spiritual resources were cross-sectionally correlated with greater anxiety ($r = .33$, $p < .05$, and $r = .20$, $p < .05$, respectively) and more physical symptoms ($r = .29$, $p < .05$, and $r = .18$, $p < .05$, respectively). Associations with spiritual coping persisted after other variables were controlled in a regression model. Researchers concluded that spiritual persons perceived war as a greater threat to their religious culture, nation, and people as a whole. Alternatively, given the severe stress of the situation, many persons may have turned to religion for comfort (as discussed earlier).

In a related study, Pargament, Ishler, et al. (1994) examined the association between religion and coping around the time of the Gulf War in a sample of 215 college psychology students at Bowling Green State University. A multi-item scale was used to assess religious coping two days (T1) before the 1990–1991 U.S.-led invasion of Kuwait and one week (T2) after the war had stopped. The pleading to God subscale was related to T1 negative affect ($r = .25$) and T1 poorer mental health ($r = .21$) before the assault, but to T2 positive affect ($r = .20$, $p < .01$) after the assault. Religious good deeds and religious discontent were also related to negative affect before assault. Religious support was related to positive affect before the assault ($r = .17$, $p < .05$) and was inversely related to global distress after the assault ($r = -.16$, $p < .05$). Religious avoidance was related to higher global distress after the assault ($r = .21$, $p < .05$). Thus, different types of religious coping may be related to mental health in different ways at different time points before and after the stressor.

Midwest Flood

Pargament, Smith, and Brant (1995) examined religious and nonreligious coping methods used by 225 persons who experienced the flooding in the Midwest in 1993. Frequency of prayer and self-rated religiousness were correlated with better overall mental health ($r = .14$ and

$r = .21$), and self-rated religiousness was related to less negative affect ($r = -.20$). Religious attendance was also associated with less negative affect ($r = -.23$), less poor physical health ($r = -.20$), and better mental health status ($r = .19$). Intrinsic religiosity was related to better mental health ($r = .14$) and less negative affect ($r = -.19$). Spiritually based coping was correlated with positive affect ($r = .15$) and better mental health ($r = .30$). Self-directing religious coping (without God's help), on the other hand, was related to poorer mental health ($r = -.17$). Collaborative and deferring styles were both related to better mental health ($r = .20$ and $r = .25$). The timing of the interviews in relationship to the flood (i.e., how long after the flood the interviews took place) was not given.

Oklahoma City Bombing

Pargament et al. (1996) interviewed 310 members of two churches in the area where the federal building was bombed in Oklahoma City six weeks after the blast. Scales of positive religious coping (PRC) and negative religious coping (NRC) were cross-sectionally correlated with stress-related growth and symptoms of posttraumatic stress disorder (PTSD). PRC was related to stress-related growth ($r = .62$) and to greater PTSD symptoms ($r = .25$) (again in the acute situation). NRC was related less strongly to stress-related growth ($r = .21$) and more strongly to PTSD symptoms ($r = .48$).

Homicide

Thompson and Vardaman (1997) surveyed 150 family members of homicide victims to examine the role that religion played in coping with the loss. The sample was mostly African American (90%) and from Atlanta, Georgia. Researchers assessed spiritually based coping, religious support, religious avoidance, religious pleading, religious good deeds, and religious discontent. Religious coping behaviors were very common and, except for religious support, were related to greater distress. Religious support (respondents' perceived support from clergy and church members) was inversely related to PTSD symptoms ($\beta = -.14$, $p < .10$) and distress ($\beta =$

−.17, $p < .05$), whereas religious pleading, religious deeds, and religious discontent were all associated with more symptoms ($p < .05$, after controls). The "pleading to God" scale was again related to greater pathology on both measures of psychological distress. Pleading or bargaining with God, however, can be viewed as a normal stage of grief in response to the loss of a loved one.

Other Life Crises

Parker and Brown (1982) examined coping behaviors among 108 medical patients (mean age 38) receiving services at four general practices in Sydney, Australia. Coping was examined in relationship to an interpersonal stressor such as the breakup of a love relationship or increased criticism by an important other. Subjects were asked to report the degree to which they would increase, decrease, or not change the listed coping behaviors and to rate whether engaging in the coping behavior would improve, worsen, or have no effect on the situation. Prayer was one of 25 coping behaviors presented to subjects. More than 40% of the subjects would increase prayer, compared to 13% who would decrease it; 56% indicated that prayer was effective, and 1% said it was ineffective. Prayer was ranked seventh highest in effectiveness among the 25 coping behaviors. Factor analysis of responses revealed that prayer loaded on the "problem-solving" factor.

Ebaugh et al. (1984) compared religious coping in response to life crises among 50 active Christian Scientists, 50 active Catholic Charismatics, and 50 active Bahais, all of whom lived in the Houston metropolitan area. Religious group leaders selected persons for each of the three groups (subjects clearly represented the more active and fully committed members). Three dimensions of crises were examined: number of crises, type of crises, and reactions to crises. Subjects cited 1,122 crises and 1,049 reactions to those crises. The number of crises was similar in all three groups. Differences were found between groups in terms of reactions to crises. Christian Scientists were less likely to seek emotional support from church members than were members of the other groups but instead engaged in positive thinking and consulted group leaders for advice. Catholics, on the other hand, tended to cope with stress by depending on emotional support from church members; Bahais sought answers and advice based on interpretation of their sacred writings.

Pargament, Zinnbauer, et al. (1998) examined bereavement and religious coping among 49 members of a Midwestern Catholic church and 196 students in an introductory psychology class who had either experienced death of a family member or friend or had experienced a personal injustice within the past couple of years. The investigators administered an anger-at-God scale, doubts-about-God scale, and several religious coping scales. Mental health was measured using Rosenberg's self-esteem scale, Spielberger's trait anxiety inventory, and the psychosocial competence scale (measure of purposeful problem-solving skills). Self-worship, religious apathy, feeling punished by God, anger at God, and doubts about God were related to negative mental health states. Religious denial was related to positive mental health. Religious denial was measured by items such as: "Wasn't upset because believed this would bring me closer to God"; "Refused to feel bad because my faith teaches that there is good in everything"; "Wasn't bothered at all because it was God's will"; and "Wasn't bothered because God has His own plan for things."

INFREQUENT USE OF RELIGION

Persons in some northern European countries (e.g., Sweden, Norway, the Netherlands) do not rely as heavily on religion when coping with stress as do persons in the United States, Canada, Egypt, and other countries. This probably reflects the relatively low rates of religious involvement in northern European countries. Pettersson (1991) reported that the average weekly church attendance in Sweden is about 2%. Rudestam (1972) reported that nearly 80% of persons in Sweden indicated "none" for degree of religiosity (vs. only about 10% who indicate none in the United States). Ringdal et al. (1995) reported that 43% of their Norwegian sample of cancer patients did not believe in

God, and 45% received no comfort from religious beliefs. In their study of 300 medical inpatients, King, Speck, et al. (1994) found that only 57% of hospitalized patients in London claimed a religious affiliation, compared to 92–98% in the United States (Princeton Religion Research Center, 1996; Koenig, Cohen, Blazer, Pieper, et al., 1992).

Cederblad et al. (1995) surveyed a probability sample of healthy community-dwelling adults from two southern Swedish communities. The sample consisted of 148 persons born between 1932 and 1947 who had three or more childhood risk factors for mental disorder. Nearly 70% were socially mobile, with white-collar or skilled jobs. Religious coping was measured by a single item, "relies on religious faith." Religion was noted as a form of coping by only 1% of the sample. Likewise, Braam, Beekman, Deeg, et al. (1997) reported that religion was salient for only 29% of depressed subjects in their Dutch sample. Thus, when religious involvement and importance are low, religious coping is less common.

DO PEOPLE WANT RELIGIOUS ISSUES ADDRESSED AS PART OF THEIR HEALTH CARE?

As we debate the positive and negative effects of religion on mental and physical health, it is necessary to consider how patients feel about having health care professionals address religious issues. If, on the one hand, religion relates to how patients cope with health problems and patients wish health care providers to address their spiritual needs, then this may be an important reason for having health care providers deal with religious issues. If, on the other hand, patients do not want their physicians or other health care providers to address spiritual or religious needs, then perhaps all such needs should be referred to clergy.

Primary Care Patients

When Koenig, Bearon, and Dayringer (1989) asked physicians in Illinois whether older patients in certain circumstances (during stress or near death) would like their physicians to pray with them, 63% said that patients would not want this. In a separate study of 72 geriatric medical patients and senior center participants from the same area, Koenig, Smiley, and Gonzales (1988) asked how they would feel about their physician praying with them during times of extreme physical or emotional distress. The responses were different from what was expected. More than half (51%) indicated "yes, very much," and 27% indicated "yes, somewhat." Fewer than 20% indicated mixed feelings about physicians praying with them, and only 5% were definitely opposed.

King and Bushwick (1994) examined the religious beliefs and preferences of 203 inpatients (all ages) at Pitt County Memorial Hospital in eastern North Carolina ($n = 120$) and at York Hospital in York, Pennsylvania ($n = 83$). The investigators found that 98% of patients believed in God, and 58% indicated that their belief was "very strong" in this regard. Almost three-quarters (73%) of the sample prayed daily or more often. When asked about whether they would like their physicians to pray with them, 48% said that they would (54% in the North Carolina sample and 40% in the Pennsylvania sample). In addition, 42% thought that physicians should ask patients about faith-healing experiences, and 77% indicated that the physician should consider their patients' spiritual needs. Thirty-seven percent of patients wanted physicians to discuss religious issues more often with them (31% in North Carolina and 47% in Pennsylvania). Most important, 80% said that their physicians had never or only rarely discussed religious beliefs.

Recall from chapter 4 the study by Oyama and Koenig (1998), who interviewed 380 family medicine outpatients in Texas and North Carolina. A significant proportion of patients (43%) were interested in knowing the religious beliefs of their doctors, and 73% felt that patients should share their religious beliefs with doctors. Finally, two-thirds (67%) of patients felt that in certain circumstances they would like their physicians to pray with them. The more religious the patient, the more likely he or she was to want to know about the religious beliefs of his or her physician and to share personal religious beliefs with the physician. Recall also that Kald-jian et al. (1998) found that 56% of HIV-positive patients in Connecticut believed that it was important to discuss spiritual needs with their physicians, and 46% thought it would be helpful to pray with their physicians.

General Population

In February 1996, *USA Weekend* magazine conducted a nationwide poll of 1,000 adults, asking whether people believed that it was good for doctors to talk to patients about spiritual faith (McNichol, 1996). Almost two-thirds (63%) of the respondents indicated that it was good for doctors to talk to patients about these matters (60% of persons ages 18–34 and 67% of those ages 55–64). Only 10% of respondents, however, indicated that their doctor had talked to them about their spiritual faith as a factor in physical health (similar to the 20% reported by King and Bushwick, 1994).

While not accustomed to doing this, many health care professionals may be at least open to addressing the religious needs of patients. In Koenig, Bearon, and Dayringer's (1989) survey of family physicians and general practitioners in Illinois, investigators inquired about the appropriateness of addressing religious or spiritual issues with older patients in the context of a medical visit. Ninety-two percent felt that the physician may address religious issues with patients under certain circumstances: 88% thought this was appropriate if the patient requested it, 82% if the request was implied, and 66% even if no request was made by the patient. Only 31% of physicians felt that the religious needs of the older patient should be left entirely up to the clergy. More than one-third of physicians (37%) had prayed with patients, and 89% indicated that they believed this had helped the patient.

SUMMARY AND CONCLUSIONS

When patients themselves are asked how they cope with physical health problems and other major life stressors, they frequently mention religious beliefs and practices. This is true for both medical and psychiatric patients. In certain parts of the United States, between one-third and one-half of patients report that religion is the most important strategy used to cope with the stress of medical illness and health problems. Religious beliefs and behaviors are particularly important for coping among African Americans, the elderly, and women. Religious coping appears to increase as the severity of the medical condition and the level of distress increase, perhaps as persons turn to religion for comfort as their health becomes less and less under their control.

Religious behaviors are used for coping not only by persons who are acutely stressed (i.e., "foxhole" religion) but also by many people who are dealing with the day-to-day stresses of life. Religious and spiritual coping strategies appear related to better mental health and faster adaptation to stress (particularly in the long run), although some religious beliefs and attitudes are associated with worse health outcomes. In some areas of the world (northern Europe in particular), religious coping is an infrequent response to stress, even in the face of life-threatening medical illness. This does not, however, diminish the positive effects that religious coping may have on physical and mental health among people who use it (Ringdal, 1996; Braam, Beekman, Deeg, et al., 1997).

In the United States, surveys of primary care patients and the general population indicate that the majority of patients would like their physicians to address religious or spiritual issues in the context of a medical visit. Currently, only a small proportion of physicians do so (about 10–20%). Health professionals tend to be less religious than patients and therefore may not value religious or spiritual practices as much as patients do. Nevertheless, a majority of physicians believe that it is appropriate for physicians to address religious issues in the health care setting and that these issues cannot be left entirely up to the clergy. These conclusions, however, are based upon a limited number of studies conducted primarily in the Midwest and in the southeastern United States. Research on physician and patient attitudes toward inclusion of religion in the patient-physician relationship are needed in other areas of the country, especially in the western and northeastern United States, and in other, less religious parts of the world.

PART III

RESEARCH ON RELIGION
AND MENTAL HEALTH

6

Well-Being

I N LATER CHAPTERS WE EXAM-
ine the relationship between religious
involvement and negative mental states
such as depression, anxiety, schizophrenia, and other disorders. In this chapter, however, we explore religion's connection with well-
being—the positive side of mental health.
Synonyms for well-being include happiness, joy,
satisfaction, enjoyment, fulfillment, pleasure,
contentment, and other indicators of a life that
is full and complete.

Well-being is not a condition that one
achieves after reaching some type of threshold
of good feelings. Rather, it exists on a continuum, ranging from states of very low well-being
(including severe depression and hopelessness)
to those of very high well-being (genuine happiness) that are sustained over time. Rather than
simply existing to avoid pain, humans strive
to experience pleasure, joy, completeness, and

meaning. In his book *The Pursuit of Happiness*,
David Myers (1993) notes that Aristotle (384–
322 B.C.) argued that happiness is the "supreme
good" and that "all else is merely a means to
its attainment" (p. 19). Likewise, the American
psychologist William James (1890) wrote that
"how to gain, how to keep, how to recover happiness is in fact for most men at all times the
secret motive of all they do" (p. 19). How does
religion contribute to (or distract from) well-
being?

In order to answer this question, we first
examine nonreligious predictors of well-being
and then explore the connection between these
predictors and religion to try to understand
why and how religion might influence happiness. We then review the research, discussing
cross-sectional, prospective cohort, and intervention studies of the relationship between religion and well-being.

PREDICTORS OF WELL-BEING

According to a review by W. Wilson (1967), persons with the most advantages have the highest well-being and greatest happiness. In other words, the "happy person emerges as a young, healthy, well-educated, well-paid, extroverted, optimistic, worry-free, religious, married person with high self-esteem, high job morale, modest aspirations, of either sex and of a wide range of intelligence" (p. 294).

In Diener's (1984) more recent review of studies that examine predictors of well-being, he reported that no single variable explains a large proportion of the variance. Rather, well-being is determined by a large number of different factors, including biological forces (genetic influences that transmit capacity for happiness), developmental influences (extent to which basic emotional needs are met during infancy and childhood), positive and negative life events during adulthood, and current situational factors.

Contrary to most expectations, income or wealth is a poor predictor of happiness (Myers & Diener, 1996). Increases in income have not been associated with proportional increases in well-being. Campbell (1981) found that between 1946 and 1978, real income in the United States rose dramatically; this was not, however, associated with an increase in average well-being (in fact, well-being declined slightly). Although wealthier people were happier than those who were poor for every year of the study, influences of income on happiness occurred primarily at very low incomes, and, once basic needs were met, there was no proportional increase in happiness with further increase in income. Interestingly, education is not associated with well-being once income is controlled.

Age is inconsistently associated with well-being. Many early studies reported that young persons were happier than older persons (Diener, 1984). More recent studies, however, have not demonstrated such age effects. Younger persons may experience higher levels of joy, but older persons have higher levels of life satisfaction and in general tend to have more positive judgments about their lives.

A number of well-designed epidemiological studies have shown that marital status influences well-being. Married persons report greater happiness than never-married, divorced, or separated persons (Andrews & Withey, 1976). In fact, Glenn and Weaver (1979) found that marriage was the strongest predictor of well-being after education, income, and occupational status were controlled. The effects of marital status by itself, however, appear to be relatively small. More relevant are family and marital satisfaction, which appear to be strong correlates of well-being in numerous studies (Diener, 1984).

As far as gender is concerned, women report more negative affect than men but also tend to experience greater joy, so the two largely neutralize each other. There is an interaction with age, however, in that younger women are happier than younger men, but this association reverses in later life (Diener, 1984). Nevertheless, gender differences in well-being are not very great at any age (quite unlike the situation for depression; see chapter 7).

After controlling for confounders (education, income, urban residence), race exerts a small but significant effect on well-being that is at least partly dependent on age and gender. In the United States, African Americans in general report a lesser sense of well-being than whites; this trend reverses in later life, however, when older African Americans tend to be happier than older whites (Campbell et al., 1976).

While unemployment is associated with unhappiness, homemakers are not less happy than women with salaried jobs.

Health is the strongest predictor of well-being in both younger and older populations. One meta-analysis on well-being and health revealed a consistent correlation of approximately 0.32; correlations were particularly strong in women (Diener, 1984). Well-being has been more strongly related to measures of subjective health than to objective measures (i.e., disease checklists or physician ratings) (Diener, 1984).

Activities are associated with greater happiness and well-being, particularly among the elderly, although the causal direction of this relationship remains uncertain. A popular theory of successful aging (called Activity Theory) argues that active involvement creates happiness (Maddox, 1963; Graney, 1975), although this relationship is likely heavily confounded by physical health and income. When these variables are controlled, the relationship with activity disappears (Bull & Aucoin, 1975). Furthermore, only certain activities may be associated with well-being, whereas others are not (Kozma & Stones, 1978).

Numerous studies have demonstrated a positive relationship between well-being and social support. Both longitudinal (Bradburn, 1969; Graney, 1975) and intervention studies (Fordyce, 1983) have shown that increasing social contacts is associated with increasing well-being. A meta-analysis by Okun et al. (1984) of 115 studies found that social activity predicts about 2 to 4% of the variance in well-being (after other covariates are controlled). Studies also show that while some social contacts (friends) are associated with greater well-being, other social contacts (relatives) may not be (Mancini & Orthner, 1980).

While 2 to 4% of variance in well-being may seem pretty small, recall that no one sociodemographic factor predicts a large amount of the variance in subjective well-being. In fact, all sociodemographic factors combined probably predict less than 10% of the variance (Andrews & Withey, 1976). Not surprisingly, psychological factors (such as optimism, purpose in life, high self-esteem, extroversion) predict a much larger proportion of the variance in well-being (Diener, 1984; Myers & Diener, 1996). These variables, however, may actually be components of well-being, rather than independent variables that *lead to* greater happiness.

Personal control (or degree of perceived choice) is a strong predictor of happiness (Myers & Diener, 1996). In contrast, persons with no control over their lives—such as prisoners, nursing home patients, or the poverty stricken—have the least sense of well-being. Likewise, persons with an internal locus of control (a tendency to attribute outcomes to oneself rather than to external causes) seem to have a greater sense of well-being than those with an external locus (Diener, 1984; Sundre, 1978). While religion (i.e., depending on God as agent of con-

trol) on the surface appears to involve an external locus of control, most studies that examine this relationship have found the opposite (i.e., religious involvement is related to a greater *internal* locus of control; this finding is discussed in the next section).

RELIGION AND PREDICTORS OF WELL-BEING

Religious involvement may promote certain behaviors or attitudes that increase happiness, satisfaction, and general well-being. Such associations do not "explain away" the effects of religion on well-being but simply provide an explanation of *how* religion accomplishes this end.

Marital Status

Numerous studies have shown that religious persons are less likely to divorce or separate and are more likely to have intact, stable families (see chapter 13). For example, in their 28-year follow-up of 5,286 persons who participated in the Alameda County Study, Strawbridge, Cohen et al. (1997) found that married persons who attended religious services at least once per week in 1965 were almost 80% more likely than less frequent attenders to stay married to the same person (OR 1.79, 95% CI 1.36–2.35).

Health

Persons with high religious involvement are less likely to abuse alcohol and drugs (see chapter 11); experience less hypertension (chapter 17), heart disease (chapter 16), stroke (chapter 18), cancer (chapter 20), and disability (chapter 22); and live longer (chapter 21). Better physical health invariably translates into a higher level of well-being, given the strong association between physical and mental health.

Activities

Most religions promote activities such as attendance at religious services, participation in prayer and scripture study groups, volunteer activities, religious pilgrimages, and active involvement in social and community life. This makes it more difficult for religious persons to be sedentary and uninvolved. Religious activities may be a particularly important source of well-being for older adults (Cutler, 1976).

Social Support

Religious institutions typically promote and even prescribe socialization among members of the congregation ("love thy neighbor as thyself"). Many studies show that persons who participate in religious activities, whether attending religious services or participating in prayer or Bible study groups, have larger support networks, more social contacts, and greater satisfaction with support (Ellison & George, 1994; Bradley, 1995; Idler & Kasl, 1997a; Koenig, Hays, et al., 1997; see also chapter 15).

Optimism

Many religious beliefs promote optimism and positive thinking (Peale, 1952) (see chapter 14). For example, Sethi and Seligman (1993, 1994) studied 623 members of nine major religions in the United States, divided into fundamentalists (Orthodox Judaism, Calvinism, and Islam), moderates (conservative Judaism, Catholicism, Lutheranism, and Methodism), and liberals (Unitarianism, reform Judaism). They found significant differences among groups in terms of religious influence in daily life, religious involvement, and religious hope, which were all significantly greater (all $p < .00001$) among fundamentalists. Fundamentalists were also much more optimistic than members of liberal religions, with moderates lying in between ($F = 14.8$, $p < .0001$). Greater optimism was observed for both positive events ($p < .0001$) and negative events ($p < .05$). When analyses were controlled for income, sex, and education, the findings persisted. In the second part of the study, investigators selected tape-recorded sermons and typical hymns and prayers for each religion as suggested by church leaders. They found more optimism in the fundamentalists' religious materials and religious services than

in liberals' religious materials and services, with moderates' materials falling in between ($p < .00001$). When these factors were controlled for at the individual level in the first part of the study, fundamentalism dropped out as a predictor of optimism. Investigators concluded that the differences in optimism stem partly from the religious material to which persons are exposed and partly from greater religious involvement and influence.

Hope

Sethi and Seligman (1993, 1994) also found that the religiously devout were more hopeful. Numerous other investigators have reported a positive relationship between measures of religiousness and hope in a variety of clinical and nonclinical settings (Herth, 1989; Carson, Soeken, Shanty, et al., 1990; Raleigh, 1992; Ringdal, 1996; Idler & Kasl, 1997a; Plante & Boccaccini, 1997a), although some have not (Moberg, 1984; Fox & Odling-Smee, 1995) (see chapter 14).

Purpose and Meaning in Life

Religion also provides adherents with a sense of purpose and meaning in life. Many religions teach that existence is not merely a random act of chance but rather the design of a creator who has purpose and intention and who desires human involvement in that purpose. Consequently, many studies have found a positive correlation between religious involvement and having a sense of purpose or meaning in life (Bolt, 1975; Crandall and Rasmussen, 1975; Jacobson, Ritter, et al., 1977; Gifford & Golde, 1978; Tellis-Nayak, 1982; Acklin, Brown, et al., 1983; Chamberlain & Zika, 1988; Jackson & Corsey, 1988; Richards, 1990; Ellis & Smith, 1991; Richards, 1991; Burbank, 1992; Carroll, 1993), although there are a few exceptions (Moberg, 1984; Idler & Kasl, 1997a).

Internal Locus of Control

While believing that God is in control might at first suggest an external locus of control, this is actually not the case. Most studies have found a positive and significant relationship between religious beliefs or activities and an internal locus of control (Kahoe, 1974; Kivett, 1979; Sturgeon & Hamley, 1979; Jackson & Coursey, 1988; Richards, 1990), although, again, there are some exceptions (Benson & Spilka, 1973). Religious belief gives persons a form of indirect control over their lives that reduces the need to depend on chance or powerful others (e.g., political leaders, physicians, employers). In many respects, an internalized, intrinsically motivated religious faith empowers the individual; prayer directed to an all-powerful and sympathetic God gives religious persons a tool that can be used to change their situation or acquire the strength to endure it. This counteracts feelings of helplessness, loss of control, and need to depend on others.

RESEARCH ON RELIGION AND WELL-BEING

We now turn to a review of studies that have directly examined the relationship between religion and well-being. Our systematic review of the literature uncovered 100 studies that statistically examined the relationship between religiousness and well-being. Of those studies, 79 (79%) reported at least one positive correlation between religious involvement and greater happiness, life satisfaction, morale, or positive affect. Of the remaining 21 studies, 13 found no association, 1 found a negative association, and 7 reported mixed or complex relationships. Because of the large number of positive studies, we review here only those positive studies that received a 7 or higher on our 0–10 quality rating scale (see part VIII). Studies that evaluate world religions about which we know very little in terms of their relationship with well-being are reviewed regardless of quality. Also, we review most of the studies that found no association or a negative association regardless of quality.

First, we examine cross-sectional research on the relationship between religiousness and well-being. Such studies provide no information about whether religious involvement leads to greater well-being or vice versa. Second, we re-

view prospective studies of the religion-well-being relationship. These studies provide indirect evidence about the causal nature of the relationship because they include a time element. Third, we examine intervention studies that directly test the hypothesis that religious or spiritual factors enhance well-being. We categorize the studies reviewed by whether they report a positive association, no association, or negative association between religious involvement and well-being. Studies are further subcategorized into those that involve younger adults or adults of all ages and those that study older adults, as well as those that study Christianity or Judaism and those that study other world religions. Within each subcategory, studies are discussed in the chronological order of year of publication.

CROSS-SECTIONAL STUDIES

Positive Associations

Positive Associations in All Ages. Spreitzer and Snyder (1974) examined correlates of life satisfaction among 1,323 persons under and 224 persons over age 65. Investigators analyzed pooled data from the 1972 and 1973 General Social Surveys (conducted by the National Opinion Research Center at the University of Michigan). The dependent variable, life satisfaction, was measured by a single question, as was church attendance (measured on a 1–9 scale) and nine other covariates. Church attendance was significantly related to greater life satisfaction in those under age 65 ($r^2 = .33$, $p < .05$), but, surprisingly, not in those over age 65.

Hadaway and Roof (1978) examined the relationship between religious commitment and quality of life, using data from Campbell et al.'s Quality of American Life survey. This survey, conducted by the University of Michigan's Survey Research Center, involved a national probability sample of 2,164 persons from across the United States. Importance of religious faith was significantly correlated with "worthwhileness of life" ($p < .001$); 58.9% of those who indicated their faith was "extremely important" reported high worthwhileness, compared with only 34.6%

of those whose faith was "not at all important." In fact, importance of faith was the strongest predictor in a model that included number of friends, marital status, age, education, health, income, and race. Worthwhileness was also predicted by church/synagogue membership ($p <$ .001) and by religious attendance; church attendance was the second strongest predictor, behind number of friends, in a regression model that did not include importance of religious faith. Correlations were strongest in persons with lower incomes. Investigators concluded that religion provided two benefits: meaning and purpose in life and a sense of belonging to and participating in a fellowship of like-minded believers.

Ortega, Crutchfield, et al. (1983) examined race differences in personal well-being in a random sample of 4,522 persons of all ages from urban, rural, and isolated rural communities in northern Alabama. Investigators oversampled persons who were physically disabled, elderly, women, and African American. Single item measures of happiness, general life satisfaction, and relative life satisfaction were administered. Religious measures were frequency of attendance (at least monthly vs. less frequent) and frequency of contact with church-related friends in nonchurch settings. Investigators controlled for education, income, age, marital status, health status, and place of residence, using regression analyses. Results indicated that elderly African Americans reported significantly higher life satisfaction and happiness than elderly whites. Informal interpersonal contact was the strongest predictor of life satisfaction. Contact with friends mediated this relationship only when friendships had the church as their locus. The presence of church-related friends was more strongly related to life satisfaction than was race itself. Investigators concluded that the greater life satisfaction of the African American elderly was largely the result of their greater contact with church-related friends.

St. George and McNamara (1984) explored the relationship among religion, race, and psychological well-being, using pooled data from the General Social Surveys conducted between 1972 and 1982. While each of the nine surveys sampled approximately 1,500 persons age 18 or older, the focus here was on persons ages 25–54. Well-being was assessed in terms of global happiness, excitement with life, subjective health, and satisfaction with four aspects of life (community, nonwork activities, family life, friendships, and health). Religious involvement was measured by strength of religious identification (SRI) and church attendance.

Among white males ($n = 1,343$), SRI was significantly related to four measures of well-being, with correlations ranging from $\beta = .08$ ($p < .01$) to $\beta = .12$ ($p < .001$). Among white women ($n = 1,570$), SRI was related to seven measures of well-being, with correlations ranging from $\beta = .09$ ($p < .01$) to $\beta = .15$ ($p < .001$). Among African American men ($n = 144$), SRI was related to six measures of well-being, with correlations ranging from $\beta = .20$ ($p < .01$) to $\beta = .41$ ($p < .001$). Among African American women ($n = 188$), SRI was related to global happiness only ($\beta = .17$, $p < .01$).

Church attendance (coded in reverse) was correlated with five measures of well-being from $\beta = -.11$ ($p < .05$) to $\beta = -.19$ ($p < .01$) in white males ($n = 1,853$), three measures of well-being from $\beta = -.12$ ($p < .01$) to $\beta = -.18$ ($p < .01$) in white women ($n = 2,024$), five measures of well-being from $\beta = -.13$ ($p < .05$) to $\beta = -.25$ ($p < .001$) in African American men ($n = 205$), and four measures of well-being from $\beta = -.14$ ($p < .05$) to $\beta = -.27$ ($p < .001$) in African American women ($n = 244$). Analyses were controlled for age, education, income, and occupational prestige. Investigators concluded that religious participation is more important for well-being in African Americans than in whites (because of the size of the betas, presumably), and that strength of religiousness is more important for African American men, while church attendance is more important for African American women.

Glik (1986) compared general well-being in three samples: 93 volunteers from "New Age" or metaphysical healing groups (MHG), 83 from charismatic Christian healing groups (CHG) (largely Pentecostal), and 137 primary care (PC) medical patients from a local HMO in Baltimore. CHG members had significantly less education and were less likely to have professional occupations than MHG or PC members ($p < .001$), and both CHG and MHG had lower incomes than PC. CHG were also older than MHG or PC groups (70% over age 46 vs. 40% and 28%, respectively). Subjects were interviewed three times over six months, and researchers assessed sociodemographic and social factors, measures of physical, psychological, social and behavioral health, religious attitudes and beliefs, and healing behaviors. Results at Time 1 indicated that physical well-being, general well-being, positive mental health symptoms, and illness/wellness behavior were all highest in the CHG group, lower in the MHG group, and lowest in PC group ($p < .001$). There was no significant difference in severity of physical health problems among the three groups, but, after covariates were adjusted, significant differences persisted at $p < .001$ for all outcome variables except illness/wellness behavior.

Recall Reed's (1987) survey of 300 adults with and without terminal illness (see chapter 5). Group 1 consisted of 100 terminally ill hospitalized patients with incurable cancer; Group 2 consisted of 100 nonterminally ill hospitalized patients with other medical problems; and Group 3 consisted of 100 healthy nonhospitalized persons free from any serious illness. The three groups were matched on age, gender, years of education, and religious background. Religiousness was measured by a 10-item Spiritual Perspective Scale (SPS). Well-being was assessed by Campbell's 9-item Index of Well-being (IWB). IWB scores were similar in each group, ranging from 10.3 to 10.4 (scores on this index ranged from 2.1 to 12.6). There was a significant positive relationship between SPS scores and IWB scores, but only in terminally ill patients (Group 1) ($r = 22$, $p < .02$, uncontrolled).

Pollner (1989) used data from a national sample of 3,072 adults (pooled from 1983 and 1984 General Social Surveys) to examine relationships between religion and life satisfaction. Religious variables were religious experience, image of God, and religious attendance. Life satisfaction variables were general happiness, marital happiness, life excitement, and life satisfaction. Religious experience (termed "divine relations") was measured by closeness to God, frequency of prayer, and closeness to a powerful spiritual force. Images of God were measured and categorized as follows: (1) God as ruler (king, judge, master), (2) God as source of remedy for human problems (healer, liberator, redeemer, creator), and (3) God as someone to relate to (friend, lover, mother, father, spouse). Regression analyses revealed a positive relationship between global happiness and church attendance ($\beta = .09$, $p < .01$) and between global happiness and divine relations ($\beta = .15$, $p < .01$). The latter relationship persisted even after researchers controlled for church attendance ($\beta = .11$, $p < .01$). Divine relations was also significantly correlated with life satisfaction, life excitement, and marital happiness, all $p < .01$, whereas church attendance was significantly related only to marital happiness ($\beta = .06$, $p < .01$). Perception of God as ruler was correlated negatively with global happiness ($\beta = -.16$), whereas perception of God as healer or liberator was associated with greater life satisfaction ($\beta = .03$); perceptions of God in relational terms was unrelated to any of the four well-being measures.

Interactions between variables were also examined. The positive relationship between divine relations and marital happiness was restricted primarily to those with few other social relationships. The association between divine relations and life excitement was largely restricted to married persons (contrary to expectations). Finally, the association between divine relations and well-being was greatest among those with less education. Image of God also affected the association between divine relations and well-being. The relationship between divine relations and global happiness was significantly stronger among those who viewed God as ruler (king, judge, master). On the other hand, the relationship between divine relations and marital happiness was significantly stronger among those who viewed God as healer, liberator, or redeemer. An important conclusion from this study was that one's image of God (i.e., beliefs about God) may impact the relationship between religious experience and well-being.

Christopher Ellison and his team have conducted some of the best work on the relationship between religious involvement and well-being among persons in the general population.

Ellison, Gay, et al. (1989) studied the relationship between religion and life satisfaction, using data from a national random sample of persons age 18 or over in the United States (1983 General Social Survey). Life satisfaction was assessed by four domain-specific measures (single items assessing finances, health, family, and friends), with the resulting scale ranging from 4 to 24. Religious commitment was measured by (1) type of affiliation, (2) strength of affiliation, (3) organizational religious activities (frequency of attendance and membership in church-related organizations), and (4) devotional intensity (frequency of prayer and closeness to God). "Sociability" was assessed by intensity of sociability and social affiliation (quality and quantity of secular voluntary association and social interaction). Results of regression analyses indicated that life satisfaction was related to Baptist religious affiliation ($\beta = .11$ for Southern Baptist and $\beta = .08$ for other Baptist, both $p < .05$), frequency of attendance ($\beta = .08$, $p < .05$), and devotional intensity ($\beta = .12$, $p < .01$). Devotional intensity was the third strongest predictor of life satisfaction, behind marital status ($\beta = .14$) and income ($\beta = .13$). Note that the relationship between life satisfaction and religious attendance was significant even after controlling for sociability.

Ellison and Gay (1990) used data from a random sample of 2,107 adults who participated in the 1979–1980 National Survey of Black Americans to examine the relationship among region of the country, religious commitment, and life satisfaction. Well-being was measured by a single four-level global life satisfaction item. Investigators found that church attendance (assessed by a single item on a 1–5 scale) was associated with greater life satisfaction ($\beta = .05$, $p < .05$), even after controlling for denominational affiliation, self-rated religiosity, demographic and social factors. Religious affiliation was also related to life satisfaction (Fundamentalist affiliation, in particular, $\beta = .22$, $p < .01$), although frequency of prayer and self-rated religiosity were not after controlling for attendance and affiliation. Because of the high correlation between religious variables, it is difficult to identify from this study which dimension of religiousness is most important for life satisfaction.

Using data from a national probability sample of 997 subjects (1988 General Social Survey), Ellison (1991) examined the relationship among religion, life satisfaction, and traumatic events. Religious variables included affiliation, church attendance, divine interaction (closeness to God and frequency of prayer), and existential certainty. The last variable was measured using a three-item scale that assessed doubts about faith because of evil, conflicts with science, and feeling that life has no meaning—variables designed to "tap the strength and durability of religious faith without reference to specific articles of religious doctrine." Subjective well-being was assessed by asking about satisfaction with community life, nonworking activities/hobbies, family life, friendships, and health or physical condition (five-item scale) and about personal happiness (three-item scale).

Life satisfaction and personal happiness were associated with church attendance ($r = .14$ and $r = .19$), divine interaction ($r = .09$ and $r = .12$), and existential certainty ($r = .18$ and $r = .17$). Regression analysis revealed that religious variables accounted for 5–7% of the variance in life satisfaction scores. Significant relationships were found between greater life satisfaction and existential certainty ($p < .001$), nondenominational Protestant affiliation ($p < .001$), Mormon or Jehovah's Witness affiliation ($p < .05$), liberal Protestant affiliation ($p < .05$), and divine interaction ($p < .05$) (but not church attendance). Personal happiness was positively related to greater existential certainty ($p < .01$) and negatively related to being Catholic ($p < .05$). Overall, religious variables accounted for 2–3% of the variance in personal happiness (recall, though, that most studies find that all social and demographic factors *combined* account for less than 10% of the variance in well-being).

Gee and Veevers (1990) examined religious involvement and life satisfaction in Canada, using data from a probability sample of 6,621 Canadians who participated in the 1985 Canadian General Social Survey. Religious affiliation and attendance were assessed and used to form three categories: unaffiliated (no religious affiliation), affiliated (affiliated but attending services less than once a week), and actively affiliated (affiliated and attending services once a week or more). Life satisfaction was measured using a seven-item satisfaction scale involving six life domains. Among men, 50.6% of actively affiliated were "very satisfied" with life in general, compared with 41.4 percent of unaffiliated ($p < .01$). Among women, 52.5% of actively affiliated were very satisfied, compared with 44.1% of unaffiliated ($p < .01$). Greater satisfaction was particularly evident in terms of satisfaction with job, housing, finances, and family relationships, whereas the effect weakened for satisfaction with health and friendships. Analyses were controlled for gender only.

Poloma and Pendleton (1990,1991) surveyed a random sample of 560 persons living in and around Akron, Ohio. They examined the relationships between well-being (life satisfaction, negative affect, happiness, existential well-being) and prayer experience, orthodoxy of belief, frequency of church attendance, born-again status, frequency of prayer, relationship with God, and church activities. Religious satisfaction was the strongest correlate of existential well-being ($p < .001$) and of life satisfaction to a borderline degree ($p = .06$). When religious domains and covariates were controlled, after removing religious satisfaction from the model, the strongest correlates of well-being (life-satisfaction and happiness) were frequency of prayer (negatively related) and prayer experience (positively related). The negative relationship between frequency of prayer and well-being may have resulted from the fact that persons going through difficult life circumstances were more likely to pray. This hypothesis suggests the difficulty of interpreting cross-sectional relationships in terms of causality.

When Poloma and Pendleton considered type of prayer (conversational, petitional, ritual, and meditative prayer), they found that conversational and meditative prayer were more strongly related to well-being than was ritual prayer. Ritual prayer was associated with greater negative affect (feeling sad, lonely, depressed, tense), whereas meditative prayer was related to greater existential well-being, and conversational prayer was related to greater happiness. When level of religious commitment was controlled, however, most relationships between prayer variables and well-being disappeared.

Reed (1991) analyzed data collected on a probability sample of 1,473 adults who participated in the 1984 General Social Survey. Religious affiliation was categorized into strong (very strong) and weak (somewhat strong and not very strong). Dependent variables were single-item measures of overall happiness, family satisfaction, health satisfaction, and life excitement. Uncontrolled bivariate analyses demonstrated that general happiness, family satisfaction, and life excitement were all significantly related to strength of religious affiliation ($p \leq .001$). Analyses involving general happiness were then stratified by six demographic variables: class, age, education, income, religion, and sex. Associations were particularly strong in the upper social class and among persons over age 65, the more educated, those with incomes over $25,000, Catholics, and women.

Levin, Chatters, and Taylor (1995) examined the relationship between religiousness and life satisfaction among 1,848 African Americans, using data from the National Survey of Black Americans. The mean age of the subjects was 42; 62% were female, 79% were living in urban areas, and average income was less than $9,000. Organizational religious activities were assessed by five items, nonorganizational religious activities by four items, and subjective religiosity by three items. The dependent variable, life satisfaction, was assessed by three items. Covariates included a four-item physical health status measure. Structural equation modeling (LISREL) was used to examine relationships among the variables. Investigators found that organizational religious activities were associated with both better health and greater life satisfaction ($p < .01$). A statistical model of the relationships was developed in the first half of the sample and then replicated in the second. When the researchers controlled for age, gender, education, marital status, employment status, geographical region, urbanicity, and, in particular, health status, organizational religious activities remained significantly associated with life satisfaction in both halves of the sample ($\beta = .26$, $p < .05$, and $\beta = .24$, $p < .01$). Subjective religiosity was also significantly related to life satisfaction in both subsamples in uncontrolled analyses ($r = .32$, $p < .05$, and $r = .38$, $p < .01$), but not in controlled analyses. Associations between organizational religiosity and life satisfaction were present in all three age groups (under age 30, 30–55, and over age 55). This study utilizes state-of-the-art statistical methodology to demonstrate the association between well-being and religious involvement in African Americans of all ages, a relationship that was found to be independent of physical health status.

Ringdal (1996) examined the relationship among religiosity, quality of life, and survival in 253 cancer patients in Norway. Religiosity was assessed by two questions: What can you tell about your religious beliefs (believe in God, don't believe, don't know)? and Have your religious beliefs been of support to you after you became ill with cancer (very good, some, no)? Scores on these two items were summed to create a religiosity scale ranging from 2–6. Using regression analysis, religiosity was significantly related to general life satisfaction ($\beta = .23$, $p < .001$) and less hopelessness ($\beta = 0.17$, $p < .02$).

Positive Associations in Older Adults.   In one of the first studies to examine the relationship between religiousness and well-being in older adults, Moberg (1956) surveyed 219 persons age 65 or over residing in seven old age homes in the Minneapolis-St. Paul area. Personal adjustment was measured by the Burgess-Cavan-Havighurst Attitudes Inventory. Religious activity was assessed by 11 items (church membership, present attendance, present attendance compared to age 55 attendance, age 12 attendance, positions or church offices held, listening to religious radio, frequency of reading the Bible, frequency of reading other religious books, private prayer, saying grace at meals, frequency of family prayers). Religious activities were positively related to adjustment ($r = 0.59$, standard error = .04, highly signifi-

cant). The sample was also divided into those with high, medium, and low religious scores. Subjects with high religious scores ($n = 86$) reported higher personal adjustment than those with low religious scores ($n = 41$). Nineteen low-religious persons were then matched with 19 high-religious subjects by sex, marital status, number of living children, education, present employment, club activities, and self-ratings of health. Personal adjustment scores for religious and nonreligious subjects differed by a significant degree (28.3 vs. 16.3, $p < .01$). Unlike most researchers of that period, Moberg controlled for other covariates (by matching).

Moberg and Taves (1965) next analyzed data on 5,000 persons age 60 or over who participated in several large surveys in Minnesota, Missouri, North Dakota, and South Dakota. Subjects were divided into (1) officers and committeemen in church or other religious organization, (2) other church members, and (3) nonchurch members. Personal adjustment was again measured by the Burgess-Cavan-Havighurst Attitudes Inventory (happiness, enjoyment, or satisfaction with health, family, friendships, employment status, religion, usefulness, and aging). In each of the surveys, personal adjustment was significantly higher among subjects in categories 1 and 2 than among those in category 3. This was particularly true in the largest survey ($n = 1,340$ Minnesota residents), where the effect persisted at $p < .001$ after stratifying (controlling) analyses by sex, age, education, marital status, home ownership, social participation, changes in social participation, self-ratings of health, and concept of age. Among 40 comparisons of personal adjustment among the three groups, investigators found only three reversals of the hypothesized pattern of higher adjustment among church members and church leaders.

Edwards and Klemmack (1973) surveyed a random sample of 507 persons age 45 or older who were living in a four-county area of Virginia. Most were white Protestants. The researchers' aim was to reexamine the relationship between religion and life satisfaction after controlling for multiple covariates. The dependent variable was measured using a 10-item Life

Satisfaction Index; 22 hypothesized correlates were also measured, including intensity of involvement in church-related organizations or activities. Regression analysis revealed that church-related activities were the third strongest correlate of life satisfaction ($\beta = .14, p < .05$) (behind income and perceived health). Note that participation in voluntary organizations other than church was not related to life satisfaction (confirmed by Cutler).

Cutler (1976) examined two random national samples of elderly persons (over 65) to assess the association between membership in different types of voluntary associations and psychological well-being. He studied 16 types of voluntary associations in one analysis ($n = 438$) of elderly participants in the 1974 and 1975 General Social Surveys (GSS). In the second analysis, he examined 17 types of voluntary associations participated in by 395 older persons that were surveyed as part of the 1972 American National Election Study. Only membership in church-affiliated groups was a significant predictor of life satisfaction and happiness (after other covariates and membership in other types of associations were controlled). Almost three-quarters (73%) of older adults in the General Social Surveys belonged to one or more voluntary associations: 49% belonged to church-affiliated groups (most common), 18% to fraternal groups (next most common), and 9% to veterans groups. It is evident from this study of two random national samples that religious involvement is common among older adults and may be uniquely associated with greater well-being.

Singh and Williams (1982) examined the relationship between religious attendance and "satisfaction with health" (a proxy for well-being) among the elderly. Investigators analyzed pooled data on persons age 65 or over ($n = 1,459$) from six General Social Surveys conducted between 1973 and 1978. A single item (seven-point scale) assessed satisfaction with health and physical condition. Religious attendance and 11 other covariates (including social memberships, alcohol use, smoking, and hospital admissions in past five years) were examined as predictors of health satisfaction. Multivariate

analysis revealed that the strongest predictor of health satisfaction among all variables assessed was religious attendance.

Beckman and Houser (1982) systematically surveyed 719 white Los Angeles County women ages 60–75 to examine the consequences of childlessness on the social-psychological well-being of older women. Half the women were widows, and half were currently married and living with their spouse. The sample was stratified into those who were currently childless and those who had living children. Subjects completed the Philadelphia Geriatric Center Morale scale, the Zung Depression scale, the Dean Social Isolation scale, and a social interaction measure. Religiosity was measured by a single item in which the women rated their degree of religiousness on a 1–5 scale. Age, education, socioeconomic status, income, religion, siblings, fertility status, and employment status were controlled using multiple regression. Investigators found that among the childless widowed ($n = 114$) and the parent widowed ($n = 138$), religiosity was significantly related to well-being ($\beta = .27, p < .01$, and $\beta = .22, p < .05$). Religiosity and quality of social interaction were the strongest predictors of well-being in these two groups, although the former was unrelated to well-being in married childless or married parent women.

Doyle and Forehand (1984) examined data from a national sample of 2,306 persons ages 40–96 years (surveyed by Louis & Harris for the National Council on Aging) to examine the association between life satisfaction and religion among middle-aged and older adults. Importance of religion was measured using a single variable that was self-rated on a 1–3 scale. Life satisfaction was measured using the 18-item Neugarten Life Satisfaction Index. Regression models were run for groups ages 40–54, 55–64, and 65 or over, controlling for nine covariates. Among persons ages 40–54 years ($n = 1,029$), there was a positive association between importance of religion and life satisfaction ($\beta = .18$, likely significant, but no p value reported); religion was the second strongest predictor of life satisfaction behind "loneliness a problem." In persons ages 55–64 ($n = 552$), religion was only weakly correlated with life satisfaction ($\beta = .04$). Among those age 65 or over ($n = 567$), importance of religion was related to life satisfaction at about the same level as social involvement ($\beta = .08$), and the relationship was weaker than that for poor health, loneliness, or financial problems. The association between religion and life satisfaction was not discussed in the paper.

Usui et al. (1985) examined predictors of life satisfaction in a random sample of 704 adults age 60 or over and living in Jefferson County, Kentucky. Life satisfaction was measured by the 13-item Neugarten Life Satisfaction Index. Frequency of church attendance was associated with greater life satisfaction ($\beta = .12$, $p < .01$, after controlling for 15 other covariates).

Harvey et al. (1987) studied factors related to morale in a random sample of 11,071 Canadians over age 40 who participated in the 1978–1979 Canadian Health Survey. Morale was assessed by a single item that measured happiness and by Bradburn's Affect Balance Scale. Importance of religion was measured using a single item with three response categories (important, somewhat important, and of little or no importance). Religious importance was related to greater happiness in all four income-sex groups ($p < .001$), and was a significant predictor of positive affect in low-income men and women. Income and gender were the only variables controlled.

Lee and Ishii-Kuntz (1987) examined the relationship among social interaction, loneliness, and emotional well-being in a random sample of 2,872 persons age 55 or over and living in Washington State. Attendance at religious services was correlated with loneliness (four-item scale) and well-being (seven-item morale scale). When marital status, health, friends, and neighbors were controlled, the positive relationship between church attendance and loneliness was reduced to nonsignificance in both men and women. After the authors controlled for 10 other covariates, including social variables, religious attendance was significantly and positively related to well-being ($p = .02$) in men ($n = 1,321$), but, unlike in most other studies, not in women.

Levin and Markides (1988) explored the connection between religious attendance and psychological well-being in a probability sample of 375 middle-aged and 375 older Mexican Americans (middle and older generations from the same family). Life satisfaction was assessed with Neugarten's 13-item index. Regression analyses of this largely Catholic population revealed that frequent church attendance was significantly related to greater life satisfaction for middle-aged women ($p < .01$) and older women ($p < .05$), after researchers controlled for age, marital status, income, education, subjective health, and functional status. No relationships were found for the men.

McGloshen and O'Bryant (1988) explored the relationship between religious attendance and psychological well-being among 226 recently widowed older women (widowed 7 to 21 months prior to interview). Positive affect was measured using the Affect Balance Scale. Frequency of religious attendance and 18 covariates were examined in a regression model that accounted for 22% of the variance in positive affect and 18% of the variance in negative affect. Religious attendance was related to greater positive affect ($\beta = .19$, $p < .01$). Religious attendance and physical health were the strongest predictors of positive affect in this sample (both $\beta = .19$). Interestingly, attendance was unrelated to negative affect. As have other studies, this study found that religious attendance appears more strongly related to positive affect (i.e., well-being) than to negative affect.

Koenig, Kvale, and Ferrel (1988) examined the relationship between religion and well-being among 836 persons age 55 or older and living in the midwestern United States. Included in the sample were senior center participants, church and synagogue members, retired nuns, and medical outpatients. The multi-item Springfield Religiosity Schedule was used to assess organizational religious activities (ORA) (2 items), nonorganizational religious activities (NORA) (3 items), and intrinsic religiosity (IR) (10 items). ORA, NORA, and IR were all significantly and positively related to great morale at correlations ranging from $r = .16$ to $r = .26$. After the authors controlled for the effects of physical health, social support, and financial status, relationships with morale remained significant for all three religious dimensions ($p <$

.0001). The effects were greatest in women (17% of explained variance in well-being) and persons age 75 or older (25% of explained variance).

O'Connor and Vallerand (1989) examined the relationship between religious motivation and life satisfaction among 176 elderly French-Canadians in Quebec. While the quality rating given this study was 6 (slightly below our cutoff of 7), we decided to include it here because of its international relevance. The sample was drawn from nursing homes in the greater Montreal area (83% women, mean age 82). Four types of religious motivation were assessed (intrinsic religiosity, self-determined extrinsic religiosity, nonself-determined extrinsic religiosity, and amotivational religiosity) on the basis of a Religious Motivation scale developed by the investigators and translated into French. Life satisfaction was measured by a French translation of Diener's Satisfaction with Life Scale. Intrinsic religiosity was positively related to life satisfaction ($r = .25$, $p < .001$), self-esteem ($r = .30$, $p < .001$), and meaning in life ($r = .31$, $p < .001$) (uncontrolled). Other studies of Canadians have reported significant relationships between religious measures and well-being (Harvey et al., 1987; Gee & Veevers, 1990; Jamal & Badawi, 1993; Krause, 1993; Frankel & Hewitt, 1994).

Coke (1992) examined correlates of life satisfaction among 166 African Americans ages 65–88 in New York (87 males, 79 females). Religiosity was measured by a single self-rated religiosity item and by a single item that asked about hours per week of church participation. Other covariates included adequacy of income, self-rated health, family role involvement, self-reported annual income, and years of education. Life satisfaction, the dependent variable, was measured by Diener's five-item life satisfaction scale. Bivariate correlations were strongest for life satisfaction and self-rated religiosity in both sexes and for life satisfaction and "hours of church participation" in males (but not females). Using multiple regression, Coke found that self-rated religiosity was the strongest predictor of life satisfaction among all the correlates assessed. It was the only predictor in men ($p < .01$) (explaining 27% of the total variance

in life satisfaction) and was stronger than self-rated health in women ($p < .01$) (explaining 10% of the variance).

Krause (1992) examined the relationship among stress, religiosity, and psychological well-being in a sample of 448 African Americans over age 60 who participated in the American Changing Lives Survey. Structural equation modeling was used to analyze the data. Religiosity was assessed using measures of self-rated religiosity, personal religious activity, and church attendance (four questions total). Outcomes included emotional support, personal control, self-esteem, and depressed affect, each assessed by two or three questions. Subjective religiosity was significantly related to emotional support ($\beta = .31$, $p < .01$) and to self-esteem ($\beta = .26$, $p < .05$), but not to personal control or to depressed affect. Church attendance, on the other hand, was unrelated to any of the four outcomes. Krause concluded that subjective religiosity affects psychological well-being among elderly African Americans primarily by bolstering feelings of self-worth.

Krause (1993) examined the relationship between religiousness and well-being next in a sample of 709 persons age 55 or older who participated in the World Values Survey (only data from United States and Canada were included in this report). Religious measures included organizational religiosity (3 items), subjective religiosity (3 items), and religious beliefs (12 items); life satisfaction was measured by 3 items. Using structural equation modeling (LISREL), Krause found a positive relationship between a second-order religiosity factor (global religious orientation based on five religious dimensions) and life satisfaction ($\beta = .16$, $p < .01$), as well as a positive relationship between subjective religiosity and life satisfaction ($\beta = .26$, $p < .05$).

Positive Associations in Younger Adults

Jewish. Anson, Carmel, et al. (1990) surveyed a random sample of members of a religious ($n = 105$) and a nonreligious ($n = 125$) kibbutz in Israel. The two kibbutzim were located in similar regions, were of similar size, and had both been established about 45 years previously. Religious variables were kibbutz type (religious vs. secular), self-rated religiousness (very observant to completely secular), religious commitment (rated-self in comparison to other members of kibbutz), religious practice scale (observance of nine religious practices), frequency of private prayer, and degree of comfort derived from religion during times of stress. Investigators found that membership in a religious kibbutz was associated with greater well-being and fewer physical symptoms and seemed to act as a buffer against stressful life events. Kibbutz type was strongly related to religious practice and self-rated religiosity, but not to comfort derived from religion, private praying, or religious commitment (variables controlled using regression models). This is an important study because the design (comparison of well-being between members of religious and secular kibbutzim) controlled for many social factors that would otherwise be difficult to take into account.

Muslim. Jamal and Badawi (1993) examined religiosity's effect on moderating job stress among 325 Muslim immigrants in North America. Participants were paid members of the Islamic Society of Canada and the United States. Self-rated religiousness was assessed on a 1–10 scale. Outcomes were satisfaction with job, job motivation, organizational commitment, psychosomatic problems, happiness in life, and turnover motivation. Multiple regression analyses (including only job stress, religiosity, and interactions between the two) revealed that religiosity was significantly and positively related to fewer psychosomatic symptoms, more happiness in life, greater job satisfaction, greater job motivation, more organizational commitment, and less turnover motivation (all $p < .05$). Interactions between job stress and religiosity were all significant for these outcomes, indicating that religiosity was a buffer against the dysfunctional consequences of job stress. Analyses were largely uncontrolled.

No Association

Because we could find relatively few studies that reported no association between religious involvement and well-being ($n = 12$), we review *all* of those here regardless of study quality. As in earlier sections, we present these studies chronologically by year of publication. Because many involve small, nonrepresentative samples and/or weak measures of religious involvement (e.g., affiliation, membership), we also provide study quality ratings after we describe the study.

No Association in Younger Adults/All Ages. Bulman and Wortman (1977) surveyed a convenience sample of 29 rehabilitation patients with paraplegia or quadriplegia. Researchers used the Poppleton and Pilkington religious attitude scale to assess religious involvement. Regression analyses revealed that persons who coped better were those who blamed themselves, not others, for their health problems. Self-blame was significantly related to better coping, and religiousness was associated with self-blame, but there was no direct relationship between religious attitude and happiness or coping (quality rating 5).

Zautra et al. (1977) surveyed 454 subjects age 18 or over in Salt Lake City, Utah (all Mormons). Assessment of religious participation was based on whether respondent mentioned a religious activity when asked what he or she did on a typical day. Dependent variables included perceived quality of life (measured by an established scale), psychiatric symptoms measured by the 22-item Langer Psychiatric Screening Inventory, negative affect measured by the Affect Balance scale, recent life events measured by Holmes and Rae checklist, social participation measured by an established scale, and performance in life concerns. Factor analysis, not multiple regression, was used to examine how variables related to each other. Religious participation was highly correlated with social participation ($r = .61$) and increased family responsibility ($r = .23$) but was not associated with happiness or value preferences (quality rating 6).

Chamberlain and Zika (1988) surveyed 188 women involved in a study of personality factors and well-being in New Zealand. The mean age of the sample was 29; almost all subjects were married and white; the majority had children; and 73% were middle class. Well-being was measured using the Life-3 (life satisfaction) and the 20-item Affectometer-2 that assessed positive and negative affect. Religiosity was measured using two King and Hunt subscales (Orientation to Growth and Striving and Salience Cognition) that are similar to intrinsic religiosity scales. Religiosity was uncorrelated with positive or negative affect but was positively associated with greater life satisfaction ($r = .17$, $p < .05$). When measures of purpose and meaning in life were controlled, the association between religiosity and life satisfaction diminished to nonsignificance. This is not surprising, however, since the way religiosity increases life satisfaction may be by providing purpose and meaning in life (quality rating 6).

Feigelman et al. (1992) examined happiness in Americans who have given up religion. Using pooled data from the General Social Surveys conducted between 1972 and 1990, investigators identified more than 20,000 adults for their study. Subjects of particular interest were "disaffiliates"—those who were affiliated with a religion at age 16 but who were not affiliated at the time of the survey (disaffiliates comprised from 4.4% to 6.0% of respondents per year during the 18 years of surveys). "Actives" were defined as persons who reported a religious affiliation at age 16 *and* a religious affiliation at the time of the survey (these ranged from 84.7% to 79.5% of respondents per year between 1972 and 1990). Happiness was measured by a single question that assessed general happiness (very happy, pretty happy, not too happy). When disaffiliates ($n = 1,420$) were compared with actives ($n = 21,052$), 23.9% of disaffiliates indicated they were "very happy," as did 34.2% of actives. When the analysis was stratified by marital status, the likelihood of being very happy was about 25% lower (i.e., 10% difference) for married religious disaffiliates compared with married actives. Multiple regression analysis revealed that religious disaffiliation explained only 2% of the variance in overall happiness, after marital status and other covariates were controlled. Investigators concluded that there was little relationship between religious disaffiliation and unhappiness (quality rating 7).

No Association in Older Adults.   Moberg (1953) examined the relationship between church membership and personal adjustment in 219 elderly residents of seven nursing homes in Minneapolis-St. Paul, Minnesota. Personal adjustment was measured by the Burgess-Cavan-Havighurst Attitudes Inventory. Church members in the sample ($n = 132$) had higher mean personal adjustment scores than nonchurch members ($n = 87$) (28.4 vs. 23.3, $p < .01$). Differences persisted in both men and women and in all cases where members were contrasted to nonmembers within categories of age, nativity, place of residence, years of schooling, marital and family status, self-rating of health, participation in social organizations, and verbal self-rating of happiness. To test this association further, 53 church members were matched with 53 nonmembers on sex, present employment, club participation, marital status, number of living children, education, and self-rated health. This reduced the mean personal adjustment score of church members to 26.8 and increased that of nonmembers to 24.9, a statistically nonsignificant difference. When two more matching factors were added (nativity and institution in which subject resided), sample size was reduced to nine persons in each group. Differences on mean adjustment scores between the two groups declined even further to 24.1 for church members and 24.2 for nonchurch members. Moberg concluded that church membership by itself is unrelated to personal adjustment in old age (quality rating 6).

Toseland and Rasch (1979) examined correlates of life satisfaction in a national probability sample of 871 persons age 55 or over. Investigators looked at 31 predictors of life satisfaction (assessed by semantic differential scale), including an indicator of "religious participation." A description of the religious variable was not given, since it was not a focus of the study. Religious participation as a predictor of life satisfaction dropped out of the analysis ($p = $ ns) when other variables were controlled (quality rating 6).

Steinitz (1980) examined the relationship between religious involvement and well-being using pooled data from the 1972–1977 General

Social Surveys, a probability sample of 1,493 persons age 65 or over. Religiosity was measured by four items that inquired about church attendance, strength of affiliation, belief in afterlife, and confidence in organized religion. Six single items assessed happiness, self-rated health, excitement in life, and satisfaction with city, family, and health. Church attendance was related to happiness ($r = .11$, $p < .01$), self-rated health ($r = .09$, $p < .01$), excitement ($r = .18$, $p < .01$), satisfaction with family ($r = .10$, $p = .05$), and satisfaction with health ($r = .11$, $p < .01$). Relationships for church attendance were particularly strong in women and whites, where significant relationships were found for all six well-being variables. Strength of denominational affiliation was weakly related to satisfaction with city and satisfaction with health ($p < .05$) but was related to no other well-being measures. There were no associations between measures of well-being and confidence in organized religion. Belief in life after death was significantly related to excitement in life ($r = .29$, $p = .05$) and satisfaction with city ($r = .16$, $p = .05$).

Since church attendance was more important than other religious measures in predicting well-being, and since that factor might be influenced by the health of subjects, the investigator stratified analyses by self-reported health. The association between church attendance and well-being was significant only among persons in poor or fair health. Analyses did not control for other covariates, although the researcher stratified for race, sex, and subjective health. Despite the positive associations found, the author concluded that "Contrary to earlier findings, the data here demonstrate that religious older people do not have consistently greater feelings of well-being nor a better Wetanschauung than less religious older people" (p. 66). On the basis of the data reported, however, this conclusion appears incorrect. Finding significant associations only among those in poor or fair health does not automatically mean that frequency of church attendance measures only the effects of physical activity. Another explanation for this finding is that those who force themselves to attend religious services may benefit in terms of greater happiness and life satis-

faction than those who allow their limitations to keep them at home (quality rating 6).

Leonard (1982) examined the relationship between "belief in an afterlife" and life satisfaction in a probability sample of 320 adults age 60 or over who participated in a General Social Survey (year unknown). The investigator examined 23 psychosocial and health predictors of life satisfaction (measured by a five-item scale). Belief in afterlife (the only religious variable examined) was unrelated to life satisfaction (quality rating 4).

Magee (1987) surveyed 150 retired nuns ages 71–85 in New York in order to explore the relationship between religious activity and life satisfaction. Life satisfaction was measured using Neugarten's Life Satisfaction Index. The investigator found that 30.7% of nuns expressed high life satisfaction, 50% moderate life satisfaction, and 19% low life satisfaction. Multiple regression was used to identify predictors of life satisfaction. The only religious variable measured was "holding an administrative or governance position in one's congregation before retiring." This variable was significantly related to greater life satisfaction ($p < .05$) when list-wise regression was used, but the association disappeared when step-wise regression was employed to analyze the data (quality rating 5).

Walls and Zarit (1991) studied the relationship between informal support provided by churches and well-being in 98 elderly African Americans in central Pennsylvania. Well-being was measured using the Philadelphia Geriatric Center Morale Scale. Religious involvement was measured using King and Hunt's Dimensions of Religion scale (personal religiosity) and Moberg's Social Integration of the Aged in the Church scale (organizational religiosity). Regression analysis revealed that perceptions of social support from church, but not personal religiosity or involvement in organized religious activity, predicted well-being (quality rating 6).

Francis and Bolger (1997) examined religion and psychological well-being in a convenience sample of 55 retired civil servants in Wales, United Kingdom. Religious involvement was measured by single items of frequency of prayer and frequency of religious attendance. Positive affect was measured using Bradburn's Affect Balance Scale. Positive affect was associated with prayer ($r = .17$) and church attendance ($r = .12$); neither correlation was statistically significant (analyses uncontrolled). The investigators concluded that there was no association between religion and well-being (quality rating 3).

Negative Associations

Few studies have found a negative association between religious involvement and well-being; we could locate only one. Maranell (1974) examined the relationship between religiosity and personality adjustment in 109 college students. Of the eight different types of religiousness measured, two dimensions were consistently related to mental pathology (superstition and ritualism). The author found no relationship between emotional pathology and church orientation, altruism, fundamentalism, theism, idealism, or mysticism. Maranell concluded that religious persons are likely to be less well-adjusted than nonreligious persons. If multiple statistical comparisons were taken into account, however, the significant findings would vanish (quality rating 4).

PROSPECTIVE COHORT STUDIES

Prospective cohort studies that examine the relationship between religion and well-being have typically been of higher quality than cross-sectional studies. Because of their importance, particularly in providing information about causality, we review all the studies we located; study quality ratings are included only when they are less than 7.

Positive Associations in Samples of All Ages

In one of the longest longitudinal studies on record, Willits and Crider (1988) examined the relationship between religion and well-being among men and women as part of a 37-year prospective cohort study. This investigation involved 2,806 sophomores in 75 rural high schools in Pennsylvania in 1947 who were followed up in 1984. Questionnaires were mailed to the 2,009 subjects who were still alive or locatable. A total of 1,650 men and women in their early fifties completed follow-up questionnaires. Both parent and adolescent religiosity were assessed in 1947. Parent church or Sunday school involvement was measured by yes-no responses. An "adolescent participation index" was created on the basis of the summation of yes-no responses to questions about attendance at church, Sunday school, and church socials. In 1984 religious attendance was measured on a six-point scale and religious belief on a five-point scale based on agreement or disagreement with five items concerning belief in God as a controlling or caring force. The dependent variable, well-being in 1984, was measured by overall life satisfaction and satisfaction with community, job, and marriage.

Cross-sectional analyses in 1984 revealed that church attendance and religious beliefs were significantly related to overall life satisfaction ($r = .13$ and $r = .10$, $p < .001$) and to satisfaction with community ($r = .12$ and $r = .09$, $p < .001$); these associations persisted after controlling for gender, income, and other religiosity measures. Longitudinal analyses revealed that adolescent religious participation and parent religious attendance in 1947 were not related to overall life satisfaction in 1984, once gender, income, and other religiosity measures were controlled. Adolescent religious participation in 1947, after researchers controlled for other variables, *was* significantly related to job satisfaction in 1984.

Recall Tix and Frazier's (1997) prospective study of patients who received renal transplants ($n = 239$) and their significant others ($n = 179$) (see chapter 5). Subjects were surveyed 3 and 12 months after surgery (T1 and T2). T1 and T2 measures assessed religious coping, life satisfaction, and psychological distress. Results of multiple regression models indicate that religious coping at T1 was related to greater life satisfaction at T1 and T2 for patients and significant others and to less psychological distress at T1 for significant others. Religious coping at T1, however, did not predict life satisfaction or psychological distress at T2 after T1 satisfaction or distress was controlled. When analyses were stratified by denomination, however, religious coping was associated with psychological outcomes in Protestants but not in Catholics. Among Protestant patients, T1 religious coping was significantly associated with T2 life satisfaction when T1 life satisfaction was controlled ($\beta = .20$, $p < .05$, $n = 59$). Among Catholic significant others (but not patients), on the other hand, T1 religious coping predicted increased psychological distress at 12 months when T1 distress was controlled ($\beta = .27$, $p < .05$, $n = 34$).

Positive Associations in Older Adults

Graney (1975) examined the relationship between happiness and social participation in a four-year prospective cohort study of 60 elderly women selected from the rosters of a metropolitan Housing and Redevelopment Authority project. The investigator administered the Affect Balance Scale and nine questions on social participation, including a question about church attendance. Cross-sectional analysis revealed that religious attendance was related to positive affect ($r = .33$, $p < .01$), an association that was stronger for women ages 66–75 years ($r = .67$, $p < .01$) than for women ages 82–92 years ($r = -10$, $p = $ ns). Religious attendance at baseline, however, only weakly predicted positive affect (happiness) over time ($r = .14$, $p = .07$, entire sample). No covariates were controlled (quality rating 6).

Blazer and Palmore (1976) examined the relationship between religion and well-being in a 20-year prospective study of 272 volunteers. These subjects were ages 60–94; 67% were white; 52% were female; and 90% were Protestant. The religion subscale of the Chicago Inventory of Activities and Attitudes assessed religious activities such as attending church, listening to religious radio/TV, and reading Bible/devotional books. Religious attitudes were measured by asking respondents to indicate agreement or disagreement to statements describing the importance of religion and the comfort they derived from religion.

At Round 1 (1955–1959), religious activities were related to happiness ($r = .16$ overall, $r = .26$ in men, and $r = .25$ in persons over 70), feeling useful ($r = .25$ overall, $r = .34$ in those with manual occupations, and $r = .32$ in those over 70), and personal adjustment ($r = .16$ overall, $r = .33$ in manual occupations, and $r = .28$ in males). Religious attitudes, while unrelated to happiness, were positively related to usefulness ($r = 0.16$ overall, $r = .24$ for manual occupations). These cross-sectional correlations increased from Round 1 to Round 7 of the study, suggesting the increasing importance of religion for well-being among subjects as they grew older (however, this result may also have been caused by study dropouts). All correlations were statistically significant and controlled by stratifying analyses by age, sex, and occupation. The investigators conducted no longitudinal analyses involving relationships between religion and well-being but only repeated cross-sectional analyses.

Markides (1983) examined the relationship between religiosity and life satisfaction in a four-year prospective cohort study involving a probability sample of older Mexican-Americans (70%) and Anglos (30%) from San Antonio, Texas. Subjects were initially surveyed in 1976 (T1) ($n = 510$) and again in 1980 (T2) ($n = 338$). Religious variables included church attendance, self-rated religiosity, and private prayer, each assessed using a single item. The dependent variable, life satisfaction, was measured using Neugarten's 13-item Life Satisfaction Index. After controlling for sex, age, marital status, and education, the author found that T1 church attendance correlated positively with T1 life satisfaction among both Mexican Americans ($\beta = .51$, $p < .05$) and Anglos ($\beta = .52$, $p < .05$). T1 self-rated religiosity and private prayer were correlated with greater T1 life satisfaction for Anglos only ($\beta = 1.85$, $p < .05$, and $\beta = 1.58$, $p < .05$, respectively). T2 attendance and T2 private prayer were correlated with T2 life satisfaction ($\beta = .39$, $p < .05$, and $\beta = .93$, $p < .05$, respectively) in Mexican Americans; in Anglos, only T2 church attendance was associated with T2 life satisfaction ($\beta = .98$, $p < .05$). As in the Blazer and Palmore study, investigators performed cross-sectional analyses at T1 and T2 but did not examine the longitudinal relationship between T1 religious variables and T2 life satisfaction.

Musick (1996) examined the relationship between religious involvement and subjective health (similar to Singh and Williams's 1982 study that examined satisfaction with health). The investigator utilized data from a three-year prospective investigation of 4,162 randomly selected persons age 65 or over who participated in the EPESE survey at its North Carolina site. Of the original 4,162 subjects surveyed in 1986 (Wave I), 2,623 were resurveyed in 1989 (Wave II). Regression (residualized change analysis) was used to examine 1986 predictors of 1989 subjective health in the African American and the white subsamples. For 1,421 African Americans, Wave I religious devotion (private prayer/Bible reading) was significantly related to greater Wave II subjective health ($\beta = .07$, $p < .01$). Because African Americans with higher levels of functional impairment also spent more time in devotional activities, the effect of devotion on subjective health did not appear until functional impairment was controlled; the opposite dynamic, however, was present for church attendance. Religious attendance, initially related to subjective health, dropped out as a predictor after functional disability (impaired activities of daily living) was controlled.

While there was no main effect for either Wave I devotion or Wave I attendance among 1,202 whites, there was a significant interaction between both religious measures and functional impairment on subjective health ($\beta = .06$, $p < .05$, and $\beta = .09$, $p < .001$). In other words, among those with high levels of functional impairment at Wave I, both high devotional activity and high religious attendance were related to better perceptions of physical health at Wave II. Thus, religious activity may have led to more positive evaluations of health status among Caucasians who were disabled (suggesting greater well-being in the presence of health problems, given the close link between well-being and subjective health). See also Idler (1987).

No Association in Older Adults

Carp (1974) examined the relationship between church attendance and adjustment among 133 elders relocated from their homes to a new living situation (elder housing). Subjects were assessed prior to relocation and then again 18 months and eight years thereafter. Outcome variables at the eight-year follow-up were self-ratings of happiness, peer ratings of popularity, and administrator ratings of adjustment. Among 27 predictors assessed at either baseline or 18-month follow-up, church attendance was the second strongest predictor of adjustment as judged by administrator evaluations. Attendance was not, however, one of the primary predictors of happiness as rated by subjects themselves or of popularity as rated by their peers. Level of statistical significance (p value) for associations was not reported.

Markides et al. (1987) conducted an eight-year follow-up of their 1976 cohort in 1984. Cross-sectional analyses using multiple regression were again performed for data collected in 1976 (T1, $n = 511$), 1980 (T2, $n = 338$), and 1984 (T3, $n = 254$). There were 230 respondents who participated in all three waves of data collection. The following cross-sectional associations between religious attendance and life satisfaction are listed by year of survey: in 1976, $\beta = .09$ ($p < .05$) for the 511 participants at T1, and $\beta = .03$ (ns) for the 230 subjects at T1 who participated at all three waves; in 1980, $\beta = .15$ ($p < .01$) for the 338 subjects at T2, and $\beta = .13$ (ns) for the 230 subjects at T2 who participated at all three waves; and in 1984, $\beta = .08$ (ns) for the 254 subjects at T3, and $\beta = .06$ (ns) for the 230 subjects at T3 who participated in all three waves. In other words, among subjects who participated in all three waves of data collection ($n = 230$), there was no association between religious attendance and life satisfaction at any time point.

Comparable correlations between self-rated religiosity and life satisfaction were as follows: in 1976, $\beta = .10$ ($p < .05$) for the 511 subjects, and $\beta = .05$ (ns) for the 230 in all three waves; in 1980, $\beta = .08$ (ns) for the 338 subjects and

$\beta = .03$ (ns) for the 230; and in 1984, $\beta = .07$ (ns) for the 254 subjects and $\beta = .09$ (ns) for 230. Again, no relationship at any time point was found between self-rated religiosity and life satisfaction among subjects participating in all three waves of data collection. Correlations between private prayer and life satisfaction were as follows: in 1976, $\beta = .07$ (ns) for 511, and $\beta = .04$ (ns) for 230; in 1980, $\beta = .13$ ($p < .05$) for 338, and $\beta = .14$ ($p < .05$) for 230; and in 1984, $\beta = -.04$ (ns) for 254, and $\beta = -.04$ (ns) for 230. Again, the same pattern largely persists.

The authors note that, among dropouts, means on life satisfaction, religious attendance, and functional health were all much lower than those for participants. They concluded that the associations (particularly with church attendance) lose their significance over time because dropouts (because of death or serious illness) were less frequent attenders who also reported lower levels of functional health and life satisfaction. As in the 1983 study, these are all cross-sectional comparisons, not longitudinal analyses. As with the Steinitz study, these findings do not rule out the possibility that the relationship between religious involvement and life satisfaction may simply be greatest among persons with medical illness and may diminish among those who are healthy. In other words, the buffering effects of religious involvement on well-being may be greatest for those experiencing health-related stressors (see Strawbridge et al., 1998).

No Association in Samples of All Ages

No studies were found.

Negative Association

No studies were found.

INTERVENTION STUDIES

In contrast to the many cross-sectional and prospective cohort studies we found, we could locate only a few clinical trials that examined the effects of a spiritual intervention on emotional well-being. Beutler et al. (1988) conducted a prospective randomized clinical trial of 120 volunteers in the Netherlands who had high diastolic blood pressures. While the focus of the study was blood pressure, investigators also examined well-being as an outcome variable. Three groups of 40 persons each were formed. Group 1 subjects received a healing intervention consisting of laying on of hands; Group 2 received a healing intervention at a distance by "thought projection"; and Group 3 was the control group. The groups were treated once a week for 20 minutes in the morning for 15 consecutive weeks. Twelve known healers experienced with laying on of hands or healing at a distance were selected from societies of paranormal healers. Results indicated that 83% of Group 1 subjects who had received the physical laying on of hands reported slightly to much improved well-being, compared with 43% of Group 2 subjects and 41% of Group 3 subjects ($p < .001$).

O'Laoire (1997) assigned 90 adults ("agents") to pray for the needs of 406 people ("subjects"). Agents were assigned to either a directed prayer group or a nondirected prayer group. Subjects were randomly assigned in a double-blinded fashion to one of three groups: being prayed for with directed prayer (A), being prayed for with nondirected prayer (B), or receiving no prayer (C). Agents prayed for their subjects 15 minutes daily for 12 weeks. Outcome measures included the Coopersmith self-esteem inventory, state-trait anxiety questionnaire, Beck depression inventory, Profile of Mood States, and perceived change in physical health, emotional health, intellectual health, spiritual health, relationships, and creative expression. Results indicated no difference in 11 outcome measures between groups A and B (prayed for) and group C (controls); that is, those prayed for did not do better than those who were not. The prepost scores on the well-being measures for subjects (groups A and B) and for agents of prayer, however, revealed that the agents of prayer (those who were praying for subjects) experienced greater improvements in well-being than did the subjects of prayer ($p < .05$–$p < .0001$).

Matthews, Marlowe, et al. (2000) examined the effects of intercessory prayer on physical health and psychological well-being in 40 patients (mean age 62 years, 82% female) with moderately severe rheumatoid arthritis. Subjects were randomly assigned to either a three-day in-person prayer intervention (including six hours of instruction and six hours of direct-contact prayer in the form of Christian laying on of hands) ($n = 26$) or to the control group ($n = 14$). After six months, control subjects were crossed over to receive the intervention and followed up for six months. A single clinician, blinded to group status of subjects, assessed all subjects prior to the intervention and at 3, 6, 9, and 12 months postintervention (or 3 and 6 months postintervention for the control group). Existential well-being was assessed with Palouzian and Ellison's Spiritual Well-being Scale as one of the outcome variables. Preliminary results indicate that both number of tender joints and patients' perceptions of the degree of arthritis-related disability (assessed using the Modified Health Assessment Questionnaire) at six months were significantly better in the prayed-for group compared to the control group. The results with regard to existential well-being are pending at this time.

SUMMARY AND CONCLUSIONS

We first examined the characteristics of persons with high well-being and life satisfaction and found that such persons were often healthy and active, had plenty of social support, were married, had high internal locus of control, had a strong sense of purpose and meaning, and were hopeful and optimistic. We then examined the relationship between these characteristics and religious involvement and found that religious persons have many of these characteristics. We then reviewed studies that have directly examined the relationship between religious involvement and measures of well-being, happiness, and life satisfaction. We divided our review of this research into cross-sectional, prospective/longitudinal, and intervention studies. We then categorized studies into those that found a positive association, those that found

no association, and those that found a negative association, and further into studies of younger and older adults, and studies of different religious groups, and organized these by year of publication.

Many studies have examined the relationship between religious involvement and psychological well-being. While the vast majority of these are cross-sectional studies, a number of important prospective cohort and intervention studies are reviewed. Almost 80% of the 100 studies that have statistically examined the religion-well-being relationship report a positive correlation between religiousness and greater happiness, life satisfaction, morale, or other measure of well-being. Populations have included younger and older adults, African Americans and Caucasians, men and women, Christians ($n = 67$), Jews ($n = 1$), and Muslims ($n = 1$). Thirteen percent of studies reviewed ($n = 13$) reported no association, and 7 percent reported mixed or complex findings. Only one study found a negative correlation between religiousness and mental adjustment/well-being, and this study was conducted in a small, nonrandom sample of college students. In the vast majority of studies, religious involvement was positively correlated with greater well-being.

Because most studies have been cross-sectional, more prospective cohort studies are needed to carefully assess religious and well-being variables, control for confounding factors, and follow subjects for a sufficient period of time to allow for changes in well-being to occur. Such studies are especially needed in high-risk populations, where religious behaviors may be particularly important for well-being. While prospective studies can provide information about causal order, there will always be doubt concerning religion's effects on well-being until clinical trials demonstrate that making people more religious increases their happiness, life satisfaction, or morale. A few studies, as reviewed, have already attempted this, with more or less success. The difficulties in designing, carrying out, and interpreting the results of such experimental studies are formidable (see chapters 31 and 32).

7

Depression

EPRESSION IS THE MOST common and treatable of all mental disorders. Approximately 330 million people around the world suffer from depression, and unfortunately only 10% receive adequate treatment. At least 800,000 suicides occur each year as a result of depression, which has a lifetime mortality rate of nearly 15% (Editorial, 1998b). According to Christopher Murray, head of epidemiology at the World Health Organization, by the year 2020 unipolar major depression will be the world's second most debilitating disease, surpassed only by cardiovascular disease. In the United States, the lifetime prevalence of major depression is 10–25% in women and 5–12% in men. At any given point in time, 5–12% of women and 2–3% of men meet the criteria for major depression (American Psychiatric Association, 1994). The lifetime prevalence of major depression in the United States has increased dramatically with each successive birth cohort between 1936 and 1975, and the age of onset is lowering, with younger adults being affected more often than ever before (Editorial, 1998b).

Treatment for depression is on the rise in the United States. Pincus et al. (1998) found that visits to physicians for depression were up from 11 million in 1985 to 20.4 million in 1993–1994. Visits that included treatment with an antidepressant medication were up from 5.3 million in 1985 to 12.4 million in 1993–1994. In 1988, physicians in the United States wrote 1.5 million prescriptions for fluoxetine hydrochloride (Prozac). By 1997, that number had increased almost sevenfold to 9.9 million prescriptions, with total sales exceeding $1.4 billion (Morrow, 1998). By the year 2002 the sales of Prozac alone (which makes up only 40% of the antidepressant market) are projected to reach $2.3 billion. The worldwide market for antidepressants was $7 billion in 1998 and was expected to increase by more than 50% by 2003 (Editorial, 1998b). People with depression are also at increased risk for use of hospital and medical services and for early death from physical causes (Koenig, Shelp, et al., 1989; Covinsky et al., 1999).

Religion is a variable not commonly included in standard epidemiological discussions of depression. However, clinical observations and systematic research since Kraeplin (1899) suggest that depression and religion are somehow related. The cumulative weight of 100 years of investigation of the religion-depression relationship has yet to be fully summarized, reviewed, and critiqued.

Our discussion of this topic is divided into four sections. First, we review the existing research on the prevalence of depression and depressive symptoms among members of different religious groups (e.g., Jews, Catholics, Protestants, and Pentecostals). Second, we examine the research on the relationship between level of religious involvement and depression. Third, we examine research on the role that religion plays in helping people cope with life stressors, thereby buffering them from depression. Fourth, we look at the existing quasi-experimental and experimental research on religion and depression (psychotherapy studies, in particular).

RELIGIOUS AFFILIATION
AND DEPRESSION

Epidemiologists have long observed that members of certain religious groups are at increased risk for mental disorder (e.g., Sanua, 1992). In such studies, the prevalence of depressive symptoms or depressive disorder among members of a religious group is compared with that in the general population. Because the U.S. population is approximately 60% Protestant and 26% Catholic (Kosmin & Lachman, 1993), Christian populations usually become a sort of de facto comparison group in such studies (at least those conducted in the United States). The religious constitution of the hidden comparison group differs from culture to culture; in cultures where the general population is mostly Muslim, or Hindu, or Buddhist, the conclusions we draw here may not generalize.

Jews

In the United States, Jews represent approximately 2–3% of the population (Kosmin & Lachman, 1993). Studies since the 1880s from around the world have suggested that Jews experience an elevated risk for depressive disorders (Levav, Kohn, Golding, et al., 1997). Sanua (1992) reviewed a large group of epidemiological and clinical studies related to mental disorders, including depression, among Jews. Citing a variety of cross-sectional studies (Bart, 1968; Figelman, 1968; Fernando, 1975; Cooklin et al., 1983), Sanua concluded that people of Jewish descent appear to be at increased risk for depression. Even when researchers examine the conditions of patients admitted to psychiatric hospitals, Jews tend to have higher rates of depressive disorder than non-Jews (Malzberg, 1973; Cooklin et al., 1983; Flics & Herron, 1991). As Levav, Kohn, Golding, et al. (1997) point out, however, studies that use clinical populations are subject to a variety of biases, particularly those relating to the propensity to seek mental health care.

More recent studies that use community samples and rigorous sampling methods, however, also indicate that Jews are at increased risk for depression. Community-based epidemiological studies find that Jews have an approximately twofold risk of major depression compared to members of other religious groups (e.g., Ross, 1990; Yeung & Greenwald, 1992; Kennedy, Kelman, et al., 1996; Levav, Kohn, Golding, et al., 1997). For example, Levav, Kohn, Golding, et al. (1997) found the lifetime and period prevalence of major depression for Jews was 1.5 to 2 times that of non-Jews in two large, random regional samples after they controlled for covariates.

Is the association between Jewishness and depression causal? In a two-year prospective study of 1,855 older community-dwelling adults in New York, researchers found that Jews were 1.4 times more likely than Catholics and more than four times as likely as members of other faiths to score high on the Center for Epidemiological Studies Depression (CES-D) scale (Kennedy, Kelman, Thomas, et al., 1996). Among subjects who were not depressed at baseline but became depressed by the two-year follow-up, Jews were significantly overrepresented. Being Jewish remained a risk factor even after researchers controlled for six other correlates of depression. In contrast, Idler and Kasl (1992) reported that Jews had a lower risk of developing depression than did Catholics during a three-year follow-up of 2,812 older adults from New Haven, Connecticut (a finding that persisted after the authors controlled for baseline levels of depression and a variety of covariates). Most studies, however, find that Jews—men and women, young and old—have an elevated lifetime and period prevalence of major depression and are also more likely to remain depressed over time than are depressed people of other faiths. Risk for depression among Jews is associated with many of the standard risk factors for depression (including poor subjective and functional health, lack of social support, and gender). Jews of Eastern European descent appear particularly vulnerable to depression (Kennedy, 1998).

It is also important, however, to acknowledge the fact that Jews—especially Jews of Eastern European descent—may be more willing to admit to negative affects (Glicksman, 1991), creating a potential response bias. Finally, the elevated prevalence of depression in Jews may be a trade-off for their reduced rates of alcohol abuse and dependence. In their analysis of data from the New Haven and Los Angeles Epidemiologic Catchment Area (ECA) sites, Levav, Kohn, Golding, et al. (1997) compared the prevalence of depression and alcohol abuse and dependence among Jewish and non-Jewish men and women. They found that excess depression among Jews was present only in Jewish men (not in Jewish women), and alcohol use and dependence were lower only in Jewish men. Jewish and non-Jewish women had roughly equal rates of both depression and alcohol abuse and dependence. The combined prevalence of both depression and alcohol abuse and

dependence was not significantly different for Jewish and non-Jewish men.

Furthermore, alcohol use among Jewish men was higher in Los Angeles (the less traditional Jewish community) than in New Haven (the more traditional Jewish community). The usual 2:1 female-male ratio for depression was found in the more secular Jewish community of Los Angeles (where alcohol abuse and dependence among Jewish men were fairly high), whereas the female-male ratio was approximately 1:1 in the more conservative Jewish community of New Haven (where alcohol abuse and dependence among Jewish men were low). Since more conservative Jews tend to avoid excess use of alcohol, conservative Jewish men with a propensity toward psychopathology might be at increased risk for depression instead of alcohol abuse or dependence, whereas liberal Jewish males may be more likely to express psychopathology in terms of substance abuse.

Catholics

Catholics constitute approximately 26% of the American population (Kosmin & Lachman, 1993). The existing studies are quite inconsistent regarding the relationship between Catholicism and depression. Miller, Warner, et al. (1997) reported the results of a 10-year prospective study of 60 mothers and 151 of their children. At the 10-year follow-up, the mothers' religious affiliation was determined. Investigators found that Catholic mothers had a lower rate of depression both at baseline and at follow-up. Catholic mothers were also somewhat less likely than other mothers to have children diagnosed with major depression at baseline and at follow-up. Likewise, studying a sample of adults whose relatives were undergoing coronary artery bypass grafts, VandeCreek, Pargament, et al. (1995) found that Catholics had significantly lower levels of depressive symptoms than non-Catholics.

Other studies report either no association or a positive association between Catholicism and depression. Ross (1990) examined denominational differences in self-rated depressive symptoms. After controlling for a variety of covariates (including level of religious involvement, age, gender, race, marital status, education, income, and willingness to express feelings), Catholics had slightly higher depression scores than Protestants. Likewise, Sorenson et al. (1995) reported higher depression scores among unwed Catholic mothers than among unwed Protestant mothers. Park, Cohen, et al. (1990) found that Catholic women scored lower than Protestant women on measures of depression in one study, but not in a second study (see also Hertsgaard & Light, 1984). Other studies that used small samples of recently bereaved adults (Sherkat & Reed, 1992), nursing home residents (Commerford & Reznikoff, 1996), and undergraduate students (e.g., Schafer, 1997) also found Catholicism unrelated to depression scores.

Even in the best studies—those involving large samples drawn regionally or nationally—results are inconsistent. Levav, Kohn, Golding, et al. (1997) reported that Catholics in the New Haven and the Los Angeles sites of the ECA survey had prevalence rates of depressive disorder that were approximately 50% those of Jews. Likewise, Jones-Webb and Snowden (1991) found that among the 1,947 African American adults in their cross-sectional, nationally representative survey, only 11% of African American Catholics scored in the clinical range on the CES-D scale. Rates of depression were substantially higher among African American Protestants and African Americans of other faiths (whose depression rates ranged from 21% for Protestants to 43% for non-Western religions). In that study, the association of Catholicism with lower rates of depression persisted after researchers controlled for seven demographic and geographic variables (including socioeconomic status, marital status, age, and sex). Among the 1,747 white respondents, however, no denominational differences in the presence of depressive illness were found (rates of depression ranged from 14% to 16% for all faiths).

Pentecostals/Fundamentalists

Pentecostals constitute approximately 2–5% of the U.S. population (Kosmin & Lachman,

1993). Some evidence suggests that members of Pentecostal faiths are at increased risk for major depression. Meador et al. (1992) examined cross-sectional data from 2,850 adults in North Carolina who were involved in the Duke ECA study (one of five sites, along with New Haven and Los Angeles, chosen to help assess the prevalence of psychiatric disorders in the American population). Meador et al. (1992) found that members of Pentecostal churches had rates of major depression that were three times higher than those of non-Pentecostals. This difference persisted after researchers controlled for a variety of covariates, including gender, age, race, socioeconomic status, unexpected life events, and social support.

Another report that used the same data set (Koenig, George, Meador, Blazer, & Dyck, 1994) compared the rate of depression among Pentecostals to that for members of other Christian faiths. The sample was split into "baby boomers" (born between 1945 and 1966) and middle-aged and older adults (born between 1889 and 1944). The six-month and lifetime risk of depressive disorders for Pentecostal baby boomers was found to be considerably higher than the risk for baby boomers from other conservative denominations or mainline Christian denominations. These differences persisted after sex, race, physical health, and socioeconomic status were controlled. On the other hand, Pentecostalism was not associated with depression in middle-aged or older adults.

Koenig, George, Meador, Blazer, and Dyck (1994) speculated as to whether the association between Pentecostalism and depression among baby boomers reflected a causal effect. They concluded that Pentecostalism either (a) leads to higher rates of depression; (b) attracts members who are more likely to be depressed; or (c) is associated with some third variable (related to both Pentecostalism and depression) that was uncontrolled or poorly controlled. The authors concluded that, of these three explanations, (b) was the most likely, given (1) the aggressive evangelistic outreach of Pentecostals to persons in lower socioeconomic classes and other groups at high risk for mental disorder (e.g., alcoholics, drug addicts) and (2) the positive, optimistic, hopeful message that often draws these people into Pentecostal congregations. Meador et al. (1992) speculated that Pentecostals, like Jews, might have higher levels of emotional expression.

No Affiliation

Currently, approximately 8% of the U.S. population claim no religious affiliation (Kosmin & Lachman, 1993). People with no affiliation appear to be at greater risk for depressive symptoms than those affiliated with a religion. In a sample of 850 medically ill men, Koenig, Cohen, Blazer, Pieper, et al. (1992) examined whether religious affiliation predicted depression after demographics, medical status, and a measure of religious coping were controlled. They found that, when relevant covariates were controlled, men who indicated that they had "no religious affiliation" had higher scores on the Hamilton depression rating scale (an observer-administered rating scale) than did men who identified themselves as moderate Protestants, Catholics, or nontraditional Christians.

The association between lack of religious disaffiliation and depressive symptoms is particularly strong among African Americans. In a sample of 537 African American males, Brown and Gary (1987) found that men who were not affiliated with a religion had higher CES-D scores than men who were affiliated (17.0 vs. 11.8). This significant difference persisted after the authors controlled for church attendance, age, income, education, marital status, and employment status. Ellison (1995) examined religious affiliation and depression in 2,956 adults who participated in the North Carolina site of the ECA survey. Depressive symptoms were assessed using the Diagnostic Interview Schedule. Among white respondents, absence of religious affiliation did not predict depressive symptoms. Among African American respondents, however, people who were not affiliated with a religion scored significantly higher on depressive symptoms. This relationship remained significant (though weakened) after controlling for numerous covariates.

Explanations

Aside from methodological reasons for the relationship between religious affiliation and depression (e.g., selection biases, response biases, and differential test validity for certain religious or ethnic groups), other explanations exist as well. These include genetic explanations, sociological explanations, lifestyle differences, differential exposure to historical events (e.g., the Holocaust or World War II), and differences in religious or spiritual practices (Kennedy, 1998). We focus here on two explanations that relate to aspects of religion per se.

Religious Marginalization. The first of these explanations is a sociological one. Some researchers theorize that the elevated risk of depression among Jews, at least in the United States, is related to the marginalization of Jewish people. Research supports the hypothesis that religious marginalization—being of a different religion than those in one's surrounding culture—creates social conditions that foster depression. Rosenberg (1962) conducted a cross-sectional survey with a sample of high school juniors and seniors (495 Catholics, 405 Protestants, and 121 Jews) and found that children reared in neighborhoods where others were similar to them in terms of religious affiliation (e.g., Jewish adolescents raised in traditionally Jewish neighborhoods) had significantly lower levels of depressed affect than did adolescents raised in religiously dissimilar neighborhoods. Likewise, Williams and Hunt (1997) found that Muslims who lived in Scotland were nearly four times as likely to report significant depressive symptoms as were non-Muslims. While approximately 50% of the elevated risk resulted from differences in the social and psychological conditions of Muslims and non-Muslims (e.g., greater stress, lower standard of living, and lack of social support), Muslims still had twice the risk of depressive symptoms as non-Muslims after such factors were controlled. Similar findings have been reported for Ashkenazi Jews in various Israeli neighborhoods (Rahav et al., 1986).

Differences in Religious Involvement. Another explanation for the differences in rate of depression across religious groups is the level of religious involvement. For example, Jews possess religious attitudes, beliefs, and practices that distinguish them from the members of other religions. Research on large, representative samples shows that Jews' rates of participation in public religious activities, participation in informal religious groups, and strength of conservative beliefs about the Bible are lower than those of any other large religious group in the United States (Musick & Strulowitz, 1998). Could these differences in religious involvement by themselves explain the relationship between religious affiliation and depression? We now turn our focus to whether religious involvement predicts depressive symptoms or depressive disorder.

RELIGIOUS INVOLVEMENT AND DEPRESSION

We retrieved more than 100 published studies that explored the religion-depression relationship in some fashion, including 22 prospective cohort studies (see part VIII). In general, we find that greater religiousness is associated with less depression, although this is not always the case. The most likely methodological explanation for the lack of consistency in results is sampling error (Hunter & Schmidt, 1990). The second most likely explanation is that the relationship changes depending on how religiousness is measured. In the section that follows, we attempt to find consistency in the literature by examining specific aspects of religious involvement.

Measures of General Religious Involvement

Many studies have examined the relationship between depression and multi-item measures of religious belief and behavior. We refer to these multi-item measures as indicators of "general religious involvement" because they lump together public religious involvement (e.g., frequency of church attendance), private religious involvement (e.g., frequency of private prayer), and religious salience (e.g., self-rated importance of religion) into a single measure. Such

measures tend to be quite reliable, since the measurement errors associated with each individual item tend to cancel each other out when the items are aggregated (Schmidt & Hunter, 1996).

Multi-item measures of religious involvement are consistently negatively correlated with measures of depressive symptoms and affect (Brown & Gary, 1987, 1994; Fehring, Brennan, et al., 1987; Morse & Wisocki, 1987; Brown, Ndubuisi, et al., 1990; Pressman et al., 1990; Strayhorn et al., 1990; Brown, Gary, Greene, et al., 1992; Bienenfeld et al., 1997; Kendler et al., 1997; Ferraro, 1998). The zero-order correlations between these measures and depression are in the range of $r = -.07$ to $r = -.40$, with a central tendency around $r = -.20$.

When covariates are controlled, the associations between general measures of religious involvement and depression adjust downward to some degree. For example, after controlling for age, marital status, geography, race, and obesity, as well as for religious salience and strength/comfort from religion, Ferraro (1998) found that scores on a three-item measure of general religious practice were still negatively associated with depressive symptoms, but at a lower magnitude than generally reported ($\beta = -.08$, $p < .01$). It is not surprising, though, that when other measures of religious involvement or importance are controlled simultaneously, the strength of the association between general religiousness and depression declines (Fehring, Brennan, et al., 1987; Brown & Gary, 1994) because of the high correlation between religious variables.

Several explanations exist for the weak relationship between general measures of religious involvement and depression. Foremost among these is that some religious activities may be *positively* related to depression, whereas other religious activities are *negatively* related to depression, each relationship canceling the other out to some degree if different religious variables are combined into a single index, particularly in a cross-sectional analyses (Koenig, Hays, George, et al., 1997). For example, private religious activities such as prayer often increase when stress increases as the person attempts to cope with a difficult situation or problem, resulting in a positive relationship between private religious activity and stress/depression. Alternatively, activities such as church attendance may decrease when depression increases, resulting in a negative relationship between public religious activity and depression. Combining private and public religious activities into a single measure, then, tends to cancel out the association of each with depression in cross-sectional analyses.

One way to get around this problem is to disaggregate items in a combined religious measure and to include these together in a regression model as separate variables. This is also problematic, as noted earlier, since different religious variables are often highly correlated. When these different but highly correlated variables are included in a single regression model, they must "fight" for common variance in the dependent variable (depression). This problem is called *multicollinearity*. For example, Koenig (1998b) found in a sample of 455 adults that religious attendance was strongly correlated with intrinsic religiosity ($r = .44$) and with religious coping ($r = .49$); likewise, private religious activities were strongly correlated with intrinsic religiosity ($r = .47$) and with religious coping ($r = .50$), and religious coping was strongly related to intrinsic religiosity ($r = .66$). Including several of these highly correlated religious variables into the same regression model will weaken or eliminate the correlations between some of the religious variables and depression.

We recommend that each religious dimension be examined separately concerning its relationship to depression (in separate regression models). Three dimensions of religion are commonly recognized: organizational religious activities, nonorganizational religious activities (private religious activities such as prayer, Scripture study), and subjective religiousness (e.g., self-rated religiousness, importance of religion, intrinsic religiosity). Other, less widely recognized religious constructs are specific religious beliefs and religious coping (the use of religion as a way of handling stress). We now review studies that have examined the relationships between each of these religious dimensions and depression.

ORGANIZATIONAL RELIGIOUS INVOLVEMENT

The most common and easiest way to measure religiousness is to assess participation in public, social, or organizational religious activities (ORA), often determined by single-item measures of attendance at religious services, membership in religious organizations, or short scales that combine two or more single-item measures of such involvement. Measures of organizational religiosity are readily included in large surveys, but the variance in responses is not very great because nearly half of the population attends religious services on a weekly basis (Schmidt & Hunter, 1996). Also, such measures cannot accurately capture the religiousness of highly religious people who are not able to participate in religious congregations because of physical health problems (Idler & Kasl, 1997b).

Despite these psychometric limitations, most studies that have assessed the relationship between ORA and depression report inverse relationships. Of studies that examined the cross-sectional association of ORA (usually frequency of church attendance), more than 85% found fewer depressive symptoms in the more religiously active (Brown & Prudo, 1981; Hallstrom & Persson, 1984; Hertsgaard & Light, 1984; Spendlove et al., 1984; Idler, 1987; Koenig, Moberg, & Kvale, 1988; Maton, 1989; Nelson, 1989b; Idler & Kasl, 1992; Sherkat & Reed, 1992; Wright, Frost, et al., 1993; Brown & Gary, 1994; Koenig, 1995a; McIntosh & Danigelis, 1995; Sorenson et al., 1995; Thearle, Vance, & Najman, 1995; Commerford & Reznikoff, 1996; Kennedy, Kelman, et al., 1996; Braam, Beekman, van Tilburg, et al., 1997; Koenig, Hays, George, et al., 1997; Mosher & Handal, 1997; Koenig, Pargament, & Nielsen, 1998; Musick & Strulowitz, 2000; Strawbridge, Shema, et al., 1998; Husaini et al., 1999). Persons actively involved in religious community are also less likely to be diagnosed with depressive disorders or to score in the clinical range on dichotomized measures of depression (Hallstrom & Persson, 1984; Koenig, Moberg, & Kvale, 1988; Kennedy, Kelman, et al., 1996; Braam, Beekman, van Tilburg, et al., 1997; Strawbridge, Shema, et al., 1998). Only a few studies have reported weak or nonexistent associations between ORA and depression (for example, Siegel & Kuykendall, 1990; Schafer, 1997; Musick, Williams, et al., 1998).

When demographic, psychosocial, and health status are controlled, the association between ORA and depression is reduced to some degree, usually yielding standardized regression coefficients in the range of beta = −.10 to beta = −.18 (Spendlove et al., 1984; Idler, 1987; Sherkat & Reed, 1992; McIntosh & Danigelis, 1995; Commerford & Reznikoff, 1996; Braam, Beekman, van Tilburg, et al., 1997; Koenig, Pargament, & Nielsen, 1998; Musick, Williams, & Jackson, 1998; Husaini et al., 1999; Strawbridge, Shema et al., 1998). Well-controlled studies using depressive diagnoses or depressive symptom thresholds as the dependent variable suggest that lack of ORA increases the odds of experiencing a significant depression by 20 to 60 percent (Spendlove et al., 1984; Braam, Beekman, van Tilburg, et al., 1997; Koenig, Hays, George, et al., 1997).

The largest drop in strength of the ORA-depression relationship occurs when social support, health status, and functional disability are added to models. If controlling for social support and physical health status reduces the size of the correlation between ORA and depression, this does not mean that there exists only a weak relationship between religious activity and depression. Rather, it may mean only that we have controlled for the mechanism by which ORA helps to reduce depression (i.e., by increasing social support and/or improving physical functioning).

Longitudinal studies on the relationship between ORA and depression tend to confirm cross-sectional findings (Maton, 1989; Idler & Kasl, 1992; Kennedy, Kelman, et al., 1996; Koenig, George, & Peterson, 1998; Musick, Koenig, et al., 1998; Musick & Strulowitz, 2000). Furthermore, Musick and Strulowitz (2000) have found that ORA predicts the future development of depressive symptoms differently depending on one's religious affiliation. In a seven-year prospective study of 8,866 randomly sampled Americans, Musick and Strulowitz esti-

mated the effects of attendance at formal and informal religious activities on somatic retardation symptoms of depression and depressed affect. Formal religious involvement was measured by attendance at religious services and participation in church- or synagogue-related social events; informal organizational religious involvement was assessed by frequency of participation in other religious groups.

Zero-order correlations between the depression and ORA variables at baseline were small ($r = -.04$ to $r = -.06$). The longitudinal effects, however, were more considerable. When sociodemographic variables and baseline levels of somatic-retarded depressive symptoms, physical health, and several measures of social support were controlled, investigators found that involvement in formal religious activities at baseline significantly predicted fewer somatic-retarded depressive symptoms at the seven-year follow-up for most groups of Christians. Similar findings were found when depressed affect was examined. Among Jews ($n = 192$), however, formal religious involvement at baseline predicted greater somatic-retarded depressive symptoms and depressed affect at follow-up. In contrast, participation in informal church groups was associated with lower levels of depressive symptoms in Jews but higher levels of depressive symptoms in Christians. The investigators attributed these findings to the different psychosocial resources provided by each type of organizational religious activity for Christians and Jews in modern culture. Thus, while ORA may deter depression, by no means does it do so in a "one size fits all" fashion.

NONORGANIZATIONAL RELIGIOUS ACTIVITY

Studies have also investigated the relationship between private religious activities (private prayer, reading of scripture, watching or listening to religious broadcasts) and depressive symptoms. Measures of private religious activity (NORA) have typically been single-item indicators (Hallstrom & Persson, 1984; Spendlove et al., 1984; Pargament, Ensing, et al., 1990; Sherkat & Reed, 1992; Commerford & Reznikoff, 1996; Koenig, Hays, George, et al., 1997; Shafer, 1997; Koenig, Pargament, & Nielsen, 1998; Musick, Koenig, et al., 1998), although some researchers have employed multi-item measures (Koenig, Kvale, & Ferrel, 1988; Mosher & Handal, 1997; Strawbridge, Shema, et al., 1998; Husaini et al., 1999).

Most studies find that NORA is only weakly related to depression. Both zero-order and multivariate associations tend to be small, regardless of whether NORA is measured with single or multiple items (Hallstrom & Persson, 1984; Spendlove et al., 1984; Koenig, Moberg, & Kvale, 1988; Pargament, Ensing, et al., 1990; Sherkat & Reed, 1992; Commerford & Reznikoff, 1996; Koenig, Hays, George, et al., 1997; Shafer, 1997; Strawbridge et al., 1998; Koenig, Pargament, & Nielson, 1998). Of course, there are exceptions to this general trend, with some studies finding more sizable inverse associations between NORA and depressive symptoms (Idler, 1987, in men; Mosher & Handal, 1997).

Longitudinal studies also report inconsistent results. Koenig, George, and Peterson (1998) found that frequency of private religious activity was not significantly related to speed of remission of depression among 87 older adults hospitalized for medical illness. In contrast, Kendler et al. (1997) found, in their study of 1,902 female twins, that personal devotion (including frequency of prayer to God) was inversely related to depressive symptoms ($\beta = -.09$, $p < .0001$, after controlling for multiple covariates). High personal devotion also appeared to buffer the effects of stressful life events ($p < .01$, when controlling for multiple covariates), prompting the authors to conclude that religious devotional activities are "associated with less of a response to the depressogenic effects of stressful life events" (p. 325).

In cross-sectional studies that show no association or a positive association between NORA and depression, it is important to remember that people often increase prayer and other private religious activities in response to negative life situations or uncontrollable stress and decrease such activities when life returns to normal, giving the false impression in the short run that NORA is associated with poor mental health. Given the few longitudinal studies, the short follow-up periods, and the weak religious measures used (typically single-item measures where 80% of the sample chooses one or two of the three or four response options), it is difficult to come to any firm conclusions about the NORA-depression relationship.

RELIGIOUS SALIENCE AND MOTIVATION

Religious Salience

As with NORA, studies typically use single-item measures to assess self-rated religiousness and importance of religion (e.g., Levin & Markides, 1985; Ross, 1990; Sorenson et al., 1995; Ferraro, 1998; Koenig, Pargament, & Nielsen, 1998). Many cross-sectional studies that utilized single-item measures of subjective religiousness (SR) reported small bivariate associations with depressive symptoms. These weak relationships are not surprising, since, as noted before, single-item measures with three or four response options usually contain low amounts of variance (Schmidt & Hunter, 1996).

On the other hand, some studies find that single-item measures of religious salience are rather good predictors of low depression risk, particularly in longitudinal studies (Rabins, Fitting, Eastham, & Zabora, 1990; Ross, 1990; Braam, Beekman, Deeg, et al., 1997; Shafer, 1997). For example, Ross (1990) found that, when relevant covariates were controlled, a single-item measure of strength of religious belief was associated with reduced depressive symptoms in a sample of Illinois residents ($\beta = -.12$). Rabins and colleagues (1990) at Johns Hopkins examined emotional adaptation during a two-year prospective study of 62 highly stressed caregivers of patients with Alzheimer's disease or end-stage cancer. Investigators found that a single item assessing self-reported strength of religious beliefs significantly predicted positive affect ($p < .0001$, after controlling for covariates).

In a one-year follow-up of 177 older adults in the Netherlands, Braam, Beekman, Deeg, et al. (1997) also found that subjects who indicated that a strong religious faith was "not important" in their lives (low religious salience) were almost three times more likely to become depressed than those who indicated high religious salience (OR 2.66, 95% CI 0.95–7.55, p = ns). Among the 48 subjects who were depressed at baseline, those who indicated low religious salience were almost six times more likely to experience persistent depression than those who indicated high religious salience (OR 5.91, 95% CI 1.48–23.6). The effect was especially strong among women ($n = 24$), where 100% of those with low religious salience had persistent depression, compared with 50% of those with high religious salience ($p < .01$).

Religious Motivation

Following Allport (1950), social scientists distinguish between extrinsic religious motivation (a strictly utilitarian motivation for being religious) and intrinsic religious motivation (finding religion valuable in and of itself). Multi-item scales that measure intrinsic and extrinsic religious motivation include those by Allport and Ross (1967), Hoge (1972), and Feagin (1964). Extrinsic religiousness is often found to be positively related to depression. The correlations between extrinsic religiosity and depressive symptoms have typically been in the $r = .03$ to $r = .25$ range, with a central tendency around $r = .15$ (Watson, Morris, et al., 1988, 1989; Nelson, 1989a; Rosik, 1989; Park et al., 1990; Genia & Shaw, 1991; Rigby et al., 1993). Thus, people who are motivated to be religious because of the benefits that religion brings (e.g., social prestige, friends, affirmation of one's lifestyle) are at greater risk for depression.

In contrast, multi-item measures of intrinsic religious motivation usually correlate negatively with depression. These correlations have typically been in the range of $r = -.05$ to $r = -.36$, with a central tendency around $r = -.20$ (Watson, Morris, 1988, 1989; Nelson, 1989a; O'Connor & Vallerand, 1989; Pargament, Ensing, et al., 1990; Park et al., 1990; Genia & Shaw, 1991; Park & Cohen, 1993; Rigby et al., 1993; Wright et al., 1993; Koenig, 1995a; Commerford & Reznikoff, 1996). Thus, people experience lower levels of depressive symptoms if they are motivated to be religious because they believe being religious is worthwhile in and of itself.

The intrinsically religious are also only about 55% as likely as extrinsics to receive a diagnosis of major depression (Spendlove et al., 1984), although controlling for health, income, and education reduces the difference to some degree. Medically ill adults who score high on intrinsic religiousness are also somewhat less likely to be diagnosed with depression than those with low scores (Koenig, Moberg, & Kvale, 1988).

Longitudinal research on religious salience, religious motivation, and depression is limited. In an eight-week prospective study, Park et al. (1990) administered Feagin's six-item IR and six-item ER scales to 83 introductory psychology students who had indicated that religion was either fairly or extremely important to them (44 Catholics, 39 Protestants). Among Catholics, baseline IR (T1-IR) was positively related with Time 2 (T2) depression (.58, $p < .001$) in the bivariate analysis, but the finding disappeared in the multivariate analysis. T1-ER was unrelated to T2 depression in both bivariate and multivariate analyses for Catholics and Protestants. Among Protestants, on the other hand, while T1-IR was unrelated to T2 depression in the bivariate analysis, it was significantly and inversely related to T2 depression in the multivariate analysis. There was also a significant interaction between negative life stress (NLEs) and T1-IR on T2 depression among Protestants; as T1-IR scores decreased, the positive relationship between NLEs and T2 depression increased (indicating stress buffering). This effect was especially strong ($p < .001$) for uncontrollable life stress. In this prospective study, then, greater intrinsic religiousness predicted less depression over time and buffered the negative effects of life stress (particularly uncontrollable life stress) on depression. This was true only for Protestants, however, not for Catholics (just as Tix & Frazier, 1997, had reported).

Similarly, Koenig, George, and Peterson (1998) found that, among 87 depressed older adults hospitalized for medical illness, scores on a 10-item intrinsic religious motivation scale predicted speed of remission from depression. After researchers controlled for multiple sociodemographic, medical, and psychosocial covariates, a 10-point increase on the intrinsic religious motivation scale (approximately one standard deviation) was associated with a 70% increase in speed of depression remission (Figure 7.1). Among subjects whose level of physical disability stayed the same or worsened during the one-year follow-up (i.e., their physical illnesses did not respond to medical treatments), speed of remission from depression increased by more than 100% for every 10-point increase on the intrinsic religiosity measure.

Thus, the available data on religious salience, religious motivation, and depression lead to several conclusions. First, extrinsic religious motivation—being involved in religion for its potential to confer temporal benefits—is associated with a greater risk of depressive disorder and a higher degree of depressive symptomatology. Second, religious salience and intrinsic religious motivation tend to be negatively related to depressive symptoms. Finally, in studies that examine whether levels of religious salience or intrinsic religiousness predicts longitudinal change in depressive symptoms after controlling for relevant covariates—the best nonexperimental evidence for causality that scientists have—these variables appear to prevent depression and/or speed recovery. Further studies, however, are clearly needed.

RELIGIOUS BELIEFS

Do religious beliefs per se have any causal association with depression? This question is difficult to answer because most research on the topic is cross-sectional. Carey (1974), Hallstrom and Persson (1984), Kroll and Sheehan (1989); Alvarado et al. (1995); Koenig (1995a); and Schafer (1997) all found that single-item measures of belief in God (or in a personal God), belief in Jesus as God's divine son, and belief in an afterlife were associated with lower levels of depressive symptoms or better adjustment. For example, Hallstrom and Persson (1984) reported significantly lower rates of depressive disorder among those who believed in God, a finding that persisted after the authors controlled for multiple covariates. Among those with major depression, 26.7% said they did not believe in God, compared with 10.9% of those without depression. Note, however, that only 68% of the Swedish sample believed in God, providing at least some variance in response. Low variance in response has been a problem in many studies in the United States, where the vast majority of the population has traditional beliefs (e.g., 96% believe in God, 90% in heaven) (Princeton Religion Research Center, 1996).

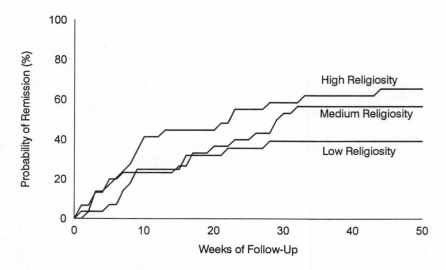

FIGURE 7.1 Kaplan-Meier survival curves for remission of depression by intrinsic religiosity (sample subdivided into thirds based on Hoge scale scores). From Koenig, George, & Peterson (1998), *American Journal of Psychiatry* 155, 536–542. Used with permission.

Some investigators report little or no association between religious beliefs and depression. Mosher and Handal (1997), Schafer (1997), and Musick and Strulowitz (2000) found that conservative beliefs about the Bible, belief in Heaven and Hell, and belief in life after death were unrelated to depressive symptoms. Likewise, using a factor score represented by four items assessing conservative religious belief (belief in God, belief in a God who rewards and punishes, literal belief in the Bible, belief in being "born again"), Kendler et al. (1997) found that conservative religious belief was unrelated to depressive diagnoses in a sample of 1,902 female twins from Virginia. Again, however, failure to demonstrate a significant relationship in some of these studies may be the result of the low variance in responses.

On the other hand, Koenig, Pargament, and Nielsen (1998) found that the content of religious belief has a lot to do with how well older medical patients cope with their physical health problems. Studying a sample of 577 patients over age 55 who were hospitalized with acute medical illness, investigators found that, while benevolent reappraisals of God were associated with lower depression scores, patients' appraisals of God as punishing or as without power to affect their situations or their beliefs that demonic forces were involved were all positively related to depression scores.

In summary, the research findings are mixed on whether religious beliefs per se are predictors of depression. No large prospective studies have examined the relationship between religious belief and depression (with the exception of Musick & Strulowitz, 2000, who examined conservative beliefs about the Bible only). Clearly, more serious construct validity work is needed before high-quality studies can be designed to compare different beliefs systems in an appropriate way and thereby answer the question of whether the content of faith really makes a difference.

RELIGIOUS COPING

Responding to the well-known association between stressful life events and depression, researchers have examined the roles that religion plays in moderating this relationship. In general, studies have used one of two approaches. The first approach looks at the "main effect" of religious coping on depression. The second approach looks for statistical evidence that stressful life events and religious involvement interact in their effect on depressive symptoms or depressive disorder.

Religious Coping and Depression

In recent years, the association between religious coping and depression has been studied intensively in medical settings. Koenig, Cohen, Blazer, Pieper, et al. (1992) developed a three-item index of religious coping (RCI) to be administered in an interview format. The RCI assesses the extent to which an individual uses religion in general to cope with stress. Cross-sectional research indicates that scores on the RCI tend to be inversely correlated with self-report and clinician-rated measures of depression (Koenig, Cohen, Blazer, Pieper, et al., 1992; Koenig, Cohen, Blazer, Kudler, et al., 1995). This inverse relationship is particularly strong for the cognitive symptoms of depression but weakens with somatic symptoms (Koenig, Cohen, Blazer, Kudler, et al., 1995). In some studies, the inverse association of RCI scores and depression is more modest (Koenig, 1995a; Grosse-Holtforth et al., 1996; Koenig, Weiner, Peterson, et al., 1998).

Longitudinal research suggests that the link between RCI scores and depressive symptoms might indeed be a causal one. Koenig, Cohen, Blazer, Pieper, et al. (1992) found that scores on the RCI at baseline were inversely related to depressive symptoms at follow-up an average of six months later in a sample of 202 elderly medical inpatients. This longitudinal effect persisted ($\beta = -.18$, $p = .01$) after the authors controlled for baseline levels of depression, extent and nature of medical illness, and a variety of other physical health and sociodemographic variables. Some evidence suggests that religious coping might help to deter depression in medical settings by conferring more adaptive health control beliefs (Grosse-Holtforth et al., 1996).

Pargament has examined the effects on depression of specific religious activities that people use to cope with stressful life situations (Pargament, Ishler, et al., 1994; Belavich & Pargament, 1995; Brant & Pargament, 1995; Pargament, Smith, & Brant, 1995; Pargament, 1997; Koenig, Pargament, & Nielsen, 1998; Pargament, Zinnbauer, et al., 1998; Pargament, Koenig, & Perez, 2000). Through a programmatic series of studies, Pargament has begun to identify the specific cognitive and behavioral elements of religious coping that relate to mental health and adjustment. In what is perhaps their most comprehensive look at the elements of religious coping to date, Pargament's team administered scales for assessing 22 different aspects of religious coping to a group of 577 medically ill older adults (Koenig, Pargament, & Nielsen, 1998; Pargament, Koenig, & Perez, 2000). Participants were asked to indicate the extent to which they used these cognitive and behavioral religious methods for coping. Investigators also administered an 11-item scale for assessing depression, along with several other measures of mental health. Using a series of regression equations, Pargament and colleagues found that certain types of religious coping (e.g., seeing God as benevolent, collaborative religious coping, religious helping, and seeking the support of clergy and church members) were inversely related to depressive symptoms (when age, race, sex, education, and severity of medical illness were controlled). These results suggest that some forms of religious coping—particularly those that involve interpreting stressful life circumstances in terms of God's love, developing a sense of working "with God" to solve problems, and giving and receiving support from other religious people—may facilitate adaptation to severe life stressors.

Koenig, Pargament, and Nielsen (1998) also found that some types of religious coping were positively related to depression. These included seeing God as punitive, demonic reappraisals, reappraisals of God's power, passive religious deferral, self-directed religious coping, dissatisfaction with one's religion and congregation, and pleading for direct intercession from God. These forms of coping may be "red flags" for greater psychological distress. The magnitude of the associations between these religious coping methods and depressive symptoms was on the order of $\beta = .20$. Other studies by Pargament and colleagues have reported a similar pattern of results (see Pargament, 1997).

The work of Pargament and his colleagues sheds much light on the cognitive and behavioral mechanisms that help to explain the relationships between certain measures of religious involvement and depression. Their research suggests that the particular ways that people engage religious beliefs in the process of coping with stressful life events might be critical to understanding how religious beliefs and practices prevent or bring on depression. Interpreting one's circumstances in terms of God's love and benevolence and seeking comfort through productive engagement with God, one's congregation, and the clergy all predict less depression in the aftermath of stressful life events. Conversely, interpreting one's stressful circumstances in terms of God's impotence, God's malevolence, or one's own sinfulness, surrendering control over one's circumstances solely to God, and experiencing conflict with God or one's religious community all correlate with more depressive symptoms in the setting of serious medical illness and other life stress.

Religion as Deterrent or Moderator of the Stress-Depression Relationship

Other studies have addressed the stress-depression relationship by statistically examining the interaction between religion and stress in their relationship to depressive symptoms. Does the association between religious involvement and depression change as a function of the amount and/or type of life stress that one has encountered (as in the Park et al., 1990, study described for intrinsic religiousness)? The focus here is not so much on the "main effect" of religious involvement as a predictor of depression but, rather, on the interaction between stress and religious involvement. In other words, as stress increases, does the association between religion and depression weaken or strengthen; does religion facilitate coping better at lower or higher levels of stress?

Most studies that have examined the interaction of stress and religious involvement find at least partial support for a stress-moderating effect (Idler, 1987; Brown & Gary, 1988; Friedrich et al., 1988; Maton, 1989; Park, et al., 1990; Siegel & Kuykendall, 1990; Idler & Kasl, 1992; Pargament, Ishler, et al., 1994; Kendler et al., 1997; Strawbridge, Shema, et al., 1998; Bickel et al., 1998). For example, Kendler et al. (1997) found that, as stressful life circumstances increased in their sample of 1,902 female twins, the negative relationship between personal religious devotion and depressive symptoms became stronger ($\beta = -.04$, $p < .01$). Personal conservatism or memberships in a conservative religious denomination had no such moderating effect on the relationship between stressful life events and depression.

On the other hand, some cross-sectional research suggests that certain life stressors may make highly religious people more vulnerable to depression. Strawbridge, Shema, et al. (1998) assessed organizational and nonorganizational religious involvement among 2,537 residents of Alameda County, California. They also asked respondents two questions about depressed mood and loss of interest; a yes response to either question was interpreted as indicating depression. Investigators obtained a history of the types of stressors experienced during the previous 12 months. Using interaction terms to examine whether religious involvement moderated the relationship between stressful life events and depression, researchers found that for people who had encountered family stressors (e.g., abuse, marital problems, caregiving burdens, and child problems), organizational and nonorganizational religious involvement were associated with a greater likelihood of depression. For NORA, a positive association with depression was found for those having child problems ($\beta = .09$, $p < .05$); for ORA, positive associations with depression were found for those experiencing physical or emotional abuse from a family member ($\beta = .15$, $p < .05$), stress of caregiving for a spouse, parent, or grandchild ($\beta = .21$, $p < .05$), and marital problems ($\beta = .20$, $.05 < p < .10$). Conversely, for people who reported having encountered nonfamily stressors (e.g., financial problems, neighborhood problems, health problems, chronic illness, or disability), organizational and nonorganizational religious involvement were both

associated with a significantly lower likelihood of depression.

Thus, research that examines the cognitive and behavioral ways that people use religion to cope with life's crises has helped us to better understand the dynamic and transactional nature of the relationship between religion and depression. The fact that most of this research is cross-sectional in nature, however, makes it difficult to conclude that some methods of religious coping deter depression or that others exacerbate it. The same applies to cross-sectional research that suggests that religious activities are more effective in coping with some stressors and less effective with others.

QUASI-EXPERIMENTAL AND EXPERIMENTAL RESEARCH ON RELIGION AND DEPRESSION

So far, this chapter has reviewed cross-sectional and longitudinal studies that examine the religion-depression relationship. This observational research is considered nonexperimental because no variables were experimentally manipulated, thus leaving open the question of causality. We turn now to quasi-experimental and experimental research that has examined the role of spiritual activities or religiously oriented psychotherapies in reducing depressive symptoms.

Quasi-Experimental Studies

At least three studies (Morris, 1982; Griffith, Mahy, et al., 1986; O'Laoire, 1997) have examined whether intense, discrete religious experiences designed to facilitate spiritual growth lead to a reduction in psychological symptoms (including depression). Griffith, Mahy, et al. (1986) conducted prepost assessments on a group of 16 members of a Baptist church in Barbados that encouraged a practice called "mourning," a five-day spiritual ritual involving seclusion, limited diet, and extended periods of prayer and mystical experiences. Prior to engaging in this activity and at the conclusion of this activity, mourners were assessed on the Symptom Check List-90 (SCL-90). These Yale investigators found that subjects who underwent the mourning exercise had significant prepost score reductions on every subscale of the SCL-90, except the somatization subscale. In particular, subjects dropped more than a standard deviation (d = 1.16) on the depressive symptoms subscale.

Morris (1982) conducted psychological assessments on 24 people with chronic illness before and after they made pilgrimages to Lourdes, France, in search of physical healing. Subjects were administered the Beck Depression Inventory (BDI) immediately prior to the pilgrimage, one month after the pilgrimage, and 10 months after the pilgrimage. Morris reported significant reductions in depressive symptoms from the first assessment (mean score = 7.2) to the second assessment (mean score = 1.0) and from the first assessment to the third assessment (mean = 0.8). A mean BDI score of 7 indicates mild depressive symptoms. Thus, across the 10-month follow-up period, these religious pilgrims went from mild depressive symptoms to virtually no symptoms.

A third study yielded somewhat provocative results concerning the efficacy of intercessory prayer. Recall from chapter 6 that O'Laoire (1997) randomly assigned 90 people (referred to as "agents") to pray for the needs of 406 subjects. Agents were assigned to either a directed prayer group or a nondirected prayer group. Subjects were randomly assigned to either a directed prayer, a nondirected prayer, or a no-prayer control group. Agents prayed for their subjects for 15 minutes daily for 12 weeks. Three agents prayed for each subject. Prior to beginning the study, both subjects and agents completed measures of depression, anxiety, and self-esteem. Interestingly, scores on well-being variables improved for both the subjects and the agents of prayer during the 12-week period. This finding is not surprising, since many prepost studies find a decrease on scores of dysfunction with no intervention at all. What was surprising, however, was the comparison of agents and subjects on the well-being scores. The agents of prayer actually had greater improvements in well-being than the subjects of prayer.

Given the amount of energy currently devoted to examining the health benefits of inter-

cessory prayer, the spotty track record of positive results in such studies, and the theological conundrums raised by putting intercessory prayer "to the test," O'Laoire's results are provocative. Regardless of whether intercessory prayer affects the health of those prayed for, it may at least have psychological benefits for those doing the praying. Koenig, Pargament, & Nielsen, (1998) reported similar findings in their cross-sectional study of 577 older hospitalized medical patients. They found that "religious helping" (e.g., praying for others, encouraging others spiritually) was correlated with fewer depressive symptoms and higher quality of life.

The three studies reviewed above are quasi-experimental. The lack of control groups (i.e., people who did not participate in the mourning experience, physically disabled people who did not go on the pilgrimage, or agents who did not participate in prayer) seriously limits the validity of any causal conclusions about the relationship between these spiritual experiences and depression. However, the data are consistent with the hypothesis that depressive symptoms are highly sensitive to religious activities.

Adjunctive Religious Psychotherapies

Using a more traditional experimental design, patients with depression are randomly assigned to either a religious treatment condition or a control group, and outcomes are compared. Azhar and Varma (1995a, 1995b) examined the effects of religious psychotherapy as an adjunct to standard psychological care for the treatment of depression in one study and bereavement in another. In the first study, a group of 64 highly religious Muslim patients in Malaysia with dysthymia were randomly assigned to one of two treatment conditions. In the second study, 30 highly religious Muslim patients who were experiencing bereavement were likewise randomly assigned to religious treatment or control groups. The control condition in both studies consisted of weekly supportive psychotherapy plus psychotropic medication. The religious psychotherapy condition consisted of weekly supportive psychotherapy plus psychotropic medications along with weekly sessions of religious psychotherapy. Religious psychotherapy involved discussions of religious issues specific to the patients and the prescription of religious practices (such as reading verses from the Holy Koran and prayer). Patients in religious treatment groups, then, received 12 to 20 additional 45-minute sessions of religious psychotherapy as an adjunct to standard psychotherapy and pharmacological intervention (see Varma, Zain, & Kerian, 1997, for a complete review).

Patients in the religious psychotherapy groups experienced a greater reduction of depressive symptoms (measured by the Hamilton depression scale) in both studies. In the first depression study, differences between the treatment and the control groups were significantly different at three months but not at six months. In the bereavement study, a statistically significant difference emerged by six months (but was not present during the first three months). While these results are supportive of the general hypothesis that religious involvement speeds remission from depression, it is impossible to determine whether the differential efficacy in these two studies results from the religious content of the additional psychotherapy per se or simply from the additional psychotherapy. In other words, could these results simply stem from the well-documented dose-effect relationship in psychotherapy, which holds that more treatment leads to greater improvement?

Accommodative Religious Psychotherapies

At least five studies have now compared the effectiveness of religious-oriented and secular psychotherapy in the treatment of depression. In these studies, researchers randomly assigned religiously committed depressed Christian patients (mostly students scoring in the clinical range on measures of depression) either to a standard form of psychotherapy or to religious psychotherapy. The standard forms of psychotherapy against which religious psychotherapy has been tested include cognitive therapy (Pecheur & Edwards, 1984), cognitive-behavioral therapy (Propst, 1980; Propst, et al., 1992), and rational-emotive therapy (Johnson & Ridley, 1992; Johnson, DeVries, et al., 1994). In each

study, approximately one-half of patients received a religious version of the standard secular therapy.

The first of these studies was conducted by Propst (1980), who examined the effects of religious and nonreligious imagery as used in cognitive therapy with 44 mildly depressed religious subjects selected from an undergraduate class of 300 students. Subjects were randomly matched into four groups: (1) nonreligious imagery group ($n = 11$), (2) religious imagery group ($n = 9$) (received same therapy as first group except used religious Christian imagery instead of standard secular images), (3) therapist-led discussion group ($n = 13$), and (4) a wait-list control (WLC) group ($n = 11$). Subjects met for one-hour during group therapy sessions two times per week for four weeks. Postintervention assessments performed at the termination of therapy revealed that 14% of the religious imagery group and to 60% of the nonreligious imagery group ($p < .05$), 60% of the WLC group ($p < .05$), and 27% of the nondirected therapist-led discussion group subjects remained depressed. After six weeks, there was no significant difference among the three treatment groups. This initial study provided evidence that religious imagery works at least as well as other group therapy techniques for treating mild depression in religious college students and may speed remission of depression in religious subjects.

Next, Propst et al. (1992) compared the effectiveness of religious-based cognitive-behavioral psychotherapy (RCBT) to (1) traditional secular therapy (CBT), (2) ordinary pastoral counseling (PCT), and (3) a no-therapy WLC group. A total of 59 mild to moderately depressed religious patients (mean age 40) were randomized to each of the four treatment groups. RCBT used Christian religious rationales and arguments to counter irrational thoughts, along with religious imagery. Subjects were assessed before treatment, at termination of treatment, and at three and 24 months after termination. The intervention groups received eighteen 50-minute sessions over 12 weeks. Results indicated that only the RCBT group had significantly lower self-rated scores on the Beck Depression Inventory than the WLC group on posttreatment evaluation ($p < .001$), although the CBT and PCT groups also experienced similar trends in that direction ($p = .02$ for CBT vs. WLC and $p = .02$ for PCT vs. WLC). With regard to observer-rated scores on the Hamilton Depression Rating scale, only the RCBT group and the PCT group scored significantly lower than the WLC group ($p < .05$ for both comparisons); the CBT group did not score significantly lower than the WLC group at treatment termination. When the proportions of subjects in the three treatment groups that experienced "meaningful change" in depressive symptoms are compared, we find that only the PCT group (80%, $p < .001$) and the RCBT group (68.4%, $p < .05$) were significantly different from the WLC group (27.3%). By 3 months and 24 months posttreatment, there were no significant differences among the treatment groups (RCBT vs. CBT vs. PCT).

Therapist effects were evident during the course of the study, but not in the direction expected. Subjects in the RCBT group who received RCBT from nonreligious therapists scored significantly lower on posttreatment BDI scores than did either the WLC group ($p < .001$) or subjects in the CBT group who received CBT from nonreligious therapists ($p < .02$); similar findings were present for scores on the HDRS. At three months after study termination, subjects who received RCT from nonreligious therapist did significantly better than subjects who received RCT from religious therapists ($p < .05$). In summary, religious subjects with mild to moderate depression who received RCBT recovered faster from depression then did subjects who received secular CBT (better immediate posttreatment results); surprisingly, nonreligious therapists achieved better results using RCBT then did religious therapists using RCBT.

The rationale behind the religious treatment approaches in the psychotherapy studies described (Propst, 1980; Pecheur & Edwards, 1984; Johnson & Ridley, 1992; Propst et al. 1992; Johnson, DeVries, et al., 1994) is the principle of accommodation (Johnson & Ridley, 1992). The principle of accommodation states that secular approaches to psychotherapy can and should be translated into the language of religious clients (a) to make religious clients more open to value change, (b) to make the treatments understandable to religious clients, and (c) to improve compliance, satisfaction, and mental health outcomes. Researchers interested in accommodative forms of religious counseling have developed religious versions of standard cognitive-behavioral techniques such as cognitive restructuring, cognitive coping skills, and rational-emotive therapy. These religious techniques, including "biblical counter-challenges" and "scriptural justification for rational thinking," are thought to be theoretically equivalent to standard cognitive-behavioral therapies (Propst, 1996) but more amenable to the religious worldview of religious clients. Researchers interested in accommodative forms of religious psychotherapy have also developed religious methods of delivering such interventions, such as prayer and religious imagery (Propst, 1996). We again stress that nonreligious therapists can deliver such religious interventions just as effectively as religious therapists (Propst et al., 1992).

McCullough (1999) conducted a meta-analytic review of the results of the religious psychotherapy studies performed to date. Since all five studies reported pretreatment and posttreatment scores using the Beck Depression Inventory (BDI), he aggregated the differences in the treatment efficacy between the religion-accommodative therapies and the standard cognitive-behavioral treatments. McCullough found a mean weighted effect size of $d = .18$ ($p = .34$), suggesting that conservative Christian clients who participated in religion-accommodative therapies did not experience significantly greater symptom reduction than those who received standard psychotherapy. He concluded that, since religion-accommodative psychotherapy is certainly no worse than standard cognitive-behavioral psychotherapy, clients who desire such a religious approach to psychological care should probably be given the opportunity to receive it (McCullough, 1999).

Thus, quasi-experimental research suggests that some forms of religious activity can lead to substantial reductions in depressive symptoms. Several studies also indicate that religiously oriented psychotherapies might, compared to standard approaches to psychological treatment, lead to faster remission of depressive symptoms. Additional research is needed to determine whether religion-accommodative psychotherapies differ from standard psychotherapies in effectiveness when patients are followed over longer periods of time.

SUMMARY AND CONCLUSIONS

Research on religion and depression supports five conclusions. First, the data on religious affiliation and depression suggests that two religious groups—Jews and people who are not affiliated with any religion—are at elevated risk for depressive disorder and depressive symptoms. These findings have been replicated across a number of large, well-designed studies.

Second, some aspects of religious involvement are indeed associated with less depression. People who are involved frequently in religious community activity and who highly value their religious faith for intrinsic reasons may be at reduced risk for depression. Even when these persons experience depression, available research suggests that they recover more quickly from it than those who are not religious. Conversely, people who are involved in religion for reasons of self-interest or extrinsic gain are at higher risk for depression. While the longitudinal data do not definitively prove causal inference, they do provide considerable circumstantial evidence in support of causality. Certainly, the existing evidence is strong enough to encourage further inquiry, through either prospective cohort studies or clinical trials.

Third, certain measures of religious involvement—particularly private religious activities and religious beliefs—are not as strongly related to depression as are organizational religious activities or intrinsic religious commitment. The fact that certain aspects of religion are consistently associated with a lower risk for depression, while others are not, may help researchers build theories to explain how religion affects this disorder. Since most of the research is based upon cross-sectional studies and seldom utilizes sophisticated measures of religious belief or private practice, further research, especially prospective studies that assess multiple dimensions of the religious variable, is needed to sort out these complex relationships. The results of such research may facilitate the design of future strategies for depression screening, prevention, and treatment in religious and nonreligious settings.

Fourth, religious involvement plays an important role in helping people cope with the effects of stressful life circumstances. Some forms of religious coping are related to a lower likelihood of depression during or after stressful life events, while others appear to be "red flags" for greater depression risk. Furthermore, although religious activities buffer against the deleterious effects of some psychosocial stressors (particularly health and financial stressors), they may exacerbate the effects of others (family-related stress); such conclusions, however, are again based largely on cross-sectional studies.

Fifth, prospective cohort studies and quasi-experimental and experimental research all suggest that religious or spiritual activities may lead to a reduction in depressive symptoms and that religiously accommodative psychotherapy is at least as effective as secular psychotherapy for depression. These findings are consistent with much of the cross-sectional and prospective cohort research that has found less depression among the more religious.

8

Suicide

IN 1996, NEARLY 31,000 PEOPLE in the United States committed suicide, making suicide the ninth leading cause of death for Americans. Experts recognize that this figure is probably an underestimate, since many "accidental" deaths and many of those reported as due to "natural causes" may be disguised suicide (Garland & Zigler, 1993). Suicide is the third leading cause of death among people ages 15–24. Recent data have shown a sharp rise in the rate of completed suicides among U.S. adolescents since 1950 (Wagner, 1997). The problem of suicide is particularly serious among adolescent males, since males commit suicide five times more frequently than females. In 1995, the suicide rate for males ages 15–24 was 23.4 per 100,000, and suicide accounted for 16% of all deaths for males in that age group—a rate that has quadrupled since 1950 (Ghosh & Victor, 1994).

The problem of adolescent suicide has been further delineated by the national school-based Youth Risk Behavior Survey (1995). This survey of a nationally representative sample of more than 11,000 students in grades 9–12 assessed suicidality through a variety of measures and found that 27% of students had seriously considered attempting suicide and 16.3% had made specific plans to end their lives during the 12 months preceding the survey. Furthermore, of the 16%, approximately one-half (8.3% of all respondents) indicated that they had actually attempted suicide. Two percent of students indicated that they had made a suicide attempt that required medical attention. Generalizing from these nationally representative data to the entire nation, it appears that a staggering 276,000 high school students in the United States made at least one suicide attempt that required medical attention in the 12 months prior to the study.

Given the prevalence of suicidal thoughts

and attempts and of completed suicide, and of the costly consequences of suicide in terms of person-years of life, many researchers over the past 100 years have examined the associations between religious involvement and suicide. In the present chapter, we review this large body of research.

AGGREGATE VERSUS INDIVIDUAL DATA

Summarizing the research on religion and suicide is challenging because of the wide variety of research designs, measures, and theoretical frameworks that have been used to investigate the relationship. Studies have typically employed one of two major designs; some have used individuals as the unit of analysis, whereas others have used aggregate data, such as suicide rates for cities, states, counties, or nations, as the unit of analysis. Studies that employ these two designs address two different kinds of questions. Studies that use aggregate data typically examine sociological variables that are useful for predicting *rates* of suicide. Studies that use individual observations are useful for examining qualities of individual persons (e.g., personality, attitudes, social functioning, physical health, and mental health) that might be useful for predicting and understanding suicide. It is not safe to assume that findings about suicide generated using aggregate level data (i.e., suicide rate) would be replicated if one were to analyze individual data. Making such overgeneralizations is what some researchers have called the *ecological fallacy*. As we review the research in this chapter, we distinguish individual-level studies from those that use aggregate-level data and attempt ourselves to avoid the ecological fallacy.

This review of research takes us through a wide body of literature, from sociology to psychology to medicine. We examine the research on the relationship between religious affiliation (denomination) and completed suicide, suicide attempts, suicidal ideation, and attitudes toward suicide. Of particular interest is research on the associations between *level of religious involvement* and these four suicide measures.

DURKHEIM AND HIS LEGACY

Without a doubt, the most important figure in the history of research on religion and suicide is Emile Durkheim. More than a century ago, Durkheim's (1897) book *Suicide* argued that suicide was primarily a sociological phenomenon, rather than an individual psychological one. Durkheim's goal was to demonstrate that many human phenomena, including both religion *and* suicide, were best understood as sociological events, rather than as characteristics of individuals. In *Suicide*, Durkheim presented data that suggested that the suicide rates in different population groups (e.g., nations, provinces, counties) were directly related to the characteristics of the social groups themselves, rather than to the characteristics of the persons who made up those social groups.

For these reasons, Durkheim posited that religion and suicide might be intimately connected. He suggested that societies with higher levels of integration (including religious and family integration) would have lower suicide rates. Because Durkheim theorized that the Roman Catholic Church fostered greater degrees of religious integration than did Protestant churches, he expected that predominantly Catholic countries would have lower suicide rates than Protestant ones. Through a series of arguments and the presentation of tables and tables of statistical data, Durkheim made a strong case for the value of religious integration as a deterrent to suicide. Summarizing this argument, he notes:

We see why, generally, religion has a prophylactic effect upon suicide. It is not, as has sometimes been said, because it condemns it more unhesitatingly than secular morality, nor because the idea of God gives its precepts exceptional authority which subdues the will, nor because the prospect of a future life and the terrible punishments there awaiting the guilty give its proscriptions a greater sanction than that of human laws. . . . If religion protects man against the desire for self-destruction, it is not that it preaches the respect for his own person to him with arguments *sui generis*; but because it is a society. . . . The details of dogmas and rites are secondary. The essential thing is that they be capable of supporting a sufficiently intense collective life. (pp. 169–170)

Durkheim's intellectual paradigm for understanding the religion-suicide connection reigned supreme through the first half of the twentieth century, and his basic conclusions went largely undisputed. However, as we shall see, researchers who have pursued the religion-suicide relationship have come a long way since Durkheim.

RELIGIOUS AFFILIATION AND SUICIDE

Suicide Rates

Since Durkheim's initial formulation, his theoretical work has often been a starting point for empirical inquiries into the nature of the religion-suicide relationship (Stack, 1992a). Some of these studies have used rather limited statistical methods that have led to invalid conclusions (Gargas, 1932; Gibbs, 1961). Several studies have found that population aggregates, such as U.S. counties, that have higher percentages of Roman Catholics also have lower suicide rates (Faupel et al., 1987; Joubert, 1995; Skog et al., 1995). Two studies that used individual-level data (Becker et al., 1987; Goss & Reed, 1971) found that Protestants were overrepresented among both people who attempted suicide and those who completed it.

The relationship between Catholicism and Protestantism and suicide rate, however, has been called into question at both the individual (e.g., Beit-Hallami, 1975) and the aggregate levels (Pope, 1976; Bainbridge & Stark, 1982; Bankston et al., 1983; Stark, Doyle, & Rushing, 1983; Day, 1987). Many later studies based on analyses of country-level, state-level, and county-level data have found that, after relevant confounders are controlled, geographic areas that are predominantly Roman Catholic do not have lower suicide rates than predominantly Protestant areas (Templer & Veleber, 1980; Stack, 1980b, 1981; Breault, 1986; Wasserman & Stack, 1993; Burr et al., 1994). In fact, one time-series study that used U.S. data from 1940 to

1984 found that the years in which the percentage of Roman Catholics in the population was high preceded years in which suicide rates rose (Yang, 1992), suggesting a *positive* relationship between Catholic affiliation and suicide (although Catholic affiliation here may have been nominal in many cases).

Other investigations have found that the suicide rates in the U.S. states are negatively related to the percentage of Jews who reside in the state (Bailey & Stein, 1995; Lester, 1996a; for individual-level findings see Danto & Danto, 1983) and positively related to the percentage of residents who are not affiliated with a religion (Joubert, 1995). Another study found that states' percentages of Baptists and Mormons were negatively related to suicide rates over a 14-year period from 1976 to 1989 (Gruenewald et al., 1995). In an aggregate sample of suicide rates from 71 nations, Simpson and Conklin (1989) found that the percentage of Muslims was negatively correlated with suicide rate, even after the authors controlled for a large variety of socioeconomic variables. Finally, Levav and Aisenberg (1989a, 1989b), using Israeli data, found that Muslim Arabs and Christians had lower suicide rates than did Jews during the years 1976–1985.

Attempting to make sense of the relatively large set of studies that employ aggregate data to examine the effects of religious affiliation on suicide is a formidable task. Very different conclusions emerge when slight changes are made in statistical controls or population aggregates sampled, leading to the impression that these studies yield few consistent findings about the religious affiliation-suicide relationship. However, taken as a whole, the existing data on religious affiliation and suicide seem to suggest two important conclusions. First, the uniquely suicide-deterrent aspects of Catholicism appear to have waned toward the close of the twentieth century (perhaps because of an increasing number of nominal Catholics). Second, many religions, including Protestant sects and Islam, appear to have lower suicide rates at the aggregate level. As we will see later, the Durkheimian tradition of comparing the suicide rates of various religious groups has been supplanted by a more fruitful line of research that examines the effects of degree of religious *involvement* on suicide.

Attitudes toward Suicide

Compared to the inconsistent findings on the relationship between religious affiliation and suicide rate, the data on religious affiliation and attitude toward suicide are clearer. In general, Catholics are less tolerant of suicide than are non-Catholics (Singh et al., 1986). Bagley and Ramsay (1989) and Johnson, Fitch, et al. (1980) found that members of conservative Protestant groups and Catholics had more negative attitudes toward suicide than did members of less conservative denominations or Jews. In particular, people who do not belong to any religious denomination are more accepting of suicide than those who do belong (Siegrist, 1996).

Suicidal Ideation

As with completed suicide, religious affiliation is a relatively poor predictor of suicidal thoughts (i.e., serious consideration of suicide in the present or past) (Harkavy-Friedman et al., 1987; Stack & Lester, 1991). However, Bagley and Ramsay (1989) found that mainline Protestants and Mormons were considerably less likely than members of other religious groups to report past suicidal ideation. Also, in a group of university students, Murray (1973) found that students who were Catholic reported having had less suicidal ideation in the past than did Protestants or others. Students who indicated that their affiliation was something other than Catholic or Protestant were significantly more likely to indicate having had previous thoughts about suicide.

Suicide Attempts

At the individual level, religious affiliation appears to exert a rather modest influence on suicide attempts (Harkavy-Friedman et al., 1987). In a survey of 473 high school students, Conrad (1991) found no differences in self-reported history of suicide attempts as a function of religious preference (i.e., Catholic, Protestant, Jewish, other, none). Bagley and Ramsay (1989) also found no denominational differences among respondents who reported past suicide attempts. A variety of other studies have examined the association of religious affiliation with attempted suicide, but most of these studies were conducted in clinical settings and failed to control for the distribution of religious groups in the surrounding populations.

RELIGIOUS INVOLVEMENT AND SUICIDE

Despite the considerable effort that has gone into exploring the effects on suicide rates, suicidal ideation, and attitudes toward suicide of membership in a particular religious denomination, interest in this question has waned considerably in the century that has passed since Durkheim's important book. Instead, the major focus in the last quarter of the twentieth century was on whether level of religious involvement, rather than membership in a specific religious faith or denomination, has a suicide-deterring effect (see also Stack, 1992a).

Stack (1983a) has suggested a variety of mechanisms by which involvement in religion might deter suicide. These include: (a) encouraging beliefs in an afterlife and in a responsive, loving God; (b) conveying purpose and self-esteem; (c) providing role models for coping with stress and crisis; (d) offering resources for reframing life's struggles and difficulties; and (e) offering a social hierarchy, that runs counter to the socioeconomic hierarchy in which many religious people find themselves in a one-down position. Indeed, some religions even place a special emphasis on people who are at socioeconomic disadvantage. In addition, many religions disapprove strongly of suicide. Together, Stack (1983a) argues, the resources that religion offers work to deter suicide among people who are involved in religion.

Completed Suicide

Many studies, often conducted by sociologists, have examined the association of suicide rates with national or other aggregate-level indicators of religious involvement. Most of these studies find that the percentage of people involved in religion in a given geographic area (county, state, or nation) is inversely proportional to that area's suicide rate (Breault & Barkey, 1982; Hasselback et al., 1991; Trovato, 1992; Krull & Trovato, 1994; Martin, 1984; Neeleman et al., 1997). Breault and Barkey (1982), for instance, found that the 1970 suicide rates for 42 nations could be predicted by only three sociological variables—political integration (measured by number of deaths due to political violence), family integration (measured by marriage and divorce rates), and religious integration (measured by ratio of religious newspapers and books to all newspapers and books). Together, these three measures of social integration accounted for nearly 79% of the variability in suicide rates. Moreover, each of the three integration measures accounted for unique variance in suicide rates.

Bainbridge and Stark (1981) reported strong negative correlations between church membership and suicide rates for 78 large metropolitan areas in the United States during the early decades of the twentieth century. Bainbridge (1989) also found that rates of church membership were negatively associated with suicide rates in a cross-sectional survey based on data from 75 U.S. metropolitan areas with populations of more than 500,000 in 1980. However, unlike Breault and Barkey (1982), Bainbridge found that the religious involvement-suicide association was reduced to nonsignificance when measures of social integration (particularly, divorce rates and relocation rates) were controlled (see also Lester, 1987a).

In one of the few longitudinal studies, Stack (1992b) examined the association between religious involvement and suicide rates in Finland during the years 1952–1968. In this study, the investigator used a time-series design to examine the effects of divorce, unemployment, and religiousness on suicide rates in later years. Stack found that the years in which Finland's production of religious books was high were likely to be followed by years with low suicide rates (particularly for women, but also for men). Interestingly, the rate of religious book produc-

tion was strongly correlated with divorce rates ($r = .72$), suggesting that in years when religious book production was high, divorce rates were fairly low. Stack took this high correlation as evidence that religious book production and divorce were indicators of a third, latent variable that is reflected in both high divorce rates and relatively low production of religious books: individualism.

Using a statistical technique called factor analysis, Stack showed that the latent variable measured both by religious book production and rate of divorce was itself a significant predictor of suicide rates (see also Stack, 1985). Stack's analyses are important because of their suggestion that religious involvement might be negatively associated with suicide rates (at least in studies that use aggregate data) because such involvement reflects a communally oriented society, as Durkheim had argued. Stack (1983b) completed similar analyses on time-series data for the United States for the years 1954–1978 and found more robust associations between religious involvement and suicide rates for both males and females.

In contrast, Fernquist (1995–1996) failed to find even a zero-order relationship between percentage of religious book production and suicide rates for the elderly in nine European countries over the years 1975–1989. Stack (1991), using time-series data for Sweden, also failed to find a correlation between religious book production and suicide rates. In a cross-sectional study using data from 25 nations, Stack (1983a) found an inverse association between religious book production and suicide rates for women only. The association between religious book production and suicide rates for men was not significant (see also Stack, 1983c).

Only a handful of studies have examined the relationship between religious involvement and completed suicide at the individual level. However, among these few studies, the relationship found is uniformly negative. In an early case-control study, Breed (1966) compared a group of men who committed suicide in New Orleans to a group of sex- and race-matched controls. Among the men who committed suicide, informants reported that approximately 62% attended church two times per year or less.

Among the nonsuicidal controls, only about 25% of the men were reported to attend church this infrequently.

Comstock and Partridge (1972) followed more than 50,000 adult residents of Washington County, Maryland, for six years. During this six-year follow-up, the suicide rate among people who attended church once or more per week was 0.45 per 1,000. Among people who attended church less than once a week, the suicide rate was 0.95 per 1,000. Thus, people who attended church regularly were less than half as likely to commit suicide during the six-year follow-up. In a 16-year study of the residents of religious and secular Israeli kibbutzim, Kark, Shemi, et al. (1996) found that the risk of dying by suicide during the 16-year period was four times higher among members of secular kibbutzim than among members of religious kibbutzim (these kibbutzim had been matched on a variety of psychosocial and demographic variables). Finally, Wandrei (1985) found that, among a sample of women who had recently attempted suicide, those who were affiliated with no religion and those who did not view the church as a resource were significantly more likely to go on to kill themselves during the following five years.

Suicide Attempts and Suicidal Behavior

People who adhere to religious beliefs—particularly religious proscriptions against suicidal behavior—appear to be at lower risk for suicidal acts (Nelson & Farberow, 1980; Ferrada-Noli & Sundbom, 1996). In their cross-sectional survey of 34,129 adolescents, Donahue and Benson (1995) found inverse correlations between public religious involvement/salience and history of suicide attempts (zero-order correlations ranged from −.05 to −.11). Similar results were obtained by Conrad (1991) and by King et al. (1996) when they used a two-item measure of religious involvement (i.e., affiliation with any religion and at least yearly religious attendance).

Not all studies, of course, find negative relationships between religious involvement and suicidal behavior (e.g., Levav, Magnes, et al., 1988; Bagley & Ramsey, 1989). In a survey of 679 adults from Calgary, Canada, Bagley and Ramsay (1989) found that people with high levels of religiousness were actually more likely to have reported past suicide attempts ($r = .11$). Investigators explained this surprising finding by examining religious differences among people who had attempted and those who had not attempted suicide in the past. Those who had attempted suicide were also more likely to have left the church in which they were raised and to have joined a fundamentalist religion. The researchers contended that these moves to more fundamentalist religions reflected a substantial reorientation of the individuals' values and beliefs that followed the suicide attempts. However, because data were collected retrospectively, these speculations could not be tested.

Although some studies of clinical populations find that religious involvement is inversely related to suicidal and self-destructive behavior (e.g., Nelson, 1977), others do not (Corder et al., 1974; Kirk & Zucker, 1979). For example, Kirk and Zucker (1979) conducted a case-control study involving 20 African American men who had made a clinically significant suicide attempt in the past six months and 20 men from the same neighborhoods who reported never having made a suicide attempt or seriously contemplated suicide. In this small sample, Kirk and Zucker did not find that those who attempted suicide had significantly lower rates of church attendance than nonattempters. In a sample of adolescent psychiatric patients, Marks and Haller (1977) found that girls who had made suicide attempts attended church substantially less often than did nonsuicidal girls. However, they found no such difference among boys.

Suicidal Ideation

Most studies reveal a robust negative correlation between religious involvement and suicidal ideation (Salmons & Harrington, 1984; Levav, Magnes, et al., 1988; Bagley & Ramsay, 1989; Schneider et al., 1989; Kandel et al., 1991; Long & Miller, 1991; Zhang & Thomas, 1991; Schweitzer et al., 1995; Shagle & Barber, 1995; Zhang & Jin, 1996). In some studies, associations between religiousness and suicidal ideation persist even after variables such as self-esteem, life stress, and depression are controlled (De Man, Balkou, & Iglesias, 1987; Zhang & Thomas, 1991; Shagle & Barber, 1995; Zhang & Jin, 1996). In other studies, the association between religious involvement and suicidal ideation disappears when variables such as neuroticism are controlled (Lester & Francis, 1993).

In their survey of adolescents selected from public schools in 460 different communities in the United States, Donahue and Benson (1995) administered three self-report measures of religious involvement (frequency of attendance at religious services, hours in the average week spent attending services or programs at a church or synagogue, and importance of religion in one's life) and a single measure of suicidal ideation. All three religious measures were inversely correlated with suicidal ideation.

Other research suggests that religiousness is not related to history of suicidal ideation in people with handicaps and physical disabilities (Cameron et al., 1973) or in police officers (Beehr et al., 1995). A study that employed a sample of older adults found no association between religious involvement and suicidal ideation (Mireault & De Man, 1996). Whether these null results are simply the result of sampling error or point to specific populations for whom religious involvement is, in fact, *not* related to suicidal ideation, remains to be explored.

Attitudes toward Suicide

Religious people are considerably more intolerant of suicide than are less religious people. The former report less tolerance and approval of suicide (Steininger & Colsher, 1978–1979; Hoelter, 1979; Singh, 1979; Johnson, Fitch, et al., 1980; Ostheimer, 1980; Feifel & Schag, 1980–1981; Minear & Brush, 1980–1981; Best & Kirk, 1982; Singh et al., 1986; Lee, 1987; Bagley & Ramsay, 1989; Diekstra & Kerkhof, 1989; Monte, 1991; Stack & Lester, 1991; Stack & Wasserman, 1992; Stack, Wasserman, & Kposowa, 1994; Stein et al., 1992; LoPresto et al., 1994–1995; Kaplan & Ross, 1995; Seidlitz et al., 1995; Stack & Wasserman, 1995; King,

Hampton, et al., 1996; Siegrist, 1996; Neeleman et al., 1997; Neeleman et al., 1998), greater moral objection to suicide (Ward, 1980; Ellis & Smith, 1991), and greater belief that suicide should be prevented (Bascue et al., 1982). In one study, the effects of religious involvement on suicide attitudes was stronger for men than for women (Stein et al., 1989).

SUMMARY AND CONCLUSIONS

Recent major reviews on the prediction and prevention of suicide (Van Egmond & Diekstra, 1989; Ghosh & Victor, 1994; Kehoe & Gutheil, 1994; Wagner, 1997) pay little attention to the relatively large literature that shows an inverse relationship between religious involvement and suicide (84% of 68 studies; see part VIII). In spite of this neglect, the research on religion and suicide yields several tentative conclusions.

First, a century of research has failed to find any robust, consistent evidence that people with particular religious affiliations are at greater or lesser risk of suicide, although members of conservative Protestant sects and Muslims tend to have lower rates than other groups. Second, religious involvement (measured by frequency of religious attendance, frequency of prayer, and degree of religious salience) is negatively associated with suicide, suicidal behavior, suicidal ideation, and tolerant attitudes toward suicide across a variety of samples from many nations. This consistent negative association is found in data from population aggregates as well as from individual-level data. While we do not yet fully understand why religious involvement is inversely related to suicide, religion's effects are likely mediated by psychological factors such as depression, self-esteem, and moral objections to suicide, as well as by social factors such as lower divorce rates and increased social support.

Finally, it is surprising to see how little of the research on religion and suicide is longitudinal in nature. Several studies of population aggregates use time-series data, and several studies on actual suicide and attempted suicide use longitudinal designs, but by far, the majority are cross-sectional or case-control studies. This prevents us from confidently asserting cause-effect relationships. Studies that examine attempted and actual suicide, however, are limited by the fact that these events occur so infrequently. Very large, expensive, long-term prospective projects would be required to acquire sufficient power to detect an effect. Such studies may be more feasible in psychiatric populations, where the suicide risk is many times higher than in the general population; extrapolating findings to the general population, however, then becomes problematic.

9

Anxiety Disorders

I N T H I S C H A P T E R , W E F I R S T present an overview of anxiety states and disorders, discussing definitions and classification, economic and clinical consequences, and etiology. We then review research that examines the relationship between religion and anxiety and explore the use of religious beliefs and practices in the prevention and management of anxiety symptoms and disorders.

DEFINING ANXIETY

Anxiety is a normal emotion associated with the anticipation of a potentially threatening event. Normal, day-to-day anxiety serves a useful purpose by preparing our bodies and minds for perceived stresses that we must confront (e.g., the proverbial "flight or fight response"). However, for a number of people, anxiety is a contin-uous part of their lives as it becomes prolonged and excessive beyond that needed for optimum functioning.

When exaggerated worry and tension persist over time even though no immediate or specific physical or emotional threat exists, anxiety can evolve into a full-blown psychiatric disorder. Such a disorder can leave a person feeling anxious most of the time without apparent reason. The anxious feelings may be so uncomfortable that the person stops or modifies her everyday activities in order to avoid the anxiety. Some people may experience occasional bouts of anxiety so intense that it terrifies and immobilizes them (National Institute of Mental Health, 1997). Major classifications of anxiety disorder include (1) generalized anxiety disorder, (2) panic disorder and/or agoraphobia, (3) other phobia, (4) obsessive-compulsive disorder, and (5) posttraumatic stress disorder. A brief overview of each disorder now follows.

Generalized Anxiety Disorder

Generalized anxiety disorder (GAD) refers to anxiety that is much more intense and generalized than the normal anxiety most people have. GAD involves chronic, exaggerated worry over largely normal, day-to-day experiences and often has no major stressor connected with it. Having this disorder means anticipating disaster and worrying excessively about health, money, family, or work much of the time. As noted, the source of the worry is often hard to pinpoint.

People with GAD are unable to shake their concerns, even though they usually realize that their anxiety is more intense than the situation warrants. GAD sufferers cannot relax, have trouble falling or staying asleep, and may experience trembling, twitching, muscle tension, headaches, irritability, sweating, or hot flashes. They may also feel lightheaded, out of breath, or nauseated and are more easily startled than other people. GAD can be associated with chronic fatigue, difficulty concentrating, and depression, from which it may be difficult to distinguish.

Panic Disorder

People with panic disorder have overwhelming feelings of terror that strike suddenly and repeatedly with little or no warning. They can't predict when an attack will occur, and many develop intense anxiety between episodes, worrying when and where the next one will occur. A panic attack typically begins with a sudden onset of heart palpatations, breathlessness, sweating, and feelings of weakness, faintness, or dizziness. Tingling or numbness of the hands and feelings of being flushed or chilled are also common. Some panic disorder sufferers experience chest pain or smothering sensations during an attack and also may experience a sense of unreality, fear of impending doom, or fear of loss of control. Many believe they are having a heart attack or stroke, losing their mind, or on the verge of death. Attacks can occur any time, day or night, even during nondream sleep. While most attacks last only a couple of min-

utes, occasionally they can go on for up to 10 minutes or longer.

Panic disorder is surprisingly common, affecting almost 6 million Americans, and is twice as common in women as in men (Wittchen & Essau, 1993). It can appear at any age—in children, adolescents, adults, or the elderly—but most often begins in young adults. Not everyone who experiences panic attacks will develop panic disorder; many people have one attack but never have another. Panic disorder requires that a person have at least four panic attacks within a single four-week period or have one or more attacks followed by a period of at least one month of persistent fear of having another attack (*Diagnostic and Statistical Manual of Mental Disorders*, 4th edition). Panic disorder is often accompanied by agoraphobia, the fear of leaving one's house, being in a crowd, or going grocery shopping (agoraphobia means "fear of the marketplace"). Agoraphobia involves fear of being in any situation that might provoke a panic attack or from which escape might be difficult if an attack were to occur.

Other Phobic Disorders

A phobia is fear of a particular object or situation. Many people experience specific phobias, which are intense, irrational fears centered on a specific place, activity, or thing (e.g., closed-in places, heights, escalators, tunnels, highway driving, water, flying, and injuries involving blood; National Institute for Mental Health, 1997). Specific phobias aren't just extreme fear; they are irrational fear. People with phobias often realize that their fears are irrational but are unable to control the fear before it brings on a panic attack or severe anxiety.

Specific phobias strike more than one in 10 Americans, or 25 to 30 million people (National Institute for Mental Health, 1997). No one knows just what causes them, though they seem to run in families and are a little more prevalent in women. Phobias usually first appear in adolescence or young adulthood. They start suddenly and tend to be more persistent than childhood phobias. When children have specific phobias—for example, a fear of animals—those fears usually disappear over time, though they may continue into adulthood. No one knows why they persist in some people and disappear in others.

Social Phobia.   Social phobia is an intense fear of becoming humiliated in social situations or of embarrassing oneself in front of other people. It often runs in families and may be accompanied by depression or alcoholism. Social phobia typically starts in early adolescence or even younger. The most common social phobia is a fear of public speaking. Sometimes social phobia involves a general fear of social situations, such as parties. More rarely, it may involve a fear of using a public restroom, eating out, talking on the phone, or writing in the presence of other people, such as signing a check. Although this disorder is often thought of as shyness, the two are not the same (National Institute for Mental Health, 1997). Shy people can be very uneasy around others but do not experience extreme anxiety when anticipating a social situation and do not necessarily avoid circumstances that make them feel self-conscious. In contrast, social phobics may not be shy at all and can be completely at ease with people most of the time. However, particular situations, such as walking down an aisle in public or making a speech, can give them intense anxiety.

Underrecognition of social phobia remains an issue of concern, and, consequently, patients are often treated inappropriately. The reason for this is that social phobia frequently occurs simultaneously with other psychiatric disorders, including other anxiety disorders, depression, alcohol abuse, and personality disorders (Fones et al., 1998). Given the degree of disability caused by social phobia, whether "pure" or comorbid, there is need for improved education of doctors, clergy, and patients regarding its diagnosis and treatment.

Obsessive-Compulsive Disorder

Obsessive-compulsive disorder (OCD) is characterized by anxious or disturbing thoughts or rituals that appear out of the individual's control. The disturbing thoughts or impulses are called *obsessions*, and the rituals that are performed to try to prevent the obsessions are called *compulsions*; hence the term obsessive-compulsive disorder (National Institute for Mental Health, 1997). People with OCD usually receive no pleasure in carrying out the rituals they are forced to perform, which provide them with only temporary relief from the discomfort caused by the obsession. These persons are often preoccupied by thoughts of violence and fear that they might harm someone close to them, or they may spend long periods of time touching things or counting and recounting things to make sure they have done so perfectly. They also may have persistent thoughts of performing sexual acts that are repugnant to them or may be troubled by thoughts that are against their religious or spiritual beliefs (National Institute for Mental Health, 1997).

OCD strikes men and women in equal numbers and afflicts roughly one in 50 people in this country (National Institute for Mental Health, 1997). It can appear in childhood, adolescence, or adulthood but usually first shows up in early adolescence or young adulthood. A third of adults with OCD experience their first symptoms as children. The course of the disease is variable—symptoms may come and go, they may ease over time, or they can grow progressively worse. Evidence suggests that OCD is at least in part an inherited disorder. Depression or other anxiety disorders may accompany OCD, and many people with OCD have eating disorders (National Institute for Mental Health, 1997). People often try unsuccessfully to use alcohol or drugs to calm themselves. If OCD grows severe enough, it can keep the sufferer from holding a job or from carrying out normal responsibilities at home.

Posttraumatic Stress Disorder

Posttraumatic stress disorder (PTSD) is another debilitating condition that can occur soon or even years after the patient witnesses a terrifying or unusually traumatic event. People with PTSD have persistent frightening thoughts and memories of their ordeal and feel emotionally numb, especially with people to whom they were once close (National Institute for Mental

Health, 1997). PTSD, sometimes referred to as "shell shock" or "battle fatigue" during wartime, was first brought to public attention by war veterans. However, recent research has demonstrated that PTSD can result from any number of traumatic incidents, such as kidnapping, serious accidents (car or train wrecks), natural disasters, violent attacks, or being held against one's will (National Institute for Mental Health, 1997). The specific event that triggers PTSD must be something life-threatening to the individual or someone close to him or her; PTSD may also occur after one witnesses mass destruction, such as an earthquake or a plane crash.

Whatever the triggering event, some people with PTSD repeatedly relive the trauma in the form of nightmares and disturbing recollections called "flashbacks." People with PTSD also experience sleep problems, depression, feelings of detachment or numbing, irritability, and violent aggression. They may lose interest in things they used to enjoy and have trouble showing affection toward people they care about. PTSD can occur at any age, including childhood, and is often accompanied by depression and/or substance abuse (National Institute for Mental Health, 1997).

CONSEQUENCES OF ANXIETY DISORDER

Anxiety disorders are extremely common in modern society (Schatzberg, 1991). Indeed, it has been estimated that as many as 26.9 million Americans will develop diagnosable anxiety disorders at some point in their lifetime (Regier et al., 1993), and symptoms of anxiety in the general population are even more prevalent (Olfson et al., 1996). Anxiety disorders are associated with a variety of adverse psychological and physical health consequences. For example, panic disorder is frequently associated with major depression, substance abuse, impaired quality of life, and suicide (Katerndahl, 1996). Rates of suicide attempts among individuals with panic disorder are surprisingly high—as high as 20%, which exceeds the 15% rate among individuals with major depression (Hirschfeld,

1996). People who suffer from anxiety often turn to alcohol to relieve their symptoms (Kushner et al., 1990).

Marcus and colleagues (1997) recently conducted a nationwide survey of more than 20,000 households and found that those with self-reported anxiety had nearly fourfold greater disability (mean = 18.0 days spent in bed per year) than respondents who reported little or no anxiety (mean = 4.8 bed days). The authors of this study concluded that self-reported anxiety in combination with other medical conditions may be associated with extensive functional disability.

The high prevalence of anxiety disorders and their associated comorbid conditions and functional disabilities exact a high cost on our society. In 1990, the estimated direct and indirect costs to society of anxiety disorders totaled $46.6 billion, or approximately one-third of all mental health costs. Nearly three-quarters of this amount is due to lost productivity (DuPont et al., 1996).

CAUSES OF ANXIETY DISORDER

Other than PTSD, where vivid recall of a traumatic event may trigger severe anxiety, the etiology of many anxiety disorders remains poorly understood. The role of genetic factors is not yet fully known, although there is a clear familial aggregation (Gorwood, 1998). Twin studies have found genetic factors to be at least as important as environmental factors for some anxiety disorders, such as panic disorder and phobias. Some have suggested that anxiety disorders are related to a deficiency in the endogenous opioid system that many be congenital or acquired (Sher, 1998). Challenge studies have demonstrated that individuals with panic disorders and social phobias have a sensitivity to certain compounds, such as carbon dioxide, cholecystokinin, lactate infusions, or caffeine, which may trigger anxiety attacks (Bourin et al., 1998). Serotonergic pathways likely play a major role in anxiety disorders (Nutt et al., 1998). In addition, dopaminergic function and striatal dopamine uptake appear reduced in some anxiety disorders. There is also evidence of cardio-vascular and adrenergic abnormalities.

ANXIETY AND RELIGIOUSNESS

Freud has argued that religion's focus on punishing wrong or sinful thoughts or deeds can lead to excessive guilt (Freud, 1907, 1927). Such guilt can increase anxiety and generate neuroses. Others have argued that religion often buffers against and relieves anxiety (Bergin, 1983). We now examine the evidence for each argument.

On the one hand, Spellman and colleagues (1971) found that individuals who had recently undergone a sudden religious conversion ($n = 20$) experienced significantly higher anxiety than individuals who had become religious gradually over time ($n = 20$) (both groups were picked for the study by local ministers). Although Steketee and colleagues (1991) found no differences in religiosity or religious affiliation between 33 OCD patients and 24 patients with other anxiety disorders, they did find that religiosity in OCD patients was significantly related to severity of OCD symptomatology ($r = .40$, $p < .04$, uncontrolled). In particular, religiosity was correlated with total guilt ($r = .37$, $p < .05$) and interpersonal harm guilt ($r = .37$, $p < .05$) in these patients.

Recall that Zeidner and Hammer (1992) also reported a positive relationship between religious or spiritual coping and increased anxiety (chapter 5). These investigators conducted a cross-sectional survey of 261 Jewish northern Israelis who experienced missile attacks during the Gulf War (55% women, 48% single, mean age 29). They measured a number of coping activities and resources, including "increased engagement in religious activities" and use of "spiritual/philosophical" resources. State anxiety and personal stress symptoms were assessed using standard scales. Investigators found that both high levels of religious activities and use of spiritual resources were correlated with greater anxiety ($r = .33$, $p < .05$, and $r = .20$, $p < .05$, respectively) and more physical symptoms ($r = .29$, $p < .05$, and $r = .18$, $p < .05$, respectively). Associations persisted after other variables

were controlled in a regression model. The investigators concluded that spiritual persons were more likely to perceive war as a threat to their religious culture, nation, and people than those who were less spiritual. Alternatively, given the severe stress that many were experiencing, a number of persons may have turned to religion for comfort during this traumatic period in their lives (i.e., anxiety may have led to religion, rather than religion to anxiety).

Finally, Dhawan and Sripat (1986) conducted a study of 40 undergraduate students in Northern India to examine the moderating effect of religiosity on experimentally induced death anxiety. Subjects were divided into high ($n = 20$) and low religiosity ($n = 20$) groups on the basis of their scores on Bhushan's scale (an Indian religiosity scale). Fear of death was experimentally induced by exposing subjects with high and low religiosity to death threat cards. Investigators found that, compared to unexposed subjects, subjects in the experimental group had greater need for affiliation with others after exposure to the death threat cards (as predicted). Religiosity, however, did not moderate the effect of experimentally induced fear of death on affiliation (i.e., religiosity did not reduce fear of death and consequently decrease the subjects' need for affiliation).

On the other hand, research has found that whether one's religious orientation is *intrinsic* (i.e., religion chosen as an end in itself) or *extrinsic* (i.e., religion chosen in order to achieve other ends) may be a key factor in determining whether religiousness has positive or negative effects on anxiety. For example, Baker and Gorsuch (1982) administered an intrinsic-extrinsic measure of religious orientation and a standard anxiety scale to a group of 52 participants in a religious wilderness camp in southern California. They found that trait (dispositional) anxiety was negatively correlated with intrinsic scores ($r = -.33$, $p < .05$) and positively correlated with extrinsic scores ($r = .35$, $p < .01$). They also found that other negative psychological constructs, including lack of self-sentiment (i.e., poor social integration), ego weakness (i.e., inability to balance one's emotional forces), and paranoia (i.e., suspicious insecurity), were positively correlated with extrinsic religiousness but negatively correlated with intrinsic religiousness.

A negative correlation between intrinsic religiousness and anxiety and a positive correlation between extrinsic religiousness and anxiety has been confirmed in other studies (e.g., Sturgeon & Hamley, 1979; Bergin et al., 1987; Tapananya et al., 1997). Tapananya and colleagues (1997) conducted an investigation of the relationship between intrinsic religiousness and worry in a sample of elderly Buddhists from Thailand who were living in Canada and a group of elderly Canadian Christians. This study found an overall inverse relationship between worry and intrinsic religious orientation in both Buddhists and Christians. Interestingly, like many of the studies of Christian populations discussed earlier, Buddhists who were more extrinsic in their religious orientation were found to be even more prone to worry than extrinsic Christians.

Investigators explained the significant difference in worry between extrinsic Buddhists and extrinsic Christians as the result of differences in belief systems; Christianity allows for redemption from a forgiving God at any stage of the life cycle, whereas Buddhism offers no help from a personal savior but only the promise of enlightenment. The Buddhist who does not achieve enlightenment before death will not be liberated from samsara, or the cycle of death and reincarnation. The researchers concluded, "Therefore, for Buddhists higher levels of worry might be associated to a greater extent with the realization that their extrinsic religious behavior does not help in alleviating individual responsibility or guilt" (p. 80).

Although measures of intrinsic and extrinsic religiousness may help to explain the mixed findings regarding the religion-anxiety relationship, studies show that other aspects of religion may also influence anxiety. Hertsgaard and Light (1984) surveyed a random sample of 760 women on farms in North Dakota and found that women who attended church more than once a month scored significantly lower on anxiety and depressive symptoms (as measured by the Multiple Affect Adjective Check List) than those who attended less often ($p < .0001$, with numerous other variables controlled in a regression model). In this study, Catholic and Lutheran women scored significantly higher on anxiety and depression scales than did women of other faiths.

Koenig, Ford, and colleagues (1993) examined the relationship between religious involvement and anxiety disorders among 2,969 young, middle-aged, and elderly adults in North Carolina. Among young adults (18–39 years), rates of anxiety disorder were lower among frequent church attenders, mainline Protestants, and those who considered themselves born-again Christians. In contrast, anxiety disorder was more frequent among younger adults who were affiliated with fundamentalist Pentecostal religious groups, those with no religious affiliation, and those who frequently watched religious television programs or listened to religious programs on the radio. Koenig and colleagues also found that among middle-aged adults (40–59 years), social phobia was less common among frequent church attenders and among those who considered themselves born again. However, this relationship could largely be explained by the greater social support enjoyed by frequent attenders. Investigators concluded that "a pattern of both positive and negative relationships [exists] between religion and anxiety disorder that is most evident among young adults age 18 to 39, and weakens with age as dynamic factors increase the complexity of these relationships" (p. 321).

One drawback of many studies in this area is their cross-sectional nature, which limits our ability to sort out causation and to identify dynamic changes in religiousness and anxiety that only longitudinal data can reveal. A positive cross-sectional correlation between religious involvement and anxiety may mean that religious activities lead to increased anxiety or guilt. On the other hand, it may also mean that anxiety acts as a stimulus for prayer and other religious activities, which over time help to relieve anxiety and guilt. Indeed, when Williams and colleagues (1991) followed 720 randomly selected adults longitudinally to examine the effect of religious attendance on "psychological distress," they found that frequency of attendance at Time 1 (baseline) was significantly (and inversely) related to psychological distress at

Time 2 (two years later). This relationship remained robust even when adjusted for sociodemographic variables ($p < .01$). More important, when examining the interactions among religious attendance, stressful life events, and psychological distress, the investigators found that frequent religious activity buffered against the negative mental health consequences of negative life stress that occurred during the two-year follow-up period.

DEATH ANXIETY AND RELIGIOUSNESS

Anxiety and fear of death are closely related. "Fear" is usually associated with a very specific threat, whereas anxiety is often nonspecific. The predominant distress associated with death is the fear of the unknown (Pressman et al., 1992). Fear of death, then, is not so much a fear as a ubiquitous anxiety state about an existential fact of life.

As with other types of anxiety, research on the relationship between religious beliefs and death anxiety reveals mixed results (Thorson & Powell, 1989). Some studies show that religious beliefs and commitment are related to specific aspects of death anxiety but not to the total construct as generally defined. For example, the dimension of death anxiety sometimes referred to as "fear of the unknown" has been related to religious motivation (Thorson & Powell, 1989). Other studies show different relationships, depending on the aspect of religion assessed and the dimension of death anxiety examined.

Gartner and colleagues (1991) reviewed research on the relationship between religious involvement and death anxiety. Six studies found less fear of death among subjects who were more religious (Young & Daniels, 1980; Richardson et al., 1983; Smith et al., 1983; Tobacyk, 1983; Aday, 1984; Westman & Canter, 1985). Three studies found more fear of death in religiously involved subjects (Beg & Zilli, 1982; Florian et al., 1984; Dodd & Mills, 1985). Finally, five studies found no relationship between religious commitment and death anxiety

(Muchnik & Rosenheim, 1982; Mahabeer & Bhana, 1984; Rosenheim & Muchnik, 1984; Kunzendorff, 1985; Dahawn & Sripat, 1986).

A more comprehensive review reveals that the majority of studies find that those who are more religiously active or committed experience lower levels of death anxiety. For example, Templer (1972) found that religiously involved persons had lower anxiety about death, and, of those who were affiliated with a religion, the most religious had the least death anxiety. In a study of elderly Catholic Germans, Wittkowski, and Baumgartner (1977) found that those who were the most religious had less anxiety about death. Likewise, Florian and Kravetz (1983) found that Jews who were more religiously involved had less fear of personal death than Jews who were only moderately religious or nonreligious. Similarly, Minear and Brush (1980) found a significant inverse relationship between death anxiety and belief in an afterlife. A similar relationship is found in clinical samples. Gibbs and Achterberg-Lawlis (1978) reported that terminally ill cancer patients who were more religious had less anxiety about death than did less religious patients, and Kaczorowski (1989) found that cancer patients with high levels of spiritual well-being had lower levels of anxiety.

Because some studies have reported finding no relationship between religiousness and death anxiety (Muchnik & Rosenheim, 1982; Mahabeer & Bhana, 1984; Rosenheim & Muchnik, 1984; Kunzendorff, 1985; Dhawan & Sripat, 1986), more recent research has focused on how different dimensions of religiousness relate to different aspects of death anxiety. For example, Thorson and Powell (1990, 1991) found that those who were older and who scored higher on intrinsic religiousness (Hoge scale) had significantly less anxiety about death. On the other hand, in a sample of older adult men, Thorson and Powell (1989) found that only two of 25 statements on a questionnaire about death anxiety—"I am not at all concerned over whether or not there is an afterlife" and "I am looking forward to a new life after I die"—correlated with scores on the Hoge scale ($r = -.41$, $p < .001$, and $r = .55$, $p < .001$, respectively). Thus, intrinsic religiousness appeared in that study to relate only to specific aspects of death anxiety.

When Alvarado and colleagues (1995) explored the relationship of eight separate religious variables to both death anxiety and death depression, they found that people with the lowest levels of death depression had greater strength of religious conviction and greater belief in an afterlife. People with less death anxiety also were found to have greater strength of religious conviction. Paradoxically, these same individuals were less likely to believe that the most important aspect of religion is that it offers the possibility of life after death. Indeed, people who believed that the most important aspect of religion is that it offers the possibility of life after death had both higher death depression and death distress. This finding suggests that people who are more anxious or depressed by the prospect of death may try to become more religious in an attempt to allay their fears. However, such an approach is not a guaranteed remedy. "Perhaps, faith, belief, and commitment must come first before one experiences a lowering of death discomfort," the investigators concluded (p. 204).

Another possibility is that the relationship between religious involvement and death anxiety is not linear. Leming (1980) surveyed a random sample of 372 relatively well-educated residents of Northfield, Minnesota, nearly half of whom had experienced the death of a friend or family member within the past year. Religiousness was assessed by 10 items selected from various religion scales; fear of death was assessed by Leming's 15-item Death Fear Scale. Religiosity (religious experience, belief, and ritual) was significantly and inversely related to fear of death, although when the relationship was plotted it suggested an inverted-U type pattern. Leming concluded that this finding provided support for Homan's Thesis, which suggests that religiosity may serve the dual function of "afflicting the comforted and comforting the afflicted" (p. 358). A careful examination of Leming's plots, however, demonstrates relatively weak support for this hypothesis (since most of the curve sloped downward), and others have failed to replicate the inverted-U type rela-

tionship between anxiety and religious involvement (Koenig, Ford, et al., 1993).

Although there is substantial evidence that religion may play a role in relieving death anxiety, the evidence also suggests that both "religion" and "death anxiety" are complex, multidimensional phenomena. More research is needed to address how and in what context religion might be applied to the treatment of death anxiety and specific anxiety disorders. A brief overview of the limited research on this topic is presented in the next section.

RELIGIOUS AND SPIRITUAL INTERVENTIONS IN ANXIETY DISORDERS

If religious beliefs or practices, particularly intrinsic religiousness, can somehow buffer against stress and reduce the likelihood of experiencing anxiety, might such factors be used as therapeutic tools in the treatment of anxiety disorders? Unfortunately, there have been few studies to date on the use of religious interventions for this purpose (McCullough, 1999).

Among studies that have examined the efficacy of religious and spiritual interventions for treating anxiety problems, most have employed meditation as a relaxation technique. Indeed, several meditation studies suggest that such interventions can significantly reduce anxiety in individuals with either mild or severe anxiety problems. For example, Carlson et al. (1988) conducted a randomized controlled trial to determine the effects of devotional meditation (DM) on physiological state and psychological stress. DM consisted of a period of prayer and quiet reading and pondering of biblical material. This technique was compared to progressive relaxation (PR). The interventions were delivered in six sessions of 20 minutes each over a two-week period. Subjects, who were 36 undergraduates at a Christian liberal arts college in the Chicago area, were randomly assigned by sex to either DM, PR, or a wait-list control group (WL). Heart rate and skin temperature were assessed, and electromyogram (EMG) was used to monitor tension in four muscle groups.

Subjects completed a variety of standard anxiety, tension, and emotional adjustment scales. Results indicated that subjects in the DM group experienced reduced muscle tension in two of four sites, whereas subjects in the PR group experienced increased tension in two of four muscle sites. Postintervention assessment revealed that anger and anxiety scores were significantly lower in the DM group compared to the PR group or the WL control group, although no physiological differences were observed.

Not all studies, however, have confirmed these results. Elkins et al. (1979) conducted a randomized clinical trial involving 42 members of a Baptist church in Tennessee (mean age 34). Subjects were randomly assigned to one of three groups: 10 days of deep muscle relaxation training (DMR), 10 days of training in prayer (P), or no treatment (C). Prayer was either traditional petitionary prayer (50%) or reflective prayer (50%). Outcomes were measures of muscle tension in the frontalis muscle group by EMG and state anxiety as assessed with a standard scale. Subjects in the DMR group experienced significantly greater reduction of muscle tension than did those in the prayer group or the control group. DMR subjects also experienced a significantly greater reduction in anxiety than the control group but not a significantly greater reduction compared to the prayer group. There were no significant differences in either muscle relaxation or anxiety between the prayer and the control groups, and type of prayer (reflective vs. intercessory) was also unrelated to outcome.

One study has examined the effects of Buddhist meditation as a treatment for anxiety disorder. Kabat-Zinn and colleagues (1992) administered a meditation intervention to 22 individuals who met DSM-III criteria for generalized anxiety disorder or panic disorder with or without agoraphobia. The meditation-based program consisted of weekly two-hour structured classes on relaxation and stress reduction and a 7.5-hour mostly silent meditation retreat in the sixth week of the eight-week intervention. This study found a statistically significant and clinically important reduction in anxiety and in frequency of panic attacks in 20 of the 22 patients treated with the meditation-based inter-

vention. A three-year follow-up of 18 of the 22 patients showed that reductions in anxiety and panic attacks achieved through meditation were maintained among those who complied with the meditation regimen (Miller et al., 1995).

In addition to meditation, a few studies have employed more explicit religious interventions. These studies, however, have involved primarily religious clients. For example, Azhar and colleagues (1994) found that in a group of deeply religious Muslim patients, religious psychotherapy used in conjunction with standard psychotherapy and antianxiety drugs was more effective in reducing generalized anxiety than were standard psychotherapy and antianxiety drugs alone. The religious psychotherapy consisted of having the subjects discuss specific religious issues, reading from a holy text, and encouraging prayer and meditation. This study suggests that, at least for highly religious individuals, overtly religious psychotherapy can be used as a tool to reduce anxiety (if done in conjunction with traditional treatments).

Another form of religious intervention for anxiety problems might be participation in a religious pilgrimage. Nearly 20 years ago, Morris (1982) conducted a prospective cohort study of 24 persons with serious, chronic physical illness who made a pilgrimage to the healing shrine at Lourdes, France. Subjects were assessed during the month preceding the pilgrimage (T1) and at one month (T2) and 10 months (T3) after return. Subjects received Spielberger's State-Trait Anxiety Inventory at all three time points. Morris found a significant lessening of both state and trait anxiety from T1 to T2 ($p < .01$) and from T1 to T3 ($p < .01$) and a significant decrease in state anxiety from T2 to T3 ($p < .05$). The relationships remained significant when the subjects were stratified by sex. Since there was no control group to use for comparison, however, these results are difficult to interpret.

Are religious approaches for treating anxiety effective only with the very religious, or can they be applied more broadly to moderately religious or nonreligious individuals? At present, we simply don't know. Recall that Alvarado and colleagues (1995) concluded that forcing oneself to become more religious or to attend religious services more frequently is not a guaranteed remedy for reducing anxiety. More research is needed to determine whether more sensitive forms of religious or spiritual encouragement, depending on the individual's baseline level of religious or spiritual belief, might help in the treatment of anxiety problems.

SUMMARY AND CONCLUSIONS

Anxiety disorders are a public health concern because they are prevalent and because they tend to be chronic and disabling. These conditions are associated with a host of other negative emotional and physical health consequences, including depression, alcohol abuse, and suicide. While anxiety is a normal, even necessary emotion for dealing with life's uncertainties, if allowed to persist unchecked it can seriously affect quality of life and even physical health.

While one study has found that religiousness is associated with severity of symptoms in obsessive-compulsive disorder, the preponderance of evidence suggests that religion as a whole, especially intrinsic religiousness, tends to buffer against anxiety. Part of the difficulty in demonstrating consistent negative relationships between anxiety and different dimensions of religious involvement is that anxiety itself may be a stimulus for prayer and other religious activities. When people are anxious or fearful, they often cry out to God for relief and may plunge into religious activities for both comfort and distraction. This creates the illusion that anxious people involve themselves in religious practices and also gives the impression in some cross-sectional studies that religion is either unrelated or positively related to anxiety.

Religious involvement may be especially important in protecting persons with serious medical illness from experiencing anxiety related to dependency, loss of control, and end-of-life issues. Although the very limited evidence to date suggests that religious interventions are most helpful in treating religious individuals with anxiety, other spiritual-based interventions, such as meditation, may be useful for treating anxiety in more secular populations.

Schizophrenia and Other Psychoses

IN THIS CHAPTER, WE EXAMINE how religion relates to schizophrenia and other psychotic disorders, symptoms, traits, and tendencies. Before delving into these associations, we provide an overview of psychotic disorders, describing the different types of psychoses and emphasizing their health and economic consequences.

PSYCHOTIC DISORDERS

Psychotic disorders are a group of mental illnesses characterized by an imbalance of brain neurotransmitters (dopamine, in particular) that causes symptoms such as paranoia (fear that someone intends to harm or injure the person), delusions (fixed, false beliefs from which the person cannot be dissuaded), hallucinations (sounds, sights, or sensations that are perceived, yet are not real), and abnormal thought processes (e.g., looseness of associa-

tions, tangentiality, circumstantiality, or flight of ideas). Psychotic disorders may also be associated with disorders of affect (difficulty expressing emotion); persons with chronic psychosis may be unable to express emotion, express too much emotion, or express emotion inappropriate to the circumstances. The psychotic person is often described as having lost contact with reality. Lay terms such as "insane" or "crazy" typically apply to persons with these disorders.

TYPES OF PSYCHOTIC DISORDER

Schizophrenia

The Diagnostic and Statistical Manual of Mental Disorders, 4th edition (DSM-IV; 1994), provides a comprehensive description of schizophrenia, its subtypes, and related mental disorders, along with criteria for diagnosis. Schizophrenia is a chronic, often lifelong psychotic disorder that typically begins in young adulthood (most often between ages 16 and 30). The illness is characterized by "positive" and "negative" symptoms. Positive symptoms include hallucinations (particularly auditory hallucinations), delusions (bizarre paranoid or persecutory ideas), and disorganization (of thought, speech, and/or behavior). Negative symptoms include a flattening of affect (the person's face appears immobile or unresponsive), alogia (poverty of speech manifested by brief, empty replies), and avolition (inability to initiate or persist in activities). Social withdrawal is perhaps the earliest symptom of the disorder. Schizophrenics often demonstrate problems functioning in interpersonal relations, work, education, and self-care but are not usually violent or dangerous unless the psychosis is out of control. To justify a diagnosis of schizophrenia, symptoms must be present for at least six months. The prevalence of schizophrenia is between 0.2% and 2.0% of persons in the general U.S. population; it affects approximately one in 100 people worldwide.

Delusional Disorder

A diagnosis of delusional disorder requires the presence of one or more nonbizarre delusions (fixed, false beliefs) that lasts for a period of one month or more. Other mental disorders that have delusions as a symptom (e.g., schizophrenia, substance intoxication or withdrawal, mania, psychotic depression, dementia, or delirium) must be ruled out. The nonbizarre nature of the delusions helps distinguish this disorder from schizophrenia. No amount of rational argument can convince the person that his belief is untrue (hence, the term "fixed"). The prevalence of delusional disorder in the general population is about 0.03%. Delusions fall into several categories:

- Erotomanic (belief that a particular someone is in love with the person)
- Grandiose (belief that the person has a great but unrecognized talent or insight, has a special relationship with a very important individual, or is a very important person, such as Jesus or Moses)
- Religious (belief that the devil or other

spirits are watching, influencing, or tormenting the person)
- Jealous (belief that the person's spouse is unfaithful; Othello syndrome)
- Persecutory or paranoid (belief that the person is being conspired against, followed, watched, drugged, or maliciously plotted against)
- Somatic (belief that the person is emitting a foul smell or odor, is infested by insects or parasites, or has a misshapen body part or a malfunctioning organ)
- Mixed or unspecified type

Devout religious beliefs may be viewed by some as delusional. Indeed, such beliefs are often fixed (the person cannot be dissuaded from them) and may be viewed by unbelievers as having no basis in reality (i.e., as being false). The important differentiating factor is that the beliefs of those who are not psychotic are *culturally sanctioned* (i.e., they are shared by the majority of members of the social group to which the person belongs).

Brief Psychotic Disorder

This disorder involves the sudden onset of "positive" psychotic symptoms such as delusions or hallucinations, which last at least one day but less than one month (e.g., Jim Bakker, during his federal trial, briefly became psychotic). When the condition remits, there is a complete return to normal functioning. The brief episode of psychosis is usually precipitated by a severe psychological or social stressor but can occur in the absence of such a stressor. Again, DSM-IV emphasizes that brief psychotic disorder needs to be distinguished from "culturally sanctioned" responses, such as seen in religious ceremonies, where persons may report hearing voices. In the latter case, symptoms do not usually persist and are recognized by the majority of those within the subculture as being normal. The prevalence of brief psychotic disorder in the general population is lower than that of either schizophrenia or delusional disorder.

Psychotic Disorder Caused by a Medical Condition

Also sometimes called delirium, psychotic symptoms, particularly visual hallucinations, can result from an underlying medical condition. The underlying medical condition can be an infection, metabolic or electrolyte imbalance, or brain disease. Hallucinations can be visual, olfactory, gustatory, tactile, or auditory. Delusions may be somatic, grandiose, religious, or persecutory. It is essential to identify the underlying medical condition so that it can be adequately treated, since untreated delirium has a high mortality rate.

Substance-Induced Psychotic Disorder

Prominent hallucinations or delusions can occur as a direct physiological result of ingestion of a drug, alcohol, or a prescribed medication or from exposure to some type of toxic chemical. These psychotic symptoms can occur either during intoxication with the substance or during withdrawal from the substance.

CONSEQUENCES OF PSYCHOSIS

Psychotic disorders, particularly those that are chronic, disrupt people's lives in many ways. They impair the ability to work. Social relationships are almost impossible to develop and maintain. Fear, anxiety, and confusion are common associated emotions. Consequently, the suicide rate among persons with schizophrenia is high (second only to that for people with depression). Approximately 50 percent of persons with schizophrenia have attempted suicide, and 10 percent successfully kill themselves within a 20-year period (Kaplan & Sadock, 1988b).

Chronic Disability

Most schizophrenic patients cannot work; between one-third and two-thirds of the homeless have schizophrenia (Kaplan & Sadock, 1988b). Before psychotropic medication was available, many schizophrenics had to be institutionalized in state hospitals. With appropriate treatment, many are now able to live in the community. Nevertheless, schizophrenic patients occupy nearly 50 percent of all mental hospital beds today in the United States.

Comorbid Psychiatric Disorders

Substance abuse (cocaine, marijuana, alcohol) is common among schizophrenics and may lead to a worsening of the underlying illness (due to noncompliance with antipsychotic therapy) and early mortality (due to both natural causes and suicide). Depression is also common in schizophrenics whose work, social lives, and inner world have been completely disrupted. Schizoaffective disorder is a psychiatric disorder characterized by symptoms of both schizophrenia and major depression, requiring treatment of both disorders.

COST OF SCHIZOPHRENIA

Schizophrenia has both direct costs (for disease treatment) and indirect costs (social, psychological, and work losses experienced by patients and families). Costs to the patient include suffering, loss of productivity, and increased mortality. Costs to the family include suffering and loss of productivity. Costs of treatment include costs of medications, rehabilitation services, day hospitals, inpatient facilities, and outpatient care. In the United States, the costs of all mental illnesses are estimated to be $103.7 billion (1985 dollars); schizophrenia alone accounts for $22.7 billion, making it the most costly of all mental illnesses (Williams & Dickson, 1995). The direct costs of mental health care alone exceed $10,000 per year per patient (Dickey et al., 1996).

CAUSES OF SCHIZOPHRENIA

The cause of schizophrenia is largely unknown, although almost all theories on its origins are biological, suggesting that schizophrenia is an organic disorder of the brain. There is a substantial hereditary or genetic component, since the risk of the disorder is about 10 times greater among persons who have a first-degree relative with schizophrenia (Kaplan & Sadock, 1988b). Genetics probably explain at least 70% of the risk (Kendler, 1988).

Findings from Positron Emission Tomography (PET) and Magnetic Resonance Imaging

(MRI) indicate that schizophrenics have both functional and structural brain abnormalities, especially in the frontal cortex and the thalamus. Schahram Akbarian, at the University of California-Irvine, has demonstrated abnormalities in nerve cell populations in the prefrontal cortex of schizophrenic patients, which suggests an abnormality of embryonic brain development (NARSAD, 1998).

The dopamine hypothesis suggests that schizophrenia results from hyperactivity of the dopaminergic systems (i.e., there are excessive amounts of the neurotransmitter dopamine in certain parts of the brain), which explains the effectiveness of antipsychotic drugs that bind to dopamine receptors. Nutritional deficiencies, obstetrical complications that cause neonatal brain damage, and viral infections may also increase the risk of schizophrenia (NARSAD, 1998). Interestingly, a 15-year follow-up study of 45,570 Swedish army recruits found that using marijuana on more than fifteen occasions increased the risk of developing schizophrenia to six times the risk for less frequent users or nonusers (Bromet et al., 1995).

Studies of monozygotic (identical) twins suggest that environmental influences (stress, relationship with parental figures) also play a role, although probably more in the expression of the disease than in the cause. On the basis of data from twin studies, environmental and familial factors account for less than 25% of the risk (Bromet et al., 1995).

RELIGIOUS AFFILIATION AND PSYCHOSIS

Is there a relationship between religious affiliation and psychotic disorder? Some studies have compared prevalence rates of schizophrenia or other psychotic symptoms among members of different religious groups. While such research has not been very helpful in elucidating the relationship between religiousness and psychosis, it is a place to start.

Protestants versus Catholics

Flics and Herron (1991) surveyed 152 patients in three psychiatric units in New York City hos-

pitals. Regression analysis was used to identify predictors of "premorbid adjustment" (used as a proxy for prognosis). Researchers found that Protestants in the sample had the largest percentage of schizophrenics; Jews had the largest percentage of affective illnesses; and Catholics had the largest percentage of personality disorders, adjustment disorders, and brief reactive psychoses. Catholics and Jews had higher levels of premorbid adjustment than Protestants or members of other religious groups. It is not surprising that Protestants, who were more likely to have schizophrenia (a disorder with a poor prognosis), had worse premorbid adjustment scores than Jews, who were more likely to have depression (a disorder with a much better prognosis).

Fundamentalists

Buckalew (1978) examined the association between religious affiliation and mental disorder in 1,323 first-admission adult patients at Central State Hospital in Georgia. The denominational breakdown of the sample was Baptist (68%), Methodist (21%), Pentecostal/Holiness (3%), Presbyterian (2%), Church of God/Christ (2%), Catholic (2%), and Episcopal (1%). There was no difference in proportion of persons with psychiatric disorder among the different religious groups; individual disorders, however, did vary ($p < .01$). Neuroses and affective disorders were more common but schizophrenia was less common among affiliates of Pentecostal/Holiness groups then among members of other denominations.

Catholic Clergy

Moore (1936) examined rates of psychiatric disorder among Catholic clergy, surveying all Catholic mental hospitals, state hospitals, city hospitals, county sanitaria, and private institutions in the United States (77–100% response rate). Among priests in 1935 ($n = 30,250$), 135 were admitted to mental hospitals, for a rate of 446/100,000. Among nuns/sisters in 1935 ($n = 122,220$), 593 were admitted to psychiatric hospitals, for a rate of 485/100,000. Among brothers in 1935 ($n = 7,408$), 31 were admitted to mental hospitals, for a rate of 418/100,000. These rates were compared to the admission rates for members of the U.S. Navy (357/100,000), members of the U.S. Army (740/100,000), citizens in New York in 1934 (600/100,000), and citizens in Massachusetts in 1934 (591/100,000). The difference in rates of psychiatric hospitalization between Catholic clergy and the other groups was significant ($p < .001$), suggesting lower rates of mental illness among Catholic clergy. Nevertheless, Moore found a hospital admission rate of 4,118/100,000 among cloistered, exclusively contemplative nuns. The rates of admission for schizophrenia was especially high in this group, being 5 times greater than expected. The investigator concluded that there was a tendency for prepsychotic schizophrenics to seek admission to certain religious orders.

Kelley (1958) later reexamined the rate of psychiatric hospitalization among all women religious in the United States in 1956. Kelley studied 357 private and public hospitals with psychiatric facilities and compared women religious with women in the general U.S. population during that year. Kelley found that the hospitalization rate for women religious was less than that for other women (320/100,000 vs. 358/100,000, $p = .02$). For those with diagnoses of schizophrenia, the rate was 194/100,000 for women religious versus 260/100,000 for women in the general population ($p < .001$). Kelly concluded that schizophrenia was not more common among women religious.

Jews

Flics and Herron (1991) reported that Jews had the greatest percentage of affective illnesses compared to other religious groups in their sample and were more likely to seek mental health services (Sanua, 1989), which enhanced their prognosis. In that study, however, only a small percentage of Jews had schizophrenia (compared to Protestants).

Trappler et al. (1995) examined 15 severely ill patients who attended an orthodox Jewish community-based mental health clinic in Brooklyn, New York. These patients (a) had experienced either a psychosis, a major depressive episode, or a manic episode within the past year, (b) were in weekly treatment, and (c) were receiving psychotropic medication. All subjects were born Jewish but had little religious involvement until they returned to Orthodox Judaism in later adulthood. These "cases" were compared with 14 mental health clinic patient controls who had also returned to Orthodox Judaism in adult life but who were experiencing only adjustment disorders and were not receiving psychotropic medications (i.e., had milder disorders). The study found that the 15 subjects were less likely than the controls to experience gratification from adhering to religious rules (47% vs. 100%, $p < .01$), to have a caring mother (60% vs. 100%) or father (40% vs. 79%), to have a family connected to the community (13% vs. 85%), or to have been sent to Jewish day school or summer camp (20% vs. 71%) (all $p < .05$). Trappler and colleagues concluded that "subjects' ability [referring to severely ill patients] to internalize religion and make effective use of a close community support system to buffer them against stressful life events appeared to have been influenced by genetic or environmental factors before their religious conversion." The patient sample, however, was small and highly selective.

A number of other studies have compared Jews with non-Jews on rates of psychiatric disorder. A consistent finding in the literature is that the rates of depression and manic-depressive illness are higher among Jews than among non-Jews but that schizophrenia is less common in Jews (particularly Western Jews) than in non-Jews (Miller, 1979; Cooklin et al., 1983; Sanua, 1989, 1992; Levav et al., 1993; Bilu & Witztum, 1997). While not as common as among Christians, religious delusions do occur among Jews (Clark, 1980), and there is some evidence that delving into Jewish mysticism may be associated with the development of psychosis (Greenberg et al., 1992).

No Denominational Affiliation

Bohrnstedt (1968) surveyed 3,700 freshman college students at the University of Wisconsin (1,815 females, 1,851 males), comparing Catholics (22%), Protestants (54%), Jews (19%), and those with no religious affiliation (5%) on MMPI scales. The study found that male students with no religious affiliation had higher scores on hypochondriasis, depression, hysteria, psychopathic deviation, lack of interest, paranoia, schizophrenia, hypomania, and social introversion (although the observed differences were small). Similar patterns were observed among females, and the observed differences were larger.

Other Religious Denominations

Armstrong et al. (1962) compared the religious beliefs of 121 "normals" and 88 psychotic patients at a state psychiatric facility. The investigators constructed a religious attitude scale to measure the subjects' religious beliefs. Among Catholic males, "normals" had significantly higher religious belief scores than patients (136 vs. 114, $p < .05$). Among conservative Protestant males, there was a weak trend in the opposite direction (100 vs. 114, p = ns). Among Catholic females, normals also had higher religious belief scores than patients (143 vs. 125, $p < .05$), and there was a trend in the same direction among conservative Protestant females (110 vs. 106, p = ns). However, in the liberal religious group (Unitarian), the findings were in the opposite direction; normals had much lower religious belief scores than did psychotic patients (14 vs. 80, $p < 0.05$) (but only six psychotic patients were Unitarian).

Spencer (1975) studied 50 Jehovah's Witnesses with schizophrenia who had been admitted to Western Australian Mental Health Service Psychiatric Hospitals during a 36-month period between 1971 and 1973. There were three times more schizophrenics (1.83/1000 vs. 0.61/1000) and nearly four times more paranoid schizophrenics (1.4/1000 vs. 0.38/1000) in the Jehovah's Witnesses group than among other persons living in the country ($p < .001$, analysis uncontrolled). Spencer concluded that either Jehovah's witnesses tend to be prepsychotic individuals who then break down when pressures are placed on them by aggressive proselytizing or being a Jehovah's Witness itself induces stress that precipitates psychosis.

Ullman (1988) examined psychological well-being among 40 converts to traditional and non-traditional religious groups. The subjects had converted two months to 10 years prior to the study, and they were evenly distributed among Jews, Catholics, Baha'i, and Hare Krishna groups. The study found that Jewish and Catholic converts were more likely to have a history of seeking outpatient psychiatric help than were Baha'i or Hare Krishna converts (32% vs. 5%, $p < .025$). However, Baha'i and Hare Krishna converts were more likely than Jews or Catholics to have had psychotic episodes that required psychiatric hospitalization (25% vs. 5%, $p < .025$) and were more likely to have experienced a chaotic lifestyle prior to conversion (75% vs. 40%, $p = .01$).

These studies suggest that persons from non-traditional religious groups may be at higher risk for psychosis or schizophrenia, although this conclusion remains controversial. It is also likely that certain religious groups may draw persons with psychotic tendencies into their membership, giving the false impression that such membership somehow induces these disorders.

RELIGIOUS BACKGROUNDS OF SCHIZOPHRENICS

Asking persons with chronic mental illness about their experiences with religion may further elucidate the relationship between religion and psychosis. Wilson and colleagues (1983) surveyed 72 schizophrenics recruited from the inpatient services at two psychiatric hospitals in North Carolina (68% men, 49% African American, 82% low SES) and compared them to 109 normal persons from the same area without histories of mental health problems or substance abuse (44% men, 16% African American, 13% low SES). Researchers found that the fathers of the subjects were less likely to be involved in their children's religious instruction than were the fathers of the controls (19% vs. 35%, $p < .05$). Parents of schizophrenics were also less likely to practice family devotions regularly (8% vs. 32%), were more likely to teach that God is punitive and harsh (73% vs. 30%), and were more likely to teach religion in an authoritarian manner (40% vs. 14%). Schizophrenics themselves were less likely to regularly read the Bible (26% vs. 49%, $p < .01$), to say grace at meals (51% vs. 80%, $p < .01$), and to have a religious conversion experience before age 21 (63% vs. 78%, $p < .01$). These results suggest that schizophrenics experience less religious nurturance as children and participate less regularly in religious devotions as adults. Cases and controls in this study, however, were very different, and these differences were not controlled for; furthermore, the survey results concerning parents' religious behavior were based on self-report by hospitalized schizophrenics whose perception and recall may have been affected by their illness.

RELIGIOUSNESS AS A CAUSE OF SCHIZOPHRENIA OR OTHER PSYCHOSIS

Some mental health specialists maintain that religiousness can facilitate the development of schizophrenia. As noted earlier, the psychiatrist Wendell Watters (1992) argues that devout religious beliefs contribute to the development of schizophrenia in persons born with a limited capacity to adapt. Watters claims that religious teachings interfere with the process of "related individuation" because the schizophrenogenicity of western Judeo-Christian culture acts through the family to make it difficult for parents to be effective catalysts for their offsprings' growth processes (pp. 140–146). We examine research that addresses this possibility.

Wootton and Allen (1983) reviewed the literature on dramatic religious conversions and schizophrenic decompensation, suggesting a relationship between the two. Dramatic and sudden religious conversions are contrasted with a milder and more gradual turn to faith which occurs, according to Leon Salzman (1953), "in the course of real maturing . . . after a reasoned, thoughtful search" (p. 178). William James (1902) noted that the "sick soul" is a more likely candidate for sudden conversion than the "healthy minded" person. While not presenting

any original research, Wootton and Allen (1983) review the ideas and case reports of other authors, including Christensen, Docherty, Salzman, James, Beit-Hallahmai, and Maslow. Recall that Wilson et al. (1983) found that schizophrenics were actually less likely then normal persons to have religious conversion experiences, especially before their twenty-first birthdays.

There is little doubt, however, that delusions and hallucinations seen in acute schizophrenia and schizotypal personality disorder frequently have religious content (Smith, 1982). Cothran and Harvey (1986) performed a case-control study with 18 manic and 23 schizophrenic cases admitted consecutively to a state psychiatric facility in New York (vs. 53 normal controls). Of the subjects, 17 were nondelusional (9 manic, 8 schizophrenic), 11 were delusional without religious content (5 manic, 6 schizophrenic), and 13 were delusional with religious content (4 manic, 9 schizophrenic). Of the 24 delusional patients, then, 13 had some religious content to their delusions (54%). Religious delusions were equally prevalent in both manic-depressives and schizophrenics. Patients with religious delusions reported high religiosity but less identification with fundamentalist type beliefs and less support for organized religion than did nondelusional patients and normal controls. These findings do not support the hypothesis that religious content in psychotic delusions results from the patient's being more fundamentalist or religiously active.

Other investigators have observed that strongly held religious belief is often present among persons with premorbid schizophrenia (Dittes, 1971; Clark, 1981; Spero, 1983; Margolis & Elifson, 1983). These observations, however, are based on anecdotal clinical experience, single case reports of acutely psychotic patients, or studies of first-year psychology students, not on systematic research conducted in population-based samples. We now review some of the studies that have examined the relationship between religiousness and psychosis.

Recall that Armstrong et al. (1962) compared the religious beliefs of 121 "normal" patients to those of 88 psychotic patients at a state psychiatric facility. For the majority of the Catholic and Protestant subjects, religious beliefs were stronger among normals than among psychotic patients (although this relationship was reversed among Unitarians). Richek et al. (1970) administered the MMPI to 166 college students, examining the association between the religious subscale of the MMPI and other MMPI scale scores. Investigators categorized students into religious females ($N = 78$), nonreligious females ($N = 21$), religious males ($N = 45$), and nonreligious males ($N = 22$); students were further categorized into high- and low-dogmatic subjects using the Rokeach D scale. Among religious males, those in the high-dogmatic group scored "significantly" lower than those in the low-dogmatic group on three MMPI clinical scales: hypochondriasis, psychopathic deviate, and schizophrenia. Among religious females, in contrast, high-dogmatic subjects were more depressed, more psychasthenic, and more anxious (but not more schizophrenic). The statistical significance of these findings is not clear since few details are given in the report—no percentages, no numbers, and no significance levels or description of the statistical tests.

Francis and Pearson (1985) surveyed 132 15-year-olds at secondary schools in Oxfordshire, England. Religiosity was measured using an Attitude toward Religion Scale developed by the authors. Personality traits were measured using the Junior and Adult Eysenck Personality Questionnaires (JEPQ and AEPQ). The study revealed that psychoticism on the JEPQ and the AEPQ was inversely related to religiosity ($r = -.16$, $p = .05$, and $r = -.22$, $p = .01$, respectively), as Nias (1973) and Powell and Stewart (1978) had found. After controlling for gender, the relationship disappeared with the JEPQ but persisted with the AEPQ. In a later study, Francis et al. (1992) analyzed 50 consecutive admissions to a 12-month-long Christian residential rehabilitation program for female drug abusers in Great Britain. Patients were assessed using the Eysenck Personality Questionnaire and Attitude toward Christianity scale. Christian attitudes were unrelated to neuroticism, extroversion, or Lie scale scores but were significantly

and inversely related to psychoticism ($r = -.23$, $p < .05$).

It is important to be careful when interpreting MMPI scale 8 (schizophrenia) or EPQ psychoticism scores to diagnose schizophrenia or the presence of psychotic symptoms. In the absence of high scores on scale 6 (paranoia), scale 7 (psychasthenia), or scale 9 (mania), it is difficult to interpret scale 8. This is especially true in nonpsychotic samples. Likewise, the psychoticism scales on the EPQ deal more with psychopathic tendencies (just plain meanness or lack of sensitivity) than they do with psychotic symptoms per se.

Feldman and Rust (1989) conducted two case-control investigations to determine the association between religiosity and schizotypal thinking. The first study examined a sample of 31 acute schizophrenics at four psychiatric wards in London hospitals (13 men, 18 women) and a sample of 70 men and 70 women at London University (controls). A second study involved 36 chronic schizophrenics (25 men, 11 women) at St. Mary's Hospital and 10 normal controls matched for age. Researchers administered the Rust Inventory of Schizotypal Thinking to both study populations. In the first study, religiosity was measured by two items: (1) "without my religion I would be lost" and (2) "religion is not particularly important to me." In the second study, religiosity was measured using a scale consisting of 12 agree/disagree items that asked about belief in God.

In the first study, the correlation between religiosity and schizotypal thinking in 140 normal controls was $-.17$ ($p = .03$); that is, religious controls were significantly less likely than less religious controls to demonstrate schizotypal thinking. This finding replicated the results of two other studies by these investigators that showed a significant negative relationship between religiosity and schizotypal thinking; one study involved 315 young persons in Hong Kong, and the other involved 608 Venezuelan university students. Among acute schizophrenics, the correlation between religiosity and schizotypal thinking was 0.15 ($p = $ ns).

In the second study, the correlation between religiosity and schizotypal thinking in chronic schizophrenics was 0.11 (p = ns). Overall religiosity level was not significantly different for chronic schizophrenics and normal controls matched for age. However, the positive nonsignificant correlations in acute and chronic schizophrenics were both significantly different from the negative correlation for normal controls in the first study. On the basis of this result, the authors concluded that religious thought is of a different nature in normals and in schizophrenics and suggested that the processes leading to the development of religious beliefs may be different in schizophrenics and in normals. Unfortunately, the authors inaccurately concluded, "Our results generally support a connection between religious experience and factors associated with the etiology of schizophrenia" (Feldman & Rust, 1989, p. 592), which in fact their data did not.

Sheehan and Kroll (1990) surveyed 52 psychiatric patients on a psychiatric ward at the University of Minnesota hospital in Minneapolis. Of the patients, 31% had major depression, 21% had bipolar disorder, 19% had schizophrenia, and 8% had personality disorder. Only 23% thought their illness could have resulted from sinful acts, 10% believed they were in the hospital because they had sinned (mainly patients with borderline personality disorder or bulimia), and 19% believed they needed penance before they could improve. Depressed patients averaged one sin-related item, compared with two sin-related items for schizophrenics (p = ns). From this study we can conclude that only a minority of acutely hospitalized psychiatric patients believe that religious factors are a cause for their illness, and schizophrenic patients are no more likely to believe so than are other psychiatric patients.

Neeleman and Lewis (1994) conducted one of the few studies that have linked psychotic illness with greater religiosity. These investigators compared religious beliefs and attitudes of psychiatric patients with those of orthopedic patients at two university hospitals in London, England. The following four groups were formed: (1) depressed psychiatric outpatients (n = 26), (2) suicidal patients (n = 26), (3) psychotic outpatients with chronic schizophrenia (n = 21), and (4) consecutive patients seen at an orthopedic clinic (controls) (n = 25). Religiosity was measured by a 16-item questionnaire that included: seven questions about religious practices and experiences and nine questions about religious beliefs and attitudes. Psychotic schizophrenics and depressed patients were more likely to have had a personal religious experience compared with controls (48% vs. 38% vs. 17%, respectively, p = .05). Schizophrenic patients in particular, and psychiatric patients more generally, were more likely to hold religious beliefs and to receive comfort from religion than were the orthopedic controls. Even when other factors such as race and age were taken into account by using regression analysis, significant differences in religious belief between psychiatric patients and orthopedic controls persisted (p < .005). The cross-sectional nature of this study prevents our determining whether greater religiousness prior to illness onset led to the illness or whether psychotic schizophrenics turned to religion as a source of comfort after their illness developed.

In summary, then, the evidence linking religiousness and schizotypal thinking, psychoticism, psychosis, or schizophrenia is inconsistent. All of the studies reviewed provide no information about causality. Schizophrenia may be characterized by a certain type of hyperreligiosity; conversely, chronically mentally ill adults often turn to religion for comfort. Finally, religious beliefs and expressions of religiousness in schizophrenics and psychotic persons may be quite different from those in normal persons.

SCHIZOPHRENIA AND DEMONIC POSSESSION

While mental health professionals have tried to show that religious beliefs somehow contribute to the development of schizophrenia, some Christian fundamentalists have maintained that the bizarre behaviors of schizophrenics and psychotic persons are due to demonic possession. Possession was also a concern in the fifteenth and sixteenth centuries, when persons with chronic mental illness were occasionally burned at the stake because they were thought to be witches or sorcerers. McAll (1982) reports a high prevalence of "possession states" among patients with schizophrenia. If demonic possession plays a role in etiology, then exorcism might be a possible treatment. Not surprisingly, however, exorcism has not been helpful in the treatment of schizophrenia or other psychotic illnesses. McAll notes, that while some patients exhibit less dramatic and violent manifestations of psychosis following exorcism, they invariably remain schizophrenic and require pharmacologic treatment for their illness. In a comprehensive review of the subject, the Duke University psychiatrist William P. Wilson (1998) has described the differences he perceives between demonic possession and schizophrenia. According to Wilson, the possessed person does not have the affective changes (blunting of affect), the disturbances of thought (looseness of association), or the ambivalence usually seen in schizophrenia. It is clear, then, that the presence of evil does not characterize the schizophrenic state (Peck, 1983).

In our opinion, the primary influence of Judeo-Christian beliefs and practices on schizophrenia and other psychotic disorders is in providing comfort, hope, and a supportive community to individuals who must cope with their emotionally devastating, largely biological illnesses.

RELIGION AS A SOURCE OF COMFORT AND HOPE

Carson and Huss (1979) conducted an intervention study with 20 Christian schizophrenic patients in a state mental hospital. The intervention was weekly prayer and Scripture reading conducted one on one by a student nurse for 10 weeks. The focus of prayer and Scripture readings was God's love and concern for each individual and the worth of each individual to God. Student nurses and patients were assessed at the beginning and at the end of the 10-week project. Student nurses experienced several benefits—a greater sensitivity to others, a strengthening of their religious beliefs, and a greater sense of being hopeful, realistic, and empathetic. Patients became more verbal about what bothered them, acted out their anger and

frustration more, and were more willing to take risks in expressing their inner feelings. Patients who received the intervention were also more likely than control patients to express a desire for change in their lives and for a more normal life. Compared to the controls, patients who received the intervention became more articulate, showed more appropriate affect, and complained of fewer somatic symptoms. While these results are encouraging, the investigators did not make random assignments to groups and did no statistical tests, affecting the validity of the study findings.

Breier and Astrachan (1984) examined characteristics of all patients registered at the Connecticut Mental Health Center who committed suicide between 1970 and 1981 ($n = 38$). They formed four groups of patients: Group 1 comprised 20 patients with schizophrenia who committed suicide; Group 2 comprised 18 nonschizophrenic patients who committed suicide; and there were two schizophrenic nonsuicidal control groups (81 "randomly" selected patients [Group 3] and 20 sex-matched patients [Group 4]). Comparing Groups 1 and 3, the authors found that schizophrenics who committed suicide were more often without a religious affiliation or affiliated with non-Protestant religious groups than were nonsuicidal schizophrenics (40% vs. 10%, $p < .05$). This small study suggests that religious affiliation may help prevent suicide in schizophrenics.

Lindgren and Coursey (1995) performed a clinical trial that examined the effect of a spiritual intervention on 28 patients with serious mental illness (19 with schizophrenia) at three psychosocial rehabilitation centers. All patients expressed an interest in spirituality at the start of the study. A four-session course (1.5 hours per session) was developed and administered as the intervention. The intervention was a psychoeducational program designed to help patients utilize their spiritual beliefs to foster healthy self-esteem; it was administered in four 1.5-hour sessions. Five to six people were in each of the three experimental groups and five to six people in each of the three wait-list control groups. Once the intervention was completed in the experimental group, the intervention was applied to the control group. Significant differences were found on the Spiritual Support Scale before and after the intervention in both groups, but there were no significant differences in depression, hopelessness, self-esteem, or purpose in life between intervention and control groups. Researchers noted that 47% of these seriously ill patients indicated that spirituality/religion had helped "a great deal," 60% indicated that religion/spirituality had impacted "a great deal" on their lives, 57% prayed daily, and 76% thought about God or spiritual/religious matters daily.

Wahass and Kent (1997) examined ways that patients with auditory hallucinations cope with the hallucinations. The subjects were 33 Western (British) and 37 non-Western (Saudi Arabian) inpatients and outpatients with schizophrenia. Saudi Arabian patients were more likely than British patients to use religion (praying, reading the Koran/Bible, listening to religious cassettes) (43% vs. 3%, $p < .01$, uncontrolled) to cope with hallucinations, whereas the British were more likely to use distraction or physiologically based approaches. Religious coping by schizophrenics, then, may vary in different parts of the world.

Prospective Cohort Studies

Prospective studies provide more information about the relationship between religious involvement and schizophrenia. Chu and Klein (1985) prospectively followed 128 African American schizophrenic patients consecutively admitted to seven hospitals and mental health centers of the Missouri Division of Mental Health. Patients (65 urban and 63 rural subjects) were interviewed on admission, discharge, and either a year after discharge or on readmission (if this occurred before one year). Urban patients were significantly less likely to be rehospitalized if they said prayers once daily (vs. more often). They were also less likely to be hospitalized if their families encouraged them to continue religious worship while they were in the hospital ($p < .001$). For both urban and rural patients, there were fewer rehospitalizations if the family was Catholic and more rehospitalizations if the family had no religious affiliation ($p < .025$). These findings are particu-

larly notable given that the most costly form of treatment for schizophrenia is acute hospitalization (Knapp & Kavanagh, 1997).

In the largest investigation to date, Verghese et al. (1989) conducted a two-year prospective study of 386 schizophrenic patients ages 15–45. These patients, whose illness had lasted two years or less, were seen in 1981 at psychiatric outpatient clinics in India. Health outcomes deteriorated among patients who reported a decrease in religious activities at the baseline evaluation ($p < .001$, uncontrolled). Investigators concluded, "If these associations are confirmed, it is possible to plan some intervention programs, such as changing the attitudes of others to the patient, and giving more importance to various types of religious activity. Religiosity is important in Indian culture and the increase in religiosity that was related to better outcomes in the present study could be a means of effectively handling the anxiety of the patient" (p. 502). To our knowledge, this is the only major prospective study of a large sample of schizophrenic patients.

RELIGIOUS COMMUNITIES AS SOURCES OF CARE

If increased religiousness and religious involvement helps schizophrenics cope better with their illness, and if a mission of the Church is to minister to less fortunate members of society, might religious communities play a role in meeting the needs of persons with schizophrenia or other chronic mental disorders? The following study underscores the contribution that religious communities can make. Katkin et al. (1975) recruited volunteers from the community to work with community mental health center patients in Cincinnati, Ohio. They asked volunteers to spend a couple of hours per week to ensure that the schizophrenic patients took their medication, to evaluate the patients for decompensation, to help the patients find housing and jobs, and to give supportive counseling. After one year, the recidivism rate for the 36 chronic schizophrenic patients in the study was 11% in the group treated by volunteers and 34% for a control group of 36 patients treated with traditional aftercare ($p \leq =.05$). The volunteers decreased their visits to once a month in the second year. After two years, the recidivism rate was 33% in the treated group and 56% in the control group.

Because of its success, the volunteer program was repeated. In the second round, volunteers saw patients weekly for the first four months and once every two weeks thereafter; both the intervention and the control groups were seen monthly by a psychiatrist, and both received medication. This time the recidivism rate after one year for 11 schizophrenics (seven men and four women) who had been randomly assigned to the treatment group was 9%, and the rate for 11 control group members was 37%. This study has clear implications concerning the impact that church volunteers might have on quality of life and health service needs of persons with chronic mental illness.

SUMMARY AND CONCLUSIONS

Schizophrenia and psychotic disorders are common, disabling, isolating, frightening, and costly illnesses that have an enormous impact on the quality of life of patients and their families. Given the considerable influence of genetic loading and other biological factors on the etiology of schizophrenia (70% or more), it is unlikely that religious factors contribute much to cause the disease or negatively impact its course. Denominational differences found among inpatient samples probably indicate either socioeconomic influences on admission rates or some other methodological bias. There are no prospective data on religious involvement as a predictor of new cases of schizophrenia, and this lack seriously limits what conclusions can be drawn. While religious delusions are quite frequent among psychotic patients, many studies show that religiousness is not associated with schizotypal thinking, psychotic symptoms, or psychotic personality traits in the general population. In fact, a number of studies show a significant inverse relationship between religiousness and psychotic tendencies.

What can be said more definitively (on the basis of prospective data) is that religion provides a powerful source of comfort and hope for many persons with chronic mental illness. Religious or spiritual interventions may help these persons utilize their spiritual resources to improve functioning, reduce isolation, and facilitate healing. By mobilizing volunteers from within the congregation, religious communities can play an important role in helping to meet the emotional and practical needs of persons with schizophrenia or other chronic mental illness. This role may become increasingly important as societal resources to care for these persons diminish.

11

Alcohol and Drug Use

LCOHOL ADDICTION AND other drug problems exact an enormous cost from society in terms of physical disease and mental suffering, disturbed social order, and lost productivity. In this chapter we define alcohol and drug problems and examine their clinical and social consequences, as well as possible etiologic factors. Religious beliefs and practices may play an important role in the prevention of serious alcohol and drug problems and in the rehabilitation of abusers. We explore these possibilities, along with the possibility that religion may lead to, exacerbate, or interfere with recovery from substance abuse problems.

CATEGORIZING ALCOHOL AND OTHER DRUG PROBLEMS

Clinicians use two major systems for classifying alcohol and other drug problems: the interna-

tional diagnostic system published by the World Health Organization (WHO) entitled the International Classification of Disease: Tenth Revision: Clinical Descriptions and Diagnostic Guidelines (ICD-10, 1992), and the system used primarily in the United States, the Diagnostic and Statistical Manual of Mental Disorders, Fourth Edition (DSM-IV; 1994). Both classification systems provide categories for substance use syndromes in which individuals develop impaired control over alcohol or drug intake and/ or experience symptoms of withdrawal and tolerance with chronic heavy intake.

Recent research provides overwhelming evidence that alcohol and drugs not only interfere acutely with normal brain activity but also have long-term effects on brain metabolism and functioning (National Institute for Drug Abuse, 1998). At some point, these changes in central nervous system activity can lead to a compulsive craving for drugs, that is, a preoccupation that becomes so overwhelming that the user becomes impaired in her ability to exercise restraint in their consumption (National Institute on Alcohol and Alcoholism, 1997; Pickens & Johanson, 1992).

As continued craving leads to chronic intake of the substance, the user may develop physical dependence in addition to psychological craving and dependence. A hallmark of physical dependence is tolerance (i.e., a need for more and more of a substance to achieve a desired effect and/or the experience of withdrawal symptoms if substance intake is reduced or stopped). True dependence on alcohol or other drugs often involves a combination of physical and psychological factors (Fritzche, 1998), and those with both psychological craving and physical dependence suffer far more problems than those with only psychological craving (Schuckit et al., 1998).

At the end of the substance use spectrum is long-term addiction, which is defined as repeated failures to refrain from alcohol or drug use despite prior resolutions to do so (Heather, 1998). Soon, the addict's time, resources, and energy are focused more and more on acquiring, using, and recovering from alcohol or drugs (Miller, 1998). As a result, he begins to neglect the other dimensions of life, including home, family, work, and play. Despite their best intentions, without adequate intervention, addicts are often doomed to repeated cycles of short-term abstinence, only to be followed by even greater periods of excessive consumption and despair.

CLINICAL AND SOCIAL CONSEQUENCES

The abuse of alcohol and illicit drugs ranks among the leading health and social concerns in the United States today. Chronic alcohol consumption, for example, is associated with an increased risk of both morbidity and mortality, including liver disease, cancer, cardiovascular problems, accidental deaths, suicides, and homicides (Chick & Erickson, 1996). Because the liver, the primary site of alcohol metabolism, can be severely damaged by heavy alcohol consumption, cirrhosis deaths are typically used as an indicator of abusive alcohol consumption patterns in populations. Although mortality from chronic liver disease and cirrhosis has been declining steadily in the United States since the early 1970s, cirrhosis is still ranked as the ninth leading cause of death in this country, causing more than 26,000 deaths a year (National Center for Health Statistics, 1989).

Alcohol dependence and other psychiatric disorders, especially depression and anxiety, occur together at significantly higher than chance rates (Lynskey, 1998). The increased risk of psychiatric disorder explains in part why suicide rates are so high among those who regularly abuse alcohol and other drugs (Tondo et al., 1999). Indeed, one-fifth to one-third of the increased death rate among alcoholics is explained by psychiatric disorder–related suicide (Berglund & Ojehagen, 1998). In the adolescent populations, driving while intoxicated is an important cause of injury, disability, and premature death (Augustyn & Simons-Morton, 1995). Individuals admitted to hospital emergency rooms with violence-related injuries are more likely to have been drinking prior to the event and to report more frequent heavy drinking and alcohol-related problems than those admitted to the same emergency room during the same time period with injuries from other causes (Cherpitel, 1997).

Similarly, misuse and abuse of drugs is associated with increased risks of morbidity and mortality (Bravender & Knight, 1998), as well as of psychiatric problems (Kosten et al., 1998). As with alcohol, drug abuse is associated with higher levels of depressive symptoms and greater risk for suicide (Windle & Windle, 1997). Among adolescents, drug use is also a significant risk factor for early sexual activity (Rosenbaum & Kandel, 1990), which increases the risks for early pregnancy and sexually transmitted diseases.

Finally, alcohol and other drug problems adversely affect not only users but also those around them. The National Institute on Drug Abuse (NIDA) estimates that 7.6 million babies (18.6%) were exposed to significant amounts of alcohol during gestation, and there are currently 28.6 million children of alcoholics in the

United States. In California alone, approximately 18% of children live with a parent who has used illegal substances during the past year (Young, 1997).

PREVALENCE AND ECONOMIC COSTS

According to the National Household Survey of Drug Abuse, approximately 111 million persons age 12 or over, or about 51% of the age 12 and over population, are current alcohol users in the United States. Of these, about 31.9 million (15.3% of the population) engage in binge drinking, and about 11.2 million Americans (5.4% of the population) are heavy drinkers (National Institute for Drug Abuse, 1997).

Additionally, 13.9 million Americans (6.4% of the U.S. population age 12 or older) are current users of illicit drugs, meaning that they reported using an illicit drug in the month prior to the survey (National Institute for Drug Abuse, 1997). About 62 million people in the United States age 12 or older (29% of the population) are current cigarette smokers (National Institute for Drug Abuse, 1997). This makes nicotine, the addictive component of tobacco, the most heavily used drug in the United States (besides alcohol).

Society pays an enormous economic cost as a result of the heavy use and misuse of alcohol and other drugs. These costs result from decreased productivity of the abusers; increased taxes to pay for treatment, education, and law enforcement; and increased need for health services, which results in higher medical costs and insurance rates. In 1992, the economic cost to U.S. society of alcohol abuse and alcoholism was estimated at $148 billion (Harwood et al., 1998). It is estimated that 45% of costs are borne by alcohol abusers and/or members of their households, 39% by government, 10% by private insurance, and 6% by victims of alcohol-related trauma (motor vehicle crashes plus crime victims).

Like alcohol abuse, use of other drugs for nonmedical reasons brings specific, well-recognized consequences and costs. This increased burden to society results from costs related to the health consequences of drug abuse; costs related to increased criminal behavior by drug users (including those resulting from violence to others, increased need for law enforcement, and costs of confinement in prison); and costs related to job losses, family impoverishment, and subsequent reliance on welfare or other elements of society's safety net (Swan, 1998). Not surprising, then, the economic cost of drug abuse in the United States was an estimated $97.7 billion in 1992, bringing the total cost for substance abuse in 1992 to $246 billion. This total represents $965 for every person in the United States in 1992. The per-person cost for drug abuse alone was $383 (Harwood et al., 1998).

Alcohol and drug use are having a significant social and economic impact on other countries, as well. For example, a recent study conducted in Canada found that there were 33,498 deaths and 208,095 hospitalizations attributed to tobacco, 6,701 deaths and 86,076 hospitalizations due to alcohol, and 732 deaths and 7095 hospitalizations due to illicit drugs in 1992. The study also found that 21% of all deaths, 23% of all years of potential life lost, and 8% of all hospitalizations were the result of substance abuse (Single et al., 1999).

ETIOLOGY OF ALCOHOL AND DRUG ABUSE

The causes of alcohol and drug abuse are complex and multifactorial. Recent research suggests that both biological factors (including genetic characteristics and temperament) and family environment are important etiological factors that predict substance abuse (Weinberg et al., 1998). Other variables, such as behavior problems, absence of supportive parents, having a parent as a role model for substance abuse, and peer influence, also confer significant risk for alcohol and drug use or abuse among adolescents (Petraitis et al., 1998; Yang et al., 1998). Poor academic achievement is also a significant predictor of substance abuse; debate continues on whether it is a cause or result of substance abuse (or both) (Guagliardo et al., 1998).

RELIGION AND SUBSTANCE ABUSE

The history of alcohol and drug abuse is intertwined with religion, and societal views on these behaviors often have their roots in spiritual or religious perspectives (Miller, 1998). In Jewish and Christian Scriptures, for example, the drinking of wine is assumed to be part of ordinary life, and its virtues are even extolled. The central sacramental observances in both Judaism and Christianity involve the use of wine. Other religions have assigned sacred uses to other drugs as well, including tobacco (Wilbert, 1991) and hallucinogens, such as peyote (Wiedman, 1990). On the other hand, many religions, such as Islam, strictly forbid the use of alcoholic beverages or other drugs (Akabaliev & Dimitrov, 1997), and other religious groups strongly advise against their use (Lyon et al., 1976; Phillips, Kuzma, et al., 1980).

Religion has also impacted our views of the problems associated with alcohol and drug abuse. Although Judeo-Christian teachings approve of light to moderate alcohol use, there is a clear and consistent biblical denunciation of drunkenness—the use of alcohol in a manner that causes impairment or harm (Miller, 1998). It is this excessive use or abuse of alcohol that is often denounced by religious teaching as "sinful" (Advisory Council on Church and Society, 1986). Use of drugs that inflict harm or increase risk of harm to oneself or others is also placed in this category (Miller, 1995).

Given these long-standing connections between religion and substance use, and the important roles of religious and spiritual perspectives in shaping our moral understanding of addiction, epidemiological researchers have long been interested in the relationship among religion, alcohol, and drug use problems in populations. In a highly acclaimed and widely quoted epidemiological study, Hirschi and Stark (1969) surveyed 4,077 public school students in central California and found that religiosity was unrelated to delinquent behavior, including alcohol and drug use. This report, which directly contradicted a number of earlier studies (e.g., Bales, 1946; Straus & Bacon, 1953; Thorner, 1953; Skolnick, 1958; Cisin & Cahalan, 1968), "quickly became the accepted word

on the subject, frequently cited and widely reprinted" (Stark et al., 1982, p. 5).

Hirshi and Stark's (1969) initial conclusion, however, turned out to be an aberration. Later research (including a study by Stark himself, 1996) has consistently found that there is a negative relationship between religion and alcohol or drug use and abuse. Gorsuch and Butler (1976) comprehensively reviewed the literature to assess factors predisposing adolescents to the use and abuse of drugs. They found that, in the many studies examined, whenever religion was included in an analysis, it predicted lower use of illicit drugs regardless of whether the research was conducted prospectively or retrospectively and whether the religious variable was defined in terms of membership, active participation, personal importance of religion, or religious upbringing.

The inverse relationship between religious participation and substance use or abuse has been demonstrated in a variety of population groups across religious denominations and age. The literature base on this topic is too extensive to be covered here, although information about many of these studies can be found in part VIII. The following review presents a sampling of some of the more methodologically rigorous studies.

RELIGION AND SUBSTANCE ABUSE IN ADOLESCENTS

Virtually all drug addicts begin their use during the teen years (MacDonald, 1984), and, among adolescents, the two most commonly used drugs are alcohol and marijuana (not counting nicotine). Research has shown that more than 90% of America's youth try alcohol by the time they are seniors, and a third of high school seniors report having been drunk during the previous month (Johnson et al., 1998). Almost one in four American college students report having used marijuana during the past year (Bell et al., 1997). Although much less frequent than marijuana use, the use of other illicit drugs such as cocaine, amphetamines, and tranquilizers is still alarmingly high among American teenagers (Johnson & O'Malley, 1998).

Because of the high levels of use and abuse of alcohol and other drugs by teens and the consequences that result, researchers have long sought to identify factors that might prevent or protect youth from being tempted to use these substances. Among the factors most extensively examined is religion, primarily because of its value as a source of social control (McIntosh et al., 1981).

In a study involving data from 2,066 Canadian adolescents, Adlaf and Smart (1985) examined the relationship between drug use and several measures of religion, including religious affiliation (Protestant, Catholic, or none), religiosity (very religious, moderately religious, not particularly religious), and frequency of church attendance (never to very frequent). They found that Catholic students were less likely than Protestants or nonaffiliated students to have used marijuana, nonmedical, or hallucinogenic drugs during the previous year. Religiosity and church attendance variables both had strong negative relationships with drug use. Students who reported they were very religious were less likely to have used alcohol or other drugs during the previous year than were students who indicated they were not particularly religious: 61% versus 80%, respectively, for alcohol use, 8% versus 39% for marijuana use, 6% versus 31% for nonmedical prescription drug use, 2% versus 22% for hallucinogenic drug use, and 10% versus 20% for medical drug use. Similarly, students who attended religious services very frequently were less likely to use drugs than were students who never attended church or who attended infrequently: 62% versus 77%, respectively, for alcohol use, 11% versus 36% for marijuana use, 10% versus 28% for nonmedical drug use, 3% versus 21% for hallucinogen use, and 12% versus 21% for medical drug use.

Further evidence that religion may be a protective factor against drug use among youth was reported by Hadaway and colleagues (1984), who explored the relationship between religion and drug use in a sample of more than 23,000 white high school students from 21 public high schools in Atlanta, Georgia. In this study, Hadaway and colleagues included multiple measures of religion, including frequency of church attendance, parental attendance at religious services, self-rated importance of religion, respondents' belief that God answers prayers, an index of religious orthodoxy, and a denominational variable divided into Protestant, liberal Protestant, and Catholic.

This study found a moderate to strong negative relationship between all religion measures and both attitudes toward drug use and actual self-reported use ($\gamma = -.27$ to $-.57$). Among those who said that religion was extremely important to them, 52% had not used alcohol, 83% had not used marijuana, and 97% had not used other illicit drugs during the previous year. In contrast, among those who said religion was not important to them, 21% had not used alcohol, 47% had not used marijuana, and 75% had not used other illicit drugs during the previous year.

Lorch and Hughes (1985) reported similar results from a survey of 13,878 students in grades 7 though 12 in six school districts in Colorado. They examined the relationship between alcohol and drug use and six dimensions of religion—religious membership, degree of religious fundamentalism or liberalism, frequency of church attendance, personal importance of religion, a combination of church attendance and religious importance, and a combination of fundamentalism/liberalism and importance of religion. Church membership was inversely related to alcohol and drug usage. Students who were church members had a significantly lower rate of usage compared to nonmembers in the all drug categories except one—heavy use of cocaine.

Of all six religious variables, church attendance yielded the highest zero-order correlations for almost all measures of substance use, with the combination of church attendance and importance of religion showing the second highest zero-order correlation. Importance of religion by itself was third. However, when investigators controlled for the influence of other dimensions of religion, as well as for gender and grade in school, they found that "importance of religion" had the strongest inverse correlation with substance of use. On the basis of these results, investigators concluded that "this implies that the controls operating here are deeply internalized values and norms rather than those that may come just from fear associated with church ideology or peer pressure coming from interaction with others of one's religious group" (Lorch & Hughes, 1985, p. 207).

Amoateng and Bahr (1986) provide further evidence to support the hypothesis that religion deters drug abuse. These investigators analyzed data from a national survey of more than 17,000 high school seniors, examining the impact of a number of factors on adolescents' use of alcohol and drugs, including parents' education, mother's employment status, number of parents in the household, religiosity, religious affiliation, gender, and race. Investigators found that religious affiliation was related to drug use, with Mormons using alcohol and marijuana much less often than other groups. Baptists and fundamentalists also had usage rates lower than those of other denominations. Conversely, students who reported no religious affiliation had the highest rate of marijuana use. Among all the religious denominations, however, degree of personal religiosity had the most consistent inverse relationship with drug use. Students most committed to their religion were the least likely to report either marijuana or alcohol use ($p < .001$, after adjusting for multiple covariates). Interestingly, none of the three family variables—parents' education, mother's employment status, or number of parents in the household—had any effect on student alcohol use, although students who lived with both parents were slightly less likely to use marijuana than students who lived in one-parent families.

Hardert and Dowd (1994) examined the relationships between four "socialization" variables and alcohol and marijuana use in a sample of high school and college students who resided in middle-class suburbs of Phoenix, Arizona. Socialization variables were sociodemographic factors (gender and educational level), intrapersonal variables (personality and attitudes and values), interpersonal values (peers' values, peers' use of drugs, and parents' values), and contextual factors (communication with teachers, exposure to violence at school, and fear of nuclear attack). Investigators also measured class in school (high school vs. college), gender, and religiosity, because of previous studies that

had suggested these factors play a role in drug use.

College students were six times more likely to use both alcohol and marijuana than were high school students. However, after controlling for class in school (college versus high school), two peer variables—peer drug use and peer attitudes about drugs—emerged as the strongest predictors of both alcohol and marijuana use. Interestingly, not being religious produced a significant additional increase in likelihood of marijuana use for both high school and college students but did not appear to affect alcohol use (other than indirectly through communication with teachers, peer use, or hedonism). Hardert and Dowd (1994) concluded that "perhaps religiosity and other 'conventional' systems of thought become more of an insulator against deviance as the substance in question is perceived as becoming more illicit" (p. 901).

Among the most extensive studies of drug use in adolescents or young adults to date, two different investigative teams have reported evidence that links religious involvement with lower levels of substance abuse. Amey et al. (1996) surveyed a random national sample of 11,728 senior high school students in 130 high schools around the country (*Monitoring the Future Survey: A Continuing Study of Values and Lifestyles of Youth*). Religiosity was measured by affiliation, religious importance, and religious attendance. The dependent variable was use of a variety of substances (cigarettes, alcohol, marijuana, and other drugs, including LSD, cocaine, amphetamines, barbiturates, tranquilizers, heroin, other narcotics, and inhalants). Religious involvement was inversely related with use of all substances. The odds ratios from logistic regression models for frequent church attendance were 0.71 for cigarettes (29% lower), 0.55 for alcohol (45% lower), 0.67 for marijuana (33% lower), and 0.79 for other drugs (21% lower). For religious importance, the odds ratios were 0.75 for cigarettes (25% lower), 0.45 for alcohol (55% lower), 0.78 for marijuana (22% lower), and 0.88 for use of other drugs (12% lower). All of these controlled associations were strong and statistically significant except for the relationship between religious importance and use of other drugs. Significant inter-actions were found for race and affiliation, race and religious attendance, and race and religious importance on alcohol use; for race and affilia-tion and race and religious importance on mari-juana use; and for race and religious attendance on use of other drugs. These interactions sug-gested that religion is more of a deterrent for drug use among whites than among African Americans.

Bell and colleagues (1997) examined the per-sonal background and college characteristics of 17,952 students who attended 140 American colleges. Investigators used a detailed 20-page survey to ask students about their illicit drug use, as well as other high-risk behaviors, health issues, and other factors considered to be im-portant predictors of substance abuse. Al-though the study was primarily about alcohol use, the survey also included questions about illicit drug and tobacco use. Drugs included in the survey were marijuana, "crack" and other forms of cocaine, barbiturates, amphetamines, tranquilizers, heroin and other opiates, LSD and other hallucinogens, anabolic steroids, and tobacco products.

Investigators found that almost 25% of stu-dents reported having used marijuana in the past 12 months. Because the use of other illicit drugs was uncommon, with none being used by more than 5% of the students, the investigators decided to limit the remainder of their analyses to examining the correlates of marijuana use. Characteristics that predicted higher marijuana use were being single, being white, spending more time at parties and socializing with friends, spending less time studying, participat-ing in high-risk behaviors such as binge drink-ing, cigarette smoking, having multiple sexual partners, perceiving parties as important, *and* perceiving religion and community service as unimportant. After controlling for the effects of other variables (both college and student characteristics), importance of religion and community service remained significant pre-dictors for not using marijuana. Students who stated that religion was "not very important" had nearly three times the risk of using mari-juana of students who said religion was very

important to them (adjusted OR = 2.7, 95% CI 2.3–3.2).

In summary, research on adolescent and young adult drug use suggests that there is a clear inverse relationship between various mea-sures of religion (attitudes, beliefs, affiliations, behaviors) and alcohol or drug use. Young per-sons who frequently attend religious services, who report that religion is very important in their lives, and who belong to denominations that prohibit or discourage drug use are less likely to be involved with drugs than are those who are less religious. Peer association may be one of the mechanisms by which religion exerts its effect on drug use in adolescents. However, other mechanisms may be involved and are dis-cussed later in this chapter.

RELIGION AND SUBSTANCE ABUSE IN ADULT POPULATIONS

Like studies in adolescents and young adults, studies of middle-aged or older adult popula-tions consistently find an inverse relationship between religious involvement and substance use/abuse. For example, in an early NIH-sup-ported study comparing characteristics of ab-stainers and heavy alcohol drinkers in a nation-wide sample of 2,746 adults, Cisin and Cahalan (1968) found that more abstainers than infre-quent, moderate, or heavy drinkers participated in church activities.

In a later national study of problem drinking among 1,561 American men ages 21–59, Caha-lan and Room (1972) found that, out of 30 independent variables tested as possible pre-dictors of alcohol problems, only 10 signifi-cantly predicted "current" problems with alco-hol. Among these 10 variables, two religious variables were ranked sixth and seventh: conser-vative Protestant religious affiliation and atten-dance at religious services. Both predicted fewer current alcohol problems. Results indi-cated that there were relatively few abstainers from alcohol and many heavy drinkers among Catholics and liberal Protestants. In contrast, among Jewish men, most drank at least a little, but few drank heavily. Among conservative

Protestant denominations (i.e., those favoring complete abstinence), there was a high percentage of abstainers. However, among the few conservative Protestants who did drink heavily or binge, more reported that they suffered "high consequences" from their drinking behavior than did heavy drinkers affiliated with other religious groups (Catholics, liberal Protestants, or Jews).

Similarly, Khavari and Harmon (1982) examined data from a survey of 4,853 persons from a variety of occupations, including college students, members of labor unions, military reservists, and housewives. They reported a "powerful relationship" between degree of religious belief and consumption of both alcohol and psychotropic drugs, with marked differences in alcohol and drug intake between the "very religious" and those who said they were "not religious at all." Use of alcohol, marijuana, hashish, amphetamines, and tobacco were all significantly greater in nonreligious group. On the basis of these results, Khavari and Harmon (1982) concluded that "drug treatment personnel may do well to closely scrutinize the possibility of enlisting the addict's religion as an aid in the overall treatment strategy" (p. 855).

Koenig and colleagues (1994b) examined the associations between religious variables and alcohol abuse or dependence among 2,969 persons ages 18–97 in North Carolina. Religious variables included frequency of Bible reading, prayer, and church attendance; time spent watching or listening to religious television or radio; and importance of religion, religious denomination, and identification as "born again" Christian. Recent (past six months) and lifetime DSM-III alcohol disorders were significantly less common among weekly churchgoers and among those who considered themselves born again. Those who frequently read the Bible or prayed privately also were less likely to have had recent alcohol problems, although this relationship did not hold for lifetime alcohol problems.

Interestingly, alcohol disorders were more common among those who frequently watched or listened to religious television or radio programs. Finally, lifetime alcohol disorders were more prevalent among members of Pentecostal denominations than among members of other Christian denominations (perhaps because of the more aggressive proselytizing by this religious group among the lower classes).

Thus, research from a variety of populations suggests that adult alcohol and drug use, like adolescent substance abuse, may be influenced by religion. Greater religious importance, frequent church attendance, and private religious practices (e.g., prayer and Bible reading) all predict less alcohol and drug use and abuse in adults. Further, membership in a religious denomination that strongly denounces alcohol and drug use usually also predicts less substance use and abuse.

POSSIBLE EXPLANATIONS

What is it about religious involvement that influences alcohol and drug abuse? As previously discussed, adolescents who are more religiously involved are also less likely to associate with peers who drink and use drugs, which is perhaps the most powerful predictor of alcohol or drug use known (Burkett & Warren, 1987). According to the peer influence model, religion's effects on alcohol and drug use are largely indirect. A number of studies, however, suggest that religious commitment may also have direct effects on alcohol and drug use by instilling moral values and character and by enhancing psychological well-being.

Instilling Moral Values

Evidence that religion may directly influence substance use by serving as a moral compass comes primarily from studies that have looked at why people choose not to drink. For example, Burkett (1980) conducted a study of 323 high school students to correlate attitudes about drinking and drinking habits with several measures of religiousness, including affiliation, church attendance, degree of satisfaction derived from church activities, and the extent to which the students considered themselves very religious. Students were also asked about the orthodoxy of their religious beliefs and whether they believed that drinking was a "sin." Three measures of religiousness significantly predicted alcohol use among these adolescents: Protestants (rather than Catholics), the highly religious, and those who believed that drinking was a sin were significantly more likely than others to abstain from drinking.

Hughes and colleagues (1985) examined the relationship among religious involvement, drinking practices, and attitudes toward alcohol among the members of a church in Southampton, England. Church members who completely abstained (teetotalers) reported that their childhood upbringing and the teachings of the Bible were the main factors that led them to abstain. Interestingly, only a small proportion of the teetotalers cited other reasons, such as health, the cost of alcohol, seeing the adverse effects of drinking on others, the taste of alcohol, or the availability of cheaper health insurance for teetotalers.

In a detailed examination of the social and psychological factors responsible for drinking behaviors among young girls, Coombs and colleagues (1985) interviewed 197 girls ages 9–17 who lived in the Los Angeles area. Investigators were particularly interested in why these young girls chose to abuse drugs and alcohol. Four hypotheses were tested: (1) deprivation (i.e., broken homes and economic hardship), (2) personal deficiency (i.e., lack of emotional maturity or having specific character traits that promote unhealthy behaviors), (3) youth culture (i.e., the belief that everybody's doing it), and (4) family pathology (i.e., detrimental interactions between family members or lack of parental rewards, role modeling, belief systems, or controls).

Surprisingly, the results indicated that deprivation (family breakup or low-income status) was not significantly related to alcohol use in this sample. There was stronger evidence that youth culture played a role in promoting drinking behavior. "Peer approval" was rated as very important by a large number of the girls who drank than compared to girls who did not. Getting together and discussing personal problems with friends was also more characteristic of girls who drank than of abstainers. However, family

pathology was the strongest predictor of drinking behavior. In particular, family religious values and participation in church-related activities were "highly significant factors" distinguishing between alcohol users and nonusers. In fact, only two of nine measures of family religiousness failed to reach statistical significance. The importance of the father's belief in God proved to be the most influential factor ($p < .001$). However, attendance at church or synagogue and other related activities (as reported by both parent and child) also significantly differentiated alcohol users from nonusers. Indeed, the more a girl participated in such activities, the less likely she was to use alcohol; 61.5% of abstainers attended weekly services, compared to 46.3% of past drinkers and 41.6% of current drinkers ($p < .01$). Finally, although the father's religious beliefs appeared to be more influential than the mother's beliefs in affecting daughters' alcohol use, mother's attendance at services was more influential than father's attendance in this regard.

To test the hypothesis that religion can directly influence alcohol consumption via strong moral messages, Bock and colleagues (1987) examined the use and misuse of alcohol between 1972 and 1980, across a variety of religious denominations, using data collected from a random national sample of 4,278 American adults. Religious variables included strength of religious identification, frequency of church attendance, and membership in a church organization; alcohol consumption was measured by asking respondents, "Do you use alcohol?" and "If so, do you sometimes drink more than you should?" Analyses were controlled for a number of demographic variables including age, sex, race, area of residence (urban vs. rural), income, region, and education. Results indicated that the moral message of respondents' religious affiliation increased with increasing religious involvement. Members of churches that prohibited alcohol use had a higher rate of abstinence, and religious commitment was a better predictor of abstinence among members of those churches (Conservative Protestants, in particular).

In addition to indirectly influencing alcohol and drug use by influencing peer interactions, then, religion may play a direct role in discouraging alcohol use among both adolescents and adults by supporting a moral code of conduct. The more one is exposed to religion, through either worship services or personal religious activities (particularly in denominations that prohibit alcohol use), the more this moral code is reinforced.

Religion and Psychological Well-Being

Another way that religion might reduce the risk of alcohol and drug use is by increasing psychological well-being. Although only a few empirical studies have been conducted in this area, the existing literature suggests that religion reduces the need for alcohol and other drugs by making people less susceptible to stress, increasing their coping skills, or both.

Krause (1991) examined survey data from a national sample of 1,607 people ages 60 years or older to identify factors associated with the use of alcohol in later life. The relationship between coping resources and alcohol use was also examined and included assessment of two religious resources—frequency of church attendance and personal religiosity (measured by importance of religion, frequency of watching or listening to religious programs, and frequency of seeking spiritual comfort to deal with problems). Greater health problems were related to a greater probability that older adults would refrain from drinking alcohol ($\beta = .170$, $p < .001$). As health difficulties became more bothersome, religious involvement tended to intensify ($\beta = .087$, $p < .05$), suggesting that religion was being used as a method for coping with health problems. Increased subjective religiosity was, in turn, related to a greater probability that elderly people in the sample would not drink alcohol ($\beta = .336$, $p < .05$).

Conversely, increased financial difficulties were associated with lower levels of subjective religious involvement ($\beta = -.184$, $p < .001$) and greater levels of alcohol consumption ($\beta = -.062$, $p < .05$). Although the reasons for the diminished subjective religiosity among those with greater financial problems was not clear, Krause speculated that older adults in this sample who faced financial problems were more likely to consume alcohol and less likely to avail themselves of religious involvement as a means of coping. Although initially Krause found that older African Americans were as likely to abstain from alcohol as whites, when other factors were controlled the data revealed that African Americans were significantly more likely than whites to abstain ($\beta = .180$, $p < .05$). Further analysis revealed that the reason elderly African Americans were more likely to abstain from alcohol was their increased subjective religiosity ($\beta = .240$, $p < .05$).

Another significant finding in this study was that women were significantly more likely than men to abstain from drinking ($\beta = .296$, $p < .05$). Again, the bulk of the indirect effect of gender ($\beta = .125$) on alcohol abstinence involved subjective religiosity ($\beta = .108$, $p < .05$). As with race, a significant part of the relationship between gender and abstinence could be attributed to the fact that women in the sample had higher levels of subjective religiosity than did men. Furthermore, although women were more likely to experience financial difficulties than men, they were still were more likely to abstain from using alcohol than men because of their consistently higher levels of subjective religiosity ($\beta = .321$, $p < .001$).

On the basis of these results, Krause (1991) concluded that "the data suggest that older women and African-Americans are especially likely to have strong subjective religious commitments and that people with high levels of subjective religiosity are particularly likely to abstain from drinking alcoholic beverages" (p. 143). In attempting to explain why increased financial problems caused decreased subjective religiosity, Krause suggested that older people who experience financial problems may become more distrustful in general, and, regardless of specific religious doctrine, religious involvement tends to be based on both trust in God and trust in humanity. This study did not find that attending formal church services was a replacement for subjective religiosity, since church attendance did not have an independent effect on drinking behavior.

In another study of an elderly population, Alexander and Duff (1991) examined correlates of life satisfaction among adults living in two retirement communities. Investigators interviewed 156 individuals, assessing demographic characteristics, living arrangements, perceived health, social relationships and activities, life satisfaction, religiosity, death anxiety, drinking patterns and history of alcohol use, attitudes toward drinking, and perceptions of alcohol use in their community. Of these, 75 respondents lived in a secular retirement community, and 81 lived in a religious retirement community.

Investigators found the communities differed significantly on all variables except perceived health. As expected, there was a higher rate of alcohol use in the secular community than in the religious community (53% in the secular community drank weekly, compared to 30% in the religious community). Residents in the religious community also had higher life satisfaction, lower levels of death anxiety, and higher levels of social activity than did residents of the secular community ($p < .01$, uncontrolled).

In summary, persons who are religiously involved—whether adolescents, young adults, or older adults—are less likely to use, abuse, or become dependent on alcohol or other drugs.

RELIGIOUS AND SPIRITUAL INTERVENTIONS FOR TREATING ALCOHOL AND DRUG PROBLEMS

If religious involvement is protective against initial alcohol or other drug use, might it also be utilized as method of treating those whose lives have been devastated by such addictions? Research has shown that religious involvement tends to be low among people in treatment for substance abuse (e.g., Kroll & Sheehan, 1989; Brizer, 1993). Might it be possible to treat substance abuse problems by involving individuals in religious or spiritually based programs?

Fostering religious or spiritual beliefs in substance abusers may provide a transcending mechanism for bolstering therapeutic expectations and outcomes (Levin, 1994). Thoresen (1997) argues that religious or spiritual interventions can help people find meaning, direction, and purpose in life. Along these same lines, the Harvard psychiatrist George Vaillant (1983) notes,

In the treatment of addiction, Karl Marx's aphorism "religion is the opiate of the masses" masks an enormously important therapeutic principal. Religion may actually provide a relief that drug [and alcohol] abuse only promises. . . . First, alcoholics and victims of other seemingly incurable habits feel defeated, bad, and helpless. They invariably suffer from impaired morale. If they are to recover, powerful new sources of self-esteem and hope must be discovered. Religion is one such source. Religion provides fresh impetus for both hope and enhanced self-care. Second, if the established alcoholic is to become stably abstinent, enormous personality changes must take place. It is not just coincidence that we associate such dramatic change with the experience of religious conversion. Third, religion, in ways that we appreciate but do not understand, provides forgiveness of sins and relief from guilt. Unlike many intractable habits that others find merely annoying, alcoholism inflicts enormous pain and injury on those around the alcoholic. As a result the alcoholic, already demoralized by his inability to stop drinking, experiences almost insurmountable guilt from the torture he has inflicted on others. In such an instance, absolution becomes an important part of the healing process. (p. 193)

Although some interventions have occasionally included a spiritual component among several other treatment modalities, only a few have specifically utilized spiritual treatments in rehabilitation programs for alcohol or drug problems. We now present an overview of research that examines the effectiveness of three types of religious or spiritual interventions: (1) church-based interventions, (2) 12-step programs, and (3) meditation.

Churches and Substance Abuse Rehabilitation

Most early church-based substance abuse programs were run by Protestant churches. Since the 1960s, however, the Catholic Church has become increasingly involved in providing treatment and rehabilitation services to substance abusers. Although churches stressed religious values and the importance of faith in God, they often adopted more secular approaches to treatment (Muffler et al., 1992). Today, many of these church-based substance abuse programs are confined to sponsoring Alcoholics Anonymous and Narcotics Anonymous meetings and services. Some congregations, however, offer a broader range of social services and referrals in conjunction with ministries to the homeless (Muffler et al., 1992).

Unfortunately, only a few of these church-based programs for substance abusers have been thoroughly evaluated (Gorsuch, 1995). Muffler and colleagues (1992) evaluated four programs, two that were supported by mainline churches and two that were supported by conservative churches, and found that "these programs have demonstrated successful outcomes comparable to secular treatment regimes" (p. 594). However, investigators were unable to ascertain whether the religiousness of participants changed or played a role in mediating outcomes.

Hess (1977) reported that Teen Challenge, a program that explicitly bases its treatment on conservative Christian religious doctrine, has a differential retention rate that varies with the religiousness of the person coming into the program. Interestingly, three of four participants (75%) who were not initially religious successfully graduated from the program, compared to only one of five (20%) who had attended church regularly at 12 years of age. Because this was an explicitly religious program, it is likely that some aspect of religiousness changed in the first group. However, persons in the second group (i.e., those who had attended church regularly at age 12), may have had an ineffective experience with religion in the past, making it difficult for them to use religion as a tool for successful recovery.

Joining certain religious cults may also aid in recovery from alcohol and drug problems. Galanter (1982a) examined alcohol and drug use among persons who were participating in two cults—the Unification Church ("Moonies") and the Divine Light Mission. He found that one-third of those who joined these cults reported a decrease in their frequency of substance abuse.

Twelve-Step Fellowships

Twelve-step fellowships seek to help people with alcohol or drug problems (Trice & Staudenmeier, 1989; Scott, 1993), and recently have begun reaching out to those with other problems that involve excessive dependence or addiction (e.g., gambling and overeating). Alcoholics Anonymous (AA), the original 12-step program, is explicitly based on spiritual principles. These principles include dependence on a self-defined Higher Power, self-examination, prayer and meditation, and assistance to others (Carroll, 1993). Steps 10, 11, and 12, in particular, are seen as most important for spiritual growth and maintenance of sobriety (Alcoholics Anonymous, 1976, pp. 59–60):

Step 10. Continued to take personal inventory and when we were wrong promptly admitted it.

Step 11. Sought through prayer and meditation to improve our conscious contact with God *as we understood Him*, praying only for knowledge of His will for us and the power to carry that out.

Step 12. Having had a spiritual awakening as the result of these steps, we tried to carry this message to alcoholics and to practice these principles in all our affairs.

Twelve-step programs have burgeoned in the past few decades and today are considered by many to be one of the most successful methods for ending substance abuse and preventing relapse (Emrick et al., 1993). Studies have concluded that active AA membership enables 60–68% of alcoholics to drink less (or not at all) for up to a year, and 40–50% achieve sobriety for many years (Emrick et al., 1993). Not all experts, however, are so positive about AA programs.

After reviewing the research, Peele (1990) concluded that standard AA programs have not demonstrated their efficacy. He based this conclusion on three early studies that compared involvement in AA with involvement in other treatment programs and found no difference or better results in the other treatment programs or with no treatment (Ditman et al., 1967; Brandsma et al., 1980; Vaillant, 1983). Since Peele's review, a number of other studies have examined the effects of involvement in AA or similar programs on treatment outcomes.

Alford and colleagues (1991) found that the positive effects of involvement in AA, while short-lived in men, persisted for at least two years or more in women. In this study, 157 chemically dependent male and female adolescents who had been enrolled in an AA or Narcotics Anonymous (NA) program were followed for two years after treatment. At six-month follow-up, of those who had completed treatment, 71% of male subjects and 79% of female subjects were abstinent or essentially abstinent, compared to only 37% of males and 30% of females who did not complete treatment ($p < .005$ for both males and females). At one-year follow-up, however, abstinence rates for males who had completed treatment were similar to those for male noncompleters (48% vs. 44%). At the end of the two-year follow-up period, there was no significant difference between male completers and noncompleters.

In contrast, 70% of females who completed treatment were still abstinent or nearly abstinent at one-year follow-up, compared to only 28% of females who did not complete treatment ($p < .01$). At the two-year follow-up, the percentages declined somewhat, although they remained significantly different for treatment completers and noncompleters. Unfortunately, investigators did not include an untreated control group for comparison. Since all subjects were at least temporarily in treatment, the noncompleters did not reflect the natural history of untreated substance abuse. Considering the pretreatment histories of these adolescents (who had used substances several times per week to every day for an average of 17 months), however, the researchers concluded that "subjects who completed this AA/NA-oriented treatment program demonstrated remarkable changes in their chemical use and general behavioral functioning" (p. 125).

Some AA practices may be more important than others in alcoholic rehabilitation, helping to explain some of the differences in treatment outcome reported in the literature. Montgomery and colleagues (1995) found that, while posttreatment frequency of AA attendance was not predictive of drinking outcomes, the extent to which patients became involved in AA did predict longer sobriety. Carroll (1993) studied AA members who attended meetings in northern California to assess the relationship between abstinence from alcohol and increased "purpose in life." The Purpose in Life (PIL) test was administered to 100 AA members, who also answered questions that assessed the extent to which members practiced Steps 11 and 12 of the 12-step program (those that emphasize spiritual practices). The extent to which participants practiced Step 11 was significantly correlated with PIL scores ($r = .059$, $p < .001$), whereas practice of Step 12 was not. Length of sobriety and PIL scores were also significantly correlated ($r = .31$, $p < .001$). The number of AA meetings attended was also correlated with longer sobriety ($r = .25$, $p < .01$), purpose in life ($r = .24$, $p < .01$), and fewer relapses ($r = -.27$, $p < .01$). Carroll concluded that practicing Step 11 (seeking through prayer and meditation to improve conscious contact with God, praying for knowledge of God's will and for the power to carry it out) was especially important for developing purpose in life and for affecting length of sobriety.

Meditation

Meditation-based interventions have been reported in a number of studies (e.g., Alexander et al., 1994; Taub et al., 1994) to reduce levels of alcohol or drug abuse. Gelderloos and colleagues (1991) reviewed 24 studies on the benefits of Transcendental Meditation (TM) in treating and preventing substance abuse and dependence. These studies covered noninstitutionalized users, participants in treatment programs, and prisoners with histories of heavy alcohol or drug use. All studies showed positive effects for the TM program. Reviewers indicated that the positive results from some of these studies could have been due to self-selection or responder bias. Nevertheless, longitudinal studies with random-assignment and more objective measures also showed positive results. The authors concluded that TM simultaneously addressed several factors that underlay chemical dependency, providing not only immediate relief from physical distress but also long-range improvements in well-being, self-esteem, personal empowerment, and other areas of "psychophysiological" health.

RELIGION AND EXACERBATION OF SUBSTANCE ABUSE

By inducing guilt and suppressing aggressive or sexual drives, religion may in some cases lead to or worsen problems with substance abuse. The evidence from systematic research to support this assertion, however, remains rather meager. Studying 50 male patients admitted to the Topeka, Kansas, VA hospital for treatment of alcoholism, Walters (1957) reported that a larger proportion of these alcoholics had parents who were both members of the same church than did a control group of men chosen from the medical, surgical, neurological, or psychiatric wards of the same hospital (66% vs. 48%, respectively). Mothers of alcoholics were also more involved in religious activities than were mothers of control group members (66% active vs. 50% active) (perhaps in order to cope with the behaviors of husbands who were also much more likely to be alcoholic). The author did not provide statistical comparisons or take into account control variables. Social class may have had a considerable influence on the findings given that both religion and substance abuse are more common in the lower classes. Furthermore, persons with religious backgrounds may have been more likely to seek substance abuse treatment than those without religious backgrounds (as the author readily admits).

Zucker et al. (1987) conducted a prospective study of 61 male alcoholics from an inpatient alcohol treatment program at the Bronx, New York, VA hospital. The method of assessing

religiosity was not specified, although it was correlated with religious attendance ($r = .65$), which was also measured but not examined in its relationship to alcohol use. Religious patients had more antialcohol attitudes on admission, but, when changes in attitudes toward alcohol were examined 4 weeks later, the least religious patients were more likely to change to antialcohol attitudes. Note, however, that the least religious patients started from a lower baseline and had greater room for change in attitudes. Religious patients were also more likely to have prior admissions for detoxication and rehabilitation and so probably already had fairly set attitudes. Finally, a selection effect may also have been operating, since persons with strong religious attitudes who continue to problem drink may be a unique breed.

Finally, Waisberg and Porter (1994) examined the relationship between purpose in life and treatment outcome in a clinical trial that involved 95 inpatients with substance abuse problems. The 55 patients (89% alcoholics) in treatment Program A focused on skill acquisition—group therapy, medical information, relaxation training, assertiveness training, marital therapy, exercise, nutrition, spiritual aspects, goal planning, viewing films, and attending family programs for substance abuse. The 40 patients (73% alcoholics) in treatment B Program focused on direct teaching of spiritual values, including confrontation of patients by staff and fellow alcoholics. Subjects in Programs A and B were compared to 36 people on a waiting-list control group. Purpose in life increased significantly and to the same degree for subjects in both treatment programs; Program A had lower dropout rates and a higher proportion of abstinent subjects after treatment, however. Patients in Program A were significantly older, had higher yearly incomes, and were less likely to have legal problems than persons in Program B (factors that may have favored successful abstinence). Furthermore, subjects in Program A also had their spiritual needs addressed, which contaminated the secular intervention.

Other than these three studies, however, most of the nearly 150 studies on the relationship between religious involvement and substance abuse suggest less substance abuse and more successful rehabilitation among the more religious (see part VIII).

SUMMARY AND CONCLUSIONS

Alcohol and drug use problems have a substantial adverse impact on individuals and society as a whole. Because these problems are so difficult to treat, researchers have explored a host of psychosocial factors that might be used as tools in the war against alcohol and drug abuse. To date, there are nearly a hundred studies suggesting that religion may be a deterrent to alcohol or drug abuse in children, adolescents, and adult populations. The greater a person's religious involvement, the less likely he or she will initiate alcohol or drug use or have problems with these substances if they are used. Religious participation may reduce alcohol and other drug use by a number of mechanisms, including reducing the likelihood of choosing friends who use or abuse substances, instilling moral values, increasing coping skills, and reducing the likelihood of turning to alcohol or other drugs during times of stress. Finally, although much further research is needed, formal church-based programs, nonchurch-based 12-step fellowships, and private spiritual practices can have a significant impact on the rehabilitation of persons with substance abuse problems.

12

Delinquency

IN 1948, J. EDGAR HOOVER STAT-
ed flatly that "In practically all homes
where juvenile delinquency is bred there
is an absence of adequate religious training for children . . . most of them have never
been inside a church" (Hoover, 1948, pp. 33–
35). In 1998, the Rev. Eugene Rivers appeared
on the cover of *Newsweek* magazine as part of
a story entitled, "God vs. Gangs: What's the
Hottest Idea in Crime Fighting? The Power
of Religion" (Leland, 1998). This chapter
presents an overview of delinquency, including
definitions, risk factors, and social and economic consequences, with a primary focus on
the relationship among religion, delinquency,
and later criminality. We also examine the potential efficacy of religious or spiritual-based
programs for preventing and controlling delinquency.

DEFINING DELINQUENCY

Delinquency is problem behavior, especially by
the young, that is against the basic principles
of society or is harmful to society (i.e., is antisocial) or is in violation of the law. Problem behaviors tend to start at relatively early ages, around
age 9 or 10, particularly in boys, and may be
marked by the onset of stubborn behavior and
minor covert acts such as frequent lying or
shoplifting. These behaviors tend to be followed, around ages 11–12, by acts of defiance,
minor aggression, and property damage (Huizinga, 1994). In time, more serious forms of
delinquency may ensue, such as violent behavior (e.g., fighting or assault) and chronic
resistance to authority figures, including truancy, staying out late at night, and running
away.

CONSEQUENCES OF DELINQUENCY

In 1992, an estimated 1 million juveniles in the United States were charged with approximately 1.5 million delinquent acts, a 26% increase over the number of cases reported in 1987. In addition, a disproportionate increase occurred in violent offenses (56%) and in weapons offenses (86%) among people under age 18 years (Snyder & Sickmund, 1995). In 1996, an estimated 2.9 million juveniles were arrested, an almost threefold increase in just four years; juveniles accounted for 19% of all arrests (Snyder, 1997).

Most juveniles who are arrested, whether male or female, have committed not serious or violent crimes but rather property crimes or status offenses (e.g., drinking while under age or using illicit drugs). Indeed, juvenile delinquents make up a far greater proportion of all property crime arrests (33%) than of either violent crime arrests (18%) or drug arrests (8%) (Federal Bureau of Investigation, 1994). In 1992, the juveniles comprised 49% of those arrested for arson, 45% of those arrested for vandalism, and 44% of those arrested for motor vehicle theft (Snyder & Sickmund, 1995).

Although the juvenile property crime arrest rate in 1992 was five times greater than the juvenile violent crime arrest rate (Snyder & Sickmund, 1995), more and more violent crime involves young offenders. Indeed, juvenile arrests for violent crimes increased 50% from 1988 to 1992, twice the increase for those age 18 years or older. Persons most likely to be victimized by juveniles were also young, between 12 and 19 years of age (Federal Bureau of Investigation, 1994; Rennison, 1998). With regard to the types of violent crimes juveniles commit, juvenile arrests in 1991 included 3,400 arrests for murder, 6,300 arrests for rape, 44,500 arrests for robbery, and almost 70,000 arrests for aggravated assault (Dilulio, 1994).

Given population growth projections and the trends in juvenile arrests over the past decade, criminologists expect that the rate of juvenile arrests for violent crimes will more than double between 1990 and the year 2010 (Allen-Hagen, 1991). Statistics also indicate that violent juvenile female offending is on the rise and that the increase for girls is greater proportionately than that for boys. Between 1988 and 1992, the number of girls under age 18 arrested for all violent crimes increased 63%, whereas the number of boys under age 18 arrested for violent crimes increased 45% (Coordinating Council on Juvenile Justice and Delinquency, 1996).

CAUSES OF DELINQUENCY

What causes juvenile delinquency? There is no single cause of delinquency and violence. Delinquents, especially chronic delinquents, exhibit a variety of social and psychological deficits in their backgrounds. These deficits (or risk factors) stem from breakdowns in five influential domains in juveniles' lives: neighborhood, family, school, peers, and individual characteristics (Hawkins & Catalano, 1992). Risk factors, such as community disorganization, availability of drugs and firearms, and persistent poverty, make children more prone to delinquent behavior than if those factors were not present. Additionally, when a child's family life is filled with violence, problem behaviors, poor parental monitoring, and inconsistent disciplinary practices or maltreatment, the child's risk of delinquency increases. Youth who exhibit combinations of these deficits in several areas of their lives are at the highest risk for delinquency (Huizinga & Menard, 1989).

In sum, there are many risk factors for delinquency and violence. These factors often occur simultaneously, exacerbating one another and making them more difficult to ameliorate. Identifying the factors that are most prevalent in a community is the essential first step toward developing effective programs to prevent or control delinquent behavior (Kumpfer et al., 1996).

COSTS OF DELINQUENCY

How much does juvenile delinquency cost? There is no clear, simple answer to this question. Although many studies over the past few years have tried to quantify the total direct and indirect costs of all crime (adult and juvenile) to government and society, the results have varied. However, all of these studies have concluded that the national cost is in the tens to hundreds of billions of dollars annually.

Some costs of crime (such as the government's direct cost of fighting crime) can be readily estimated. For example, in 1988, federal, state, and local government agencies spent more than $150 billion to fight crime. This figure includes the costs for police, prosecution, courts, probation, and incarceration (Fadaei-Tehrani, 1990). Since a disproportionate share of crime is committed by juveniles (albeit mostly older juveniles), the cost for fighting juvenile crime is considerable.

Other costs cannot be easily measured. Many crimes go unreported; from 1993 to 1998 only about half of violent crimes were reported to police (Rennison, 1998). Other crimes go undetected. The total costs to society of these unreported and undetected crimes are not recorded. Also, some costs, such as those for shoplifting and vandalism, are simply transferred by manufacturers and retailers to consumers in order to cover the victims' costs for crime prevention activities or losses from crime.

Nevertheless, it has been estimated that personal crime generates $105 billion annually in property and productivity losses and medical expenses (Miller et al., 1996). Another recent study found that the typical career criminal causes $1.3–$1.5 million in costs to society; a heavy drug user costs $370,000–$970,000; and a high-school dropout costs $243,000–$388,000. Even after eliminating duplication caused by counting twice each crime committed by individuals who are, for example, both heavy drug users and career criminals, the overall estimate of the monetary value of saving a single high-risk youth is $1.7–$2.3 million (Cohen, 1998). On a national scale, extrapolated to the estimated 1 million juveniles in the United States who were charged with approximately 1.5 million delinquent acts in 1992, the economic cost of delinquency is certainly enormous.

PREVENTING AND CONTROLLING DELINQUENCY

The past century has witnessed a number of approaches to the prevention and treatment of delinquency. Some approaches have emphasized focusing on physiological, psychological, and other individual characteristics; others have focused on the structure of the family; still others have considered the structure of social relations within the broader society. More recent approaches have attempted to conceptualize an integrated complex of factors that includes community characteristics (Sullivan & Wilson, 1995).

As briefly discussed, researchers have identified a number of positive (protective) and negative (risk factor) characteristics associated with delinquency that may be present or lacking in communities, families, schools, peer groups, and individuals. These factors either equip a child with the skills and capacity to become a healthy, productive individual or expose that child to potential involvement in crime and violence. Among the factors that appear to provide some protection against delinquency is religious involvement. Although it is still not clear what aspects of religious involvement are the most protective against delinquency, there is a growing body of research suggests that religious involvement may steer young people away from peer groups, attitudes, and behaviors that put them at greater risk for committing delinquent or criminal acts. The remainder of this chapter discusses that research.

RELIGION AND DELINQUENCY

Religion has long been considered by some to be a deterrent to crime because it promotes social control and encourages the development of moral character and the acceptance of societal norms and values (Davis, 1948; Erikson, 1966; Fitzpatrick, 1967). However, this notion was disputed by Hirschi and Stark (1969), who reported, because of their finding that church attendance and belief in supernatural sanctions were unrelated to self-reported delinquency, that religiosity and delinquency were virtually unrelated. This finding became, for some, the conclusion to a long-debated relationship between personal religiousness and delinquency.

However, because such findings were counterintuitive, some researchers persisted in studying this relationship. As they refined their measurements of religiousness and further delineated how aspects of religiousness related to various forms of delinquency, these later studies demonstrated that religiousness in adolescents is, in general, negatively correlated with delinquent behavior.

Delinquency and Religious Denomination

Early studies on the relationship between religious denomination and delinquency suggested that, among youth who express a religious preference, Jews have the lowest rates of juvenile delinquency, with Protestants intermediate and Roman Catholics highest (Hersch, 1936; Glueck & Glueck, 1950; Wattenberg, 1950). Attempting to interpret these denominational differences on rates of delinquency, investigators have generally concluded that they result from differences in the social class of members of these major denominations. In other words, denominations such as Catholicism, which draw many members from lower socioeconomic levels, have the highest delinquency rates (Robison, 1960). The low rate of delinquency among Jews is explained as a joint effect of high socioeconomic status and high family integration.

Taken as a whole, however, youth that are more religiously involved tend to have significantly lower rates of delinquency than the nonreligious. For example, Rhodes and Reiss (1970) examined the relationship between religious orientation and delinquent or truant behavior among a regional sample of more than 20,000 junior and senior high school students. They found, as previously reported, that, among those who indicated a religious affiliation, Jews and nonfundamentalist Protestants had the lowest rates of delinquency. White female and African American male Catholics had the highest rates of delinquency among the religiously affiliated. Baptists and fundamentalist

Protestants had higher rates than nonfundamentalist Protestants.

More notable, however, was the finding that white males with no religious preference had almost twice the delinquency rate of white males with any religious affiliation. This finding persisted even after the researchers controlled for other risk factors, including parents' occupational status and religious participation and family structure (one-parent vs. two-parent homes). This $2:1$ adjusted rate also held for nonreligious African American males compared to religious African American males. Interestingly, the overall delinquency rate for both nonreligious and religious girls was very low. This study suggests that merely having a religious affiliation, regardless of whether one is a "true believer" or a frequent participant, may be a significant deterrent to delinquent behavior.

An inverse relationship between religious affiliation and deviant behavior in adolescents was confirmed by a more recent study by Tenant-Clark and colleagues (1989), which examined the impact of participation in "occult" practices among 50 teenagers, all of whom had substance abuse problems and 25 of whom were in treatment. The teenagers were given a three-part questionnaire that assessed their self-esteem, belief and participation in the occult, and drug and alcohol use. Apart from their occult participation, they were also asked a number of questions about their religious affiliation, beliefs about religion, strength of their religious convictions, and involvement in religious activities.

Investigators found a significant relationship between substance abuse and occult participation ($r = .56$). High occult participants were also likely to have low self-esteem, negative feelings about school, poor self-concept, and little desire to be considered a "good person." They were also much more likely than occult nonparticipants to harbor negative feelings about religion, have a high tolerance for deviance, have negative feelings about the future, experience few social sanctions for drug use, and feel that others were blaming them for their problems.

In other words, adolescents who participate in the occult have often rejected traditional forms of religious expression. Adolescent occult participation and traditional religious involvement seldom coexist, and occultism may be a rebellion against the family's religion and societal norms.

Church Attendance and Delinquency

Participation in traditional forms of religion may deter delinquent behavior. The evidence for this is based primarily on cross-sectional studies that use frequency of church attendance as the measure of religious involvement. For example, Higgins and Albrecht (1977) analyzed data from a survey of approximately 1,400 high school students on the relationship between respect for the juvenile court system and delinquent behavior. Two items about religion—church attendance and church affiliation—were included in the questionnaire. When the investigators analyzed the relationship between these two items and 17 delinquency-related items in the questionnaire, they found a modest to moderately strong negative relationship between frequency of church attendance and each of the 17 delinquent behaviors (for the composite delinquency measure, the γ was −.48). Although this negative relationship between church attendance and delinquency was consistent across all racial groups (whites and nonwhites), it was greatest for white males (−.57).

In a later report, Ellis (1985) reviewed the literature on church attendance and delinquency. Ellis found 31 relevant studies, the vast majority of which reported that frequent church attenders committed less crime than did infrequent attenders. All but five studies (84%) reported a significant inverse relationship between church attendance and crime. Even among the five studies that did not report a significant inverse relationship, the direction of the relationship was still negative; that is, religious attendance was inversely related to delinquency.

Despite the findings by Ellis (1985) and others (e.g., Johnson, Spencer, et al., 1997) that the majority of studies report an inverse relationship between church attendance and delinquency, controversy continues over this issue. Some have argued that the religion-delinquency relationship exists only with certain types of

antisocial behaviors or within certain denominational groups but not others. It has also been argued that the effects of religion on delinquency are mediated either directly or indirectly through more proximate social controls (e.g., peers and family). The following sections explore some of these issues.

Religious Salience and Delinquency

As early research on the relationship between religion and delinquency evolved, some researchers recognized the need to include religious salience, or the importance of religion to an individual, as one of several measures of religiosity. An early study by Middleton and Putney (1962) found that religious salience, as well as religious ideology (belief in God) and religious attendance, were all negatively related to antiascetic actions or victimless crimes. That is, adolescents who were more religious were less likely to engage in activities such as gambling, smoking, petting, and drinking than were those who were less religious. However, no significant differences were found between the religious and the nonreligious in terms of antisocial actions (crimes involving victims).

Stark and colleagues (1982) operationalized what might be called an "ecological" measure of religious salience by computing church membership for Standard Metropolitan Statistical Areas (SMSAs) in the United States. Assessing religious variables as well as involvement in delinquent activities, these investigators analyzed data from a nationally representative sample of tenth grade boys who attended 87 different high schools. Investigators found that there was a high level of religiousness in the majority of students in most states throughout the United States, except in Oregon, Washington, and California, which they referred to as a "secular peninsula." When the researchers analyzed the effects of moral climate on delinquency, they found that delinquency was consistently lower in the more religious communities than in secular communities. On the basis of these results, Stark and associates concluded that they had discovered a possible explanation for religion's inverse relationship with delinquency: Religion is inversely associated with delinquency *only* when it is part of widely accepted social values and norms that prohibit such behavior. In other words, religion lowers one's risk of delinquency only if it is reinforced by prevailing social norms, that is, by one's surrounding community. This is known as social control theory.

However, a number of more recent studies have since challenged this notion. Of particular note is Benda's (1995) survey of more than 1,000 high school students in rural Arkansas and in urban Baltimore, Maryland. Benda asked students about their religiousness (using eight separate religion variables) as well as about their involvement in property crimes, crimes against other people, and status offenses (e.g., truancy or staying out late). He also asked them about their use of alcohol and other drugs, degree of attachment to parents, commitment to finishing school and getting a job, degree of monitoring by their parents, and beliefs about stealing and obeying laws. In direct contrast to Stark et al.'s (1982) assertion, it was only after Benda (1995) factored out elements of social control theory that the effect of religiousness on crimes against other people became statistically significant. In other words, if elements of social control are not factored out of the analysis, they mask the significance of the relationship between religiousness and crimes against others.

The finding that at least some of religion's effects on delinquency are independent of social control is also supported by a study by Chadwick and Top (1993) on a population of Mormons (LDS). To test the theory that religion is negatively related to delinquency only in a highly religious climate, Chadwick and Top surveyed more than 2,000 LDS youth living in widely scattered communities along the East Coast of the United States and compared their data to data previously collected in three highly concentrated, conservative LDS communities in southern California, Idaho, and Utah. Investigators found that religiousness had a strong negative relationship to delinquency in both the religiously conservative and the nonreligiously conservative environments. Furthermore, a multivariate analysis of the data revealed that, although peer pressure was the strongest factor that influenced delinquency, religiousness also made a significant independent contribution.

Benson and Donahue (1989) produced similar results when they analyzed data obtained from a nationally representative sample of high school seniors from 1976 to 1985. This study found that religion was a stronger predictor of delinquency than was a variety of other factors traditionally believed to have a strong influence on preventing delinquency. These investigators examined the prevalence of cigarette smoking, alcohol use, marijuana use, and truancy among seniors from more than 125 high schools throughout the United States. They then analyzed the relationship between these delinquency variables and 10 separate social and demographic characteristics, including region of the country, type of school (public vs. parochial), gender and race, the presence of a father at home, parents' educational level, mother's employment status, importance of religion, college plans, hours worked per week during the school year, and number of "nights out" for fun and socializing during the week.

In their multivariate analysis, Benson and Donahue found that the number of nights per week that seniors reported that they "went out for fun and recreation" was the single strongest positive predictor of delinquent behaviors. However, religiousness and plans to graduate from a four-year college were the two most powerful negative predictors. None of the other variables showed the strength and consistency that number of nights out for fun and recreation, religiousness, and college plans did in "reducing" cigarette use, binge drinking, and monthly marijuana use.

The relationship between religion and delinquency, then, results from more than just peer and community influences. Although these influences are important, religion may also reduce delinquency by promoting positive moral values. Such values play a critical role in helping youths resist the temptation by peers to engage in delinquent behaviors.

Religion and Type of Delinquent Behavior

Is religion salient for only certain types of delinquency? Ellis's (1985) early review of the literature found that, among studies that separated criminal offenses into victimless and victim-related crimes, the strength of the relationships between religion and delinquency was greater for victimless crimes. In one of these reviewed studies, Burkett and White (1974) interviewed approximately 850 high school students about their frequency of church attendance and involvement in delinquent acts. They also asked the students about their acceptance of certain moral values, their acceptance of worldly authority, and their belief in the possibility of supernatural sanctions (e.g., going to heaven or hell).

This study, conducted in the Pacific Northwest (part of the "secular peninsula"), found that religious participation is more strongly associated with belief in the supernatural than with the development of moral values and acceptance of conventional authority. Further, although the data analysis revealed a strong inverse relationship between church attendance and alcohol ($\gamma = -.36$) and marijuana use ($\gamma = -.32$), there was only a weak inverse relationship between church attendance and other forms of delinquent behavior.

However, recent studies that used more comprehensive measures of religiousness have tended to contradict, or at least modify, these findings. Recall that Benda's (1995) survey of youths found that, contrary to earlier reports, the data did not support the notion that religiousness is predictive of only victimless crimes. Rather, in the final analysis, Benda found that religiousness was inversely related to adolescents' committing both victimless and victim-related crimes. Similar results were reported by Fernquist (1995). This investigator interviewed approximately 180 students from four separate colleges about their past and present involvement in various types of delinquency (both victimless and victim-related), as well as their frequency of prayer and church attendance. He also asked the students about their peer associations and their parental attachment (both maternal and paternal). As a whole, increased religiosity was associated with lower levels of both victimless and victim-related delinquency, even when other variables were controlled. However, the relationship was weaker for victim-related delinquency ($R^2 = .37$) than it was for victimless

delinquency ($R^2 = .54$). For both types of crime, the strongest and most significant impact came from peer associations.

Interestingly, Fernquist found that males were more likely to commit victim-related delinquent acts than were females, yet they were no more likely to commit victimless crimes than females. Also, although strong attachment to one's mother had a negative relationship to delinquency, it was only marginally significant. Paternal attachment had no significant association with either type of delinquency. These findings replicated those of an earlier study by Sloane and Potvin (1986), which reported that both church attendance and religious influence were strongly and negatively related to a variety of delinquent acts, including skipping school, running away from home, having sex, drinking alcohol, using marijuana and other drugs, trespassing, and committing acts of vandalism, stealing, and fighting (whether as an individual or as part of a gang). On the basis of these results, Sloane and Potvin (1986) concluded that the "association between religion and delinquency . . . is not confined to certain offenses or to certain groups or social contexts" (p. 104).

It is significant that Stark (1996), who had coauthored the 1969 article with Hirschi in which the authors concluded that religion was "irrelevant to delinquency," revised his initial conclusion 27 years later after analyzing results from a random national sample of 11,995 high school seniors. He concluded that religious communities have moral and ethical teachings that discourage many forms of deviant or illegal conduct and that most studies show less crime and juvenile delinquency among the more religious.

Finally, Wallace and Forman (1998) analyzed data on a random sample of 5,000 students from 135 high schools across the United States (part of the University of Michigan's Monitoring the Future Project) to determine the relationship between religious involvement and delinquent behaviors. Religious variables included religious importance and religious attendance. Outcome variables were behaviors such as carrying a weapon to school, engaging in interpersonal violence, drinking while driving, riding while drinking, cigarette smoking, binge drinking, and using marijuana. Religious importance was inversely related to carrying a weapon to school ($p \le .05$), interpersonal violence ($p \le .01$), driving while drinking ($p \le .001$), riding while drinking ($p \le .001$), binge drinking ($p \le .001$), and using marijuana ($p \le .001$). Except for carrying a weapon to school, frequency of religious attendance was even more strongly inversely associated with delinquent behaviors and substance use (all at $p \le .001$). These relationships persisted after adjusting for demographic factors (race, gender, parents' education, family structure, urbanicity, and region). Trend analyses using data from 1976 to 1996 indicated that these relationships have existed over time.

Thus, much of the largely cross-sectional research to date suggests that religion may have a persistent and significant impact on delinquency, including delinquency that harms other people. Although the mechanisms by which religion exerts its buffering influences against delinquency are not yet fully understood, peer influence plays a significant role. On the other hand, as we have seen, not all of religion's effects on individual behavior can be explained by external influences (such as peers).

RELIGION AND LONG-TERM CRIMINALITY

What about the long-term effects of religion on deviant behavior? A recent study by Evans et al. (1995) extends the findings of an inverse relationship between religion and delinquency in adolescents to adult criminality. These investigators looked at the relationship between adult criminality and four measures of religiousness—frequency of religious activities, daily influence of religion in one's life, beliefs in and fears of punishment or damnation (hellfire) by God, and general religiousness. They also examined other potentially confounding factors, such as denominational conservatism, interpersonal religious networks, and social environment variables.

Researchers found, surprisingly, that three of the four measures of religiousness—general religiousness, religious beliefs of punishment, and religious influence (salience)—were unrelated to adult criminality. Furthermore, members of more conservative religious denominations did not commit crimes less frequently than did members of liberal denominations. By contrast, religious activities (i.e., attending religious services, reading religious material, and listening to religious TV and radio broadcasts) were significantly related to less adult criminality. This inverse relationship persisted when social environmental variables were controlled for. Perhaps most important, this relationship persisted over a wide range of crimes, not just victimless crimes, and was independent of social and religious contexts. Thus, involvement in religious activities may significantly decrease the risk of adult criminality, as it may for adolescent delinquency. More longitudinal studies, however, are needed to establish the causal nature of these relationships.

RELIGIOUS/SPIRITUAL-BASED PROGRAMS FOR PREVENTING OR CONTROLLING DELINQUENCY

Despite the historical importance of religious groups as unique and powerful social institutions within communities, the influence of these institutions in preventing or controlling juvenile delinquency among youth has drawn limited attention from social scientists and criminologists. One of the few exceptions is the economist Richard Freeman (1986), who concluded that participation in the African American church helps inner-city African American male youth escape from the world of poverty, drug use, and crime. Analyzing survey data collected from 2,358 young African American males from the most poverty-stricken areas of Boston, Chicago, and Philadelphia between 1979 and 1989, Freeman found that church attendance had significant negative effects on deviant activities among at-risk youth, including alcohol and drug use. This inverse relationship with deviant behavior persisted after the researcher controlled for "religious attitude" and numerous sociodemographic factors (e.g., family income, family structure, family disruption, family size, and residence in public housing).

What is it about church participation that may help to protect against delinquency? One possibility is that religion teaches youths to have empathy for others. For example, a recent investigation by O'Donnell and colleagues (1995) found that involving adolescents in prosocial activities can significantly lower their risk for delinquency. Prosocial behavior, or altruism, involves making sacrifices for others with little or no expectation of reward (Batson, 1987). Most religious traditions promote altruistic behavior as a means of achieving inner peace and redemption.

To assess the effects of prosocial behavior on delinquency, O'Donnell and colleagues analyzed longitudinal data collected annually in the Seattle, Washington, area on "urban" children from the time they enter first grade until they are teenagers. This is a multiethnic population of children most of whom live in economically disadvantaged or working-class families and who are at significant risk for becoming involved in delinquent or violent behavior.

Investigators analyzed data on 808 children ages 12–13 and 13–14 years (and their parents). They also examined data from the Teacher Child Behavior Checklist, which was completed by teachers when the same children were ages 10–11 and 12–13 years. In addition to information on academic standing and achievement, these surveys assessed degree of early aggressive behavior, ethnicity, socioeconomic status (i.e., family income), mobility (i.e., how often their family moved), and family composition.

From this sample of 808 children, the investigators selected 52 boys who had been rated by their teachers when they were 10 or 11 years old (i.e., in the fifth grade) as being very "aggressive." The researchers then used measures taken from five scales—(1) prosocial involvement, (2) family bonding and family management practices (i.e., how rules are set and enforced), (3) school bonding (i.e., participation) and school achievement, (4) social norms against substance abuse, and (5) interaction with antisocial peers—to attempt to predict which boys would continue to be aggressive or would become involved in delinquent behavior when they were in high school.

In the initial analysis, investigators found to their surprise that none of the five scales predicted later delinquent behavior, and only two of the other factors—being poor and moving frequently—accurately predicted later involvement with drugs. However, more detailed analyses revealed that specific items on the scales significantly predicted later aggressive or delinquent behavior. In particular, prosocial skills, school bonding and achievement, family bonding and management practices, and norms against substance abuse, when included with measures of antisocial involvement in a regression model, predicted whether the boys would later become involved in delinquent behavior or substance abuse. Furthermore, involvement in "prosocial" activities appeared to inhibit later delinquent involvement rather than substance abuse, whereas norms against substance abuse appeared to inhibit both delinquency and substance abuse, as did school bonding and achievement. Investigators concluded that high levels of prosocial skill, school bonding and achievement, and antisubstance abuse norms may protect at-risk aggressive boys from later involvement in delinquent behaviors. They further suggested that the ability of these factors to discriminate between aggressive boys who were and were not involved in later problems could be promising for the development of interventions to prevent later involvement in multiple problem behaviors.

Although not conducted with adolescents, a study by Johnson, Larson, et al. (1997) suggests that religious involvement can ameliorate as well as prevent deviant behavior. This study followed prison inmates in four New York State prisons for two years to determine whether participation in a Prison Fellowship (PF) program while incarcerated had any effect on the inmates' adjustment in prison. It also examined the inmates' recidivism rates, or postrelease arrests, as a function of PF participation. PF is a nonprofit religious program for institutionalized prisoners that provides opportunities for group Bible study, spiritual development seminars, and life-plan seminars. Prisoners can participate in all three kinds of activities or several times in only one.

Investigators selected 201 former inmates from the four prisons who were PF program participants and matched them with 201 inmates who did not participate in PF. Matching was done on the basis of seven factors: age, race, religious denomination, county of residence, military discharge, minimum sentence, and initial security classification (low, medium, or high). In other words, each PF-program participant was matched with a non-PF participant who closely resembled him on these seven factors.

Results indicated that both groups were similar on their initial adjustment to prison, with each committing similar amounts and types of institutional infractions. Analyzing the effect of PF participation on recidivism, Johnson and colleagues also found no difference between the two groups: 37% of PF inmates and 36% of non-PF inmates were arrested during the one-year follow-up period. Level of PF participation in Bible study groups, however, did significantly predict recidivism rates. PF inmates in the high-participation category (10 or more Bible studies) were significantly less likely than non-PF inmates to be arrested during the follow-up period (14% vs. 41%, $p < .05$). Prospective studies that examine the impact of prisoner involvement in religious groups during incarceration are now under way to determine whether such participation impacts behavior either during prison stay or after release.

SUMMARY AND CONCLUSIONS

The causes of delinquency are multifaceted. Individual, familial, community, and societal factors interact in various ways to produce such behavior. There is growing evidence that affiliation with religion may help protect against delinquent behavior and attitudes among youth. Further evidence suggests that such effects persist even if there is not a strong prevailing social control against delinquent behavior in the surrounding community.

Although some studies have found that religion is salient only to delinquent behaviors that do not directly harm others (i.e., victimless offenses), there is mounting evidence that religious involvement may lower the risks of a broad range of delinquent behaviors, including both victimless crimes and those that involve harm to individuals. Religious involvement in youth, then, may significantly lessen the risk of later adult criminality.

There is also growing evidence that religion can be used as a tool to help prevent high-risk urban youths particularly from engaging in delinquent behavior. Religious involvement may help adolescents learn "prosocial behavior" that emphasizes concern for others' welfare. Such prosocial skills may give adolescents a greater sense of empathy toward others, which makes them less likely to commit acts that harm others. Similarly, once individuals become involved in deviant behavior, it is possible that participation in specific kinds of religious activity can help steer them back to a course of less deviant behavior and, more important, away from lives as career criminals.

13

Marital Instability

THIS CHAPTER PROVIDES AN overview of marital instability, its personal and societal costs, and its relationship to religious beliefs and practices. We also look at the possible role of religion in increasing marital stability and explore the mechanisms by which religion might do so. Finally, we examine the potential role of religious interventions in either preventing marital problems or addressing them once they occur. To begin this chapter, we define marital instability and review its effects on mental and physical health.

DEFINING MARITAL INSTABILITY

Marital instability is defined as ongoing conflict in marriage because of communication problems, disagreements about parenting or gender roles, financial difficulties, untrustworthiness, infidelity, or alcohol and drug abuse (Kitson & Sussman, 1982; Albrecht et al., 1983; Bloom et al., 1985). Marital conflict often arises early on in a marriage merely because one partner, or perhaps both, had unrealistic expectations about marriage before their wedding and suddenly finds himself living with someone he barely knows and has little in common with (Nock, 1987).

Whatever the cause of marital conflict, if left unresolved it can ultimately result in marital separation or divorce. Indeed, separation and divorce are often the result of years of discord and unhappiness in a marriage (Rasmussen & Ferraro, 1979). The decision to separate or divorce often is made unilaterally by one spouse over the strenuous objections of the other. The nonconsenting spouse, as well as the seldom consulted children, often suffers dire emotional consequences as a result of this decision. Many experts believe divorce is the second most traumatic life event that can occur for most people, after the death of a child or parent (Everett & Everett, 1994).

PERSONAL CONSEQUENCES OF MARITAL INSTABILITY

On an individual level, marital instability affects both the spouses and their children in a variety of ways. The emotional stress has direct effects on mental health and indirect effects on physical health. There is evidence that the indirect effects of marital instability on physical health may be mediated by immune system changes. We now discuss these topics in greater detail.

Marital Instability and Mental Health

Quite naturally, people undergoing marital disruption experience a great deal of emotional turmoil and stress. For some, this emotional upheaval subsides once the divorce is finalized. However, the majority of research suggests that the emotional and psychological consequences linger long after the legal proceedings are over. Exposure to this prolonged period of emotional distress as a result of separation or divorce can make people vulnerable to a host of adverse psychological consequences, including depression (Perlin & Johnson, 1977; Meneghan & Lieberman, 1986; Cohen & Brook, 1987; Baydar, 1988; Bruce & Kim, 1992; Amato & Keith, 1991), alcohol and drug abuse (Duncan, 1978; Long & Scherl, 1984; Burnside et al., 1986; Gfellner, 1994), and even suicide (Crumley, 1979; Stack, 1980a; Carlson & Cantwell, 1982; Maris, 1985; Stack & Wasserman, 1993).

For example, Merikangas and colleagues (1985) examined the association between depression and marital adjustment in 45 married inpatients with primary recurrent unipolar major depression and their spouses as compared with 45 age- and religion-matched nonpatient control couples from the same geographical area. Mean age of both groups was approximately 37 years. The participants completed a questionnaire that covered the following 10 aspects of their marriage: individual development, parental family situations, psychosocial history, courtship, premarital and marital sexual activity, the impact of children on their marriage, work and social activities, use of leisure time, medical history, and attitudes about role behavior in marriage. From this study, three factors emerged that distinguished the families of origin of patient couples and normal couples: mental illness in parents or siblings, divorce and/or separation, and a death in the family. Furthermore, twice as many children of the patient couples had serious medical or psychiatric illness as were found in the children of normal couples. In an analysis of a national sample of adults in the United States, Stack and Wasserman (1993) also found much higher rates of alcohol consumption and suicide among divorced and separated persons compared to those who are married.

Children who experience a parental divorce are also more likely to have emotional problems (Baydar, 1988) and to engage in delinquent or antisocial behavior than are children from intact families (Farrington et al., 1988; Farrington, 1990). This is particularly true for adolescents. A number of empirical studies have documented a positive relationship between marital disruption and increased psychopathology in both clinical (e.g., Porter & O'Leary, 1980; Snyder et al., 1988) and nonclinical (e.g., Wierson et al., 1988; Forehand et al., 1991) adolescent populations. Like their parents, children exposed to divorce are significantly more likely to experience depression and to commit suicide than are children from intact families (McCall & Land, 1994). For example, C. A. King and colleagues (1995) found that parents of adolescents in a psychiatric inpatient population reported less marital satisfaction and more conflicts over child rearing than did parents of adolescents who were not being treated for psychiatric problems. This same study also found that marital conflicts over child rearing were associated with a more distant father-adolescent relationship and more severe school behavior and spare time problems, as well.

Marital Instability and Physical Health

Compared to married or single people, those who have experienced a divorce or separation also have greater vulnerability to a variety of acute and chronic physical illnesses, including infectious diseases, respiratory illness, digestive system illness, and severe injuries. Verbrugge (1979) found that the formerly married (widowed, divorced, or separated) not only had higher rates of acute conditions but, when they experienced these conditions, higher amounts of work loss and disability. Lilienfeld and colleagues (1972) also found, in an earlier study, that divorced individuals of either sex (both white and nonwhite) had significantly higher risk for almost every type of terminal cancer than did married individuals. In fact, divorced males had double the incidence of respiratory cancers, a fourfold increase in throat cancer, and more than a 50% increase in cancer of the digestive system, peritoneum, and urinary tract compared to married men.

Researchers have long noted significantly higher rates of premature death among the divorced compared to the married and the never married. Lynch (1977), for example, reviewed mortality data from the National Center for Health Statistics on all deaths that occurred in the United States over a two-year period and found, that both white and nonwhite divorced men had double the premature death rate from cardiovascular disease of married men. The premature death rate for white divorced men due to pneumonia was seven times that of their married counterparts. The premature death rate from hypertension and cardiovascular disease for divorced men was double that of married men, and the suicide rate for divorced white men was four times higher than that for married men.

Increased mortality for the divorced, particularly divorced men, has been found in other developed countries, as well. Hu and Goldman (1990) analyzed marital-status-specific death rates for 16 developed countries and found several consistent and striking patterns. First, in all countries, the excess mortality of unmarried men greatly exceeded that of married men. Second, in all but three of the 16 countries—Portugal, Taiwan, and France—divorced men had the highest death rate among the three unmarried groups studied (single, widowed, and divorced). An increased mortality rate in divorced women (compared to that for married, single, or widowed women) was also found in about half the countries. Finally, in almost all of the 16 countries, widowed and divorced people (both men and women) in their twenties and early thirties experienced the highest mortality risks, which were sometimes 10 times higher than those of married persons of the same age. In the majority of these countries, the relative mortality rates of the three unmarried groups (single, widowed, and divorced) had increased over the past two or three decades.

Other studies demonstrate health benefits for married persons. In an analysis of 20,000 white women ages 18–55, Aanson (1988) found that married women were significantly less prone to physical illness than single women and that marriage was more important to health status than other demographic risk factors such as age, education, and family income. Furthermore, Wilson and Schoenborn (1989) found that divorced men and women had 50% greater risk for activity restrictions due to illness or injury than did married men or women of the same age.

Children exposed to marital instability also experience an increased risk of physical health problems. Dawson (1991) found that children exposed to marital disruption were significantly more likely to develop asthma and had a 20–30% greater risk of injury than children living in intact families. More ominously, people exposed to divorce as children also may be more prone to premature death than adults who are not (Friedman, Tucker, et al., 1995).

Marital Instability and Immune Status

Is there a connection between the emotional and psychological problems caused by marital instability and the poorer physical health that divorced or separated people experience? There is evidence that the emotional trauma of divorce may cause physical health problems by impairing the body's immune system (Kiecolt-Glaser et al., 1987). These researchers found that women separated from their spouses for one year or less had poorer immune function in five out of six immunological assays than had married control subjects (Kiecolt-Glaser &

Glaser, 1988). Another study by Kiecolt-Glaser, Newton, and colleagues (1996) found that the degree of a husband's withdrawal in response to his wife's negative behavior significantly impacted the wife's norepinephrine and cortisol levels. That is, increases in a husband's emotional withdrawal was associated with increases in his wife's norepinephrine and cortisol levels. Norepinephrine and cortisol are stress hormones that, when elevated chronically over time, can cause both cardiovascular and immune system problems (see chapter 19). Conversely, high frequencies of positive behaviors by husbands were associated with lower levels of epinephrine and higher prolactin levels in their wives. There was no relationship, however, between wives' behaviors and their husbands' hormone levels.

SOCIAL AND ECONOMIC COSTS OF MARITAL INSTABILITY AND DIVORCE

Since the 1950s, the United States has witnessed unparalleled changes in the patterns of family dissolution. The most rapid changes, however, have been fairly recent. The ratio of divorced persons to married persons increased by 34% during the 1960s and more than doubled in the 1970s (U.S. Bureau of Census, 1978). Between 1970 and 1992, the number of currently divorced individuals nearly quadrupled, from 4.2 million in 1970 to 16.3 million in 1992 (Saluter, 1992). Although the divorce rate leveled off in the 1990s, it remains at a persistently high level.

As previously noted, a growing body of research has found that marital disruption and divorce often set into motion a cascade of events that can dramatically alter the course of both spouses' lives, as well as those of their children. Unfortunately, the personal consequences and costs of separation and divorce may have a significant spillover effect onto the rest of society (Larson et al., 1995). The costs of divorce are generally believed to adversely affect society in several ways. First, many divorced and separated adults, particularly men, use psychological and psychiatric counseling services at much higher rates than do married persons (Rednick & Johnson, 1974; Hirschfeld & Cross, 1982; Bruce & Kim, 1992). In an early study, Verbrugge (1979) found that divorced individuals tended to be insitutionalized for mental health disorders at much higher rates than were those who were married. Divorced individuals also had a significantly higher number of physician visits per year compared to married people (Verbrugge, 1979). Studies have also found that separated and divorced men have higher acute hospitalization rates—an indication of more serious and expensive health problems—than do married, widowed, or single men (Verbrugge, 1979; Schoenborn & Morano, 1987).

Finally, young children or adolescents who experience the breakup of their parents' marriage are disproportionately likely to have adjustment or achievement problems later in life (Zill et al., 1993) or to become involved in risky sexual behavior (Seidman et al., 1994), both of which can have substantial personal and social costs in terms of lost potential income, risk of early pregnancy, and risk of sexually transmitted diseases. These children are significantly more likely than children from intact families to experience poverty (Lamison-White, 1992). They are also at significantly greater risk of going through a divorce themselves when they become adults (Amato, 1988; Glenn & Supancic, 1984), thus, perpetuating the negative social consequences of marital instability.

Another way that marital instability adversely affects society is through increased utilization of social services. For example, divorced and separated mothers often do not receive financial support from their spouses, causing them to become one of the fastest growing groups of welfare and Medicaid recipients (Committee on Ways and Means, U.S. House of Representatives, 1993). Indeed, the majority of women experience a substantial decline in standard of living after divorce, an average one-third decline in economic status (Weitzman, 1985). Berk and Taylor (1984) found that many divorced and separated women relied on public assistance to obtain health and mental health services and were twice as likely as married women to be uninsured.

Therefore, the personal problems experienced by both adults and children are most immediately felt by the health care and social-welfare systems. The lower level of private insurance coverage for many divorced and separated mothers, compounded by their increased risk for both physical and mental illness, translates into an additional burden on society because these women are disproportionately reliant on state and federal aid. Also, the reduced educational achievement of children of divorce, as well as their increased risk of delinquent and risky behavior, has a significant impact on all Americans. These children may grow up to be underemployed or unemployed or, worse, incarcerated for criminal behavior. Thus, marital disruption has a significant negative impact on both the national economy and the criminal justice system.

CAUSES OF MARITAL INSTABILITY

Over the years, researchers have found a variety of causes for marital instability. The most frequently cited contributors to marital instability include exposure to divorce as a child, premarital sex and pregnancy before marriage, young age at first marriage, short length of courtship before marriage, premarital cohabitation, membership in a racial minority group, low socioeconomic status, and the influence of economic cycles (see Larson et al., 1995, for a review of this literature).

To determine which factors have the greatest impact on marital stability, Glenn and Supancic (1984) analyzed data from seven national surveys conducted during the 1970s and early 1980s. The variables they studied in relation to divorce and separation included time of marriage, race, age at first marriage, frequency of attendance of religious services, religious preference, region of residence, kind of community (rural vs. urban), education, income, and occupation. Of these 10 variables, the three strongest predictors of divorce and separation were race, age at first marriage, and low frequency of attendance at religious services.

Thus, as research on marital stability has progressed over the years, it has become apparent that, although religion is not the only factor that affects marital stability, it is nevertheless one of many factors that may play an important role in keeping people from dissolving marriages. Chan and Heaton (1989) studied factors that predict willingness to stay in a marriage among 1,595 women (ages 15–44 years) and found that, on the one hand, many of the same factors associated with marital stability also were positively correlated with delayed divorce. The wife's age at marriage, the age of the youngest child, the wife's religion, the region of residence, and metropolitan residence all had substantial effects on delayed divorce. On the other hand, the effects of racial minority membership, parental divorce, premarital pregnancy, and low socioeconomic status (SES) were relatively small in that study.

RELIGION AND MARITAL INSTABILITY

An inverse relationship between involvement in religious activities and marital instability was first postulated on the basis of the observation that participation in religious activities was waning at about the same time that divorce rates were surging (Shrum, 1980). Early research confirmed this relationship, using simple measures of religious activity, such as the frequency of church attendance. Religiously active individuals may have stronger marriages because of both greater exposure to antidivorce proscriptions and a greater sense of personal commitment to marriage.

One of the first empirical studies to confirm an inverse relationship between church attendance and marital instability was by McCarthy (1979), who analyzed data collected in the 1973 National Survey of Family Growth. According to this study, 17% of couples who attended church once a year or less were separated or divorced after five years of marriage, compared to only 7% of the couples who attended church at least once a month. This same study found that after 15 years of marriage, 37% of infrequent churchgoers were no longer married, compared to only 14% of frequent (once a month or more) churchgoers.

Similar findings were reported by Shrum (1980), who analyzed data collected in six social surveys of primarily Protestant and Catholic populations conducted between 1972 and 1977. He found that the principal indicator of religious commitment was frequency of church attendance and that more frequent religious attendance was clearly associated with a decreased probability of divorce ($\chi^2 = 161.7$, $p < .001$, uncontrolled). To determine whether the relationship between frequency of church attendance and marital instability would disappear when other factors were controlled, Shrum (1980) introduced five additional control variables into the analysis: education, level of family income, age at first marriage, age, and marriage cohort (created by subtracting age at first marriage from age). This multivariate analysis found that the relationship between church attendance and marital stability could not be explained by the indirect effects of these five control variables but rather resulted from some more direct influence of religion on marital stability.

Other studies suggest that the direct effects of religious commitment on marital stability stem from greater personal commitment to the marriage. Larson and Goltz (1989) analyzed data from a random survey of 179 married couples who were living in Edmonton, Canada, that inquired about how often they attended church and their level of personal and structural marital commitment. In this study, personal commitment was defined as the commitment to stay in a marriage no matter what the cost; structural commitment was defined as the commitment to marriage in general because of social proscriptions. After controlling for demographic variables (e.g., education and income), the researchers found that personal commitment was positively related to church attendance for both husbands ($r = .26$) and wives ($r = .22$). Structural commitment, likewise, was significantly correlated with church involvement for both husbands and wives. In other words, the more frequently husbands and wives attended church, the more personally and structurally committed they were to staying married. The inverse relationship between formal religious involvement and marital instability, then, may result from

religion's emphasis on personal commitment to marriage and its proscriptions against divorce.

Other studies also suggest that both religious belief and religious activity play a role in maintaining marital stability. Call and Heaton (1997) analyzed data on 4,587 married couples who participated in Wave I (1987–1988) and Wave II (1992–1994) of the National Survey of Families and Households (NSFH) to determine the relationship between religious involvement and marital stability. The NSFH is the largest and most detailed study of factors related to marriage and family life ever conducted in the United States. Religious variables measured were religious affiliation, concordance of religious affiliation between spouses, religious attendance, and religious belief ("The Bible is the answer to all important human problems"). Using regression modeling, investigators examined predictors of the log-odds of separation/divorce. Several covariates were controlled for, including marital duration, race, parental divorce, previous divorce, full-time employment, education of wife and husband, number of children, birth interval, and wife's age at marriage.

Analysis of the results indicated that persons with no affiliation or in mixed-faith marriages had the greatest likelihood of divorce or separation. The wife's attendance and difference in attendance between wife and husband both predicted divorce or separation. The husband's religious belief was initially positively related to separation or divorce, although this effect diminished to nonsignificance when the wife's marital commitment or the wife's attitude toward nonmarital sex was entered into the model. In the final model, the wife's religious belief (but not the husband's) predicted less separation or divorce. When all religious and control variables were entered into the model, the wife's religious attendance, the difference between the wife's and the husband's religious attendance, and the wife's religious belief predicted separation or divorce ($\beta = -.08$, $p < .05$, $\beta = .12$, $p < .01$, and $\beta = -.20$, $p < .05$, respectively). Investigators concluded that religious involvement has "more than trivial affects on marital stability and should not be omitted from models of marital stability" (Call and Heaton, 1997, p. 391).

In a related study, Wilson and Musick (1996)

analyzed data on a subsample of 5,648 participants in the NSFH who were married and whose spouses completed secondary questionnaires to determine the impact of religion on marital dependency. Marital dependency refers to the extent to which either spouse believes his or her life would be worse should the marriage end. Investigators found that religious affiliation (contrasted with no affiliation) increased the likelihood of marital dependency, as did membership in more conservative Protestant denominations (especially those self-identified as fundamentalist). They also found that greater frequency of church attendance was significantly associated with increased marital dependence.

These studies suggest that religious commitment, measured by frequency of church attendance and religious belief (especially the wife's), contributes to marital stability by increasing personal commitment and marital dependency. The evidence also suggests that religiously committed individuals may be more inclined not only to stay in a marriage but also to take steps to better the marriage (Larson & Goltz, 1989).

Religious Heterogamy and Marital Stability

Another line of inquiry in this field has to do with religious heterogamy, that is, marriages in which spouses have different denominational affiliations. Early studies of interfaith marriages reported lower levels of marital satisfaction and adjustment (Glenn, 1982; Heaton, 1984; Ortega et al., 1988). Studies also suggested that heterogamous marriages were more likely to end in divorce (Bumpass & Sweet, 1972; Bahr, 1981; Call & Heaton, 1997).

Heaton and Pratt (1990) studied the relationship between marital satisfaction and three types of religious homogamy—denominational homogamy, frequency of church attendance homogamy, and belief in the Bible homogamy—among 13,017 households in the 1988 NSFH study. Investigators found that marital satisfaction tended to increase with increases in religious involvement. Of the three religious homogamy variables, denominational homogamy was the strongest predictor of marital satisfaction. Homogamous church attendance frequency also contributed to marital satisfaction, but the relationship was not significant. There was also no statistically significant relationship between homogamous beliefs about the Bible and marital satisfaction. Thus, religious denominational homogamy was the primary predictor of marital happiness in this nationwide study.

Shehan and colleagues (1990), however, reported that religious homogamy did not have a significant effect on marital happiness for a group of Catholics. In this study, Shehan and colleagues examined data collected as part of the General Social Surveys conducted by the University of Chicago in the 1970s and 1980s. The sample included 1,753 respondents, representing 412 Catholics in interfaith unions and 1,341 Catholics in homogamous marriages. Catholics involved in heterogamous marriages were just as happy in their marriages as were Catholics in homogamous marriages. Indeed, approximately two-thirds of each group reported high marital happiness. There were interesting differences, however, between Catholics in heterogamous and those in homogamous marriages. Catholics in homogamous marriages were more likely than those in interfaith marriages to report frequent attendance at mass, whereas Catholics in interfaith marriages were younger and more likely to have preschool children in the home. The investigators noted that these religious and age differences between heterogamously and homogamously married Catholics were potentially important because they may reflect a tendency for heterogamous marriages involving Catholics to be less stable.

A later report by Lehrer and Chiswick (1993) more clearly supports the notion that religious heterogamy is associated with marital instability. These researchers again used data from the 1987–1988 NSFH to examine the role of religious homogamy as a predictor of marital stability (i.e., the probability of marital dissolution). They found that, with the exception of Mormons and of people with no religious affiliation, marital stability was remarkably similar across the various types of homogamous marriages. Homogamous Mormon marriages and those marriages in which neither spouse reported a religious affiliation had the highest and lowest levels of marital stability, respectively. (Using the same data set, Wilson and Musick [1996] had found that that the effect of marital homogamy on religious dependence was strongest in those self-identified as religious fundamentalists.)

Religious heterogamy, on the other hand, was associated with a higher likelihood of marital dissolution. However, the magnitude of this destabilizing effect depended on the differences in religious belief and practice between members of the couple. Interestingly, among Protestant and Catholic couples who achieved homogamy through conversion of one of the partners, Lehrer and Chiswick found that marital stability was at least as strong as in those marriages that involved two members who had the same religious denomination before marriage.

Religious intermarriage comes in different shades and degrees, and heterogamous marriages between those whose religions are significantly different in practice and beliefs (e.g., Protestants and Catholics) may be more unstable than those between people whose faiths share many common beliefs and practices (e.g., Methodists and Lutherans). In addition, there is evidence to suggest that religious conversion to achieve homogamy may have a beneficial effect on marital stability. It should be noted that over the past few decades some religious denominations have moved closer in terms of beliefs and practices, and heterogamous marriages between individuals in such nearly identical denominations presents little additional risk for marital instability.

One recurrent explanation for the greater degree of marital instability among heterogamous marriages is that persons who marry partners of faiths different from their own are either less religious than those who marry homogamously or are at risk of becoming less religious (Heaton, 1984). According to this explanation, it is the low level of religiosity of the spouses in heterogamous marriages, rather than the heterogamy itself, that increases marital discord and decreases barriers to divorce.

RELIGIOUS INVOLVEMENT AND MARITAL ADJUSTMENT

In addition to its association with greater personal commitment to marriage, religion has also been found to promote marital stability by facilitating adjustment to marriage. A variety of studies over the past several decades have found that increased religiousness is associated with better marital adjustment (e.g., Albrecht, 1979; Schumm et al., 1982; Bahr & Chadwick, 1985).

Only within the past two decades has greater understanding about these relationships begun to emerge. In one study, for example, Wilson and Filsinger (1986) analyzed data obtained from a survey of 190 married Protestant couples who were living in a Southwestern metropolitan area. The survey included a multidimensional measure of religious involvement that included 37 items. These items measured the couples' degree of religious ideology (e.g., conservative or liberal), religious experience (e.g., repentance or forgiveness), ritualistic involvement (e.g., frequency of church attendance), religious knowledge, and religious morality. Marital adjustment was measured by asking the couples about their degree of agreement on issues of importance to the relationship, satisfaction with and commitment to the relationship, engaging in activities together, and satisfaction with expressions of affection and sex. Socioeconomic status, length of marriage, and number of children were also measured and controlled in the analysis.

Investigators found a consistent pattern of significant positive relationships between several dimensions of religiousness and marital adjustment. Specifically, the higher the couples' level of church participation, reported religious experience, and conservativeness of religious beliefs, the better their marital adjustment. These three dimensions of religiousness also predicted the degree of each couple's agreement on issues of importance to the relationship, satisfaction with and commitment to the relationship, and pursuit of joint activities. On the other hand, religiousness was not related to partners' expressions of affection with their mate. Because this study was conducted in a largely Protestant sample who attended church fairly frequently, the authors emphasized that they could not generalize their conclusions to those who do not attend church regularly or who are not religious. However, because they found that the relationship between religion and marital adjustment was robust across several different measures, the authors encouraged future researchers to explore this relationship in other populations.

In a later study, Roth (1988) explored the underlying reasons for the relationship between religion and marital adjustment by looking at subjective "inner experiences." Specifically, she asked 147 married people who attended church in southern California about their existential well-being (EWB) and religious well-being (RWB). She also asked questions about their degree of marital satisfaction, cohesion, consensus, and expression of affection. EWB was defined as an individual's sense of self, that is, knowing who one is and what one needs to do. RWB was defined as one's beliefs about God and one's sense of being in a relationship with God. Roth found a significant relationship between EWB and all four marital adjustment subscales ($p < .001$). Although RWB scores often showed a significant relationship to the marital adjustment subscale scores, the correlations were smaller than those for EWB. On the basis of these results, Roth suggested that a religious belief alone is not enough to ensure marital stability. Rather, such beliefs need to be integrated into one's self-concept.

This conclusion is at least partially supported by an earlier study in which private prayer was found to have a significant correlation with marital adjustment. In this study, Gruner (1985) examined the relationship between private religious devotional practices and marital adjustment in a sample made up of members of several different religious groups, including members of a sect, a conservative-evangelical denomination, a liberal denomination, and an institutional-authoritarian denomination (i.e., Roman Catholicism). Private devotional practices that were assessed included prayer and Bible reading at home. The respondents were also asked about other potentially confounding factors, such as age, length of marriage, social class, and race. Gruner found that for those involved in sects (primarily Pentecostal Protestants), roughly half reported high marital adjustment. Among conservative-evangelical Christians (e.g., Southern Baptists), reports were more evenly distributed among high, medium, and low levels of marital adjustment (about one-third for each). Among liberals and Catholics, only about a quarter in each group reported high marital adjustment, with the remaining three-quarters almost evenly divided between low and medium marital adjustment.

In assessing the relationship between prayer and marital adjustment, Gruner found that, on the one hand, most liberal Christians and Catholics did not use prayer at all when addressing marital adjustment problems. On the other hand, 50% of those affiliated with a sect reported using prayer frequently to address marital adjustment problems. Those affiliated with evangelical religions also reported high use of prayer when dealing with marital adjustment problems. Examining the relationship between prayer and marital adjustment across all the religious groups, the investigators found that a significantly greater percentage of those who scored high on marital adjustment also used prayer extensively in connection with marital adjustment problems compared to those who scored low on marital adjustment (53% vs. 17%, respectively, $p < .001$, uncontrolled). Further, an even greater percentage (59%) of those who read the Bible extensively to deal with marriage problems reported high marital adjustment. In contrast, only 12% of those who read the Bible extensively to deal with marriage problems were among those who reported low marital adjustment ($p < .001$, uncontrolled). Thus, there was a fairly strong relationship between both prayer and Bible reading and marital adjustment.

Conversely, a significantly greater percentage of those who scored low on marital adjustment reported never using prayer to deal with marital problems compared to those who scored high on marital adjustment (43% vs. 15%, respectively). Likewise, among those scoring the lowest on marital adjustment, 45% reported never reading the Bible to deal with marital problems; in contrast, 22% in the high marital adjustment category reported never reading the Bible.

These studies further support the idea that, like personal commitment to marriage, a strong commitment to religious practice and ideals can enhance marital stability. However, it is the internalization of these practices and beliefs that may be most important, and this internalization process may be influenced by private devotional prayer and scripture reading. Again, however, since most of these studies are cross-sectional, any suggestions about direction of effect must be made cautiously.

RELIGION AND MARITAL SATISFACTION

Marital satisfaction may be one result of successful marital adjustment. Studies that have looked at religion as a predictor of overall marital satisfaction, however, have reported mixed results. Edmonds (1967) developed a Marital Conventionalization Scale (MCS) to measure the extent to which spouses might be describing their marital situation in socially desirable rather than realistic terms. He and his colleagues found some support for the hypothesis that relationships between measures of religiousness and marital adjustment were influenced by biased reporting (Edmonds et al., 1972). In other words, empirical relationships between measures of religiousness and marital satisfaction may be found partly because religious respondents give socially desirable answers or give answers they believe the researchers want to hear.

In another study, Glenn and Weaver (1978) analyzed data collected from three U.S. national surveys to estimate the effects of 10 independent variables, one of which was church attendance, on marital happiness. The data were from a probability sample of persons ages 18–59 (997 men and 1,281 women, all married and all white). Marital happiness was assessed by asking, "Taking things all together, how would you describe your marriage—very happy, pretty happy, or not too happy? The religious variable, church attendance, was significantly related to marital happiness in men ($p < .0001$) and women ($p = .0003$) after seven other major predictors of marital happiness were controlled. The authors minimized these findings, arguing that "more conventional" persons were both more likely to attend church and more likely to report happy marriages. In this particular study, however, investigators did not mea-

sure or control for social desirability or marital conventionalization but simply referred to the work of Edmonds et al. (1972) to support their argument.

In contrast, after analyzing data from two surveys conducted in husbands and wives in Kansas, Schumm and colleagues (1982) concluded that the positive relationship between religion and marital satisfaction was not due only to marital conventionalization. In this study, the researchers randomly surveyed 83 rural and 98 urban families on three items of marital satisfaction—degree of satisfaction with their spouse, degree of satisfaction with marriage, and quality of the relationship with their spouse. They also measured marital conventionalization. Respondents were asked about the importance of church and religion in the quality of their life, as well as about the importance of these two religious variables (i.e., church and religion) compared to other factors, including family, friends, community, leisure and recreation, housing, financial security, work, and education. In the uncontrolled analysis, Schumm and colleagues found that the marital conventionalization argument was "at least partly valid" in explaining the association between religion and marital satisfaction. However, further analysis revealed that religiousness was an important predictor of marital satisfaction, even among those who scored low on marital conventionalization. The investigators concluded that the positive association between religiousness and marital satisfaction was real.

To complicate things further, a study by Booth and colleagues (1995) reported that, although religion did not enhance marital satisfaction, marital satisfaction did enhance religiousness. This study assessed the impact of changes in religiosity on marital quality (and vice versa), using longitudinal data from a sample of 1,008 married persons. While increases in religiosity significantly decreased the probability of the partners considering divorce, increases in religiousness did not enhance marital happiness or interaction or decrease the type of conflict or problems commonly thought to cause divorce. Analyzing the reciprocal relationship between marital satisfaction and religiousness, researchers found that an increase in either marital happiness or marital interaction was associated with an increase in two of five religious measures—the extent to which religion influenced daily life and the frequency of church attendance. Researchers concluded that "the link between religion and marital quality is both reciprocal and weak."

The debate about the impact of religion on marital satisfaction is far from settled. While religion can play a significant role in enhancing marital adjustment, evidence to link increased religiousness to increases in marital satisfaction is less plentiful. Other research, however, suggests that religion plays an important role in the marital adjustments and satisfactions of those who stay married a long time.

RELIGION AND LONG-TERM MARRIAGES

Although most of the studies we cite in this section are small and dependent on personal accounts, they do point to religion as one of a number of key ingredients in successful long-term marriages. Sporakowski and Hughston (1978) interviewed 40 couples who had been married 50 years or more to determine the most important factors behind their happy marriages. This study found some variations in responses between husbands and wives. Wives mentioned "importance of religion" most frequently as a key ingredient in a happy marriage, followed by love, give and take/talking things through, home/family/children, the idea that it takes two to make a marriage work, and understanding/patience, in that order. In contrast, husbands mentioned "it takes two to make a marriage" most frequently, followed by honesty and trust, give and take, the belief that marriage is for life, and the importance of religion, in that order. The investigators noted, however, that even though the spouses mentioned the key factors with different frequencies, the top five key ingredients were essentially the same for both men and women.

In a more recent study, Robinson and Blanton (1993) found that intimacy, commitment, communication, congruence, and similar religious orientation were the factors cited most

consistently as contributing to marital satisfaction among 15 couples who had been married more than 30 years. In a follow-up report on the same sample, Robinson (1994) asked these couples to discuss their perceptions of the strengths of their marital relationship. Most of the individuals in this study, who had been married between 35 and 48 years, emphasized that their religious faith was one of the important assets in enhancing their marital relationship. Indeed, some of the respondents indicated that religion was "primary" in their marriage and enhanced other key aspects of marriage, including intimacy, commitment, and communication. They also stated that their faith provided them with moral guidance, facilitated decision making, and helped minimize marital conflict.

Finally, Kaslow and Robinson (1996) studied 57 couples who had been married between 25 and 46 years to determine their perceptions of the factors that contributed most to their marital satisfaction and longevity. Love, mutual trust, mutual respect, religious beliefs, loyalty and fidelity, mutual give and take, similar philosophy of life, enjoyment of shared fun and humor, shared interests, and shared interests in their children were the most frequently cited factors; each was endorsed by more than 50% of respondents.

Religion, according to these subjective reports, appears to be an important factor that contributes to ongoing marital satisfaction and longevity. Religion may also be synergistic with other important factors related to marital satisfaction and stability, such as intimacy, commitment, communication, and shared values. Future research needs to clarify the relationship between religion and the other factors that affect marital satisfaction.

RELIGION AS AN INTERVENTION FOR MARITAL INSTABILITY

Research on the use of religion as an intervention for marital problems is relatively new, with most studies consisting of anecdotal accounts with primarily religious clients (e.g., Stewart & Gale, 1994; Sperry & Giblin, 1996). It is difficult, then, to draw any conclusions based on empirical evidence regarding the efficacy of religious interventions for marital problems.

Supportive evidence can be found in research that explores the relationship between religion and success rates of efforts at marital reconciliation. For example, Wineberg (1994) used data from the 1987–1988 NSFH to examine the prevalence of successful marital reconciliations among white women and the predictors of such reconciliations. In about 30% of cases where women attempted to reconcile their marriages, the woman was still with her husband one year after the reconciliation began (the end of the study period). The probability of a successful attempted reconciliation varied. Women who had the same religious denominational affiliation as their spouses had a significantly higher probability of having a successful reconciliation than women from mixed-faith marriages. Additionally, as Lehrer and Chiswick (1993) discovered, a change in religious affiliation in connection with the marriage (i.e., to achieve religious homogamy) was also associated with a significantly greater probability of successful reconciliation.

Although this study does not illuminate how religion might be employed specifically as an intervention in dealing with marital instability, it does provide useful information on the factors that go into successful marital reconciliation. The fact that religion plays a major role in enhancing marital reconciliation for the minority of couples who are successful (indeed, 70% of couples who attempted reconciliation failed) indicates that this is a fertile area for future research.

Regardless of the role of religion in marital reconciliation, many couples with marital problems often seek advice from their clergy (e.g., Benner, 1992), and clergy often report that family problems are the most frequent and difficult counseling issues they must address (Wasman et al., 1979). Weaver, Koenig, and colleagues (1997) have called for greater research on how marital and family therapists might collaborate with clergy in addressing marital problems. Because marital and family therapists themselves have the highest rates of religious involvement of any mental health profession, Weaver and

colleagues suggested that these professionals are in a unique position to provide continuing education for clergy in this important area. They noted, however, the unfortunate lack of research, training, and collaboration between the two vocations, despite the role religion might play in promoting marital stability.

SUMMARY AND CONCLUSIONS

Marital instability extracts a heavy toll by increasing susceptibility to mental and physical health problems for spouses and children. There is evidence that the mental health problems brought about by the stress of divorce may impact physical health through a number of mechanisms, including psychoneuroimmunological ones. The greater susceptibility of those experiencing marital instability to physical health problems may be serious enough to affect mortality. On a societal level, the personal consequences of divorce lead to significantly higher use of mental and physical health care resources. The social welfare system also bears the consequences of marital instability.

Researchers have become increasingly interested in the role religion plays in promoting marital stability. A variety of studies find a consistent positive relationship between religious involvement and marital stability, and there is additional evidence to support a connection between religious activity and marital adjustment and/or satisfaction. This may be the result of the increased personal commitment that religiously involved people have to each other and to their marriage, although other factors such as religious homogamy, religious proscriptions against divorce, and existential and spiritual well-being also play a role. Qualitative studies find that those who have enjoyed satisfying long-term marriages often cite religion as a key factor in their success. Moreover, they often report that religion helps to strengthen other factors that are key ingredients to a satisfying marriage.

Finally, although there is evidence that religion can play a key role in both preventing marital problems and helping couples with significant problems to reconcile, research is needed to delineate how religion might be used as an intervention for marital problems. Are religious interventions valuable only for those who are already deeply religious, or might they also be helpful for moderately religious or even nonreligious couples? Perhaps greater collaboration among marriage and family therapists, clergy, and researchers will help answer some of these questions.

14

Personality

PERSONALITY AND RELIGION have long been associated (James, 1902), and personality may influence whether persons naturally gravitate toward or move away from religious involvement. According to Cloninger (1987), personality exists along three dimensions that are genetically influenced and biologically determined: (1) from low to high novelty seeking (dopamine mediated), (2) from low to high reward dependence (norepinephrine mediated), and (3) from low to high harm avoidance (serotonin mediated). The person who is low novelty seeking (conservative), high reward dependent (socially gregarious), and high harm avoidance (fearful or anxious) may seek refuge and find great comfort in religion (Koenig, 1994a). On the other hand, the novelty-seeking person who has low reward dependence and low harm avoidance may shy away from religion because it is too constricting and inhibiting. In turn, religion may affect the development of personality, moderating or suppressing certain traits (high novelty seeking and low harm avoidance) while promoting the development of others (reward dependence) (Boomsma et al., 1999).

In this chapter, we are primarily interested in how personality relates to mental and physical health and how religion affects this relationship. Before we explore how religion impacts the dimensions of personality that relate to health, we examined personality itself and the way different mental health specialists have understood it.

WHAT IS PERSONALITY?

Standard textbooks typically define personality as a set of human psychological characteristics that is more or less consistent across situations. For example, Maddi (1989) defines personality as the "stable set of tendencies and characteristics that determine those commonalities and differences in people's psychological behavior (thoughts, feelings, and actions) that have continuity in time and that may not be easily understood as the sole result of the social and biological pressures of the moment" (p. 8).

For many years, similar definitions of personality have propelled the field of personality psychology toward the study of enduring personality traits. However, in recent years, personality theorists have proposed that personality can be best understood at three levels (McAdams, 1995, 1996). The first of these levels refers to personality traits and dispositions. Traits and dispositions are more or less enduring dimensions of personality that differ across people but that are thought to have a strong genetic component and to be more or less continuous across the lifespan. Although theorists have posited the existence of between three and 21 traits that constitute the "basic," irreducible features of human personality (Maddi, 1989), the most compelling modern framework for conceptualizing personality has been the "Big Five" model championed by Norman (1963) and, more recently, by McCrae and Costa (1990) and by John (1990). This "Big Five" model categorizes relatively stable personality traits into one of five overall dimensions: (1) openness to experience; (2) conscientiousness; (3) extraversion/introversion; (4) agreeableness; and (5) neuroticism or negative affectivity. Each of these five dimensions probably subsumes a broad variety of lower-order traits, or facets.

A second level at which personality can be conceptualized is the level of strivings or goals (Emmons, 1999). Goals are the regulatory mechanisms that guide behavior to achieve certain outcomes (Austin & Vancouver, 1996). Goals, strivings, and other "personal action constructs" tend to be developmental in nature and rather malleable as a result of changing life circumstances. If traits describe what a person "has," then goals and strivings describe what a person is "trying to achieve in life."

A third level at which personality can be conceptualized is at the level of identity. Identity, or the life narrative, is the relatively coherent story or set of stories that people in modern societies use to bring coherence and unity to their lives (McAdams, 1995, 1996; McAdams et al., 1997). The usual method for assessing people's life narratives is to submit case material or data from semistructured interviews to intensive content analysis (e.g., McAdams et al., 1997).

With this general understanding of the meaning of personality, let us examine the relationship among personality variables, religion, and health. Psychologists and other behavioral scientists have examined literally hundreds of personality variables as potential predictors of health and well-being (Stroebe & Stroebe, 1995). This chapter focuses on the associations of religion with three personality variables that have consistently been shown to influence physical health and well-being: hostility, hope and optimism, and control.

HOSTILITY

Hostility is a more or less enduring pattern of suspiciousness, resentment, frequent anger, and cynical mistrust of others. Research on hostility and physical health was pioneered by Redford Williams and his colleagues at Duke University (e.g., Williams et al., 1980; Barefoot, Dahlstrom, & Williams, 1983; Williams, 1989). They discovered that hostility was a particularly toxic aspect of the Type A behavior pattern (which is defined as a set of traits that involves a sense of time urgency and extreme competitiveness, in addition to angry aggression). Studies in the 1980s demonstrated that hostility was as good as and often superior to measures of Type A behavior as a predictor of coronary heart disease (CHD). People high in hostility experience two to four times the risk of CHD of people who score low on this trait (Barefoot et al., 1983; Chesney et al., 1988). In a recent meta-analysis of 45 prospective studies, Miller and colleagues (1996) found that measures of hostility, including the widely used Cook-Medley Hostility [Ho] scale (Cook & Medley, 1954), were independent predictors of all-cause mortality, even after controlling for potential covariates and confounding variables.

Religion and Hostility

Research is beginning to accumulate on the relationship among religion, anger and hostility (Tennison & Snyder, 1968; Heintzelman & Fehr, 1976; Acklin et al., 1983; Geist & Daheim, 1984; Morse & Wisocki, 1987; Strayhorn et al., 1990; Koenig, Siegler, Meador, et al., 1990; Kark, Carmel, et al., 1996). Much of this research has examined correlations between religious involvement and standard measures of hostility, such as the manifest hostility scale of the Multiple Affect Adjective Checklist (MAACL; Zuckerman & Lubin, 1965), the Buss-Durkee hostility inventory (Buss & Durkee, 1957), and the Cook-Medley Ho Questionnaire (Cook & Medley, 1954). In general, investigators find that religious involvement is associated with lower hostility, less anger, and reduced aggressiveness.

In such studies, religious involvement has been assessed with a wide range of measures, including church attendance (e.g., Acklin et al., 1983; Hertzgaard & Light, 1984), intrinsic religiousness (Acklin et al., 1983), religious coping (Koenig, Siegler, Meador, et al., 1990), transcendent meaning (Acklin et al., 1983), orthodox religious belief (Heintzelman & Fehr, 1976), and mixed measures of religious involvement (Tennison & Snyder, 1968; Morse & Wisocki, 1987; Strayhorn et al., 1990). Unfortunately, most of this research is cross-sectional in nature and tells us nothing about whether greater religiousness leads to less hostility or less hostility leads to greater religiousness. Furthermore, almost all the studies depend on self-report, leaving open the possibility that religious persons may not admit to aggressive or hostile behaviors as readily as others (although there is no scientific evidence to support this claim).

Surveying a nationally representative sample of 1,030 American adults, Gorsuch and Hao (1993) examined the relationship among religiousness, forgiveness, and hostility. Participants completed 25 questions about behaviors they engaged in (positive and negative) when someone deliberately did something wrong to them. They were also asked about their motives for the positive and negative actions and were given the opportunity to cite justifications for

not forgiving. The 25 items were factor analyzed and yielded four factors. Three of these factors measured forgiving attitudes and behaviors, while a fourth factor measured hostility, resentment, and an apparently smug, self-justified willingness to retaliate against others. Participants also completed a variety of religious measures that formed a personal religiousness factor (assessing the personal importance of religious beliefs) and a religious conformity factor (measuring certainty about religious beliefs and conformity to the teachings of their religion).

Results indicated that people who scored higher in personal religiousness had higher forgiveness scores and lower hostility scores ($r = -.18$, $p < .0001$). There was no relationship between religious conformity and forgiveness or hostility, suggesting that the personal importance of one's religious beliefs, and not the conformity to the religion per se, is the aspect of religion most closely linked with lower hostility. Since one might expect conformity to religion, in particular, to predict socially desirable responses (i.e., subjects might fail to admit to hostile behaviors and thus bias the association), it is interesting that the inverse relationship was found with personal religiousness, not with religious conformity.

Using a very different measure of religious involvement, Kark and his associates (1996a) surveyed 300 members of five secular kibbutzim and 300 members of five matched religious kibbutzim (located in the Beit She'an and Jordan valleys and in the eastern lower Galilee). The samples were very similar on a variety of demographic variables, including age and gender. Participants completed several measures, including a 35-item version of the Cook-Medley Ho scale. Even after the results were adjusted for gender and sense of coherence, people living in the religious kibbutzim were only about half as likely as people living in the secular kibbutzim to report high levels of hostility (odds ratio = 0.52). In a later study, Kark, Shemi, et al. (1996) found that both men and women living in religious kibbutzim experienced significantly lower mortality during a 16-year follow-up period compared to members of matched secular kibbutzim. These studies are important because the measure of religious involvement—that is, membership in a religious versus a secular kibbutz—was more objective, rather than determined entirely by self-report.

At least one study has failed to find a relationship between religious involvement and hostility (measured with the MAACL). In this study, Hertsgaard and Light (1984) assessed hostility, along with a number of demographic and psychosocial variables, in 760 women from the rural Midwest. Investigators found that rural women who attended church at least once a month did not differ in hostility from women who attended church less than once a month. It is not clear whether this single discrepant finding resulted from sampling error, inadequate measurement of religious involvement, or some other factor. It is likely, however, that the vast majority of rural women attend church more than once per month, making this categorization of the religious variable a rather insensitive measure. Almost 50% of women (rural and urban) attended religious services once a week or more, according to national Gallup polls conducted around that time, and persons living in rural areas attended even more frequently (Princeton Religion Research Center, 1982). Nevertheless, investigators have generally found that greater religiousness is associated with lower levels of hostility.

OPTIMISM AND HOPE

Optimism, Hope, and Health

Optimism is defined as an enduring tendency to expect good personal outcomes in the future (Scheier & Carver, 1993; Segerstrom et al., 1998). People who are optimistic expect that efforts to achieve certain desirable outcomes will eventually pay off. Pessimists, on the other hand, rarely expect things to go their way. Even if they expend considerable effort, pessimists are more likely to doubt that their efforts will result in beneficial outcomes.

Hope is related to optimism. C. R. Snyder, who has done more than any other researcher to advance our understanding of hope, defines it as a "cognitive set that is based on a reciprocally derived sense of successful (a) agency (goal-directed determination) and (b) pathways (planning of ways to meet goals)" (Snyder, Harris, et al., 1991, p. 570). In other words, people who have high levels of hope tend to have high levels of determination to reach their goals *and* perceive themselves to have high-quality options for obtaining those goals. According to Snyder, hope is distinct from optimism in that it involves not only consideration of personal agency but also positive expectations that viable pathways exist for accomplishing a given goal (Snyder et al., 1996).

Considerable research demonstrates that hope and optimism are associated with better mental health; some studies use these variables as *proxies* for mental health. Optimism and hope have been associated with better psychological adjustment in both clinical samples (e.g., Carver & Gaines, 1987; Ringdal, 1995; Schulz et al., 1996) and nonclinical samples (Robinson-Whelen et al., 1997; Scioli et al., 1997; Sumi, 1997; Segerstrom et al., 1998). Furthermore, people with high levels of optimism appear to use more adaptive coping methods (Aspinwall & Taylor, 1992).

Measures of hope and optimism are also correlated with indices of physical health and functioning. There is evidence that hopelessness and pessimism predict self-reported health problems (Robinson-Whelen et al., 1997; Scioli et al., 1997; Sumi, 1997). High levels of optimism, by contrast, are related to better physiological and functional measures of physical health. For example, Peterson et al. (1988) conducted a 35-year prospective study of 99 Harvard University graduates to examine the effects of pessimistic attitudes on physical health outcomes. CAVE techniques were used to analyze data from open-ended responses to questions in 1946 about difficult wartime experiences (average age of respondents was 25). Physical health was assessed by physical examinations performed at five-year intervals. A pessimistic explanatory style significantly predicted poor physical health at ages 45 ($p < .001$), 50 ($p < .10$), 55 ($p < .05$), and 60 ($p < .02$) (after controlling for initial physical and mental health). These investigators concluded that a pessimistic explanatory style predicts physical health 25 to 35 years later.

In a study of men who underwent coronary artery bypass graft (CABG) surgery, Scheier et al. (1989) found that those who had high levels of optimism prior to surgery had fewer enzyme and EKG changes indicative of myocardial infarction during surgery. Indeed, optimists recovered quicker and experienced less functional disability for at least six months after surgery. There is also evidence that hopelessness is an independent risk factor for progression of artherosclerosis (Everson, Kaplan, et al., 1997) and that pessimism and hopelessness predict lower survival in some groups of cancer patients (Ringdal, 1995; Schulz et al., 1996).

Finally, catastrophizing—a tendency to expect the worst when bad events occur—is related to all-cause mortality even in young, healthy individuals (Peterson, Seligman, Yurko, et al., 1998). Pessimistic attitudes may in some way impact the physical body's ability to respond to illness. In a prospective study of first-semester law students, Segerstrom et al. (1998) examined whether optimism early in the semester would predict immune functioning later in the semester. Investigators hypothesized that the first semester of law school would be a stressful time for students, possibly leading to decrements in immune functioning. They found that students who were optimists at the beginning of the semester (as measured by the Life Orientation Test) had better immune functioning eight weeks later, even after researchers controlled for initial levels of immune function.

Thus, hopeful, optimistic people are more likely to avoid depression and anxiety, cope more adaptively with stress, experience fewer physical health problems, and perhaps even live longer once they develop diseases such as cancer. It is important, then, to examine the relationships among religion, optimism, and hope.

Religion, Optimism, and Hope

A limited amount of research has examined the relationships among these variables. Studies have focused on three groups of people: healthy individuals, disabled persons or those under significant life stress, and patients with chronic or terminal illness.

Healthy Individuals. In general, religious involvement is associated with higher levels of hope and optimism in healthy individuals. Carson, Soeken, and Grimm (1988) administered a state-trait hope inventory and measures of spiritual well-being (including subscales for assessing both religious well-being and existential well-being) to a group of 197 university nursing students. Investigators found that hope was positively related to both religious well-being and existential well-being, although the association was somewhat stronger between hope and existential well-being than between hope and religious well-being. In another study, Zorn (1997) investigated the predictors of hope in a sample of 169 noninstitutionalized older adults. The mean age of the respondents was 75.4 years. Religious well-being, along with social support and physical health, was significantly and positively related to hope. Dember and Brooks (1989) reported similar findings.

Ressler (1997) recently developed a measure to assess the multifactorial construct that he called "Jewishness." On the basis of a preliminary factor analysis, Ressler found that a 10-factor solution best described his measure of Jewishness. These factors were (1) interest in Israel; (2) interest in broad Jewish topics; (3) commitment to religious traditions; (4) holiday celebration; (5) Jewish organizational activism; (6) propinquity to other Jews; (7) antiestablishment Jewish organizational activism; (8) personal belief in God; (9) belief that Jews are obligated to excel; and (10) secular community activism. Ressler found that three of these subscales—holiday celebration, Jewish organizational activism, and personal belief in God—were significantly related to a 10-item measure of optimism. Using multiple regression, Ressler found that holiday celebration and Jewish organizational activism remained significant predictors of optimism after other variables were controlled. Interestingly, the Ressler study suggests that participation in Jewish community life and the observance of religious holidays were most important for optimism in this Jewish sample, although belief in God was strongly related to both activities.

Recall from chapter 6 that Sethi and Seligman (1993) examined the aspects of religion that were most strongly related to optimism among Christian groups in the United States. Members of nine major religious denominations ($n = 623$) completed self-report measures of optimism and religiousness. Religiousness was measured by influence of religion in daily life ("To what extent do your religious beliefs influence whom you associate with?"), religious involvement ("How often do you attend religious services?"), and religious hope ("Do you believe your suffering will be rewarded?"). Respondents were also categorized as fundamentalist, moderate, or liberal on the basis of their religious affiliation.

On the main measure of optimism (a difference score obtained by subtracting people's attributions for a series of negative hypothetical events from their attributions for a series of positive hypothetical events), the mean score for fundamentalists (including Orthodox Jews, Muslims, and Calvinists) was 2.09 (SD = 1.10). The mean score for moderates (including Catholics, conservative Jews, Methodists, Lutherans, and Methodists) was 0.48 (SD = 1.27). The mean score for liberals (including reform Jews and Unitarians) was −0.07 (SD = 1.60). Fundamentalists were significantly more optimistic than liberals, but moderates were not significantly different from either fundamentalists or liberals.

In a second study described in the same report, Sethi and Seligman coded the optimism and pessimism expressed in typical prayers and hymns of each of the nine religions from which respondents were drawn. They then used multiple regression techniques to examine whether the fundamentalism-optimism association was mediated by personal religiousness and/or the optimism expressed within each religion. When religious influence in daily life, religious involvement, religious hope, and the level of hope in the prototypical prayers and hymns were controlled for, fundamentalism no longer predicted optimism. Investigators concluded that the relationship between fundamentalist

religious orientation and optimism was largely the result of the greater intensity of religious involvement and the greater emphasis placed on hope contained in fundamentalist liturgy.

Disabled or Stressed Persons. Religion is also related to greater optimism and hope in people experiencing high levels of life stress and appears to be even more important for this group than for those without stress. Surveying 2,812 older adults in the Yale Health and Aging Study, Idler and Kasl (1997a) found that public religious involvement (measured by attendance at religious services) was significantly related to optimism and positive affect among elders with high levels of disability (after controlling for depression, self-rated health, negative affect, somatic complaints, and interpersonal complaints) but was weakly or unrelated to optimism in participants with little or no physical disability. Private religiousness (measured by a two-item scale that asked how deeply religious the person was and how much strength and comfort he or she received from religion), however, was unrelated to optimism in controlled analyses for either the high- or low-disability groups.

Other studies report similar results among people who were undergoing major life stress. Sanders (1979–1980) administered the MMPI and Grief Inventory Scale to 102 newly bereaved persons (who had lost a spouse, child, or parent) and 107 nonbereaved individuals. Additional measures administered to both samples included a single-item measure of frequency of church attendance. While frequency of attendance was not significantly associated with levels of grief, it was positively related to self-reported optimism. Similar findings have been reported by others in recently bereaved people (see Bohannon, 1991).

Medically Ill Persons. Several studies suggest that religious involvement is associated with hope and optimism among persons with cancer. Mickley, Soeken, et al. (1992) administered measures of intrinsic and extrinsic religious orientation, existential and religious well-being, and hope to a group of 175 women with various stages of breast cancer. Hope was significantly related to intrinsic religiousness ($r = .36$), religious well-being ($r = .44$), and existential well-being ($r = .73$). When other variables were controlled using regression, existential well-being was the only religious variable significantly related to hope (although intrinsic religiousness and religious well-being may have had positive effects on hope through existential well-being). Cotton et al. (1998) similarly reported a significant correlation between spiritual well-being and loss of hope in a sample of 87 women with breast cancer ($r = -.62$), and Ringdal (1996) found a two-item measure of subjective religiousness negatively related to hopelessness in a sample of 253 hospitalized cancer patients ($\beta = -.17, p < .03$) after controlling for age, sex, level of education, and prognosis.

This review suggests that religion, optimism, and hope are significantly and positively correlated; only a few studies have not supported such a relationship (Moberg, 1984, and Fox & Odling-Smee, 1995, found no association). Among people who are undergoing significant life stress, the relationship between religion and optimism and hope is especially strong. The religious or spiritual dimension is also an important predictor of optimism and hope among cancer patients (see chapter 20). Research is needed with more refined measures of these variables to understand the cognitive and affective pathways through which religion and spiritual variables influence optimism and hope (or vice versa).

CONTROL

People have a fundamental need for control over their life circumstances. When persons have control, they are generally happier and more alert to potentially health-relevant problems; they take more preventive measures, engage in more productive efforts at coping with life stressors, and seek more information when they encounter stressors. For these reasons, sense of personal control is related to better mental and physical health (Lefcourt & Davidson-Katz, 1991; Shapiro et al., 1996).

Conceptualizing and Measuring Locus of Control

The concept of control has been of great importance to the field of health psychology. For the past 30 years, the aspect of control that has received the most attention has been locus of control (Rotter, 1966; Shapiro et al., 1996). Rotter (1966) conceptualized locus of control as either *internal* (meaning that the person believes he or she is the primary causal agent that controls his or her life and circumstances) or *external* (meaning that powerful outside forces, fate, or other powerful persons are believed to be the primary causal agents responsible for the person's circumstances).

As the concept of locus of control was refined and studied further, researchers developed measures of locus of control that assess perceived control over specific aspects of life. For example, Wallston et al. (1978) developed the Multidimensional Health Locus of Control Scales to assess factors that people believe are responsible for their health. This scale consists of three subscales: internal, powerful others, and external chance. People who score high on the internal dimension perceive their health to be primarily influenced by their own actions. People who score high on the powerful others dimension believe that authority figures (e.g., physicians and health professionals) are primarily responsible for their health. Finally, people who score high on the external chance dimension believe that good health is completely a matter of luck (fate) and that nothing can be done to influence health to any great degree.

Locus of Control and Health

Researchers have repeatedly shown that people with an internal locus of control experience better health. Persons with a high internal locus of control become aware of changes from the status quo more quickly than do externals (Lefcourt et al., 1974). Some investigators have hypothesized that this ability to "catch on" might alert them to changes in their health more quickly, thereby allowing them to intervene before minor problems become serious ones. Internals are also more likely to take care of themselves when they are healthy (thereby preventing future problems). For example, they have better attitudes toward exercise and seat belt use and are less likely to smoke. Internals also have consistently more upbeat, optimistic moods than do externals (see Benassi et al., 1988). When under stress, internals are also less likely to succumb to psychological symptoms (Solomon et al., 1988). When they receive news that they have an illness, people with an internal locus of control are more likely to take positive steps to cope with the illness. As might be expected, the better health and health maintenance activities of internals translate into longer survival (Reid & Zigler, 1981; Lefcourt & Davidson-Katz, 1991; Shapiro et al., 1996). Of course, an internal locus of control is not always a good thing to have. When one's circumstances are definitely *not* under one's control, then the desire to obtain control can become counterproductive and lead to poor adaptation. Overall, however, an internal locus of control is a personality characteristic that typically predicts better mental and physical health.

Religion and Locus of Control

At first glance, one would expect religious involvement to be positively related to an external locus of control or control by powerful others. A hallmark of many forms of religious belief is the idea that a supreme being or higher power possesses and exerts control over the affairs of the world. Indeed, one would predict that religious involvement might be related to a lower internal locus of control.

The association between religiousness and locus of control has been studied in some detail. Several studies have found that religiousness is associated with a higher—not lower—internal locus of control. For example, Strickland and Schaffer (1971) examined the association of Rotter's I-E scale and an intrinsic-extrinsic religious orientation scale in a sample of 114 adolescent and adult church members. They found that people who reported higher intrinsic religious motivation scored higher on internal locus of control than those with lower intrinsic religiousness. Pargament, Steele, and Tyler (1979) found that frequent church attendance

was associated with weaker beliefs in control by chance and in personal control; intrinsic religious motivation, however, was associated with stronger beliefs in personal control, weaker beliefs in powerful others, and weaker beliefs in control by chance. In another early study, Kivett et al. (1977) found that intrinsic religiousness was significantly and positively related to internal locus of control in a sample of middle-aged and older adults. Finally, Furnham (1982) found that Church of England clergymen who were identified as "fundamentalist" on a fundamentalist-liberal theology scale had higher scores on measures of internal locus of control than did liberal clergymen.

Some studies have not found a relationship between religious involvement and internal locus of control. Friedberg and Friedberg (1985) reported that religiousness and locus of control were unrelated in a sample of 143 undergraduate students. Likewise, Richards (1991) found that degree of spiritual experience during prayer was not correlated with internal locus of control in a sample of 345 healthy adults who were participating in a spiritual growth program. However, Richards (1991) did find that subjects with high levels of spiritual experience during prayer scored lower on measures of belief in control by powerful others and in control by chance. Using a different method of assessing locus of control, Loewenthal and Cornwall (1993) had 74 British adults assign causes to 38 hypothetical life events. The participants were free to assign causality to (a) God, (b) powerful others, (c) luck, or (d) self and could assign causality for each of the 38 scenarios to as many of these four agents as they pleased. Nonreligious subjects were no more likely than the religious to assign causality to self, powerful others, or luck. Similarly, in a small clinical study involving 28 cancer patients, religiousness and locus of control were unrelated (Tebbi et al., 1987).

In what is perhaps the most extensive examination of religious involvement and locus of control to date, Watson, Milliron, et al. (1995) administered measures of intrinsic and extrinsic religious motivation, religious problem-solving styles, "internal-external" locus of control, and beliefs in "chance" control, "powerful others" control, and "personal" control to 467 undergraduate college students. Intrinsic and extrinsic religious motivation were unrelated to either beliefs in personal control or internal locus of control. However, those with intrinsic religious motivation were less likely to believe in either the "chance" locus of control or the "powerful others" locus of control ($r = -.13$ and $r = -.10$, respectively, both $p < .05$). Conversely, extrinsic religious motivation was correlated with stronger beliefs in "chance" control and in "powerful others" control ($r = .22$ and $r = .24$, respectively, both $p < .001$).

Religious Coping Style and Locus of Control. Two groups of researchers (Pargament, Kennell, et al. 1988; Watson, Milliron, et al., 1995) have moved beyond static measures of religious involvement such as frequency of church attendance and religious motivation to try to understand how various forms of control beliefs are related to styles of religious coping. In these studies, participants completed measures of their beliefs in internal control, personal control, control by chance, and control by powerful others. They also completed Pargament, Kennell, et al.'s (1988) religious problem-solving scales, which include measures of (a) the extent to which people use a *self-directing* religious style for solving problems (e.g., "God gives me the skills to solve problems myself"), (b) the extent to which people use a *deferring* religious problem-solving style (e.g., "I wait on God to instruct me about what I should do"), and (c) the extent to which people use a *collaborative* religious problem-solving style (e.g., "God is a partner who gives me guidance and strength").

Pargament and colleagues (1988) found that the self-directing religious problem-solving style was associated with higher personal control ($r = .33$, $p < .001$), and not with chance control ($r = .08$, $p = $ ns). The deferring religious coping style was negatively related to personal control ($r = -.44$, $p < .001$) and positively related to chance control ($r = .18$, $p < .05$). The collaborative religious coping style was negatively associated with personal control ($r = -.16$, $p < .01$) and uncorrelated with chance control ($r = -.06$, $p = $ ns). After the researchers controlled statistically for the other two religious problem-solving styles, the correlation between collaborative coping and personal control actually became positive ($r = .25$, $p < .001$), and the association with chance control became negative ($r = -.17$, $p < .05$).

Thus, the self-directing religious problem-solving style appears to be most strongly associated with an internal locus of control, and the deferring style appears to be most strongly associated with an external locus of control. The most interesting aspect of the study, however, was that the collaborative religious problem-solving style was associated with lower internal locus of control in the bivariate analyses, but, when its associations with other religious coping styles were controlled, it became significantly associated with a higher internal locus of control.

While these results are intriguing, Watson, Milliron, and colleagues (1995) could not replicate them. They found that Pargament's measures of religious problem-solving style were largely uncorrelated with measures of beliefs in chance, powerful others, and personal control, as well as Rotter's global measure of internal/external locus of control. Indeed, no correlation between a measure of religious problem-solving style and locus of control exceeded $r = |.10|$.

Belief in God as a Locus of Control. A final dimension of locus of control relevant to this topic is a small but interesting literature on beliefs in God as a locus of control. In the Loewenthal and Cornwall (1993) study described earlier, 74 British adults were instructed to assign causes to 38 hypothetical life events. While religious participants were no more likely than nonreligious to assign causality to self, powerful others, or luck, they were more likely to assign causality to God for matters of health or life and death. Pargament, Steele, et al. (1979) also found that church attenders and people high in intrinsic religious motivation had stronger beliefs in God as a locus of control than did nonchurch attenders or people low in intrinsic religious motivation (see also Jackson & Coursey, 1988). As might be expected, the deferring and collaborative religious problem-solving styles are related to stronger beliefs in God as a locus of control, while the self-directing religious coping style is related to weaker beliefs in God's control (Pargament, Kennell, et al., 1988).

How are beliefs in God as a locus of control related to health and well-being? Only a few studies have addressed this question. Attributing causality to God for one's health problems (which is similar but still different from believing in God as a locus of control) has been related to *slower* recovery and *poorer* psychological adjustment in some prospective studies (Agrawal & Dalal, 1993; Pargament, 1997). However, standardized measures of belief in God as a locus of control predict little unique variance in measures of coping and purpose in life after internal locus of control and other measures of religious involvement are controlled (Jackson & Coursey, 1988). Interestingly, one study found that belief in God's control were related to lower anxiety for Caucasians but to greater anxiety for Koreans (Bjorck, Lee, et al., 1997). Unfortunately, beliefs in God as a locus of control have not yet been studied in sufficient detail for us to understand whether the construct is truly distinct from belief in other forms of locus of control and, if so, whether it is related to better or worse physical health and well-being.

SUMMARY AND CONCLUSIONS

This chapter has focused on associations between religious involvement and three personality variables that are relevant to physical health and well-being—hostility, hope and optimism, and control. People who are high in religious or spiritual involvement tend to have low levels of hostility and high levels of hope and optimism. These findings are quite robust and suggest that low hostility and high hope and optimism might be two mechanisms by which religious involvement conveys positive effects on health and well-being.

The literature on religion and locus of control is not as straightforward. While many studies find that people who are intrinsically religious have a higher internal locus of control, these findings are not universal. What is clear, however, is that intrinsic religious motivation is not correlated with an external locus of control. Indeed, certain religious problem-solving styles (i.e., particularly the collaborative style) may allow religious people to maintain an internal locus of control and *simultaneously* sustain the belief that God is also in control. This combination of internality and trust in God may be a particularly strong combination of control beliefs that helps religious people maintain health and recover more quickly and effectively from life stress. Conversely, people who maintain a deferring, passive religious problem-solving style have high beliefs in God as a locus of control and low belief in internal control—a pattern that may portend poor psychological adjustment and poor physical health (particularly where individual effort might facilitate problem solving). Further studies are needed in populations that have no control over health outcomes (e.g., the severely disabled or nursing home patients) and where failed efforts to control one's situation may increase distress.

The three health-relevant personality variables reviewed here—hostility, hope and optimism, and locus of control—have been shown to predict both mental and physical health. There exist many other personality variables that influence or are influenced by health and/or religion. The present chapter has provided only a small sampling of the many ways that religion, personality, and health are related.

15

Understanding Religion's Effects on Mental Health

IN THIS CHAPTER WE EXAMine why and how religion influences mental health. We are assuming here that religion does influence mental health, thus making a leap to causal inference. While the cross-sectional and prospective data are overwhelmingly consistent with and supportive of such a leap, the number of intervention or experimental studies are as yet too few to conclude without doubt that religion *causes* better mental health. With this note of caution, we proceed. The effects of religious involvement on mental health as discussed in chapters 5 through 14 are first summarized. We then review factors that previous research in the psychological, social, and behavioral sciences have found to influence adult mental health. These determinants of mental health are then linked to religion in order to understand how religion directly and indirectly influences mental health. A theoretical model helps guide this discussion

and provides hypotheses that can be tested in future studies. As in most of this book, we focus primarily on Western religious traditions.

SUMMARY OF RESEARCH FINDINGS

A comprehensive list of studies examining the relationship between religion and each of the mental health outcomes discussed in this chapter can be found in part VIII. The percentages noted here largely pertain to the studies in that list, unless otherwise noted.

Greater Well-Being

Religious beliefs and practices are consistently related to greater life satisfaction, happiness, positive affect, morale, and other indicators of well being. In chapter 6, we observed that nearly 80% of the 100 studies that examined the association between religion and well-being reported at least one significant positive correlation between these variables. While the correlations reported by many studies are modest, they typically equal or exceed correlations between well-being and other psychosocial variables, such as social support.

Greater Hope and Optimism

With few exceptions, 80% or more of the studies reported a positive association between religiousness and greater hope or optimism about the future. No studies have been published that show that religious persons are less optimistic than those without religious faith. Where there is belief in the miraculous or supernatural, there is always hope. Even the threat of death itself cannot easily destroy the confidence of a person who believes in a new and better life in the hereafter. Having greater purpose, meaning, and sense of coherence in life also provides a powerful boost for hope and optimism.

Greater Purpose and Meaning

The religious person lives in a world that has purpose and meaning. Many believe in a purposeful creator who has a *will* for humanity: "Thy will be done in earth, as it is in heaven" (Matthew 6:10, KJV). This often includes a belief that each person plays a vital and important part in the Divine plan. It is not surprising, then, that 15 out of 16 studies located in our literature review reported a statistically significant association between greater religious involvement and a greater sense of purpose or meaning in life.

Greater Self-Esteem

According to Watters (1992), "it is difficult to understand how any family can perform this task [help a child develop autonomy and actualize her human potential] if it is influenced to any degree by the teachings of the Christian church, since that institution's teachings are uncompromisingly antithetical to the development of self-esteem" (p. 51). This is not, however, what the research shows. Of the 29 studies

that have looked at the relationship between religion and self-esteem, primarily in Judeo-Christian populations, 16 (55%) reported *greater* self-esteem among the more religiously involved. Of the remaining 12 studies, 10 reported no association, one reported a negative association, and two reported mixed results. According to a recent study by Neal Krause (1995) at the University of Michigan's School of Public Health, feelings of self-worth "tend to be lowest for those with very little religious commitment" (p. 236). Religious beliefs and teachings, by discouraging both excessive pride and self-condemnation, may foster a healthier view of the self that is more in line with reality (Koenig, 1994a).

Better Adaptation to Bereavement

Religious faith can help cushion the emotional blow associated with loss of a loved one. In our review, we found 17 studies that quantitatively examined the relationship between religious involvement and adaptation following bereavement. Almost half of these studies ($n = 8$) reported better adaptation among those who were more religious; five studies reported no association; one study found a negative association; and three studies reported mixed or complex results. Particularly important are the results of Azhar and Varma (1995a), who conducted a clinical trial that showed that, when religious psychotherapy is added to secular treatment for bereavement, improvement occurs significantly faster. All major religious traditions have rituals that facilitate grieving and adaptation to loss. Indeed, funerals have long included religious ceremonies designed to ease the grief of loved ones.

Greater Social Support

The need to help and support others is encouraged by virtually every one of the world's major religions (Coward, 1986). Of the 20 studies we located that quantitatively examined the relationship between religious activity and social support, 19 reported at least one statistically significant relationship between a religious variable and greater social support. The remaining single study reported mixed results. In that study of 98 older subjects recruited from African American churches in urban areas of central Pennsylvania, Walls and Zarit (1991) found that 50% of the subjects indicated that their closest friends were family members, while 40% of subjects indicated that their closest and most important friends were members of their church. Not surprisingly, family members were significantly more likely than church members to provide emotional support, instrumental support, reliable support, nurturance, and reassurance of worth. Note that this was a comparison of church-related and family support, and it does not diminish the fact that church members provide a huge amount of support for aging African Americans. Other studies have also found that the majority of supportive nonfamily relationships of older Americans (whether African American or white) are found among persons they meet at church (Koenig, Moberg, & Kvale, 1988).

Less Loneliness

Religious beliefs and practices, particularly when they include active participation in religious community, can help relieve loneliness and counteract isolation. Unfortunately, few high-quality studies have directly examined the relationship between loneliness and religious involvement. We found 10 such studies: four reported less loneliness among those who were more religious, three found no association, and two reported mixed results, and one study found greater loneliness among the more religious. Only one of these 10 studies, however, received a quality rating above 6, and we now describe that study.

Lee and Ishii-Kuntz (1987) conducted a telephone survey of a random sample of 2,872 persons age 55 or over who were living in the state of Washington. Frequency of church attendance was the only religious variable, and outcomes were a four-item loneliness scale and a seven-item morale scale (both developed by the study investigators). Among men, religious attendance was significantly and positively related to greater morale after researchers controlled for 10 other covariates, including a host of social variables. Church attendance was also inversely

related to loneliness in both men ($r = -.06$, $p \geq .01$) and women ($r = -.07$, $p < .01$). After marital status, health, friends, and neighbors were controlled, the relationship between church attendance and loneliness lost its statistical significance in both genders. Note, however, that investigators controlled for marital status, friends, and neighbors in their analysis of the attendance-loneliness relationship. By doing this, they may have controlled for the *mechanism* by which religious attendance relieves loneliness. In other words, frequent attendance may relieve loneliness because it increases the number of one's friends and neighbors and improves the likelihood that one will be married and stay married. Further studies, however, are clearly needed to assess the relationship between religion and loneliness.

Less Depression

We found 101 studies that examined the relationship between level of religious involvement and depression, eight of which were clinical trials. Of the 93 cross-sectional or prospective studies, 60 (65%) reported a significant positive relationship between a measure of religious involvement and *lower* rates of depression or depressive symptoms; 13 studies reported no association; four reported greater depression among the more religious; and 16 studies reported mixed findings (positive associations with some religious variables and negative associations with others). Among denominational studies, Jews (six out of six studies) and Pentecostals (two out of two studies) had more depression than comparison groups. Of the 22 prospective cohort studies that examined the relationship between religion and depression, 15 (68%) found that greater religious involvement predicted lower rates of depression over time. Finally, eight clinical trials have examined the effects of religious interventions on speed of recovery from depression. Five of these eight studies showed that depressed patients receiving religious interventions recovered significantly faster than subjects in comparison or control groups. Thus, there is growing consensus in the literature that the religiously active are less likely to become depressed and less likely to stay depressed.

Fewer Suicides

Most Western religious traditions (Judaism, Christianity, Islam) teach that suicide is wrong. Consequently, one would expect lower rates of suicide among the more religiously active and committed. This is indeed the case. We located 105 studies that quantitatively assessed the relationship between religion and suicide (completed suicide, attempted suicide, or attitude toward suicide). Of those, 37 compared suicide rates/attitudes by religious denomination and 68, by level of religious involvement.

Eight of the denominational studies compared Jews with member of other religious denominations; four studies showed lower suicide rates (or more negative attitudes toward suicide) among Jews, two studies showed higher suicide rates/positive attitudes among Jews, and two studies found no difference between Jews and members of other religious groups. Thirty studies compared suicide rates and attitudes in Catholics with members of other religious groups (usually Protestants, but also Jews in three studies); nine studies found lower suicide rates (or more negative attitudes toward suicide) among Catholics, six studies found higher suicide rates in Catholics, and 13 studies showed no differences between Catholics and members of other religious groups. One study showed that Protestants made more suicide attempts than members of other religious groups, and one study showed that Mormons and Baptists had lower suicide rates than members of other religious groups.

More interestingly, of the 68 studies examining suicide rates and attitudes by level of religious involvement, 57 (84%) found less suicide and more negative attitudes toward suicide in the more religious; nine studies showed no relationship; and two studies reported mixed results. No studies found higher suicide rates or more positive attitudes toward suicide among the more religious (with the exception of Bagley and Ramsey, 1989). Thus, in studies that correlated suicide with some measure of religious belief or activity (i.e., religiousness), the vast majority found an inverse relationship between religion and suicide. Furthermore, all 11 studies (100%) that examined attitudes toward "as-

sisted suicide" maintained this pattern of results.

Less Anxiety

Given the concern about whether religion fosters neurosis, many studies have examined the correlation between religion and anxiety. These studies have either assessed general anxiety or anxiety related to a specific situation (i.e., death anxiety). Our review identified 76 studies that examined the religion-anxiety relationship, including seven clinical trials. Of the 69 cross-sectional and prospective studies, 35 (51%) reported significantly less anxiety or fear among the more religious; 17 reported no association; seven reported mixed or complex results; and 10 reported greater anxiety among the more religious. Of the 17 studies that reported no association, 16 were cross-sectional studies, and 12 did not control for other variables in the analyses. Of the 10 studies that found greater anxiety among the more religious, two compared anxiety between religiously affiliated and unaffiliated subjects; three examined prayer or religious coping and anxiety in cross-sectional analyses (anxious persons may have turned to prayer or religion *because* of their anxiety); and three studies were conducted among HIV-positive patients, psychiatric patients with obsessive-compulsive disorder, or persons who had suddenly converted to a different religious faith. Of the seven clinical trials, six reported significant benefit in terms of anxiety relief from religious interventions. In summary, the majority of the studies we reviewed found less anxiety and fear among the more religiously involved, including 80% of the five prospective cohort studies and 86% of the clinical trials.

Less Schizophrenia and Fewer Other Psychoses

Relatively few studies have examined the relationship between religion and psychotic symptoms or chronic mental disorders such as schizophrenia. We found 16 studies (10 cross-sectional, one prospective, three denominational, and two clinical trials) that examined this relationship. Four of the 10 cross-sectional studies found *less* psychosis or fewer psychotic tendencies among the more religiously involved; three studies reported no association; and two studies reported mixed findings. The tenth study found religious beliefs and practices more common among 52 depressed and 21 schizophrenic psychiatric inpatients than among 26 orthopedic control patients. One of the largest studies was a two-year prospective cohort study that followed 386 schizophrenic patients seen at psychiatric outpatient clinics in Madras and Vellore, India. Worse outcomes were seen among patients who reported a *decrease* in religious activities at the baseline evaluation ($p < .001$, uncontrolled).

The three small denominational studies reported complex findings. Jews were found to have more depression, whereas Protestants tended to have more schizophrenia; Jehovah's Witnesses in Australia were more likely to have schizophrenia than were persons in the general Australian population; and Baha'i and Hari Krishna were more likely to have psychotic episodes that required hospitalization than were Jews or Catholics.

Of the clinical trials that utilized religious interventions, one study of 28 psychiatric patients with serious mental illness (19 with schizophrenia) involved administration of a psychoeducational program designed to help patients utilize their spiritual beliefs to foster healthy self-esteem. No significant improvements in self-esteem or depressive symptoms were observed following the intervention (although no worsening was seen, either). In the second study, 20 schizophrenics who received weekly prayer and Scripture reading from student nurses demonstrated notable improvements in mental state and functioning. In general, then, religious involvement, particularly in mainstream religious groups, is either unassociated with psychotic tendencies or inversely related to them.

Less Alcohol and Drug Abuse

Religious persons are less likely to abuse alcohol and/or to take illicit drugs. With regard to alcohol use, we located 95 studies that quantitatively examined the religion-alcohol relationship (including nine studies that compared denominations). Of the 86 studies that examined religiousness, 76 (88%) reported significantly lower alcohol use or abuse among more religious subjects (including eight of nine prospective cohort studies); six studies reported no association, two studies reported a positive relationship with alcohol use or abuse, and two studies reported mixed results. Of the nine denominational studies, six found more alcohol use or abuse among Catholics, and the remaining three found less alcohol use or abuse among Jews and Mormons. More than half ($n = 40$) of the 76 studies that found less alcohol use or abuse among the more religious were conducted on adolescents or college students.

Religiousness is also associated with less frequent use of illicit drugs, again especially in younger persons. We found 56 studies that quantitatively tested this relationship. Of those 56 studies, 52 examined the relationship between religiousness and drug use (four compared drug use among members of different religious groups). As with alcohol abuse, most studies (48 out of 52) found significantly less drug use among the more religious; two studies reported no association, and one study reported mixed results and one, greater drug use. Most studies that found a relationship between greater religiousness and lower drug use (42 of 48) were conducted on adolescents or college students. Less frequent alcohol and drug abuse during adolescence and the teenage years likely affects the health and success of these young persons throughout the remainder of their lives.

Less Delinquency and Crime

Given the lower rates of alcohol and drug abuse among the more religious, one would expect and indeed finds lower rates of delinquency and crime in this group. We identified 36 studies that had quantitatively examined this relationship (and one denominational study). Of those 36 studies, 28 (78%) found significantly lower rates of delinquency or crime among the more religious, six studies found no association, one study found mixed results, and one found a positive association with delinquency. The last study compared attitudes toward God, Jesus, and the Bible of 28 nondelinquent actively religious youth (chosen for the study by their ministers) and 52 incarcerated juvenile delinquents (Scholl & Beker, 1964). Interestingly, delinquent youth were significantly more likely than nondelinquent youth to agree to the statement "Every word of the Bible is literally true" ($p < .001$). Delinquents were also more likely to agree to the statements "When I pray, I usually ask God to help my family" and "God is powerful and controls our life" (both $p < .02$). In perhaps the best and most definitive study on this topic, Stark (1996) analyzed data from a national random sample of 11,995 high school seniors and found that those who attended religious services more regularly were significantly less likely to get into trouble with the law. Correlations were robust in all areas of the country except the Pacific Northwest (known as the "secular peninsula").

Greater Marital Stability

Divorce and separation are significant predictors of poor mental health and suicide (Rossow, 1993) and have been linked to impaired immune system function (Kennedy, Kiecolt-Glaser, et al., 1988) and increased use of health services (Joung et al., 1995). Not only does a stable and satisfying marriage enhance the quality of life for the marital partners; it also increases the likelihood that the emotional needs of the couple's children will be met. These developmental influences will likely impact the emotional stability of the children throughout adulthood. We know that children of divorced or separated parents are at greater risk of having children as teenagers, conceiving and bearing children outside marriage, themselves becoming divorced when married, and having significant emotional problems in adult life (Chase-Lansdale et al., 1995). Children of divorce are also at higher risk for health problems, including pneumonia, tonsillitis, and repeated ear infections (Mauldon, 1990). In the year

2000, 47% of American families were expected to be single-parent homes (Bureau of the Census). Families in which the father is absent are nine times more likely than two-parent homes to have annual incomes of less than $10,000 (U.S. Congress Report, 1989). We also know that children raised in single-parent homes are at higher risk for juvenile delinquency and for drug and alcohol abuse (Zill & Schoenborn, 1990; Zill et al., 1993; Hope et al., 1998; Neher & Short, 1998).

Our review of the literature uncovered 38 studies that quantitatively examined the relationship between religiousness and marital happiness or stability. Of those 38 studies, 35 (92%) found greater marital happiness or stability among the more religious or those with similar religious backgrounds (denominational homogamy). One study found no association between marital instability and denominational homogamy. The remaining two studies reported mixed results, and both dealt with domestic violence or abuse. In the first of these studies, Brutz and Allen (1986) surveyed 290 Quaker spouses and found that religious participation was associated in both husbands and wives with *lower* levels of both communication violence (any verbal or nonverbal act, short of physical contact, that is intended to produce emotional pain in another) and ordinary physical violence. A similar association between global commitment to Quaker beliefs and testimonies and violence was found for wives, but not for husbands. For husbands, lower levels of violence were associated with higher global commitment only for communication violence. Physical violence rates for husbands with high global commitment, however, were higher than those for husbands with low global commitment.

In the second study, Ellison, Bartkowski, et al. (1996) analyzed data from a survey of 2,242 men and 2,420 women age 19 or older (1987–1988 National Survey of Families and Households). Denominational homogamy was unrelated to domestic violence in men. However, men who held much more conservative theological views than their partners were at increased risk for violence. Women, however, were less likely to perpetrate domestic violence if (1) they attended religious services one or more times per month or (2) they and their partner were either both conservative Protestant or both Catholic (i.e., homogamously affiliated).

While there is some concern about increased domestic violence in families where marital partners differ substantially in religious belief, more than 90% of studies show greater marital happiness, lower rates of divorce and separation, and greater family stability among the more religious. This fact invariably affects the health of both marriage partners and the future physical and mental health of their children.

We now examine general factors that tend to shape psychological health. We then discuss how religious beliefs and practices might influence mental health through these established biological, psychological, and social pathways.

FACTORS THAT INFLUENCE MENTAL HEALTH

Many variables influence susceptibility to mental health problems. Most important among these are genetic factors (inherited strengths and weaknesses), early childhood experiences, traumatic experiences in adulthood, cognitive appraisal of stressors, availability of coping resources to moderate stress, and specific coping behaviors mobilized to facilitate adaptation.

Heredity and Biological Factors

Genetic factors largely determine temperament, which in turn determines a person's emotional setpoint or level of sensitivity. An emotionally sensitive person may have great need for attention, support, and nurturance during infancy and later childhood, a need that may continue into adulthood. Such an individual may be easily traumatized in early life by acts of commission (things done to the child by parents or peers), acts of omission (emotional needs neglected by parents), or simple situational stressors (stressful situations or events not related to the actions of others). Particularly important is the "fit" of the infant's temperament and the parent's temperament (typically the mother, although both parents clearly have

an influence). For example, a poor outcome is probable if an emotionally sensitive and needy infant is born to an emotionally distant or otherwise preoccupied parent. The infant's unmet emotional needs from this particularly critical life stage are likely to influence her personality development and emotional neediness throughout life.

Besides determining temperament, genetic factors may be at least partly responsible for a number of psychiatric disorders, including melancholic depression, bipolar disorder, schizophrenia, obsessive-compulsive disorder, panic disorder, and attention deficit disorder. These conditions have been linked to biochemical and structural changes in the brain and are quite responsive to biological therapies. Temperamental factors and stressful life events often interact with psychiatric disorders to trigger their expression or influence their course.

Developmental Factors

Childhood losses, deprivations, or abuse (physical, emotional, or sexual) also affect later susceptibility to mental health problems. A child teased by peers, parents, or teachers because he or she is overweight, uncoordinated, or otherwise different from others will experience lasting emotional scars that may be difficult to overcome. The child who loses a parent, sibling, or other loved one to death or divorce may struggle with this loss for many years. Cultural and societal influences also leave their mark on the individual. Growing up during a world war or economic recession can influence emotional development in many different ways. Thus, each of us moves into adulthood with some degree of psychological baggage that will influence our relationships and color our future experiences.

Training received during childhood from parents and teachers also influences how a person responds to situations in adult life and has an enormous effect on decisions that affect one's use of drugs or alcohol, relationships with peers, compliance with authority, education and professional training, premarital and extramarital sexual activity, relationship with spouse, rearing of children, and caring for aging parents.

Stressful Life Events and Traumatic Experiences

Successes, failures, gains, and losses impact people differently depending on the person's temperament and personality, childhood training, prior life experiences, and social relationships. Events that threaten those elements that give meaning and purpose to life (e.g., family, work, material possessions, social status, or physical independence) can be particularly devastating to one's mental health and well-being. How one person responds to such threats will also contribute to one's later susceptibility to mental health problems. We are now discovering that each episode of severe stress or depression in adulthood may cause permanent changes in the brain that lower the threshold for future episodes of emotional illness (see chapter 18). Likewise, use of drugs or alcohol in response to life stress or depression likely exacerbates the situation, leading to neurological and other physical health changes that, in turn, adversely affect mental health.

Cognitive Appraisal

Negative life events or circumstances do not automatically and directly affect mental health. Events must first be cognitively processed in order to give meaning to them. The way people view and think about events in their lives has a lot to do with the emotions that follow (Beck, 1976). "Cognitive appraisal" is a term used to describe the thought processes that give positive or negative meaning to life events. Prior experiences and future goals heavily influence cognitive appraisal.

For example, if one sees a deer that has recently been hit by a car lying alongside the road, several emotional reactions may occur, depending on the person's background, experiences, and goals or needs. A starving person may experience great delight at the possibility that his hunger will soon be relieved. A deer hunter may experience excitement because the presence of the animal means that there are numerous deer in the area to hunt. A young child who has never seen a deer before may experience curious interest and wonder at this large animal. A

sensitive person who has previously been traumatized by having hit a deer with his or her car may experience fear or anxiety. A lover of wildlife may experience sadness or anger at such a sight. Finally, the homeowner on whose property the deer is lying may be upset because the county animal control has not yet removed the remains, which are creating a horrible stench that will ruin the homeowner's outdoor party that afternoon.

Thus, the same event can provoke a range of different emotions, depending on the meaning of the event to the person. Again, the meaning of an event is determined by cognitive appraisal; the person thinks about what has happened and relates it to his or her own personal needs, goals, and experiences. If someone repeatedly appraises events in a negative way (seeing the glass as half empty rather than half full), this will create negative feelings that can build up, eventually reduce quality of life, and possibly lead to emotional disorder.

Worldview can also greatly impact the cognitive appraisal of life events. A purely scientific worldview sees little purpose or meaning in events, which are viewed as occurring at random and without connection, sees people as primarily self-focused and as competing with one another for scarce resources, and sees nature and the universe as cold, impersonal, and threatening. Such a "realistic" worldview evokes a different cognitive appraisal of events than does a worldview that conveys a sense of coherence (Antonovsky, 1979). A sense of coherence sees order and meaning in events; sees others as working together toward a common goal; sees nature and the universe as personal, "friendly," and safe; and believes that good can be extracted from even the worst of life experiences. Such a positive worldview helps people weather the "slings and arrows of outrageous fortune" by imbuing these events with meaning and fitting them into an understandable framework that yields comfort and hope.

Coping Resources

Particularly important for maintaining mental health are coping resources that help people adapt to or overcome life stressors. Coping resources include financial resources, education, physical health, supportive social relationships, and altruism (the capacity and motivation to reach out and help others). Socioeconomic status, whether measured by income, occupation, or education, is a strong, consistent, and independent predictor of mental and physical health (Adler et al., 1993). Financial resources and education increase the number of options for coping with a stressor. Physical health status (particularly the physical ability to care for oneself) is one of the strongest predictors of mental health and well-being at any age, but particularly in later adulthood (Koenig & George, 1998). Vigorous health also expands the number of coping strategies. Social support has been shown to buffer stress, reduce the risk of depression, and speed recovery from depression (George et al., 1989; George, 1992). When bad things happen, then, it always helps to have friends, money, and good health.

Coping Behaviors

Coping behaviors are things that people do in response to stressful life changes. Some of these behaviors are ultimately destructive to self and others, such as alcohol or drug use, extramarital sexual activity, or other addictive-type behaviors. Positive coping behaviors are life enriching, character building, and growth enhancing. An example of a positive coping behavior is altruism. Reaching out to and encouraging others in worse circumstances is a powerful antidote to depression and other negative emotions caused by stressful life events. Altruistic behaviors help to meet others needs, distract one from one's own problems, and promote feelings of usefulness, purpose, and well-being (Krause et al., 1992).

MODELING THE EFFECTS OF RELIGION ON MENTAL HEALTH

A theoretical model is needed to illustrate how and why religious beliefs and practices might influence mental health. Models help researchers develop research questions, choose appropriate study designs to answer those questions,

understand and interpret research findings, and organize a body of knowledge that can be understood more generally for education purposes. A model of the religion-mental health relationship should:

- Do justice to the complexity of the mechanisms involved (since religion's effects are likely conveyed through multiple influences that interact with one another)
- Be overinclusive rather than leave out possible mechanisms (since the field is young and much is yet to be learned)
- Be simple enough to be understood by professionals from a wide variety of disciplines (to encourage multidisciplinary study of the subject)
- Consider that the effects of religion may accumulate over time and vary in influence at different stages of the life cycle.

The model in Figure 15.1 illustrates hypothesized pathways by which religion can influence mental health. Religious beliefs and activities may have a direct impact on emotional well-being by arousing wonder, awe, joy, or peace during worship, hymns, prayer, practice of religious rituals, or spontaneously in natural settings (e.g., a sunset, a quiet pond, a mountain, or an ocean scene). Such religious experiences range from those that are hardly noticeable to those that are profoundly meaningful, joyful, and life changing.

Perhaps even more powerful in their cumulative effect than direct influences, however, are the indirect effects of religion on mental health mediated through genetic or biological factors, developmental experiences, stressful events during adulthood, cognitive appraisal of events, coping resources, and coping behaviors. It is to these indirect influences that we now turn.

Genetic and Biological Factors

Religion can influence heredity if religious persons selectively mate with others from the same religious group. Such inbreeding increases the risk of genetically transmitted psychiatric disorders (depression in Jews or bipolar disorder in the Old Order Amish). Religion may also influence fetal development in utero. If reli-

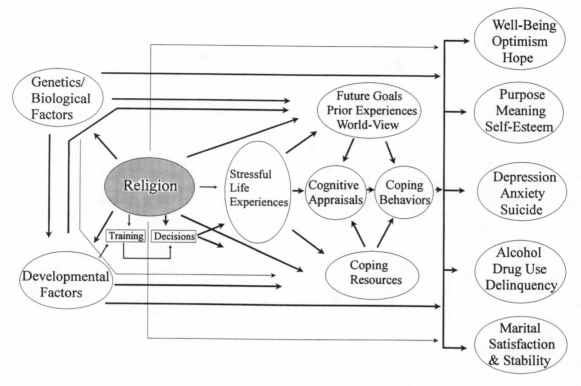

FIGURE 15.1 Theoretical model of religion's effects on mental health.

gious mothers are less likely to drink alcohol, use drugs, smoke cigarettes, or carry sexually transmitted diseases such as AIDS, then this will likely have a direct biological impact on the developing fetal brain, fostering normal and healthy development. By contrast, religious beliefs that encourage avoidance of prenatal care may increase the risk of brain damage both in utero and during delivery. Anything that interferes with normal brain development or causes brain injury increases the likelihood of future neurological and psychiatric disorder (including attention deficit disorder and retardation) and the associated social and psychological problems.

Religion may also act against the force of natural selection, increasing the survival of those who are less biologically or psychiatrically fit (i.e., those with genes that transmit depression and other psychiatric illnesses, such as schizophrenia, that could impair reproduc-

tion). Persons with psychiatric illness who would have ordinarily died by suicide or been so disabled by their illness that they are unable to form relationships and attract sexual partners may be helped to cope with illness more effectively through religion and live long enough to pass on their genetic traits to progeny. In this instance, religion promotes the propagation of persons with genetic predispositions to psychiatric disorder (but also possibly equips them with the tools to cope with that disorder).

Developmental Factors

As noted previously, early life experiences have a major impact on future susceptibility to mental disorder. The religiousness of parents may affect their availability and motivation to meet the emotional needs of children. If the parent has a history of mental disorder and his religiousness helps him to cope better with that

disorder, then the parent will be more emotionally available to meet the needs of his children.
Likewise, if there are major stressors in the parent's life and his religious faith enhances his
coping, then he will be more able to nurture.
Furthermore, if that parent turns to religious
faith, instead of alcohol, drugs, or sexual promiscuity, for comfort, this will further affect his
availability to meet others' emotional needs.

Religious beliefs stress the importance and
value of children and emphasize the high priority of family. This increases the motivation of
religious parents to spend time with and energy
on their children. Most religious traditions
strongly emphasize childhood training, stress-
ing values, character, and generosity toward
others. Religious beliefs further encourage the
avoidance of alcohol and drugs, delinquent behaviors, and premarital sexual activity, all of
which can lead to stressful experiences and
mental health problems for children and adolescents during their teen years and later. Finally, religious marriages tend to be happier
and more stable, reducing the likelihood of divorce, separation, and family turmoil that can
adversely affect the nurturing and the psychological development of children. Of course, extreme or rigid religious beliefs may lead to the
physical abuse of children and spouses, which
can increase vulnerability to emotional problems.

A person's image of God also forms early
in life (Fowler, 1981). Both childhood training
about God and the child's relationship with her
parents can influence that image. If she is taught
that God is all-powerful, all-knowing, present
everywhere, personal and friendly, just, fair,
and, especially, understanding, forgiving, and
merciful, then the image of a powerful and loving personal God will be instilled. This image
is reinforced if the parent is also understanding,
forgiving, and merciful toward the child and
meets the child's emotional needs. The child
will then see God as a powerful friend who can
be trusted and relied on, particularly in times
of distress. By contrast, if the child is taught
that God is distant, uninterested, unforgiving,
and punishing, ruling by fear and intimidation,
then she will absorb an image of God as a powerful dictator to be feared and pacified. This im-

age will be further reinforced if the parent is a
strict and unyielding disciplinarian, demanding
and harshly punishing and seeking to trap the
child in her mistakes. Likewise, if the parent is
absent or emotionally unavailable when needed, the child may have problems trusting others
and, in particular, trusting God to meet her
needs when she is older. Thus, the ability to
use religion successfully as a coping behavior
in adult life may be heavily dependent on the
image of God that one develops in childhood.

Stressful Events and Circumstances

Religious beliefs and practices may reduce the
frequency of negative life events and stressful
circumstances in adulthood. The decisions people make on a daily basis help determine
whether they will experience stress in their lives.
If religious beliefs enable people to make better
decisions, this will help them avoid stress that
could lead to emotional problems. For example,
suppose that a man has an opportunity to have
an extramarital affair with a coworker. His religious beliefs help him decide not to have the
affair, which would otherwise lead to a broken
marriage or at least cause major stress for his
wife and children. Likewise, a woman executive
may be tempted to avenge a slight by a colleague
by returning the insult. Her religious beliefs,
however, may encourage her to forgive that
colleague. Failure to do so might have created
further stress and resentment that could have
led to depression and perhaps even loss of her
job.

The same model applies to decisions on
whether to use alcohol or drugs, spending time
nurturing one's marriage or family life, balanc-
ing work with play, placing value on material
possessions, and many other aspects of living
and relating to others. Religion discourages
stealing, cheating, and risky behaviors that are
likely to lead to accidents or misfortunes and
encourages prosocial decisions that benefit
family and community. Thus, religious beliefs
and commitment to those beliefs help people
make wise decisions and avoid unnecessary
stressors that can reduce well-being and precipitate emotional problems.

Physical Illness as a Stressor

For many people, particularly as they grow older, the primary stressor they face is physical illness. Chronic pain, uncomfortable physical symptoms (e.g., constipation, insomnia, incontinence, or difficulty with memory), changes in physical appearance, restrictions in diet and activity, disability and dependency—these are but a few of the physical health problems that reduce well-being and interfere with activities and relationships that give meaning and purpose to life. Health problems create enormous psychological and social stress. Religious beliefs and activities, because of their possible influences on health and health behaviors (see Part IV), may help maintain and promote physical health. Furthermore, religion may be an important strategy for coping with the stress caused by health difficulties.

Cognitive Appraisal of Stressful Life Events

Besides reducing the frequency of negative life events, religion may also provide a cognitive framework that enables a healthier appraisal of those stressors that do occur. By promoting a positive and coherent worldview, religious belief and commitment help people interpret losses in a more optimistic manner that is non-threatening to the self.

Religion and Self-Esteem. Religion provides a basis for self-esteem that is independent of individual productivity, talent, physical appearance, or relationships with others. By attaching their hopes and dreams to religion, people may be better prepared to detach themselves from material possessions or personal relationships when these are lost. In other words, if a person's self-esteem is rooted in religious faith, he may view other losses as less significant threats to his happiness. Religion provides a focus outside the individual and discourages excessive preoccupation with self or excessive dependence on others to meet all of one's personal needs. Rather than being centered on one or the other, personal identity becomes rooted both within the individual and within the faith community and its shared traditions.

Religion, Worldview, and Sense of Control. The Western religious worldview sees the universe as friendly and, even more important, as personal. Every human is significant and plays a vital role in the great plan of the Divine. The Divine is viewed as resembling a person and as responding in a personal way. According to this tradition, the Divine wishes to be known and to be involved in people's lives. Nothing can happen that is out of God's control. God is seen as a loving and caring father who is all-powerful, all-knowing, and ever-present and who, in particular, responds to prayer. This last point is extremely important in understanding how religion facilitates adaptation to serious, uncontrollable life events. By praying to God, the religious person believes she can *influence* her situation. No longer is she out of control. She is now empowered with the capacity to directly communicate with the source of all control and change. Religiously devout people believe that their prayers will be answered in God's timing and in God's way, either by reversing the situation or by facilitating adaptation and personal growth that will ultimately bring deeper joy and fulfillment. If one relies and depends on a higher power, one feels less pressure to control circumstances and to worry about results. This way of appraising stressful life situations cognitively may relieve anxiety and counteract feelings of hopelessness and despair, even in the most desperate of circumstances.

Religion and Suffering. In today's world, pain and suffering are often seen as having no purpose or meaning but rather as destructive and humiliating, to be escaped at all cost. This attitude only magnifies suffering. Most religions teach that suffering should be expected, can be useful, and may be overcome. If events involving loss or change are seen as having meaning and purpose, they will be easier to bear. According to Victor Frankl (1959), a Viennese psychiatrist and a survivor of a German concentration camp, the search for meaning is the primary motivator in life. Religion provides a worldview that keeps meaning, purpose, and hope alive. Even Freud (1930) noted that "only religion can answer the question of the purpose of life. One can hardly be wrong in concluding that the idea of life having a purpose stands and falls with the religious system" (p. 25).

Coping Resources

Religion can enhance resources that facilitate coping, such as health, education, socioeconomic status, social support, and altruistic activities. Religion's effects on promoting physical health have already been discussed and are discussed further in Part IV.

Socioeconomic Status.   While religiousness is often inversely related to education level and income (because the poor, lacking other resources to fall back on, often turn to religion), religious involvement can promote education and professional success. For example, devout religious faith may help a teenager avoid a pregnancy that would require her to quit school and end her education. Similarly, religion may prevent alcohol and drug abuse or delinquent activity that would likewise derail one's future education and professional development. Religious beliefs also emphasize the development of character, responsibility, commitment, social skills, and honesty, all of which facilitate professional success.

Social Support.   As noted earlier, religiousness is related to greater social support and satisfaction with that support. Persons who actively involve themselves in religious community are more likely to make social contacts that develop into supportive friendships. This promotes social integration and reduces alienation and anomie. Religious communities also provide shared human experiences, beliefs, and values that bind the community together.

A problem often occurs for older adults who need to relocate to a different area of the country in order to be closer to their children. Such moves may quickly result in social isolation, as friendship ties in their old community are broken and adult children, busy with their own lives, have little time for their aging parents. Ties to a religious denomination can facilitate this transition by almost immediately providing a group of like-minded believers in the same faith in the new community. For example, a devout Lutheran in California can join a Lutheran church community in his new home in Pennsylvania. The prayers, hymns, and religious rituals will remain largely unchanged, and church activities will provide opportunities to meet and get to know others. Forming new friends and social contacts may be particularly difficult for older persons who are out of the workforce or whose physical health problems prevent them from participating in activities that foster the growth of social relationships. Many of these problems can be overcome by involvement in the religious community, which can provide the emotional support needed to cope with life problems and can prevent depression and stress from overcoming the individual. Religious organizations also provide rituals for dealing with loss and death that facilitate mourning and mobilize support from the community.

Coping Behaviors

When a life event is cognitively appraised as involving loss or negative change, coping behaviors are mobilized to correct the situation or reduce the stress associated with it. Many religions encourage active problem solving to a point and then advocate acceptance and turning the problem over to God, as in the serenity prayer: "Lord, grant me the ability to change the things I can, accept the things I can't, and the wisdom to know the difference." After a person has done everything possible to change a situation, accepting the inevitable can reduce stress (Koenig, Pargament, & Nielsen, 1998).

Also at this time, shifting one's focus from oneself to others in worse circumstances may be an effective coping strategy, especially for the person with chronic health problems. Most religions, and the Judeo-Christian religious tradition in particular, encourage members to make the effort and time to reach out to those in greater need. Religion promotes a sense of accountability and responsibility to others in the community. In fact, the most important source of volunteers in the United States is religious organizations. Koenig, Pargament, and Nielsen (1998) have demonstrated that stressed persons with medical illness who reach out to others by praying for them or encouraging them spiritually (i.e., "religious helping") are less depressed, have a better quality of life, and experience more psychological growth when going through stressful life circumstances than those who do not extend themselves to others. Conducting a clinical trial to examine the benefits of intercessory prayer, O'Laoire (1997) found that persons who prayed for others actually experienced improvements in well-being that were superior to changes in the subjects of the prayer. Thus, religion may provide persons with a powerful coping resource that encourages them to reach out and help others. This benefits not only those who reach out but also the entire community.

NEGATIVE INFLUENCES ON MENTAL HEALTH

We have been primarily discussing the positive effects of religion on mental health. Religion may also have negative influences (as noted in chapter 4). These may be categorized broadly into effects on (1) number and type of stressful experiences, (2) attitudes and cognitive processes, and (3) coping resources/behaviors.

Effect on Number and Type of Stressful Experiences

Excessive devotion to religious practices or religious social activities can lead to the neglect of loved ones and disruption of family life. The devoutly religious person may become so involved in his personal religious life of prayer, Scripture study, or other spiritual activities that he neglects spouse, children, or other dependents. Spending excessive time at church-related social or volunteer activities instead of meeting the emotional needs of family members can create an unhappy home life that increases stress for all involved. Excessive devotion to religious activities can likewise lead to neglect of job responsibilities, resulting in financial stress that affects the religious person and those he supports. This can become a particular problem when one spouse is more religious

than the other and often creates bitterness and resentment in the less devout partner.

Rigid interpretations of religious Scriptures may lead to mental or physical abuse of spouse or children. For example, Scriptures may be taken out of context to justify violence against a nonsubmissive wife, particularly, as noted earlier, when there is a disparity in the religious backgrounds of husband and wife (Ellison et al., 1999). Likewise, religious beliefs may be used to justify excessive corporal punishment of children for minor offenses, or outright abuse through physical beatings, withdrawal of nourishment, or withholding of medical care (Ellison, 1996).

Effect on Attitudes and Cognitive Thought Processes

Religion can promote rigid thinking, overdependence on laws and rules, and disregard for personal individuality and autonomy. In susceptible individuals, religion may foster excessive guilt over real or imagined "sins" that may be used by unscrupulous religious leaders to control or dominate the person. Religious dogma may also be used to ostracize or alienate those whose beliefs differ even slightly from those of the rest of the group. Religion can be used to judge others, conceal anger or aggression, promote a self-righteous attitude, or justify lack of sensitivity to the individual needs and life circumstances of others. Finally, religious practices (e.g., repetitive prayer or confession) may be used to conceal obsessive or compulsive acts, thus delaying the seeking of professional treatment.

Effect on Coping Resources and Behaviors

As noted, excessive reliance on religious rituals or counsel may delay seeking necessary treatment for mental health problems, leading to a worsening of a psychiatric disorder and the possible development of complications. Religious persons may have conflicts about taking antidepressant or antianxiety drugs, feeling that their religious faith should be sufficient to overcome negative emotions. While religious beliefs

and practices may often be very helpful in relieving mild to moderate symptoms of depression
or anxiety, more severe or advanced psychiatric
symptoms may require biological therapies
(Koenig, Cohen, Blazer, Kudler, et al., 1995).
Some religious professionals or church-based
counselors do not refer persons soon enough
for medical treatment, with dire consequences
(i.e., suicide or homicide). As noted in chapter
4, involvement in religious cults can promote
excessive emotional dependence on a single
leader, isolation from family, and alienation
from the greater community.

As indicated in the previous research summary, however, these negative consequences of
religion tend to occur less often than the beneficial effects conveyed by a strong personal faith
and active involvement in religious community
life, particularly when these occur within an
established religious tradition.

SUMMARY AND CONCLUSIONS

In this chapter we overviewed research on the
relationship between religion and various mental health states, emphasizing caution with regard to causal inference. In the majority of studies, religious involvement is correlated with:

- Well-being, happiness, and life satisfaction
- Hope and optimism
- Purpose and meaning in life

- Higher self-esteem
- Adaptation to bereavement
- Greater social support and less loneliness
- Lower rates of depression and faster recov-
  ery from depression
- Lower rates of suicide and fewer positive
  attitudes toward suicide
- Less anxiety
- Less psychosis and fewer psychotic tenden-
  cies
- Lower rates of alcohol and drug use or
  abuse
- Less delinquency and criminal activity
- Greater marital stability and satisfaction.

We identified and discussed factors influencing
mental health, including genetic and biological
factors, developmental factors (including childhood training), stressful life events in adulthood, cognitive appraisal of events, coping resources, and coping behaviors. We developed
a theoretical model for how religion might directly and indirectly influence mental health
acting through established biopsychosocial
pathways. We ended the chapter with a discussion of the possible negative effects of religion
on mental health, which result from it potential
for increasing life stress, adversely affecting attitudes and cognitions, and impairing coping resources. We concluded that, for the vast majority of people, the apparent benefits of devout
religious belief and practice probably outweigh
the risks.

PART IV

RESEARCH ON RELIGION AND PHYSICAL DISORDERS

16

Heart Disease

EARLY 60 MILLION PER-sons in the United States have one or more cardiovascular diseases (American Heart Association, 1999a). Cardiovascular disease is by far the most common cause of death for persons in the United States; it claimed 959,227 lives in 1996, compared to 539,533 deaths from cancer, 94,948 deaths from accidents, and 31,130 deaths from AIDS (American Heart Association, 1999a). Cardiovascular diseases include heart disease, hypertension, peripheral vascular disease, and stroke. In this chapter we focus on heart disease and its relationship to religion; we deal with hypertension and stroke in chapters 17 and 18, respectively. There are a number of behavioral, psychosocial, and physiological mechanisms by which religious beliefs and practices may influence cardiovascular function, and the primary purpose of this chapter is to better understand these influences. First, we

review the different types of heart disease, their prevalence, and their impact on health. Second, we explore the relationship between heart disease and health behaviors, psychological stress, emotional disorder, and social factors. Third, we explore the reasons that religious beliefs and practices and heart disease might be related and explore the mechanisms by which this association could occur. Fourth, we review research on the relationship between religion and heart disease, focusing on coronary artery disease. Finally, we examine the effects of psychosocial and religious or spiritual interventions on cardiovascular morbidity and mortality.

TYPES AND PREVALENCE OF HEART DISEASE

Types of Heart Disease

Heart disease can be divided into coronary artery disease, hypertensive heart disease, rheumatic heart disease, valvular heart disease, infective endocarditis, arrhythmias and conduction disorders, congenital heart disease, congestive heart failure, and cardiomyopathy.

Coronary artery disease (CAD) is a condition in which one or more of the arteries that supplies the heart with blood become narrowed because of atherosclerotic plaque or vascular spasm. When the heart does not get enough blood because of this narrowing, the clinical manifestations are chest pain or myocardial infarction (irreversible death of heart muscle).

Hypertensive heart disease results from years of work by the heart to pump blood against the increased vascular resistance associated with systolic or diastolic hypertension. The heart adapts to this increased vascular resistance by concentric hypertrophy, or enlargement. If there is coexisting myocardial ischemia from CAD (which is often the case), then the blood supply to the enlarged heart muscle may become insufficient. This results in decreased contractility of the left ventricle of the heart and may ultimately end in heart failure.

Valvular heart disease can result from several causes, including degenerative calcification of heart valves, dysfunction of the muscles that open and close the heart valves, infective endocarditis (infection of the heart valves caused by bacteria or viruses), and rheumatic fever (a streptococcal bacterial infection of childhood that releases toxins into the bloodstream that damage the heart valves). Examples of valvular heart diseases include aortic stenosis (narrowing of the valve that allows blood to flow out of the left ventricle), aortic regurgitation (in which the valve does not close correctly, allowing blood from the major arteries to flow back into the heart), mitral stenosis (a narrowing of the valve that separates the left atrium from the left ventricle, preventing blood from flowing into the left ventricle), mitral regurgitation (in which blood flows back into the left atrium when the left ventricle contracts instead of flowing out into the arterial system), tricuspid stenosis (a narrowing of the valve that separates the right atrium from the right ventricle) or regurgitation, and pulmonary valve disease (a dysfunction of the heart valve that allows blood flow from the right ventricle into the blood vessels that go to lungs for oxygenation).

Arrhythmias and conduction disturbances result from abnormal transmission of electrical impulses in the heart that time the contraction of the atria and the ventricles. The heart works best when contraction of the atria and the ventricles occurs in perfect sequence. Arrhythmias include ectopic beats from the atria (premature atrial contractions) or ventricles (premature ventricular contractions), rapidly contracting atria (supraventricular tachycardia or atrial fibrillation), and the most dangerous, rapidly contracting ventricles (ventricular tachycardia). Ventricular tachycardia may progress to ventricular fibrillation and sudden death. Cardiac arrhythmias interfere with the normal sequencing and timing of contraction of atria and ventricles, resulting in decreased blood flow out of the heart. When electrical conduction between the atria and ventricles is disrupted, partial or complete heart block can result. Heart block can cause a dangerous slowing down of the heart rate, and sometimes even cause asystole, the complete cessation of cardiac contractions.

Congestive heart failure occurs when the heart is unable to pump sufficient blood out into the circulation to meet the needs of the body. Because of this weakness, blood backs up into the lungs (making breathing difficult), into the liver (causing gastrointestinal discomfort), and in the peripheral tissues (causing swelling of legs and feet). Heart failure is often the end result of other heart diseases such as coronary artery disease, hypertensive heart disease, valvular heart disease, chronic cardiac arrhythmias, idiopathic cardiomyopathy (a diffuse or generalized disorder of the heart muscle without a known cause), alcoholic cardiomyopathy (damage to the heart muscle due to excessive alcohol use), or congenital heart disease (disorder of the heart muscle, valves, or anatomy present at birth). The most common causes of heart failure are hypertension and coronary artery disease.

Prevalence

Coronary artery disease is by far the most common form of heart disease, with 12 million

Americans, or 7.2% of all persons age 20 years or older, affected (American Heart Association, 1999b). Almost 5 million people in the United States have signs and symptoms of congestive heart failure. Rheumatic heart disease and congenital heart disease affect approximately 1.8 million and 1 million persons, respectively (American Heart Association, 1999b). Because of its great prevalence, we focus here on coronary artery disease.

MORTALITY, MORBIDITY, AND COST

Mortality

In 1996, coronary artery disease caused 476,124 deaths in the United States, making it the single largest killer of men and women in this country (American Heart Association, 1999c). It is estimated that 1.1 million Americans will experience a myocardial infarction (heart attack) in 2000, and one-third of these people will die. Most of those deaths will occur within one hour of onset of symptoms and before the victim reaches the hospital (usually from cardiac arrest due to ventricular fibrillation). Almost 15% of persons who die from CAD are under age 65, and 80% of such persons die during their first attack. Men and women have similar death rates from CAD, although more women (42%) than men (24%) will die within one year of a myocardial infarction (American Heart Association, 1999c). African Americans have near equal incidence of but higher death rates from CAD than whites.

Morbidity and Disability

Approximately 21% of men and 33% of women will have a second heart attack within six years of the first one, and 21% of men and 33% of women will be disabled by congestive heart failure. Approximately 6.2 million persons have chest pain (angina) related to CAD. Almost two-thirds of persons fail to make a complete recovery following a heart attack. Many persons after a myocardial infarction are at increased risk for stroke and the disability associated with that

condition (American Heart Association, 1999b, 1999c).

Economic Impact

Among persons discharged from the hospital in 1996, approximately 2,258,000 had a diagnosis of CAD. For persons under age 65, the average cost in 1996 of a hospital admission for a coronary event was well over $20,000 (American Heart Association, 1999c).

RISK FACTORS FOR CORONARY ARTERY DISEASE

There is a hereditary component to CAD, and persons with a family history of atherosclerotic heart disease are at increased risk. Likewise, the presence of hypertension or diabetes increases the likelihood that atherosclerosis will occur throughout the vascular system, including the coronary arteries.

Environmental factors also play a major role in the development and progression of CAD. These environmental factors include health behaviors and psychosocial stressors. Health behaviors that increase the risk of CAD and myocardial infarction are cigarette smoking, high cholesterol level, physical inactivity, obesity, and alcohol abuse. We now examine each of these health behaviors.

Cigarette Smoking

Cigarette smoking has been causally linked to coronary artery disease. Vlieststra and colleagues (1986) followed 4,165 smokers with angiographically confirmed coronary artery disease for five years as part of the Coronary Artery Surgery Study (CASS). Mortality and cardiac events during this period were compared for those who continued to smoke ($n = 2,675$) and those who quit ($n = 1,490$). Continuing smokers experienced a significant 55% greater risk of dying than did smokers who quit. Excess mortality in continuing smokers (compared to those who quit) was primarily due to acute myocardial infarction (7.9% vs. 4.4%, respectively) and sudden death (2.8% vs. 1.5%, respectively).

In a six-year study of 119,404 women ages 30–55 years, persons who smoked 25 or more cigarettes per day had 5.5 times more fatal and 5.8 times more nonfatal myocardial infarctions than women who smoked fewer than 25 cigarettes per day or not at all (Willett et al., 1987). The increased risk of CAD induced by cigarette smoking was particularly high among women who were older, had a family history of myocardial infarction, were of higher relative weight, or had hypertension, hypercholesterolemia, or diabetes.

Barry and colleagues (1989) studied 65 patients with chronic stable coronary disease and a positive exercise tolerance test (24 smokers and 41 nonsmokers). Subjects underwent continuous ambulatory monitoring (4,968 total hours) to determine the amount of ischemic ST segment changes during daily life. Ischemic episodes occurred three times as often and lasted 12 times as long (24 minutes vs. two minutes per 24 hours) in smokers as in nonsmokers. These differences remained statistically significant after the investigators controlled for standard covariates.

Hasdai and colleagues (1997) examined the effects of cigarette smoking on long-term outcome after successful percutaneous coronary revascularization. Four groups were examined: nonsmokers ($n = 2,009$), former smokers who had stopped before the procedure ($n = 2,259$), quitters who stopped smoking after the procedure ($n = 435$), and persistent smokers who smoked before and after the procedure ($n = 734$). Results were based on an average follow-up time of 4.5 years. Persistent smokers had a 76% greater risk of death and 108% greater risk of myocardial infarction than did nonsmokers. Persistent smokers also had a 44% greater risk of death than did quitters. These are just a few of the studies that have established cigarette smoking as a cause of CAD.

Cholesterol

High serum cholesterol, particularly the low-density lipoprotein (LDL) fraction, has been associated with increased risk for CAD. Serum cholesterol plays a major role in the pathogenesis of atherosclerosis, the underlying disease process in CAD. Studies have shown that the lipid composition of the diet (intake of foods high in cholesterol and saturated fatty acids) is associated with serum cholesterol and risk of coronary death (Shekelle et al., 1981). Furthermore, studies have shown that drugs that lower total serum cholesterol by decreasing LDL levels can reduce the risk of CAD morbidity and mortality in persons with high LDL levels (Lipid Research Clinics, 1984), providing strong evidence for a causal role for cholesterol in the etiology of CAD.

In a six-year follow-up study of 356,222 middle-aged men never hospitalized for myocardial infarction (MRFIT study), Stamler et al. (1986) found a continuous, graded, strong relationship between serum cholesterol and age-adjusted CAD death rate. This was true regardless of smoking status or blood pressure. They concluded that the relationship between serum cholesterol and CAD was not a threshold one (i.e., one affecting only those with levels above 200 mg/dl) but a continuously graded one that powerfully affects risk for middle-aged men. Elevated serum cholesterol is also an independent risk factor for CAD in persons age 65 or older (Benfante & Reed, 1990; Corti et al., 1997). Total serum cholesterol, however, is not as good a predictor of CAD as total cholesterol/HDL ratio. The risk of CAD for men with total cholesterol/HDL ratios of less than 3 is 0.32 compared to 3.11 for men with ratios 9 or higher; the comparable risks for women are 0.59 and 2.98, (with average being 1.00) (Kinosian et al., 1994).

Exercise and Weight Control

While physical inactivity and obesity are reported risk factors for CAD (Blackburn & Jacobs, 1988; Centers for Disease Control and Prevention, 1993; Keys et al., 1972), the evidence is weaker than that for cigarette smoking or serum cholesterol. After reviewing the research in this area, Barrett-Connor (1985) concluded that the inconsistent association between obesity and atherosclerosis does not support the hypothesis that obesity causes CAD, despite its biological plausibility. A more recent study, however, has provided data to support that hypothesis. Manson et al. (1990) examined the relationship between obesity and incidence of nonfatal and fatal CAD during an eight-year follow-up of 115,886 women ages 30–55 years. For increasing levels of the Quetelet index (weight in kilograms divided by height in meters squared), the relative risk of CAD adjusted for age and cigarette smoking increased in a linear fashion ($p < .00001$). The authors concluded that even mild to moderate obesity increases the risk of CAD in middle-aged women.

Katzel et al. (1995) examined whether weight loss or aerobic exercise was more important in obese middle-aged and older men in determining CAD risk. The findings underscored the importance of weight loss. Investigators randomized 170 subjects to a nine-month diet-induced weight loss program, a nine-month aerobic exercise training program, or a weight-maintenance control group. For the group that lost weight, fasting glucose concentrations decreased by 2% and insulin levels by 18% and, after a glucose tolerance test, by 8% and 26%, respectively. Aerobic exercise did not affect fasting glucose or insulin concentrations but did increase subjects' insulin level following a glucose tolerance test by 17%. Finally, for the group that lost weight but not for the group that did aerobic exercise, HDL cholesterol level increased by 13% and blood pressure decreased compared to controls. The authors concluded that diet-induced weight loss is preferred over aerobic exercise to improve CAD risk factors in overweight men who are middle-aged or older.

Alcohol Abuse

While some research suggests that low levels of alcohol consumption may be protective against CAD (by inhibiting platelet aggregation and by raising HDL cholesterol levels), the opposite is true for high levels of alcohol use. Heavy alcohol consumption has been associated with excess CAD mortality and sudden coronary death

(Deutscher et al., 1984). In fact, the most common cause of excess mortality among male alcoholics is coronary death (Rosengren, Wilhelmsen, et al., 1987; Denison et al., 1997). Because of the excess number of sudden cardiac deaths, it is thought that rapid drinking predisposes the drinker to fatal disturbances of cardiac rhythm. In one of the largest studies to date, Hanna et al. (1997) examined the relationship between drinking and heart disease among 18,323 males and 25,440 females in the 1988 U.S. National Health Interview Survey. They found that heart disease was significantly more common among men who reported having more then five drinks per day and in women who reported having more than two drinks per day. They concluded that the protection from heart disease that drinking affords occurs *only at low levels* of drinking.

Thus, while low or moderate alcohol consumption is associated with some protection against CAD, chronic heavy alcohol consumption is associated with a variety of cardiovascular disorders, including stroke from alcohol-induced hypertension, congestive heart failure from alcoholic cardiomyopathy, and sudden cardiac death from ventricular arrhythmias.

Interactive Effects

Cigarette smoking and heavy alcohol use lead to and exacerbate hypertension (Gitlow et al., 1986; Maheswaran et al., 1986; Mann et al., 1991; Sawicki et al., 1996), hypercholesterolemia (Imamura et al., 1996), and diabetes (Wicks et al., 1974; Muhlhauser, 1994; Sawicki et al., 1996), acting synergistically to increase CAD risk.

New Germ Theory

Conventional cardiovascular risk factors, however, fail to completely explain the variations in prevalence and severity of CAD. Recent research has suggested that infection of coronary arteries by cytomegalovirus (Nieto et al., 1996; Zhou et al., 1996) or by Chlamydia pneumoniae (Gupta & Camm, 1997; Davidson et al., 1998;

Hooper, 1999) may contribute to as many as 50% of all cases of CAD.

PSYCHOSOCIAL STRESS AND CORONARY ARTERY DISEASE

A major independent risk factor for CAD is psychological stress. The heart has held symbolic significance as the center of human emotion throughout modern history. Consider, for instance, the following phrases: "Have a heart!" (a plea for compassion) and "He broke my heart" or "He died of a broken heart" (signifying the depth of emotional distress over a lost relationship). For centuries the heart was viewed as the source of emotion, perhaps because of the heaviness one feels in the chest when experiencing psychological pain. Recent research has increasingly demonstrated that there is indeed a very close connection between the emotions and the heart.

Depression and Heart Disease

Glassman and Shapiro (1998) and Musselman, Evans, et al. (1998) recently reviewed in the *American Journal of Psychiatry and the Archives of General Psychiatry* the research on depressive disorder and heart disease. Since the 1970s, investigators have compared mortality rates among depressed patients with that of the general population. Glassman and Shapiro report that nine out of 10 studies found increased cardiovascular mortality among the depressed. Even when community-dwelling populations are examined and followed prospectively, the relationship between depression and mortality persists (after smoking and other risk factors are controlled).

Depression and Development of CAD

A relationship has also been documented between depression and the development of ischemic heart disease (Anda et al., 1993; Aromaa et al., 1994; Barefoot & Schroll, 1996; Prigerson et al., 1997; Ford, Mead, et al., 1998). Within the past few years, several studies have followed depressed and nondepressed subjects who were initially free of CAD. Most found an increased risk of ischemic heart disease among depressed persons. We now review some of the more notable studies.

Anda et al. (1993) conducted a 12-year prospective study of 2,832 Americans ages 45–77 years as part of the National Health Examination Follow-up Study. At baseline, 11% of the cohort had depressed affect; 11% also reported moderate hopelessness, and 3% reported severe hopelessness. A total of 189 fatal cases of ischemic heart disease was observed during the follow-up period. After adjusting for other risk factors, subjects with depressed affect had a 50% greater risk of death from CAD (relative risk = 1.50, 95% CI = 1.0–2.3). For those with moderate hopelessness at baseline, there was a 60% increased risk of death (relative risk = 1.60, 95% 1.0–2.5). For those with severe hopelessness, the risk of death was increased by 110% (relative risk = 2.10, 95% CI 1.1–3.9). The investigators concluded that depressed affect and hopelessness may play a causal role in both fatal and nonfatal CAD. "Hope deferred makes the heart sick," says Proverbs 13:12.

As part of a survey of the Baltimore Epidemiologic Catchment Area funded by the NIMH, Pratt et al. (1996) conducted a 13-year prospective study of 1,551 subjects without myocardial infarction (MI) who were first assessed in 1981. The diagnosis of major depression at baseline in 1994 increased the risk of MI by more than 100% (odds ratio 2.1, 95% CI 1.2–3.7), a finding that was independent of other coronary risk factors. Likewise, in a four-year prospective study of middle-aged men in California, Everson et al. (1997) found that those who felt hopeless or felt like failures (indicating high levels of despair) had a 20% increase in measurable atherosclerosis compared with other participants. This risk is equivalent to comparing the risk for a one-pack-a-day smoker to that for a nonsmoker.

Finally, Ford, Mead, et al. (1998) prospectively followed 1,190 male medical students from Johns Hopkins University from 1948 to 1964. The students were assessed annually for cardiovascular disease endpoints such as development of coronary heart disease and myocardial infarction. During the 40 years of follow-up, the cumulative incidence of clinical depression was 12%. Subjects who developed clinical depression did not differ from nondepressed subjects in terms of baseline blood pressure, smoking status, physical activity, obesity, or family history of coronary artery disease. Multivariate analyses showed that men with clinical depression were more than twice as likely to develop CAD (relative risk [RR] 2.1, 95% CI 1.2–3.6) and twice as likely to develop a MI (RR 2.1, 95% CI 1.1–4.1) during the follow-up. The investigators concluded that clinical depression was an independent risk factor for CAD.

Thus, there is growing evidence from these studies, and from a number of other large prospective studies performed in different areas of the United States by different investigators, that depression increases the risk of developing CAD.

Depression and Outcome of CAD

In studies that examine subjects who already have ischemic heart disease, *outcomes* are decidedly worse if depression is present. Frasure-Smith, Lesperance, and Talajic (1993) conducted a six-month prospective study of 222 patients who met the criteria for acute myocardial infarction between 1991–1992 at the Montreal Heart Institute. The Diagnostic Interview Schedule was used to make diagnoses of major depression at baseline. Among the 35 patients with major depression, six died during the six-month follow-up (17%), compared with six of the 187 nondepressed patients (3%). Regression analysis demonstrated that major depression significantly predicted death rate after controlling for warfarin administration, number of close social contacts, Killip class, previous MI, and number of close friends. After adjusting for other factors, the hazard ratio for major depression was 3.96 (95% CI 2.25–4.63, $p =$ .047). The findings were attributed to an alteration in platelet function and changes in autonomic tone (see later discussion).

A number of other studies have also documented higher mortality following acute MI among depressed patients (Ahern et al., 1990; Ladwig et al., 1991; Barefoot, Helms, et al., 1996). This increased mortality risk exists for at least 18 months following acute MI (Frasure-

Smith, Lesperance, Talajic, et al., 1995). Depression also appears to increase the risk of nonfatal serious cardiac events in subjects with CAD (e.g., acute MI, arrhythmias) (Kennedy, Hofer, et al., 1987; Carney, Rich, et al., 1988; Barefoot et al., 1996). There is little doubt, then, that emotional disorder increases the risk of both fatal and nonfatal cardiac events in persons with ischemic heart disease.

Depression also interferes with return to normal function following acute MI. Stern and Pascale (1979) followed 68 post-MI patients for one year after their discharge from George Washington University Medical Center to assess their psychological adjustment. Of those who scored as depressed on the Zung Depression Scale immediately postinfarct, 70% remained depressed throughout the year after discharge. These patients were more likely to fail to return to work, to fail to function sexually, and to experience higher hospital readmission rates than were nondepressed subjects.

Physiological Mechanisms

The mechanism by which depression worsens CAD is thought to involve hyperactivity of the sympathoadrenal system, which results in changes in autonomic tone that increase the risk of fatal cardiac arrhythmias (Veith et al., 1993). In addition, depressed patients are found to have significant abnormalities of platelet function, including an increased propensity for platelets to aggregate (Musselman, Tomer, et al., 1996). Depressed patients with CAD also have diminished heart rate variability that adversely affects cardiac prognosis (Carney, Freedland, et al., 1995). Finally, the alteration of cholesterol and lipids in depressed patients could lead to the development of CAD or worsen its prognosis.

Psychological Stress and Heart Disease

Besides depressive disorder, psychological stress is also associated with an increased risk for CAD. Smith, Allred, et al. (1989) conducted two experiments with introductory psychology students (148 subjects in Study 1 and 79 in

Study 2). The investigators examined how efforts to secure positive outcomes or avoid negative outcomes influenced systolic blood pressure (SBP), diastolic blood pressure (DBP), and heart rate (HR). They found significantly higher SBP, DBP, and HR in male subjects under stress. Cardiovascular reactivity increased as magnitude of incentive for success increased. This study shows the acute effects that psychological stress can have on blood pressure, even in healthy college students.

Examining a community sample, Rosengren, Tibblin, et al. (1991) prospectively followed 6,935 middle-aged men for 12 years. The investigators examined the relationship between psychological stress and the occurrence of nonfatal MI or fatal MI. Six percent of the men with low stress ratings at baseline experienced a fatal or nonfatal MI, whereas 10% of the men with high stress ratings experienced coronary events (OR = 1.50, 95% CI 1.20–1.90). This 50% increase in risk persisted after the researchers controlled for age and other risk factors.

Emotions associated with psychological stress, especially anger and hostility, have been associated with increase risk of MI (Diamond, 1982). Wenneberg, Schneider, Walton, MacClean, Levitsky, Mandarino, et al. (1997a) conducted an experiment in which subjects performed six minutes of mental arithmetic tests under time pressure. There was a positive correlation between collagen-induced platelet aggregation and outwardly expressed anger, pointing to a physiological mechanism by which anger may precipitate a coronary event.

Degree of perceived personal control may also affect susceptibility to acute cardiac ischemia, but not in the way one might expect. Seeman (1991) surveyed 119 men and 40 women ages 30–70 who had been referred for angiography to San Francisco Bay area hospitals for suspected CAD. Subjects completed questionnaires the day before cardiac catheterization, including a measure of personal mastery. Covariates included age, sex, income, education, hypertension, cholesterol, smoking, angina, diabetes, family history of CAD, hostility, and Type A behavior. The dependent variable was angiographically documented coronary atherosclerosis. The investigator found that CAD score was significantly higher among those with *high* mastery (692.3 vs. 584.1, $p < .05$, uncontrolled). After other risk factors were controlled, mastery continued to predict CAD score ($\beta = 0.20$, $p = .03$). The author concluded that a strong sense of personal mastery (or "internal" control) is independently associated with greater CAD over and above other traditional risk factors. The reason for this finding may lie in the patterns of physiological arousal that occur in response to environmental stimuli. Those with a greater need for personal control may experience greater activation of the sympathetic, adrenal, and pituitary axis when such control is threatened, producing excess amount of catecholamines and corticosteroids that increase heart disease risk. Thus, being able to give up control, particularly in uncontrollable life situations, may help reduce psychological stress.

In addition to the physiological mechanisms described, psychological stress may further increase risk of heart disease through its negative effects on the immune system (see chapter 19). An impaired immune system, in turn, may be less able to prevent or contain infections by organisms like cytomegalovirus or C. pneumoniae, which have been implicated in the etiology of coronary atherosclerosis (Zhou et al., 1996; Hooper, 1999).

Social Factors and Heart Disease

Just as depressive disorder and psychological distress increase the risk of CAD and adversely affect cardiovascular outcomes, social support may reduce CAD by improving coping, preventing depression, and counteracting psychological stress. After reviewing the evidence pertaining to psychosocial variables and CAD, both King (1997) and Anderson, Deshaies, et al. (1996) concluded that a lack of social ties predicts greater CAD mortality, and strong social support reduces this risk.

Reviewing the research on the role of psychosocial factors in the etiology and course of CAD, Greenwood et al. (1996) identified 14 studies that examined coronary disease, psychological stress, social support, social isolation, and life change events. They concluded that both life stress and social support influenced CAD, with social support having a greater influence than psychological stress. In this review, psychosocial factors had a stronger impact on the course of CAD than on the development of the disease (i.e., initial incidence). We now briefly examine some of the studies identified by Greenwood et al. (1996).

Seeman and Syme (1987) compared the relative impact of different types of social support on CAD risk as measured by degree of coronary atherosclerosis. Regression analysis was used to examine biological and social predictors of coronary atherosclerosis in 119 men and 40 women who underwent coronary angiography. Results indicated that network instrumental support and feelings of being loved were more important than network size or "problem-oriented" emotional support in predicting low CAD risk. Investigators concluded that the *quality* of social support is more important than the quantity.

Williams, Barefoot, et al. (1992) examined the effects of social and economic resources on cardiovascular mortality among 1,368 patients with CAD. Researchers examined patients who underwent cardiac catheterization between 1974 and 1980, following them through 1989 and estimating survival time until cardiovascular death. Among the predictors of survival were marital status and presence of a confidant. Unmarried patients without a confidant had an unadjusted five-year survival of 50%, compared with a survival rate of 82% among patients who were married, had a confidant, or both. When other covariates were adjusted, the risk of dying for unmarried subjects without a confidant was 3.3 times greater (95% CI 1.8–6.2, $p < .0001$) than that for married subjects with a confidant. Investigators concluded that low levels of social resources, independent of other prognostic factors, identified CAD patients at high risk for mortality.

In a six-year prospective study, Orth-Gomer et al. (1993) examined "attachment" (emotional support from very close persons) and "social integration" (support provided by an extended network of friends) on the incidence of MI and death from CAD among 736 middle-aged men in Gothenborg, Sweden. Investigators found that both attachment ($p = .07$) and social inte-

gration ($p = .04$) were lower in men who went on to experience negative CAD outcomes. Even when multiple other risk factors were controlled in a logistic regression model, significant effects persisted. Smoking and lack of social support were the two main risk factors for CAD in this population. In an earlier study, Orth-Gomer and Unden (1990) reported that lack of social support or social isolation was an independent predictor of mortality in Type A men but not in Type B men. In that study, the 10-year CAD mortality experience of socially isolated Type A men was 69%, compared with 17% for Type A men who were socially integrated. This replicated previous findings reported by Blumenthal et al. (1987) on social support, Type A behavior, and CAD. In summary, the combination of Type A personality type and social isolation is highly lethal among patients with CAD.

Woloshin et al. (1997) examined the impact of social support on health outcomes in 734 patients with chronic CAD. Adequacy of tangible support was assessed by asking respondents (1) if they needed help at home because of health problems and (2) if these needs were being met. Subjects who perceived that they needed more help were 3.2 times more likely to die, and those needing *much* more help were 6.5 times more likely to die than were subjects with no perceived need. Investigators concluded that adequacy of tangible support was an important prognostic factor for patients with CAD. Frasure-Smith (1991) conducted an experimental study that examined the effects of social support on reinfarction among 461 men followed for five years. Subjects in the intervention group received supportive visits from a nurse during periods when they reported high stress. Subjects in the control group who did not receive supportive visits experienced significantly more cardiac events than did supported subjects.

Social support also affects outcome of surgical treatment for CAD. Oxman et al. (1995) followed 232 older patients an average of six months after they underwent elective CABG surgery. Twenty-one deaths occurred during the follow-up. Lack of participation in social or community groups was a significant predictor of mortality, independent of other biological risk factors.

Thus, social support—particularly high-quality, emotionally satisfying support—affects both the onset and the outcome of CAD. Anything that increases social support, then, will likely influence cardiac health.

WHY SHOULD RELIGION AND CORONARY ARTERY DISEASE BE RELATED?

Consider the risk factors for onset and progression of CAD that we have reviewed—hypertension, diabetes, cigarette smoking, high serum cholesterol, physical inactivity and obesity, heavy alcohol use, depressive disorder, psychological stress, and lack of social support. As we saw in earlier chapters and will see in later ones, religious beliefs and behaviors are inversely related to many of these risk factors. Religious involvement has been associated with lower blood pressure (chapter 17), less cigarette smoking (chapter 24), more exercise (Strawbridge et al., 1997), less alcohol use (chapter 11), less depression and faster recovery from depression (chapter 7), improved coping with stress (chapter 5), greater well-being (chapter 6), and greater social support (chapter 15). There are reasons why devout religious beliefs and practices might influence the onset and course of CAD. Unfortunately, few studies have carefully examined this relationship.

RESEARCH ON RELIGION AND CORONARY ARTERY DISEASE

We now review research that examines the relationship between religion and CAD. First, we explore rates of CAD among members of different religious groups and attempt to understand why these variations occur. Second, we examine the relationship between degree of religiousness and the development and course of CAD.

Religious Affiliation

The first studies that examined the relationship between religion and CAD explored differences across religious groups. Unfortunately, such studies provide little information about the effects of religiousness on heart disease; we review them here primarily for historic reasons.

Jews. Dreyfuss (1953) examined rates of MI in three groups of Jews drawn from a sample of 412 patients hospitalized in Israel with acute MI: Jews who came from Europe, called Ashkenazi Jews; Jews from Spain and other western Mediterranean countries, called Sefardi Jews; and Jews from Eastern Mediterranean countries (e.g., Kurdistan and Iran), called Oriental Jews. The investigators found a smaller than expected percentage of Oriental Jews (5%) with MI given their representation in the general population (12–26%) but a larger than expected percentage of Ashkenazi Jews. The author observed that, while Oriental Jews belong to a lower social class and have a more primitive way of life, they are less likely to smoke and have lower rates of hypertension. Religious differences in orthodoxy between the two groups were not discussed.

Epstein and Boas (1955) examined the relationship between cultural background and CAD among 506 male and 398 female members of the Garment Worker's Union in New York City; all subjects were over 40 years of age. Some 36% of the men and 51% of the women were from Italian backgrounds, and 54% of the men and 35% of the women were Jewish. Diagnosis of CAD was based on clinical symptoms and ECG changes. The prevalence of CAD was higher in Jewish men and women than in Italians. After age 50, in particular, Jewish men experienced consistently higher CAD rates than Italian men. The overall prevalence of CAD among Jews was 17%, compared to 7% for Italians ($p < .01$). This difference was independent of calorie or fat intake.

Epstein, Simpson, and Boas (1956) next reported on a subgroup of their original sample of garment factory workers in New York City. They found that Jewish men ($n = 153$) and women ($n = 85$) obtained a larger proportion of their total fat intake from animal sources than did Italian men and women (80% vs. 68% for men and 78% vs. 63% for women, $p < .01$). Jews also had a higher prevalence of hypercholesterolemia and a higher rate of CAD than

Italians, even though they consumed equal amounts of fat (but dissimilar amounts of *animal fat*). This study was one of the first to demonstrate a possible role for animal fat in the etiology of CAD.

Epstein, Arbor, et al. (1957) reported a third time on their garment worker sample in New York City. This time they examined an expanded group of 683 men and 592 women, plus 183 male and 272 female family members. They found that Jewish men had twice the rate of CAD of Italians, but found no difference in the rates for women. Jewish men and women had slightly higher serum cholesterol levels than Italians (237 vs. 209 for men and 249 vs. 226 for women), but serum phospholipid levels were similar. There were no differences in blood pressure or in the prevalence of diabetes mellitus. The overall prevalence of CAD among Italian men was related to serum cholesterol, blood pressure, and body weight. In contrast, these variables exerted no appreciable effect on the prevalence of disease in Jewish men, leaving the reason for the higher rates of CAD in this group a mystery (genetic factors?).

Friedman and Hellerstein (1968) examined correlates of CAD in a sample of 2,342 attorneys from Cleveland and Detroit. A law professor independently rated the stress level of different legal specialties and ranked subjects into four groups based on the quality of the law school they attended. Subjects were also classified as Jewish or non-Jewish. Coronary disease was measured by three questions: "Do you have (1) coronary disease, (2) myocardial infarction, or (3) angina pectoris?" A yes answer to any of these questions indicated the presence of coronary disease. The investigators found that CAD was unrelated to the stress level of legal specialty but was significantly lower in Group I (e.g., Harvard and Yale) law school graduates than in Groups III and IV graduates. Among lawyers in the 40–59 age bracket, Jews had significantly more CAD than non-Jews (13.2% vs. 3.3%, $p < .01$, uncontrolled).

Medalie, Kahn, Neufeld, Riss, Goldbourt, Perlstein, et al. (1973) prospectively followed a random sample of 10,056 male adult government and municipal employees in Israel who were first assessed in 1963. They presented data on the prevalence, incidence, and mortality from ischemic heart disease for this group. The five-year MI incidence (including sudden death) was 44 per 1,000. The authors concluded that the MI incidence of 8.7/1,000 per year was high compared to that in samples studied in other countries. The number of subjects in this study who died from acute MI, however, was extremely low, resulting in a case-fatality rate of 16% during an average 2.5 years of observation. Recall that 24% of American men today die within one year of acute MI (American Heart Association, 1999c).

In an earlier study, Shapiro, Weinblatt, et al. (1969), reporting on the incidence of MI among white males insured for medical care in New York, found, as had other studies before it, that Jews had a higher MI rate than members of other religions. The age-adjusted incidence was 6.6 per 1,000 for Jews, 5.0 for Protestants, and 4.5 for Catholics. Like Medalie and colleagues, however, they found that Jews were less likely to die from MI within 48 hours (24/100 Jews vs. 33/100 Protestants vs. 38/100 Catholics). No explanation for the finding was given, although prompt seeking of medical care may have been a factor.

Catholics and Protestants

Wardwell et al. (1963) conducted a case-control study of 32 white male survivors of acute myocardial infarction in Middlesex County, Connecticut, and 32 age-matched white male controls. The rate of acute MI was nearly four times higher in Protestants than in Catholics (an observed/expected ratio of 2.00 for Protestants vs. 0.58 for Catholics). The rate of acute MI was also increased in persons whose parents were of different religious affiliations (denominational heterogamy). The investigators concluded that, "As Rousseau phrased it, 'forced to be free,' the Protestant cannot avoid personal responsibility for life's decisions nor can he assuage feelings of guilt in the confessional" (Wardwell et al., 1963, p. 158).

Wardwell et al. (1964,1968) soon reported similar findings in three larger epidemiologic studies in Connecticut. The first study involved an expanded sample of the investigators' 1963

Middlesex County Heart Study; the larger sample included 87 cases with MI and 435 controls. The observed-to-expected (O/E) ratio among Protestants was 1.34, compared with 0.66 in Catholics (and 1.11 in Jews). For subjects whose parents represented a mixed (Catholic and Protestant) marriage, the O/E ratio was 2.38, compared with 0.51 if both parents were Catholic, 1.27 if both parents were Protestant, and 1.32 if both were Jewish. In the second study, the Midtown Manhattan Study, 16 cases with acute MI were compared to 128 controlled subjects who were free of heart problems. The O/E ratio among Protestants was 1.57, compared with 0.68 for Catholics. In that study, there was no association between rate of MI and similarity of parents' religious affiliation. The third study examined 176 randomly selected persons from the population. Again, the O/E ratio for Protestants (1.41) was higher than that for Catholics (0.72), and there was no association between rate of MI and parents' religion.

Next, Wardwell and Bahnson (1973) examined 114 patients hospitalized whose first MI occurred between 1963 and 1965 in Southeastern Connecticut and compared them to the sickest 114 patients among other admissions to the same hospitals. MI rates in these two groups were then compared with those for a group of 145 age-matched healthy controls. This time, investigators found that Catholics were somewhat more likely to have MI than Protestants. The distribution of Catholics, Protestants, and Jews among the cases was 53%, 32%, and 12%, respectively; among the hospital controls it was 51%, 40%, and 3%; and among the healthy community controls it was 45%, 50%, and 3% ($p <$ .001, uncontrolled).

Other studies have found no differences in CAD across religious affiliation. Winkelstein et al. (1958, 1969) found little or no differences in the frequency of Protestant and Catholic affiliation in a group of female patients hospitalized with CAD and in healthy controls in Buffalo, New York. Likewise, Skyring et al. (1963) found no differences in religious affiliation among persons dying with CAD compared with controls. Ross and Thomas (1965) surveyed 1,272 medical students at Johns Hopkins, obtaining information on their religious preference and

on the presence of CAD in their fathers. The fathers of Protestant and Catholic students had similar rates of coronary heart disease, although the rate among fathers of Jewish students was somewhat higher (227/1,000 in Jews vs. 195/1,000 in Protestants and 208/1,000 in Catholics).

According to unpublished data from the Tecumseh Community Health Study, the prevalence of coronary disease among Catholic males was lower than that for Protestants, although the number of Catholics in the study was small. Cholesterol levels did not differ among Catholics and Protestants, and there was no difference in CAD prevalence among Catholic and Protestant females (Marks, 1967).

Brown and Ritzmann (1967) studied 2,921 persons over age 65 who received electrocardiograms (ECG) at the Portland Veteran's Hospital. Only 133 patients were found to be free of heart disease both by ECG and by clinical evaluation. These were defined as cases and were compared with 100 control patients over age 65 with CAD as defined by the new New York Hospital Association (NYHA) criteria. Among the disease-free cases, 81 (61%) were Protestants, 20 (15%) were Catholic, Jewish, Greek Orthodox, or Islamic, and 32 (24%) had no religious preference. Among the controls, 47% were Protestants, 31% Catholic or of other religious faiths, and 22% had no religious preference. The investigators concluded there was no association between CAD and lack of religious affiliation. Likewise, Winkelstein and Rekate (1969) compared religious affiliation in 123 white female hospitalized patients ages 50–80 with a history of pregnancy. Of these, 59 women had CAD, and 64 had other diagnoses. The two groups did not differ in the percentages that belonged to three religious groups (Catholic, Protestant, or Jewish).

Lehr et al. (1973) examined 12 social and 12 biological precursors of CAD in a prospective study of 679 white men ages 40–49 who worked as industrial employees in the San Francisco Bay area. Parents' religious conservatism was determined by ranking the men according to the religious affiliation of their parents. Congregationals, atheists, Christian Scientists, Episcopalians, Jews, and Presbyterians were defined as liberal; Lutherans, Roman Catholics, members of the Reformed church, small-body Protestants, and Baptists were defined as conservative. Investigators found that "parental religious difference" was second only to high blood pressure in predicting six-year coronary events. Subjects whose mothers were affiliated with liberal religions and whose fathers were associated with conservative religions had the highest rate of CAD. On the other hand, subjects whose mothers were affiliated with conservative religions and fathers with liberal religions had the lowest rate of CAD. The findings were independent of education level.

Investigators attributed this finding to the "success" ethic hypothesis. The Protestant work ethic and the emphasis on personal responsibility for achievement (stressed by conservative fathers) may have increased the psychological pressure on the sons to achieve, leading to higher rates of MI. The authors also note that "the Jewish emphasis on occupational achievement resembles in many ways the Protestant ethic" (Lehr et al., 1973, p. 25). This explanation, however, is not entirely consistent with the data presented in this study, since Judaism was categorized as a liberal religion, and Catholicism was categorized as conservative. The authors did not consider that conflict at home, arising from the parents' different religious views, might also have been influential. Alternatively, mothers with more liberal religious views may not have emphasized religious values as strongly as mothers with conservative views, thus providing their sons with fewer faith resources to utilize when faced with stress in adult life.

In the most recent study to compare mortality rates from CAD across major religious groups, Watson (1991) examined the percentage of Roman Catholics in 24 "Christian" countries in Western Europe (obtained from the Europa World Year Book, 1990). He correlated these percentages with CAD mortality rates per 100,000 for each country (obtained from the World Health Statistics Annual, 1987). The correlation between the percentage of the population that was Catholic and CAD mortality was $-.59$ ($p < .001$, uncontrolled). In other words, the higher the percentage of Catholics found in a country, the lower that country's death rate

from CAD. Socioeconomic factors, however, were not taken into account.

Mormons

Lyon, Wetzler, et al. (1978) studied the death rate among Mormons in Utah from 1969 to 1971, and found that Mormons had 35% lower mortality from CAD than the general U.S. population of white men, while mortality among non-Mormon men in Utah occurred at the same rate as the U.S. population. Mormon men also had lower mortality from hypertensive heart disease. Mormon women experienced lower mortality from rheumatic heart disease than did non-Mormon women in Utah. Mormons' avoidance of tobacco and alcohol may have played a role in these findings.

More recently, Enstrom (1989) prospectively followed 9,844 religiously active California Mormons (53% were high priests and 47% were wives of high priests), comparing disease-specific mortality rates in that group with those of a control population of 3,119 non-Mormon adults in Alameda County. Mormons had fewer cardiovascular diseases and lower mortality rates. For high priests, the all-cause standard mortality ratio (SMR) was 47 and for the controls was 100 (53% less); likewise, the Mormons' SMR for cardiovascular disease was only 52 (48% less). For wives, the SMR was 66 for all causes and 64 for cardiovascular disease. Among the controls in Alameda County, white participants, regardless of religious affiliation, who attended church weekly, did not smoke cigarettes, exercised, and slept regular hours had an all-cause SMR of 38 (vs. 39 for Mormons with similar health behaviors) and a SMR of 49 for cardiovascular deaths (vs. 37 for Mormons). Thus, much of the health benefit that Mormons enjoy can be explained by their positive health behaviors and regular religious involvement.

Seventh-Day Adventists

Phillips, Lemon, et al. (1978) prospectively followed 24,044 California SDAs for a period of six years. CAD mortality rates for SDAs in age groups 35–64 and 65 and over were 28% and 50% those of age-matched persons in the general California population. About one-half of the reduced risk was the result of not smoking, and the remainder could be attributed to other aspects of SDA belief and lifestyle. Risk of fatal CAD for SDA nonvegetarian males ages 35–64 was three times greater than that for vegetarian men ($p < .01$), suggesting that diet explains at least part of the remaining risk. This effect persisted after the investigators controlled for six other CAD risk factors. The beneficial effect of a vegetarian diet, however, was considerably weaker among women and persons over age 65.

Phillips, Kuzma, and colleagues (1980) next reported the results of a 16-year prospective cohort study of 22,940 California SDAs and a 12-year prospective study of 112,726 California non-SDAs. Both groups were initially assessed in 1960. All subjects were white and over age 35 in 1960. Mortality ratios for the two groups were compared, and a Health Habit Index assessed the extent to which subjects adhered to 16 SDA-prescribed health behaviors. The SDAs, had a CAD mortality ratio of 0.66 for men (34% lower than controls) and 0.98 (no significant difference) for women. The mortality ratio among SDAs for cerebrovascular disease was 0.72 for men and 0.82 for women, (both $p < .01$); for other circulatory diseases the ratio was 0.64 in men and 0.92 (not significant) in women. The risk of fatal CAD among men was strongly and inversely related to scores on the Health Habit Index in younger subjects; the strength of that relationship, however, decreased with increasing age. The association was present even among the SDAs who did not smoke; again, elements of the SDA lifestyle other than not smoking may be important determinants of SDA's lower CAD mortality.

Examining SDAs outside the United States, Webster and Rawson (1979) compared the health status of 779 SDAs in New South Wales, Australia, with that of 8,363 non-SDAs referred by their general practitioners and 9,825 non-SDAs from the general Sydney population. The SDAs had lower systolic blood pressure and diastolic blood pressure, lower plasma cholesterol, greater lung ventilatory capacity, and less obesity than non-SDAs. With increasing age, however, the SDA's breathlessness, heart dis-

ease, hypertension, and use of diuretic treatments approached that of the comparison groups (possibly because of the deaths of high-risk individuals among the non-SDAs). SDAs faired significantly better on 22 of 25 health measures. Blood pressure and serum cholesterol were not only lower in adult life but rose less as the subjects aged than did those of the comparison groups.

Looking at the effects of diet on CAD mortality, Snowdon et al. (1984) examined meat consumption as a predictor of 20-year mortality from CAD among 25,153 California SDAs. Meat consumption was related to greater CAD mortality in both men and women, an effect not due to confounding by dairy products, obesity, marital status, or cigarette smoking. The association between meat consumption and fatal CAD was stronger in men than in women; overall, it was strongest in younger men (as Phillips et al. had reported in their six-year follow-up of this sample). For men ages 45–64 years, there was a threefold difference in risk between those who ate meat daily and those who did not eat meat.

Examining CAD risk factors within the SDA community itself, Frazer et al. (1992) followed a cohort of 27,658 male and female SDAs for six years. In addition to finding a lower risk of CAD in this population compared to other population groups, investigators reported that lack of exercise, obesity, and cigarette smoking were all significantly related to coronary events. They concluded that the epidemiology of ischemic heart disease in SDAs was qualitatively similar to that seen in other population groups.

Thus, it is clear that Mormons and Seventh-Day Adventists experience substantially less ischemic heart disease than do persons in the general population. This is probably a result of a healthier diet and positive health behaviors, which are largely based on religious beliefs and commitment to those beliefs. In addition, these close-knit religious communities place high priority on strong family life and promote supportive relationships among members, thus providing protection from many psychosocial stressors. Such factors likely work together to reduce the risk of heart disease in these groups.

Other World Religions

Gupta et al. (1997) surveyed all occupants of randomly selected villages in Rajasthan, India, assessing 3,148 adults age 20 or over. Diagnoses of CAD were based on past medical records, responses to a World Health Organization questionnaire, and changes found on EKG. In addition, subjects were asked about their participation in religious prayer and yoga (30% of the sample were involved in these activities). Multivariate analysis revealed that persons involved in religious prayer or yoga were more than 70% less likely to have CAD (odds ratio = 0.28, 95% CI = 0.08–0.95), a finding that was independent of other CAD risk factors.

Gopinath and colleagues (1995) surveyed a random sample of 13,560 adults in Delhi, India, examining risk factors for CAD. Diagnosis of heart disease was based on (1) a clinical history, supported by evidence that the subject had been treated in a hospital or at home or (2) EKG evidence of ischemic changes. The prevalence rate of "silent" CAD based on EKG evidence was highest among Muslims (89.5/1,000) and Sikhs (87.3/1,000), intermediate among Hindus (60.0/1,000), and lowest among Christians (25.0/1,000). Sikhs also showed the highest rate of myocardial infarction in (15.5/1,000) and angina pectoris (31.8/1,000). The authors concluded that the wide variations in the prevalence of CAD in these different religious groups could not be explained on the basis of conventional risk factors alone.

These studies demonstrate that rates of CAD vary across religious affiliation. Health practices, type of religious community, and possibly genetic factors largely determine the risk of heart disease in these broad religious groups. This research, however, tells us very little about the effects of "religiousness" on ischemic heart disease, since religiousness varies tremendously within each religious group. Religious affiliation for many people may be in name only (nominal) and have little impact on the way they think or live their lives. For others of the same affiliation, religious beliefs and practices may be very important and direct daily decisions. We now examine how degree of *religiousness* affects CAD risk.

RELIGIOUSNESS AND CORONARY ARTERY DISEASE

In contrast to the many denominational studies cited, few investigations have focused on the association between level of religious involvement and coronary heart disease.

Medalie, Kahn, Neufeld, Riss, and Goldbourt et al. (1973) examined biological and psychosocial factors associated with developing a first myocardial infarction within five years of the initial examination among 10,059 Jewish immigrant males (the Israeli Ischemic Study). All subjects were age 40 or older and worked as civil servants or municipal employees in Israel. Although no actual data on religion are reported, the authors indicate on the last page of the article that "The results of the sociological questionnaire will be the subject of a separate publication but it might be added here that one of the factors which stood out was the inverse relationship between the degree of religiosity and the 3-year incidence of myocardial infarction—in other words, the more religious developed fewer infarcts" (Medalie, 1973, p. 346). The study reporting these results was published in Hebrew, and is thus inaccessible.

In a literature review published a few years later, Kaplan (1976) referred to preliminary results from the Israeli Ischemic Study. He indicated that the age-adjusted rate of CAD in that cohort of 10,059 Jewish men was 29 per 1,000 among Orthodox Jews, 37 per 1,000 among traditional Jews, and 56 per 1,000 among nonreligious Jews (data based on a personal communication from Jack Medalie). Kaplan also noted that the age-adjusted rate of CAD for men in the 1967–1969 Evans County Cardiovascular Study was significantly lower for "church-goers" than for "non-church-goers" but provided no details.

A decade passed before another report appeared in the literature on the relationship between religiousness and CAD, and again it focused on Jews. Friedlander et al. (1986) compared a sample of 454 men and 85 women who had experienced their first myocardial infarction with a control group of 295 men and 391 women without heart disease who were living in Jerusalem. Some 51% of the men and 50%

of the women with MI defined themselves as secular, compared with 21% of the men and 16% of the women in the control group. After adjusting for the effects of age, ethnicity, education, smoking, physical exercise, and body mass index, investigators found that secular subjects had a significantly higher risk of MI than did the orthodox subjects (OR = 4.2, 95% CI 2.6–6.6, for men and OR = 7.3, 95% CI 2.3–23.0, for women). In other words, the risk of MI among secular men was more than four times greater than that for religiously orthodox men; among secular women, the risk of MI was more than seven times that of orthodox women. The relationship with religiousness persisted in a subsample of cases examined two or three months following the acute phase of the MI, even after the researchers controlled for plasma cholesterol, HDL cholesterol, and hypertension.

Reporting the 23-year follow-up results from the Israeli Ischemic Study, Goldbourt, Yaari, et al. (1993) noted that religious orthodoxy was significantly related to death rates from CAD. Religious orthodoxy was measured by three items: religious versus secular education, self-definition as orthodox, traditional, or secular, and frequency of synagogue attendance. The most orthodox group experienced a lower mortality rate from CAD (38 vs. 61 per 10,000) and from other causes (135 vs. 168 per 10,000) than did nonbelievers. The risk of death from CAD among the most orthodox believers during the 23-year follow-up was 20% lower than that for less orthodox Jews or nonbelievers (see Figure 16.1). These results remained significant after the researchers controlled for age, systolic blood pressure, cholesterol, smoking, diabetes, body mass index, and baseline CAD.

Finally, Oxman et al. (1995) examined the effects of religious attendance, importance of religion, and support derived from religion on six-month mortality rates for 232 older adults following elective coronary artery bypass graft (CABG) surgery. The vast majority of participants were either Protestant (63%) or Catholic (25%). Only 5% of persons who attended religious services at least every few months died compared to 12% of those who never or rarely attended services ($p = .06$, uncontrolled). None

of the persons who described themselves as deeply religious ($n = 37$), died, compared with an 11% mortality rate for other subjects ($p = .04$, uncontrolled). Six percent of those who obtained strength or comfort from religion died, compared to 16% of those who received no strength or comfort from religion ($p = .01$, uncontrolled). When other variables were controlled, including previous cardiac surgery, severity of ADL impairment, age, and social participation, persons who did not obtain strength or comfort from religion were three times more likely to die than those who depended on their religious faith (OR = 3.25). Even more striking, subjects who neither depended on religion for strength or comfort nor participated in social groups had a mortality risk more than 14 times that of persons who depended on religion and were involved in social groups (OR = 14.3) after biological and other risk factors were controlled.

Thus, it appears that religiousness is independently associated with a lower risk of myocardial infarction, a lower death rate from CAD, and longer survival following surgery for CAD. This statement, however, is based on only a few studies, primarily among Jews in Israel. Because of the public health implications of such a conclusion, further research is essential to examine this relationship more closely in other populations, and, if results are replicated, to seek a better understanding of the mechanisms involved.

PSYCHOSOCIAL AND SPIRITUAL INTERVENTIONS FOR HEART DISEASE

A number of studies have evaluated psychological, social, and spiritual interventions to prevent or treat coronary heart disease. Intervention studies tell us something about the causal direction of effects that cross-sectional and even prospective studies cannot.

Frasure-Smith and Prince (1989) examined outcomes of 461 post-MI male subjects during a seven-year follow-up period. These men were randomized to either a program that lowered stress scores or to a control group. Subjects

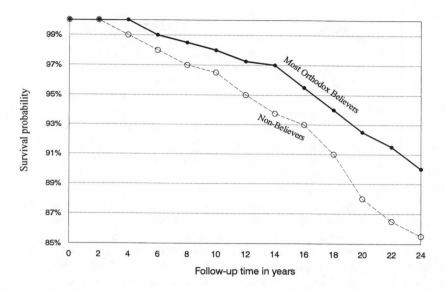

FIGURE 16.1 Kaplan-Meier life table curves demonstrating mortality from CHD among Jewish orthodox believers and nonbelievers based on a sample of 10,059 civil servants and municipal employees. Differences remain significant after blood pressure, diabetes, cholesterol, smoking, weight, and baseline heart disease are controlled (adapted from Goldbourt et al., 1993).

involved in the stress reduction program experienced a reduction in cardiac deaths of almost 50% during the one-year intervention. This reduction in cardiac mortality was the result primarily of a drop in out-of-hospital deaths (i.e., sudden death) and persisted until six months after the stress reduction program ended (after which mortality curves approached each other). Overall, however, there were fewer recurrences of MI among the treated group throughout the seven-year follow-up period ($p = .043$).

Leserman et al. (1989) examined the efficacy of the Relaxation Response (RR) (elicited by meditation or repetitive prayer) in preparation for cardiac surgery. Investigators randomly assigned 27 cardiac surgery patients (mean age 68) to either educational information plus RR or to educational information only (controls). The group that practiced RR had a lower incidence of supraventricular tachycardia ($p = .04$), but there were no differences in systolic or diastolic blood pressures or in heart rate. On the Profile of Mood States, the RR group experienced significantly greater reductions in ten-

sion and anger than did the education-only group. Patients who performed RR, however, had significantly higher "tension" scores and "anger" scores at the start of the study than did the education-only subjects, leaving open the possibility that "regression to the mean" may have explained the results. Furthermore, a single unblinded nurse collected both questionnaire information and helped experimental patients practice RR.

Ornish and coworkers (Ornish et al., 1990; Gould et al., 1992) conducted two randomized, controlled clinical trials to determine the effects of a low-cholesterol, low-fat, vegetarian diet, moderate aerobic exercise, and stress management on the geometric dimensions, shape, and fluid dynamic characteristics of coronary artery stenoses. During the course of these studies, the control groups demonstrated a significant worsening of coronary artery stenosis and stenosis flow reserve. In contrast, the intervention groups experienced significant improvement of coronary artery stenosis and improved stenosis flow reserve. These are some of the first studies to demonstrate that a psychosocial intervention can actually *reverse* the anatomical changes associated with coronary artery disease. Regression of even severe coronary atherosclerosis was seen after only one year and without drug therapy (Ornish et al., 1990).

Burell (1996) conducted a randomized clinical trial in Sweden that evaluated the effects of a behavioral intervention on prognosis following coronary artery bypass graft (CABG) surgery. A total of 261 subjects (mean age 58) had undergone CABG three to 12 months prior to participating in the study. Of these 128 subjects were randomly assigned to a behavioral intervention group that received one year of the intervention, followed by five or six booster sessions during years 2 and 3 of the study. The other 133 subjects were assigned to a routine-care control group. Subjects in the intervention group were subdivided into small groups of 5–9 persons who underwent three-hour group sessions every third week during the first year (17 sessions). Six of the sessions involved education about CAD and how psychological factors influence well-being; the subjects were given homework to observe their health behaviors (eating, alcohol, smoking) and coronary-prone behaviors (Type A behaviors, depression, anxiety). The remainder of the group sessions focused on modifying coronary-prone activities by encouraging new reactions and behaviors—less impatience, irritation, hostility, depression, and stress and more "reflecting on spiritual issues" (Burell, 1996, p. 298). The results of the study, assessed five to seven years after CABG, showed a significant difference in total mortality between the intervention and the control groups (7 vs. 16 deaths, $p = .02$). Subjects who received the intervention also spent fewer days than control subjects in the coronary care unit (243 vs. 416 days). Both Type A behavior and depression were significantly reduced among subjects who received the behavioral intervention.

Zamarra et al. (1996) conducted a clinical trial to test the hypothesis that a stress reduction intervention that uses transcendental meditation (TM) reduces exercise-induced myocardial ischemia among patients with known CAD. Twenty-one patients with known CAD were re-cruited from a Buffalo, New York, Veterans Administration Hospital and assigned either to TM ($n = 12$) or to a wait-list control group ($n = 9$). Investigators did not indicate whether assignment was random. Two subjects in the TM group and three in the control group did not complete the study, leaving a final sample of 16 (10 intervention, six controls). The TM group received 10 hours of basic instruction and follow-up, including personal instruction for 60 minutes initially and 30 minutes twice a week for the first month and monthly thereafter. Subjects were instructed to practice TM for 20 minutes twice daily. The intervention was conducted over six to eight months. After eight months, the TM group had a 14.7% increase in exercise duration ($p = .01$), an 11.7% increase in maximal workload ($p = .004$), and an 18.1% delay of onset of ST depression ($p = 0.03$), whereas control subjects showed no substantial changes in these outcomes. In addition, the TM group showed significantly greater reduction in rate-pressure products after three and six minutes of exercise than did the controls ($p = .02$).

In a related study, Wenneberg, Schneider, Walton, MacClean, Levitsky, Salerno, et al. (1997) examined the cardiovascular effects of TM in 39 normotensive males and an equal number of controls. The investigators reported an average 9 mmHg drop in diastolic blood pressure ($p < .04$) after four months among those in the TM group. No differences were found in the cardiovascular responses to stressors of the TM group and the control group. Alexander, Robinson, et al. (1994) comprehensively review studies that examine the effects of TM and other methods of relaxation and meditation on cardiovascular risk factors, morbidity, and mortality.

There is increasing evidence, then, that psychosocial and spiritual interventions directed at reducing psychological stress, improving health behaviors, and increasing social support benefit prognosis in CAD.

Controversial Reports and Studies

Kowey et al. (1986) describe the fascinating case of a prayer-meeting cardioversion in an article in the *Annals of Internal Medicine*. On the morning before planned electrical cardioversion, an elderly patient with atrial fibrillation summoned her daughters and Baptist minister to conduct a prayer meeting in her hospital room. After direct supplication that "this evil rhythm leave her body," a nurse with a direct view of the cardiac monitor reported that at *that moment* the patient reverted to normal sinus rhythm. Atrial fibrillation did not recur. This remarkable report illustrates the effect that mind and spirit can have on cardiac functioning; it is, however, only a single case. Research studies could be designed to test hypotheses suggested by this report.

Perhaps the most extraordinary study in recent times is the Byrd study. The cardiologist Randolph Byrd (1988) conducted a double-blind clinical trial in the coronary care unit at San Francisco General Hospital that involved 393 patients randomized to either an intercessory prayer group ($n = 192$) or a control group ($n = 201$). Neither doctors nor patients knew which patients were being prayed for, and the people praying for the patients did not know the patients. Intercessory prayer of the petitionary type and to the Judeo-Christian God was employed. Patients in the intercessory prayer group experienced fewer episodes of congestive heart failure (8 vs. 20, $p < .05$); needed fewer diuretics (5 vs. 15, $p < .05$); experienced fewer cardiac arrests (3 vs. 14, $p < .05$) and fewer pneumonias (3 vs. 13, $p < .05$); and were prescribed fewer antibiotics (3 vs. 17, $p < .005$); in addition, no one in the intercessory group was intubated (vs. 12 in the control group, $p < .05$). After controlling for other variables, members of the prayed-for group required less respirator support and fewer medications ($p < .0001$). This is a highly controversial study whose results cannot be explained by any known psychosocial or physiological mechanism. Replication of this study is essential before the scientific community can begin to consider these findings more seriously, and at least three research groups are currently attempting to replicate these findings in cardiac patients. Herbert Benson's group from Harvard Medical School is currently conducting a study to replicate the findings of the Byrd study. Prior to undergoing

CABG surgery, a total of 1,800 patients will be randomly assigned to either an intercessory prayer group or a no-prayer group, and subsequent outcomes will be compared. The results of this study will be available in early 2002.

SUMMARY AND CONCLUSIONS

Cardiovascular disease (including heart disease, hypertension, peripheral vascular disease, and stroke) accounts for about 1 million deaths per year in the United States, nearly double the number caused by cancer. In this chapter we focused on coronary artery disease (CAD), a condition that affects more than 7% of persons over age 20 in this country and is responsible for more than 2 million acute hospital admissions each year. Risk factors for CAD include medical conditions such as hypertension and diabetes, family history, and other factors such as cigarette smoking, poor diet, high serum cholesterol, little or no exercise, excessive weight, and alcohol abuse. These factors interact, magnifying and synergistically increasing the risk. Psychiatric illnesses, especially depression, and psychological stress also increase the risk of CAD. Because social factors help to prevent depression and relieve stress, group support lowers the risk of CAD and may improve prognosis.

Because of the strong link between religious beliefs and activities and many risk factors for CAD, there is ample reason to hypothesize a relationship between religion and heart disease. Rates of CAD vary across different religious groups. Some studies show that Jews and, to a lesser extent, Protestants are at higher risk than Catholics. Most studies show that Mormons and Seventh-Day Adventists are at lower risk. It is likely that diet, health behaviors, and quality of social and family life account for much of this lowered risk. While studies on this topic are few, degree of religious involvement also appears to be an important influence on risk of myocardial infarction, mortality from CAD, and survival following coronary artery bypass graft surgery. Psychosocial, behavioral, and spiritual interventions are now being designed to help improve CAD prognosis and possibly even reverse coronary artery lesions.

17

Hypertension

THIS CHAPTER REVIEWS RE-search on the relationship between religious involvement and blood pressure, examines studies on the application of specific religious or spiritual practices to the treatment of hypertension, and discusses a few church-based hypertension control programs. We begin with an overview of hypertension, including its classification, etiology, health consequences, and economic cost.

DEFINING HYPERTENSION

Hypertension is defined as a sustained or chronic elevation in blood pressure. Previously it was felt that persons with systolic pressures within the range of 160 to 170 mm Hg (millimeters of mercury) had an acceptable blood pressure and were not at unusual risk. However, more recent evidence suggests that systolic pressure should be less than 140 mm Hg and dia-stolic pressure less than 90 mm Hg to reduce the risk of cardiovascular disease (Alexander, Schlant, et al., 1998).

Unfortunately, there is no specific clinical sign or symptom that provides evidence for high blood pressure. Most cases are found during routine physical examinations. Sadly, however, many people become aware of their hypertension only after they have had a stroke or a heart attack, which is why this disease is often referred to as the silent killer. Some nonspecific symptoms may include headaches, dizziness, nosebleeds, chest pain, or ankle swelling. Even in persons who feel well, the clinical consequences of high blood pressure can be serious.

CAUSES OF HYPERTENSION

Although there is usually no known cause, hypertension can be influenced by a person's lifestyle. For example, a diet high in salt can elevate blood pressure, especially in African Americans because of the enhanced ability of their kidneys to retain salt (National Heart, Lung, and Blood Institute, 1997). This genetic trait is very useful in very hot climates where sweating is common and water may not be readily available; salt retention by the kidneys can also lead to water retention, helping to prevent dehydration, and is especially useful when people spend long hours working under the hot tropical sun. Now, however, as many people lead more sedentary lives, there is still a tendency to consume high amounts of dietary salt, even though the body does not need it, thereby increasing the risk of hypertension.

Other hereditary factors besides salt retention play a role in predisposing certain individuals to the development of hypertension. Except for a few rare forms, hypertension appears to be a complex trait that does not follow the classic Mendelian rules of inheritance attributable to a single gene locus. Rather, it appears to be a polygenic and multifactorial disorder in which the interaction of several genes with each other and with the environment is important. Potential candidate genes suggested by recent experimental data include those that affect various components of the renin-angiotensin-aldosterone system, which influences the actions of the kidneys, the kallikrein-kinin system, and the sympathetic nervous system (National Heart Lung and Blood Institute, 1997).

Other factors known to induce or aggravate high blood pressure include cigarette smoking, heavy alcohol use, diabetes, and the use of certain medications, such as oral contraceptives. In particular, psychological and social stress (job strain, anxiety, depression, emotional distress), by increasing catecholamines and cortisol (Raikkonen et al., 1996), are thought to have significant influences on blood pressure (Schnall et al., 1992; Cesana et al., 1996; Landsbergis et al., 1996; Jonas et al., 1997). Thus, hypertension is likely due to the interaction of genetic factors, lifestyle, and environmental factors.

TYPES OF HYPERTENSION

High blood pressure in which the exact cause is unknown is referred to as *essential hypertension* *or primary hypertension* and usually begins in the second or third decade of life. This is the most common form of hypertension. Without blood pressure measurements or continuing aggravating symptoms, the person with essential hypertension is usually unaware that his blood pressure is elevated. Stress, anxiety, depression, and anger may all contribute to the development or worsening of essential hypertension (Boutelle et al., 1987; Kulkarni et al., 1998).

Malignant hypertension is a form of hypertension that, once diagnosed, progresses very rapidly and is accompanied by severe vascular damage. It may even result in sudden death.

Benign hypertension is a type of hypertension that progresses very slowly. The basic disease process may reach the same endpoint as malignant hypertension but at a much slower rate.

Renal hypertension is defined as hypertension that results from kidney disease or disease of the arteries that supply blood to the kidney. It results from the excessive excretion of a humoral substance called renin that is produced by the kidney and causes severe constriction of the renal arteries. This leads to increased salt and water retention by the kidneys.

CONSEQUENCES AND COSTS OF HYPERTENSION

Hypertension is the most common cardiovascular disorder. It affects about 20% of the adult population in many countries. It is associated with coronary heart disease, stroke, congestive heart failure and chronic renal failure and is one of the major risk factors in 20–50% of all deaths in the United States (National Heart Lung and Blood Institute, 1997). Hypertension is a major risk factor for coronary artery disease, and the incidence of both conditions increases with age. Consequently, the majority of individuals over 65 years of age with coronary artery disease probably also have hypertension. Some authorities predict that, because of the increasing size of the elderly population, there will be a doubling in the prevalence of hypertension in the next century (National Heart, Lung, and Blood Institute, 1997).

The incidence of hypertension in the United States has increased dramatically in recent years. Currently, as many as 50 million Americans have high blood pressure, with 2 million new cases occurring each year. On the other hand, over the past 10 years there has been more than a 50% reduction in incidence of serious complications related to hypertension (National Heart, Lung, and Blood Institute, 1997), largely due to improved pharmacological treatments.

Hypertension is a pervasive public health problem with enormous medical as well as economic consequences. As noted earlier, it is a significant contributor to coronary heart disease (CHD), stroke, congestive heart failure, and other cardiovascular disorders. As noted in chapter 16, cardiovascular disease is the leading cause of death in the United States, claiming nearly 1 million lives annually and accounting for more than 40% of all deaths. In economic terms, the annual direct and indirect costs of CAD and stroke are approximately $259 billion, or $492,444 per second, in the United States alone. Reduction of blood pressure has been shown to reduce stroke risk by up to 40% in hypertensive populations (American Heart Association, 1999).

TREATMENT OF HYPERTENSION

Although there is strong evidence that pharmacologic treatment of hypertension can save lives by lowering blood pressure, concerns persist about the potential adverse side effects of such treatments. Subtle metabolic changes due to drug treatment that may go unnoticed by the patient and that could offset the beneficial effects of blood pressure reduction include hyperglycemia, hypokalemia, hypercholesterolemia, and hypomagnesemia.

In terms of the risk-to-benefit ratio, the potentially adverse effects of pharmacologic treatment, including reductions in quality of life and the expense of medication, assume a greater importance for patients with milder forms of hypertension. The role of nonpharmacologic approaches in the treatment of essential hypertension, then, must be explored vigorously. Indeed, for many people with less severe forms of hypertension, nondrug therapies may be the treatment of choice.

Behavioral or psychosocial treatments for mild to moderate hypertension include stress reduction, dietary change, and alterations in lifestyle. Because research into the efficacy of these factors has implications for both treatment and primary prevention, social epidemiologists have long shown interest in the effects of socioenvironmental and intrapsychic determinants of blood pressure level. Among the psychosocial factors shown to correlate with hypertension is involvement with religion. The rest of this chapter discusses the relationship between religion and the development, course, and treatment of hypertension in various populations.

RELIGIOUS INVOLVEMENT AND BLOOD PRESSURE

In recent years, a growing number of epidemiological studies have found a significant correlation between the degree of religious involvement and blood pressure. In general, these studies suggest that individuals who report higher levels of religious activity experience a lower risk for hypertension. In one of the earliest studies, Scotch (1963) examined the relationship of hypertension to psychosocial and lifestyle factors among rural and urban Zulus in South Africa. Scotch interviewed 548 randomly selected people in rural areas and 505 people in urban areas. During interviews, subjects' blood pressure was measured several times, their height and weight were determined, and a number of questions were asked concerning education, income, and degree of religiousness. A diastolic blood pressure of greater than 90 mm Hg was the criterion used to define hypertension.

Among rural dwellers, Scotch found that the frequency of church attendance was negatively correlated with hypertension ($p < .001$). Additionally, urban women who belonged to Christian churches had less hypertension than those who were not churchgoers ($p < .02$). Urban men who belonged to Christian churches, however, had slightly higher rates of hypertension than nonmembers ($p < .10$). Thus, among rural dwellers, religious commitment was negatively related to hypertension among both men and women; among urban dwellers, church affiliation was negatively correlated with hypertension for women and positively (but weakly) correlated for men. The researchers explained the tendency for male urban-dwelling church members to have higher rates of hypertension by noting that only a small number of churchgoers in the urban population were men. Therefore, they posited, these men were "deviant" from the more "normal" men who spent Sunday mornings playing sports or involved in other activities. They speculated that hypertensive men tended to become church members because they were seeking through the church to cope with psychosocial problems that may have been related to their development of hypertension.

In a later study, Graham and colleagues (1978) analyzed data from the Evans County Cardiovascular Epidemiologic Study (ECCPS), a survey funded by the National Institutes of Health and conducted in Georgia in the late 1960s. This study examined the relationship between a variety of sociological factors, including religious involvement and blood pressure, in 771 white community-dwelling males. The investigators found a consistent association between frequent church attendance and lower age-standardized systolic and diastolic blood pressure. This association was present among smokers ($t = 1.886$, $p < 0.005$) and nonsmokers ($t = 1.585$, $p < 0.06$), as well as among white-collar ($t = 1.627$, $p < 0.06$) and blue-collar ($t = 1.999$, $p < 0.025$) workers in the sample. Although these data were cross-sectional and care must be taken in drawing conclusions about causal relationships, the consistency of the data among different demographic groups is noteworthy.

In a follow-up report, Larson, Koenig, and colleagues (1989) reanalyzed the data for the original 771 subjects who participated in ECCPS to examine the relationship among blood pressure, frequency of church attendance, and importance of religion. Individuals in the original survey identified as having had a history of

hypertension or heart disease, however, were eliminated from this analysis, leaving 401 individuals from the original ECCPS for this analysis. Investigators this time found only a weak, nonsignificant trend toward lower blood pressures among those who attended church more frequently compared to infrequent attenders. The relationship between "importance of religion" and blood pressure followed the same pattern but again did not reach statistical significance. However, when the two items were combined and analyzed in relation to blood pressure, more notable differences emerged. Indeed, for those with high frequency of attendance and for whom religion was important, diastolic pressures were significantly lower than for those with low frequency of attendance and for whom religion was not important (after socioeconomic status, body mass index, smoking status, and age were controlled). Systolic pressures followed the same trend but again did not reach statistical significance after covariates were controlled.

Interestingly, for nonsmokers, there was almost no difference in blood pressures between those for whom religion was important and those for whom it was not, with or without adjustment for covariates. For smokers, on the other hand, diastolic blood pressure was significantly lower for those for whom religion was important compared to those for whom it was not. This suggests that religion helped to protect smokers in the former group from high diastolic blood pressures. The same relationship was found for systolic pressure. Associations between religious importance and both diastolic and systolic blood pressures were statistically significant after adjusting for covariates. Among smokers, those for whom religion has *low* importance experienced a 4.3 times greater likelihood of having abnormal systolic and 7.1 times greater likelihood of having abnormal diastolic pressure than did those for whom it was of *high* importance.

The ECCPS, however, was conducted in Georgia, the center of the Bible Belt in the United States. Perhaps results were affected by the location of the study in a very religious part of the country, where social norms encourage religious involvement. Studying a northeastern population, Lapane et al. (1997) surveyed two large population-based random samples of 2,442 and 2,799 persons in Pawtucket, Rhode Island. Investigators compared the health status of church members with that of nonmembers. While church members were more likely to be 20% overweight, 48% had never smoked (vs. 35% of nonmembers) ($p < .001$) and, after adjusting for other risk factors, the average diastolic blood pressure of church members was again significantly lower than that of nonmembers ($p = .017$); no differences in systolic blood pressure were noted. For unclear reasons, religious involvement appears more strongly related to diastolic than to systolic blood pressures in numerous studies.

In one of the largest and most detailed studies to date, Koenig, George, Cohen, et al. (1998a) examined the relationship between blood pressure and religious activities in a probability sample of 3,963 persons age 65 years or older who participated in the Duke EPESE survey. Participants were asked whether their doctor had ever informed them that they had high blood pressure and whether they were currently taking medication for high blood pressure. After the interview, systolic and diastolic blood pressures were measured following a standard protocol. Data were available for three waves of the survey (1986, 1989–1990, and, 1993–1994). Analyses were stratified by age (65–74 and those over 75) and by race (whites and African Americans) and were controlled for age, race, gender, education, physical functioning, body mass index, and, in longitudinal analyses, blood pressure from the previous wave. Cross-sectional analyses revealed small (1–4 mm Hg) but consistent differences in measured systolic and diastolic blood pressures between frequent (once a week) and infrequent (less than once a week) church attenders. Lower pressures were also observed among those who frequently prayed or studied the Bible (daily or more often) (see Figure 17.1). Blood pressure differences were particularly notable in African American and younger elderly, in whom religious activity at one wave predicted blood pressures four years later.

The most striking finding in this study was that among participants who both attended religious services and prayed or studied the Bible frequently, the likelihood of having a diastolic blood pressure of 90 mm Hg or higher was 40% lower than that for participants who attended services less than once per week and prayed or studied the Bible less than once per day (OR 0.60, 95% CI, 0.48–0.75, $p < .0001$, after adjusting for covariates). Among participants told they had high blood pressure, religiously active persons were more likely to be taking blood pressure medication; this could not, however, explain the differences in blood pressure observed. While most religious activity was associated with lower blood pressure, those who frequently watched religious TV or listened to religious radio actually had higher blood pressures (although these differences were small and largely due to confounding by ethnicity).

Religious Involvement, Ethnicity, and Hypertension

A lower rate of hypertension among the more religiously committed has been found not only in persons of different age and socioeconomic status but also in various ethnic populations. Stavig and colleagues (1984) investigated economic, social, and psychological factors that might influence hypertension among 1,757 Asians and Pacific Islanders who lived in California. This study found that 18.3% of Asians and Pacific Islanders had hypertension, compared with, 19.8% of the general population in California. Investigators also found that hypertension was positively correlated with increased consumption of high-calorie, high-fat American food, which increased body weight and contributed to the development of hypertension. Hypertension was also positively correlated with increased alcohol consumption and lower educational status. Several measures of social support also predicted hypertension. In particular, the number of close friends available to provide support was inversely related to hypertension. Another measure of social support that Stavig and colleagues analyzed was the extent of community and/or religious involvement. Individuals with no religious affiliation had rates of hypertension almost double those of subjects with

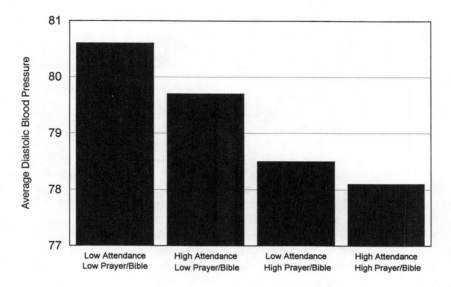

FIGURE 17.1 Relationship between religious activities and diastolic blood pressure ($n =$ 3,632). Association significant at $p < .0001$ (analyses weighted and controlled for age, sex, race, smoking, education, physical functioning, and body mass index).

religious affiliations (29.3% vs. 15.0%, respectively, adjusted for age, sex, and body mass index, $p < .01$). When eight other covariates were controlled in a multiple regression model, religious affiliation still predicted lower rates of hypertension ($\beta = -.13$, $p < .05$). The effect was greatest at age 25 and declined slightly as subjects increased in age (as biological causes began to account more and more for elevations in blood pressure).

Studying a group of 75 recent immigrants to the United States, Walsh (1980) found evidence that religion may play a role in reducing the risk of hypertension by increasing social support. A number of studies indicate that recent immigrants are at increased risk for cardiovascular disease due to high levels of stress. Walsh hypothesized that recent immigrants would be an ideal group in which to measure the effects of religious involvement on the development of hypertension. In other words, he wanted to determine if religion could have a protective effect against hypertension in this at-risk population. Religious variables measured were church attendance and importance of religion.

Although this study did not find a significant

relationship between religious involvement and blood pressure, it did find a relationship between the immigrants' degree of assimilation into American society and their blood pressure. That is, the more they were assimilated, the less likely they were to have hypertension. Moreover, Walsh found that church attendance had a strong impact on the assimilation/blood pressure relationship. Those who attended church more frequently were less likely to experience feelings of alienation and uprootedness and, thus, also less likely to experience tension and distress. Consequently, those who attended church more frequently were more likely to assimilate and become citizens ($\chi^2 = 3.85$, $p = .05$). Involvement in a religious community may have ameliorated the negative effects on blood pressure of the increased distress associated with immigration.

In a later study, Hutchinson (1986) found similar results after examining blacks who lived in St. Vincent, West Indies. In this study, information on age, sex, ethnicity, church attendance, marital status, educational level, and number of children was collected for 144 men and 213 women selected randomly from households on the island. In addition, two blood pressure readings were taken and averaged for each individual. The subjects also were asked a number of questions about their health status. Analyses revealed that men who did not attend church had significantly higher blood pressures than men attending church frequently. No relationship, however, was found for women.

To explain why church attendance was unrelated to blood pressure in women, Hutchinson (1986) suggested that it "may be due to the fact that the vast majority of women do attend church [74%] and these women do have normal pressures. Therefore, there was not enough deviation to demonstrate that variation in blood pressure [among women] is related to frequency of church attendance" (p. 77). Hutchinson speculated that an increased level of social support through marriage and church attendance may protect men from hypertension.

Religious participation may be particularly valuable for enhancing social integration in certain ethnic groups. For example, Livingston et al. (1991) evaluated the potential role that social integration plays in explaining variations in blood pressure among African Americans. In this study, which examined a random sample of 1,420 adults in Maryland, social integration was defined in terms of five variables: employment, marriage, church affiliation, group affiliation, and having someone to talk to when necessary. Investigators conducted separate multiple regression analyses that examined the relationship between social integration and blood pressure in men ($n = 587$) and women ($n = 833$), controlling for age, education, income, hypertension medication status, exercise, daily physical activity, alcohol consumption, salt consumption, cigarette smoking, and body mass index. Among men, 64.7% of the subjects said that they had no church affiliation; 55.1% of the women so reported. After the researchers adjusted for the covariates listed earlier, church affiliation was found to be significantly related to lower systolic ($\beta = -4.90$, $p = .04$) and lower diastolic ($\beta = -6.51$, $p = .0003$) blood pressures in men; church affiliation was also significantly related to lower systolic ($\beta = -4.01$, $p = .07$) and diastolic ($\beta = -5.32$, $p = .0006$) blood pressures among women. The investigators concluded that social integration, especially affiliation with a church, contributes to lower blood pressure in African Americans.

No Association

A small number of studies report a weak, absent, or positive association between religiousness and high blood pressure.

Levin and Markides (1985) surveyed three generations of Mexican Americans in the San Antonio area, interviewing a total of 1,125 persons (375 in each generation—young, middle aged, and elderly). Frequency of religious attendance and self-rated religiosity were assessed. Respondents were also read a list of seven chronic diseases and asked whether they had any of them. Among older persons ($n = 203$), investigators found a relationship between hypertension and self-rated religiosity. Thirty percent of the "less than very religious" group had self-reported hypertension, compared to 43% of the "very religious" group ($p < .05$, uncontrolled). Investigators speculated that religious behavior may be a risk factor for stress-related illness, perhaps resulting from the tendency of certain religious groups (such as Calvinists) to induce high anxiety among their members. The researchers also suggested that religion may increase the risk for emotional problems that stem from guilt, such as depression. These ideas, however, were an attempt to explain a finding discovered after the fact. Investigators had no preexisting hypothesis to make them suspect such a finding before doing the statistical analysis and therefore were forced to interpret a serendipitous finding post hoc.

Koenig, Moberg, and Kvale (1988) surveyed 106 consecutive medical outpatients ages 56–94 from Springfield, Illinois. Investigators examined the relationship between hypertension and organizational religious activity (ORA), nonorganizational religious activity (NORA), and intrinsic religiousness (IR). Being hypertensive was defined as having two or more recorded blood pressures of 160/90 mm Hg or higher or receiving antihypertensive treatment. Analyses were stratified by sex. There was no relationship between hypertension and ORA, NORA, or IR among women ($n = 77$). Among men ($n = 29$), the same was true except that there was a trend for men with hypertension to score lower on IR than men without hypertension (mean rank 9.9 vs. 15.7, respectively, Z score = 1.75, .05 < p < .10, uncontrolled).

Finally, Brown and Gary (1994) surveyed 537 African American men in Norfolk, Virginia, examining the relationship between religious involvement and physical illness. Religious involvement was measured by a 10-item religiosity scale, frequency of religious attendance, and religious affiliation. Physical health was measured by self-reported presence of hypertension, cigarette smoking, or alcohol use. No relationship was found between religious variables and hypertension (in uncontrolled analyses), although men who were more religiously involved were less likely to smoke cigarettes, less likely to drink alcohol daily, and less likely to experience depression. It is interesting that both studies that found no relationship between religious involvement and hypertension measured hypertension by self-report, a notoriously unreliable method of identifying the disease.

Religious Denomination and Blood Pressure

Studies have also investigated blood pressure differences across religious denominations. They have found for the most part, as Stavig and colleagues (1984) reported, that the religiously affiliated experience a lower risk of hypertension than the nonaffiliated. However, this research also suggests that there are differences among religious groups. For example, Armstrong and colleagues (1977) found that Seventh-Day Adventists (SDA) in western Australia (n = 418) had significantly lower blood pressure than nonvegetarian non-Adventists (n = 290) (p < .001). In this study, increased consumption of eggs, tea, or coffee was associated with increased blood pressure among SDAs. Controlling for alcohol, tobacco, tea, coffee, or egg consumption, socioeconomic status, and physical activity could not explain the significant blood pressure differences between SDAs and non-SDAs. While investigators still attributed the differences to dietary factors (intake of animal protein, animal fat, salt, or some other dietary component), they did admit that "Religious commitment, the habit of resting one day in seven, or other social characteristics of SDAs could affect BP" (Armstrong et al., 1977, p. 449).

Another study compared the health status of 779 SDA volunteers in New South Wales, Australia, to 8,363 persons referred by general practitioners and 9,825 volunteers (who, combined, "probably represent the overall Sydney population"). In that study, Webster and Rawson (1979) found that SDAs were less likely than non-SDAs to have systolic and diastolic hypertension. SDAs also tended to have better respiratory capacity, better cholesterol and blood urate profiles, and less obesity, sleeplessness, and depression than did the non-SDA comparison group. With increasing age, the differences in breathlessness, heart disease, hypertension, and use of diuretic therapy between SDAs and non-SDAs decreased, which, according to the authors, could have been a result of the natural attrition (death) of those in the more high-risk non-SDA group. Investigators concluded that "the lifestyle of the Seventh-Day Adventist is conducive to lessened morbidity, delayed mortality, and decreased call on health services compared with the general population" (Webster & Rawson, 1979, p. 417).

In a study that compared SDAs and Mormons, Rouse and colleagues (1982) found that both male and female SDAs had lower systolic blood pressure than male and female Mormons, and female SDAs had lower diastolic blood pressure than did the female Mormons. These findings were again attributed to the vegetarian diet of SDAs. Interestingly, two studies of vegetarian and nonvegetarian subjects—Trappist monks and Benedictine monks, respectively— reported findings that conflicted with Rouse and colleagues' explanation, showing instead that the vegetarian Trappists had higher mean blood pressures than the nonvegetarian Benedictines (Groen et al., 1962; Caffrey, 1969). Differences in blood pressure among similarly tightknit religious groups, then, are likely due to many factors besides diet.

Investigations of other religious denominations have also reported differences among groups. In one study, Ross and Thomas (1965) found that among female medical students who were attending Johns Hopkins University, Protestants had lower mean blood pressures than did either Catholic or Jewish medical students. When the investigators reran their analysis using only Jews and Gentiles (Protestant and Catholics combined) as their comparison groups, Jews again were found to have significantly higher blood pressures than Gentiles. In an earlier study, which compared strict orthodox Jews (Yemenites) with other Jews, Toor and colleagues (1954) found that the Yemenites had significantly lower mean blood pressures than did the other Jews.

Blood Pressure in Clergy

If degree of religious involvement is key to the relationship between religion and hypertension, one might expect that those who make a lifelong commitment to religion as a profession will have lower blood pressures than persons in the general population. One of the earliest studies to compare blood pressures of a group of clergy with those of persons in the general population was reported by McCullagh et al. (1960). These investigators examined the physical health status of 44 Trappist monks in Kentucky and Massachusetts (77% were over age 50). While the monks had lower serum cholesterols because of their avoidance of animal fat, they were not protected from either atherosclerotic vascular disease or hypertension. In fact, the data suggested that arterial hypertension may have been more frequent in this group (48%) than in men of similar age in the general American population (although no actual comparison was made).

Another study of clergy, by Locke and King (1980), however, reported different findings. Examining the causes of death for 5,207 male clergy of the American Baptist convention, these investigators found that they had a significantly lower rate of mortality due to hypertension and heart disease (standardized mortality ratio = 61) than did men in the general population. (The disparity was almost 40%.) Similar findings were reported by Timio et al. (1988), who conducted a 20-year prospective study of blood pressure in 144 nuns who belonged to a secluded monastic order and in 138 laywomen controls. While average blood pressures in the two groups were equal at the start of the study, blood pressures increased over time only in the laywomen; mean slope of the regression line was 0.89 in the nuns and 2.17 in the laywomen ($p < .0001$, adjusting for education, race, weight, body mass index, smoking, family history of hypertension, serum cholesterol and triglycerides, and 24-hour urinary sodium excretion). Although the finding was attributed to the nuns' being isolated from the stresses of society, religious belief and commitment may have also played a role.

Coupled with the findings on degree of religious activity and hypertension, it appears that a higher degree of religious involvement is inversely related to high blood pressure. Only a few studies have suggested otherwise. Unlike other conditions, this disease does not impair mobility and often has no symptoms or signs whatsoever. It is unlikely, then, that high blood pressure prevents religious involvement, but rather the other way around.

MECHANISMS OF RELIGION'S EFFECT ON BLOOD PRESSURE

By what mechanism or mechanisms might religion protect against high blood pressure and its health consequences? As with heart disease, most investigators attribute the lower risk for hypertension in religious groups such as Seventh-Day Adventists and Mormons to the promotion of healthy lifestyle practices (e.g., vegetarianism, abstinence from alcohol and tobacco) (Lyon, Wetzler, et al., 1978; Phillips, Kuzma, et al., 1980; Brown & Gary, 1994). Other explanations may also exist, as we have suggested.

After reviewing 20 studies on the relationship between religion and hypertension, Levin and Vanderpool (1989) posited the healthy lifestyle theory as well as several additional explanations for the inverse relationship. They proposed that a salutary effect of religion on blood pressure might result from some combination of a variety of biological, social, psychological, and behavioral factors, including:

- Promotion of beneficial healthy lifestyle behaviors
- Hereditary predispositions in particular groups
- Healthful coping and social support effects of religious practice
- Beneficial psychodynamics of particular religious belief systems, religious rites, and faith.

Because religious practices pervade human society and because hypertension is a common and serious problem that religion may help to prevent, Levin and Vanderpool (1989) suggested that "the question of whether characteristics or functions of religion can indeed lower or prevent high blood pressure is both scientifically and clinically intriguing." They also emphasized that if the salutory effects of religion are going to be found anywhere, they will be found in hypertension studies, since religion is related to many factors likely to affect blood pressure. We now examine further research studies that support two of the hypothesized mechanisms—social support and psychodynamics.

Religion as a Source of Social Support and Social Integration

The dimension of religious involvement that increases social support can influence level of psychological stress as well as lifestyle risk factors for hypertension, such as smoking and drinking. For example, Gottlieb and Green (1984) examined the relationships among social structure, stress, social support, lifestyle behavior, and health status and found that, for both men and women, church attendance and marriage were associated with less smoking and less alcohol use. Frequent church attendance was characteristic of both men and women nonsmokers in the study and was negatively related to monthly alcohol consumption for both sexes. Men who were former smokers also were likely to be frequent church attenders. Additionally, women nonsmokers and former smokers and those of both sexes who drank less alcohol were likely to be married. These two findings suggest that religious teachings and family responsibility are likely to affect substance use and abuse (which are known to influence blood pressure).

Such findings are also consistent with other studies showing that religion-mediated social support is associated with lower morbidity (Ferraro & Koch, 1994; Commerford & Reznikoff, 1996).

Religion, Self-Esteem, and Susceptibility to Stress

Religious beliefs and practices also tend to be associated with higher self-esteem, which may, in turn, promote a healthier lifestyle and/or reduce stress. Psychosocial stress can lead to repeated blood pressure elevations, which eventually lead to sustained hypertension (Kulkarni et al., 1998). Thus, any factor that can protect against psychological stress may help prevent the development of hypertension.

Krause and Van Tran (1989) analyzed data from the National Survey of Black Americans to determine the interrelationships among religious involvement, self-esteem, mastery (feelings of personal control), and stressful life events. Investigators found that stressful life events exerted a large and statistically significant impact on both self-esteem and mastery. As exposure to stressful events increased, particularly for older African Americans, there was a decline in feelings of positive self-worth ($\beta = -.34$; $p < .001$), as well as a diminished sense of personal control ($\beta = -.25$, $p < .001$). In contrast, as the subjects' involvement in public religious activities and church increased, there was a significant increase in self-esteem ($\beta = .37$, $p < .001$). To a lesser extent, increased private religious activity/subjective religiosity also increased feelings of personal control ($\beta = .20$; $p < .05$). Thus, while stress tended to erode feelings of mastery and self-esteem, these negative effects were offset by religious involvement. These data also suggested that religiousness might exert a beneficial effect on self-esteem and mastery even in the absence of life stress.

Further evidence for religion's ability to buffer stress effects comes from a study by Shams and Jackson (1993), who examined the effects of religiousness on the psychological stress created by unemployment. Investigators interviewed employed ($n = 69$) and unemployed ($n = 71$) male Asian Muslims who were living in Britain about their overall psychological well-being and the strength of their religious values. Analyses revealed that unemployment was inversely related to psychological well-being, particularly for middle-aged individuals. Stronger religious values, however, were associated with greater well-being in the overall sample ($p < .01$, when researchers controlled for age and employment status). There was also a significant interaction between religiosity and employment status. For the unemployed group (average length of unemployment 3.5 years), higher religiosity scores were associated with greater psychological well-being ($r = .37$, $p < .001$), whereas the association in the employed respondents was not significant. Investigators concluded that strong religious belief may help the unemployed retain a sense of self-worth despite their jobless status. If religious involvement can help reduce stress and increase self-esteem, then this may be one mechanism by which it keeps blood pressure low.

RELIGIOUS PRACTICES AND REDUCTION OF HYPERTENSION

Few clinical trials have examined whether traditional religious or spiritual beliefs and practices can reduce blood pressure in persons with hypertension. Nevertheless, some studies suggest that meditation or repetitive prayer may elicit the relaxation response (RR), an integrated physiological reaction that is the opposite of the "stress response" (Benson, 1977, 1996). Repeated elicitation of RR is associated with a reduction in muscle tension, a reduction in the activity of the sympathetic branch of the autonomic nervous system, a reduction in the activity of the anterior pituitary/adrenocortical axis, and, consequently, a lowering of blood pressure, heart rate, and oxygenation (see Delmonte, 1985, and Benson, 1996, and for complete reviews of this literature).

Meditation.   In the mid-1970s, Blackwell et al. (1976) studied seven hypertensive patients who were given standard antihypertensive medication in addition to learning transcendental med-

itation (TM), a Hindu-based mind-focusing practice. Patients were seen weekly and took their own blood pressure several times daily. After 12 weeks of TM, six subjects showed psychological changes and reduced anxiety scores. More important, six of the seven patients had significant reductions in clinic-measured blood pressures. On six-month follow-up, four subjects continued to show psychological benefits, and two experienced further significant blood-pressure reductions (as measured at home and in the clinic) attributed to TM.

In another study where meditation was combined with yoga (a Hindu and Buddhist religious practice), Patel and North (1975) randomly assigned 34 hypertensive patients either to six weeks of treatment with yoga relaxation methods plus biofeedback or to a control therapy (general relaxation). Both groups showed a reduction in blood pressure (from 168/100 to 141/84 mm Hg in the yoga-treated group and from 169/101 to 160/96 mm Hg in the control group). The difference between groups was highly significant. The members of the control group were then trained in yoga relaxation, and their blood-pressures dropped further to the same level as the other group. In a follow-up study, Patel and Datey (1976) obtained similar results in a group of 27 hypertensive patients.

Sundar and colleagues (1984) studied 25 patients with essential hypertension, 20 of whom were not given any antihypertensive treatment (Group A); the other five subjects had to be put on antihypertensive drugs before they could be included in the study (Group B). These patients were then taught how to perform "Shavasana" yoga, which has meditation as its major component. After six months of Shavasana therapy, both mean systolic and mean diastolic pressures in both groups fell to an extent that was statistically significant. Group B patients also experienced a significant reduction in need for antihypertensive drugs. In 65% of group A patients, blood pressure could be controlled with Shavasana only. However, blood pressure rose significantly to pre-Shavasana levels among patients who stopped practicing yoga.

In contrast, Pollack et al. (1977) found no significant change in blood pressure in a group of patients who practiced transcendental meditation (TM) for six months, although there were small reductions in systolic blood pressure and pulse rate early in the trial that disappeared after six months. Likewise, Hafner (1982) studied 21 patients with essential hypertension who were randomly allocated to a group that received eight one-hour sessions of meditation training, to a group that performed meditation plus biofeedback-aided relaxation, or to a no-treatment control group. Although this study found significant falls in systolic and diastolic blood pressures after both training programs, overall reductions in blood pressure were not significantly greater in either program than for the control group. Meditation plus biofeedback-aided relaxation produced falls in diastolic blood pressure earlier in the training program than did meditation alone. While all patients practiced mediation regularly between training sessions, the amount of practice did not correlate with the amount of blood pressure reduction after training.

Leserman et al. (1989) conducted a study in which 27 cardiac surgery patients (mean age 68) were randomly assigned either to a group that received educational information plus training in the relaxation response (RR) or to a group that received educational information only. The experimental group did not achieve lower systolic or diastolic blood pressures than the control group, despite the fact that the RR group experienced significantly greater reductions in tension and anger than the education-only group. Further analyses revealed that the subjects in the RR group had significantly higher "tension" and "anger" scores on admission to the study than did subjects in the education-only group, increasing the likelihood of "regression to the mean" in the former group.

More recent, larger, and better-controlled studies that employed meditation as an intervention for hypertension report more positive results. For example, Sudsuang and colleagues (1991) studied the effects of two months of Dhammakaya Buddhist meditation in 52 male college students and compared their serum cortisol levels, serum total protein, blood pressure, pulse rate, and pulmonary ventilation to those of 30 control group students who were not

taught meditation skills. In the meditation group, the serum cortisol showed a significant decrease ($p < 0.001$) after three weeks, whereas there was no change in cortisol levels among members of the control group. At six weeks, cortisol levels were still significantly lower among those who were able to meditate successfully each time (i.e., achieve a state of tranquility) (group A meditators), whereas cortisol levels among those who did not always meditate successfully (group B meditators) were similar to premeditation levels. In both group A and group B meditators, blood pressure decreased significantly after three weeks ($p < 0.01$). At six weeks, however, group A meditators maintained lower blood pressures, while the inconsistent group B meditators experienced a slight increase in blood pressure (which was still significantly lower than baseline levels).

Another recent study has found similar results for transcendental meditation (TM). Schneider, Staggers, et al. (1995) conducted a randomized, controlled, single-blind trial of TM in a group of 111 African Americans ages 55–85 with mild hypertension (blood pressures equal to or less than 179/104 mm Hg). Subjects were randomized to a group that did three months of TM, a group that did progressive muscle relaxation exercises, or a control group that received only education about lifestyle modification. Investigators found that TM reduced systolic pressure by 10.7 mm Hg ($p < .0003$) and diastolic pressure by 6.4 mm Hg ($p < .00005$); progressive muscle relaxation lowered systolic pressure by 4.7 mm Hg ($p = .0054$) and diastolic pressure by 3.3 mm Hg ($p < .02$). The control group experienced no significant changes in systolic or diastolic blood pressures. The difference in the reductions achieved by the TM group in both systolic blood pressure ($p = .02$) and diastolic blood pressure ($p = .03$) were significantly greater than those in the progressive muscle relaxation group. These findings were confirmed in two follow-up clinical trials (Alexander & Selesnick, 1996; Wenneberg et al., 1997b).

Meditation-based spiritual practices have the potential (at least in the short term) to treat high blood pressure, particularly in cases of mild to moderate hypertension. It remains to be determined, however, whether Western-based spiritual interventions involving petitionary prayer or other religious practices can have similar effects.

Nonlocal Healing.   Nonlocal healing methods typically involve agents who pray for or send positive mental thoughts toward subjects who are located at a distance; agents who are praying for subjects typically don't know the subjects, and subjects don't know that they are being prayed for by agents. The mechanism of effect is unknown. Miller (1982) conducted a double-blind study in which eight "healers" used remote mental healing in attempt to treat 96 hypertensive patients ages 16–60. The healing treatment used by healers involved (a) a relaxation step, (b) attunement with a higher power or infinite being, (c) visualization and/or affirmation of the patient in a state of perfect health, and (d) expression of thanks to God or to the source of all power and energy. Neither doctors nor subjects knew which patients received the mental healing treatments. Normal medical treatment was continued in all cases, and improvement was judged by changes in the diastolic and systolic blood pressure, heart rate, and weight. The subjects in the healer-treated group showed significant improvement in systolic blood pressure compared to the control group, but there was no significant difference in change in diastolic blood pressure, pulse, or weight between the groups. Interestingly, four of the healers achieved a 92.3% improvement rate in their total group of patients, compared with a 73.7% improvement in the control group.

In a later double-bind study of nonlocal healing, Beutler and colleagues (1988) randomly assigned 115 patients with hypertension to receive 15 weeks of paranormal healing by laying on of hands ($n = 40$), paranormal healing at a distance ($n = 37$), or no paranormal healing ($n = 38$). Neither patients nor investigators knew which patients received the paranormal healing and which did not. From week to week patients who received healing at a distance experienced a successively greater lowering of diastolic blood pressure (average 1.9 mm Hg) compared to controls, but on paired comparisons these differences were not statistically significant. After 15 weeks, all three groups had significantly lower systolic and diastolic blood pres-

sure ($p < .05$). However, neither treatment was significantly better than the other treatment or no treatment.

RELIGIOUS COMMUNITIES AS SOURCES OF HYPERTENSION CONTROL

Church-based interventions have long been considered effective in the treatment of chronic illnesses that affect African Americans (Ferdinand, 1997), primarily because of the central role the church plays in African Americans' social support networks. Given the high (40%) rate of hypertension among African Americans, there has been increasing interest in the effectiveness of churches as blood pressure control centers. Most of the studies to date on the efficacy of church-based programs have been conducted in the African American community.

For example, Kumanyika and Charleston (1992) analyzed data from the Baltimore Church High Blood Pressure Program, which offered a behaviorally oriented weight control program that consisted of eight weekly two-hour diet counseling and exercise sessions. The investigators analyzed measurements of pre- and postprogram weight and blood pressure for 184 African American and three white women ages 18–81 years who participated in the program in, 1984–1986 (88 were taking antihypertensive medication, and 99 were not). The mean systolic/diastolic blood pressure (SBP/DBP) reduction during the program was 10/6 mm Hg in the group treated with antihypertensive medication and 5/3 mm Hg in the untreated group ($p < 0.001$ for all pre/post comparisons). Final SBP was <140 mm Hg for 74% of all participants, compared to 52% at the start of the study. Final DBP was <90 mm Hg in 92% compared to 65% at the start. Percentage changes in blood pressure were significantly correlated with percentage changes in weight. At six-month followup ($n = 74$), weight loss during the eight-week program had been maintained or exceeded by 65 percent of participants, and net weight change at eight months from baseline ranged from −28 to +4 pounds. Such church-based programs, then, may help initiate long-term behavioral changes that positively influence weight and blood pressure.

Also evaluating the efficacy of an education intervention for hypertension among people attending African American churches, Smith (1992) trained six registered nurses from six inner-city African American churches to administer the intervention. The intervention, which provided information about the nature of and management strategies for hypertension, was administered to 32 individuals. Data were collected before, immediately after, and three months after the intervention. Smith found a statistically significant difference in knowledge between pre- and postintervention assessments. No significant changes, however, were noted in blood pressure readings or sodium intake.

In a more recent follow-up study, Smith, Merritt, et al. (1997) trained church health educators to teach 97 African American subjects with hypertension how to manage their condition. Using a pretest/posttest design, investigators collected data on knowledge, social support, and blood pressure at baseline (pre), immediately postintervention (post1), and three months postintervention (post2). This study too found a significant increase in knowledge scores on pre- and postintervention assessments. Education, age, and number of years with hypertension explained 49% of the variance in knowledge about hypertension. Systolic blood pressure and mean arterial BP (MAP) decreased significantly from pre to post1 and post2 assessments (SBP, $p < 0.0001$; MAP, $p < 0.0001$). Diastolic blood pressure significantly decreased from pre to post1 measurements ($p = 0.008$) but not from pre to post2 assessments. Finally, the investigators found significant relationships between social support and both DBP and MAP.

Thus, it appears that church-based weight control and blood pressure education programs can have a significant impact on both treatment and prevention of hypertension in African Americans and probably in others as well.

SUMMARY AND CONCLUSIONS

Hypertension is a common, life-threatening disorder that can lead to coronary heart disease, stroke, congestive heart failure, diabetes, and renal dysfunction. Currently, as many as 50 million Americans have high blood pressure, and 2 million new cases are discovered each year. Given the rapidly expanding population of elderly in this country, the prevalence of hypertension may increase dramatically in this century.

Although pharmacologic treatment of hypertension can save lives by lowering blood pressure, concerns persist about the potential side effects of such treatments. Because of these concerns, there is increasing interest in nonpharmacologic approaches to the treatment of hypertension, particularly for people with only mild to moderate disease. Among nonpharmacologic methods for treating hypertension are psychosocial approaches such as increasing social support and reducing stress. There is also growing evidence that involvement in organized religion can not only provide individuals with greater social support but also enhance their sense of self-esteem and help reduce the negative consequences of stress on blood pressure.

Of the 16 studies that have examined the relationship between level of religious involvement and blood pressure, 14 (88%) found lower blood pressure among the more religious (see Appendix); diastolic blood pressures, in particular, are lower among religious than among nonreligious subjects. Furthermore, certain religious practices, such as meditation, may directly lower blood pressure by inducing a relaxed state. Finally, given the success that church-based hypertension intervention programs have had in African American populations, there is reason to explore the effectiveness of such programs in a variety of populations, including Hispanics, Native Americans, and the elderly.

18

Cerebrovascular Disease and the Brain

WEBSTER'S DICTIONARY defines the brain as "the mass of nerve tissue in the cranium of vertebrate animals, an enlarged extension of the spinal cord: it is the main part of the nervous system, the center of thought, and the organ that receives sensory impulses and transmits motor impulses" (from Guralnik, 1980, p. 171). Indeed, the brain is the center of human thought, personality, emotion, feeling, and will and mediates all sensory experience and motor activity. In other words, everything we think, feel, and do has its origins in the brain and the central nervous system. One might even argue that all spiritual experiences are a result of (or at least possible because of) brain activity. For this reason, it is important to explore the relationship among religious beliefs, experiences, and brain function, both normal and abnormal.

In this chapter, we first examine the relationship between religion and cerebrovascular disease. The emphasis is primarily on stroke, given its widespread prevalence and its devastating consequences. We then explore links between temporal lobe epilepsy and religiousness, which leads to a discussion of the relationship between religious experience and brain functioning. This topic is controversial and highly speculative. We balance what could become an excessively reductionistic approach with a more sensitive view that considers alternative, more holistic processes.

CEREBROVASCULAR DISEASE

We begin this section by reviewing the types, causes, and consequences of cerebrovascular disease. Transient ischemic attacks, stroke, and vascular dementia are the most common types of cerebrovascular disorder. These disorders result from (1) a narrowing or other dysfunction of the arteries that supply the brain with nutrients and oxygen, (2) diseases that affect the heart, which pumps blood through these arteries, or (3) other diseases that reduce blood flow to the brain (such as massive blood loss or infection that causes a marked drop in blood pressure). If it persists long enough, the reduction of blood flow to the brain can lead to dysfunction and even death of parts of the brain. This, in turn, can lead to temporary or permanent motor paralysis, sensory dysfunction, or disorders of swallowing, speech, and balance. If blood flow is restored and neurological deficits disappear, then the event is called a *transient ischemic attack*. If blood flow is not restored before death of brain tissue occurs, then the neurological deficits will be permanent; this is called a *stroke*. Brain cells do not regrow or regenerate and once lost are permanently gone. Rehabilitation helps train other areas of the brain to take over the function of brain areas that have died. If a person experiences enough strokes, either large ones or lots of small ones, memory and higher cortical functions, including language abilities, orientation to surroundings, ability to perform motor functions, and personality, can be affected; this is called *dementia*.

Transient Ischemic Attacks (TIAs)

TIAs result from a temporary reduction in blood flow to a part of the brain. A person may become dizzy and fall, lose vision in one eye, develop weakness in an arm or leg, or experience some other temporary loss of function. This dysfunction typically lasts less than 24 hours, after which there is a complete return to normal functioning. TIAs have been reported by 2.7% of men ages 65–69 and 3.6% of men ages 75–79; rates are similar in women (1.6% of women ages 65–69 and 4.1% of women ages 75–79) (American Heart Association, 1998). A TIA is a frightening experience, since it often heralds an impending stroke. The risk of stroke in persons who have had one or more TIAs is increased by about 10 times (American Heart Association, 1999a).

Stroke

By far the most common cerebrovascular disorder is stroke. Strokes are categorized as either ischemic, in which there is reduced blood supply (80% of all strokes), or hemmorrhagic, in which a blood vessel bursts and bleeds into or around the brain. According to the American Heart Association (1999b), 4.4 million Americans alive today have had strokes (almost 2% of the U.S. population). Stroke is the third leading cause of death in the United States, after heart disease and cancer, and results in more than 160,000 deaths per year. Every 53 seconds someone in the United States suffers a stroke, and every three minutes someone dies from one. Data from the National Heart, Lung, and Blood Institute suggest that 600,000 people suffer new or recurrent strokes each year (American Heart Association, 1999b). While the percentage of persons dying from stroke fell by 13.3% between 1986 and 1996, the actual numbers of stroke deaths increased by 6.9%, a result of the increase in the elderly population, which is at high risk for stroke. Almost three-quarters (72%) of people who suffer a stroke are over age 65. The incidence of stroke is almost 20% higher for men than for women. In 1996, the death rates per 100,000 for stroke in the United States were 62.8 for white men and 93.3 for African American men; figures for white and for African American women were 59.0 and 78.9, respectively.

Stroke is the leading cause of long-term disability in the United States and accounts for more than one-half of all patients hospitalized for acute neurological disease (American Heart Association, 1998). Of the more than 4.4 million stroke survivors who are alive today in the United States, about 1.0 million have severe disability as a result of their stroke (American Heart Association, 1999b). Almost three-quarters of stroke survivors cannot work, nearly one-third need help caring for themselves, and more than 15% need to be institutionalized. More than one-third of stroke survivors die within a year of their first stroke, and two-thirds die within twelve years of the event (men have a worse prognosis then women). For persons under age 65 hospitalized with a stroke, the average cost from hospital admission to discharge is about $18,000 for an average length of stay of seven days (American Heart Association, 1998). The cost of care plus loss of earnings due to stroke in the United States was estimated more than 20 years ago at between $7.5 and $11.2 billion per year (Feigenson, 1979), and that figure has risen considerably since then. Thus, stroke is a common, deadly, disabling, and costly illness.

Dementia

After Alzheimer's disease, frequent strokes are the most common cause of dementia (10–20% of all dementias) (Kaufman, 1990). Multi-infarct or vascular dementia is characterized by an incremental loss of ability to perform mental and physical activities caused by repeated small or large strokes that cause the death of increasing amounts of brain tissue. It is often difficult to distinguish dementia caused by Alzheimer's disease from that caused by multiple strokes, and the two are often present in the same individual. When possible, it is important to differentiate these two types of dementias, since control of blood pressure and antiplatelet drugs can help prevent repeated strokes and thus halt the progressive nature of multi-infarct dementia. Dementia places an enormous burden on family members and is the most common cause for nursing home placement in this country.

CAUSES OF CEREBROVASCULAR DISEASE

A number of well-known risk factors exist that increase the likelihood of stroke (American Heart Association, 1999a). Foremost among preventable risk factors is high blood pressure. High blood pressure causes damage to cerebral arteries, leading to narrowing, occlusion, or bursting of these vessels. Preventing or treating high blood pressure (defined as a diastolic blood pressure of 90 or higher or a systolic blood pressure of 140 or higher) can reduce the risk of stroke. Heart disease is the second most important risk factor for stroke and is the most common cause of death among stroke survivors. Heart disease can cause either sustained ventricular arrhythmias or myocardial infarction that lead to stroke by reducing blood flow to the brain or allowing blood clots to form in the heart that embolize to cerebral arteries. Like high blood pressure, heart disease can be

prevented or treated. The next most important risk factor for stroke is cigarette smoking. The nicotine and carbon monoxide in cigarette smoke damage the blood vessels throughout the body, including those that supply blood to the brain. This is perhaps the most preventable of all risk factors.

TIAs are harbingers of impending stroke. Optimizing blood pressure and treating with either antiplatelet drugs (i.e., aspirin) or anticoagulants (i.e., warfarin) can prevent the occurrence of stroke. High red blood cell counts can make blood thicker and increase the risk of clot formation in arteries that supply the brain. While there are hereditary conditions that increase blood cell counts, one of the most common causes is cigarette smoking. Diabetes can increase risk of stroke because of the vascular damage the disease causes. The presence of both diabetes and high blood pressure dramatically increases the likelihood of stroke. Controlling blood sugar through diet, weight control, or medications can help reduce the vascular damage that diabetes causes. Excessive alcohol intake (defined as two drinks or more per day on a regular basis or as binge drinking) can increase blood pressure and/or cause heart damage (alcoholic cardiomyopathy), which may then lead to stroke. Finally, certain types of drug abuse can increase the risk of stroke. Intravenous drug abuse increases the risk of cerebral embolisms that come from clots or infections that form in the heart or peripheral arteries due to drug injection. Cocaine use can also increase the risk of stroke, perhaps because of the accompanying adrenaline surge, which dramatically increases blood pressure.

Other risk factors for stroke that cannot be changed are aging, being male or African American, and heredity. Persons with a family history of stroke must pay particular attention to avoiding some of the preventable risk factors.

PSYCHOLOGICAL FACTORS AND RISK OF CEREBROVASCULAR DISEASE

There is considerable evidence that psychological factors contribute to the development of stroke by their effects on risk factors.

High Blood Pressure

A number of early studies have linked high blood pressure with psychosocial factors such as anxiety, repressed hostility, and psychological stress (Jacob et al., 1977; Weiner, 1979; Brody, 1980; Linden & Feuerstein, 1981; Taylor & Fortman, 1983). Studies among African Americans have shown that stress is directly related to blood pressure, and social support appears to modify the effect (Barnes et al., 1997; Strogatz et al., 1997). Models have been developed to describe how stress affects blood pressure. One of these is a tripartite model with these three components: environmental stressors, individual factors that affect *the perception* of stress (including cognitive appraisal and coping resources), and the individual's genetic susceptibility (Schwartz, Pickering, et al., 1996) (see chapter 17).

Heart Disease

Studies in both animals and humans have shown that brain stimulation can provoke cardiac arrhythmias (Lown et al., 1977) by increasing sympathetic nervous system activity (as is seen in psychological stress). Environmental stresses of a variety of types can injure the heart, lower the threshold for ventricular fibrillation, and provoke malignant ventricular arrhythmias. Numerous studies in humans have documented the relationship among stress, negative psychological states, and heart disease (Lukl, 1971; Raab, 1972; Friedman, 1976; Rosengren, Tibben, et al., 1991; Steenland et al., 1997; Carney, 1998) (see chapter 16).

Cigarette Smoking

A number of studies report that psychological stress increases the desire to smoke cigarettes (Pomerleau & Pomerleau, 1991; Perkins & Gorbe, 1992), increases the likelihood of smoking during adolescence (Byrne et al., 1995), and can be linked to the physical health consequences of smoking (Colby et al., 1994). Coping strategies and social support have been shown to influence smoking behavior by providing alternative behavioral and cognitive outlets for dealing with stress (Sussman et al., 1993; Steptoe et al., 1996) (see chapter 24).

Diabetes

Psychological and social factors can affect the onset and course of diabetes mellitus (Surwit et al., 1992; Wales, 1995). Findings from different clinical investigators working in a variety of settings have documented the disruptive effects of emotional distress on diabetic control (Evans, 1985) and the development of diabetic complications (Lloyd et al., 1991). Neural and hormonal responses to emotional stress induce an energy mobilization response that diabetics (either juvenile onset or adult onset) cannot easily counterregulate (Surwit et al., 1992). For example, Inui et al. (1998) examined diabetic control (as measured by Hemoglobin A1C levels) in those exposed to a life-threatening earthquake that resulted in either severe damage to their homes or death or severe injury to relatives. Earthquake-exposed diabetics had significantly worse diabetic control than the unexposed diabetics. Other studies have shown that effective coping with chronic psychosocial stress can prevent its disruptive effects on glycemic control (Peyrot & McMurry, 1992).

Alcohol or Drug Abuse

High psychosocial stress also predicts alcohol and drug use, particularly among adolescents and teenagers (Schinke et al., 1988; Budd et al., 1985; Bruns & Geist, 1984), an effect that is moderated by coping behaviors (Wills, 1986). The relationship between stress and substance use (particularly benzodiazepines) has also been demonstrated among physicians (Jex et al., 1992), teachers (Fimian et al., 1985), and the elderly (Folkman et al., 1987). Stress may also interfere in the rehabilitation of persons with substance abuse problems, and coping behaviors directed at controlling stress and improving mood are associated with higher rates of abstinence (Hall et al., 1991).

In summary, psychological and social stress can lead to and/or adversely affect the course of hypertension, heart disease, cigarette smoking, diabetes, and alcohol or drug abuse. These influences on major risk factors for cerebrovascular disease may increase vulnerability to stroke. Despite the mounting evidence that points to such an association, there are relatively few published studies on the direct relationship between psychological stress and stroke (Schneck, 1997).

PSYCHOLOGICAL FACTORS AND STROKE

Psychological Stress

House, Dennis, et al. (1990) conducted a retrospective case-control study in which they examined the incidence of stressful events in the lives of 113 stroke survivors during the year preceding their strokes. The researchers then compared their findings to those for 109 age-matched and sex-matched controls. The likelihood that a severe, threatening event occurred in the year prior to stroke was 26% in stroke patients and 13% in controls (odds ratio 2.3, 95% CI 1.1–4.9). The authors concluded, "It therefore appears that severe life events may be one of the determinants of stroke onset" (House, Dennis, et al., 1990, p. 1024).

Rosengren, Tibblin, et al. (1991) conducted a 12-year prospective cohort study of 6,935 men ages 47–55 to examine the relationship between stress and the occurrence of cardiovascular events (myocardial infarction and stroke). During the baseline interview, men were asked whether they had experienced feeling tense, irritable, or filled with anxiety or had sleeping difficulties as a result of conditions at work or at home. Subjects were asked to rate their level of stress on a scale ranging from 1 (never experienced stress) to 6 (permanent stress during the past five years). Men with ratings of 1–4 (low stress, $n = 5,865$) were compared to those with ratings 5–6 (high stress, $n = 1,070$). After controlling for other standard cardiovascular risk factors, the investigators found that high-stress men were 80% more likely to experience a stroke during the 12-year follow-up than were low-stress men (OR 1.80, 95% CI 1.10–2.80).

Siegrist et al. (1992) conducted a 6.5-year prospective study of 416 middle-aged male blue-collar workers to examine cardiovascular and psychosocial risk factors for myocardial infarction and stroke. Multivariate logistic regression was used to examine the effects of hypertension, left ventricular hypertrophy, hyperlipidemia, and psychological stress (measured as chronic work stress) on these outcomes. Chronic stress significantly increased the likelihood of acute stroke or myocardial infarction, independent of other cardiovascular risk factors (OR 2.86–3.57).

Depression and Hopelessness

Colantonio et al. (1992) examined the likelihood of stroke among 2,812 older persons living in New Haven, Connecticut, over the seven-year period between 1982 and 1988. In the bivariate analysis, they found a significant relationship between depressive symptoms as measured by CES-D and likelihood of stroke (OR 1.23, 95% CI 1.05–1.44). When other risk factors for stroke were controlled (e.g., hypertension, prior myocardial infarction, diabetes, or smoking), the association disappeared. Thus, the higher risk of stroke among those with more depressive symptoms could be explained by the relationship between depression and other risk factors for stroke.

In the Kuopio Ischemic Heart Disease Risk Factor Study, Everson, Kaplan, et al. (1997) examined 942 middle-aged men in eastern Finland over a four-year period to determine the relationship between hopelessness and the progression of carotid atherosclerosis as measured by intima-media thickening of arteries that supply blood to the brain (a major cause of stroke). Researchers found that men who felt hopeless or felt like failures (high levels of despair) had a 20% greater measurable increase in atherosclerosis over four years. This is the same level of risk difference seen in a pack-a-day cigarette smoker and a nonsmoker. In a later report, these investigators documented an increased risk of stroke during a 29-year follow-up among those who were depressed (Everson, Roberts, et al., 1998). Depression has also been associated with greater mortality following stroke (Morris, Robinson, et al., 1993).

Thus, psychological stress and poor mental health not only are associated with risk factors for stroke (high blood pressure, heart disease, diabetes, cigarette smoking, and substance abuse) but also predict the occurrence of stroke when this relationship is examined directly. In a majority of these studies, the relationship between psychological stress and stroke persists even after other cardiovascular risk factors are controlled.

PLAUSIBLE REASONS FOR A RELIGION-STROKE RELATIONSHIP

Given the link among psychological stress, risk factors for stroke, and the occurrence of stroke, it is possible that a relationship between religious beliefs and activities and stroke may also exist. The reasons for this hypothesized relationship are the following:

- Religious beliefs and activities are associated with lower blood pressure.
- Religious beliefs and activities are associated with less CAD.
- Religious beliefs and activities are associated with lower rates of cigarette smoking.
- Religious beliefs and activities are associated with lower rates of alcohol and drug use.
- Religious beliefs and activities are associated with improved coping skills and better adjustment to stress.
- Religious beliefs and activities are associated with lower rates of anxiety.
- Religious beliefs and activities are associated with less depression and less hopelessness.

Thus, not only are religious beliefs and practices associated with fewer biological risk factors for stroke; they may also reduce psychological stress, depression, and other negative mental health states that are predictors of stroke. Consequently, we might expect an inverse relationship between religion and stroke. To our knowledge, however, only six published studies have examined this relationship.

RELIGION AND CEREBROVASCULAR DISEASE

Wassersug (1989) describes the fascinating case of an 86-year-old retired barber from an Italian Catholic family in Massachusetts. The patient suffered a massive stroke that left him with a sudden, severe right hemiplegia, making him completely bedridden and unable to move his right arm or right leg. Neurological consultation determined that, because of the patient's age and history of hypertension, there was little or no chance for neurological recovery. He and his wife spoke frequently of God during the hospitalization, convinced that God would help them. On the fifth day of hospitalization, the patient greeted his doctor with excitement, saying that he had just dreamed the night before that an angel dressed as a nurse stood at the foot of his bed and told him that he would be able to move his arm and leg when he awoke. The patient easily raised his right arm and right leg off the bed. This is the only case we could locate in the literature of a religious healing involving a stroke deficit.

Colantonio et al. (1992) examined the effects of religious factors on new-onset stroke. This is the only study that has examined the relationship between level of religiousness and stroke. During a seven-year follow-up of 2,812 persons age 65 or over living in New Haven, Connecticut, investigators identified 167 new cases of stroke. Bivariate Cox regression analysis determined that high religious attendance (defined as attending once or twice per year or more) was a significant predictor of fewer strokes (0.86, 95% CI 0.79–0.94, $p < .001$). In other words, those who attended religious services at any frequency ($n = 1,921$) were 14% less likely to have a stroke than those who never or almost never attended ($n = 637$). Religion as a source of strength (a single item rated on a 0–2 scale) and self-rated religiosity (single item on 0–3 scale) were unrelated to stroke, although there were weak trends in the expected direction. However, when hypertension, myocardial infarction, diabetes, and smoking were controlled in a multivariate logistic regression model, the significant inverse relationship between attendance and stroke disappeared. In other words, the investigators found that risk factors for stroke alone explained the relationship between religion and stroke. As we have seen, religious attendance may decrease the risk of stroke by reducing blood pressure, discouraging cigarette smoking, and lowering the risk or severity of diabetes and myocardial infarction. Thus, when investigators find that the relationship between religion and stroke disappears after controlling for risk factors that mediate the relationship, they cannot conclude that there is no relationship between religion and stroke, only that they have identified the mechanism of the effect.

Only five other published studies have examined the relationship between religion and stroke, and they focus primarily on religious affiliation, not religiousness. Friedman and Hellerstein (1968) examined cardiovascular risk factors between Jewish and non-Jewish attorneys in Cleveland and Detroit. They found that Jews ($n = 331$) were significantly less likely to have a family history of stroke than were non-Jews ($n = 1,414$) (10.7% vs. 15.2%, $p < .05$) (although Jews were more likely to have a family history of diabetes, 12.9% vs. 8.3%, $p < .01$).

Jarvis (1977) studied causes of mortality among Mormons in Alberta, Canada, between 1967 and 1975. The sample consisted of 1,169 persons who died, out of a base population of 31,085. The standardized mortality ratio (standardized by age) for cerebrovascular disease in Mormon men was significantly lower than for non-Mormons (SMR 0.71, $p < .05$); in other words, Mormon men were 29% less likely to die of cerebrovascular disease than were other men in Canada. No reduced risk was found for Mormon women.

Lyon, Bishop, et al. (1981) compared mortality rates from cerebrovascular disease (CBVD) in Utah with those for the rest of the United States and found the rates of CBVD in Utah to be significantly below the U.S. average. However, when they compared CBVD rates for Mormons and non-Mormons in Utah between 1968 and 1971, they found no significant difference between the two groups. Unlike the Jarvik study, this study suggests that Mormon affiliation is unrelated to CBVD.

Abu-Zeid et al. (1975) examined predictors of new-onset stroke that occurred between January 1970 and June 1971 in Manitoba, Canada, among 700,000 residents ages 20–64 years. During that time there were 434 new strokes. Among the significant predictors of stroke was religious affiliation. Incidence of stroke was highest among Jews, intermediate in Protestants and Catholics, and lowest among Mennonites, Hutterites, and other minority groups ($p < .025$, uncontrolled). The authors noted that Mennonites and Hutterites are conservative groups that discourage unhealthy diets, smoking, and drinking, which might help explain their low risk.

Finally, Phillips, Kuzma, and colleagues (1980) examined causes of mortality in a 16-year prospective cohort study of 22,940 California SDAs and a 12-year prospective study of 112,726 California non-SDAs. All the subjects were white and over age 35. The researchers compared mortality ratios for the two groups and found that the mortality ratio for cerebrovascular disease for SDAs was 0.72 for men and 0.82 for women (both $p < .01$). In other words, SDA men were 28% less likely to die of stroke than were non-SDA men, and SDA women were 18% less likely to die of stroke than were non-SDA women.

In summary, some evidence links religiousness to lower rates of cerebrovascular disease and stroke. The evidence is weak and somewhat conflicting, however, and clearly more research is needed to examine this association. Studies that employ more detailed and sophisticated measures of the religious variable in prospective studies are particularly needed.

RELIGION AND ALZHEIMER'S DISEASE

For years scientists have been aware of an association between depression and Alzheimer's disease. There is evidence that depression, particularly when it occurs early in life, may be a risk factor for the disease. For example, Spect et al. (1995) evaluated the strengths of the association between reported history of depression and onset of Alzheimer's disease in a large community-based sample of older persons. While they found no increased risk for Alzheimer's in those who experienced depression within 10 years of the onset of the dementia, they did find an association between Alzheimer's and depressive episodes that occurred more than 10 years before the disease appeared. Other studies have shown increased risk of Alzheimer's disease among persons who experience depression *within* 10 years of the onset of Alzheimer's symptoms (Jorm et al., 1991). Thus, any coping behavior (including religion) that reduces the risk of depression in early or later life may perhaps forestall the development of this dreaded disease.

A neuroendocrine mechanism may help explain why depression is a risk factor for Alzheimer's disease. Because it activates the hypothalamic-pituitary-adrenal axis, depression is associated with an increase in the level of blood cortisol. Increased levels of blood cortisol have now been found to lower the threshold for age-associated degeneration of hippocampal pyramidal neurons in aged rats (Sapolsky, Krey, et al., 1985; Sapolsky, 1992, 1996; Chan et al., 1996). In humans, these hippocampal neurons are severely affected in Alzheimer's disease. Studies have also shown that high plasma cortisol levels are associated with cognitive decline in older persons without dementia (Lupien et al., 1994). Repeated stress may increase cortisol that then causes atrophy of the dendrites of pyramidal neurons in the hippocampus. This involves the effects of cortisol and of excitatory amino acid neurotransmitters on neurons both during and after stress (McEwen, Albeck, et al., 1995). Magnetic resonance imaging (MRI) has demonstrated a link between atrophy of the hippocampus and stress-related illnesses such as depressive disorder and posttraumatic stress disorder (Sapolsky, 1996; McEwen & Magarinos, 1997).

Unfortunately, there have been no good epidemiological studies examining the association between prevalence or onset of Alzheimer's disease and religious beliefs or activities during earlier life. Future studies will need to consider the confounding that occurs when persons with Alzheimer's-related memory problems turn to religion as they attempt to cope with this frightening illness (Stolley & Koenig, 1995; Whitlatch et al., 1992). Patients' turning to religion when symptoms arise could disguise an inverse relationship between religiousness and Alzheimer's disease. On the other hand, Alzheimer's disease may reduce a person's capacity to tap into religious resources, given that religious beliefs are largely cognitive in nature, thus creating an artificial inverse relationship between the two (Koenig, 1994a).

BRAIN FUNCTIONS RESPONSIBLE FOR RELIGIOUS EXPERIENCE

In this section, we review studies that have attempted to link religious and spiritual experiences to activity in specific regions of the brain. This work reflects a broader area of research that attempts to explain spiritual and religious experiences in terms of neurological processes that involve the central and the autonomic nervous systems. Electroencephalograms (EEGs) and, more recently, Positive Emission Tomography (PET) and Single Photon Emission Computed Tomography (SPECT) have been used to better study and visualize brain activity during spiritual states. Quantitative MRI-PET imagery and functional MRI (fMRI) promise to provide still further resolution and quantification of brain functioning during spiritual experiences.

Some see progress in the neurosciences as a threat to the validity of many long-held religious beliefs and experiences (Bennett, 1998). According to Saver and Rabin (1997), however, "Determining the neural substrate of any of these states does not automatically lessen or demean their spiritual significance. The external reality of religious percepts is neither confirmed nor disconfirmed by establishing brain correlates of religious experience. Indeed it has been argued that demonstrating the existence of a neural apparatus sustaining religious experience can reinforce belief because it provides evidence that a higher power has so constructing humans as to possess the capacity to experience the divine" (p. 498).

D'Aquili and Newberg (1993) were among the first to comprehensively describe a neuropsychological model for spiritual or mystical states, and they have recently refined and expanded this model (Newberg & d'Aquili, 1998). These investigators trace spiritual experiences to the activation of sympathetic and parasympathetic nervous systems, which, together with the limbic system, facilitate or inhibit discrete areas of the brain responsible for mental experience.

Much research has attempted to link religiousness to activity in the temporal lobes. The temporal lobes are part of the limbic system, that part of the brain that helps generate and modulate feelings and emotions, and influences functions related to memory, sexual activity, and aggression. The limbic system evolved from subcortical brain structures and in humans has extensive connections with the cerebral cortex, that part of the brain which is said to separate human beings from other animals and is the source of much of our thought, language, art, and culture. There are also extensive connections between the limbic system and the autonomic nervous system, which, as noted earlier, may provide an organic substrate for spiritual experience (d'Aquili & Newberg, 1993).

Temporal Lobe: The "God Module?"

What scientific evidence supports the hypothesis that the temporal lobes are involved in religious or spiritual experience? Dewhurst and Beard (1970) performed several early studies of temporal lobe epilepsy (TLE), focusing on its relationship to sudden religious conversion. While religiosity in the epileptic has been recognized since Esquirol (1838), Dewhurst and Beard were the first to provide a detailed description of six conversion experiences associated with TLE. These six conversion experiences were selected out of 26 cases that involved mystical delusional experiences in a group of 69 patients with schizophrenic-like psychoses of epilepsy. As we have noted in (chapter 10), up to 50% of psychotic patients without epilepsy have religious delusions, so such a finding is not unexpected. Dewhurst and Beard go on to attribute the visions of St. Teresa, as well as the conversions of several other famous religious persons, to temporal lobe epilepsy. This study provides little evidence for a unique association between religious experience and TLE that is independent of psychiatric illness.

Waxman and Geshwind (1975) reviewed the published literature to identify an interictal behavioral syndrome characteristic of TLE. The only data provided in this article are three case reports. The distinct syndrome of interictal behavior described by these investigators included changes in sexual behavior and religiosity and a tendency toward extensive and, in some cases, compulsive writing and drawing. Among the three cases, only one patient was devoutly religious. She experienced multiple religious conversions and had a diagnosis of acute schizophrenia. In the other two cases, religion was only a marginal part of the subjects' lives.

Bear and Fedio (1977) conducted a case-control study of 48 patients separated into four groups in order to examine interictal behavior in TLE. Twenty-seven cases with TLE (15 with right TLE, 12 with left TLE) were "chosen" from five general epilepsy clinics. Twelve normal adults, comparable in age, education, geographical distribution, and socioeconomic status (all were employees of the National Institutes of Health or a state agency) and nine patients with neuromuscular disorders were selected as controls. Important sociodemographic differences were present between the groups; in particular, the normal controls were better educated than the patient groups ($p < .05$). Subjects completed the Bear-Fedio Personal Behavior Inventory, which includes items on religiosity, philosophical interests, and hypermoralism. Religiosity was defined as "holding deep religious beliefs, often idiosyncratic; multiple conversions, cosmic consciousness" (Bear et al., 1982, p. 482). In addition, subjects were rated "objectively" along the same dimensions by "a long-time observer."

According to the self-ratings, epileptic patients exhibited significantly greater religiosity than nonepileptics ($p < .001$); no differences were found between those with left TLE and those with right TLE. According to the observer ratings, the epileptic patients also had significantly greater religiosity than the nonepileptics ($p < .01$) (again without left vs. right TLE differences). Note, however, that one-third of the TLE group ($n = 9$) had a history of psychiatric hospitalization for thought disorder or affective disorder, whereas none of the control subjects had psychiatric histories. Thus, these results could have been confounded by religious delusions associated with chronic mental illness. Finally, the researchers could not exclude the possibility that the TLEs were more likely to gravitate toward religion because of other character traits, such as obsessionalism, emotionality, or hypermoralism.

In a later study, Bear et al. (1982) again examined the interictal behavior of hospitalized patients with TLE. Research assistants randomly selected subjects for the study from patients who were receiving EEGs at McLean Psychiatric Hospital. All the subjects were between the ages of 15 and 69, and this time both cases and controls were all psychiatric patients. Ten subjects were assigned to each of five groups: 10 patients with TLE (average 1.5 prior psychiatric hospitalization), 10 other epileptics (average 1.2 prior psychiatric hospitalizations), 10 schizophrenics with normal EEGs (average 1.3 prior psychiatric hospitalizations), 10 primary affective disorders (primarily bipolar type, average 1.5 prior psychiatric hospitalizations), and 10 aggressive character disorders (primarily borderline personality disorder, average 1.1 prior psychiatric hospitalizations). Subjects underwent structured interviews by two psychiatric interviewers who were unaware of the subject's assigned group. The interviewers then rated the patients on 14 general character traits. The researchers found that patients with TLE were higher on 13 of 14 character traits (including religiosity) than were the patients in the other four groups. Specifically, patients with TLE were significantly more religious than the character-disordered group ($p < .001$), the affective disorder group ($p < .05$), and the other seizures group ($p < .05$), but they were not more religious than the schizophrenic group.

In order to eliminate the possible confounding effects of psychiatric disorder, Sensky, Wilson, et al. (1984) surveyed 179 patients at neurological clinics in three London teaching hospitals. Forty-two patients were excluded because they had mental disorders or histories of psychiatric illness or substance abuse or were without EEG-confirmed epilepsy. The remaining 137 subjects were divided into groups with primary generalized epilepsy ($n = 58$), migraine ($n = 50$), and temporal lobe epilepsy ($n = 29$). Assessment included questions on religious practices, mystical experiences, and religiousness. Temporal lobe epileptics did not score significantly higher than other groups on religious measures.

Persinger (1984) surveyed 150 first-year psychology students to determine whether religious experiences were correlated with temporal lobe characteristics. Two studies were conducted. Study 1 included 108 students (56% women, 61% single, 50% Catholic) who were attending an evening course, and Study 2 included 42 students (69% women, 60% single, 45% Catholic) who were attending a day course. Students completed a Personal Philosophy Inventory test (PPI) that included questions on religious attendance, religious experiences (meditation), and items from the MMPI. Four groups were formed: (1) subjects who were not attending religious services and who had not had religious experiences ($n = 52$); (2) subjects who were not attending religious services but who did have religious experiences ($n = 8$); (3) subjects who attended religious services regularly but who did not have religious experiences ($n = 33$), and (4) subjects who attended regularly and who also had religious experiences ($n = 15$). Forty-three of the 140 items on the PPI scale were "temporal lobe relevant," on the basis of the experiences of persons with temporal lobe activity (either induced, seizure related, or tumor related). Both studies found that persons who reported religious experiences also reported more symptoms of temporal lobe activity. The reasoning here is somewhat circular, however, as religious subjects were more likely to score high on temporal lobe activity that was itself defined at least partly in terms of religious, spiritual, and paranormal experiences.

Fedio (1986) reviewed the previous research on interictal personality traits of patients with TLE. Fedio's report was more balanced in his presentation than were previous reports, and it placed less emphasis on religious characteristics. He concluded that left TLEs may be more prone to psychogenic symptoms than right TLEs and suggested that future studies compare religious interests before and after temporal lobe surgery.

In the most recent published report on this topic, Tucker et al. (1987) studied 76 cases with TLE (51 left TLEs and 25 right TLEs), comparing them to 58 control subjects (31 with primary generalized seizures and 27 with pseudoseizures). This is the largest sample of TLEs studied to date. All subjects were neurological patients, not psychiatric patients as in most previous studies. Researchers administered the MMPI, which included 12 items on religion that assessed degree of religious fundamentalism, religious belief, and religious activity. No difference in religiosity between cases and controls were found.

The Ramachandran Study

In a poster session presented at the annual meeting of the Society of Neurosciences, Ramachandran et al. (1997) described a study that compared skin conduction responses (SCRs) in three groups of people: three cases with temporal lobe epilepsy, 10 normal highly religious people, and eight normal people not screened for religiosity. The three TLE cases were selected on the basis of their responses to the Bear-Fedio (1977) Personal Inventory and Personal Behavior Survey, which is designed to diagnose the interictal behavior syndrome of TLE. Recall that this inventory includes items that assess religiousness and mystical states, possibly biasing the selection of cases in favor of those with religious and spiritual proclivities. The TLE cases and the controls read four categories of words (neutral, religious, sexual, and violent), and their SCRs were recorded. The results indicated that the eight normal subjects were highly responsive to sexual items but were minimally responsive to violent or religious words. Two of the three TLE cases were highly responsive to religious words (to the same extent as the highly religious subjects) but were minimally responsive to violent or sexual words. The third TLE case demonstrated a minimal response to sexual items, moderate response to religious items, and the greatest response to violent words.

On the basis of these findings, the investigators concluded, "These results clearly demonstrate that in TLE patients there can be selective enhancement and reduction of SCRs to very specific categories of stimuli; our patients exhibited large responses to words pertaining to religion and God with an actual decrement in responsivity to other categories that would ordinarily be evocative to normal people, such as to sexually loaded words" (Ramachandran et al., 1997). (Note, however, that temporal lobe dysfunction—usually the cause of TLE—is often characterized by decreased libido and hyposexuality during interictal periods [Kaufman, 1990, p. 332].) The researchers went on to say that a "God module" in the temporal lobes may have evolved to "encourage tribe loyalty and conformist behavior." Needless to say, this is a rather broad interpretation of the findings, which are suspect with regard to methodology and statistical significance.

Alternative Hypotheses

Rather than arising from specific areas like the temporal lobes, religious or spiritual experience may result from whole brain activity that requires the working together of many different parts of the brain (e.g., cerebral cortex, limbic system, thalamus) and the autonomic nervous system in a way similar to that described by Newberg and d'Aquili. For example, Herzog et al. (1990–1991) used PET scanning to examine regional cerebral metabolic rates during normal states and Yoga meditation in eight subjects. The investigators found that no single area, but rather the whole brain, was activated during meditation.

Another alternative hypothesis is that religious and spiritual experiences are epiphenomena that occur separate from brain or other neurological substrate. This is called a "super-empirical" explanation since it relies on the existence and functioning of such energies that have not yet been empirically verified to the satisfaction of mainstream science (Levin, 1996). A related third hypothesis is based on a concept called "emergence"—the notion that extreme complexity in biological systems can lead to a higher order of experience that cannot be explained by study of first-level phenomena (Davies, 1995). A fourth possibility is that religious or spiritual experiences are supernatural and cannot be examined using the tools of science, which are designed to study natural phenomena (an untestable hypothesis).

Concerns about Reductionism

As we attempt to explain the biological basis for religious and spiritual experiences, it is possible to become so reductionistic as to view these phenomena as simply a result of the workings of neurons and neural circuits. Thus, one might conclude that there is nothing more to spirituality than a simple biological process that has evolved through the many years of human history. From a scientific standpoint, as we understand science today, this may indeed be true. Still, there may be something more here than a study of individual parts of the whole might suggest. For example, while it is certainly true, from a biological reductionistic viewpoint, that a mother is simply a conglomeration of cells made up of atoms and molecules, she is also more than that to her husband and children. In other words, there is more to a mother than simply the biological parts that make up her body and define her as a female *Homo sapien*. The same general principle may hold true for our study of religious and spiritual experience. Even if we are able to completely explain such experiences in terms of biological processes (which is overwhelmingly likely in the future), something may be operating at a different level of organization, one that supersedes biology.

SUMMARY AND CONCLUSIONS

We have described the different types of cerebrovascular disease, examined the consequences of stroke in terms of disability and eco-nomic cost, and explored risk factors that predispose individuals to this devastating illness. We have also seen that risk factors for stroke (hypertension, heart disease, cigarette smoking, diabetes, and alcohol and drug use) are substantially influenced by psychological stress and negative mental states such as depression and hopelessness. Because religious beliefs and practices help persons cope better with stress and thereby reduce depression and anxiety, we hypothesized that greater religiousness might also help prevent stroke. Only a couple of studies have directly examined the relationship between religion and stroke, and only one study has examined the relationship between religiousness and stroke. While the results are weakly supportive of our general hypothesis, it is clear that further research is necessary.

In the second part of this chapter, we reviewed research that examines the neurological basis for religious and spiritual experience. While some reports suggest an association between temporal lobe epilepsy and religious experience, the evidence is not strong, is hampered by poor study methodology, and has been contradicted by other, carefully designed investigations. While it is likely that the temporal lobes may give rise to mystical-like emotional experiences, there are alternative explanations for religious and spiritual experiences. Alternative explanations understand such experiences as "whole brain" phenomena, as "emergent" phenomena, as "epiphenomena" (superempirical phenomena), or as supernatural occurrences not capable of being studied with the tools of natural science.

19

Immune System Dysfunction

THE IMMUNE SYSTEM IS THE body's defense against outside invaders (e.g., viruses, bacteria, fungi, parasites) and internal errors (e.g., malignant transformation). In this chapter, we explore relationships between religious beliefs and practices and immune system functioning. We examine the organs and cellular components that make up the immune system; the role and function of these components; the biological, psychological, and social factors that affect immune function; and the physical health consequences that result from impaired immunity. Second, we hypothesize how religion might influence the immune system and review the limited research that has examined the link between religious activity and immune functioning.

COMPONENTS OF THE IMMUNE SYSTEM

The immune system is made up of solid lymph organs, of vessel-like channels (lymphatics) that contain lymph fluid, and of immune cells that circulate in lymph fluid, tissues, and blood (Guyton, 1971; Gilliland, 1980).

Solid Organs

The solid organs of the immune system produce and store the circulating immune cells. Organs include the thymus, spleen, lymph nodes, and, to some degree, the liver and the bone marrow. In the newborn, the *thymus* is a large organ that lies just beneath the sternum (or breast bone) of the anterior chest. It stimulates the development of lymphocytes and other cellular components of the lymphatic system. If the thymus is removed early in life, no immune system will develop. In the adult, the thymus shrinks to a small, almost undetectable size. The *spleen* is a spongy, highly vascular organ that lies under the rib cage on the left side of the body. It acts as a large sieve that filters and screens the blood that passes through it of abnormal blood cells, bacteria, parasites and other outside organisms.

The spleen is also made up of a large number of lymphocytes and plasma cells. In many infections, the spleen enlarges in the same way that the lymph nodes enlarge in order to perform their cleansing function.

Lymph nodes are small, marble-size solid collections of lymphocytes and other cells located intermittently along the lymphatic channels. Lymph fluid (which is largely blood serum without red blood cells) must pass through lymph node sinuses lined with cells that engulf and destroy particles and foreign proteins, preventing their dissemination throughout the body. Other lymphoid tissue is found along the gastrointestinal tract (tonsils, Peyer's patches, and the appendix).

Lymphatics

The lymphatic system consists of both the solid organs of the immune system and a *system of porous channels* (lymphatics) through which lymph fluid flows from the body's intercellular spaces back into the blood stream. The lymphatics are thin-walled vessels, comparable to blood veins but not as well defined, that extend throughout the body and carry proteins and other particulate matter away from tissue spaces. This is such an important function that without this system, humans would die within twenty-four hours. While most of the fluid that filters out through the arterial capillaries is reabsorbed into the venous capillaries, about one-tenth of this fluid enters lymphatic capillaries and returns to the blood through the lymphatics, rather than through the venous system. No particulate matter (even large molecules) can be directly absorbed through the venous capillaries into the blood stream. Bacteria and other foreign organisms must first pass through the lymphatics in order to get into the blood.

If foreign organisms such as viruses or bacteria escape the lymphatics and make their way into the blood circulation, white blood cells can destroy these invaders. There are also immune cells located in the liver and bone marrow that are capable of engulfing and destroying bacteria, viruses, and other particles and of producing immune proteins to facilitate this process.

Cellular Components and Their Products

The cells in the immune system derive from primordial cells called "reticulum" cells. White blood cells (granulocytes, monocytes, and lymphocytes), tissue histiocytes, and plasma cells all develop from reticulum cells. White blood cells are mobile units that quickly circulate throughout the blood and lymphatics to areas of inflammation, destroying any infectious agent they come into contact with. White blood cells formed in the bone marrow are called granulocytes (neutrophils, eosinophils, and basophils); white blood cells formed in the lymph nodes are called lymphocytes and monocytes. Granulocytes and monocytes surround and consume invading organisms. Each granulocyte (with a life span of 2–12 hours) is capable of ingesting and killing five to 25 bacteria before it dies. Monocytes live much longer than granulocytes, and each monocyte can engulf as many as 100 bacteria before dying. Macrophages are large phagocytic cells derived primarily from monocytes and are particularly important in chronic infection because they can remove large particles and necrotic debris. With chronic infections, the concentration of monocytes in the blood can increase from 5% of all white blood cells to as high as 30%–50%.

Lymphocytes can live anywhere between 100 and 300 days. They consist of B cells and T cells. B cells make up about 10–15% of lymphocytes that circulate in the blood, 50% of lymphocytes in the spleen, and 10% of lymphocytes in the bone marrow (Haynes & Fauci, 1998). When a B cell (or B lymphocyte) sees a foreign invader or "antigen," it begins replicating and turns into a plasma cell. Plasma cells are responsible for making antibodies (also called immunoglobulins) that circulate and attach to antigens. These antibodies neutralize toxins, deactivate foreign proteins and viruses, and cause bacteria to stick together, making it easier for other immune cells to destroy them. This process is called *humoral immunity*. The most common types of immunoglobulins are IgG (present in serum at a concentration of 1200 mg/100 ml), IgA (280 mg/100 ml), and IgM (100 mg/100 ml).

T cells make up about 70–80% of lymphocytes that circulate in blood, 90% of thoracic duct lymphocytes, 30–40% of lymph node cells, and 20–30% of spleen lymphoid cells (Haynes & Fauci, 1998). T cells (or T lymphocytes) are the main effectors of *cell-mediated immunity*, or delayed hypersensitivity. Upon exposure to the foreign antigen, T cells begin to proliferate and become sensitized to the antigen. T cells are subdivided into T-helper cells, T-suppressor cells, and T-killer cells. T-helper cells act to stimulate B cell activity (formation of plasma cells and production of antibodies). T-suppressor cells suppress B cells and cell-mediated immune responses, resulting in reduced antibody production and T-killer-cell activity. Responding to antibodies on the surface of tumor cells or bacteria, T-killer cells (also called cytotoxic T cells, large granular lymphocytes, or natural killer [NK] cells) directly attack and destroy them by secretion of lymphokines and cytotoxic agents. Lymphokines initiate cell-mediated immunity reactions by activating other immune cells (e.g., macrophages). Approximately 5–10% of peripheral blood lymphocytes are T-killer cells.

Cytokines are soluble proteins produced by immune cells. These proteins are critical for normal immune system function and coordinate many immune activities. Cytokines influence gene activation that result in cellular growth and differentiation, thereby having effects on regulation of immune responses and disease processes. Almost 30 different kinds of cytokines have now been identified and their molecular structure sequenced. They are divided into three major groups: (1) immunoregulatory cytokines (e.g., interleukin-2 [IL-2], IL-4), (2) proinflammatory cytokines (e.g., IL-1, tumor necrosis factor, IL-6, IL-8), and (3) cytokines that regulate immune cell growth and maturation (e.g., IL-3, IL-7) (Haynes & Fauci, 1998). Cytokines have multiple effects throughout the body as they circulate in the blood, including fever, lethargy, decreased appetite, and stimulation of cortisol production through activation of the hypothalamic-pituitary-adrenal axis (Naitoh et al., 1988). Psychological stress itself is a strong inducer of cytokine production (Bianchi et al., 1991).

IMMUNE RESPONSE

There are two kinds of immune responses: immediate and delayed. The immediate response system, which begins within minutes of exposure to the antigen, results in acute inflammation (swelling, redness, and increased warmth or fever). Granulocytes, NK cells, monocytes, and macrophages rapidly travel to the site and begin engulfing the foreign material and other necrotic particles and activate and enable lymphocytes involved in the delayed immune response.

The delayed response system usually takes several days or longer to develop. It is characterized by development of "memory" for the foreign invader or antigen, so that subsequent exposure to the foreign antigen will result in a more rapid and vigorous response. When a foreign substance is detected in the body, B cells transform into plasma cells and begin producing antibodies. The antibodies attach to other immune cells, activating them, and to the foreign antigens themselves, making them easier to destroy. T cells proliferate and become sensitized, initiating the cell-mediated immune response that includes the production of natural killer T cells capable of directly destroying bacteria, tumor cells, and other target organisms. In addition, T cells release lymphokines that stimulate other immune cells to actively disable these antigens.

Immune cells and their interactions with foreign antigens produce many other products, including cytokines, tumor necrosis factor, and other mediators of the inflammatory response. The end result is that the foreign substance is destroyed or deactivated and the breakdown products are removed. The immune response occurs not only in response to outside invaders such as viruses, bacteria, and parasites but also to abnormal cells that arise within the body and are recognized as foreign. In chapter 20, we discuss the theory of immune surveillance as it relates to the development of malignancy.

TESTS OF IMMUNE SYSTEM FUNCTIONING

Scientists employ a number of tests to measure the function of different components of the immune system:

Tests of Immune System Function

Complete blood count with differential (neutrophils, lymphocytes, monocytes, eosinophils)

Serum levels of immunoglobulins (IgM, IgG, IgA, IgD, IgE)

Quantification of T cells, B cells, NK cells

T cell function—delayed hypersensitivity to skin tests (e.g., TB skin tests, Candida)

T cell function—proliferative response to mitogens (e.g., concanavalin A, phytohemaglutanin)

T cell function—cytokine production

B cell function—antibodies to common viruses (e.g., influenza, rubella)

B cell function—antibodies to bacterial toxins (e.g., diphtheria, tetanus)

B cell function—response to immunization with tetanus toxoid or other antigens

B cell function—IgG subclass quantification

Complement—CH_{50}, C3, C4, etc., assays

Phagocyte function—reduction of nitroblue tetrazolium

Phagocyte function—chemotaxis assays

Phagocyte function—bacteriacidal activity (Haynes & Fauci, 1998)

These tests assess the number, activity and products of the three major immune cell types: granulocytes/phagocytes, T lymphocytes, and B lymphocytes. Number of granulocytes in peripheral blood may reflect the body's capacity to deal with bacterial and viral infections. Lymphocytes proliferate in response to a variety of stimulants or mitogens, and the extent to which they do so provides a measure of lymphocyte activity and function. Number and activity of NK cells, the specialized T lymphocytes that seek out and destroy neoplastic cells and infectious agents, is another measure of cell-mediated immunity. Humoral immunity can be measured by serum immunoglobulin levels and by the number of functioning B cells and plasma cells. Blood levels of certain cytokines, such as interleukin-6, can also be assessed and used as an indicator of immune system functioning.

BIOLOGICAL FACTORS INFLUENCING THE IMMUNE SYSTEM

A number of biological factors are known to affect the immune system. These include hereditary influences, exposure to toxins, infectious diseases (like HIV infection), medications, alcohol, cigarette smoking, and marijuana use (Gilliland, 1980; *Merck Manual of Geriatrics*, 1995).

Hereditary Influences

Genetic defects can result in immunodeficiency syndromes characterized by unusual susceptibility to infection, autoimmune diseases, and lymphatic cancers. Persons who have defects in B cells (humoral immunity) may have recurrent bacterial infections. Those who have defects in T cells (cell-mediated immunity) may be unusually susceptible to viral and fungal infections.

Exposure to Toxins

Benzenes are regularly contained in volatile solvents, such as paint removers, kerosene, and degreasers, that are available commercially and domestically. Benzenes can cause aplastic anemia that, among other defects, is associated with greatly reduced number of granulocytes, which impairs the body's response to bacterial infection.

Infection

Infection with certain viruses can weaken the immune system. For example, infection with the human immunodeficiency virus (HIV) is responsible for the acquired immunodeficiency syndrome (AIDS). HIV infects a subset of helper/inducer T cells characterized by CD4 transmembrane proteins. This loss of critically important helper T cells results in significant immune system dysfunction and consequent susceptibility to life-threatening infections such as pneumocystis carinii pneumonia, fungal meningitis, disseminated candidiasis, encephalitis, and cytomegalovirus infection and to neoplasms such as Kaposi's sarcoma (Merck, 1995).

Prescription Drugs

A number of medications can impair immune function. Perhaps the most widely used drugs that affect the immune system are the corticosteroids. Corticosteroids impair wound healing and predispose to infection. In the laboratory, steroids decrease the activity of granulocytes, reduce the killing of bacteria by monocytes, and interfere with other cell-mediated immune responses. Steroids induce such a broad defect in the body's immune mechanisms that it makes the individual vulnerable to both common and unusual infections. Other, less frequently used drugs that suppress the immune system include cyclophosphamide, chorambucil, and methotrexate (Gilliland, 1980).

Alcohol

Studies in humans (Lundy et al., 1975; Bomalaski & Phair, 1982; MacGregor, 1986) and animals (Caren et al., 1983; Alcohol Effects, 1993) have documented the ways that alcohol affects the immune system. In humans, this includes specific defects in cell-mediated immunity that may be responsible, in part, for the high incidence of head and neck cancers in alcoholics (Lundy et al., 1975).

Smoking

Cigarette smoking may alter immune system activity in animals and humans (Carlens, 1976; Holt & Keast, 1977; Holt, 1987). In contrast, cessation of smoking is associated with improvements in immune function. For example, in a study of 28 light to moderate smokers ages 21–35 years, Meliska et al. (1995) examined immune function after the subjects abstained from smoking for 31 days. These subjects were compared to 11 matched controls paid to continue smoking during that period. Cessation of smoking was associated with a decrease in serum cortisol and an increase in NK cell cytotoxic activity. Cigarette smoking may also have a synergistic effect on depressing immune function in persons exposed to benzene-containing organic solvents. Moszczynski (1992) compared the immune functioning of 19 nonsmokers and 41 smokers exposed to organic solvents with that of 46 nonsmokers and 47 smokers who were not exposed. Cigarette smoking and organic solvent exposure synergistically depressed concentrations of serum immunoglobulins IgA, IgD, IgG, lysozyme, and T-lymphocyte subpopulations.

Marijuana Use

Recreational drugs such as marijuana may also adversely affect components of the immune system (Friedman, Klein, et al., 1991). The major psychoactive component of marijuana, delta-9-tetrahydrocannabinol or THC, has been shown (in vitro) to be toxic to peripheral blood lymphocytes and to inhibit natural killer cell activity against human tumor cells (Friedman, 1986). Petersen, Lemberger, et al. (1975) compared chronic marijuana smokers and matched nonsmokers on several aspects of humoral and cellular immunity. They found that the number of T-lymphocytes with respect to the ratio of T and B-lymphocytes was lower in marijuana smokers. In addition, phytohemagglutinin stimulation of lymphocytes was less effective. Finally, granulocytes in the blood of smokers contained fewer cells capable of phagocytizing yeast cells than did the granulocytes from nonsmokers.

Substance abuse involving other drugs may have both direct effects on immunity (Jaffe, 1980) and indirect effects through changes in nutrition (Chandra & Newberne, 1977).

PSYCHOLOGICAL INFLUENCES ON IMMUNITY

A growing body of research is linking psychological factors with immune system functioning. Several major reviews of this work have appeared in top-tier medical journals. Addressing this topic in the *Annals of Internal Medicine*, McEwen and Stellar (1993) examined how psychological stress may contribute to a wide range of diseases, including asthma, diabetes, gastrointestinal disorders, myocardial infarction, hypertension, cancer, viral infections, and autoimmunity and discussed immunological mechanisms by which these effects might be mediated. McEwen (1998) and Glaser, Rabin, et al. (1999) recently updated this literature in reviews published in the *New England Journal of Medicine* and the *Journal of the American Medical Association*, respectively.

A number of pathways exist by which psychological factors may affect the immune system. First, psychological stress and emotional disorders such as depression or anxiety increase the production of cortisol by the adrenal glands. They do so by stimulating the production of corticotropic releasing factor (CRF) in the hypothalamus of the brain, which stimulates the pituitary gland to produce adrenocorticotropic hormone (ACTH) or corticotropin, which activates the adrenal cortex to produce cortisol. Second, stress causes the release of catecholamines from nerve endings and from the adrenal medulla. While in the short term these stress hormones are highly adaptive (preparing the body physiologically to either fight or escape from a threat), over the long term (as in chronic depression or chronic stress) they can result in several problems: elevated blood pressure, accelerated atherosclerosis, osteoporosis due to inhibition of bone formation, cognitive impairment due to damage to hippocampal regions of the brain, and impaired cellular immunity (Rassnick et al., 1994; McEwen, 1998).

Effects of Cortisol

Irwin and colleagues have demonstrated that cortisol and biological hormones such as CRF or ACTH that stimulate cortisol production suppress natural killer cell activity and other lymphocyte functions (Irwin, Britton, et al., 1987; Irwin, Daniels, et al., 1988; Strausbagh & Irwin, 1992). A number of more recent studies have confirmed the negative effects of these stress hormones on cell-mediated immunity (Dhabhar et al., 1996; McEwen et al., 1997).

Effects of the Autonomic Nervous System

Psychological stress, acting through the locus ceruleus, stimulates the sympathetic nerves that terminate in lymphoid organs. If stress becomes chronic, sympathetic nerve stimulation may down-regulate immune functioning and reduce its responsiveness (Felten et al., 1987; Felten & Felten, 1991). Thus, both endocrine and autonomic nervous system changes induced by chronic emotional stress can impair immunity.

Depression

Persons who suffer from depression experience a number of neuroendocrine changes, including higher levels of serum cortisol. The clinical significance of such elevations is demonstrated by the fact that women with a history of depressive illness have decreased bone mineral density resulting from inhibited bone formation caused by excess cortisol (Michelson, Stratakis, et al., 1996). The dexamethasone suppression test (DST) is a common biological test for diagnosing major depression and for monitoring its response to treatment that takes advantage of depression-induced neuroendocrine changes. Patients are given 1 mg of dexamethasone (equivalent to 25 mgs of cortisol) at 11 P.M.; serum cortisols are then measured the next day at 8 A.M., 4 P.M., and 11 P.M. If depressive disorder is absent, the 1 mg of dexamethasone will suppress corticotropin (ACTH) and thereby reduce production of cortisol by the adrenal glands. Serum cortisol levels the next day will typically drop below 5 μg/deciliter. In persons with depression, however, dexamethasone will not suppress cortisol production, and serum cortisol will remain high. Might this high level of serum cortisol impair immune function?

A number of studies have now shown that persons with depressive disorder have impaired lymphocyte functioning, including reduced NK cell cytotoxicity (Kronfol et al., 1983; Schleifer, Keller, & Meyerson, 1984; Schleifer, Keller, & Siris, 1985; Irwin et al., 1987; Schleifer, Keller, & Bond, 1989; Irwin, Patterson, et al., 1990; Irwin, Smith, et al., 1992). One of the first research teams to show this was Bartrop et al. (1977), who reported impaired lymphocyte functioning in 26 persons studied two and six weeks after bereavement. Lymphocyte responses to phytohemagglutinin and concanavalin A were significantly diminished at week six in the bereaved group compared with responses in 26 controls.

Likewise, in a prospective study of 15 spouses of women with advanced breast cancer, Schleifer, Keller, Camerino, et al. (1983) found that lymphocyte stimulation in response to phytohemagglutinin, concanavalin A, and pokeweed mitogen was significantly depressed during the first two months after bereavement compared with the spouse's prebereavement levels. An intermediate level of lymphocyte functioning was found during the four- to 14-month period after bereavement. Investigators concluded that impaired immune functioning may be responsible for reports of increased morbidity and mortality after bereavement.

Psychological Stress

Psychological stress, even when it is of short duration, can induce marked changes in physiological functioning. Breier et al. (1987) stressed 10 healthy human volunteers with loud noise (100 dB) under controlled and uncontrolled conditions. The lack of control over even mildly aversive stimuli produced alterations in mood (helplessness, tension, stress, unhappiness, anxiety, depression), as well as changes in neuroendocrine and autonomic nervous system functioning in these healthy persons (elevated ACTH, higher levels of sympathetic nervous system activity, and higher electrodermal activity).

Likewise, Cacioppo et al. (1995) studied 22 older women to determine their neuroendocrine and immune responses to brief psychological stressors. Stress heightened cardiac activation, elevated plasma catecholamine concentrations, and affected cellular immune responses. Furthermore, individuals characterized by high cardiac sympathetic reactivity showed higher stress-related changes in ACTH and plasma cortisol levels.

Psychosocial stress that occurs within interpersonal relationships may likewise induce neuroendocrine and immune changes. Kiecolt-Glaser, Malarkey, Chee, et al. (1993) analyzed 90 newlywed couples to determine the relationship between negative behavior during marital conflict and immunological down-regulation. Spouses who displayed more negative or hostile behaviors during a 30-minute discussion of marital problems showed, in comparison to low-negative spouses, (1) greater decrease of NK cell activity, (2) weaker blastogenic response to two mitogens, (3) weaker proliferative responses to a monoclonal antibody to the T3 receptor, (4) larger increases in number of total T lymphocytes and helper T lymphocytes, (5) higher antibody titers to latent Epstein-Barr virus (consistent with a down-regulated immune system), and (6) larger and longer-lasting increases in blood pressure. These effects were particularly strong in women.

In a follow-up study, Kiecolt-Glaser, Newton, et al. (1996) assessed endocrine function of newlywed couples on days when they experienced conflict. Withdrawal by the husband in response to the wife's negative behavior was associated with higher norepinephrine and cortisol levels in the wives. Higher frequency of positive behaviors by the wives was associated with lower epinephrine and positive behaviors by husbands with higher prolactin levels in the wives. Norepinephrine, epinephrine, prolactin, and cortisol levels in the husbands were not associated with either the husbands' or the wives' behaviors.

Kiecolt-Glaser, Glaser, Cacioppo, et al. (1997) next examined the endocrinological and immunological correlates of marital conflict in 31 older couples (average age 67 years, married an average of 42 years). A 30-minute conflict session was followed by 15 minutes of recovery. Among wives, marital satisfaction and escalation of negative behavior during conflict showed strong relationships to endocrine changes, explaining 16–21% of the variance in changes of cortisol, ACTH, and norepinephrine. In contrast, the husbands' endocrine data again did not show relationships with negative behaviors or marital quality. Both men and women with negative behaviors during conflict, however, showed poorer immunological responses across several functional assays (blastogenic response to two T cell mitogens and antibody titers to latent Epstein-Barr virus).

Neuroimmunological changes in response to long-term naturalistic stressors have also been documented and may be even greater than changes induced by short-term stressors (Andersen, Kiecolt-Glaser, et al., 1994). Particularly sensitive in this regard are natural killer cell activity, helper/suppressor ratio, and percentage of suppressor/cytotoxic T cells. Esterling, Kiecolt-Glaser, et al. (1994) compared the effects of chronic stress, social support, and persistent alterations in NK cell response to cytokines in 14 active family caregivers of Alzheimer's patients, 17 former Alzheimer's patient caregivers (the death of whose patient had occurred at least three years earlier), and 31 control subjects. Both current and former Alzheimer's caregivers had significantly more depressive symptoms than did the controls (but the two caregiver groups did not differ from each other). Compared with the controls, the current and the former Alzheimer's caregivers demonstrated significantly poorer NK cell responses when exposed in vitro to recombinant interferon-gamma and recombinant interleukin-2 (and did not differ from each other in this regard).

After reviewing the research, Restak (1989) concluded that psychological stress—particularly uncontrollable stress—produces an elevation in plasma adrenocorticotrophic hormone (ACTH) similar to that seen in major depression. He also notes that "Attitudes, spiritual resources, hopes, and ideals can neutralize the effects of an uncontrollable stress situation" (p. 23). We now consider factors that may buffer the effects of depression and chronic psychological stress on immune system functioning.

SOCIAL INFLUENCES ON IMMUNE FUNCTION

Social support has been shown to buffer the negative impact of stressful life events, prevent the onset of depression, and speed recovery from depression (George et al., 1989; George, 1992). If social factors affect whether stressful life situations lead to emotional disorder, they may also influence neuroendocrine changes that impair immunity. In other words, greater social support may prevent the negative endocrine and immunological changes associated with stress. In contrast, social isolation may increase emotional distress and lead to physiologi-

cal changes that adversely affect immune functioning. Studies in both nonhuman primates and humans bear this out.

For example, Sapolsky and colleagues (1997) examined 70 yellow baboons in Africa to determine the relationship between hypercortisolism and social subordinance and isolation. Baboons with the lowest ranking in the troop had post-DST cortisol levels that were three times higher than the cortisol levels found in dominant baboons. Similarly, socially isolated males had elevated basal cortisol concentrations and tended to show dexamethasone resistance. Investigators concluded that social status and degree of social affiliation influence adrenocortical profiles.

This is consistent with findings from the work of Kiecolt-Glaser and colleagues (1984) who more than a decade earlier had documented reduced immune system function among hospitalized psychiatric patients who were experiencing feelings of loneliness. These investigators also found that Alzheimer's caregivers with low social support experienced greater declines in immune function than did those with high support during a one-year follow-up (Kiecolt-Glaser, Dura, et al., 1991). Baron et al. (1990) reported that among wives of cancer patients, those with higher levels of social support showed greater immunocompetence on two of three measures (NK cell cytotoxicity and phytohemagglutin stimulation) than did women with less social support. In a sample of 66 women with stage I or stage II breast cancer who had had either lumpectomies or mastectomies, Levy, Herberman, Lee, et al. (1990) found that women with higher social support had greater NK cell activity than those with low support. More recently, Esterling, Kiecolt-Glaser, et al. (1996) compared 28 current and former spousal caregivers of Alzheimer's patients and 29 control subjects. NK cell activity was again positively related to increased emotional support and tangible social support (independent of depressive symptoms).

In a comprehensive review of 81 such studies, Uchino et al. (1996) found that social support was linked to a number of physiological processes, including cardiovascular, endocrine, and immune functioning. More recently, Cohen, Doyle, et al. (1997) documented further evidence that social support and greater social involvement may increase host resistance to infectious disease through immunological mechanisms. These health benefits likely result from the stress-buffering effects of friendships and close family relationships.

HEALTH CONSEQUENCES

While there is ample research to demonstrate that depressive disorder and psychological stress impair immunity, is there any evidence that such changes result in greater susceptibility to disease? Several investigators have reviewed the health implications of stress-related immunosuppression (Dorian et al., 1986; Glaser, Rice, et al., 1987; Kiecolt-Glaser & Glaser, 1995; Rabin, 1999). We now examine specific studies of the role that stress-related immunosuppression plays in cancer, infectious disease, diabetes mellitus, and wound healing.

Cancer

Psychological stress in healthy persons may affect immune system functioning in a way that increases susceptibility to malignancy. Shekelle, Shyrock, et al. (1981) examined psychosocial predictors of death from cancer in a random sample of 2,020 middle-aged employed men followed for 17 years. Depressive symptoms were assessed during the 1958 baseline evaluation using the MMPI. By 1975, 82 men had died of cancer. After controlling for age, smoking, alcohol use, family history, and occupational status, the likelihood of dying from cancer was twice as high among men with depression at baseline (OR 2.3, $p < .001$).

More recently, Prigerson et al. (1997) reported similar results in a study of 150 future widows and widowers at the time of their spouses' hospital admission and at 1.5, 6, 13, and 25 months after their spouses' death. Traumatic grief was assessed using a grief scale and physical health by self-report and interviewer evaluation. Subjects with traumatic grief had a probability of developing a new case of cancer between the 6- and 25-month evaluations that was substantially higher than that of subjects

without such symptoms ($p < .0001$). In fact, all four cases of cancer developed in bereaved subjects who had high traumatic grief scores.

The diagnosis of cancer itself may create psychological stress that then impairs the body's ability to contain the disease. Animal models (Fisher rats) suggest that stress-induced immunosuppression of NK cell activity may contribute to the development of metastatic disease. Pain induced by surgery in these rats leads to a decrease in NK cell cytotoxicity with consequence increase in tumor metastasis (Ben-Eliyahu et al., 1991). NK cell cytotoxicity is particularly important because studies have repeatedly documented an association between reduced NK activity and tumor spread (Akimoto et al., 1986).

Studies suggest similar processes in humans. Levy, Lippman, et al. (1987) prospectively followed 75 women (mean age 52) with stage I or stage II breast cancer. They examined natural killer cell (NK) activity and psychological status of subjects at baseline and three months later as part of a National Cancer Institute protocol. Both at baseline and at three-month follow-up, there was a similar cross-sectional correlation among fatigue, lack of family support, and lower NK cell activity. Those who reported depressive fatigue-like symptoms and complained about lack of family support at baseline also tended to show a decrease in NK activity at three months ($.05 < p \leq .10$, baseline NK cell activity controlled). Reduced activity of NK cells, in turn, was associated with shorter survival (node-positive patients had lower levels of NK cell activity than did patients without metastatic disease).

Levy, Lee, et al. (1988) next examined time to death following recurrence in 36 women with breast cancer. After controlling for medical variables, including physician-rated prognosis and number of metastatic sites, these investigators found that positive affect, in particular the experience of joy, predicted longer survival after cancer recurrence. Speed of metastatic spread was also associated with negative affect in a study by Roberts, Andersen, et al. (1994), who examined disease progression in women with gynecologic cancer. Status of nodal involvement was determined 16 days after initial assessment of mood. Interviewer-assessed mood disturbance (i.e., presence of blunted, inappropriate, or depressed affect) significantly predicted number of positive nodes (explaining 14% of the variance).

Some of the best evidence that impaired immunity may lead to the progression of cancer comes from studies by Fawzy, Kemeny, et al. (1990); Fawzy, Fawzy, Hyun, et al. (1993); and Fawzy, Fawzy, Arndt, et al. (1995). This work is described in greater detail in chapter 20. Investigators randomly assigned patients with the same kind and stage of cancer to a structured group intervention designed to reduce stress (health education, teaching problem solving skills, stress management, relaxation, and enhancement of psychological support) or to a control group. Psychological, immunological, and disease change were carefully measured at baseline and at follow-up. Intervention group members experienced significant short-term reductions in psychological stress and changes in immunological functioning (increased number of NK cells and increased NK cytotoxic activity). A six-year follow-up found greater recurrence and higher mortality rate in the controls than in the subjects who received the intervention.

According to Andersen, Kiecolt-Glaser, et al. (1994), cancers related to hormonal stimulation or to the immune system may be particularly sensitive to psychological stress. These include breast, ovarian, endometrial, and prostate cancer, which are influenced by hormonal factors, and leukemias or lymphomas, which are related to the immune system. Thus, future studies that explore psychosocial influences on immune functioning among patients with these particular cancers may be most fruitful. Likewise, studies in middle-aged persons (35–65 years of age) are more likely to demonstrate associations than are studies in the very young or the very old, for whom hereditary or age-related influences are likely to dominate the development and course of cancer. See chapter 20 for more discussion of the relationship between the immune system and cancer.

Infectious Diseases

Psychological stress disrupts the finely modulated communication network that links the central nervous system and the endocrine and the immune systems (Glaser, Rabin, et al., 1999). This may predispose to or influence the course of viral, bacterial, and fungal infections. It does so by down-regulating various aspects of the cellular immune response necessary for combating infection. An example of how psychological factors may affect the course of illness is seen in HIV infection and its progression to AIDS (Kiecolt-Glaser & Glaser, 1988). In HIV infection, immune system reserve is already low, and any negative psychosocial influences are likely to be observed more readily.

Ironson et al. (1990) conducted a prospective study of men tested for HIV, examining psychological functioning and immune responses among those testing seropositive and those testing seronegative. Men testing seropositive reported significantly more acute anxiety and traumatic stress, and there was also a significant inverse correlation between self-reported anxiety and NK cell activity.

Evans, Leserman, et al. (1997) examined 93 HIV-positive homosexual men, all without clinical symptoms at study entry. Comprehensive interviews and physical examinations were conducted at six-month intervals for 42 months in order to assess stressful life events that had occurred in the preceding six months (omitting HIV-related stresses). Those with high life stress ($n = 38$) had a significantly greater risk of early HIV disease progression than did those with low life stress ($n = 55$) ($p = .03$, Relative Risk = 2.0). In other words, the risk of disease progression doubled for each stressful life event per six-month study interval. Interestingly, depression was unrelated to disease progression.

Individuals with compromised immune systems are also susceptible to viral infections other than HIV. Well known is the reactivation of herpesviruses when an infected individual is exposed to stress or experiences a weakened immune system. This is particularly true for patients with AIDS or those undergoing immunosuppressive therapy (Glaser & Kiecolt-Glaser, 1994). Likewise, Kasl et al. (1979) found that West Point cadets followed over four years were at greater risk of developing infectious mononucleosis (Epstein-Barr virus infection) if they were experiencing significant psychological stress. Subjects with the greatest psychological stress were those with a high motivation toward a military career (emphasized by their over-achieving fathers) but unable to perform well academically.

Aging itself can reduce immune system reserve and increase susceptibility to certain viral infections. This natural progression makes it easier to demonstrate the effects of psychosocial factors on immune functioning. The down-regulation of immune function with age and disease has been shown to increase the reactivation of viruses such as herpes zoster, for example (Schmader, 1996). Such down-regulation in immune functioning may be particularly prominent in older adults who are experiencing severe psychosocial stress. In a study of elderly caregivers of relatives with dementia, Kiecolt-Glaser and colleagues (1991) found that caregivers were significantly more likely than age-matched controls to experience depression, have measurable impairments in immune functioning, and report more infectious diseases, especially upper respiratory tract infections. In a later study, Kiecolt-Glaser, Glaser, Gravenstein, et al. (1996) compared 32 dementia caregivers with 32 controls matched for sex, age, and socioeconomic status. Caregivers showed poorer antibody response following vaccination than did control subjects as measured by two independent methods. In addition, caregivers had decreased in-vitro virus-specific-induced interleukin-2 and interleukin-1 beta levels. These findings suggest that chronic stress is associated with down-regulation of immune response to influenza vaccination in the elderly (this finding was confirmed by Vedhara et al., 1999).

Stress may also impair immune responses to viral infections in physically healthy individuals. Kiecolt-Glaser, Garner, et al. (1984) vaccinated 48 second-year medical students on the last day of a three-day examination series to study the effects of academic stress on students' ability to generate an immune response to hepatitis B vaccination. Students who developed an immune response (seroconverted) were significantly less stressed and anxious than students who did not seroconvert. Students who had greater social support also had stronger immune responses to the vaccine than those with less social support. A second research group has replicated these findings (Jabaaij et al., 1993).

Cohen, Tyrell, et al. (1991) more directly demonstrated the increased susceptibility of stressed persons to infection. Investigators inoculated 394 healthy volunteers ages 20–55 with a cold virus and injected an additional 26 subjects with a placebo. Psychological stress was assessed by three measures: (1) number of major stressful life events judged by the subject as having a negative impact on psychological state in the past year; (2) degree to which the subject perceived that demands exceeded his or her ability to cope; and (3) a measure of current negative affect. Clinical colds were defined as symptoms in the presence of an infection verified by isolation of virus or by increase in virus-specific antibody titer. Investigators found that both respiratory infections ($p < .005$) and colds ($p < .02$) increased in an almost linear fashion with increases in psychological stress. These results persisted after researchers controlled for age, sex, education, allergic status, weight, season of the year, number of subjects housed together, infectious status of subjects sharing same housing, and virus-specific antibody at baseline. The associations were similar for each of the five different viruses that subjects were inoculated with.

Stress increases susceptibility not only to viral infections but also to certain bacterial infections. For example, psychological stress (such as crowding) prior to and following tuberculosis infection has been shown to negatively impact the course of infection (Tobach & Bloch, 1956).

Diabetes

Studies that used animal models have found that repeated exposure to stress increases the risk of diabetes, a disease whose etiology is associated with immune dysfunction (Lehman et al., 1991). Human studies also show that family stress and instability increases the incidence and severity of juvenile-onset diabetes (Hagglof et al., 1991). Likewise, symptoms indicative of chronic stress (fatigue, irritability, depression, and hostility) have been associated with the development of insulin resistance, a major factor in adult-onset diabetes (Raikkonen et al., 1996).

Speed of Wound Healing

Psychological stress may also impair the speed at which normal wound healing occurs, acting through neuroimmunological mechanisms. Kiecolt-Glaser, Marucha, et al. (1996) evaluated 13 women caregivers (mean age 62) of demented relatives to determine whether wound healing is slowed by psychological stress. Caregiver cases were compared to 13 controls matched for age (60 years or older) and family income. Cases and controls underwent a 3.5-mm punch biopsy. Healing was assessed by photography of the wound and response to hydrogen peroxide (with healing defined as no foaming). Wounds in caregivers took significantly longer to heal (48.7 vs. 39.3 days, $p < .05$). Investigators also found that peripheral blood leukocytes of caregivers produced significantly less interleukin-1 beta mRNA in response to lipopolysaccharide stimulation.

POSSIBLE INFLUENCES OF RELIGION ON IMMUNITY

Until now, we have said nothing about the relationship between religion and immune function. It was necessary to present this extensive background information on the immune system and the factors that affect it in order to lay the groundwork for understanding the mechanisms by which religion might impact immune functioning. From our discussion, it should be clear that there are several pathways by which religious beliefs and practices could influence immunity.

First, we saw in chapter 11 that religious involvement is inversely related to alcohol abuse, cigarette smoking, illicit drug use, and high-risk sexual practices that can lead to HIV infection (see chapter 24). All these behaviors can adversely affect immune function. Second, religious beliefs and practices are associated with better adaptation to stress (chapter 5), greater well-being (chapter 6), lower levels of anxiety (chapter 9), less depression, and quicker recovery from depression (chapter 7). Given the relationship between psychological distress and impaired immunity, any factor that im-

proves coping and prevents emotional disorder is likely to benefit immune function.

Finally, religious involvement is associated with a larger and more varied social support network and to greater satisfaction with that support (chapter 15). The association between greater social support and stronger immune function is another plausible mechanism by which religious activity might reduce stress-related neuroendocrine changes that impair immunity. Despite these plausible reasons for a relationship between religion and immune function, few studies have attempted to investigate this area.

RELIGION AND STRESS HORMONES

While research examining the relationship between religious involvement and stress hormone production is almost nonexistent, two studies at least peripherally address the topic. Katz et al. (1970) conducted a cross-sectional study of patients at Montefiore Hospital in New York City. Patients were 30 women (11 Jewish, 10 Catholic, seven Protestant, two other/none) in good health who were awaiting breast biopsy for possible cancer (22 biopsies eventually turned out positive). Investigators found a correlation between cortisol production rates and types of psychological defenses used by patients. Those who employed prayer and faith ($n = 4$) tended to have lower cortisol production than those who depended on projection or displacement. This was only a descriptive study, however, and no statistical comparisons were made.

Sudsuang and colleagues (1991) conducted a clinical trial to study the effects of Buddhist meditation on serum cortisol and other biological and physiological measures. The trial included 52 men ages 20–25 who practiced Dhammakaya Buddhist meditation (similar to Zen or transcendental meditation); all were novices at this practice. Meditators were compared with 30 men of the same age group who did not meditate. Researchers nonrandomly assigned subjects to a meditation group that stayed in a monastery for two months during summer vacation or to a control group of nonmeditators that stayed at home for the summer. Physiological measures were taken before the meditation program began and at three and six weeks into the study. During the first three weeks meditators practiced four hours a day, and during the last three weeks they practiced two hours a day. Physiological measurements were obtained one hour after meditation began in the morning. Cortisol levels on follow-up were significantly reduced in meditators compared to controls ($p < .01$).

Schaal et al. (1998), at Stanford University, examined correlations between religious involvement and endocrine function in 112 women with metastatic breast cancer. The sample consisted largely of white women; the subjects' mean age was 53 years. Religious affiliations of participants were Protestant (38%), Jewish (13%), Roman Catholic (15%), other affiliations (18%), and no religious affiliation (16%). Besides affiliation, attendance at religious services and importance of religious or spiritual expression in life were also measured. Diurnal salivary cortisol levels were assessed over three consecutive days. Overall salivary cortisol levels (e.g., area under the diurnal curve) were not associated with religious expression or religious attendance, but evening (5 P.M.) cortisol levels were lower among women for whom religious or spiritual expression had greater importance ($r = .22$, $p = .01$, $n = 104$).

RELIGION AND IMMUNE FUNCTION

Study of the relationship between religious involvement and immune function is in its infancy. We could locate only three published studies and two unpublished reports that have addressed the topic.

Immunological Reaction to a Spiritual Experience

The first study focuses on religious experience rather than religious involvement and only indirectly examines the relationship between religion and immune function. Immune function here is defined as acute mobilization of immunoglobulins, which may or not have anything to do with long-term changes in the immune system. In this experimental study, McClelland (1988) analyzed the effect of motivational arousal on salivary immunoglobulin A (IgA) in students who were watching different types of movie films. The study population consisted of 132 college students who were shown either the film *Triumph of the Axis in World War II* ($n = 62$) or the film *Mother Teresa* ($n = 70$). *The Triumph of the Axis* is a documentary prepared in the United States before its entry into the war to show how the Axis powers (Germany and Italy) had deceived the allies, were persecuting the Jews, and were pursuing domination of the world. *Mother Teresa* is a documentary that presents the activities and convictions of Mother Teresa, a Roman Catholic nun who served the poorest of the poor, the diseased, and the dying in the slums of Calcutta, India. Each film was shown twice, and each sample of viewers was examined separately. McClelland found that salivary IgA immunoglobulin levels were significantly higher ($p < .025$) in the 70 persons who viewed the film on Mother Teresa—results that were replicated in two subsamples ($n = 39$ and $n = 31$). The increases were greatest among those characterized as having the relaxed affiliative syndrome (subjects who scored high on affiliation, low on need for power, and low on activity inhibition).

Religious Involvement and Immune Function

In the first attempt to examine the relationship between religious involvement and immune function, Koenig, Cohen, George, et al. (1997) conducted a prospective study of a large community sample in North Carolina to evaluate the effect of religious attendance on interleukin-6 (IL-6) and other biological indicators of immune function. The sample consisted of 4,000 randomly selected community-dwelling persons age 65 or older who were participating in the Establishment of Populations for Epidemiologic Studies in the Elderly (EPESE) project sponsored by the National Institute on Aging. Frequency of religious attendance was measured in 1986, 1989, and 1992, and plasma interleukin-6 (IL-6) levels were measured in 1992 in 1,718 subjects. Researchers hypothesized that frequent religious attendance in 1986, 1989, and 1992 would predict lower plasma IL-6 levels in 1992 (indicating a more stable immune system), a hypothesis that was generally confirmed (see Figure 19.1). After researchers controlled for covariates, however, significant differences were found only for the cross-sectional association in 1992. The likelihood that persons who attended religious services to any degree would have high IL-6 levels (>5 pg/ml) in 1992 was almost 50% lower than that for nonattenders (OR 0.51, 0.35–0.73, $p \le .001$, uncontrolled; OR 0.58, 0.40–0.84, $p < .005$, controlled for age, sex, race, education, chronic illness, and physical functioning).

Susan Lutgendorf and colleagues (personal communication) at the University of Iowa also examined religious coping and plasma IL-6 in 55 older adults ages 65–89, half of whom were voluntarily moving from their own homes to senior housing. Religious and spiritual coping were measured using the spiritual subscale of Carver's COPE scale (which asks subjects about

coping mechanisms used in times of stress, such as praying to God for help, using meditation) (Carver, Scheier, et al., 1989). Lutgendorf et al. drew samples of blood and tested them for IL-6 levels three times over four months. Levels of IL-6 averaged over all three time points were unrelated to depressed mood. However, independent of whether the seniors were moving (i.e., stress level), greater use of spiritual coping was associated with lower IL-6 (partial $r = -.26$, $p = .075$).

IL-6 plays a prominent role in the induction of the acute inflammatory response, B cell proliferation and differentiation, and regulation of protein inhibitors and bone resorption. While IL-6 levels are usually undetected until advanced age, this cytokine is a particularly important indicator of disease in the elderly and may play a key role in mediating the aging process (Ershler, 1993). High levels of IL-6 (particularly levels > 5 pg/ml) have been reported in diseases such as cancer (B cell lymphoma, multiple myeloma, head and neck cancer, Hodgkin's disease), myocardial infarction, hypertension, Alzheimer's disease, osteoporosis, rheumatoid

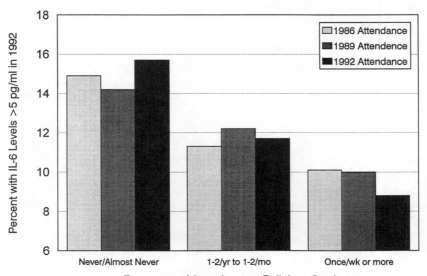

FIGURE 19.1 Attendance at religious services and interleukin-6 (IL-6) plasma levels. Adapted from Koenig, Cohen, and George (1997), *International Journal of Psychiatry in Medicine* 27, p. 242. Used with permission.

arthritis, and possibly chronic fatigue syndrome (Ur et al., 1992; Gallo et al., 1993; Manicourt et al., 1993; Blay et al., 1994; Ershler et al., 1994; Cohen, Pieper, et al., 1998). In fact, the use of anti-IL-6 antibodies to inhibit this cytokine has been suggested for therapeutic uses (Klein et al., 1992; Lu et al., 1995). The relationship found between IL-6 and religious attendance suggests that persons who actively involve themselves in religious community may have more stable immune systems. It may also help explain why they have better physical health and longer survival (see chapter 21).

Religiousness and Immune Function in AIDS/HIV Infection

Woods et al. (1999) surveyed 106 HIV-seropositive gay men to determine whether religiosity (measured as either religious activities or religious coping) is associated with less depression or better immune function in this population. Religious activities, such as prayer, religious attendance, spiritual discussions, and reading religious/spiritual literature, were associated with significantly higher CD4+ counts and CD4+ percentages (T-helper-inducer cells). The association was not confounded by subjects' becoming unable to participate in religious activity as their disease worsened and immune function decreased. Interestingly, there was no relationship between immune function and severity of depressive symptoms (researchers used multiple regression to control for self-efficacy and active coping). Religious coping (e.g., putting trust in God, seeking God's help, increasing praying) was related to lower scores on the Beck Depression Inventory ($p < .01$) and on the Spielberger Trait Anxiety Inventory ($p = .08$) but not to specific immune markers; subjects with more severe disease, however, may have turned to religion for comfort, disguising any cross-sectional association between religious coping and better immune function.

Religiousness and Immune Function in Breast Cancer

Schaal and colleagues (1998) examined correlations between religious involvement and mea-sures of immune system activity in their 112-member sample of women with metastatic breast cancer. Lymphocyte numbers and NK cell activity were measured by averaging results from two blood samples taken between 8:00 and 10:00 A.M., approximately one week apart. Functional immunity was also measured by delayed-type hypersensitivity (DTH) responses to skin test antigens. The importance of religious or spiritual expression was positively related to NK cell numbers (Spearman $r = .19$, $p = .02$), T-helper cell counts ($r = .16$, $p = .05$), and total lymphocytes ($r = .15$, $p = .05$). These effects were not mediated by the size of the patients' social networks or by cancer treatments that affected immune cell counts. Religious expression was not associated with functional immune measures (DTH). The authors concluded that, because effects were not driven by social network size, religious expression may preserve immunity in women with advanced breast cancer by some other mechanism.

FUTURE RESEARCH

In July 1999, at Duke University, we convened a meeting of 13 prominent scientists in the field of psychoneuroimmunology to brainstorm about future research studies that might expand our knowledge base about the relationship between religious involvement and immune functioning. These scientists included Robert Ader, Sheldon Cohen, Janice Kiecolt-Glaser, Ron Glaser, Ron Heberman, Bruce Rabin, Neil Schneiderman, George Solomon, and Redford Williams. Out of this meeting came several ideas that we hope will help guide future research in this area.

Future research should try to identify those components of the immune system that are most influenced by religious variables (e.g., NK cell activitiy, T cell responses, immunoglobulin production). Likewise, the specific types of religious belief or activity that have the greatest impact on immune system function need to be identified (e.g., religious attendance, religious worship, inspirational reading, meditation, ritual). Both short-term and long-term immune responses to religious involvement should be examined and immune responses compared between people who worship, pray, and sing in group settings and those who engage in these practices alone. Researchers should attempt to quantify exposure to religious beliefs and practices over the lifetime of the individual, rather than at only a single point in time. Another area to be studied is wound healing under stress in religious and nonreligious subjects. These studies should be performed in vulnerable populations—caregivers, working single mothers, the bereaved, the elderly, HIV-infected patients, the chronically ill—populations that may be at particular risk for impaired immunity (so that the effects of religious involvement may be more easily detected).

SUMMARY AND CONCLUSIONS

The immune system is our primary internal defense against foreign invaders, infectious agents, and possibly malignant cell transformation and proliferation. When the immune system encounters a pathogen, it responds by an acute-phase reaction and by formation of immunologic memory (delayed hypersensitivity). In this way, the pathogen is destroyed and a memory of the invader is encoded within the immune system to prepare the body to even more effectively combat the invader should it be encountered again.

A wide variety of biological factors (HIV infection, cigarette smoking, alcohol and drug abuse), psychological factors (depression, psychological stress), and social factors (social affiliation, social support) influence immunity. Many of these factors also relate in one way or another to religious belief and practice. Thus, there is ample theoretical justification to hypothesize a relationship between greater religiousness and better immune function.

While the research in this area is only getting started, there is some evidence that religious practices (prayer, meditation, and faith) may be associated with lower serum cortisol levels. There is also growing evidence to link religious experiences, practices, and belief with better immune function in the elderly and in persons who are HIV-positive or have AIDS. This promising area of research, however, needs much further work to ensure that confounding factors do not explain these relationships.

20

Cancer

IMPORTANCE, PREVALENCE, CAUSES, AND PREVENTION

A diagnosis of cancer probably creates more fear than any other medical condition, for in the minds of most people it evokes the image of a painful, disfiguring, and imminent death. Deaths due to cancer have risen 20% in the past 30 years (American Cancer Society, 1994). In 1999, each day more than 1,500 persons died of cancer and more than 3,300 new cases of cancer were diagnosed in the United States (American Cancer Society, 1999). Approximately 8.2 million Americans alive today have histories of cancer. Cancer causes one out of every four deaths (24%) and is exceeded only by heart disease (33%) as a cause of mortality.

Overall, cancer is the leading cause of death among young and middle-aged adults, with 150 per 100,000 Americans ages 25–64 dying each year from the disease. Cancer is the most com-mon cause of death among women ages 25–74 years: 28 per 100,000/year in women ages 25–44, 250 per 100,000/year in women ages 45–64, and 700 per 100,000/year in women ages 65–74 (National Center for Health Statistics, 1996). Cancer is the second most common cause of death among men ages 45–74: it is 300 per 100,000/year in men ages 45–64 and 1,100 per 100,000/year in men ages 65–74. Approximately 60% of the 1,221,800 persons diagnosed with cancer in 1999 were expected to die within five years (American Cancer Society, 1999). The staggering economic cost of cancer, according to the National Cancer Institute, is $107 billion per year (including medical costs, costs due to lost productivity, and mortality costs).

Prevalence of Different Types

The lifetime likelihood that a man in the United States will contract cancer is 50% (1 out of 2), and for women it is approximately 33% (1 out of 3) (American Cancer Society, 1999). Of all *new cases* of cancer diagnosed in men, 41% are prostate cancers, 13% lung, 9% colon or intestine, 7% urinary, 6% leukemia or lymphoma, 3% oral, 2% each for melanoma, stomach, and pancreas, and 14% for all others. Of all new cancers diagnosed in women, 31% are breast cancers, 13% lung, 11% colon or intestine, 6% leukemia and lymphoma, 6% endometrium, 4% each for ovary and urinary, 3% cervix, 2% each for oral and pancreas, and 15% for all others.

Of cancer *deaths* each year for men, 32% are from lung cancer, 14% prostate, 9% colon or intestine, 9% leukemia or lymphoma, 5% each from pancreas or urinary, 3% stomach, 2% each from oral cancers and melanoma, and 19% from all others. Of cancer deaths each year for women, 25% are from lung cancer, 17% breast, 10% colon or intestines, 8% leukemia or lymphoma, 6% ovary, 5% pancreas, 3% urinary, 2% each from cervix and endometrium, 1% each from oral cancers and melanoma, and 20% from all others. Clearly, the most common cause of cancer death in both men and women is lung cancer, the most preventable of all malignancies.

Causes of Cancer

Cancer has both external and internal causes. External causes include chemicals, radiation, and viruses. Internal causes include hormones, immune conditions, and inherited mutations. Several of these factors often interact, and many years may elapse between exposure and cancer onset. It may be 10 years or more before an exposure or mutation results in detectable cancer (American Cancer Society, 1999).

Lung Cancer. More than 170,000 new cases of lung cancer are diagnosed every year; these account for 14% of all new cancers and 29% of all cancer deaths. The age-adjusted death rates have increased 121% for men and 415% for women during the past 30 years. The one-year survival rate for lung cancer is up from 32% in 1973 to 41% in 1994, due largely to better treatments. The five-year survival rate, however, is still only about 14% (American Cancer Society, 1998, 1999). The primary risk factor for lung cancer is cigarette smoking.

Breast Cancer. Breast cancer is the leading cause of death among women ages 40–55, with approximately 175,000 new cases of invasive disease diagnosed and 44,000 deaths in 1999. Women who have a first-degree family member with the disease have a two-fold increase in risk compared to those without a family history; having two first-degree relatives increases the risk five-fold. Age also increases risk, and nearly 80% of women cancer patients are over age 50 at the time of diagnosis. Genetic factors also play a role. Between 5–10% of breast cancers are inherited, the result of mutations of the BRCA1 and BRCA2 genes. Between 50–60% of women with mutations at these gene sites will develop breast cancer by age 70. Previous history of breast cancer also increases the risk. A woman with breast cancer in one breast has three to four times the risk of developing it in the second breast, compared to a woman with no history of the disease. White women are slightly more likely to develop breast cancer than are African American women, but African American women are more likely to die from their cancer (due to late stage at diagnosis).

There are also several lifestyle-related risk factors for breast cancer. These include oral contraceptive use (slight increased risk), having no children or having one's first child after age 30 (slight increased risk), estrogen replacement therapy (slight increased risk), alcohol consumption (women who consume two to five drinks daily have a 50% increased risk compared with women who do not drink alcohol), obesity, high-fat diet (especially polyunsaturated fats such as corn oil, tub margarine, and saturated fats in meat), and physical inactivity (recent studies suggest that regular exercise may provide some protection against breast cancer) (American Cancer Society, 1998).

Prostate Cancer. Prostate cancer is the only malignancy more common in men than lung cancer (excluding skin cancers), and it is the second leading cause of cancer death in men (13% of all male cancer deaths). The overall five-year survival rate is 89% and the 10-year survival rate is 63%; with only local spread (60% of diagnosed cases), the five-year survival rate nears 100% (American Cancer Society, 1998, 1999). Factors that affect risk for prostate cancer are age (75% of cancers are diagnosed in men over age 65), race (risk among African Americans is about twice that in whites), family history (having a father or brother with prostate cancer doubles the risk), nationality (prostate cancer is more common in North America and in northwestern Europe), vasectomy (slight increase in risk), diet (high-fat diet increases the risk and diets high in calcium, selenium, and fruits and vegetables, especially cooked or raw tomatoes, decrease the risk), and level of physical activity (regular activity and maintenance of healthy weight may reduce risk) (American Cancer Society, 1998).

Colorectal Cancer.   Colorectal cancer is common in both men and women. It comprises about 10% of all newly diagnosed cancer cases and accounts for 10% of deaths each year. The five-year survival rate is 91% for colorectal cancer detected at an early stage before it has spread to local lymph nodes, although only about 37% are diagnosed at that stage. If the cancer has spread locally to involve adjacent organs or lymph nodes, the five-year survival rate drops to 66%. For persons with distant spread to the lung or liver, five-year survival rate is about 9%. The overall 10-year survival rate for colorectal cancer is now 55%. Risk factors include age (90% of cancers are diagnosed in persons over age 50), diet (foods high in fat and low in fiber increase risk), family history of colorectal cancer, and other genetic factors (up to 10% of colorectal cancers are caused by inherited gene mutations) (American Cancer Society, 1998, 1999).

Cervical Cancer.   Cervical cancers make up between 3–6% of cancers in women. About 20% are invasive, and the remaining 80% are cancer in situ. The number of invasive cervical cancers among women in the United States has dramatically decreased over the past 40 years, declining by almost 75%. The major reason for this has been the use of the Pap test, which allows for early detection. The five-year survival rate for

cancer in situ is 100%; for all stages of cervical cancer combined, it is 69%. Among white women, 55% of cervical cancers are diagnosed in a localized stage, compared with 43% of cervical cancers in African American women. Risk factors for cervical cancer include the following: infection with the human papillomavirus (HPV) (which is passed from one person to another by unprotected intercourse; risk is increased by having sex at an early age and by having multiple sexual partners), smoking (tobacco by-products accumulate in cervical mucus and cause damage to cells in the cervix), HIV infection (perhaps due to damage to the immune system's ability to destroy cancer cells and/or contain their growth and spread), use of oral contraceptives (very slight increased risk), and poor diet (which may increase risk) (American Cancer Society, 1998, 1999).

Prevention of Cancer

Nine types of cancer can be detected early by screening (breast, colon, rectum, cervix, prostate, testes, tongue, mouth, and skin), and these account for approximately half of all newly diagnosed malignancies. Detection results in earlier treatment, thus preventing spread. The overall five-year survival rate for cancers that are detectable by screening is 81%, a rate that could be increased to over 95% with regular screening (American Cancer Society, 1999). Approximately 30% of all deaths from cancer are due to cigarette smoking and 35% to nutrition and diet (*Healthy People 2000*, 1991); thus, nearly two-thirds of cancers are preventable.

Lung Cancer. All cancer deaths due to cigarette smoking are preventable. Smokers have ten times the risk of developing lung cancer as nonsmokers.

Breast Cancer. Self-breast examinations, regular check-ups by a physician, and periodic mammograms can help detect cancer at an early stage. Avoiding excess alcohol use, eating a healthy diet low in fats, and engaging in regular exercise may also reduce risk.

Prostate Cancer. Having regular prostate examinations (accompanied by prostate-specific antigen [PSA] test when indicated), eating a diet with plenty of fruits and vegetables, and maintaining regular exercise may increase detection or prevent its occurrence.

Stomach and Esophageal Cancers. Heavy alcohol use is responsible for many cancers of the oral cavity, esophagus, pancreas, and stomach (19,000 cases in 1998). Using alcohol in moderation can reduce the risk of these cancers.

Colorectal cancers. Eating a diet high in fiber and low in fat, as well as having regular screenings, can help reduce risk and increase early detection.

Cervical Cancer. Cervical cancer screening by routine Pap smears is essential for early detection. The American Cancer Society suggests that women avoid risk factors for cervical cancer (cigarette smoking and sexual behavior that causes exposure to HPV infection) whenever possible.

CANCER AND THE IMMUNE SYSTEM

Immune System and Susceptibility to Cancer

The *theory of immune surveillance* proposes that the cellular immune system is the body's first line of defense against cancer. This theory maintains that spontaneously arising malignant cells are kept in check by a healthy immune system (Burnet, 1970). Malignant tumors develop in an otherwise healthy human only if there is a breakdown in the body surveillance mechanism. There is some evidence to support this theory.

According to the most recent edition of Harrison's *Principles of Internal Medicine* (Fauci et al., 1998), "Animal studies have conclusively shown that the immune system can recognize and eliminate malignant tumors in vivo. Rejection of tumor cells in several animal models appears to be mediated primarily by cytotoxic lymphocytes, including cytotoxic T lymphocytes and natural killer cells" (p. 535). Natural killer (NK) cells are a subpopulation of lymphoid cells that have spontaneous cytolytic activity against a variety of tumor cells. There is increasing evidence that NK cells may play an important role in immune surveillance because of their ability

to mediate natural resistance against tumors, certain viruses, and other microbial diseases (Herberman, 1981).

Patients with HIV infection or AIDS who have seriously weakened immune systems are unusually susceptible to the cancer known as Kaposi's sarcoma. A number of other viral and bacterial infections, likely influenced by the immune system, may predispose to the development of cancer. These include hepatitis B or C virus (liver cancer), human papillomavirus (associated with more than 80% of cervical cancer cases), *Helicobacter pylori* (causes more than 50% of cases of gastric cancer), Epstein-Barr virus (nasopharyngeal cancer, B and T lymphocyte malignancies, gastric cancer, and Hodgkin's disease), human T cell lymphoma virus I (HTLV-1) (T cell lymphomas and leukemias), and herpes virus 8 (Kaposi's sarcoma). An estimated 10–20% of all cancers are a direct result of viral infection (Fauci et al., 1998, p. 1070).

There may also be an increase in malignancy among persons who take long-term immunosuppressive drugs associated with renal transplantation. One study followed 432 renal transplant patients for 11 years; 24 developed cancers, an incidence of 5.6%, which is 100 times greater than the incidence observed in age-matched controls from the general population (Ultmann & Golomb, 1980). In another study of 184 organ graft recipients who developed new cases of cancer, 60% of the cancer patients were under age 40 and lymphomas were unusually common; both of these factors (young age and tumor type) suggest that impaired immunity may have contributed to the development of malignancies (Ultmann & Golomb, 1980; Thomas, 1982).

Gelato (1996) notes that older persons have four to five times the rate of cancer of young adults, which, he suggests, may be related to the decline of immune function with aging. Older adults experience a decline in cell-mediated and humeral immune responsiveness, and T cell responses are more severely affected than B cell responses. This could account for the increased rate of cancer (which has been experimentally demonstrated in animal models) (Doria et al., 1997). While the theory of immune surveillance has been questioned and modified over the years, it remains a viable explanation for how the human body protects itself against cancer. In fact, new approaches to the treatment of cancer involve manipulating the body's immune system. Recently identified tumor antigens recognized by cytotoxic T cells may lead to the construction of chemically defined antigens for the immunotherapy of cancers (Shu et al., 1997).

Immune System Influences on Prognosis and Metastatic Spread

The immune system may also help to control the spread of malignant disease. Recall from chapter 19 Levy and colleagues' (1987) study of NK cell activity and psychosocial status in 75 women with stage I and stage II breast cancer. Reduced NK cell activity was associated with shorter survival (node-positive patients had lower levels of NK cell activity than patients with nonmetastatic disease). Reviewing the research to date, Herberman (1991) concluded that the evidence is probably more compelling for the immune system's role in the control of tumor metastasis than for immune surveillance. See chapter 19, on immune system functioning, for more studies that address this issue.

PSYCHOSOCIAL FACTORS THAT AFFECT THE ONSET AND THE COURSE OF CANCER

If psychosocial factors influence immune system functioning (as suggested in chapter 19), and immune function influences the onset or progression of cancer, what effects might psychological stress, depression, hopelessness, personality, and social isolation have on the incidence or prognosis of cancer?

Psychological Stress

Andersen, Kiecolt-Glaser, et al. (1994) have described a biobehavioral model of adjustment to cancer, illustrating the mechanisms by which psychological factors may affect the development and the outcome of cancer. Difficulty adjusting to cancer can cause subsyndromal de-

pression, which may down-regulate elements of the immune system, leading to adverse health consequences, such as increased respiratory tract and other infections and possibly metastatic spread of the tumor. In their study of women with breast cancer, Levy, Lippman, et al. (1987) found that increased stress was associated with reduced natural killer cell activity. Andersen, Farrar, et al. (1998), in a study of 116 postsurgical patients with breast cancer, also found that stress inhibited cellular immune responses (NK cell toxicity and T-cell responses) relevant to cancer prognosis.

Depression

Recall Levy, Lippman, et al.'s (1987) study of breast cancer patients, described in chapter 19. Subjects who reported depression-like fatigue symptoms at baseline showed a decline in NK cell activity three months later compared to women without these symptoms. Likewise, recall Prigerson et al.'s (1997) study, which found that new cases of cancer developed among widows and widowers who were experiencing symptoms of traumatic grief, while none developed among those without traumatic grief.

In one of the largest studies to date, Knekt et al. (1996) evaluated lung cancer risk in a random sample of 7,018 adult men and women who were free from cancer at baseline and who were followed for 14 years in the Finland Health Survey. A total of 605 cases of cancer were diagnosed during the follow-up period. The relative risk of cancer among persons who were depressed at baseline compared to those who were not was 3.32 (95% CI 1.53–7.20). In other words, depressed subjects were more than three times more likely to develop cancer than those without depression.

Hopelessness

Everson, Goldberg, et al. (1996) conducted a six-year prospective study of 2,400 middle-aged men in Finland to examine whether lack of hope was associated with death from heart disease or cancer. During the six-year follow-up, 174 of the men died, 87 from heart disease and 40 from cancer. The death rates of men with moderate and high levels of hopelessness were two and three times, respectively, those of men with low levels of hopelessness. Men with moderate or high levels of hopelessness were at increased risk of death from both heart disease and cancer. These differences remained significant after subjects were matched for blood pressure, cholesterol levels, smoking and drinking habits, social class, education, prior depression, and social isolation. High levels of hopelessness also predicted new cases of fatal cancer and heart disease in men with no history of these problems.

Personality

Certain personality factors may also increase the risk of cancer. Schulz et al. (1996) examined pessimism and age and their affects on cancer mortality in an eight-month prospective study of 238 cancer patients who were receiving palliative radiation therapy in western Pennsylvania. When followed-up eight months later, 70 patients had died. Hierarchical regression revealed an interaction between age and pessimism (as measured by the Life Orientation Test). Pessimism had a negative effect on mortality in the youngest age group (ages 30–59) ($p < .05$), but not in persons over age 60.

In a major review of psychosocial influences on cancer incidence and progression for the *Harvard Review of Psychiatry*, Spiegel and Kato (1996) concluded that there is a significant relationship between psychosocial factors (personality, depression, emotional expression, social support, and stress) and cancer incidence and progression. According to these authors, mechanisms that might mediate this relationship include diet, exercise, variations in medical treatments received, and physiological mechanisms such as psychoendocrinologic and psychoneuroimmunologic effects.

Support from Family and Friends

Strong social support may help prevent the effects of psychological stress on the onset and course of cancer. Thomas et al. (1985) examined 256 healthy elderly adults and found that those with good social support systems tended to have lower serum cholesterol levels and higher indices of immune function; these correlations remained significant after age, body mass, tobacco use, alcohol intake, and degree of perceived psychological distress were taken into account. The authors concluded that social support systems may intervene between the stressful stimulus and physiological responses to that stimulus. Likewise, Baron et al. (1990), found, in their study of social support and immune functioning among spouses of cancer patients, that natural killer cell cytotoxicity and proliferation responses to phytohemagglutinin were greater among those with high levels of social support. All six dimensions of social support as assessed by the Social Provisions Scale were strongly related to measures of immune function. Recall that Levy, Lippman, et al. (1987) found that breast cancer patients who complained about a lack of family support at baseline showed a decrease in natural killer cell activity three months later.

Social support may be particularly important for the prognosis of cancer in elderly patients who are at risk for social isolation. Goodwin et al. (1991) studied the functional status and social support networks of 799 men and women age 65 or older who were newly diagnosed with cancer. Functional limitations increased significantly with age, and increased functional limitations led to significant decreases in social support. Unfortunately, these investigators did not examine the impact of this interaction between social support and functional status on cancer survival.

Reynolds and Kaplan (1990) provide more direct evidence in this regard. These investigators examined the association between social connections and cancer incidence and prognosis during a 17-year follow-up of 6,848 adults involved in the Alameda County Study (subjects ages 18–65 were initially surveyed in 1965). Women who were socially isolated at baseline were at significantly greater risk of dying from cancer than those who were not socially isolated. While social connections were not prospectively associated with cancer incidence or mortality in men, those men with few social connections had significantly poorer cancer survival rates. Likewise, Vogt et al. (1992) prospectively followed a random sample of 2,603 members of health maintenance organizations for 15 years to examine the effect of three social support network measures on incidence of and mortality from ischemic heart disease, cancer, stroke, and hypertension. Social network measures strongly predicted both cause-specific and all-cause mortality among persons who had incident cases of ischemic heart disease, cancer, and stroke. While not all studies show a significant impact for social support on cancer survival (Cassileth et al., 1985), many do.

Support Groups

What effect might group social support have on the outcome of cancer? Studies reviewed in chapter 19 are also relevant here.

Spiegel et al. (1989) conducted a randomized clinical trial to test the effects of a psychosocial intervention on survival among 86 women with metastatic breast cancer. The psychosocial intervention lasted one year and consisted of weekly supportive group therapy meetings and self-hypnosis for pain management. At the 10-year follow-up, only three patients were still alive; death records were obtained for the 83 deceased women. The average survival time for subjects in the intervention group was 33.6 months and 18.9 months for women in the control group ($p < 0.0001$, Cox model). Interestingly, differences in survival did not become evident until eight months after the intervention ended.

Recall the studies by Fawzy's research group, mentioned briefly in chapter 19. We describe them in more detailed here. Fawzy, Cousins, et al. (1990a) conducted a randomized clinical trial involving 80 patients with malignant melanoma. Researchers assigned half of the patients to routine care and the other half to a series of six structured support groups. The support groups met weekly and were designed to help patients cope better with the illness and its effects on their families. The results of the study showed a significant decrease in depressed mood on the POMS and an increase in active coping strategies among support group members. Fawzy et al. (1990b) also evaluated

changes in immunological measures over time. Patients in the weekly support group intervention showed significant differences in immune function at the three-month follow-up. These patients ($n = 35$) showed significant increases in percentages of large granular lymphocytes, natural killer (NK) cells, and NK cell cytotoxic activity compared with controls ($n = 26$). Measures of depressive affect showed significant correlations with immune cell changes.

Fawzy, Fawzy, Hyun, et al. (1993) next reported on the effects of the support group intervention on cancer recurrence and patient survival six years later. Researchers found that the intervention group had a lower rate of recurrence (21% vs. 38%) and were significantly less likely to die during the six-year observation period (9% vs. 29%). Higher enhancement of active-behavioral coping over time predicted lower rates of recurrence and death. For a comprehensive review of studies examining the effects of psychosocial interventions (stress-management, improved psychological coping, and group support) on survival of cancer patients, see Fawzy, Fawzy, Arndt, et al. (1995). Bearing in mind the positive effects of psychosocial factors on cancer incidence and prognosis, we now examine the relationship between religion and cancer.

CANCER IN DIFFERENT RELIGIOUS GROUPS

Members of different religious groups have varying risks of developing cancer. We review research that has examined cancer rates in Jews, Seventh-Day Adventists, Mormons, Amish, Hutterites, and Christian groups in general, presenting this research in chronological order of year of publication.

Jews

The risk of cancer among Jews is complex. Jewish persons experience a decreased rate of cancer for some sites but an increased rate for others, and this cancer risk has changed over time. In 1902, a report entitled "Cancer among

Jews" appeared in the *British Medical Journal* (Correspondent, 1902). This study compared cancer death rates in Jews and non-Jews in London from 1898 to 1900. The investigation was based on data obtained from the Burial Society of the United Synagogue. Cancer death rates were reported to be lower in Jews than in non-Jews (2.1–2.4% vs. 4.7–4.9%). No statistical comparison was made, however, and there was no comment on what types of cancer were less common among Jews. Socioeconomic status was also not controlled and could have explained the differences observed.

The next report on cancer rates in Jews was by Wolbarst (1932). He conducted a case-control study of 830 cases of penile cancer in the United States, examining the effect that circumcision had on the prevalence of this condition. Cases of penile cancer were reported by 205 hospitals, including 26 Jewish hospitals, that had a combined daily census of 40,709 patients, of whom 4.4% were Jewish. The investigators did not find a single case of penile cancer in a Jew. During that same period, the United States, India, and Java reported 2,484 cases of penile cancers in uncircumcised men but only 33 cases in men who were circumcised. Wolbarst concluded that penile cancer was almost unheard of in circumcised Jews and Muslims, despite the fact that it accounts for 2–3% of all cancers in men.

That same year, Hoffman (1932) examined cancer deaths in Amsterdam, the Netherlands, between 1920–1929 ($n = 9,405$). Cancer death rates ranged from 121/100,000 per year to 142/100,000 per year. Jews had higher death rates from cancer of the liver or gallbladder (17.2/100,000 vs. 13.2 for Catholics and 12.7 for others), rectum (8.4 for Jews vs. 6.5 for Catholics and 4.9 for others), ovaries (5.0 for Jews vs. 2.0 for Catholics and 2.0 for others), and breast (11.3 for Jews vs. 9.3 for Catholics and 9.7 for others) but lower rates of cancer of the esophagus (3.6 vs. 9.5 and 7.0), larynx (same as esophagus), stomach (32.9 vs. 47.9 and 42.6), intestine (9.5 vs. 12.7 and 12.1), and uterus (3.9 vs. 10.2 and 9.8). Hoffman noted that studies of this type have found "decidedly lower mortality from cancer of the uterus in Jewish women

compared with other racial elements in the same population" (p. 153).

The following year, Bolduan and Weiner (1933) reported, in the *New England Journal of Medicine*, the results of a case-control study of 14,047 Jews and 27,186 non-Jews in New York City. Jews were more likely to die of cancer (14.6% vs. 10.8%, all types), particularly cancers of the digestive tract and peritoneum (death rates were 50% higher among Jewish men than among non-Jewish men). Likewise, breast cancer was more common among Jewish women up to age 45, after which it was less common than in non-Jews.

A few years later, Wolff (1939) examined cancer death rates among Jews in 1924–1926 and 1932–1934 in Berlin. Overall, cancer death rates were nearly the same for Jews as for non-Jews: 15.5/10,000 vs. 14.8/10,000 in 1924–1926 and 19.7 vs. 17.1 in 1932–1934. The distribution of types of cancer, however, did vary. Jewish men and women were less likely to have cancer of the esophagus, stomach, or duodenum than were those in the general population. Jewish women were less likely to have cancer of the uterus (51 observed cases among Jewish women vs. 107 expected cases), although they were more likely to have cancer of the lung, rectum, or anus, other female genital organs, and breast. Jewish men were also more likely to have cancer of the rectum, anus, or respiratory organs.

Versluys (1949) conducted a case-control study of all deaths from cancer in the Netherlands between 1931 and 1935. Higher than expected death rates from cancer were found among Jewish men and Jewish women. Jewish women had higher death rates for cancer of the breast, ovary, intestines, and kidneys but lower death rates for cancer of the cervix. Jewish men experienced higher death rates from cancers of the intestines and rectum, lung, and bladder but a lower death rate from gastric cancer. Note that several of these early studies report higher rates of lung cancer among Jewish men than among non-Jews; this pattern was reversed in later studies.

Following up on Bolduan and Weiner's report, MacMahon conducted a series of cancer mortality studies among Jews in New York City in the 1950s (MacMahon, 1957, 1960); a decade later, Seidman extended these studies (1966, 1971). In his first study, MacMahon (1957) examined the distribution of ethnic background of 1,368 white persons who died of leukemia between 1943 and 1952 in Brooklyn, New York, comparing them to the backgrounds of persons who had died from any cause in Brooklyn during the same years. Religious affiliation was obtained from cemetery of burial. MacMahon reported that roughly twice as many Jews died of acute myelogenous leukemia (2.7 to 1.0), chronic myelogenous leukemia (1.9 to 1.0), and chronic lymphatic leukemia (2.4 to 1.0) as non-Jews.

A couple of years later, MacMahon (1960) examined the distribution of deaths from all types of cancer among residents of New York City ($n = 14,356$ whites). Religious affiliation was again obtained from the cemetery of burial. He found that cancer of the cervix was 2.1 less likely in Jewish women than in Catholics and 2.6 times less likely in Jewish women than in Protestants. He also found fewer cancers of the upper respiratory tract (tongue, buccal cavity, pharynx, larynx) in Jewish men than in non-Jewish men. In addition, he found fewer neoplasms of the esophagus and liver among Jews (because of lower alcohol consumption?). On the other hand, he found higher rates of melanoma, leukemia, and Hodgkin's disease in Jews (replicating MacMahon's 1957 report), as well as of cancers of the kidney and large intestine. He explained these findings by suggesting that Jews were more likely to seek medical care and perhaps more likely to receive ionizing radiation from x-rays, which might explain the higher rates of leukemia. About this time, Newill (1961) examined 83,341 cancer deaths of white residents in New York City between 1953 and 1958. He found almost the same pattern as MacMahon: Cancers of the lung were less frequent among Jewish men and cancer of the cervix less frequent among Jewish women, but cancers of the large intestine, lymphomas, and leukemias were all significantly more prevalent in Jews than in non-Jews.

Seidman (1966) compared rates of lung cancer among Jewish, Catholic, and Protestant white men in New York City in 1940, 1949–

1951, and 1958–1962. Like MacMahon and Newill, Seidman found lung cancer death rates for Catholics and Protestants to be 50% higher than those for Jews. Compared to earlier studies, it appeared that Jews had gone from being a high-risk lung cancer group to being a low-risk group. Low rates of lung cancer were explained by the fact that Jewish men smoked fewer cigarettes. Seidman (1971) again examined age-adjusted mortality for all cancer sites among whites in New York City between 1949 and 1951. Jewish men had lower SMRs (standard mortality ratios) for all cancer sites combined than did all non-Jewish men or Catholics alone (90 vs. 105 or 110, differences that persisted at all socioeconomic levels). In contrast, Jewish women had higher SMRs for all cancer sites combined than did all non-Jewish women or Catholic women alone (112 vs. 95 or 92, differences that also persisted at all socioeconomic levels). What was not clear, however, was whether these differences (particularly among men) were entirely due to a tendency by Jews to avoid alcohol and cigarette smoking.

Examining Jews living outside of New York City, King, Diamond, et al. (1965) studied 1,754 cancer deaths among white residents of Baltimore city and county, comparing death rates among Catholics, Protestants, and Jews (determined again by funeral home of burial service) for various forms of cancer. They found no significant differences in overall rates of cancer mortality among the three religious groups, although types of cancer did vary. Lung cancer was less common among Jews, as had been reported by others. Cancers of the intestine and rectum and leukemia, in contrast to previous reports, were found to be less common among Jewish men. Jewish women, consistent with previous reports, had lower rates of cancer of the cervix and of the corpus uteri but higher rates of cancer of the lymphatic and homatopoietic tissues and of the digestive system.

Herman and Enterline (1970) and Horowitz and Enterline (1970), studying Jews and non-Jews in Pittsburgh and Montreal, respectively, also reported a lower death rate from cancer of the lung in Jewish men. These investigators concluded that the lower death rate was probably due to avoidance of cigarette smoking, given the histologic type of cancer (low rate of epidermoid and anaplastic cell types). Interestingly, in both of these studies Jewish women had significantly higher rates of lung cancer than non-Jewish females, but these cancers were not due to smoking (on the basis of histologic type).

Greenwald et al. (1975) conducted a case control study of 800 deaths of Russian-born residents of New York State who died of cancer between 1969 and 1971. Jewish or non-Jewish affiliation was determined in the usual manner (from the cemetery of burial or the religious affiliation of funeral home). Jewish men were again more likely to die of colon cancer (36 expected, 56 observed, $p < .01$) and less likely to die of lung cancer (70 expected, 54 observed, $p < .05$); Jewish women were more likely to die of cancer of the stomach or cancer of the lung but were less likely to die of cancer of the breast or cancer of the cervix.

Rosenwaike (1984) confirmed Seidman's (1966) report that Jews were changing from a high- to a low-risk group for lung cancer. He conducted a cohort analysis of lung cancer deaths among whites age 35 or over in three religious groups in New York City in 1969–1971 and 1979–1981. Seidman's data, collected in 1949–1951 and 1959–1961, were used for comparison. Rosenwaike reported that Jewish men showed markedly lower increases in lung cancer over the 30-year period than did Catholic or Protestant men, a pattern not replicated among women. Why the lung cancer rate dropped among Jewish men but not among Jewish women was unclear, although the change was attributed to reduced smoking among Jewish men.

More recently, Egan et al. (1996) conducted a population-based case-control study of 6,611 women in the United States with breast cancer to study the influence of Jewish religion on cancer risk. Rates among Jewish women were compared with those for 9,026 control women without cancer (the study was conducted by telephone interviews). Jewish women overall had a slightly increased risk of breast cancer. However, the increased risk was much higher for Jewish women with a first-degree relative with breast cancer (RR 3.78, 95% CI 1.75–8.16, $p < .001$). The effect of family history was greater in Jewish women than in women with other religious backgrounds (significance level for interaction was .05). To address the same research question, Toniolo and Kato (1996) conducted a prospective cohort study of 10,273 women enrolled between 1985 and 1991 during mammographic screening in New York City. Among Jewish women age 50 or younger with a family history of breast cancer, the relative risk was again higher in Jews than in members of other religious groups (2.33, 95% CI 1.35–4.02, adjusted for multiple risk factors). The authors found no increased risk among Jewish women without a family history or among those over age 50. The investigators concluded that certain groups of Jewish women have a higher than expected rate of mutation in breast cancer gene BRCA1.

Finally, Steinberg et al. (1998) conducted a population-based, case-control study involving eight geographic regions in the United States in 1980–1982. They compared 471 women with ovarian cancer with 4,025 controls. Jewish women were more likely than non-Jewish women to have familial ovarian cancer (OR 8.4, CI 2.6–28). The risk of having ovarian cancer was greater in Jewish women with a first-degree relative with ovarian cancer (OR 8.81) than in non-Jewish women with a first-degree relative with the disease (OR 3.01) ($p = $ ns). On the other hand, Jewish women with no first-degree relative with ovarian cancer had no increased risk of the disease over non-Jewish women.

In summary, Jewish persons appear to be at lower risk for cancers of the cervix and penis (due to male circumcision) and for cancers of the respiratory organs and the upper gastrointestinal organs (possibly due to reduced smoking and less alcohol use). They are at increased risk, however, for some types of breast cancer and ovarian cancer (likely due to genetic factors), for leukemias and lymphomas (possibly due to genetic factors or, perhaps, increased exposure to ionizing radiation from x-rays), and for cancers of the colon and rectum (cause unknown).

Seventh-Day Adventists

Seventh-Day Adventists (SDAs) are a conservative religious group (closest in theology to Mor-

302 RESEARCH ON RELIGION AND PHYSICAL DISORDERS

mons) who almost completely abstain from the use of tobacco and alcohol and, to a lesser extent, from the consumption of coffee, tea, fish, and meat. In addition to a healthy lifestyle, SDAs often have strong families and live in supportive communities.

In 1959, Wynder and colleagues were the first to examine cancer and coronary artery disease rates among California SDAs. They found lower rates of both diseases in this group compared to the general population. Their report was soon followed by a series of other articles by these investigators that indicated that SDAs have lower death rates from cancer and respiratory diseases. The studies were published in a number of prestigious journals (Lemon, Walden, et al., 1964; Lemon & Kuzma, 1966, 1969). In a report published in the *Journal of the American Medical Association*, Lemon and Kuzma (1966) indicated that only one death from lung cancer or emphysema occurred among 3,913 lifetime SDA members who had never smoked.

Phillips and colleagues conducted further studies of California SDAs in the mid-1970s and early 1980s (see Phillips, 1975; Phillips, Lemon, et al., 1978; Phillips, Garfinkel, et al., 1980; Phillips, Kuzma, et al., 1980; Phillips & Snowdon, 1983). In 1975, Phillips reported that SDA mortality rates were 50–70% of those for the general population for cancer sites unrelated to smoking or drinking. Cancer mortality in SDA physicians and non-SDA physicians, however, was equal, suggesting that the reduced risk was due to "selection" factors. After a two-year prospective study of 100,000 SDAs in California, data on 41 Adventists with colon cancer and 77 Adventists with breast cancer were reviewed. SDAs who ate meat were found to have a risk of colon cancer 2.8 times that of vegetarian SDAs, suggesting that a lacto-ovo-vegetarian diet may be protective against colon cancer. The authors speculated that the slightly reduced rate of breast cancer in SDAs was attributable to a reduced intake of fried potatoes. Phillips and colleagues later published six-year, 16-year, and 21-year follow-up studies on this cohort. While there was a close link between smoking habits and cancer rate, the researchers continued to find lower rates of cancer at sites unrelated to smoking and concluded that elements of the

SDA lifestyle other than avoidance of smoking might be important protective factors against cancer.

In 1983, both Berkel and deWaard and Jensen examined cancer rates among SDAs in the Netherlands. Berkel and deWaard (1983) examined 522 SDA who had died between 1968 and 1977 and, found that the SMR for neoplasms in that group was 0.50; in other words, the likelihood of death from cancer in this group was only 50% that faced by the general Dutch population. A prudent diet was invoked to explain the low rates of colon cancer and other malignancies.

Jensen (1983) conducted a case-control study that compared cancer risk among SDA men and non-SDA men who did not drink alcohol compared with that faced by the general Dutch population. Participants were 1,752 men identified from the files of the National League of Temperance Societies in Copenhagen, Denmark. Of the 1,752 men, 781 Adventists and 808 non-Adventists were identified (25–50% of this group may have been recovering alcoholics). Cancer morbidity was established from municipal records, the National Central Person Registry, and National Central Death Registry. Compared to the rates of cancer morbidity in the general population of Denmark, Adventists had a SMR of 0.69 (31% lower rate), whereas non-Adventist controls had rates similar to those of the general population (SMR of 1.05). When cancers related to alcohol or smoking were excluded, the cancer risk among SDAs increased to 0.93, which was not significantly different from that for men in the general Dutch population. Jensen concluded that lower rates of cancer among Adventist men could be largely explained by their abstaining from smoking and drinking. They admitted that they had examined only morbidity, however, not mortality (as had the U.S. studies) and acknowledged that cancer mortality rates might appear to be lower among SDAs because they survived longer.

In a later study, Fraser et al. (1991) analyzed prospective data on 34,198 California SDAs and found only 61 new cases of primary lung cancer during a six-year period of observation. This study did not compare lung cancer rates in

SDAs with those in the general population but did examine risk factors within the SDA community. Smoking was strongly associated with lung cancer in this population, particularly with small cell, squamous cell, and large cell cancer (RR 53.2 for current smokers and 7.1 for past smokers). In addition, there was a lower relative risk for lung cancer among SDAs who ate a lot of fruits; for those who ate fruit three to seven times/week, the risk of lung cancer was reduced by 70 percent (Relative Risk = .30). This study suggested that risk factors for lung cancer in SDAs were generally similar to those among non-SDA groups.

Mormons

The Mormons are a Caucasian religious group that has large numbers of adherents in Utah and California. Mormons' "Word of Wisdom" forbids the use of tobacco, alcohol, coffee, tea, and drugs, especially drugs that are addictive. It also stresses a well-balanced diet, use of wholesome grains and fruits, and moderation in the eating of meat. Like Seventh-Day Adventists, Mormons live in close-knit communities and emphasize family values.

Enstrom (1975) was the first investigator to compare cancer rates among Mormons with those of non-Mormons. He examined cancer death rates among 360,000 California Mormons and compared them to rates in the general California population. He found that California Mormons experienced only about one-half to three-quarters the cancer death rates of other Californians. This was especially true for cancers of the esophagus, stomach, colon, rectum, pancreas, lung, prostate, bladder, and kidney in men and for cancers of the colon, lung, breast, and uterus (cervix and corpus) in women. A number of these cancer sites were unrelated to smoking. Enstrom soon followed up this study with several others (1978, 1980, 1989) that compared cancer death rates in California Mormons with those for different populations in and outside California. He was soon joined by investigators from other research groups, including Lyon, Klauber, et al. (1976), Gardner and Lyon (1977), Gardner and Lyon (1982a), and Gardner and Lyon (1982b), who compared Mormons in Utah, to non-Mormons in Utah and to the general U.S. population.

Lyon et al. (1976) compared cancer rates for Mormons and for non-Mormons who were living in Utah with those for a national sample; data were based on 10,641 cancer deaths in Utah between 1966 and 1970. In addition to having lower rates of cancer related to smoking, Mormon women had lower rates of breast cancer ($p < .01$), less cervical cancer ($p < .00001$), and less ovarian cancer ($p < .05$). The findings left unexplained the significant differences between Mormons and non-Mormons for cancers not thought to be due to smoking or health behaviors.

In a report from the same research group published a year later, Gardner et al. (1977) examined 867 cervical cancer cases diagnosed in Utah from 1966 to 1970 (data were from a subset of subjects in Lyon's earlier report) and compared rates between Mormons and non-Mormons. The age-adjusted cervical cancer incidence rate among Utah women was 26% less than the overall rate in the United States; Mormon women had 55% less cervical cancer than non-Mormon women ($p < 0.0001$, adjusted for age) and their rate was 45% below the overall rate for the United States. The authors also reported that the incidence of syphilis and gonorrhea was significantly lower in Utah, where Mormons predominate, than in the United States as a whole. Gardner and colleagues (1982a, 1982b) then looked at the effects of religious activity level on cancer rates within the Mormon population itself and found that cancer rates were lowest among the most religiously active (measured by lay priesthood level in men and church activity in women). Studies outside the United States (i.e., in Canada) also report lower cancer rates in Mormons (Jarvis, 1977), especially for smoking-related sites.

Enstrom (1989) conducted the most recent study of cancer mortality in Mormons, an eight-year prospective study of 9,844 religiously active California Mormons and their wives, in which he compared them with 3,119 adults who were participating in the Alameda County study. Mormon men had lower death rates from all cancers (SMR 47), particularly from smoking-related cancers (SMR 15 for smoking-related vs. SMR 71 for nonsmoking cancer sites). Similarly, Mormon wives had lower death rates from all cancers (SMR 72), in particular from smoking-related cancers (SMR 41 for smoking-related vs. SMR 82 for nonsmoking cancer sites). Among the controls in the Alameda County study, white nonsmokers who attended church weekly and engaged in three health-related lifestyle practices (not smoking, getting physical exercise, sleeping regularly) had an SMR for cancer of only 13 (compared to 51 for Mormons, both sexes combined). Religiously active persons of any denomination who live healthy lifestyles, then, appear to have the same low cancer risk as active Mormons.

Hutterites

To examine the effects of inbreeding on cancer risk, Martin et al. (1980) examined cancer deaths between 1965 and 1975 among the Hutterites, an isolated religious group of about 13,000 members who live primarily in Alberta, Manitoba, South Dakota, and Washington State. The Hutterites originated in Europe in 1528 and migrated to South Dakota in the late 1800s. Members of this religious group are concerned about their health, do not smoke, and do not hesitate to seek modern medical care. Among those descended from two of the three original Hutterite colonies (S-leut and L-leut) and therefore subject to the most inbreeding, investigators discovered 29 cancer deaths in men and 23 deaths in women, which was fewer than expected ($p < .01$), given their inbreeding, compared to the rate for the U.S. white population. This finding was largely a result of the Hutterites' lower mortality from lung cancer (one death vs. 13 expected, $p < .05$) and to their lower rates of cervical cancer; only one woman in the entire Hutterite population had cervical cancer, and she did not die during the study period. However, investigators did find higher than expected rates of leukemia in this population, which was consistent with their genetic hypothesis.

Amish

The Amish are another relatively isolated religious group with a high degree of inbreeding. The religious beliefs of the Amish, founded in the Anabaptist movement of sixteenth-century Switzerland, have led to religious, cultural, and genetic isolation. The Amish diet is relatively high in fats and carbohydrates and is prepared without commercial preservatives or additives. Tobacco use has been widespread among Amish men, although it is unusual among the women. While cigarette smoking is largely discouraged, pipe and cigar smoking and tobacco chewing are more common. Drinking alcohol, while it does occur, occurs primarily within the home, and excesses are not common. The high degree of inbreeding, however, increases the risk of genetic diseases.

Hamman et al. (1981) conducted a case-control study of causes of death in 25,822 Old Order Amish people in three settlements, in Indiana, Ohio, and Pennsylvania. Death certificates and Amish census data were used to determine mortality risk (676 men and 550 women died during the study period). While Amish mortality patterns were not systematically different from those of non-Amish (SMR 0.89 for men, 1.15 for women), they differed in age, sex, and cause of death. Amish men had higher all-cause mortality rates as children but lower mortality rates after age 40, primarily because of lower rates of cancer (SMR 0.44 for ages 40–69) and cardiovascular diseases (SMR 0.65 for ages 40–69). While the authors note that site-specific differences in type of cancer were present, this information was not provided in the study report. Amish women had lower overall death rates between ages 10–39, but their death rates did not differ for ages 40–69; the SMR for Amish women was not different from that for the general population for all cancer sites combined.

Christians

Certain cancers may be less common among conservative Christians because of their health behaviors, including less risky sexual practices. In 1963, Naguib, Lundin, et al. (1966) performed a cytologic screening program for cancer of the cervix in Washington County, Maryland. Cancer detection kits were mailed to a population-based sample of 6,801 persons. The Johns

Hopkins School of Public Health had obtained personal characteristics (including denomination and religious attendance) on the study population during a separate survey earlier that year. Of the women who received kits, 5,896 were matched to their personal data; of these, 4,341 returned the cancer screening kits. Of the Pap smears that were returned, 4,290 of them were acceptable for examination. Among the 3,962 women designated "Christians," there was an inverse relationship between the frequency of religious service attendance and rates of abnormal smears or confirmed cases of cervical cancer, an association that persisted after researchers controlled for education. Among women who attended services once a week or more, the rate of suspicious or positive smears or confirmed cases was 25/2213, or 1.13%, compared with 15/426 (3.52%) for women who attended services less than twice a year or never. The authors concluded that religious attendance among Christian women was related to lower rates of cancer of the cervix because of the Christian women's more conservative sexual practices, since Kinsey et al. (1948) had found that incidence of extramarital coitus was inversely related to church activity. Naguib et al. also concluded that their findings supported the hypothesis that having multiple sexual partners is related to cervical cancer (which we now know is related to transmission of the human papillomavirus).

Dwyer et al. (1990) used county-level cancer mortality data from the National Center for Health Statistics (3,063 counties) for 1968–1970, 1971–1974, and 1975–1980 to examine the relationship between religion and cancer death. Data on religion (percentage of population with full membership and their degree of religious conservativeness) were obtained from a separate study of churches and church membership in the United States. Investigators found that religion had a significant impact on mortality rates from cancer, even after they controlled for 15 factors known to affect cancer mortality. Conservative Protestants and Mormons had the lowest mortality rates, and counties with the highest concentrations of Jews or liberal Protestants had the highest cancer mortality rates. The investigators concluded

that the general population in an area with a high concentration of religious participants may experience health benefits because of diminished exposure to or increased social disapproval of behaviors related to high cancer mortality.

Other Religious Groups

There is little information about the relationship between cancer and other world religions. We briefly review the extant research here. Jussawalla and Jain (1977) studied the relationship between breast cancer and religion in greater Bombay, India. They identified 2,130 women from the Bombay Cancer Registry who were diagnosed with cancer between 1964 and 1972. Of these women, 59% were Hindus, 14% were Muslim, 2% were Christian, 11% were Parsis (Zoroastrian), 1% were Buddhist, and 13% were affiliated with other religious groups. When they compared their data to national data on the expected rates of breast cancer for Bombay, the authors found that the breast cancer rate in women from Parsis religious backgrounds was 48.5/100,000 compared to 18.2/100,000 for non-Parsis women in India. The high rate of breast cancer among Parsis women was similar to that found among Swedish women but still considerably below the rate in the United States (62.3/100,000). The authors gave no explanation for the lower rates of breast cancer in Bombay or for Parsis women's higher rates than those of other women in Bombay.

Kessler, Kulcar, et al. (1974) compared cervical cancer rates in Muslims and non-Muslims in Yugoslavia. Cases consisted of 350 women under the age of 60, of whom 150 were Muslims and 200 were non-Muslims. Control women were selected randomly among currently hospitalized women without cervical cancer or sexually transmitted disease who were similar to the subjects with regard to age, marital status, religion, and urban or rural residence. Among Muslims, controls were more likely to report that they were strictly observant of religious ritual than were the subjects (60.0% vs. 47.7%, $p < .05$). The controls were also less likely to smoke or drink, which may explain the differences observed. The investigators found no differences between non-Muslim subjects and controls on the basis of religious observance.

More recently, Massion et al. (1995) compared the levels of urinary 6-sulphatoxymelatonin (6-SM) in eight experienced women meditators who were graduates or teachers at the University of Massachusetts Stress Reduction and Relaxation Program with those of eight women controls who did not meditate. After factoring out the nonsignificant effect of menstrual period interval, the authors found higher levels of urinary 6-SM in the meditation group ($\beta = 1.98$, $p = .02$). Because of studies linking melatonin to the treatment of prostate or breast cancer, the authors hypothesized that transcendental meditation or "mindfulness" meditation (a Buddhist religious practice) may reduce the risk of cancer of the prostate or breast or may impact positively on outcome in cancer patients. Patients with cancer, however, were not examined in this study.

REASONS FOR LOWER RATES OF CANCER IN CERTAIN RELIGIOUS GROUPS

From the studies discussed, it is evident that dietary and health practices play a major role in explaining lower rates of cancer in certain religious groups. In a review of this area, Troyer (1988) compared SDAs, Mormons, Hutterites, and the Amish on attitudes toward meat consumption, coffee and tea use, and alcohol and tobacco use and on demographic characteristics. The author examined the overall cancer risk and risk of lung cancer, other smoking-related cancers, breast cancer, cervical cancer, gastrointestinal tract cancers, urinary cancers, and juvenile leukemia in the Amish and in Hutterites. Troyer concluded that religions that provide strong directives for personal behavior result in distinctive lifestyles that affect health in additive and multiplicative ways.

Less Smoking and Drinking

Fraser et al. (1991) found that cigarette smoking was strongly associated with lung cancer, particularly small cell, squamous cell, and large cell cancer, in their study population of 34,198 California Seventh-Day Adventists. The relative risk of lung cancer among current smokers was more than 53 times greater than for nonsmokers. Likewise, Jensen (1983) concluded from his study of Dutch Adventists that reduced cancer morbidity was largely the result of abstinence from smoking and drinking. Kessler, Kulcar, et al. (1974) found that strictly observant Muslims were less likely to smoke or drink (and more than likely had fewer sexual partners) than non-Muslims, thus explaining the lower risk of cervical cancer in that group.

Better Diet

Philips (1975) concluded from their study of 100,000 SDAs that a lacto-ovo-vegetarian diet may protect against colon cancer and that a reduced intake of fried potatoes may explain the slightly reduced rates of breast cancer in SDA women. Fraser et al. (1991) found that SDAs who ate a lot of fruit faced only 30% the risk of lung cancer of SDAs who didn't.

Safer Sexual Practices

Gardner and Lyon (1977) found that rates of syphilis and gonorrhea were significantly lower in Utah, where Mormons predominate, than in the United States as a whole, which they attributed to Mormons' less risky sexual practices and fewer sexual partners. Naguib, Lundin, et al. (1966) also found an inverse relationship between religious attendance and abnormal Pap smears and cervical cancer incidence among Christian women in Maryland County, and they also suggested that frequent church attendance was associated with fewer sexual partners (and probably lower risk of HPV infection).

Thus, absence of cigarette smoking, reduced alcohol consumption, better diet, and safer sexual practices all contribute to lower cancer risk.

Genetic Factors

Genetic factors also influence rates of cancer in different religious groups. This is especially true when mating is largely confined to other members of the religious group (i.e., when inbreeding is practiced) and is particularly true for the Old Order Amish, as noted earlier. It is less true for Jews, although it is probably still influential. Recall that Egan et al. (1996) and Toniolo and Kato (1996) found that certain groups of Jewish women have higher than expected rates of breast cancer probably because they have a mutation in the breast cancer gene BRCA1.

Hygienic Practices

Religious rituals having to do with hygienic practices may also influence cancer rates. Recall the Wolbarst (1932) report that penile cancer is almost unheard of in circumcised Jews and Muslims, despite the fact that it accounts for nearly 3% of all cancers in men.

Psychosocial Factors

Perhaps most interesting is the effect that increased social support, a close and fulfilling family life, improved adaptation to stress, reduced depression, and other positive psychosocial influences associated with devout religious practice may have on reducing the risk of certain cancers. This effect may be conveyed by degree of religiousness, rather than involvement in any particular religious group.

RELIGIOUSNESS AND CANCER RISK, ADAPTATION, AND COURSE

In the first section of this chapter, we examined the importance of cancer as a cause of death and morbidity in the United States. We reviewed the different types of cancers and their impact on survival. We explored risk factors that might predispose persons to the development of cancer and discussed how cancer might be prevented by avoiding risk factors. Finally, we examined the rates of cancer in different religious groups in the United States and around the world and discussed reasons for these differences. In this section, we focus on the relationship between degree of religiousness and the development of cancer, ability to cope with cancer, and course of cancer.

RELIGIOUS INFLUENCES ON THE DEVELOPMENT OF CANCER

What effect does degree of religiousness have on either preventing or promoting the development of cancer?

Religious Attendance

Attendance at religious services, while a poor indicator of religiosity, since people go to church for many reasons other than religiousness, still seems to be an excellent measure of involvement in religious community (the social dimension of religiosity). Numerous studies have demonstrated a strong link between religious attendance and virtually every dimension of social support (see chapter 15). Given the relationship among social support, better immune functioning, and longer cancer survival, there is ample reason to suspect an inverse relationship between religious attendance and development of cancer. Only a few studies, however, have examined this relationship, and in none of these studies was it the primary research question.

Monk et al. (1962) first reported that patients with cancer of the rectum were less likely to be members of a religious body and attended services less often than controls from the same population matched for sex, race, and age. This was not true, however, for patients with cancer of the colon.

Recall that Naguib et al.'s (1966) study of 3,962 "Christian" women in a subsample of the Washington County study found that there was an inverse relationship between the frequency of religious service attendance and rates of abnormal Pap smears. This association persisted after researchers controlled for education (a good proxy for socioeconomic status). The rate of suspicious or positive smears or confirmed cases of cancer among women who attended religious services once per week or more was less than one-third that of women who attended services less than twice a year. On the other hand, Comstock and Partridge (1972) did not find lower death rates from cancer (of all sites) among frequent church attenders in their three-to-six year prospective study of the overall Washington County cohort ($n = 55,000$), although they did not report death rates from cervical cancer separately.

Enstrom (1989) reported data from a prospective study of 3,119 adults who were participating in the Alameda County study (the control group used for his study of cancer in Mormons discussed earlier). Recall that white nonsmokers (all denominations) who attended church weekly and engaged in three health-related lifestyle practices (not smoking, getting regular physical exercise, and having a regular sleep pattern) experienced an SMR of only 13 for all cancers. In other words, these individuals had reduced their chance of developing cancer by 87% compared to persons in the general population.

A report involving the same sample was published the following year by a different group of investigators. Reynolds and Kaplan (1990) presented results from a 17-year follow-up of the entire Alameda County cohort ($n = 6,848$ adults, including the 3,119 subjects examined by Enstrom). These investigators were interested in the relationship between social connections and cancer risk. The study assessed church membership and church attendance at baseline in 1965. After adjusting for age, smoking, baseline physical health, alcohol consumption, and household income using Cox proportional hazards, the researchers found that socially isolated women were at greater risk of dying from cancer (all types combined) (Relative Hazards = 2.2), and smoking-related cancers (RH = 5.7) in particular. After adjusting for age, smoking, physical health, household income, and alcohol consumption, however, the investigators found no association between church membership or attendance (once per month or more vs. less than once a month) and cancer incidence or mortality. Recall that Enstrom defined "frequent church attendance" as once per week or more; thus, Reynolds and Kaplan's (1990) categorization of religious attendance may have been too insensitive to identify an effect on cancer incidence.

The findings from these few studies, then, are mixed. Some investigators report that frequent religious attendance is associated with fewer abnormal Pap smears for cervical cancer and lower rates of cancer in general. Others find no association, possibly because their religious attendance measure was not sensitive enough or because their study design was not powerful enough (Type II error) (e.g., because of low mortality rate, short follow-up period, lack of variance in the religiousness of the sample) to detect effects.

Cancer among the Clergy

If greater religious activity can help to protect persons from cancer, then one might expect the clergy to have the lowest cancer rates of all. Taylor et al. (1959) compared the cancer mortality experience of Catholic nuns with that of women in the general population, both single and married. Three orders of Sisters (two in Massachusetts and one in New York) were involved. Mortality was examined through 1954 for Sisters born in 1870 or later. Sisters showed lower total cancer mortality than did controls between ages 20–59 but higher mortality after age 60, and their total cancer experience was about the same. The risk of cancer of the genital organs for Sisters was 22% lower than for all white women. Tuberculosis was the principal cause of the Sisters' higher mortality during the study period, and Sisters showed greater improvement in mortality rate than controls with time.

Culminating a series of studies that examined cancer risk among clergy (King & Bailar, 1968; King, 1970, 1971; Locke & King, 1980), King and Locke (1980) examined causes of death among 28,134 clergyman in five primarily white Protestant denominations between 1950 and 1960. There were 5,207 deaths during this period. Compared to cancer death rates for the nation as a whole, the SMR for clergymen was 63 (that is, members of the clergy were 37% less likely to die of cancer). This was particularly true for cancer of the lung (SMR 35) and again suggests that health behaviors probably play a major (though perhaps not exclusive) role in explaining the observed differences in cancer rates.

Ogata et al. (1984) examined the mortality rate of 4,352 Japanese male Zen priests between 1955 and 1978 (1,396 deaths). SMRs for cerebrovascular diseases, pneumonia and bronchitis, peptic ulcer, liver cirrhosis, and cancer of the respiratory organs were all significantly lower than 100 (the mortality rate for the general population). Zen priests smoke less, eat less meat and fish, and live in less polluted areas than do most other Japanese men, although their drinking habits are similar.

Thus, clergy experience lower rates of cancer than do persons in the general population, but this difference can be largely explained by health behaviors (e.g., less cigarette smoking and alcohol use, better diet, safer environment).

Intrinsic Religiosity and Religious Commitment

To what extent are religious attitudes and commitment (as distinct from church-related activity) associated with cancer risk? As reviewed in chapter 19, depression, hopelessness, stress, and pessimism impair immune functioning and may increase the risk of cancer by reducing immune surveillance. Given the relationship between intrinsic religiosity and reduced depression, anxiety, and difficulty coping, greater hope, and improved sense of well-being, one might expect an inverse relationship between degree of religious commitment and cancer incidence. To our knowledge, however, no studies have examined the association between personal religiousness and the likelihood of developing cancer over time in a population that was disease free to begin with.

HOW RELIGION MAY INFLUENCE THE DEVELOPMENT OF CANCER

Improved Health Behaviors

As many as two-thirds of cancers may be prevented by careful attention to health behaviors and diet. Studies have shown that religious activities and religious commitment are associated with lower rates of cigarette smoking, excessive alcohol use, early sexual activity, multiple sexual partners, and sedentary, inactive lifestyles. For these reasons alone, religious involvement might reduce the risk of cancer. Remember, though, before discounting this effect as simply the result of healthier living, that adherence to positive health behaviors often grows out of strength of religious belief and commitment; these are *belief-based behaviors*.

Improved Immune Surveillance

In earlier chapters, we found that the majority of research studies indicate that religiousness is related to increased social support, greater sense of well-being, lower rates of depression, reduced anxiety, and improved coping. These benefits, in turn, may reduce neuroendocrine responses to stress that impair immune system functioning and break down immune surveillance. Consequently, one might expect those with greater religiousness to be at lower risk for developing at least certain forms of cancer.

Genetic Inbreeding

Religion may increase the likelihood of cancer related to reduced genetic variability caused by selective mating within a religious group. This is particularly problematic when the religious group is small and attracts few new members from the outside. Inbreeding allows genetic mutations to express themselves more easily, thereby increasing the risk of cancer.

RELIGION AND ADAPTATION TO CANCER

Whether or not religion prevents cancer or limits its spread, religious beliefs and activities are commonly used by cancer patients to help cope with the fear, anxiety, helplessness, and loss of control that a life-threatening illness provokes. For many people, being told that one has cancer is like confronting death itself. Images of a painful, disfiguring, disabling, and sometimes humiliating death may come to mind. Every symptom of the disease that a patient experiences is often a frightening reminder of the enemy within. The treatments for cancer may be feared as much as cancer's threat to mortality. Weakness, fatigue, nausea and diarrhea, loss of hair, and other body changes are widely known and feared complications of cancer therapies. As the disease progresses, waiting for the inevitable end can be more distressing than the physical symptoms of the disease. In this state of desperation, people may (in monotheistic traditions) turn to God for comfort either for the first time or more frequently and intensely than ever before.

What does "turning to God" in the setting of cancer involve? It often follows the stages of grief in response to loss. First, there is bargaining. The person with a newly diagnosed cancer or a recurrence of a previously dormant cancer may plead with God, asking him to remove the cancer. The person may admit to real or imagined sins, agree to follow God devoutly or turn his or her life around in order to serve and please God if only God will heal the cancer and spare the patient's life. If it appears the cancer is not going away in response to such pleas, then anger may result. The person asks, "Why me?" Bitterness or resentment may develop and deepen. After a time, when it is clear that bargaining and angry protest will not get rid of the cancer, grief and depression may set in as the person struggles to adapt to and accept the situation. At this time, the person may pray to God for the strength to deal with the illness as well as for strength and courage for the family. The person may ask for relief of fear and anxiety, for peace of mind.

The sequence of events we call "turning to God" may not occur in this order. Many people, particularly those who are already religious, may as a first step immediately pray for direction, strength, and peace. Many people may continue to persistently pray for healing, retaining hope to the end that God will cure the cancer and return them to health. Others may turn to God in preparation for their death and for the life they believe will follow. We now examine what has been learned from systematic surveys of cancer patients about the role that religion and spirituality plays in their lives.

Use of Religion by Cancer Patients

Johnson and Spilka (1991) surveyed 103 women with breast cancer. The subjects were recruited from an American Cancer Society support group in the southwestern United States. Of these women, 85% reported that religion helped them cope with their cancer. The investigators examined the relationship of intrinsic and extrinsic religiousness to religious coping and found that extrinsic religiosity was unrelated to religious coping, whereas intrinsic religiousness (IR) was associated with greater involvement with clergy, belief that God was involved in the cancer, and greater satisfaction from the use of religion as a coping behavior (IR and religious coping were correlated at $r = .70$). The investigators concluded that "It is evident that religion is an extremely important resource for the majority of these breast cancer patients" (Johnson & Spilka, 1991, p. 21) and, referred to Gross's (1982) epigram, "When misery is the greatest, God is the closest."

Carver, Pozo, et al. (1993) conducted a prospective cohort study of 59 women with breast cancer. The women, recruited from the University of Miami, Florida, oncology clinic, were assessed prior to surgery and four times after surgery for one year. Acceptance, positive reframing, and use of religion were the most common coping strategies. Religion as a coping response declined from pre- to postsurgery ($p < .02$) and then stabilized.

Roberts, Brown, et al. (1997) surveyed 108 patients with gynecologic cancer on the Oncology Service of the University of Michigan Medical Center in Ann Arbor. Among these patients, 76% indicated that religion had a "serious place" in their lives. Interestingly, 49% indicated that they had become more religious since having cancer, whereas none indicated they had become less religious. The investigators concluded that patients with gynecologic cancer often depend on religious beliefs and practices to cope with the disease.

Religious Coping and Cancer around the World. To what extent do cancer patients in areas of the world outside the United States use religious beliefs to help them cope with cancer? Kesselring et al. (1986) explored the meaning of illness and its treatments with 45 cancer patients in Switzerland. They found that 17 (38%) indicated that faith in God and prayer were important sources of "experienced help." The investigators compared this proportion to a separate study of 40 Egyptian cancer patients, where 37 of 40 (92%) indicated that God or Allah was important in coping.

Ginsburg et al. (1995) surveyed 52 patients who were being treated at a regional cancer center in Ontario, Canada. An average of 45 days had elapsed since their diagnoses of lung cancer. The researchers assessed the patients' coping responses, using an open-ended format. The two most common support systems spontaneously reported by patients were family (79%) and religion (44%). These studies suggest that cancer patients in different parts of the world depend on religious faith to varying degrees.

Relationship between Religion and Spirituality and Successful Coping

Dunkel-Schetter et al. (1992) surveyed 603 cancer patients recruited from oncology practices and support groups in Los Angeles, California. About 42% had breast cancer, and 13% had gastrointestinal cancer. Religiosity was assessed with one item on reported strength of spiritual belief. Prayer was classified in the "cognitive escape-avoidance" category, along with "prepared for the worst," "wished situation would go away," "slept more than usual," "went along with fate," and similar responses). Not surprisingly, the cognitive escape-avoidance category was associated with less positive affect (POMS), greater stress, and, of course, greater strength of spiritual belief (since prayer was in the category). This was a poor analysis strategy because prayer was mixed with negative coping behaviors, ensuring a negative relationship with positive affect. Greater reported strength of spiritual beliefs, however, was significantly associated with "focus on positive" ($\beta = .35$, $p < .001$), but correlations with affect and stress level were not examined (spiritual beliefs was used as control variable only for those analyses).

In Carver, Pozo, et al.'s (1993) prospective study of 59 Florida women with breast cancer, adaptation was assessed using the Profile of Mood States (POMS). Religion as a coping strategy was significantly related to active coping, suppression of competing activities, planning, and positive reframing—all positive coping behaviors. As far as mental health outcomes were concerned, however, religion was unrelated to either optimism or distress at any of the five measurement times.

A number of investigators have documented a positive correlation between religion and successful coping in cancer patients. Acklin et al. (1983) surveyed a convenience sample of 26 patients with a recent diagnosis of new or recurrent cancer and compared them to 18 patients with nonlife-threatening illnesses (e.g., renal stones, gallbladder stones). Outcome was measured by six subscales of the Grief Experience Inventory that assessed coping and psychological well-being. No difference was found between the two groups on psychological well-being, although the cancer group scored significantly higher on transcendent meaning. In the cancer group, intrinsic religiosity (IR) ($r = .41$) and church attendance ($r = .34$) were both significantly correlated with transcendent meaning. Likewise, both IR ($r = -.34$) and church attendance ($r = -.39$) were inversely associated with anger and hostility, and church attendance was negatively related to social isolation ($r = -.32$). Among these patients, then, religious attendance and intrinsic religiosity were related to greater transcendent meaning, less anger and hostility, and reduced social isolation—all indicators of better coping.

Jenkins and Pargament (1988) reported similar findings. They surveyed 62 cancer outpatients with a single question on God's perceived control over cancer. Perceived control by God was correlated with higher Rosenberg self-esteem (partial $r = .25$, $p < .05$) and less maladjustment as rated by nurses (partial $r = -.23$, $p < .05$, with lie scale and education level controlled). The investigators concluded that higher levels of belief about God's control were related to higher levels of self-esteem and lower levels of observed behavioral upset.

Ell et al. (1989) surveyed 369 patients age 35 or older with newly diagnosed breast (55%), colorectal (25%), or lung cancer (19%) at 23 hospitals affiliated with the Cancer Management Network of the University of Southern California's Comprehensive Cancer Center. Social support was measured by a 52-item Interview Schedule for Social Interaction (which assessed availability and adequacy of ongoing close interpersonal relationships and relationships with acquaintances and less intimate friends and relatives). Mental health status was assessed by a 38-item Mental Health Inventory (MHI), which has subscales for psychological distress, psychological well-being, social functioning, and role limitations. Religious coping was measured by a four-item "active reliance on religion" measure. Religious coping was significantly related to overall mental health (MHI score) ($r = .13$, $p < .01$), especially the psychological well-being subscale ($r = .19$, $p < .001$). Religious coping was also related to both social attachment ($r = .13$, $p < .01$) and social integration ($r = .21$, $p < .001$). The researchers did not examine religion in multivariate models, since the focus of the study was on social support and control.

Musick, Koenig, et al., 1998 recently examined racial differences in the frequency of religious activities in persons with and without cancer and the relationship of these activities to depressive symptoms in a three-year prospective study of community-dwelling persons over age 65 who were living in North Carolina. They assessed 3,007 persons in 1986 and 1989 as part of the Established Populations for Epidemiologic Studies in the Elderly (EPESE) study. Religious attendance, attention to religious media (radio or television), and religious devotions were the three single-item measures of religious activity assessed. Depressive symptoms were measured using the CES-D, divided into its four subscales. Other covariates included functional impairment (measured by the Rosow-Breslau activity scale), satisfaction with social interaction, and demographics (sex, age, education, and marital status). A total of 251 subjects with cancer were identified in 1986; these persons were compared with persons with other illnesses ($n = 1,770$) and persons with no illnesses ($n = 894$).

The investigators found no differences in religious activity between cancer and noncancer patients in 1986 regardless of race. In 1989, however, African Americans who had had cancer in 1986 were more likely to report an increase in religious devotion (prayer or Bible study) than either African Americans with other illnesses ($\beta = -.25$, $p < .01$) or African Americans with no illnesses ($\beta = -.17$, $p = $ ns). This was true also for attention to religious media ($\beta = -.20$, $p < .05$, and $\beta = -.28$, $p < .01$). In contrast, African Americans with cancer were less likely than African Americans in other groups to experience an increase in religious service attendance ($\beta = .36$, $p < .001$, and $\beta = .47$, $p < .001$). Among white Americans, cancer patients were more likely than those with other illnesses or no illnesses to show an increase in attention to religious media ($\beta = -.13$, $p < .01$, and $\beta = -.13$, $p < .05$), but there was no increase in private devotion or religious attendance.

With regard to depression, attendance at religious services in 1986 predicted fewer depressive symptoms (more positive affect, in particular) among African Americans in 1989. This relationship persisted after the researchers controlled for depression in 1986 and covariates ($\beta = .17$, $p < .01$) among the 103 African American cancer patients who were still alive. There was no relationship between religious activity and depression in whites with cancer. These findings suggest that religious activities are more likely to increase and more likely to buffer against depression in African Americans with cancer than in whites with cancer.

Religion and Anxiety. Cancer patients with strong religious or spiritual beliefs also report less anxiety than those without such faith. Kaczorowski (1989) surveyed 114 patients with cancer from a New York hospice (74% women and 60% Catholic). The investigator examined spiritual well-being (SWB) and state-trait (ST) anxiety and found that SWB was inversely related to ST anxiety in all subgroups ($p < .001$, except for breast cancer subgroup, $p < .05$). When SWB and ST were broken down into their component subscales, religious well-being was inversely related only to trait anxiety ($r = -.20$, $p < .05$).

Religion and Hope. Raleigh (1992) examined sources of hope among 90 chronically ill patients who were being attended by visiting nurses in Michigan. One-half of the patients had cancer, and one-half had other chronic illnesses; all were age 65 or younger. Stategies used by cancer patients to raise their hopes were getting busy (15/45), talking to others (8/45), and prayer or religious activities (7/45). Among those with chronic illness, strategies for raising hope included getting busy (11/45), prayer or religious activities (9/45), and talking about other things (9/45). The investigator concluded that the most common reported sources of hopefulness were family, friends, and religious beliefs.

Roberts, Brown, et al.'s (1997) survey of patients with gynecologic cancer in Michigan reported that 93% of the patients believed that their religious lives helped sustain their hopes, 41% felt that their religious lives supported their self-worth, and 17% indicated that their religious lives gave their suffering meaning.

Recall from chapter 14 the work of Mickley and colleagues, who examined religiousness and spirituality and hope among women with breast cancer. In their initial study, they surveyed 175 women at two oncology outpatients treatment centers in Texas (33% within one year of diagnosis) (Mickley, Soeken, et al., 1992). Scores for hope (measured by the 19-item Nowotny Hope Scale) were correlated with intrinsic religiosity ($r = 0.36$, $p < .001$) and religious well-being ($r = .44$, $p < .001$). When variables were entered into a multiple regression model, only existential well-being predicted higher hope scores (although religious well-being may have indirectly influenced hope through existential well-being). The following year, Mickley and Soeken (1993) examined religiousness and hope in 25 Hispanic-American and 25 Anglo-American outpatients with breast cancer. In Hispanic women, hope scores were correlated with spiritual well-being ($r = .60$, $p < .01$), religious well-being ($r = .43$, $p < .01$), and

existential well-being ($r = .63$, $p < .01$), but not with intrinsic religiosity ($r = 0.22$, $p > .05$). In Anglo women, hope scores were correlated with spiritual well-being ($r = .72$), religious well-being ($r = .59$), existential well-being ($r = .71$), and intrinsic religiosity ($r = .58$) (all $p < .01$, but uncontrolled).

Thus, cancer patients say that religious beliefs and practices enable them to sustain hope; when religiousness and spirituality are measured in cancer patients, they correlate with greater hope.

Religion and Coping by Family Members of Children with Cancer

Dealing with the fact that one's child has cancer is one of the most difficult experiences a person can face. Spilka, Zwartjes, et al. (1991) conducted in-depth interviews with 265 members of 118 families who had children with cancer. They concluded that religion acted as a protective-defensive system that motivated efforts by family members to cope constructively. In a related study, Barbarin and Chesler (1986) interviewed 74 parents of children surviving with cancer. Graduate students audiotaped the interviews, typed them up, and coded them with the assistance of several raters. Open-ended questions were asked concerning the family's reliance on religious beliefs and faith for support and understanding of the illness (ranked on a 0–10 scale by raters). Religious coping was unrelated to medically related stress, quality of relationship with medical staff, number of hospitalizations, or coping effectiveness. The anger and questioning phase of adaptation to the diagnosis of cancer may be prolonged in some family members, making it more difficult for them to access religious coping resources.

Cancer Patients' Choice of Spiritual Caregiver

Highfield (1992) surveyed 23 patients and 27 nurses from two religiously affiliated hospitals at major medical centers in the southwestern United States. Of these participants, 21 were nurse-inpatient pairs ($n = 42$). The patient sample was made up predominantly of men with lung cancer. When patients and nurses were asked to rank their choice of spiritual caregiver, they ranked "family member or friend" and "personal pastor or rabbi" first; their medical physician was ranked second; psychiatrists, psychologists, and social workers were ranked last by both patients and nurses.

Sodestrom and Martinson (1987) surveyed 25 cancer patients from a nonsectarian medical center in California. They asked patients to rate their use of 15 spiritual strategies for coping with cancer. Prayer was the most frequently used spiritual strategy. When asked to name the most important persons who acted as a spiritual resource to them, 92% of the patients indicated their family, 76% a member of the clergy, 68% a friend, 48% a nurse, and 23% a physician.

In Johnson and Spilka's (1991) survey of 103 women with breast cancer, the women described experiences with home pastors and hospital chaplains: 27% of women were visited at home by their own pastor, and 56% saw their pastor when hospitalized (37% saw a hospital chaplain). Between 93% and 98% of the women were pleased with the home or hospital visits by clergy. Their satisfaction was related to the number of visits, the use of prayer, the provision of counseling, discussion of the patient's family, readings in the Bible, the clergy's perceived understanding of the patient, discussion of church affairs, and willingness to discuss breast cancer. In summary, family members and friends, clergy persons, and medical physicians are important sources of spiritual (and emotional) support for cancer patients.

RELIGIOUS INFLUENCES ON THE COURSE OR OUTCOME OF CANCER

Information about religious influences on the course of cancer comes from two sources. One source is research that has inquired about coping behaviors among long-term cancer survivors; the second source is studies that link religious beliefs and behaviors with survival. Creagan (1997), in a comprehensive review of this topic that was published in the *Mayo Clinic*

Proceedings, concluded that "A social support system and an element of spirituality and religion seem to be the most consistent predictors of quality of life and possible survival among patients with advanced malignant disease" (p. 160). Creagan also notes that "among the coping methods of long-term cancer survivors, the predominent strategy is spiritual" (p. 163).

Coping Behaviors of Cancer Survivors

Halstead and Fernsler (1994) surveyed 59 persons with cancer (51% had breast cancer) who had (a) survived five years or more, (b) were not currently receiving therapy, and (c) were not in a terminal stage of disease. The mean length of survival for members of the group was 13 years since diagnosis. "Praying or put trust in God" was ranked first as the most "often used and very helpful" coping strategy out of a list of 12 coping behaviors.

Kurtz et al. (1995) surveyed 191 women who had a variety of cancers (58% had breast cancer) and who had lived at least five years since diagnosis. Investigators reported that the best health habits and the most supportive behaviors toward other survivors were found among women with a positive spiritual outlook, as measured by a 12-item Philosophical/Spiritual View scale.

Religiousness and Survival

Studies that have directly examined the effects of religiousness on survival of cancer patients have reported mixed results. Yates et al. (1981) conducted a prospective cohort study of 71 patients with advanced cancer in Burlington, Vermont. Subjects were followed for 12 months to determine whether religious beliefs and practices at baseline predicted mortality during that period. Religious beliefs were assessed with a multi-item scale, along with religious attendance and reported importance of church and private religious activities. No religious measures were found to be related to survival. The investigators' inability to demonstrate an effect for religion on the subjects' survival may have resulted from several factors. First, this was a very religious sample, and there was little variability in religiousness (92% believed in God, 83% believed in a personal God, 80% believed in prayer, two-thirds felt close to God or nature, and about half indicated that their church was very important in their lives). Second, only 36 of 71 patients died during the 12-month follow-up, resulting in low statistical power to detect an effect. Third, the force of mortality exerted by advanced malignant disease may have overwhelmed the more subtle effects of religious variables on survival.

Ringdal et al. (1995, 1996) conducted a three-year prospective study of 253 cancer patients diagnosed in the Department of Oncology at the University Hospital of Trondheim, Norway. Religiosity at baseline was assessed by two questions: "What can you tell about your religious beliefs? (believe in God, don't believe, don't know)" and "Have your religious beliefs been of support to you after you became ill with cancer? (very good, some, no)?" While in the initial report (1995) religiousness was unrelated to survival, in the second report (1996) the investigators indicated that religiosity was significantly related to general satisfaction, to fewer feelings of hopelessness, and to longer survival (religiosity was inversely correlated with poor prognosis) ($r = -.16, p < .01$). When religiosity was included in a Cox regression without hopelessness and life satisfaction, the relative risk of dying was 0.86 ($p = .06$); in other words, greater religiousness was associated with about a 14% lower risk of dying during the three-year follow-up.

In summary, from the limited research that exists, it appears that religiousness or spirituality may have a small positive impact on the course of cancer, although no study has yet employed comprehensive measures of intrinsic religiosity or religious commitment when examining cancer outcomes.

HOW RELIGION MAY INFLUENCE THE COURSE OF CANCER

Effects on Timing of Diagnosis

While there is evidence that religious factors may delay the diagnosis of cancer (because of reliance on God alone for cure), it is more likely that greater religiousness, particularly that expressed by level of involvement in religious community, increases early diagnosis. As noted in chapter 4, certain religious groups may delay seeking medical care because of their preference for religious treatments (Christian Scientists, small fundamentalist Christian groups); nevertheless, this behavior is relatively rare. Because of the strong relationship between religious attendance and social support (see chapter 15), and the strong relationship between social support and medical compliance and screening, organizational types of religious involvement probably increase the likelihood of early cancer detection and treatment. Nevertheless, to our knowledge, there are no studies that have directly examined this possibility, so the evidence is largely inferential (see also chapter 26).

Persons with greater social support are more likely to undergo cancer screening, particularly those in high-risk groups such as older Mexican American women and older African Americans. Suarez et al. (1994) surveyed a random sample of 450 Mexican American women age 40 or older who were living in El Paso County, Texas. A social network score was assigned to each woman on the basis of a summation of (a) number of confidantes, close friends, or close relatives, (b) frequency of contact with close friends or relatives per month, and (c) church membership and church attendance. Cancer screening history was also determined during the interview. Investigators found that the two-year prevalence of Pap smear and mammography testing was significantly correlated with social network score (church variables were not examined separately). They concluded that social networks were an important determinant of cancer screening behavior in low-income, older Mexican American women.

The same appears true for older African Americans. Kang and Bloom (1993) conducted a survey of 617 African Americans age 55 or older who were living in San Francisco and Oakland. Social network was assessed using a modified version of the Berkman and Syme Social Network Index. Multiple logistic regression determined that there was a statistically significant association between social support and use of mammography and occult blood stool examination, but there was no such association with Pap smears, clinical breast examination, digital rectal examination, or sigmoidoscopy. The association between increased cancer screening and higher levels of social support could not be explained by health status, age, gender, education, type of health insurance, or regular source of care.

Thus, if the quality and size of the social network is positively correlated with increased cancer screening, then religious involvement, which is associated with a larger social network and greater satisfaction with that network, is likely to be associated with early cancer detection. Zollinger and colleagues' (1984) study of 282 Seventh-Day Adventist and 1675 non-SDA breast cancer patients in California provides some indirect evidence that supports this hypothesis. Investigators found that the probability of not having died of breast cancer 10 years after diagnosis was 60.8% in SDAs and 48.3% in non-SDAs. When stage at diagnosis was taken into account, however, the differences in survival disappeared. In other words, SDA women simply had their breast cancers diagnosed at an earlier stage than non-SDA women, possibly because they went for more frequent cancer screenings (although this was not examined directly).

Effects on Natural History of Disease

We have reviewed the few studies that have examined the effects of religiousness on the course of cancer. None of these studies, however, were designed with that research question in mind. There are a number of reasons why religiousness might affect the course of malignant disease. First, as noted, active involvement in religious community may speed diagnosis, particularly among high-risk minority populations. Second, the increased social support provided by religious communities in the form of individual and group support may extend survival in the same way that Spiegel et al. (1989) and Fawzy, Fawzy, Hyun, et al. (1993) have shown for patients with breast cancer and patients with malignant melanoma. The support

group interventions used in those studies are very similar to the type of support that church communities provide members. Small prayer or Bible study groups offer numerous opportunities in a caring and supportive environment for patients to ventilate concerns and talk about stressors. There is also opportunity for group prayer (sometimes hands-on prayer) that helps reduce the isolation and loneliness associated with cancer.

Third, religious beliefs and activities may provide a positive worldview that offers continued hope for recovery and an increased sense of control over the cancer. This may promote greater adaptation, reduce level of depression and anxiety, and provide a sense of coherence and direction that reduces helplessness, pessimism, discouragement, and the desire to give up. Greater social support and a more positive mental outlook may act synergistically to improve immune system functioning and thus help contain the disease.

Effects on Response to Treatment

No studies have yet examined the interaction between religious factors and traditional cancer treatments on the course of the disease. It is possible that the increased social support provided by religious involvement and the positive mental outlook conveyed by a religious worldview may speed the body's responsiveness to chemotherapeutic, surgical, or radiological therapies. Studies are needed to examine this hypothesis.

SUMMARY AND CONCLUSIONS

Cancer is the second leading cause of death in the United States; more than 1,500 persons die each day of the disease. The most common malignancies are those of the lung, breast, prostate, colon, cervical, and upper gastrointestinal tract, and many of these may be prevented by avoiding high-risk behaviors or detected early by active screening. Psychosocial influences, such as low levels of social support and personal characteristics such as depression, hopelessness, and pessimism can adversely affect immune mechanisms that affect the development or containment of cancer.

Certain religious groups, including Mormons and Seventh-Day Adventists, have cancer rates about one-half to two-thirds those of persons in the general population. This lower risk of cancer results at least in part from healthier lifestyles (e.g., avoidance of smoking and alcohol use, healthier diet). Adherence to healthy lifestyle practices is determined by degree of religiousness and religious commitment; these are belief-based behaviors. An emphasis on family values, strong communities, and positive worldview may also play a role in preventing the development of cancer or in promoting its early detection. Jewish persons are at increased risk for some cancers (possibly because of genetic factors), but they are at lower risk for others (because of health behaviors and religious rituals such as circumcision). Among traditional Christians, conservative Protestants have the lowest risk of developing cancer, probably for the same reasons that Mormons and Seventh-Day Adventists have low risk. Nearly two-thirds of all cancers may be prevented by healthy lifestyles.

There is evidence that degree of religiousness (whether measured by frequency of religious activity or by depth of religious commitment) may help prevent the development of cancer through a number of mechanisms. These mechanisms include better health behaviors (avoidance of cigarette smoking, excessive alcohol use, and risky sexual practices) and improved immune surveillance (because of reduced depression, improved coping with stress,

greater social support). On the other hand, devoutly religious persons may be more likely to choose people from their own religious group as mating partners. If the religious group is relatively small and attracts few new members, then inbreeding may occur, increasing the risk of genetic mutations that predispose to cancer. A lack of prospective studies that assess people prior to the development of cancer, particularly studies that assess degree of religiousness in a sophisticated way, prevents any definitive statement on the cause-effect relationship between religiousness and cancer incidence.

Once cancer develops, we know that many people utilize religious or spiritual beliefs and practices to help cope with the disease. Some studies have shown that those who use religion as a coping resource adapt better, experience less anxiety, and are more hopeful. This, in turn, may positively affect the course of cancer, given the adverse effects of uncontrolled stress on the immune system and its ability to contain malignant spread. Religious involvement may also improve the detection of cancer (due to increased social support and monitoring), and early treatment may ultimately improve prognosis. There is some evidence that religious beliefs and behaviors may improve survival and quality of life of cancer patients, both from subjective reports of survivors and from studies that directly examine the association. Future studies that examine the religion-cancer relationship should measure multiple dimensions of religious involvement and control for appropriate covariates; this will increase the likelihood of detecting such effects, should they exist.

21

Mortality

SCIENTISTS HAVE BEEN INTER-
ested in the influence of religion on
mortality for at least 130 years. The
1870s were a time when people were
turning to science to address questions regarding anything and everything. It was in 1872 that
Francis Galton, cousin of Charles Darwin and
founder of the Eugenics movement, reported
the results of a study that sought to "scientifically" examine the efficacy of prayer.

Galton began by assuming that certain
groups of people prayed more than did others.
He reasoned that if prayer were efficacious,
then prayerful people would live longer than
less prayerful people. Galton imagined that
ministers and missionaries were likely to be
highly prayerful people. Thus, when he found
that ministers did not live substantially longer
than did attorneys or physicians, Galton felt
confident that he had discovered definitive evidence that prayer was ineffective.

Galton did not stop here. He reasoned that
the members of royal families were frequently
the subject of people's prayers (e.g., "God
save the queen") and reckoned that if prayer
were efficacious in staving off death, then sovereigns would typically live longer than other people because of the many prayers said on their
behalf. Using actuarial tables, Galton demonstrated that members of the royal houses actually had lower life expectancies than did people
from other affluent sectors of English society
(including lawyers, gentry, and military officers). On the basis of the rather unremarkable
longevity of clergy and sovereigns, Galton concluded that no statistical evidence existed for
the efficacy of prayer. So went the first scientific
study of religion and mortality.

Although most social and behavioral scientists would now chuckle at the methods and
assumptions of Galton's early study, his scientific intentions were laudable: If religion (and,

in Galton's study, prayer) is related to survival, then science should be able to detect its effects. Since Galton's time, methods for studying the relationship between religion and mortality have improved. Investigations have fallen into three categories: (1) studies of the longevity of religious leaders (e.g., priests, ministers, rabbis, monks, and nuns), (2) studies of religious affiliation and mortality, and (3) studies of degree of religious involvement and mortality.

LONGEVITY OF
RELIGIOUS LEADERS

If religion confers health benefits that translate into longer life, then the people who are most involved with religion—religious leaders—should have, on average, longer lives than people who do not follow religious pursuits as a vocation. Although the reasoning behind this approach is not ironclad (many fervently religious people have sacrificed their lives for their religious convictions, and certain occupations involve greater stress than others), this approach does provide some initial evidence that religion might affect longevity. Despite Galton's initial report, these studies suggest that clergy from a variety of faith backgrounds and cultures (both Western and non-Western) do experience a lower risk of early death.

Protestant Clergy

Two decades ago, Haitung King and his colleagues completed a series of investigations into the mortality profiles of clergy from a variety of predominantly white Protestant denominations, including the Anglican, Baptist, Episcopal, Lutheran, and Presbyterian churches (King & Bailar, 1968; King, 1970, 1971; King, Zafros, et al., 1975; King & Locke, 1980; Locke & King, 1980). In general, these studies found that Protestant clergymen had lower overall mortality ratios than did other white males in the general population (e.g., King & Bailar, 1968). The standardized mortality ratios (SMRs) for Protestant clergy were approximately 70 (with a range of 69–83) in comparison to those for other white males. In other words, clergy had only 70% of the death rate of non-clergy in these studies. The effect was particularly notable among clergy under age 55.

A number of factors could explain why Protestant clergymen live longer than men in the general population. Their profession does not require physical labor, their socioeconomic status is typically high, and the quality of their medical care is probably superior to that of the general population. Moreover, a variety of poorly understand selection factors could lead different types of men into the clergy instead of into other occupations.

To determine whether elements of lifestyle might be responsible for the favorable mortality profile of clergy, King compared the mortality of American and British clergymen to that of men from a variety of other professions, including attorneys, professors, teachers, and physicians (King, 1970, 1971; King & Locke, 1980). He found that clergymen had lower mortality rates than did physicians and attorneys (also see Harding le Riche, 1985) but that their mortality rates were similar to those of professors and teachers. Clergymen and teachers had particularly low rates of death from coronary heart disease, suicide, and vascular lesions of the central nervous system. King, Zafros, et al. (1975) also reported that Lutheran and Presbyterian clergy (who are generally better educated and of higher social class than the general population) had more favorable mortality ratios than did clergymen in general. These differences in mortality were attributed to differences in social and economic background, occupational factors, and patterns of clergy behavior.

Roman Catholic Religious

Several studies have investigated the mortality of members of Roman Catholic religious orders (Madigan, 1957; Taylor, Carroll, et al., 1959; de Gouw, et al., 1995). Madigan calculated age-specific death rates for male and female Catholic religious in the United States for each decade between 1900 and 1950. Throughout that period, Catholic religious had lower mortality than did the general population (SMRs = 0.84 and 0.66 for men and women, respectively). Taylor, Carroll, and Lloyd (1959) also examined the cancer mortality of women in three Catholic religious orders in the Northeast United States. Women religious again had lower total cancer mortality than did women in the general U.S. population.

In a third study of Catholic religious orders, de Gouw et al. (1995) examined the mortality of contemplative monks who were living in 10 Trappist and Benedictine monasteries in the Netherlands between 1900 and 1994. Monks experienced 12% lower mortality during that period than did men in the general Dutch population (SMR = 0.88). This difference could not be explained by the monks' superior health upon entering the monastery or by their higher level of education.

De Gouw and colleagues also found that the mortality pattern changed over time. At the turn of the century, monks had a slightly higher mortality than did men in the general population (because they experienced a higher rate of communicable diseases from living in close quarters?). In the later decades of the twentieth century, however, monks lived longer than other Dutch males. By the decade 1985–1994, they had an SMR of 0.75, an effect that persisted after researchers controlled for education. Madigan (1957) noted a similar reduced mortality among U.S. Catholic religious during the later decades of the twentieth century. The lower SMRs experienced by Catholic clergy since World War II were attributed (at least in part) to the higher rates of lung cancer and cardiovascular disease in the general population.

Japanese Religious Leaders

Two studies have examined the longevity of religious leaders from non-Christian religions. Ogata et al. (1984) examined the mortality of 4,352 male Japanese Zen priests between 1955 and 1978. During this period, 1,396 priests died (as confirmed by death certificates). Investigators compared the SMRs of priests to those of the general male Japanese population. The all-cause SMR for Zen priests was 0.82 (an 18% lower mortality rate). Priests were particularly less likely to die from cerebrovascular diseases, pneumonia or bronchitis, peptic ulcer disease, liver cirrhosis, and cancers of the respiratory system.

Simonton (1997) examined the longevity of 1,632 Japanese men and women born between 450 and 1883 who were important cultural figures in Japanese history. Subjects were sufficiently prominent during their lifetimes to be included in at least two of three standard reference works on Japanese civilization. Information on the subjects' gender, birth date, occupation, and death date were abstracted from their entries in these reference works. Subjects had attained eminence in at least one of 14 achievement domains (politics, war, religion, economics, medicine, philosophy, nonfiction writing, fiction writing, drama, poetry, painting, sculpture, ceramics, and sword making).

Using multiple regression that adjusted for gender and for the era in which each subject lived (to control for period effects), Simonton found that religious figures and sword makers (!) lived substantially longer (3.8 and 8.5 years, respectively) than did the average eminent person. Politicians, warriors, and fiction writers all lived fewer years than did others. Even after the researchers controlled for achievement domain, individuals who ruled at the highest levels of power (i.e., emperors and shoguns) still lived shorter lives (a finding that Galton had reported many years earlier). Simonton speculated that the longevity of religious leaders was caused either by the benefits of a contemplative life or by protection from life's risks that they enjoyed and that other leaders did not have. In conclusion, then, the research consistently indicates that persons involved in full-time religious life experience a reduced risk of early death.

RELIGIOUS AFFILIATION AND MORTALITY

Researchers have also studied the mortality of laypersons within specific religious groups. To date, studies have primarily focused on Jews and on conservative Christians who abide by strong dietary and lifestyle proscriptions. Investigators have typically compared the longevity of members of these religious groups with that of the general population.

Mortality among Jews

In a study of 10,000 Jewish families conducted over a century ago, Billings (1891) discovered that Jews had a lower death rate. Years later, Bolduan and Weiner (1933) published their seminal paper on the causes of death among Jews in New York City. They reported lower death rates from tuberculosis, pneumonia, and uterine cancer but higher mortality from cancers of the breast and digestive organs.

More recent research shows that Jews experience an elevated risk of mortality from several forms of cancer but a lower risk from other forms (see chapter 20). Recall the work of MacMahon (1960), who found that death from cancers of the stomach, colon, pancreas, ovary, and kidney, melanoma, glioma, sarcoma, Hodgkin's disease, and leukemia were all more common among Jews than among non-Jews but that Jews suffered fewer deaths from cancers of tongue, oral pharynx, larynx, lung, prostate, bladder, and cervix.

Jewish men, in particular, may be at lower risk of dying from cancer of the penis (King, Diamond, et al., 1965), tongue, larynx, mouth, and lung (MacMahon, 1960; Seidman, 1966; Herman & Enterline, 1970; Horowitz & Enterline, 1970; Greenwald et al., 1975). However, they are at increased risk for fatal cancers of the colon, Hodgkin's disease, and leukemia (Seidman, 1970, 1971; Greenwald et al., 1975), according to these early studies reviewed in chapter 20.

Seidman (1970, 1971) found that Jewish women were more likely to die from many cancers than were non-Jewish women, although they were protected from death from cancer of the uterus. Greenwald et al. (1975) found higher mortality rates in Jewish women from cancers of the stomach and the lung but lower rates from cancers of the cervix and the breast. King, Diamond, et al. (1965) reported very low rates of cervical cancer among Jewish women compared to women in the general population of New York City. However, they also found higher rates of lung cancer among Jewish women than among non-Jewish women. The high rates of lung cancer could not be explained by excess smoking.

Finally, recall that Dwyer et al. (1990) used county-level data to examine the link between religious affiliation and county cancer rates in a sample of more than 3,000 U.S. counties. Even after controlling for the usual sociodemographic and health risk factors, they found that counties in which Jews were highly concentrated had higher cancer mortality rates than counties with lower concentrations of Jews. While such ecological data are provocative, they prove not that Jews themselves are more vulnerable to cancer mortality but only that people who live in counties with relatively high proportions of Jewish people have high cancer mortality rates.

Mortality among Christians

Other studies have examined mortality rates in four Christian groups with strict proscriptions against the consumption of tobacco, certain foods, and alcohol or caffeinated beverages. These groups include the Church of Latter-Day Saints (Mormons), Seventh-Day Adventists, and the Amish and the Hutterites (two sociologically and geographically isolated Christian sects in North America).

Latter-Day Saints (LDS). Recall that Dwyer et al. (1990) found that counties in which Latter-Day Saints (Mormons) were highly concentrated had lower cancer mortality rates. In part because of strict proscriptions against the use of tobacco, alcohol, and caffeine, LDS members enjoy approximately four additional years of life compared to persons in the general population (Jarvis, 1977). LDS members in countries outside North America also enjoy a favorable life expectancy (Smith, Pool, et al. 1985). This protection from early death is largely a result of lower mortality from cancer and cardiovascular disease (e.g., Enstrom, 1975, 1978, 1979, 1980; Lyon, Gardner, et al., 1977; Lyon, Wetzler, et al., 1978).

Seventh-Day Adventists (SDAs). Studies involving samples from the United States (Lemon & Walden, 1966; Lemon & Kuzma, 1969; Phillips, Lemon, Beeson, & Kuzma, 1978; Phillips, Garfinkel, Kuzma, Beeson, Lotz, & Brin, 1980; Phillips, Kuzma, Beeson, & Lotz, 1980; Phillips & Snowden, 1983; Zollinger et al., 1984), the Netherlands (Berkel, 1979; Berkel & deWaard, 1983), and Norway (Waaler & Hjort, 1981) all indicate that SDAs live longer than persons in the general population. As for Mormons, the longer life expectancy of SDAs is likely the result of positive health behaviors and healthy diet, safe sexual practices, high community cohesion, and protection from psychological stress conferred by devout religious beliefs (Troyer, 1988). These factors contribute to reduced mortality from cancer, respiratory disease, heart disease, and accidents (Jarvis & Northcott, 1987). SDAs live on average two to four years longer than persons in the general population (Berkel & deWaard, 1983).

Amish and Hutterites. The Amish are almost completely rural, live in tight-knit communities, eschew modern conveniences, and discourage alcohol and tobacco use. The Hutterites (who live in the United States and Canada) have a similar lifestyle. Neither group restricts the consumption of meat or caffeinated beverages (Troyer, 1988; Levinson et al., 1989). As noted in chapter 20, all-cause mortality is lower among Amish young women than among non-Amish young women. However, Amish mortality rates are higher than those of the general population for women age 70 and older (perhaps because younger Amish women who would have died earlier survive into old age). Amish men age 40 or older have lower all-cause mortality than non-Amish men (Hamman et al., 1981), thanks to lower death rates from cardiovascular, digestive, and respiratory disorders.

As noted earlier, Hutterite men have higher death rates from leukemia than do persons in the general population, but they have lower mortality from cancer of the lung (Gaudette et al. Morgan, 1978; Martin et al., 1980). Hutterite women have lower rates of cervical cancer than do women in the general population, probably because they have to lower rates of extramarital sex and have fewer sexual partners (Troyer, 1988).

This review indicates that members of certain religious groups experience greater longevity than do persons in the general population. While taking health behaviors into account re-

duces the survival advantage, unexplained differences remain in some studies and may be attributed to social and psychological factors. Recognize again, however, that it is the religious convictions and values of members of these religious groups that account for their health behaviors. These are belief-dependent behaviors that explain the *mechanism* by which involvement in certain religious groups impacts health. Thus, even if health behaviors and social factors could completely explain the effects of religious affiliation on mortality, this would not discount the powerful effects that religious belief and membership can have on survival.

DEGREE OF RELIGIOUS INVOLVEMENT AND MORTALITY

Some investigators have examined intensity of religious involvement (i.e., frequency of religious attendance, prayer, and other private religious activities) as a predictor of survival. Given the large number of studies, unless otherwise noted we discuss here only studies in this area, whose quality ratings are 9 or 10 (see part VIII).

Involvement in Religious Community

Seeman et al. (1987) examined the effects of church membership on mortality during a 17-year follow-up of 4,175 persons age 38 or over who were participating in the Alameda County study (which covered the San Francisco-Oakland area in California). Lack of church membership (with age, sex, race, and baseline health status controlled) predicted greater mortality for persons age 60 or over (RH 1.32, CI 1.13–1.54, $p < .05$) and for persons ages 38–49 (RH 1.82, CI 1.27–2.59, $p < .05$). While adding explanatory variables to the model (such as smoking, physical activity, weight, depression, and perceived health status) accounted for the effects in persons age 60 or over, they could not fully explain the increased risk of dying faced by persons ages 38–49 who lacked church membership (RH 1.49, CI 1.02–2.17, $p < .05$).

Goldman et al. (1995) examined predictors of mortality between 1984 and 1990 in a national probability sample of approximately 7,500 persons age 70 or over (National Health Interview Survey: Longitudinal Study of Aging). The religious variable was "proportion not attending church within the past two weeks." Lack of attendance significantly predicted a greater probability of dying during the six-year follow-up period (β from logit models $= 0.36$, $p < .05$, $n = 2,847$ for males; $\beta = 0.35$, $p < .05$, $n = 4,631$ for females), after demographics, level of physical disability, self-rated health, and medical conditions were controlled.

Strawbridge, Cohen, et al. (1997) examined the relationship between religious attendance and all-cause mortality in a 28-year follow-up of 5,286 participants in the Alameda County study (examining all ages from 18 to 65 and assessing church attendance, rather than church membership, as Seeman et al. had done). Investigators found that frequent attendance (once per week or more in 1965) was associated with a 36% reduction in mortality during the follow-up period. Interestingly, frequent church attenders were significantly more likely than less frequent attenders to have impaired mobility at baseline (35.1% vs. 24.8%). Skeptics of such studies often attribute the mortality effect of religious attendance to confounding by health status (i.e., sick people with impaired mobility are both less likely to attend church and more likely to die, thus confounding the relationship between religious attendance and mortality) (Sloan et al., 1999). This was certainly not the case in the Strawbridge, Cohen, et al. study; if anything, the opposite was true (also see Idler & Kasl, 1997b, discussed later).

After researchers adjusted for multiple measures of baseline health status (impaired mobility, chronic health conditions, perceived health) and demographic factors (gender, education, ethnicity, religious denomination), the effect of attendance on mortality dropped from 36% to 33%. Adjusting analyses further for social connections (marital status, number of close social contacts, and number of group memberships) reduced the effect to 31%. Adding health practices to the model (cigarette smoking, exercise, alcohol consumption, and body mass index) further reduced the effect to 23% (34% in women and 10% in men). Note that both baseline covariates and time-varying covariates (changes in health status, social connections, and health behaviors during the 28-year follow-up) were adjusted for in these models.

The resulting effect of frequent attendance on mortality (relative hazard $= 0.77$, 95% CI 0.64–0.93) was highly statistically significant overall, especially among women (RH 0.66, 95% CI 0.51–0.86). The effect in men lost statistical significance when baseline health conditions were controlled (RH 0.80, 95% CI 0.62–1.02). Thus, for the nearly 3,000 women in this study, attending religious services once per week or more was associated with a greater than one-third (34%) reduction in the likelihood of dying during the 28-year follow-up.

In trying to understand how church attendance might reduce mortality, Strawbridge et al. noted that frequent church attenders at baseline were less likely to smoke or drink heavily than infrequent attenders and also had a greater number of social connections than did infrequent attenders. More important, frequent church attenders were more likely to change their health behaviors for the better during the 28-year follow-up (i.e., stay married, increase number of social contacts and nonchurch community group memberships, stop smoking, and increase exercise). Baseline differences in health practices and social connections and changes in these covariates during the follow-up period, however, still did not completely explain the relationship between frequent attendance and reduced mortality. As noted, a statistically significant 23% reduction in mortality for the overall sample and a 34% reduction in mortality for women remained unexplained.

Four more recent studies have now replicated this finding. Oman and Reed (1998) prospectively followed a random sample of 1,931 residents age 55 or over who were living in Marin County, California. There were 454 deaths during the five-year follow-up period. Subjects were dichotomized into "attenders" (weekly or occasional attenders at religious services) and "nonattenders" (never attended) at baseline. Attenders experienced a relative hazard of dying of 0.64 (95% CI 0.52–0.78). In other words, persons who attended religious services were 36% less likely to die during follow-up (identical to Strawbridge et al.'s finding). When other covariates were controlled, the risk decreased to 24% (RH 0.76, 95% CI 0.62–0.94, $p = .01$); covariates included confounders such as age, sex, number of chronic diseases, lower body disability, and balance problems, and explanatory variables such as exercise, smoking status, alcohol use, weight, social functioning and social support, marital status, and depression.

At the beginning of the study, persons who attended religious services were more likely to be married (men in particular), less likely to have balance difficulties (men in particular), less likely to smoke (both men and women), more likely to do volunteer work (both men and women), less likely to be socially reclusive (both men and women), less likely to be depressed (men in particular), and more likely to be overweight. Religious attendance tended to be more protective for those with high social support than for those with low support (the opposite of what was expected). Secular forms of social support were unrelated to survival.

Koenig, Hays, Larson, et al. (1999) conducted a six-year follow-up of a probability sample of 3,968 community-dwelling adults ages 64–101 who were residing in the Piedmont area of North Carolina. The investigators sought an East Coast replication of the results of the Strawbridge et al. study, which was conducted on the West Coast. Attendance at religious services and a wide variety of sociodemographic and health variables were assessed in 1986 as part of the Established Populations for the Epidemiologic Studies of the Elderly (EPESE) program. Vital status of members was determined prospectively over the next six years (1986–1992). Time (days) to death or censoring was analyzed using Cox proportional hazards. During the median 6.3-year follow-up period, 1,177 subjects (29.7%) died. Of the subjects who attended religious services once per week or more in 1986 (frequent attenders), 22.9% died, compared to 37.4% of those attending services less than once a week (infrequent attenders). The relative hazard of dying was reduced by 46% for frequent attenders compared to infrequent attenders (RH 0.54, 95% CI 0.48–0.61) (see Figure 21.1), an effect that was strongest in women (RH 0.51,

CI 0.43–0.59) and that approximates the reduced mortality associated with wearing seatbelts (Seat Belt Safety, 1997). The effect was also present in men but was slightly less robust (RH 0.63, 95% CI 0.52–0.75).

When confounders such as demographics (age, gender, ethnicity, education) and health conditions (functional disability, number of chronic conditions, self-rated health) were controlled, the effect remained significant for the entire sample (RH 0.69, 95% CI 0.61–0.78, $p < .0001$) and for both women (RH 0.64, 95% CI 0.55–0.76, $p < .0001$) and men (RH 0.76, 95% CI 0.63–0.91, $p < .01$). When explanatory variables such as social connections (supportive confidants, satisfaction with support, amount of help received) and health practices (cigarette smoking, alcohol consumption, body mass index) were controlled, the effect persisted in the entire sample (RH 0.72, 95% CI 0.64–0.81, $p < .0001$), as well as for both women (RH 0.65, 95% CI 0.55–0.76, $p < .0001$) and men (RH 0.83, 95% CI 0.69–1.00, $p = 0.05$). The gender-attendance interaction term failed to reach statistical significance in the final model, suggesting that the effects of attendance on survival were similar for both men and women. The size of the effect (and level of statistical significance) of frequent attendance on survival, after the researchers controlled for confounders and even for explanatory variables, was substantial and equivalent to that of abstaining from cigarette smoking.

Musick, House, et al. (1999), at the University of Michigan's Institute for Social Research, reported results from a 7.5-year prospective study of a random national sample of 3,617 Americans age 25 or over who were initially surveyed in 1986 as part of the Americans' Changing Lives Study. Persons who attended religious services more than once a week were significantly less likely to die during the follow-up period (RH 0.61, $p < .01$); those who attended religious services once a week were also less likely to die (RH 0.66, $p < .05$). These analyses were controlled for socioeconomic status, health status (functional impairment, chronic health problems, self-rated health), health behaviors (weight control, physical activity, drinking, smoking),

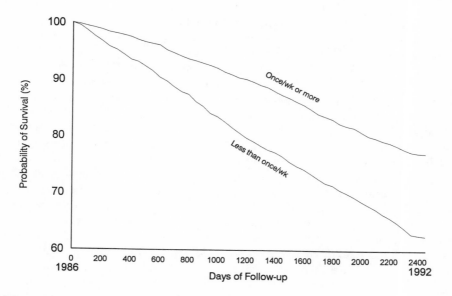

FIGURE 21.1 Religious attendance and six-year survival for 3,968 persons age 65 years or over (unadjusted Kaplan-Meier curves). From Koenig, Hays, Larson, et al. (1999), *Journal of Gerontology, Medical Sciences* 54A (7), M370–M377. Used with permission.

social integration (network size, presence of confidants, social interaction, meeting attendance, subjective social support), other religious factors (volunteering for church, private religious activity, subjective religiosity), and beliefs (concerning justice, fatalism, rewards in afterlife). Effects were greatest among those under age 60, in whom greater than weekly attendance was associated with a risk (RH) of only 0.13 ($p < .05$) and weekly attendance with a risk of 0.37 ($p < .05$).

In the largest study to date, Hummer et al. (1999) followed a random national sample of 21,204 adults from 1987 to 1995, during which 2,016 deaths occurred (documented by the National Death Index). Religious attendance was examined as a predictor of longevity. Nonattenders lived to an average age of 75.3 years, compared with 81.9 years for those who attended services once a week and 82.9 for those who attended more than once a week (an additional seven and eight years, respectively). Life expectancy estimates were similar to those conferred by sex and race. Among African Americans, average life expectancy for those who at-

tended services more than once a week was 80.1 years, compared to 66.4 years for those who never attended services (a difference of 14 years). The investigators took great care to ensure that their findings were not due to poorer health or lower socioeconomic status of nonattenders at baseline (which had been a criticism leveled at earlier studies). The investigators not only controlled for limitations to physical activity, self-reported health, and days spent in bed in the previous year but also repeated the analysis, excluding those in the sample who died between 1987 and 1991. This was done to ensure that unhealthy people in 1987 who did not attend church because of health problems would not bias the results; investigators reasoned that many of the most unhealthy people in 1987 would have died during the next four years. The results of this new analysis were similar to those obtained after controlling for demographic and health variables (with the association between religious attendance and survival remaining robust).

Thus, involvement in religious community activity has a sizable and consistent relationship with greater longevity. This has been shown by different investigators who have studied different regional samples on the West Coast and on the East Coast and several large national samples in the United States.

Finally, Glass and colleagues (1999) at the Harvard School of Public Health conducted a 13-year prospective study of 2,761 older men and women participating in the Yale EPESE study to determine predictors of survival. Social activities (church attendance; visits to cinema, restaurants, sporting events; day or overnight trips; playing cards, games, bingo; participation in social groups), productive activities (gardening, preparing meals, shopping, unpaid community work, paid community work, and other paid employment), and fitness activities (active sports or swimming, walking, physical exercise) were independently associated with longer survival after the investigators controlled for age, sex, race, marital status, income, body mass index, smoking, and functional disability, as well as history of cancer, diabetes, smoking, and myocardial infarction. Social activities reduced mortality by 19%, fitness activities by 15%, and productive activities by 23%. Great care was taken to ensure that physical health did not confound this relationship, both by controlling for physical fitness activities and productive activities and by eliminating all individuals who died during the first five years of follow-up. In an unpublished interview with the lead study investigator by Emma Ross, Thomas Glass indicated that all social activities, including church attendance, were independent predictors of mortality.

Private Religious Activities

Zuckerman et al. (1984) conducted a two-year prospective cohort study of a systematically identified group of 398 persons age 62 or over who were living in urban areas of Connecticut (quality rating = 7). A three-item index of religiousness was administered at baseline that measured religious attendance, self-rated religiosity, and religion as a source of strength and comfort. Physical illness was measured by presence of medical diagnoses and by observable physical symptoms. Twelve percent of subjects ($n = 47$) died during the two-year follow-up.

With gender accounted for in the model, there was a significant interaction between severity of physical illness and religiousness in predicting mortality ($p < .0025$). Among healthy religious men, 11% died, compared to 12% of nonreligious healthy men; among healthy religious women, 2% died, compared to 3% of nonreligious healthy women. Among physically ill religious men, 19% died, compared to 42% of sick nonreligious men; among physically ill religious women, 11% died, compared to 20% of sick nonreligious women. The odds ratio for increased risk of dying among the nonreligious in the entire sample, adjusted for health and sex, was 2.02; for physically ill persons it was 2.32 (both odds ratios are statistically significant). When individual items that make up the religion index were examined, all three were associated with lower mortality; religious attendance was related more weakly, and strength and support from religion was related more strongly.

Oxman et al. (1995) conducted a prospective study of 232 patients age 55 or over who underwent elective cardiac surgery for CABG, AVR, or both at Dartmouth Medical Center in New Hampshire. Eligible patients were those scheduled for elective surgery between November 1989 and December 1992. The final sample of 232 subjects represented 90% of eligible patients ($n = 319$) for whom surgery was not canceled or rejected and was not so urgent that it could not be carried out on an elective basis. Subjects were assessed prior to surgery and at one and six months after surgery. Religious variables measured at baseline were affiliation, attendance at services, strength and comfort drawn from religion, number of people known in the congregation, and self-rated religiousness. Logistic regression analyses identified five major predictors of mortality during the six-month period following surgery: previous cardiac surgery, severity of functional impairment, age over 70 at time of surgery, lack of participation in social groups, and low strength or comfort from religion (the same variable that had best predicted mortality among medically ill older subjects in the Zuckerman et al. study).

After adjusting for other variables (including social factors), the researchers found that subjects who did not draw strength or comfort from religion had three times greater mortality (OR 3.25, 95% CI 1.09–9.72) than those who did. Among the 72 subjects who had both high group participation and high scores on religious strength and comfort, only 2.5% died, compared with more than 21% of the 49 subjects who had no group participation and who took no strength or comfort from religion. After the researchers controlled for biomedical risk factors (previous cardiac surgery, impairment of physical functioning, age over 70), the risk of death among subjects who lacked social group participation and who drew no strength or comfort from religion was more than 14 times greater than the risk for those with both social and religious support (adjusted OR 14.3, 95% CI 2.4–86.6).

Helm and colleagues (2000) conducted a 6-year prospective study of 3,851 community-dwelling adults ages 64–101 who resided in the Piedmont region of North Carolina as part of the Duke EPESE program. Private religious activities and a wide variety of sociodemographic and health variables were assessed at baseline in 1986, and vital status of members was determined in 1992. Time (days) to death or censoring in days was analyzed using the Cox proportional hazards procedure. During a median 6.3-year follow-up period, 1,177 subjects died. Lack of private religious activity (meditation, prayer, or Bible study) was a significant predictor of mortality in healthy but not disabled subjects. After the investigators controlled for demographics and health status (including depression and stressful life events), persons with no disability and little or no private religious activity in 1986 were significantly more likely to die during the follow-up (HR 1.63, 95% CI 1.20–2.21). Even after controlling for social support and health behaviors, investigators found that lack of private religious activity continued to predict greater mortality (HR 1.47, 95% CI 1.07–2.03).

Religious Involvement and Survival among Jews

The association between religious involvement and longer survival is found not only in Christian populations. A 23-year follow-up of more than 10,000 Israeli male civil servants found that orthodox Jews were at least 20% less likely to die of coronary artery disease than were secular Jews—a statistically significant effect *after* age, systolic blood pressure, total cholesterol, cigarette smoking, diabetes, body mass index, and baseline coronary heart disease were controlled (Goldbourt et al., 1993). A 20% or greater reduced risk of death from coronary heart disease is not a weak effect. No cardiac drug that we know of can sustain an effect of this magnitude over time (Terence R. Collins, personal communication). As noted in chapter 16, religious orthodoxy in this study was measured using an index composed of three items (religious vs. secular education; self-definition as orthodox, traditional, or secular; and frequency of synagogue attendance).

Jeremy Kark, head of the cardiovascular unit at the Israel Center for Disease Control and colleagues (1996b) conducted a 16-year prospective study of 3,900 person who were living in 11 religious and 11 secular kibbutzim. The religious and secular kibbutzim were matched on geographic location, quality and type of regional hospital, number of members age 40 or older, and dates of establishment. A total of 268 deaths occurred between 1970 and 1985 (69 in religious and 199 in secular kibbutzim). Both age group and sex were taken into account by stratification, and the Cox proportional hazards procedure was used to further control for age as a continuous variable. The age-adjusted hazard ratios for secular and religious kibbutzim were 1.67 (95% CI 1.17–2.39, $p < .01$) for men, 2.67 (95% CI 1.55–4.60, $p < .001$) for women, and 1.93 (95% CI 1.44–2.59, $p < .0001$) for the entire population, with sex controlled. The causes of mortality were interesting. Men in religious kibbutzim were less likely than those in secular kibbutzim to die from coronary artery disease and circulatory disorders, whereas women were less likely to die from neoplasms. The analysis was not likely confounded by social or demographic factors, given the careful matching of religious and secular kibbutzim.

The investigators then considered the mechanism of the mortality effect by examining possible explanatory variables. Because investigators thought that risk factors such as plasma cholesterol levels, smoking, obesity, alcohol intake, exercise, and exposure to accidents might play a role, they used statistical methods to estimate the relative risk of mortality in secular and religious kibbutzim that reflected the risk factor differences between the communities (on the basis of data from another study). The analysis demonstrated that the effect of risk factor differences on mortality was on the order of 1.0 to 1.2 (negligible). Instead, the lower mortality in the religious kibbutzim was thought to result from a reduction in stress as a result of religious beliefs, highly stable marital bonding, and the close-knit family-oriented nature of these religious communities.

Studies That Find No Association

Of course, not all investigations of the relationship between religious involvement and mortality find a significant association. Idler and Kasl (1992) found that religious attendance had no effect on survival in their eight-year follow-up of 2,812 participants in the Yale Health and Aging study (men and women were examined separately). In a later report (the 12-year follow-up), however, they did find a significant unadjusted bivariate correlation ($p < .001$) between attendance and survival for men and women combined (Idler & Kasl, 1997a).

Koenig, Larson, et al. (1998) examined whether the use of religion as a source of coping was a predictor of all-cause mortality in a sample of 1,010 adult men hospitalized for medical illness. These patients were followed for an average of nine years. Subjects completed a three-item measure at baseline that assessed the extent to which they used religion to cope with their medical problems and other life stress. In both bivariate and multivariate analyses, patients who relied heavily on religion for coping did not live longer than patients who did not depend on religion. The authors proposed several reasons for the absence of an effect, including the fact that the mortality force exerted by age, medical diagnosis, and severity of physical health problems may have overwhelmed the weaker effects of psychosocial and religious variables.

RESULTS OF A META-ANALYSIS

In an attempt to resolve the disparities in studies of the relationship between religiousness and mortality, McCullough et al. (2000) identified 29 independent samples that examined the association between religious involvement and mortality. To obtain a single quantitative estimate of the size of this effect across the 29 samples, investigators conducted a meta-analytic review that incorporated data from more than 125,000 subjects. They found that religious involvement had a significant and substantial association with increased survival (odds ratio = 1.29, 95% CI 1.20–1.39, $p < .001$).

Moderators of the Religion-Mortality Association

While the 42 effect sizes obtained from the 29 studies included in the meta-analysis had a central tendency of around 1.29, they did vary considerably. One of the most important aspects of the review was the series of statistical tests that investigators conducted to identify factors related to effect size. Using these analyses, they found a number of reasons to explain the interstudy variability.

1. *Number of Covariates Adjusted.* Studies that statistically controlled for the most variables (through blocking, matching, age-adjustments, or multivariate analyses) found somewhat smaller effect sizes. It is possible, then, that at least part of the association between religious involvement and mortality is due to confounding. Few studies, however, made a distinction between covariates that were true "confounders" and covariates that were "explanatory" or "mediating" variables.

We digress for a moment to again emphasize this point. True *confounders* disguise or exaggerate a relationship between two variables; confounders typically include age, race, sex, education, and baseline health status. If confounders are controlled and no relationship is found, then there is no true association. *Explanatory* variables, however, describe the *mechanism* by which religious involvement affects health (as discussed earlier concerning health behaviors) (Koenig, Idler, et al., 1999). Explanatory variables include social support, stress level, depression, and other intervening behavioral and biological variables (e.g., smoking, hypertension). If religion increases social support, buffers stress level, reduces depression, decreases the likelihood of smoking, and lowers blood pressure, and all these variables are also related to mortality, then statistically controlling for these factors may completely account for the relationship between religious involvement and mortality. Controlling for these variables, then, may cause a negative relationship between religion and mortality to weaken or lose statistical significance. This means not that there is no relationship between religion and health but only that one has explained *how* religious involvement affects health.

To illustrate, take for example the association between a hurricane and the destruction it causes. If we "control" for the wind speed, the rain, and the waves, we are likely to find little or no association between the hurricane and destroyed buildings or other damage along the coastline. We could not, however, conclude that a hurricane has no destructive force. The same applies to religion and health, where religion acts as a convoy or proxy for a bundle of other factors (e.g., social support, health behaviors, optimism, improved coping) that likely impact health.

McCullough et al. (2000) offered evidence to suggest that confounding cannot entirely explain the relationship between religious involvement and survival. While studies that adjusted for few or no control variables tended to bias the effect size estimate downward, the mean effect size among studies that adjusted for more variables (OR = 1.23) did not differ substantially from the mean effect size for all studies (OR = 1.29).

2. *Gender.* McCullough et al. (2000) found that effect sizes for studies with a high percentage of men yielded weaker associations than did those with more women. At least two studies found significant associations between religious involvement and mortality only among women (House, Robbins, et al., 1982; Strawbridge, Cohen, et al., 1997), and a similar trend was found in several others (Kark et al., 1996b; Hummer et al., 1999; Koenig, Hays, Larson, et al., 1999).

Women generally tend to be more involved in religious practices than men. Women are more likely to attend religious services, pray privately, say religion is important in their lives, and depend on religion as a coping behavior (Koenig, Hays, Larson, et al., 1999). Thus, it is possible that religious beliefs and practices are more deeply ingrained into the social and psychological lives of women and therefore confer greater health benefits. Strawbridge, Cohen, et al. (1997) suggest that, given the much higher proportion of widowhood among older women than among men, religious institutions may fill an otherwise unmet social need for support. Similarly, Idler (1994) emphasizes a general tendency for women to seek and use social interaction to cope with stress.

3. *Measures of Religious Involvement.* Associations between religious involvement and survival were more favorable (OR = 1.43) in studies that used public measures of religious involvement (e.g., frequency of religious attendance, membership in religious groups) than in those that used private religious activities (e.g., frequency of private prayer, finding strength and comfort in one's religious beliefs) (OR = 1.04) Thus, a primary mechanism by which religious involvement may extend survival is through active participation in religious community (Kark et al., 1996b; Idler & Kasl, 1997a; Ellison & Levin, 1998).

Physical Mobility as a Confounder

As mentioned earlier, another explanation for the strong association between public religious involvement and longevity is what some have called the "proxy" effect (Levin & Vanderpool, 1987, 1989; Sloan et al., 1999). Because physical functioning is rarely measured perfectly, variables that reflect functional ability (such as religious attendance) might correlate with greater survival not because the activities themselves are conducive to better health but because the ability to engage in those activity (e.g., going to church, synagogue, or mosque) reflects a certain degree of physical health that predicts future mortality. Nevertheless, McCullough et al. (2000) found no evidence that the relationship between religious involvement and survival was substantially stronger in studies that did not control for physical health (OR 1.29 compared to 1.26).

Furthermore, while physical disability may prevent religious attendance, frequent religious attendance may also delay the onset of disability and other health problems (see chapter 22). Idler and Kasl (1997a) followed 2,812 older adults for 12 years and found that associations between church attendance in 1982 and functional disability in 1983, 1984, 1985, 1986, 1987, and 1988 were all inverse and statistically significant (after the researchers controlled for multiple confounders). In the final year of analysis (1994), the association barely failed to reach statistical significance because of the loss of power as the sample size decreased (although the size of the beta coefficient remained about the same size as the average beta coefficient for years 1983–1988).

Even more important, Idler and Kasl (1997a) found that physical functioning had only a slight impact on later attendance (most of the effect was the other way). Recall also Strawbridge, Cohen, et al.'s (1997) finding that frequent church attenders had *more* mobility problems at baseline than did infrequent attenders. It is amazing how some very ill people often make it to services every Sabbath. They arrive in wheelchairs and on walkers. We have observed this phenomenon in both the Yale and the Duke EPESE studies, which have followed thousands of community-dwelling older adults for more than a decade in Connecticut and North Carolina.

SUMMARY AND CONCLUSIONS

A substantial body of research (mostly, although not exclusively, from Western nations) reveals an association between religion and greater longevity. In this chapter, we found that religious leaders live longer than people in the general population (although perhaps not longer than teachers). We found that members of certain religious groups (e.g., Mormons and Seventh-Day Adventists) live longer than persons in the general population, particularly if the former are religiously active.

Finally, we reviewed studies that examined the association between degree of religious involvement (i.e., public and private religiousness) and survival. Involvement in religious community is consistently related to lower mortality and longer survival. Frequent religious attendance (once a week or more) is associated with a 25–33% reduction in the risk of dying during follow-up periods ranging from five to 28 years. This association appears stronger in women and is independent of confounders (age, sex, race, education, and health status). In fact, this effect is not even accounted for in most studies by explanatory variables such as social support, psychological stress, or health behaviors. While there is some evidence that functional disability can prevent religious attendance (and thus confound the relationship between religious attendance and health outcomes), religious attendance itself can also help prevent the onset and progression of physical disability.

Private religious activities (prayer and religious coping) have a more complex relationship with mortality. This relationship is confounded by the fact that, as people become sicker and closer to death, they often turn to religion for comfort and solace, thus making it appear as though religious coping activities are cross-sectionally associated with worse health and greater mortality (and disguising the health benefits that long-term practice of such activities might provide). Only careful observation and measurement over time can untangle this complex web of causation.

Francis Galton's hope was that science could be used to investigate all matters of human importance, including the relationship between religion and mortality. In the century since Galton's work, researchers have done much to illuminate the connections between religion and survival. We hope that the next century of research will shed light on exactly how religion influences physical health, what aspects of religion do so, and how these findings can be sensitively applied to clinical practice.

22

Religion and Disability

with Shelley Dean Kilpatrick

ARE FOR THE ILL AND THE disabled has historically been the primary responsibility of the religious community (Selway & Ashman, 1998). Churches founded the first sheltered workshops, hospitals, and cloisters in Europe for this purpose. The Poor Law (1601) enacted during the reign of Queen Elizabeth I put the care of the disabled into the hands of the local parishes, where it remained until the nineteenth century. This policy carried over to the British colonies and protectorates, such as Australia. Services for people with disabilities have been provided also in eastern religious communities (e.g., the care institutions created by the Buddhist emperor Asoka and the Hindu and Muslim efforts in Benares, India (1826) and Lucknow, India (1831), respectively).

On the other hand, some cultures (e.g., Northern Salteaux Indians, Jukun of Sudan, and residents of many areas of Europe in the Middle Ages) have considered disabilities to be the work of evil spirits or demons (Buscaglia, 1975; Dovey & Graffam, 1987). In some cases, people with disabilities were banned from full participation in religious communities. The ambivalent relationship between religious communities and persons with disabilities continues today. Although few religions continue to teach that disabilities have spiritual causes, religious congregations and institutions are still struggling to accommodate the needs of those with physical disabilities.

Approximately 54 million Americans live with disabilities (McNeill, 1997), and, given the growing population of older persons with disabilities in this country (Kunkel & Applebaum, 1992), that number may expand exponentially in the future (Schneider, 1999). In spite of the difficulties that religious institutions still experience in meeting the spiritual and practical needs of people with disabilities, it is worthwhile to examine the extent to which religious and spiritual involvement help prevent disability or help people cope with disability.

Research on the relationship between religion and disability has investigated six major areas:

1. The role of religious involvement in preventing disability among healthy community-dwelling adults
2. The role of religious involvement in preventing disability among high-risk populations with medical illness
3. The impact of religion on perceptions of disability and health
4. The association between religion and physical health in people with disabilities
5. The relationship among religion, well-being, and coping in people with chronic illness or disability
6. The relationship of religion to well-being and coping in caregivers of the disabled.

RELIGION AND PREVENTION OF DISABILITY IN COMMUNITY-DWELLING ADULTS

Does religion ward off disability among healthy people who live in the community? Cross-sectional studies have found inconsistent correlations between religious involvement and disability. Such studies are not very helpful, however, since different dimensions of religious involvement are likely to relate to level of disability in the opposite direction. Physical illness and mobility problems may interfere with the ability to perform some religious activities and yet promote the motivation and desire to perform others.

For example, people may decrease their attendance at religious services as their physical functioning declines; to the extent that this is going on, any observed cross-sectional associations of public religious involvement and disability would not be causal but rather result from "criterion contamination" (which occurs when a predictor variable is not causally associated with the dependent variable but rather is measuring the concept operationalized by the dependent variable). One cannot ignore, however, the fact that attendance at religious services may also play a major role in preventing the onset and/or progression of disability (see Idler studies).

Some investigators might be tempted to solve this problem by using measures of religious involvement that are less affected by physical functioning (i.e., private religious activities). Prayer, scripture reading, and other religious coping activities, however, are likely to increase as physical illness and disability worsen, biasing cross-sectional relationships in the other direction as persons turn to these private religious activities for comfort.

Confusion arises from studies that mix different kinds of religious activities as predictor variables (i.e., include public, private, and/or subjective religiosity in a single measure). Effects often cancel each other out in such combined indices. For example, Jeffers and Nichols (1961) found that a multi-item measure of religious activity was unrelated to physician ratings of physical health among a group of community-dwelling older adults, although religious attitudes were significantly related to greater disability ratings. Religious activity was measured by an index that combined church attendance, listening to religious radio/TV, reading Bible/devotional books, and engaging in other private religious behaviors, whereas assessments of religious attitudes were based on agreement or disagreement with statements about religion's importance or the extent of comfort derived from religion.

If private religious activities or religious importance increase in response to worsening health problems (as people turn to religion for comfort) and religious attendance decreases with increasing disability, then efforts to estimate the effects of these religious activities and attitudes on disability becomes hopelessly lost in cross-sectional analyses.

There are other examples. Levin and Markides (1985) examined the correlations between two measures of religious involvement (frequency of religious attendance and self-rated religiosity) and several measures of physical functioning (e.g., self-rated health, activity restrictions due to poor health, days spent in bed because of disability in the past year) in a sample of more than 1,100 Mexican-Americans from three generations (young, middle-aged, and older). Church attendance was positively related to better self-rated health ($r = .14$, $p < .01$) in older subjects, negatively related to physical activity restrictions in younger men ($r = -.15$, $p < .05$), and negatively related to physical symptoms in younger adults of both genders ($r = -.13$, $p < .01$) but especially in women ($r = -.18$, $p < .01$).

Subjective religiosity, on the other hand, was positively related to activity restrictions in older subjects ($r = .12$, $p < .05$) especially in men ($r = .21$, $p < .05$), and was positively related to bed disability days ($r = .15$, $p < .05$) in middle-aged men. In younger men, however, subjective religiosity was negatively related to activity restrictions ($r = -.26$, $p < .01$). Here we see different measures of religious involvement being related differently to different measures of physical disability in populations of different ages and genders; this mixture underscores the complex nature of interpretating the results of cross-sectional studies.

Guy (1982) surveyed 1,170 community-dwelling adults who were living in Memphis, Tennessee. Persons who attended services once a week or more and those whose church activity had increased compared to its level 15 years earlier reported higher life satisfaction ($p < .001$). As Levin and Markides had reported, Guy found a significant inverse relationship between physical disability and church attendance ($p < .001$). She also found a trend for infrequent attenders who were physically disabled and yet still maintained contact with church to have higher life satisfaction. None of these studies controlled for covariates.

More recent work by Idler and Kasl has helped to clarify the relationships between physical disability and religious variables, particularly religious attendance and subjective religiosity. Idler and Kasl (1997a) found that functional disability had a strong negative cross-sectional relationship to attendance at religious services in 2,812 community-dwelling elderly residents of New Haven, Connecticut (53% Catholic, 28% Protestant, 14% Jewish). Religious attendance, self-rated religiousness, and comfort derived from religion were measured by single items. Functional disability was measured by 15 items with a score range from 0 to

150 and by an index of physical activity (e.g., gardening, exercise, sports, walking). Regression analyses reveal that religious attendance and subjective religiosity (religiousness and comfort from religion) were related in significant and opposite directions to level of functional disability ($\beta = -.019$, $p < .001$, for attendance, and $\beta = .004$, $p < .05$, for subjective religiosity).

Attendance at religious services was also associated with better health practices—higher levels of exercise, lower rates of alcohol consumption, and lifelong abstention from smoking (all of which would likely affect future health and level of physical functioning). Higher levels of subjective religiousness were associated with never having smoked and, as others have found, with a higher weight-to-height ratio (greater obesity). More important, there was evidence that religious attendance and disability interacted in such a way that people with high levels of disability appeared to "benefit" more from religious involvement than did people with lower levels of disability. The most disabled study participants who frequently attended religious services displayed more positive affect and optimism than did disabled infrequent attenders. Attending religious services was also associated with fewer depressive symptoms, fewer complaints of physical illness, and fewer interpersonal conflicts. Again, involvement in religious community activities—but not private religiousness—was related to better physical functioning and less disability.

In one of the first true longitudinal analyses of the relationship between religious involvement and physical disability, Idler and Kasl (1997b) assessed functional disability, public and private religious involvement, health status, health practices, social activities, and well-being during a 12-year follow-up of participants in their (1997a) cross-sectional study. After controlling for baseline disability and multiple demographic and physical health covariates, the investigators found that public religious involvement (measured in 1982) predicted lower functional disability between 1983 and 1994 (betas ranging from -0.91 to -1.61). Only in the final year of follow-up, in 1994, did the relationship fail to reach statistical significance because of reduced sample size (but the size of the beta coefficient remained consistent with the effect seen in earlier years).

While disability level also affected future religious attendance to some degree (disability interfered with the ability to *get* to church), the effect was only short term. Participants decreased their attendance at religious services during the period immediately following a decline in physical functioning. This decrease was undetectable, however, three years later. The "benefits" of religious attendance on subsequent functioning were greatest for those with the greatest disability at the beginning of the study. Idler and Kasl (1997b) found that, while higher levels of physical activity, higher levels of leisure activity, more close kin, and higher levels of optimism were characteristic of religious attendees, these characteristics could not completely account for the relationship between religious attendance and later disability.

Finally, in a four-year prospective study of a national random sample of 511 persons age 65 or over in United States, Krause (1998a) examined the relationship among religious involvement, disability level, and self-rated health. Global self-rated health was measured with three items and functional disability with 14 items. Religious variables included religious coping (three items), public religious involvement (three items), and private religious activity (two items). All religious variables were assessed at Time 2, making this largely a cross-sectional analysis. Poor self-rated health was inversely related to involvement in religious community activities ($\beta = -.10$, $p < .01$) but was unrelated to private religious activities or religious coping (as usual). There was also a significant interaction between religious coping and neighborhood deterioration ($\beta = -.026$, $p < .005$), suggesting that the negative impact of living in a dilapidated neighborhood on changes in self-rated health over time was completely offset for older adults who relied heavily on religious coping strategies. No association or interaction, however, was found between religious variables and functional disability.

In summary, cross-sectional studies find an inverse relationship between religious atten-

dance and physical disability or poor health. These studies also typically find no relationship between disability level and private religious activities, subjective religiousness, or religious coping. Idler and Kasl's single longitudinal study shows that attendance at religious services is more likely to prevent the onset or progression of disability than physical disability is to prevent attendance at religious services, and they find no relationship between subjective religiousness and disability.

RELIGION AND PREVENTION OF DISABILITY IN THE MEDICALLY ILL

Other studies have examined the relationship between religion and disability in people who are at high risk for disability as a result of physical health problems, such as medical inpatients and individuals undergoing physical rehabilitation (Pressman et al., 1990; Koenig, Cohen, Blazer, Pieper, et al., 1992; Harris et al., 1995; Heinemann & Kim, 1998; Kim & Heinemann, 1998; Koenig, Pargament, & Nielsen, 1998).

Examining the relationship between religious coping and health, Koenig, Pargament, and Nielsen (1998) surveyed 577 older adults who were hospitalized with acute medical illness. They administered a variety of measures of religious involvement and religious and nonreligious coping. After controlling for age, race, sex, education, and hospital setting, the investigators found that several religious measures were related to physical health and functional ability. As studies of community-dwelling adults have found, these investigators discovered that frequent church attendance was associated with better subjective health and fewer impairments to physical functioning; again, no relationship was found between frequency of private prayer or importance of religion and disability status. Of particular interest were relationships between severity of health problems or disability and how persons used religion to cope. Those who coped by (a) understanding their illness to be a punishment or test from God, (b) understanding their health problems to be afflictions caused by demonic forces, or (c) pleading for direct intercession tended to have greater impairments in physical functioning and worse subjective health. Again, the cross-sectional nature of this study prevented investigators from determining whether these coping behaviors *led* to greater functional disability or were a *result* of greater disability.

In a prospective study that examined the role of religion in recovery from heart transplant surgery, Harris et al. (1995) interviewed transplant recipients two, seven, and 12 months postsurgery. Investigators included both objective and open-ended measures of religious beliefs and practices, the Rosenberg self-esteem scale, a measure of physical functioning (Karnofsky scale), a measure of emotional well-being (Derogatis's SCL-90), and questions about the health and emotional concerns of patients.

Over the year of the study, the number of patients who attended church frequently increased from 18% at two months to 44% at 12 months. However, during the same period, the percentage of patients who reported that religion was a significant influence in their lives declined slightly, from 46% to 37%. Patients who reported that their religious beliefs were highly influential in their lives at baseline had better physical functioning ($r = -.36$, $p < .05$), fewer health worries, and less difficulty following the medical regimen ($r = -.39$ and $-.37$, respectively; p's $< .05$) at the one-year follow-up than did other patients. Patients who regularly consulted God before making important decisions and who prayed frequently also had less difficulty following the medical regimen than did other patients ($r = -.44$, $p < .01$ and $r = -.33$, $p < .05$, respectively). Finally, patients who frequently attended religious services reported less anxiety ($r = -.33$, $p < .05$) than those who did not, and those who were active within their own congregation had higher self-esteem ($r = -.32$, $p < .05$) than those who were not active. None of these bivariate correlations were controlled.

Pressman and colleagues (1990) examined the relationship among religious belief, depression, and ambulation status in a small sample of 30 elderly women admitted for surgical correction of a hip fracture. Investigators measured religiousness with a three-item scale that included attendance at religious services, perceived religiousness, and reliance on religion (and/or God) as a source of strength and comfort. Depression was assessed with the Geriatric Depression Scale. Ambulation status was measured by assistance required and linear distance walked at discharge. Religiousness was significantly and negatively related to depression ($r = -.61$, $p < .01$) even when severity of illness was controlled. Religiosity was also positively correlated with meters walked at discharge ($r = .45$, $p < .05$), an association largely mediated by the inverse relationship between religiousness and depression. When individual items were examined, religious attendance had the strongest association with ambulation status at discharge ($r = .50$, $p < .05$).

Another study found that the effects of religious variables on disability resulted largely from better mental health status. In a sample of 156 adults in rehabilitation for either chronic or sudden onset of illness, Kim and Heinemann (1998) measured relationships among spiritual well-being, spiritual support, and spiritual dogmatism and emotional health, life satisfaction, and functional recovery. Patients were contacted during the first week of inpatient rehabilitation, during the last week of inpatient rehabilitation, and three months after release from rehabilitation. The investigators found a positive relationship between greater spirituality and better physical functioning. This relationship was tied to the fact that those with greater spirituality had greater initial levels of motor and cognitive function, life satisfaction, and emotional health.

In a final study of religious involvement and disability in medical patients, Koenig, Cohen, Blazer, Pieper, et al. (1992) examined the relationship between physical disability and religious coping (measured by a three-item Religious Coping Index). Although patients who found strength and comfort in their religious beliefs reported lower levels of depressive symptoms, no cross-sectional relationship was found between religious coping and level of disability once confounders and explanatory variables were controlled. Unfortunately, the impact of confounders and explanatory variables on the relationship between religious coping and disability was not examined separately.

NEGATIVE STUDIES

A series of studies by King, Speck, et al. (1994, 1999) have reported worse physical health outcomes among medical inpatients with strong spiritual beliefs. We now carefully analyze these studies, since their conclusions are quite different from the findings reported by other researchers.

King et al. (1994) conducted a six-month prospective study of 300 patients consecutively admitted to an acute-care hospital in London, England. A "Beliefs" questionnaire was administered to the 232 subjects who indicated a religious or spiritual belief. Subjects were asked to indicate level of agreement on a 1–5 scale to the following statements contained in the Beliefs questionnaire:

1. I need to understand why things happen to me.
2. My beliefs help me during illness.
3. Illness is a result of lack of spiritual belief.
4. My belief is weaker than it used to be.
5. Recently my beliefs have strengthened.
6. Faith in a power outside of oneself is important in healing.
7. Recently I have become less sure of what I believe.
8. Without God I would not have come through my last crisis.

Investigators wished to define beliefs broadly and appeared pleased to find no association between scores on their Beliefs questionnaire and other measures of traditional religious involvement (e.g., frequency of religious attendance, acquaintance with a religious leader).

Subjects were administered the eight-item Beliefs questionnaire both at baseline and on follow-up six months later. Hospital records of 287 patients were reviewed to determine clinical outcomes on follow-up. Outcomes were categorized as "good" if the patient was improved or completely well; outcomes were categorized as "otherwise" (poor) if the patient stayed the same or worsened. Investigators reported that 58% of the 300 patients described themselves as religious *and* spiritual, 19% as spiritual but not religious, 14% as philosophical (searching for existential meaning in life but without reference to a transcendent being), and 9% reported no belief system.

At the six-month evaluation among patients with outcome assessments who described themselves as religious or spiritual, those with good outcomes tended to score lower on the Beliefs questionnaire at baseline than did those with poor outcomes ($t = 1.76$, df $= 215$, $p = .08$). When the results were analyzed using categorical methods, patients with low Belief scores (less than one standard deviation below the mean) were significantly more likely to have "good" outcomes than those with moderate or high belief scores ($21/27$ vs. $93/191$, $p = .01$). Scores on the Beliefs questionnaire were then recategorized by dichotomizing them at the mean and entering this variable into a logistic regression model, together with three of the eight individual questions on the Beliefs questionnaire that had been associated with poor outcome in the bivariate analysis. Of the four variables, only one variable significantly predicted worse clinical outcome. Patients who agreed with the statement "Without God, I would not have come through my last crisis" were 2.4 times less likely to have a good outcome than those who disagreed with this statement ($p = .034$).

A number of methodological and interpretation problems exist with this study. First is the validity of the Beliefs questionnaire with regard to measuring religious or spiritual beliefs. The questionnaire contains several items (e.g., "I need to understand why things happen to me") that on the surface appear to have little to do with spiritual or religious belief. Furthermore, Belief scores were completely unrelated to measures of traditional religious involvement. One might argue that there should have been at least some relationship (even if weak) with other religious measures. This absence of convergent validity is disturbing. Second, the assessment of clinical outcomes by medical record review was not described; thus, we do not know who made these assessments (i.e., their qualifications) or whether they were blinded to the Belief scores of patients. Third, associations were weak, and analyses did not control for potentially relevant covariates such as age, sex, or socioeconomic status, all of which tend to be related to both health and religion.

More serious flaws, however, include the following. Investigators did not assess severity of medical illness (other than medical diagnosis) at baseline or follow-up. Other studies (see chapter 5) have shown that, as the severity of illness increases and they approach death, persons become *more* religious or spiritual, particularly when religiousness is measured in terms of personal or private religiousness (as noted earlier). Thus, greater spirituality at baseline in this study may simply have been a marker for a more advanced medical condition with a worse prognosis. Second, clinical outcomes for more than 20% of the sample ($n = 68$) who had no religious or spiritual beliefs were not examined. Outcomes for this group would be particularly interesting, since such data might either support or refute the authors' conclusions since these subjects are at the farthest end of the low-beliefs spectrum.

Finally, among subjects who completed the Beliefs questionnaire both at baseline and at follow-up, those who had good clinical outcomes were those who *increased* significantly in their Belief scores ($p = .01$), whereas those with poor outcomes did not change in Belief scores. If spiritual beliefs somehow caused worse clinical outcomes, then why were increases in those beliefs during the follow-up period associated with better clinical outcomes?

More recently, King, Speck, et al. (1999) conducted a nine-month prospective study of 250 patients (125 with heart problems and 125 with gynecological problems) admitted to a London teaching hospital. The researchers sought to examine the effects of spiritual beliefs assessed at admission on patients' clinical status nine months later. Investigators used parts of the Royal Free Interview for Religious and Spiritual Beliefs (RFIRSB) (King et al., 1995) to assess spiritual beliefs. The authors developed the RFIRSB because "The most serious drawback to published formats [of current scales] was their

Judaeo-Christian bias. We were interested in developing an interview that would measure religious, spiritual and philosophical beliefs that were not confined to any particular religious creed or school of philosophical thought" (King, Speck, et al., 1995, p. 1126). This instrument, then, was intended to capture a broad definition of spirituality, not Judeo-Christian spirituality. In this study, a subscale of the RFIRSB, the spiritual beliefs scale, was the primary measure of intensity of beliefs and consisted of five questions that subjects answered by rating their agreement on a visual analog scale ranging from 0 to 10 (total score range 0–50):

1. In respect to [spiritual/religious] belief or non-belief where would you place yourself, at present, on this scale?
2. You said that you believe in a power or force outside of yourself. How much does this influence what happens to you in your life?
3. How much can this power affect how you respond to things that happen to you? I.e., How much does it help you to cope when you are affected personally by change or other events in your life?
4. How much does this power help you to understand why things happen in the world, outside of your day-to-day activities? E.g., political events, wars, accidents?
5. What about natural disasters, like earthquakes, floods?

A total of 197 patients (79%) professed some form of spiritual or religious belief and thus were administered the spiritual beliefs scale. Christians made up the majority of these subjects (69%). Among patients with heart problems, 18% considered themselves spiritual but not religious, compared with 24% of patients in gynecological group. Nine months after admission, information from case notes was abstracted to determine clinical outcome (obtained on 202 of 250 subjects). In contrast to their earlier study, investigators appropriately noted that medical reviewers blinded to patients' spiritual beliefs performed the task of abstracting records. Outcome categories were (a) improved or completely well, (b) no change, or (c) worse clinical state or death. Logistic regression analysis revealed that patients with stronger spiritual beliefs at baseline were again more likely (OR 2.3, CI 1.1–5.1, $p = .03$, $n = 144$) to do worse (i.e., remained the same or have deteriorated clinically nine months later). Other predictors of poor outcome were male gender and sleep disturbance on hospital admission. King, Speck, et al. (1999) reported that spiritual beliefs were lower at baseline among those with more serious medical illness, ruling out the possibility that spiritual beliefs were simply an indicator of those with worse health problems. Investigators concluded that strong spiritual belief is an independent predictor of poor outcome.

As with the 1994 study, there are potential problems with the analyses and the conclusions in the 1999 study, including the following:

1. Subjects without religious or spiritual beliefs did not receive the spirituality scale (53 of 250 subjects).
2. As in the earlier study, we do not know the clinical outcome for the 53 subjects who reported no religious or spiritual beliefs (at least from what is reported in the paper).
3. We do not know the clinical outcome for 47 of the 197 subjects with spiritual or religious beliefs because they were lost to follow-up.

Consider two possibilities. First, what if the 53 subjects without religious or spiritual beliefs (who were not included in the analysis) had worse clinical outcomes? Second, what if the 47 subjects mentioned in #3 (who were not included in the analysis) had both low spiritual belief scores and worse clinical outcomes? This is certainly plausible, since the investigators reported that subjects with lower spiritual beliefs scores at baseline were sicker ($p = .05$) (and probably more likely to have worse outcomes because they were sicker). The result would be that subjects more likely to be excluded from the critical analysis of spiritual beliefs and outcome would be those with both low spiritual beliefs and poorer clinical outcomes. This would help explain why investigators found higher spiritual beliefs among those with worse outcomes—but would be an *artifact* of excluding from the analysis many subjects with low/no spiritual beliefs and poor clinical outcomes. It

would also help explain why subjects who experienced a fall in spiritual beliefs between baseline and follow-up tended to be those with the poorest clinical outcomes, which, as in the first study, makes no sense if spiritual beliefs somehow led to poorer clinical outcomes, as the investigators suggest.

Despite the weaknesses of these studies, we cannot dismiss or disregard their findings. It may be that spiritual beliefs in areas of the world where such practices are less common (as in Great Britain and Europe) have different effects on health than do spiritual beliefs in the United States. It is also possible that spirituality in the broad sense (as defined and measured by King et al. in their British studies) has different effects on health and recovery than does more traditional religious involvement.

IMPACT OF RELIGION ON PERCEPTIONS OF DISABILITY AND HEALTH

There is evidence that devout religious involvement may impact the perception of disability in persons with chronic health problems (i.e., how physically limited and restricted they perceive themselves to be). Idler (1987) examined the relationship among religious involvement, chronic illness, and disability in a sample of 2,811 elderly residents of New Haven, Connecticut, who were participating in the Yale Health and Aging project (1,139 men and 1,617 women). Public religiousness was measured by religious attendance and by the number of congregation members known; private religiousness was measured by self-rated religiousness and religion as a source of strength and comfort. Functional disability was measured by a five-category score based on the extent of impairment in performing activities of daily living, and chronic conditions were measured by aggregating self-reported health conditions. Among men, multivariate analysis revealed that, at any given level of chronic illness, those who received a great deal of comfort from religion reported less disability than those who did not receive such comfort. Religiousness, then, may have affected the perception of disability.

By providing a more positive outlook on their chronic health conditions, religious belief could have enabled the men to see themselves as less disabled than they actually were. No such pattern was found for public religiousness, nor was it found for public or subjective religiousness in women.

Musick (1996) later corroborated Idler's finding. In a three-year prospective cohort study of a stratified random sample of 2,623 persons age 65 or over in North Carolina, Musick used regression analysis to examine predictors of subjective health in African American and white subsamples. For 1,421 African Americans, baseline level of private religious devotion (private prayer or Bible reading) was significantly related to greater subjective health on three-year follow-up ($\beta = .07$, $p < .01$, using residualized change analysis), but religious attendance was unrelated to subjective health after functional impairment was controlled. Because African Americans with higher levels of functional impairment spent more time in devotional activities, the effect of devotion on subjective health could not be detected until after functional impairment was controlled. Among 1,202 whites, while there was no main effect for either baseline religious devotion or attendance on subjective health, there was a significant interaction between both private and public religious involvement and functional impairment ($\beta = .06$, $p < .05$, and $\beta = .09$, $p < .001$, respectively). In other words, high levels of functional impairment and either high devotional activity or high religious attendance at baseline were related to better perceptions of physical health on follow-up.

Another study by Idler on how persons view their health may help to explain these findings. Idler (1995) surveyed 200 randomly selected patients at an urban rehabilitation clinic who completed two instruments from the NHANES-I (a physician's examination of the client's musculoskeletal system and the patient's own self-report of pain in those same joints). Of the 200 patients, 176 whose scores were one or more standard deviations from the mean on the joint pain variable were asked to participate in a psychosocial interview. Of these, 146 consented and were interviewed. The psy-

chosocial interview included questions about social networks and support, depression, neuroticism, optimism, and body consciousness and the presentation of a set of 15 items measuring the nonphysical sense of self. Religious variables were religious activities, beliefs, and self-rated religiousness. The investigator found that the more disabled a person was, the more likely he or she was to report seeking help from religion ($\beta = .50$, $p < .05$, after self-rated religiousness, race, education, and activity level were controlled). Idler found that nonphysical sense of self was predicted by self-rated religiousness ($\beta = .23$, $p < .05$), self-rated health, and education. The investigator concluded that self-ratings of health represented broad conceptions of self in which actual physical health and abilities were deemphasized and nonphysical characteristics, including religious or spiritual self-identities, were more prominent.

SPIRITUALITY OR RELIGION, WELL-BEING, AND COPING

A number of early studies report weak and inconsistent associations between religious involvement and well-being in disabled patients. Recall from chapter 6 Bulman and Wortman's (1977) study of religion and well-being among 29 rehabilitation patients with paraplegia or quadriplegia in Chicago, in which the researchers used the Poppleton and Pilkington religious attitudes scale to assess religiousness. Regression analysis revealed that persons who coped better were those who blamed themselves, not others, for their condition. Religiousness, in turn, was positively associated with self-blame (and thus indirectly with better coping), but there was no direct relationship between religious attitude and happiness or coping.

Brooks and Matson (1982) conducted a seven-year longitudinal study that examined sociodemographic, disease-related, medical, and social-psychological factors that might affect self-concept for 103 people in the middle and later stages of multiple sclerosis (MS). Self-concept was measured using a 34-item semantic differential scale administered at two times seven years apart. Coping was assessed by a single question, "What most helps you to cope with MS?" Responses included "doctor," "religion," "family," "accepting it," "fighting it," and "not coping"; 23% of the sample chose "religion," which was second in frequency only to "accepting it" (34%).

Upon examining the relationship between types of coping and change in self-concept, however, investigators found that those who relied primarily on religion to cope with the disease experienced reductions in self-concept over time (the average decline was −0.13 units). Analyses were uncontrolled, however, and neither the statistical nor the clinical significance of a decline in self-concept of 0.13 units was provided. Furthermore, since the investigators did not indicate whether data on coping were acquired at T1 (1974) or at T2 (1981), religious coping (if measured at T2) may have been *a result of* declining self-concept (i.e., the result of the most desperate MS patients turning to religion for comfort).

More recent studies have reported positive relationships between religious involvement and well-being or coping in disabled and/or chronically ill populations. Decker and Schulz (1985) studied correlates of life satisfaction, assessing variables such as health, disability perception, social support, and perceived control, in 100 patients age 40 or older with spinal cord injuries. Self-reported religiosity was among several positive correlates of higher levels of well-being, although the statistical test and strength of the association were not reported.

Recall from chapter 6 that Reed (1987) examined the relationship between religious involvement and well-being among persons disabled with terminal cancer. Her sample included 100 terminally ill hospitalized patients with incurable cancer, 100 nonterminally ill hospitalized patients, and 100 healthy nonhospitalized persons who were free from any serious illnesses. The three groups were matched for age, gender, years of education, and religious background. Disabled terminally ill patients had significantly greater religiousness than either nonterminally ill hospitalized patients or healthy adults ($p = .02$). There was a significant positive relationship between religious involvement and

well-being, but only in disabled terminally ill patients ($r = .22$, $p < .02$, uncontrolled).

In a study of temporarily and permanently disabled patients hospitalized in India, both patients and doctors emphasized the influence of religion on recovery (Dalal & Pande, 1988). When permanently disabled patients ($n = 21$) and temporarily disabled patients ($n = 20$) were asked about the cause of their disability, they often mentioned Karma and God's will. Attributing cause to Karma or God's will tended to relate positively to psychological recovery ($r = .37$, $p < .10$, and $r = .24$, $p =$ ns, respectively). This was especially true for those who were permanently disabled ($r = .43$ and $r = .48$, respectively, both $p < .10$).

Recall from chapter 6 that Ringdal (1996) conducted a three-year prospective study of 253 patients with cancer hospitalized at the University Hospital of Trondheim in Norway. Many of these patients were seriously disabled from their cancer. Religiosity was assessed by two questions concerning importance of religious beliefs and their use in coping. Regression analyses revealed that religiosity was significantly related to life satisfaction ($\beta = .23$, $p < .001$) and feelings of hope ($\beta = 0.17$, $p < .02$).

In one of the best longitudinal studies performed to date, one that we reviewed in greater depth in chapter 5, Tix and Frazier (1997) examined the relationship between religious coping and stressful life events among 174 chronically ill patients who were receiving renal transplants. Subjects were surveyed three months after surgery (T1) and 12 months after surgery (T2). T1 and T2 measures included religious coping, psychological distress, and life satisfaction scales. Regression analyses of these data revealed that religious coping at T1 was related to greater life satisfaction at T1 and T2. Religious coping at T1, however, did not predict greater life satisfaction at T2 after T1 life satisfaction was controlled. When analyses were stratified by religious denomination, an interesting pattern emerged. Among Protestants, but not among Catholics, T1 religious coping was a significant predictor of higher T2 life satisfaction when T1 life satisfaction was controlled. The investigators concluded that their results supported the hypothesis that religious coping is associated with better psychological adjustment in chronically ill and disabled persons facing the stress of transplant surgery.

Ai et al. (1998) studied the role of religiousness in psychosocial recovery following coronary artery bypass graft surgery (CABG) (see chapter 5 for more details). One year after surgery, 151 patients indicated their level of religious involvement over the preceding 12 months, noted if they had experienced postsurgical depression, and provided information about their current level of psychological distress (12 months postsurgery). While investigators found initially that prayer was more likely in subjects who had experienced depression during the first month following CABG, after controlling for post-CABG depression, demographics, and other illnesses, prayer was associated with less current psychosocial distress ($\beta = -.11$, $t = 2.54$, $p < .05$).

Koenig, Cohen, Blazer, Pieper, et al. (1992) examined the relationship between religious coping and depression among 850 older adults with chronic health problems and disability who were admitted to the medical and neurological services of the VA Medical Center in Durham, North Carolina (see chapter 7). Religious coping was measured by a three-item index, with scores ranging from 0 to 30. The 30-item Geriatric Depression Scale (Yesavage et al., 1983) was used to measure depression. Religious coping was inversely related to depression scores ($\beta = -.14$, $p < .001$) after researchers controlled for nine other variables. The relationship was strongest for patients with more severe disability (the interaction term between disability and religious coping was statistically significant).

Koenig, George, and Peterson (1998) next conducted a 47-week prospective study of 87 depressed medical inpatients to determine whether degree of religiousness during baseline hospitalization would predict speed of remission from depression after discharge. Depressive disorder was diagnosed by a clinician using the NIMH Diagnostic Interview Schedule. Intrinsic religiousness was measured using the 10-item Hoge scale (score range 10–50). Investigators found that for every 10-point increase on the Hoge scale, there was a 70% increase in the speed of remission of depression (HR 1.70, 95% CI 1.05–2.75, $p < .05$). Among a subgroup of patients ($n = 48$) whose physical disability (measured by a 20-item activities-of-daily-living scale) was not improving or was worsening, every 10-point increase on the Hoge scale was associated with a greater than 100% increase in speed of remission (HR 2.06, 95% CI 1.02–4.15, $p < .05$). These last two studies suggest that religious involvement may help to both prevent the onset of depression and speed recovery from depression when it occurs, and this effect is particularly important for persons with persistent and protracted physical disability.

RELIGION AND ADAPTATION IN CAREGIVERS

A final set of studies examines the role that religion plays in helping the loved ones of disabled people to cope with the burdens of caregiving. Rabins, Fitting, Eastham, and Fetting (1990) studied predictors of successful adaptation among family caregivers of patients with Alzheimer's disease ($n = 32$) or cancer ($n = 30$). Caregivers who had strong religious faith reported less emotional distress ($\rho = -.24$, $p < .05$) and a more positive emotions ($\rho = .40$, $p = .001$), as measured by two multi-item scales. Attendance at religious services, however, was unrelated to these mental health variables. The subjective aspects of religious involvement, then, might be particularly important for coping among caregivers.

In a unique study of kidney transplant recipients' coping strategies, psychological adjustment and marital adjustment were measured in patients and their spouses (Vinyon, 1995). Personal adjustment was assessed with the Beck Depression Inventory and subscales of the Brief Symptom Inventory; marital adjustment was measured with the Dyadic Adjustment Scale. Coping was assessed with the Coping Strategies Inventory, which includes subscales for cognitive restructuring, emotional expression, problem avoidance, social withdrawal, and reliance on God and religion. Reliance on God and religion was one of the most common coping resources for both patients and their spouses. Men and women spouses used this resource in dealing with transplant-related stress more than did transplant recipients. Investigators found that the reliance on God and religion in coping with the transplant was correlated among married couples ($r = .49$ for female patients and $r = .54$ for male patients, $p < .01$ for both). Reliance on God and religion by male patients and their female spouses was related to higher marital satisfaction among male patients; other relationships between such reliance and patient or spousal distress were not significant.

In research that explores the spiritual aspects of the grief process for HIV-positive and HIV-negative partners of persons who had died from AIDS, Richards and Folkman (1997) found that experience of "spiritual phenomena" was both positively and negatively related to the mental health of caregivers. On the basis of a content analysis of caregivers' reports of their experiences around the time their partners died (spontaneous reports of spiritual phenomena were classified as spiritual beliefs, spiritual experiences, spiritual rituals, or self-created rituals), caregivers were classified as spiritual or nonspiritual. Note that affiliation with a religion was unrelated to report of spiritual phenomena. The two groups were compared using t-tests on coping (the Ways of Coping Scale), mood (depression and anxiety), and physical health measures (both HIV-related symptoms and general health symptoms). In this cross-sectional analysis, caregivers who made spiritual references used more positive reappraisal, planful problem solving, and confrontive coping (i.e., healthier coping strategies) than did caregivers who did not. Caregivers who made spiritual references, however, had higher levels of depression and anxiety than did those who did not. Furthermore, caregivers who reported spiritual experiences reported more HIV-related and general health symptoms than did caregivers who did not.

Note, however, that the most prevalent spiritual belief expressed in this study was spiritualism (the belief that there is a spirit that occupies the body and that leaves the body at death). Only 37% of spiritual narratives involved belief

in a higher order that governed events (i.e., God). Spiritual rituals involved blessings and personalized rituals typically at time of death, ceremonies of burial or distribution of ashes, celebrations of life, and rituals enacted privately by the bereaved partner; such rituals may or may not be related to traditional religious beliefs or practices.

In a follow-up on this sample approximately three to four years later, Richards, Acree, et al. (1999) collected both qualitative and quantitative data from 70 members of their earlier cohort of 125 caregivers regarding the presence of spiritual phenomena. Spirituality, as measured in the earlier study, had deepened in 77% of the cohort. Spirituality was identified by caregivers as a personal governing influence that provided value and direction to the caregiver. Relationships between expression of spirituality and mood, coping, and physical health symptoms were not statistically significant because of the small sample, but the investigators reported medium effect sizes.

SUMMARY AND CONCLUSIONS

In this chapter we have reviewed research on the relationship between religion and spirituality, physical disability, and the ability of patients and their caregivers to cope successfully with their own disability or chronic illness in loved ones. Both cross-sectional and longitudinal studies consistently show an inverse relationship between community religious activity (involvement in church or synagogue) and physical disability. The best longitudinal investigation to date (Idler & Kasl, 1997b) suggests that public religious involvement may help to prevent the development and progression of disability in older adults and that this effect is not overshadowed by short-term effects of disability on the capacity to participate in religious activities.

The evidence for a relationship between physical disability and religious coping or private religious activities, however, is less consistent; studies sometimes show no relationship or even a positive relationship between religious activity and disability. This is not surprising, given the complex and changing dynamics of the religion-disability relationship over time; persons increase their personal religious involvement in order to cope with health problems or worsening disability. There is also evidence that people who adopt a despairing, pleading stance toward God, who see God as punishing and vengeful, or who reframe their health problems as demonic manifestations experience greater disability (Koenig, Pargament, & Nielsen, 1998). Such religious coping strategies are "red flags" that merit clinical attention, even though they may not be causal. Some research in Great Britain suggests that "spiritual beliefs" (as distinct from traditional religious beliefs and activity) may be related to worse physical health outcomes.

Research on the association between religious involvement and mental health, well-being, and successful adaptation among those with disabilities (and those who care for them) has also been reviewed. Religious involvement may help disabled people and their caregivers avoid the negative mental health consequences associated with physical disability; it may also help them recover more quickly from depression and poor adjustment should these occur. Of particular interest is the possibility that religious involvement may affect perception of disability among those with chronic health problems. Religious people may view their physical restrictions with greater optimism and therefore experience greater hope and motivation for physical recovery.

23

Pain and Other Somatic Symptoms

IN THIS CHAPTER WE REVIEW the relationship between religious beliefs and behaviors and somatic symptoms. Somatic symptoms have been divided into pain-related and nonpain somatic symptoms. Nonpain somatic symptoms include menstrual symptoms, menopausal symptoms, gastrointestinal symptoms, and general physical complaints. We ask the question "Are religious beliefs and practices related to more or fewer symptoms of pain or other discomfort?" We first examine pain and the psychological and social factors that affect the experience of pain. If we can establish that psychological or social factors influence pain symptoms, then we may have a basis for expecting a relationship with religion also, given the link between religion and psychological and social functioning.

THE EXPERIENCE OF PAIN

Pain is an extraordinarily complex symptom that has both physiological and psychological aspects. Physiologic pain has biological causes related to inflammation around, trauma to, or physical irritation of nerves (*nociceptive* causes). These can occur anywhere along the nerve paths, from endings in the skin to nerve roots as they enter into the spinal cord to connections in the central nervous system and the brain. Physiologic pain is divided into somatic and visceral pain. Somatic pain results from activation of peripheral nerve receptors in the skin, muscles, and deep tissues of the body. It is typically described as well localized, aching, or gnawing. Visceral pain, on the other hand, results from infiltration, compression, distension or stretching of organs within the body cavity. This type of pain is often described as poorly localized and is a deep squeezing or pressure pain that may be accompanied by other symptoms such as nausea, vomiting, or sweating.

Pain is also generated by nonnociceptive causes that can be categorized as pathophysiologic (*neuropathic* pain that persists without ongoing tissue damage) and psychopathologic (*psychogenic* pain that has no physiological basis) (*Merck Manual of Geriatrics*, 1995). Pathophysiologic or neuropathic pain has biological origins within the nervous system itself and results from the abnormal processing of pain signals in the spinal cord and brain, which may be difficult to verify objectively. Psychogenic pain has no physiological or biological determinants and is entirely due to psychological causes. Neuropathic and psychogenic pain are particularly difficult to distinguish from each other because the assessment of pain is based only on a person's subjective report.

For any given level of objective or nociceptive pain there will be a wide range of reports concerning severity, depending on the setting (war, work, or home) and the personality of the individual (stoic or emotional). The person who experiences a deep wound during battle may hardly notice it because his adrenaline is flowing and his mind is focused on survival. The person at home who has only a small injury may experience and express great discomfort to family members in order to elicit nurturing. Cultural factors may influence both the perception and the expression of pain; for example, a person of Irish descent may suppress the expression of pain, whereas a person of Italian heritage may magnify the pain and communicate loudly to others that she is suffering (Zborowski, 1952). Pain pathways have multiple inputs from higher cortical systems that modulate the level of pain experienced. These higher cortical influences are greatly affected by *level of attention* given the pain. Level of attention is based largely on the *meaning* that the pain has to the individual. Suffering is different from physical pain; it is the disturbing emotional state that results from a combination of negative perceptions based on the physical, psychological, and social experiences of pain.

Understandably, pain is more common in persons over age 65, where the prevalence of pain symptoms ranges from 25–80%, depending upon the study (Hewitt & Foley, 1997). Among nursing home patients, 71% have at least one pain complaint, and 34% of these patients indicate that they are in constant pain (Ferrell, Ferrell, et al., 1990). Pain increases as persons approach death, and about two-thirds of persons have pain in the last month of life (compared to 24% of a control population) (Moss et al., 1991). Patients with cancer are particularly likely to experience pain, and about two-thirds with advanced disease experience significant pain, which reaches its greatest intensity two days before death (Foley, 1987; Morris et al., 1986).

Pain That Results from Physical Causes

Younger adults frequently complain of low back pain and myofascial pain related to acute or chronic injuries. Less frequent causes of pain include rheumatoid disorders, malignancy, and neuralgias related to nerve inflammation or irritation. Older adults often complain of pain related to osteoarthritis, which is widely prevalent in this population (44% of those over age 65) (Kane et al., 1984). Other pain syndromes in the elderly include trigeminal and postherpetic neuralgias and pain due to cancer or other clearly defined physical conditions. These pain syndromes all have a nociceptive focus (i.e., a herpes virus infection of the skin, arthritic joint, bowel obstruction, bone metastasis).

While neuropathic pain is categorized as a nonnociceptive type of pain, there are physiological reasons for the pain (i.e., it results from abnormal processing of nerve impulses). This type of pain is severe and constant and may be described by some patients as a dull ache or vise-like pressure that is accompanied by paroxysms of burning or electric shocks. The autonomic nervous system (which is also strongly influenced by emotional state) can play an important role in neuropathic pain. Examples of neuropathic pain include pain following surgical amputation of a limb (phantom limb pain), reflex sympathetic dystrophy, and certain postsurgical pain syndromes (e.g., following back operations). Neuropathic pain is frequently the most difficult to treat, and even treatment with narcotic analgesics, anesthetic blocks, and neurosurgical procedures may achieve only partial relief.

Pain That Results from Psychological Causes

Some pain is called psychogenic, because it has psychological, not physical, causes. Examples include atypical types of facial pain, low back pain (without objective findings), and other musculoskeletal complaints due to stress or other emotional cause. Pain can result from a conversion disorder, in which a psychological conflict is converted into a physical symptom. These pain complaints are *not* conscious or intentional (when they are conscious, they are called malingering). Causes for psychogenic pain include masked depression, hysterical syndromes, and somatic delusions. We do not address psychogenic pain any further in this chapter and instead concentrate on pain that results from physical causes (including neuropathic pain) and the psychological and social factors that influence it.

Pain That Results from Physiological and Psychological Causes

Often, pain complaints do not fall nicely into either physical/physiological or psychological categories. Any given level of objective physiological pain is experienced and interpreted by the person in light of that person's goals and dreams. The meaning of pain can either greatly magnify its intensity (a malignant process that is life-threatening, an arthritic condition that threatens independence) or can greatly diminish it (the joy of childbirth, pain that results from an act of valor). Chronic, unrelenting pain that is present day in and day out, pain that is disabling and that disrupts activities both inside and outside the home, and pain that interferes with sleep at night and concentration during the day invariably has psychological consequences. These psychological consequences frequently involve depression and anxiety, factors that magnify the intensity of pain further. In

turn, greater pain increases disability and worsens depression, leading to a vicious downward spiral. Common pain syndromes that result from a combination of physical and psychological causes include migraine headaches, fibromyalgia, and low back pain.

Chronic Pain and Chronic Pain Syndrome

Chronic pain, according to the International Association for the Study of Pain, is defined as pain that lasts for a period of three months or longer (IASP, 1979). Chronic pain syndrome refers to the behavioral changes that accompany long-term pain, including social isolation, loss of interest in work, and difficulty performing activities of daily living. It is not so much the pain itself as the physical disability caused by the pain that creates problems—that is, interferes with social relationships, family work roles, and self-esteem.

PSYCHOLOGICAL FACTORS AND PAIN

Much research has documented the enormous influences that psychological and social factors have on the experience of pain.

Depression and Pain

There is a strong positive correlation between depression and pain, sometimes so strong that they are difficult to distinguish. Cohen-Mansfield and Marx (1993) examined the relationship between depression and pain in a sample of 408 nursing home residents. They reported that depressed patients were more likely to have pain, independent of number of medical diagnoses and level of social support. Krause, Weiner, et al. (1994), studying 37 inpatients with chronic pain syndrome, found that depressed patients complain of significantly more pain behavior than nondepressed patients. Kelsen et al. (1995) examined the relationship between pain and depression in 130 patients with newly diagnosed pancreatic cancer. They found a significant correlation between increasing pain and increasing depressive symptoms. Overall, serious depression occurs in nearly 50% of chronic pain patients (Ruoff, 1996). Studying 67 subjects with myofascial pain disorders and 83 patients with arthritis, Faucett (1994) found that, after the researcher controlled for other factors, patients with severe depression were significantly more likely to report severe pain, conflict about pain, and less support from their social network. Likewise, Smedstad et al. (1995) found a significant relationship among pain intensity, anxiety, and depression among 238 patients with rheumatoid arthritis.

Not surprisingly, people often have difficulty distinguishing emotional from physical pain. For scientists, there is the usual "chicken-or-egg" question of whether pain leads to depression or depression leads to pain. Both likely influence each other. Von Korff et al. (1993) tried to determine the causal direction in the pain-depression relationship. They examined depressive symptoms at baseline as predictors of first onset of five common pain symptoms between 1986 and 1989 in 803 health maintenance organization (HMO) members. Compared with nondepressed patients, those with moderate to severe depression at baseline and those with chronic depression were more likely to develop headache and chest pain (adjusted odds ratios from 1.7 to 5.0) during the three-year follow-up. Magni et al. (1994) examined the time-order of effects of depression on pain and of pain on depression among 2,324 subjects in Italy. Subjects were followed for seven years. Logistic regression analysis demonstrated that depressive symptoms at baseline significantly predicted the development of chronic musculoskeletal pain seven years later (OR 2.14, depressed compared with nondepressed subjects). Among patients with pain at baseline, pain predicted only two of 20 items on the CES-D. Depression in these studies, then, was more likely to predict the development of chronic pain than vice versa.

On the other hand, Cairns et al. (1996) examined the relationship between pain and depression over time in 68 patients with acute traumatic spinal cord injury. Depression was again assessed using the CES-D; pain was assessed

using a 101-point numerical rating scale. Investigators found that changes in pain affected depression more than changes in depression affected pain. Thus, there is evidence both that depression leads to chronic pain and that pain leads to depression, a pattern expected if depression and pain have reciprocal effects.

Anxiety and Pain

McCracken et al. (1996) examined the relationship between pain and anxiety in 45 consecutive referrals to a university pain clinic. Anxiety symptoms predicted over 50% of the variance in pain severity, disability, and pain behavior. Likewise, Velikova et al. (1995) found a significant relationship between anxiety and pain in a sample of cancer patients, a relationship that persisted after age and severity of illness were controlled. Studying a sample of institutionalized elderly patients, Casten et al. (1995) examined the relationship among depression, anxiety, and pain, using multivariate modeling and path analysis. They found that, while anxiety and depression shared considerable variance, only anxiety was significantly and independently related to pain. Recall that Smedstad et al.'s (1995) study of 238 rheumatoid arthritis patients found that both anxiety and depression predicted self-reported pain. Thus, both depression and anxiety appear to influence the pain experience.

Social Support and Pain

Social support may help relieve pain by enabling people to cope better with the pain and reduce the associated depression and anxiety. Thus, social support should be inversely related to pain intensity and positively related to physical functioning. To test this hypothesis, Bradley et al. (1987) conducted a randomized clinical trial in 53 patients with rheumatoid arthritis. The intervention involved a psychological treatment and a social support program. Significant improvement in pain behavior, disease activity, and anxiety was noted posttreatment and at six-month follow-up. This social support program was particularly helpful for those with anxiety. Studying 102 women with advanced breast cancer, Koopman et al. (1998) found that the effects of social support on depressive symptoms depended on the subject's stress level. Social support was inversely related to depressive symptoms only among women who were experiencing high life stress. Finally, Jamison and Virts (1990) examined the effects of family support on treatment outcome in 181 patients who were completing an outpatient pain program. Patients with nonsupportive families tended to use more medication, reported more pain, and had lower activity levels than those with supportive families. The authors concluded that "perceived support is an important factor in the rehabilitation of chronic pain patients" (Jamison & Virts, 1990, p. 67).

Thus, it appears that both psychological and social factors influence the experience of pain. Is there any physiological basis for such effects?

Gate Theory of Pain

About 20 years ago Ron Melzack (1982), of McGill University, claimed that he had a theory that could explain the physiological mechanism by which psychosocial factors influence pain. From previous research, he knew that the severity of pain could not be entirely explained by nociceptive causes alone. Pain intensity also appeared to be affected by attention, anxiety, suggestion, and other psychosocial influences. In his "gate theory" of pain, Melzack proposed that pain signals from an injured part of the body were modulated at the spinal cord level by other, simultaneous somatic inputs and by descending influences from the brain. He proposed that a mechanism in the dorsal horns of the spinal cord acted like a gate to inhibit or facilitate transmission of pain impulses through a combination of peripheral nerve inputs and descending brain inputs. Intense stimulation of certain trigger points on the body surface was found to diminish or completely eradicate certain types of pain. Psychological influences (e.g., past experience, attention, and other cognitive activities) could also inhibit pain transmission by "closing the gate." This theory has received repeated confirmation by other investigators over the years (see Melzack, 1993, for a review).

An example of the power of the mind to reduce pain and improve outcome was provided nearly 40 years ago by Beecher (1961). Beecher describes an interesting clinical trial that involved surgical treatment for angina pectoris (pain associated with insufficient blood flow to the heart). Patients were randomized to one group that received ligation of the internal mammary artery on the theory that this would improve circulation to the heart. This operation resulted in 60–90% disappearance of pain, enhanced quality of life, and improved cardiac function on exertion as measured by electrocardiogram. The control group underwent a mock operation in which the skin was simply incised but the artery was not touched. To the investigator's amazement, outcomes were identical in both the treated and the control groups. Similar results have been obtained for more traditional coronary artery bypass surgery (Frank, 1975).

Cognitive Behavioral Treatments for Pain

The gate theory of pain has led to vigorous efforts to develop psychological treatments for neuropathic pain and other chronic pain syndromes. Some of these techniques include hypnosis, biofeedback, relaxation training, and a variety of distraction techniques. These provide the person with a greater sense of control over the pain and may reduce the need for medication. Research has shown such techniques to be quite effective (Bradley, Young, Anderson, McDaniel, et al., 1984; Keefe & Williams, 1990; Cook, 1998). For example, Rene et al. (1992) followed 40 persons with radiographically confirmed osteoarthritis for one year, assessing joint pain and physical functioning during that time. Subjects were randomized to either intervention or control groups. In the intervention group, laypersons called subjects on the telephone every month. Those who received the telephone calls reported significantly less pain ($p < .01$) and also tended to show better physical functioning than those who did not receive the calls. This study suggests that community organizations (such as churches) could help persons with chronic pain by mobilizing lay volunteers to provide supportive contacts.

RELIGIOUS VIEWS ON PAIN AND SUFFERING

Bowker (1978) notes that pain and suffering in Judaism are seen as part of the fate of mankind and the result of sin. While pain and suffering can also atone for sin, Jews are not encouraged to seek out pain or to avoid seeking help for pain. In Islam, pain may be seen as a punishment for sin and error and as a means of instruction and teaching. Like Judaism, however, Islam instructs that one may resist or fight pain because it does not ultimately belong in God's Paradise.

In Christianity, pain, suffering, and death are also seen as punishment for sin, but that the penalty can be removed through atonement and redemption. Like Jews and Muslims, Christians are not encouraged to seek pain or to avoid treatment. Christianity does teach, however, that pain and suffering can be constructive forces for personal growth and for accomplishment of a greater good. According to the medical historian Darrel Amundsen (1982), early Christian Church leaders provided several reasons for the existence of pain and suffering in the world. Clement (150–220) said that the Christian who is suffering from pain should be encouraged to ask God for (1) understanding of the reason for the pain, (2) deliverance from the pain, and, if deliverance was not possible, (3) strength to endure it. Jerome (345–419) suggested that sickness and pain can cause people to adjust their priorities. Gregory Nazianzen (330–390) concluded that pain and suffering (1) cleanse the human body, (2) test a person's virtue and character, and (3) educate the weaker, who must learn from the stronger. John Chrysostom (349–407) gave 12 explanations for suffering (among Christian leaders, in particular):

1. So that they may not too easily be exalted into presumption by the greatness of their good works and miracles
2. So that others may not have a greater opinion of them than is appropriate for mere men
3. So that the power of God may be made obvious in advancing the word preached through the efficacy of men who are infirm
4. So that their endurance may be more striking evidence that they are serving God not for a present reward
5. To demonstrate their belief in a resurrection and an eternal life
6. So that others who suffer will find consolation in their example
7. So that when exhorted to imitate them, others will be aware that they possess a similar nature
8. So that Christians may learn whom they ought to consider as happy and whom wretched, for "Whom the Lord loves He chasens, and scourges every son whom He receives" (Hebrews 12:6)
9. Because tribulation makes those who are troubled more approved, for "tribulation produces patience" (Romans 5:3)
10. So that if Christians having any blemishes, they may put them away
11. Because the Christian's crowns and rewards are thus increased
12. Because if Christians give thanks to God in the midst of their suffering, they deliver a blow to the devil (Amundsen, 1982, p. 336)

Augustine (354–430) believed that health was something good that should be sought after but reminded Christians that God promised them not health but rather eternal life in heaven where there is no pain, suffering, or fear. While he understood that it is natural for persons to pray for the removal of suffering and pain, he pointed out that they do not know the reason God has permitted their pain. Augustine believed that God allows Christians to endure suffering because it (1) heals the swelling of pride, (2) is a test and proof of patience, (3) punishes and eradicates sin, and (4) is a reminder to Christians of their mortality and of the need to rely on God.

From this review, Amundsen (1982) concluded that early Christians understood that pain could be good because it can be used by God in the lives of people for their spiritual good, particularly in those who are receptive to God's instruction. The physician's skills and medicine for relief of pain were considered blessings from God, but to put one's entire faith in them was sinful, since their ultimate efficacy came from God, who could heal without them.

Tu (1980) indicates that the role of pain in strengthening and purifying the person is common to Christianity, Buddhism, and Confucianism. The Buddhist sees pain as a defining characteristic of human life that is to be endured in a matter-of-fact manner. The Confucian views pain as a trial but also believes that a cure is both desirable and necessary for well-being. Shaffer (1978) notes that both Hinduism and Christian Science view pain as an illusion brought on by false beliefs and incorrect thinking. While the Christian Scientist concentrates on God and the good in the world, the Hindu seeks to gain understanding and attain detachment from the world (the source of pain) that is illusion.

RELIGION AND THE RELIEF OF PAIN

We have established that psychological and social influences can substantially affect the perception of pain. Herein lies the rationale for a possible relationship between religion and pain. As we saw earlier, religious beliefs provide a worldview in which pain and suffering can potentially have meaning and purpose. Anything that gives pain meaning or purpose may help reduce the suffering associated with it. Foley (1988) discusses the ways that religion may influence interpretations of personal suffering, thereby altering the perception of and ability to cope with pain. Religion may modify one's primary appraisal of negative life events such as pain, causing one to reassess the meaning of potentially stressful situations and to see them as "opportunities" for spiritual growth or learning or as part of a broader Divine plan, rather than as a threat to personal identity. As suffering is reduced, the intensity of pain and disability it causes are also affected. On the other hand, by inducing guilt or by encouraging a false hope of being miraculously cured, religion may lead to depression and disillusionment and thereby exacerbate pain. Some persons may see their pain as either just punishment for past sins or as God's will for them and may thus fail to make appropriate efforts to obtain pain relief.

Results of cross-sectional studies of relationships between pain intensity and religious variables should be interpreted with care. For example, an inverse relationship between religious attendance and pain does not necessarily mean that going to church results in less pain; instead, it may simply mean that pain prevents persons from attending religious services. Likewise, a positive relationship between prayer and pain intensity is not necessarily evidence that prayer increases pain; it may mean that people don't start praying until the pain gets really bad and other avenues of relief have failed.

Religion may influence pain intensity by affecting cultural or societal expectations, providing a distraction from the pain, "shutting the gate" through the power of belief, enhancing the ability to cope with pain, or increasing social support. We now discuss the evidence for each of these mechanisms below.

Cultural Factors

Cultural expectations may influence reactions to and focus on pain. Zborowski (1952) surveyed 103 medical patients to analyze the cultural components of responses to pain. This qualitative study compared responses to pain by Jewish ($n = 31$), Italian ($n = 24$), Irish ($n = 11$), and "old American" ($n = 26$) male veterans at the Kingsbridge VA Hospital in the Bronx, New York. While Jewish patients were reluctant to take pain medication because they feared the medication might be addictive, Jewish culture allowed them to be demanding and complaining, using their pain to control interpersonal relationships within their families. Both Italians and Jews were free to talk about their pain, complain about it, and manifest their sufferings by groaning, moaning, and crying without shame. Old Americans (largely of English descent) and the Irish tended to minimize pain and to avoid complaining or evoking pity; if the pain became too strong, they withdrew from others.

Distraction

Praying to God or meditating may take one's mind off one's pain. Rosenstiel and Keefe

(1983) reported a positive association between level of pain intensity and the "diverting attention and praying" factor of the Coping Strategies Questionnaire (CSQ). These investigators surveyed 61 chronic low back pain patients referred to the behavioral physiology lab at Duke University for behavioral treatment of pain. Chronic low back pain had been present in the subjects for at least six months (the average was six years). Factor analysis indicated that "diverting attention" and "praying or hoping" items loaded together on the same factor. When examined in a regression model, this factor was cross-sectionally related to *greater* pain level ($p < .001$) and greater functional impairment ($p < .05$).

Keefe et al. (1990) conducted another cross-sectional study of 62 chronic low back pain patients referred to the pain management program at Duke University. The subjects' mean duration of pain was seven years. The diverting attention and praying factor of the CSQ was again positively related to pain and accounted for 9% of the variance in reported pain. Likewise, Tuttle et al. (1991) surveyed 181 chronic pain patients (mean age 42) using the CSQ; praying and hoping were again cross-sectionally related to greater reported pain. Finally, in a different patient population, Fry (1990) examined fears experienced by 178 homebound elderly persons who were receiving Meals-on-Wheels in western Canada. Four major categories of fears were discovered: (1) physical pain and suffering, (2) risk to personal safety, (3) threat to self-esteem, and (4) uncertainty of life beyond death (or "supernatural concerns category"). He also examined four major categories of coping responses, one of which was prayer. In this cross-sectional analysis, prayer was again related to greater physical pain and suffering ($r = .28$, $p < .01$).

One may conclude from these four cross-sectional studies that pain and physical suffering are more common among persons who use prayer as a coping behavior. Is this because people who pray focus more on their pain and thereby intensify it? Or, are people more likely to pray as their pain becomes more severe (a stress mobilization effect)? Longitudinal studies are essential for sorting out this cause-effect relationship.

In the only prospective study to look at this relationship, Turner and Clancy (1986) examined 74 chronic low back pain patients who were participating in a treatment study in Seattle, Washington. The sample consisted of 47 men and 27 women ages 20–65. Chronic low back pain was defined as persistent low back pain lasting for six months or more. The Coping Strategies Questionnaire, the same measure used by Keefe's and Tuttle's groups, was administered, and subjects also completed a pain diary, the Sickness Impact Profile, and the Beck Depression Inventory. Patients completed all instruments before being randomly assigned to a wait-list control group, a CBT group, or an operant behavioral therapy group. The praying or hoping subscale of the CSQ was the third most commonly used coping strategy among the six cognitive strategies examined. Factor analysis again indicated that the "diverting attention" and "praying or hoping" subscales loaded together on a single factor. This factor was, as others had found, significantly and positively related to average pain level ($p < .01$). On longitudinal analysis, however, increased use of the praying or hoping strategy was significantly related to decreases in reported pain intensity (change from Time 1 to Time 2) ($r = 0.21$, $p < .05$).

Turner and Clancy (1986) concluded: "That increased Praying or Hoping following treatment was associated with decreased pain ratings suggests that the positive relationship between the Diverting Attention and Praying factor and pain may be due to the ineffectiveness of distraction techniques, and not to the ineffectiveness of praying and hoping" (p. 362). These results also suggest that prayer is mobilized as a coping strategy in response to pain and may over time help to reduce pain.

Power of Belief

As noted earlier, the power of belief—believing that God or a higher power will reduce or eliminate the pain—may provide a descending input from the brain that "shuts the gate" in the dorsal horn of the spinal cord at the level of pain entry. Research has only indirectly examined such a possibility.

Heiligman et al. (1983) describes pain relief in a patient who reported a religious visitation. The case was a 68-year-old African American woman who made no requests for pain medication after a partial colectomy for resection of a carcinoma. The absence of pain was attributed to protective angels. Although she had been aware of the presence of angels since childhood, before her "knowing of the Lord" surgery had required the usual postoperative analgesia. Psychological testing revealed that she was relaxed and comfortable and fully in touch with reality. In attempting to explain this phenomenon, Heiligman et al. suggested five factors that may influence the perception of pain: (1) the expectation of pain, (2) anxiety about recovery, (3) anxiety as a personality trait, (4) vigilance as a coping behavior, and (5) an internal locus of control. This patient had little expectation of pain and little anxiety about recovery. The belief that there were protective angels watching over her minimized her anxiety and her need for vigilance. The angels also represented a completely externalized locus of control.

In a related study, Florell (1973) randomized 44 orthopedic injury patients to one of two groups: either daily chaplain visits or no visits. Chaplain visits in the intervention group lasted 15 minutes each day. The control group received "business as usual." Patients who received the visits needed less "PRN" pain medication, made fewer calls on nursing time, and experienced less pain and stress (all $p < .05$) than control patients.

Kabat-Zinn et al. (1985) examined the effects of "mindfulness meditation," a Buddhist meditative technique, as a pain intervention in patients at two hospital clinics in Massachusetts. Subjects were 90 chronic pain patients who underwent a 10-week Stress-Reduction and Relaxation Program (SRRP). Investigators reported a statistically significant reduction in pain symptoms, mood disturbance, and psychological symptoms after the intervention. Pain-related drug utilization decreased, and self-esteem increased. Improvement was independent of sex, source of referral, and type of pain. A comparison group of patients in the regular pain clinic ($n = 21$) and referrals to the SRRP from the pain clinic ($n = 21$) did not show similar improve-

ment after traditional treatment protocols. At 15-month follow-up, the experimental group had maintained improvements for all outcomes except for one measure of pain.

Coping with Pain

By affecting a person's adjustment to pain, religious beliefs and practices may relieve (or exacerbate) anxiety and depression that worsens pain. Cronan et al. (1989) surveyed a random sample of 382 community-dwelling persons in San Diego County who had musculoskeletal complaints to determine the prevalence of unconventional remedies for arthritis in this metropolitan community. Mean age of subjects was 52 years, 31% had college degrees, 86% were white, and 57% had arthritis. Investigators determined the frequency of prayer for coping with musculoskeletal pain and the perceived helpfulness of prayer. About 84% used unconventional remedies for arthritis. Prayer was the most common unconventional method used (44%), after which came bedrest (33%), nonprescribed exercise or swimming (33%), relaxation (33%), and whirlpool or hot tub treatments (29%). Almost 61% of those who used whirlpools or hot tubs reported that these were very helpful, whereas 54% of those who used prayer said it was "very helpful" (it was the second most helpful in a field of 19 unconventional treatments).

Yates et al. (1981) examined the relationship between religion and pain in 71 patients with advanced cancer (mean age 59) at a regional cancer center in Burlington, Vermont. The sample was highly religious; 92% believed in God, 83% believed in a personal God, 80% believed prayer was helpful, two-thirds felt close to God or nature, and about half indicated that church was very important in their lives. Religious beliefs (measured by a multi-item scale) were significantly related to one of four measures of well-being ($r = .41$) and to lower pain level ($r = -.29$). Considering church and religion important was correlated with two measures of well-being ($r = .31$ and $r = .24$) and with lower levels of pain ($r = -.33$). Church attendance was related to three measures of well-being ($r = .32–.35$) and to lower levels of pain ($r = -.24$). Closeness to God was related to two measures of well-being ($r = .33$ and $r = .43$), to reduced presence of pain ($r = -.29$), and to lower levels of pain ($r = -.25$). Closeness to God was inversely related to the presence of pain as well as the intensity of pain.

Koenig, Weiner, et al. (1998) surveyed 115 chronic care nursing home residents (mean age 79, 44% women) to examine the relationship among pain, depression, and social support. Subjects were assessed using the Mini-Mental State Exam, the Barthel Index (a measure of physical functioning), the Cumulative Illness Rating Scale, the Geriatric Depression Scale, a validated social support scale, the three-item Religious Coping Index, and a self-reported measure of physical pain. Religious coping was related to greater social support ($p = .01$), more severe medical illness ($p = .04$), and better cognitive functioning ($p = .02$) (with multiple covariates controlled). The relationship between religious coping and depression was weak in the bivariate analysis ($r = -.15$, $.05 < p < .10$) and weakened further ($r = -.12$) when covariates were controlled. While there was an inverse relationship between average physical pain level during the one-month follow-up period and religious coping ($r = -.10$), this relationship did not reach statistical significance when covariates (e.g., functional status, depression, social support) were controlled. Since religious coping was significantly more common among those with severe medical illness, this behavior may have been mobilized in response to increasing physical symptoms. The positive effects of religious coping on pain, then, may have again been disguised by persons' turning to religion as physical illness worsened or pain symptoms increased.

Social Support

There are no studies that have specifically examined the relationship among religious activities (other then religious coping), social support, and pain intensity. There is plenty of evidence to suggest a link between social support and indicators of religious involvement such as attendance at services (Ellison & George, 1994; Bradley, 1995; Idler et al., 1997a), private reli-

gious activities (Koenig, Hays, George, et al., 1997), subjective religiousness (Idler et al., 1997a), and religious coping (Koenig, Cohen, Blazer, Pieper, et al., 1992; Idler et al., 1997a; Koenig, Weiner, et al. 1998). This is especially true for medically ill older adults, the majority of whose closest friends come from their church congregation (Koenig, Moberg, & Kvale, 1988). Does this greater social support among the religious translate into lesser or greater experiences of pain?

As we saw earlier, some investigators report an inverse relationship between social support and pain (Bradley, Young, Anderson, Turner, et al., 1987; Jamison & Virts, 1990). On the other hand, Gil et al. (1987) found that increased satisfaction with social support was associated with higher levels of pain behavior in 51 patients with chronic pain. The investigators explained this finding as resulting from positive reinforcement from the social environment when subjects engaged in pain behavior. Thus, it is difficult to predict what effect religion-related social support might have on pain threshold and disability resulting from pain.

The only study that provides even indirect evidence concerning this association is the Yates et al. (1981) examination of patients with advanced cancer, described earlier. Recall that frequency of church attendance was related to greater well-being on three of four measures ($r = .32$–$.35$, $p < .005$) and to less pain ($r = -.24$, $p < .05$). This suggests that religion-related social support may indeed be associated with less pain, although further studies are clearly needed.

NONPAIN SOMATIC SYMPTOMS

Besides pain, there are a number of other physical complaints that people experience and often present to doctors. These symptoms range from hot flashes associated with menopause, to gastrointestinal symptoms such as nausea, dyspepsia, diarrhea, or constipation, to fatigue and tiredness, to nonspecific complaints. For many of these somatic symptoms, no physical cause can be found. Medically unexplained physical symptoms are the main clinical problem in 20–

84% of primary care visits (Cummings & Follette, 1968; Kroenke & Mangelsdorff, 1989; Verhaak & Tijhuis, 1994; Peveler et al., 1997). Kroenke and Mangelsdorff (1989) reviewed the medical records of more than 1,000 patients who attended an internal medicine clinic over a three-year period. In 84% of cases, causes for the primary physical complaints could not be identified. After carefully reviewing these patients' records, the authors concluded that in nearly three-quarters of cases, symptoms were probably due to psychosocial factors.

More than 60% of visits to primary care physicians may be the result of physical complaints that have no organic basis. Persons with psychological disorders such as depression or anxiety may present to the doctor with physical complaints because these are more acceptable than emotional symptoms (which carry a stigma to both patients and physicians). In fact, 40–80% of depressed patients present primarily with physical complaints (Wilson et al., 1983; Bridges & Goldberg, 1985; Kirmayer et al., 1993). Bear in mind, however, that depression and anxiety also tend to amplify physical symptoms that do have a physiological basis.

Because of the strong relationship between psychological stress and somatic symptoms, there may also be a relationship between religion and somatic symptoms. On the one hand, if religious beliefs and practices encourage repression of psychological conflict, then such conflict may result in increased somatic symptoms. On the other hand, if religion helps people to cope better with stress and to resolve problems more effectively, then unexplained somatic complaints might be fewer among the more religious. Unfortunately, most studies do not differentiate medically explained somatic symptoms from those that are unexplained.

RELIGIOUS AFFILIATION AND SOMATIC SYMPTOMS

Are somatic complaints (menstrual symptoms, chronic fatigue, gastrointestinal symptoms, general medical symptoms) more prevalent among members of certain religious groups?

Acheson (1960) surveyed 2,320 male veterans diagnosed between 1953 and 1957 with regional enteritis, chronic colitis, other enteritis, or ulcerative colitis. The proportion of such cases among non-Jewish whites, African Americans, and Jews was calculated. Ulcerative colitis and regional enteritis were four times more common in Jews than in the other groups. Recall also from chapter 20 that Jewish men have an increased risk of intestinal cancer. Gastrointestinal complaints among Jews may be more common than in members of other religious groups, but these symptoms often have real causes.

Rosenberg (1962) asked the question "Does a Catholic child raised in a Protestant neighborhood . . . show more symptoms of anxiety and depression than one reared in an environment inhabited by his coreligionists?" (pp. 1–2). The author surveyed a stratified random sample of high school juniors and seniors in 10 high schools in New York State. The sample consisted of 495 Catholics, 405 Protestants, and 121 Jews. The study found that children reared in dissimilar neighborhoods in terms of religious affiliation were more likely to manifest low self-esteem, depressed affect, and psychosomatic symptoms.

De Figueiredo and Lemkau (1978) studied religious activity and psychosomatic symptoms in a stratified random sample of community-dwelling persons in Goa, India. The sample consisted of 80 Christians and 80 Hindus of similar education, occupation, and income. Approximately 43% of Hindus attended temple once per week (high attendees); 54% of Christians attended church every week. The researchers also examined private worship at home (prayer or scripture reading) (rated high in 50% of Christians and 65% of Hindus). A 23-item psychosomatic symptom scale asked questions about sleep, mood, concentration, and other items and was dichotomized into high and low psychosomatic categories. The researchers found that Christians and Hindus had similar levels of psychosomatic symptoms.

Polit and LaRocco (1980) examined the relationship between menopausal symptoms and religious affiliation in 167 women ages 40–60 years who lived in the greater Boston area. The majority of subjects were married, had two children, were employed full-time, and had completed high school but had not attended college. Religious denomination was unrelated to number or type of menopausal symptoms. Likewise, Rothbaum and Jackson (1990) examined menstrual attitudes and symptoms in 18 orthodox Jewish "ritual bath" (Mikvah) attendees, 23 orthodox Jewish non-Mikvah attendees, 35 Protestants, and 45 Catholics. Researchers found no difference in menstrual symptoms among the four groups.

Chaturvedi and Bhandari (1989) assessed complaints of somatic symptoms among 31 psychiatric outpatients in Bangalore, India. Subjects were patients who (1) volunteered a complaint of pain or other somatic symptom, (2) had no organic pathology on detailed physical examination, (3) had a duration of illness greater than six months, (4) had previously been treated by a general practitioner or other physician, and (5) had more than two somatic symptoms for which no organic basis could be found. Hindus were more likely than Muslims to recall that they had been told by their physicians that physical illness accounted for their symptoms ($p < .005$). The researchers concluded that Hindus were more likely to demonstrate "denial," since they were more likely to report being told they had physical illness when this was not the case.

In general, there is little consistent evidence to link religious affiliation with greater or lesser likelihood of reporting unexplained somatic symptoms.

ORGANIZATIONAL RELIGIOUS ACTIVITY

While there was no difference in psychosomatic symptoms between Christians and Hindus in De Figueiredo and Lemkau's (1978) study, discussed earlier, a relationship between religious attendance and symptoms did emerge within each group. High scores on measures of psychosomatic symptom were less common among Christian men and Christian women with high religious attendance than for those with low

attendance (2.5% vs. 15.0%, $p = .016$, and 2.5% vs. 32.5%, $p = .0002$, respectively). Among Hindus, this relationship held for women (10.0% vs. 50.0%, $p = .001$), but not for men.

Ness (1980) surveyed 51 members of a Pentecostal church (Church A) and 54 members of a mainline Protestant group (Church B), both located in Northeast Harbour, Newfoundland. Church B had experienced a decline in membership from 100 to 54 members prior to this 1973 study due to Church A members splitting from Church B to establish their own congregation. Somatic complaints were assessed using the Cornell Medical Index. Differences in somatic symptoms among men in the mainline church were related to their level of religious attendance—but in a different direction than expected. Among men in Church B ($n = 24$), somatic symptoms were positively related to frequency of church attendance ($r = .43$, $p < .05$) and testimonials ($r = .42$, $p < .05$); no association with somatic symptoms was found in women ($n = 30$). This mainline church, however, was declining in membership and dying out. In the Pentecostal church (which was more active and growing), somatic complaints were positively correlated with glossolalia and possession behavior in women ($n = 28$) (both $r = 0.25$, $p < .05$), but not in men ($n = 23$), and were unrelated to religious attendance in either men or women.

PRIVATE RELIGIOUS ACTIVITIES

In contrast to their finding on the impact of different levels of attendance at religious services, De Figueiredo and Lemkau's (1978)'s study of 80 Hindus and 80 Christians in India reported that psychosomatic symptoms were more common among those with high rather than low levels of private religious activities (prayer and scripture reading). This was true for Christian men (15.0% vs. 2.5%, $p = .007$) and women (30.0% vs. 5.0%, $p = .0005$) and for Hindu men (30.0% vs. 2.5%, $p = .02$), but not for Hindu women. Again, the cross-sectional nature of this study prevents causal inferences.

SUBJECTIVE RELIGIOSITY AND RELIGIOUS COMMITMENT

Shaver et al. (1980) examined religiousness and the incidence of physical complaints among readers of *Redbook* magazine. A 97-item questionnaire was published in the September 1976 issue of *Redbook*, and readers were invited to mail their answers to the editors before the end of the month. More than 65,000 replies were received. A random sample of 2,500 of these replies was studied. The sample consisted of women with a median age of 31; 96% white, 23% were Catholic, 70% were Protestant, and 60% were high school graduates. Of the respondents, 27% considered themselves very religious, 56% were moderately religious, and 16% were only slightly or not religious. Religiousness was related to 12 somatic symptoms in a curvilinear fashion (i.e., an inverted U); the very religious and the antireligious had the fewest symptoms.

McIntosh and Spilka (1990) examined the relationship between somatic symptoms and religiousness in 69 undergraduate students at universities in Colorado and Georgia and in seven adult members of a Protestant church in Denver, Colorado. All participants were volunteers who identified themselves as Christian and as moderately interested in religion. Somatic symptoms were assessed using a 57-item symptom checklist that indicated the number of days each problem had been experienced in the previous month. Intrinsic religiosity (IR) was assessed using a scale developed by Allport and Ross (1967). IR was inversely related to overall sickness score ($r = -.26$, $p < .05$) and positively related to regularity of bowel movements ($r = .20$, $.05 < p < .10$). In addition, those with higher IR tended to experience fewer general somatic symptoms, digestive symptoms, mild nausea, vomiting, runny nose, dizziness, chest pain, shortness of breath, mononucleosis, fatigue, bladder infection, asthma attack, twitching, and ulcer ($p = .01–.10$, but there were literally hundreds of statistical comparisons for only 76 subjects).

Jamal and Badawi (1993) studied 325 members of the Islamic Society of North America to determine the association among religiosity, mental health, and psychosomatic symptoms. The sample was 86% male, and 46% had graduate educations and advanced degrees. Self-rated religiousness was rated on a scale of 1–10. Multiple regression analyses (including job stress, religiosity, and interactions between the two) revealed that religiosity was again related to significantly fewer psychosomatic symptoms.

RELIGIOUS INTERVENTIONS TO REDUCE SOMATIC SYMPTOMS

The best way to test of the relationship between religiousness and medically unexplained somatic symptoms would be to conduct a clinical trial in which a religious or spiritual intervention was applied to one group but not to a control group. A change in somatic symptoms among subjects randomized to the intervention group compared to control subjects would help prove whether religion and spirituality increase or decrease symptoms.

In an attempt at such a study, Carson and Huss (1979) examined the effects of a religious intervention in a sample of 20 Christian patients with schizophrenia at a state mental hospital. The intervention was weekly prayer and scripture reading, conducted one on one by a student nurse over 10 weeks. The focus of the prayer and the scripture readings was God's love and concern for each individual and each person's worth to God. A psychological assessment tool was administered at the beginning and at the end of the 10-week project. Compared to control subjects, those receiving the intervention complained of fewer somatic complaints. While there are numerous concerns with the study design (nonrandom assignment to group [student nurses volunteered for the prayer group], use of a nonvalidated measure for assessing change in symptoms, and the absence of statistical tests), the attempt is laudable in this chronically ill population with few other resources.

SUMMARY AND CONCLUSIONS

In this chapter we examined the relationship among religious involvement, pain, and other somatic symptoms. We found that psychological and social factors strongly influence the experience of physical pain. The "gate theory" of pain suggests a physiological mechanism for producing this effect. Because of the strong relationship between religiousness and psychosocial factors, a similar association may exist between religion and pain. We examined the way different religious groups view pain and suffering and how these views might affect the experience of pain. Several cross-sectional studies have shown a positive relationship between prayer and greater pain intensity level, perhaps because religion is mobilized as a coping behavior after other methods of pain relief have failed. When patients are followed over time, however, one study shows that prayer may ultimately reduce pain intensity. While only a few studies have examined the relationship between religiousness and pain level, the evidence suggests an inverse relationship between pain intensity and both religious beliefs and religious attendance. While this conclusion is tentative and based upon relatively weak correlations observed in only a few studies, it is consistent with other

research that finds better mental health and greater social support (factors known to be inversely related to pain) among the more religious.

In a similar way, certain religious beliefs and activities appear to be related to fewer nonpain somatic symptoms. This relationship is present in studies of Christians, Hindus, and Muslims. As with pain, there is a positive relationship between somatic symptoms and private religious activities such as prayer and scripture reading in cross-sectional studies. Nevertheless, when a clinical trial examined the effects of prayer and scripture reading in schizophrenics over time, psychosomatic symptoms were reduced. These findings suggest that private religious activities may be mobilized to deal with pain and nonpain somatic symptoms but that over time the ultimate effects of such religious activities may be beneficial. Again, this is a highly tentative conclusion based on limited studies. To our knowledge, there are no studies that have examined the associations between religious beliefs and activities and psychosomatic syndromes such as chronic fatigue syndrome or fibromyalgia.

24

Health Behaviors

TAKING RESPONSIBILITY FOR self-care is particularly important in an age of health promotion and disease prevention. The promotion of healthy lifestyles has been the major emphasis of the U.S. Department of Health and Human Services over the past decade (*Healthy People 2000*, 1990), and with good reasons. The rising number of persons in the United States with disability and chronic health problems is threatening to overwhelm our ability to provide medical services to this population. While the number of severely disabled persons over age 65 is only about 3 million at present, this figure is expected to rise to nearly 12 million in the next 35 years (Kunkel & Applebaum, 1992). The cost of providing health services is already increasing at an astronomical rate, despite the introduction of managed care, and this problem will surely worsen as the elderly population nearly doubles in the next three or four decades. A

recent report in the journal *Health Affairs* projected national health expenditures in the United States to rise from $1.1 trillion in 1998 to more than $2.1 trillion by 2007 (Smith, Freeland, et al., 1998). Annual Medicare expenditures will increase from $203.1 billion to $415.6 billion over the same period. Unfortunately, the reduction of health care expenditures that resulted from the widespread enrollment of persons in managed care programs has pretty much topped out, and significant additional savings from this source are unlikely. While government surpluses growing out of a vigorous economy may help, they will be too little too late.

Writing in the journal *Science*, the gerontologist Edward Schneider (1999) projects two scenarios for the health care and housing needs of older Americans in the years 2030–2050. In Scenario 1, Medicare costs would rise slowly as major advances in disease prevention and treatment lead to improvements in health and reduced functional disability for many people. The vast majority of older adults would remain in their homes with assistance from home health services, and those with severe disability who need more intensive care would receive it in nursing homes and assisted living facilities, which would increase modestly in number.

In Scenario 2, Medicare costs would grow rapidly over the next two decades and then accelerate even more rapidly (if levels of support for research, prevention, and treatment remain at the current level) as 76 million baby boomers begin reaching age 75 in 2021. The near exponential growth of Medicare would produce great strain on the federal budget and result in (a) a requirement that seniors pay more of their health care costs through higher premiums, and deductibles, with more exclusions, (b) a change in Medicare to a needs-based program open only to the poor elderly, or (c) health care rationing on the basis of age, in which older adults would be declared ineligible for an increasing number of necessary medical services that would be available only to younger persons. Prospects for obtaining housing and care services under Scenario 2 could be even more dismal. Nursing homes and assisted living facilities would be seriously strained trying to care for the needs of over 10 million severely disabled elders. According to Schneider, older adults without financial resources, relatives, or friends to care for them might be forced to live out the end of their lives on city streets and in parks.

Many expensive chronic health problems can be prevented if people pay attention to healthy lifestyles when they are younger. At any age, greater attention to diet, smoking, and exercise patterns could reduce rates of our most widespread illnesses, heart disease, and cancer (Ornish et al., 1990). Until recently, however, self-care activities did not receive much attention. Medicare paid for most of the acute medical services that people needed, and reimbursement to health providers for such services was virtually unlimited. People lived as they wanted, and when they got sick they simply went to the doctor to receive treatment for their health problems. Doctors then treated these problems as an automobile mechanic might fix a problem

with a car, and people then went right back to their usual lifestyles. As the number of individuals in need of medical care has increased, along with an explosion in the expensive technology and pharmaceuticals that are essential to modern medical care, costs have skyrocketed and are now beginning to limit the health services that we can expect to receive. This reality is forcing Americans to pay attention to the kind of lifestyle they choose to live and to the kind of health behaviors they decide to engage in. We now examine different health practices and how they influence health.

Diet, Weight Control, and Exercise

Dietary factors contribute to the development of coronary heart disease, some cancers, hypertension, stroke, diabetes, and atherosclerosis—the leading causes of death in this country (*Healthy People 2000*, 1990). The primary problem in the U.S. diet is the high consumption of foods that are rich in fat (36% of total calories on average) and low in complex carbohydrates and dietary fiber. The healthy diet is low in fat, saturated fat, and cholesterol and rich in vegetables, fruit, and grain products.

More than a quarter (26%) of the U.S. adult population is overweight, and, according to a report from the Centers for Disease Control and Prevention (1997), obesity is a major public health problem. The direct health care costs attributable to obesity in the United States in 1995 were $52 billion (6% of total health care expenditure), including the costs of diabetes mellitus, endometrial cancer, breast cancer, colon cancer, gallbladder disease, hypertension, osteoarthritis, and coronary heart disease related specifically to obesity (Wolf & Colditz, 1998). Obesity is a particularly difficult problem for African American and Hispanic women, of whom 44% and 37% are overweight, defined as being 20% over ideal body weight (see Guggenheim, 1981, for a weight table).

Regular physical exercise is associated with lower rates of colon cancer, stroke, and back injury (*Healthy People 2000*, 1990). It is also helpful in preventing or managing heart disease, hypertension, diabetes, osteoporosis, obesity, and emotional disorders such as depression and anxiety. People who are physically inactive are about twice as likely to develop coronary artery disease as are those who engage in regular physical activity (Powell et al., 1987) and have about the same level of risk as persons who smoke cigarettes, have high blood pressure, or have high serum cholesterol levels. Despite this, fewer than 10% of Americans exercise in the way recommended. Recommended exercise uses large muscle groups for 20 minutes or longer (e.g., running, walking, swimming, bicycling) at least three days per week, performed at 60% or more of a person's cardiorespiratory capacity (Caspersen et al., 1986).

Cholesterol

As noted in chapter 16, cholesterol is a major component in the pathological process that underlies vascular atherosclerosis, the main cause of coronary artery disease, peripheral vascular disease, and cerebrovascular disease. Studies have shown that the intake of foods high in cholesterol and saturated fatty acids is associated with high serum cholesterol levels and the health consequences that follow (Shekelle, Raynor, et al., 1981). Furthermore, drugs that reduce serum cholesterol have been shown to slow down the process of atherosclerosis and to decrease cardiovascular mortality and morbidity (Lipid Research Clinics, 1984). Careful attention to diet and avoidance of foods high in cholesterol and saturated fatty acids can help reduce serum cholesterol and help prevent many of the nearly 1 million deaths per year in the United States that result from vascular disease.

Cigarette Smoking

In 1935, Raymond Pearl first documented the high death rates associated with tobacco smoking. It took nearly 30 years, however, before smoking was recognized as a major public health problem (Advisory Committee, 1964). Cigarette smoking is responsible for between 15% and 20% of all deaths in the United States (nearly 400,000 per year), including 21% of coronary heart disease deaths, 87% of lung cancer deaths, 30% of cancer deaths in general, and

almost all deaths from chronic bronchitis and emphysema (Office on Smoking and Health, 1989). Given that over 25% of the population smokes regularly, it is the single most preventable cause of death and disease in this country (Cigarette Smoking, 1996). There is some evidence that cigarette smoking is declining in the United States; 40% of Americans smoked in 1965, compared to 29% in 1987 and 25% in 1990. Cigarette smoking among younger adults, however, appears to be on the rise; smoking among teenagers has increased by as much as 2% per year since 1992, when 19% of high school seniors reported that they smoked (Johnston, O'Malley, et al., 1996).

Drugs and Alcohol

The costs to society of alcohol and drug abuse are staggering. In 1983, these problems cost Americans almost $115 billion, largely because of lost productivity. This figure does not include the problems that result from drug and alcohol misuse, such as violent crime, murder, and motor vehicle accidents. Alcohol is involved in nearly half of all deaths from motor vehicle crashes, suicides, and homicides (Perrine et al., 1989). Alcohol and drug abuse are significant problems for nearly 25% of adolescents in this country and are often responsible for school failure, unwanted pregnancy, and delinquency. Alcohol and drug use increase the risk of transmitting HIV infection, increase the likelihood of birth defects when used in pregnancy, and are the primary cause of cirrhosis, the ninth leading cause of death in the United States.

Sexual Practices

The percentage of adolescent girls ages 15–19 who have had sexual intercourse has increased from 30% in 1970 to more than 50% in 1988; by age 20, 75% of women have had sexual intercourse (*Healthy People 2000*, 1990). Out-of-wedlock pregnancy, often a result of sexual activity among adolescents, is largely responsible for the nearly 25% of American children age 6 or younger who live below the federal poverty level, typically in single-parent homes (U.S. Congress, 1989). Unmarried motherhood is also associated with a significantly higher infant mortality rate. In 1983, the infant mortality rate in married white women was 7.8/1000, in married African American women 14.1/1000, in unmarried white women 13.1/1000, and in unmarried African American women 19.6/1000 (Centers for Disease Control, 1990).

Nearly 12 million cases of sexually transmitted diseases (STDs) occur each year in the United States. STDs include gonorrhea, syphilis, genital herpes, chlamydia, cytomegalovirus, chancroid, Hepatitis B, human papillomavirus (implicated in cervical cancer), and HIV infection. Sexual promiscuity increases the risk of STDs. Among sexually active women ages 15–19, almost 60% have had two or more sexual partners, and 7% have had 10 or more partners (National Committee for Adoption, 1985). It is not surprising that approximately 25% of sexually active teenagers are infected with one or more STDs (*Healthy People 2000*, 1990). Besides AIDS, other serious complications of STDs include pelvic inflammatory disease, sterility, ectopic pregnancy, blindness, cervical cancer, fetal and infant death, birth defects and mental retardation.

Depending on the survey, somewhere between 50% and 82% of men and 26% and 70% of women have had at least one extramarital affair (Vaughan, 1998). The more conservative figures are from Kinsey's work, done in the 1940s and the early 1950s (Kinsey et al., 1953). Like sexual promiscuity in adolescence, extramarital affairs increase the risk of STDs, and the greatest victims are usually the unsuspecting faithful marital partner and innocent children.

Safe Driving and Avoidance of Risk-Taking Behaviors

Unintentional injuries kill approximately 100,000 people each year and are the fourth leading cause of death in the United States. Motor vehicle crashes account for about half of these deaths; falls are the second most common cause, followed by poisoning, drowning, and fire (Committee on Trauma Research, 1988). Many persons are disabled, often permanently, by unintentional injuries, the cost of which in

1985 exceeded $158 billion (Rice & MacKenzie, 1989). Alcohol and drug use are often involved in unintentional injuries. Reducing driving speed, using seat belts, carefully supervising children, and engaging in fewer risk-taking behaviors may all decrease the number of unintentional injuries.

Sleep Patterns

Sleep is essential for human survival and therefore is carefully regulated by a number of interconnecting systems located in the brain stem. Sleep has numerous functions, including restoration and preservation of homeostasis. Prolonged sleep deprivation leads to disorganization, hallucinations, delusions, and cognitive impairment. Shorter periods of sleep deprivation can increase daytime fatigue and irritability. Most persons require six to nine hours each night in order to function adequately. Inability to sleep not only causes disturbances in mental functioning but may often result from psychiatric disturbances, such as depression or anxiety disorder. All people have a normal sleep-wake cycle or biorhythm; if this is disturbed by irregular or inconsistent sleep times, psychological and physiological problems are likely to result (Kaplan & Sadock, 1988a).

RELIGION AND HEALTH BEHAVIORS

In this chapter, we focus on the relationship between religion and health-promoting behaviors such as good dietary habits, maintenance of low serum cholesterol levels, weight control, exercise, abstinence from cigarette smoking, safe sexual practices, safe driving, avoidance of risk-taking behaviors, and regular sleep habits. We have already addressed the problem of alcohol and drug use in chapter 11. Considerable research exists on many of these topics and is reviewed. For some of these topics, however, no scientific studies exist that attempt to establish a link between healthy practices and religion. For these practices, we make hypotheses and suggest research studies to test for such relationships.

DIET

Diet can be heavily influenced by religious affiliation, particularly when religious groups have rules about the types of food that members are allowed to eat. These dietary prescriptions and proscriptions can often be traced back to sacred religious texts.

Seventh-Day Adventists

SDAs abstain from alcohol, tobacco, and drinks that contain caffeine. They also avoid biblically proscribed meats such as pork, and some SDAs are complete vegetarians. SDAs also frequently avoid hot spices and highly refined foods. A study of food and nutrient intake among vegetarian SDA women in southern California documented a diet that was higher in folate, thiamin, vitamin C, and vitamin A; lower in total fat, saturated fatty acids, and cholesterol; and higher in dietary fiber than that of nonvegetarian Methodist women (Hunt et al., 1988). Dietary factors (avoidance of meat, coffee, and fried foods) may help explain the reduced cancer mortality rate among SDAs, which is 50–70% lower than the rate for the general population for cancer sites unrelated to smoking or drinking (e.g., colon cancer, breast cancer) (Phillips, 1975; Phillips & Snowdon, 1983). Avoidance of meat and adherence to a healthy vegetarian diet may also help to explain the reduced death rates from coronary artery disease among SDAs (Phillips, Lemon, et al., 1978).

Mormons

Mormons are encouraged by their religious doctrines to abstain from alcohol, cigarettes, caffeinated beverages, and any habit-forming drugs. They often make their own bread from whole grains, prepare their own canned products, and avoid refined and highly processed foods. Mormons typically do not abstain from meat, however, and their meat consumption is actually rather high. Death rates from cancer and CAD, as in SDAs, are considerably below those of the general population.

Jews

Orthodox Jews follow the Mosaic code (Leviticus 11, and Deuteronomy 14) that emphasizes avoidance of pork and adherence to a kosher diet, which includes the temperate use of alcoholic drinks. The avoidance of pork may have had health benefits even during the early Hebraic period, since it likely reduced the transmission of trichinosis and other parasites. Low rates of alcoholism also characterize this religious group.

African Americans

McClelland et al. (1998) examined fruit and vegetable consumption among 3,737 rural African Americans from 50 churches in 10 rural North Carolina counties. The average intake of fruits and vegetables was 3.7 daily servings, which is below the recommended 5-A-Day guidelines (Dietary Guidelines, 1995). Fruit and vegetable intake was particularly low among younger African Americans and among males.

Buddhists

Some Buddhists follow a modern vegetarian diet that is high in carbohydrates (providing 63% of calories in men and 50% of calories in women), has a high ratio of polyunsaturated to saturated fatty acids, and has a moderate fat content (25% for men and 30% for women). Rice and soybeans are the primary sources of protein in the diet. Consequently, blood concentrations of cholesterol, glucose, and uric acid are all favorably lower (Pan et al., 1993).

SERUM CHOLESTEROL

As noted earlier, high levels of serum cholesterol have been linked to the development of atherosclerotic cardiovascular disease, the primary cause of death for both women and men in the United States. Are members of certain religious groups at greater or lower risk of having high cholesterol levels?

Jews

Several early studies found higher serum cholesterol levels among Jews than among non-Jews. Schaefer et al. (1953) reported on studies of hypercholesteremia in 250 men and 250 women consecutively admitted to Mount Sinai Hospital in New York City. These investigators found that a higher percentage of Jews than non-Jews had hypercholesterolemia (21% vs. 9%, respectively).

Epstein, Carol, et al. (1956) surveyed 250 male and 166 female garment factory workers from New York to determine their 24-hour diet histories. In addition to examining their dietary histories, the investigators analyzed the relationship between diet and atherosclerosis. Researchers found that Jewish men and women both had lower caloric intake (2,188 and 1,782, respectively) than Italian men and women (2,312 and 1,962, respectively). Jewish men and women received a larger proportion of their total fat intake from animals sources than did Italians (80% vs. 68% for men and 78% vs. 63% for women, $p < .01$). Jews also had a higher prevalence of hypercholesterolemia and higher levels of coronary artery disease than did Italians, even though they took in equal amounts of fat. The major dietary difference was the higher amounts of animal fat consumed by Jews.

Genetic factors may play a role in determining cholesterol levels for members of religious groups in which there are high rates of inbreeding (e.g., certain Jewish subgroups and certain Christian subgroups). For example, Torrington and Botha (1981) conducted a case-control study of 26 families with hypercholesterolemia in South Africa and compared them to persons in the general population. These investigators reported that 20 of the 26 families were affiliated with the Dutch Reformed Church, compared with only 5% of the general population. The authors attributed this clustering of cases to genetic inbreeding.

Friedlander et al. (1987) examined the relationship between religious observance and plasma lipids and lipoproteins among 673 17-year-old Jewish residents of Jerusalem. Religious observance was determined by asking subjects' parents to self-rate their degree of religiosity by administering a six-item scale that asked whether the families observed religious commandments, kept kosher, traveled on the Sabbath, attended synagogue, observed Jewish rituals, and considered themselves orthodox, traditional, or secular. On the basis of their scores on this scale, parents were categorized as orthodox Jews, traditional Jews who observed some rules, and secular Jews who were nonobservant. The researchers found that plasma cholesterol, triglyceride, and LDL levels were all higher in youth from secular families than in youth from orthodox Jewish families, independent of sex, origin, social class, body mass index, and season (using regression analysis). The results were also independent of parental lipid phenotype and both offspring and parental environmental influences. Dietary factors were not excluded as a possible cause. The investigators concluded that their findings may help explain the lower incidence of coronary artery disease observed among members of orthodox Jewish religious groups (see chapter 16).

Trappist Monks

Barrow et al. (1960) studied two religious communities, a Trappist ($n = 80$) and a Benedictine monastery ($n = 70$). The Trappist community was known for its lacto-ovo-vegetarian diet, which has a low fat content. Benedictine community members had health habits identical to those of the Trappist monks, except for their diet. On average, Trappists derived 26% of their calories from fat, whereas Benedictines received a much larger 45% of their calories from fat. As a result, investigators found that the Trappists had significantly lower average serum cholesterol levels (205 mg%) than did Benedictines (236 mg%). Furthermore, levels of free cholesterol, esterified fatty acids, phospholipids, total lipids, and cholesterol beta fraction were all significantly lower in members of the Trappist community than in Benedictines. The investigators concluded that levels of serum lipids vary with age and dietary intake of fat.

In contrast to other reports, McCullagh and Lewis (1960) found that, while monks had lower serum cholesterol levels because of their low consumption of animal fat, they were not protected from either atherosclerotic vascular disease or hypertension. In fact, the data suggested that arterial hypertension was more frequent in Trappist monks than in other men of the same age in the U.S. population (although the researchers do not provide these statistical comparisons in their report). The investigators concluded that diets low in animal fat and low serum cholesterol levels are not by themselves sufficient to offset the development of atherosclerotic vascular disease. While such studies tell us little about how religion and cholesterol relate to each other, they do show that dietary practices adhered to by different religious groups may help explain differences in serum cholesterol levels and cardiovascular mortality.

Seventh-Day Adventists

Studies in SDAs have found that members of this religious group have lower serum cholesterol levels (and lower cardiovascular mortality) than persons in the general population. Walden et al. (1964) compared serum cholesterol levels of 145 white SDAs in Loma Linda, California, with those of 433 non-SDAs who were living in New York City. The SDA men had mean serum cholesterol levels that averaged 13% less than those of the men in New York City. Among SDA women, mean cholesterol levels averaged 21% lower than those for age-matched women in New York City. The authors attributed these differences primarily to diet.

West and Hayes (1968) surveyed 3,260 SDAs in the Washington, D.C. area. They matched 233 SDA vegetarians with 233 nonvegetarians and compared their cholesterol levels with those of 4,244 persons in metropolitan New York City. The mean serum cholesterol level of the SDA vegetarians was 185, and that for the SDA nonvegetarians was 196 ($p < .01$); both vegetarian and nonvegetarian SDAs had significantly lower serum cholesterol levels at all ages than did the non-SDAs in New York City.

Finally, Fonnebo (1992a) compared risk factors for coronary artery disease in SDAs and non-SDAs. Only 10% of SDAs were smokers ($p < .001$), and their average serum cholesterol level was 0.86 (CI 0.59–1.13) mmol/liter lower in men and 0.48 (CI 0.25–0.71) lower in

women. In this study, ex-SDAs had a risk factor level significantly higher than that of SDAs who complied with the SDA lifestyle.

These studies provided some of the first epidemiological evidence on the effects of diet on serum cholesterol. While adherence to the dietary prescriptions indirectly reflects the intensity of religious belief and commitment, it provides little direct evidence of whether religious beliefs and practices, apart from dietary habits, influence serum cholesterol level. There is some evidence that certain types of religious practices, such as meditative prayer, may help reduce serum cholesterol directly through neuroendocrine mechanisms (for reviews of this literature, see Cooper & Aygen, 1978; Delmonte, 1985; and Alexander, Robinson, et al., 1994).

WEIGHT CONTROL

To what extent does religion influence body weight and body weight control? On the one hand, religious doctrines that promote respect for the body may promote efforts to keep body weight at an optimal level. On the other hand, social activities sponsored by religious groups, such as potluck dinners, bazaars, and prayer or Bible study meetings, often involve food. We examine what studies have found.

Gottlieb and Green (1984) conducted a telephone survey of a random sample of 3,025 persons between ages 20–64. The researchers eliminated 552 persons from the sample because of poor health. They then examined five health practices (smoking, exercising, alcohol use, weight maintenance, and sleep habits), along with other variables such as income, education, age, life events, and social network. Of the social network indicators, church attendance and marriage were significantly related to health practices. Church attendance was characteristic of men and women nonsmokers and was negatively related to alcohol use as well. In addition, church attendance was characteristic of men who were former smokers and women with unfavorable weight.

Lapane et al. (1997) surveyed a population-based random sample of 2,442 in 1981–1982 and one of 2,799 persons in 1983–1984, all of whom resided in Pawtucket, Rhode Island. Investigators compared church members with nonmembers on a variety of health factors and found that church members were more likely to be 20% overweight, a finding that persisted after age, sex, and ethnicity were controlled ($p < .01$)

Ferraro (1998) examined religion and body weight in a probability sample of 3,497 adults who were participating in the 1986 Americans' Changing Lives (ACL) survey. The investigators also analyzed another data set of statewide U.S. ecological data on religiosity and weight. Four dimensions of religiosity were assessed: religious practice (attending church, reading religious material, watching religious TV/radio), religious identity (importance of religion), religious coping (frequency of seeking spiritual comfort or support for problems), and affiliation. Body mass index was assessed using the Quetelet Index (weight in kg divided by height in meters squared). Obesity was defined as weight one standard deviation (SD) above the mean (by gender); a "slight" person was defined as someone whose weight was one SD below the mean. Covariates taken into account in the analyses were socioeconomic status, age, race, marital status, and region of the country.

States with a higher proportion of persons with no religious affiliation had lower rates of obesity. The percentage of Baptists in states was positively associated with obesity. The highest body weight was found among Pietistic and Fundamentalist Protestants; Jews and non-Christians had the lowest weight. These differences disappeared, however, when demographic characteristics were controlled. Obesity was also associated with higher levels of religious practice, with underweight persons scoring lower on religious practice (these relationships persisted after covariates were controlled). Religious activity, however, moderated the effects of obesity on depression. While obese persons were more depressed than others, if they were also religious they were significantly less likely to be depressed than nonreligious obese persons.

Oman and Reed (1998), studying 1,931 persons over age 55 from Marin County, Califor-

nia, also found that persons who attended religious services weekly or more often were more likely to be overweight but less likely to be depressed than less frequent attenders. In this study, frequent attenders, despite being overweight, were also significantly less likely to die during the five-year follow-up.

In most American religious groups, satisfying the physical appetite is one biological desire against which there are no proscriptions, unlike those for sexual and other oral gratifications (e.g., smoking, alcohol use). Practical considerations, such as the ready availability of food and the absence of rules against eating (and, in many cases, actual social pressure to partake), may "outweigh" the more general though less emphasized teaching to respect one's body as a "temple of the Holy Spirit." If there are more obese persons among the religiously active, then churches may be an ideal place for instituting weight control programs.

Church-Based Weight Reduction Programs

Some churches have taken the lead in helping members lose weight and maintain that loss by using spiritual principles similar to those taught by 12-step programs like Alcoholics Anonymous. Recall from chapter 17 the report by Kumanyika and Charleston (1992) on their experience with the Baltimore Church High Blood Pressure Program, a behaviorally oriented weight control program that consisted of eight weekly two-hour counseling and exercise sessions. Both pre- and postprogram weight and blood pressure measurements were obtained on 185 African American and three white women. Of the participants, 88 were taking antihypertensive medication, and 99 were not. Both the medicated and the nonmedicated groups lost the same average amount of weight (i.e., six pounds). The mean systolic/diastolic blood pressure was reduced by 10/6 mmHg in the medicated group and 5/3 mmHg in the nonmedicated group ($p < .001$ for pre-post comparisons). The final systolic blood pressure was <140 mmHg in 74% (vs. 52% initially), and diastolic blood pressure was <90 mmHg in 92% (vs. 65% initially). During a six-month follow-up of 74 of the original 187 women in the program, 65% maintained or exceeded the weight loss they had achieved while participating in the program.

First Place is another spiritually based weight-loss program that has helped thousands of persons around the world from Protestant, Roman Catholic, and Pentecostal religious backgrounds (Lewis & Whalin, 1998). Participants meet weekly in small support groups where there is a focus on prayer and scriptural reading, on learning to cook using low-fat recipes, and on including exercise as a part of daily activities. First Place also uses Bible verses to help inspire members to lose weight. These spiritual practices and group support help to relieve the anxiety and loneliness that often lead to overeating.

EXERCISE

To what extent are religious individuals more or less likely to exercise than their secular peers? Recall from chapter 23 McIntosh and Spilka's (1990) survey of 76 undergraduate college students and adult church members. Intrinsic religiosity was assessed using Allport and Ross's 20-item scale. Investigators found that exercise was inversely related to intrinsic religiosity ($r = -.23$, $p < .05$). In other words, the more intrinsically religious subjects tended to exercise less often. However, intrinsic religiosity was positively related to other health habits, such as taking vitamins and avoiding alcohol, and abstaining from cigarette smoking. The researchers also found that intrinsic religiosity was negatively related to an overall sickness score ($r = -.26$, $p < .05$), as measured by the presence or absence of 57 different physical symptoms.

Oleckno and Blacconiere (1991) surveyed 1,077 college students at Northern Illinois University to determine the relationship of religiosity to wellness and other health-related behaviors and outcomes. The sample was 59% women, 87% white, and 55% Catholic. Using the Health-Promoting Lifestyle Profile, six dimensions of wellness were examined, including self-actualization, health responsibility, exercise, nutrition, interpersonal support, and stress management. A two-item religiosity index ("How often do you attend religious services?" and "How religious are you?") was administered and dichotomized into high and low categories for analysis. In contrast to McIntosh and Spilka's report, Olekno and Blacconiere found that regular exercise was more common among the highly religious ($F = 7.1$, $p = .008$). Gender was the only covariate controlled in the analysis (although all subjects were college students of similar age and other characteristics).

Spiritual-Based Exercise Programs

Prayer Walking, a movement begun in the mid-1980s, is an activity popularized by Linus Mundy after he discovered that vigorous walking and hiking were more relaxing if combined with prayer. This combination of physical exercise and prayer seemed to relieve his anxiety and help motivate him to lose weight. He wrote a book about the practice (Mundy, 1997) that received national attention, including articles in the *Washington Post* and in popular magazines (Hull, 1997). Other spiritual practices that may be combined with prayer in group settings include walking, singing religious hymns, worshiping, and chanting, adding the additional benefit of fellowship to help maintain compliance with the regimen. No research studies have yet assessed the benefits of such practices.

CIGARETTE SMOKING

A number of studies have examined the relationship between cigarette smoking and religious affiliation, practice, and commitment. If cigarette smoking is less common among those more religiously involved, then this will impact positively on physical health in a major way, especially with regard to lung cancer, chronic pulmonary disease, hypertension, and coronary artery disease.

Religious Affiliation

Adelekan et al. (1993) examined the psychosocial correlates of tobacco and cannabis use among 636 undergraduate students in Nigeria

(137 Muslims and 483 Christians). The researchers found no differences in cigarette smoking or cannabis use between Muslims and Christians.

Ahmed et al. (1994) examined the association between religiousness and cigarette smoking in a representative sample of 266 noninstitutionalized African American women ages 18–44 who were living in Norfolk, Virginia. Pentecostals were significantly less likely to smoke cigarettes (16.7% vs. 40.4% for Baptists, $p < .01$) and significantly more likely to have quit smoking (60.0% vs. 22.0%, $p < .01$). Religiosity was measured by a 10-item scale that examined religious values and attitudes, religious radio listening or TV viewing, and church-related religious activity; none of these religious measures, however, was related to smoking status. When a logistic regression was used to control for other variables, non-Pentecostals were 3.64 times more likely to be current smokers than Pentecostals and only 0.12 times as likely to have quit (both $p < .01$).

Ndom and Adelakan (1996) conducted two cross-sectional surveys using 10% random samples of second and fourth-year university students to determine the psychosocial correlates of substance use among undergraduates at Ilorin University, in Nigeria. The study involved a total of 649 subjects in 1988 and 859 subjects in 1993. Investigators examined the lifetime use of cigarettes, alcohol, and drugs such as marijuana. Again, no differences in cigarette smoking or cannabis use among Christians and Muslims were found.

Mullen et al. (1996) examined cigarette smoking and religious denomination in a random sample of 985 persons age 35 in Western Scotland. Among men, approximately 24% of Protestants were smokers, compared to 40% of Catholics and 37% of nonreligious ($p < .05$). Among women, 36% of Protestants were smokers, as were 49% of Catholics and 55% of nonreligious ($p < .001$). These differences, however, disappeared when "class effects" were controlled.

Thus, there is little difference in the percentages of Catholics and Protestants or of Christians and Muslims who smoke cigarettes. Pentecostals are less likely to smoke than are Christians from other religious denominations. As we learned in chapter 20, cigarette smoking is significantly less common among Seventh-Day Adventists and Mormons than among persons in the general U.S. population. In general, however, religious affiliation appears to have little impact on the likelihood of smoking (except among Pentecostals, Mormons, and Seventh-Day Adventists).

Religious Attendance

Does attendance at religious services influence the rate of cigarette smoking?

Parfrey (1976) surveyed a random sample of undergraduates at University College in Cork, Ireland, to examine the effect of religious attendance on cigarette and other drug use. Of the 444 respondents, 79% of the men and 90% of the women attended religious services once a week or more. About 84% of the men and 94% of the women believed in God. There were no statistically significant differences between believers and nonbelievers in the rate of cigarette smoking. Frequency of church attendance, however, was inversely related to both marijuana use and cigarette smoking, particularly among men ($p < .001$, both comparisons, uncontrolled).

Hundleby et al. (1982) surveyed 100 boys and 131 girls in the ninth grade in Ontario, Canada; most of the students were Catholic. Religious activity was measured by frequency of prayer, participation in choir or youth groups, attendance at religious services, and attendance at religious services without parents. Religious activity was inversely correlated with tobacco use ($r = -.16$, $p < .05$, uncontrolled), but not with use of alcohol, pain killers, tea or coffee or marijuana. The investigators concluded that "Religious behavior did not emerge as a clear correlate [of overall adolescent drug use]." Hundleby (1987) later expanded his study to include 1,008 ninth-grade boys and 1,040 girls. Frequency of tobacco and marijuana use in the past six months was assessed. This time, religious activity was inversely related to both cigarette smoking ($r = -.22$ for girls and $r = -.11$ for boys, both $p < .01$) and marijuana use ($r = -.15$ for boys and $r = -.16$ for girls, both $p < .01$).

Gottlieb and Green (1984) conducted a national U.S. telephone survey of more than 3,000 persons ages 20–64. They eliminated 552 persons from the sample for reasons of poor health. Cigarette smoking, other health practices, and church attendance were then examined. Church attendance was more frequent among men and women nonsmokers, particularly former smokers who were overweight. These investigators concluded that the reduction in cigarette smoking resulted from the subjects' acceptance of religious teachings and from their sense of family responsibility.

Gmur and Tschopp (1987) surveyed 532 heavy smokers in Switzerland and examined factors related to their successful discontinuation of smoking. The average age of the subjects was 38 years for men and 34 years for women. Subjects were assessed prior to treatment by a "faith healer" named Hermano and four months (40.0% continued not to smoke), 12 months (32.5%), five years (20%), and 12 years (15.9%) later. Researchers compared those who remained nonsmokers for 12 years ($n = 73$) with those who continued to smoke for 12 years without interruption ($n = 31$). High alcohol consumption, markedly addictive smoking, and rare attendance at church predicted subjects' continued smoking or relapse. The authors concluded that church attendance may help persons to stop smoking and to avoid relapse.

Thorne et al. (1996) surveyed 990 noninstitutionalized persons age 62 or older living in Youngstown, Ohio. While they found no association between religious activity and alcohol use or exercise, they did find a significant inverse relationship between cigarette smoking and church attendance ($p = .01$) and nonchurch-related religious participation ($p < .001$, uncontrolled).

Recall Lapane et al.'s (1997) survey of two samples of 2,442 and 2,799 persons ages 18–64 who were living in Pawtucket, Rhode Island. Almost one-half (48%) of church members never smoked cigarettes, compared with 35% of nonmembers ($p < .001$), a difference that persisted after researchers adjusted for other risk factors, such as age, sex, and ethnicity.

Koenig, George, Cohen, et al. (1998b) examined the relationship among religious activities,

current cigarette smoking, and number of pack-years smoked for 3,968 community-dwelling persons age 65 or over who were living in North Carolina. Religious activities included attendance at religious services, private religious activities (prayer or Bible study), and listening to religious radio or watching religious television (single items measured each activity). This six-year prospective study involved in-person interviews in 1986, 1989, and 1992. Attendance at religious services was significantly and inversely related to current cigarette smoking in all three surveys. In the initial survey, in 1986, approximately 8% of persons who attended religious services at least once per week currently smoked, compared to more than 25% of those who never attended religious services. These associations persisted after researchers controlled for age, sex, race, education, alcohol use, and health status using logistic regression; persons who attended religious services at least once per week were 25% less likely to smoke cigarettes than those who attended less frequently ($p < .001$). Frequency of religious attendance among smokers was also inversely correlated with number of cigarettes smoked ($p < .01$) and total number of pack-years smoked ($p < .0001$), when other variables were controlled.

Private Religious Activities

In the Koenig, George, Cohen, et al. (1998b) study just cited, frequency of prayer and Bible study was inversely related to current smoking in 1989 and 1992 but not in 1986. However, private religious activities in 1986 predicted lower rates of smoking in 1989, after researchers controlled for smoking status in 1986 ($p = .05$). Thus, persons who prayed or studied the Bible regularly in 1986 were less likely to smoke in 1989. Private religious activities were also significantly related to number of pack-years smoked ($r = -.17, p < .0001$), although this relationship weakened when covariates were controlled (partial $r = -.04, p < .05$). The strongest effect was seen among persons who both attended religious services at least once a week and who prayed or studied the Bible at least daily. After researchers controlled for covariates (age, sex, race, education, alcohol use, and health status), these persons were almost 90% more likely not to be currently smoking than were those less involved in these activities (OR = 1.88, $p < .0001$) (see Figure 24.1).

In this study, watching religious TV or listening to religious radio was associated with an increased likelihood of current smoking in the 1992 cross-sectional analysis (although no relationship was found in 1986 or 1989). Number of cigarettes smoked, however, was inversely related to frequency of religious media viewing; the association reached statistical significance in 1989 and 1992 (partial $r = -.12$ and $-.16$, controlled). Although religious media viewing was inversely related to number of pack-years smoked in 1986 ($r = -.12, p < .0001$), this association disappeared when covariates were controlled (partial $r = -.01$, $p = $ ns). Thus, private prayer and Bible study appear to be stronger deterrents to cigarette smoking than do listening to religious radio or watching religious television.

Personal Religiousness

A number of studies have examined the relationship between personal religiousness (or religious commitment) and cigarette smoking. We divide these studies into those involving adolescents or college students and those involving adults.

Adolescents or College Students. Examining the relationship among the degree of professed religious belief, cigarette smoking, and use of other drugs, Khavari and Harmon (1982) surveyed 4,853 persons from various occupations, including college students, members of labor unions, military reservists, and housewives in Milwaukee, Wisconsin. The median age of the subjects was 21.7 years, and the range was 12–85 years; 53% of the subjects were men, 89% were white, and 45% were Catholic. Degree of religious conviction was assessed by the question "How religious are you?" Possible responses were "very religious" (13%), "moderately religious"

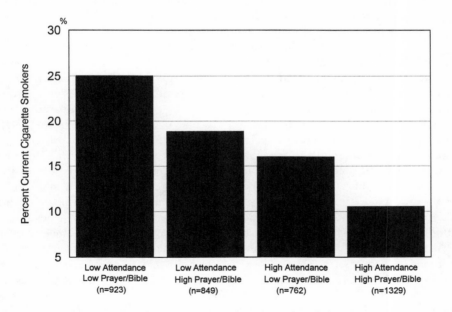

FIGURE 24.1 Relationship among cigarette smoking, religious attendance, and prayer and Bible study. High attendance = once a week or more; low attendance = less than once a week. High prayer and Bible study = once a day or more; low prayer and Bible study = less than once a day.

(44%), "slightly religious" (29%), and "not religious at all" (14%). When comparing the "very religious" and the "not religious at all" groups, researchers found significant differences in the use of marijuana ($p < .01$) and hashish ($p < .01$) and in the rate of cigarette smoking ($p < .01$) (analyses uncontrolled).

Newcomb et al. (1986) examined the relationship between religiousness and use of cigarettes and other substances among 791 adolescents in grades 7–9 in Los Angeles, California. Of the subjects, 64% were white, 15% were African American, 13% were Hispanic, and 8% were Asian. The average uncontrolled correlation between low religiosity and the five classes of substance studied (cigarettes, alcohol, cannabis, hard drugs, and nonprescription medications) was 0.13 (compared with $r = 0.41$ for peer drug use). Method of measuring religiosity was not given, nor was the individual correlation between religiousness and cigarette smoking provided.

Torabi (1990) examined cigarette smoking and strength of religious belief in 405 Midwestern American Christian and 406 Turkish Muslim undergraduates. Among American students, only religious belief ($p = .06$) and sibling smoking status differentiated smokers from nonsmokers. Among Turkish students, age, grade level, low religious belief ($p = .01$), father's smoking, and siblings' smoking were all predictive of smoking status. When discriminant function analysis was used to differentiate smokers from nonsmokers in the combined sample, only religious belief, age, and college grade level discriminated smokers from nonsmokers.

Oleckno and Blacconiere (1991) examined religiosity and cigarette smoking in 1,077 college students at Northern Illinois University (59% of the subjects were women, 87% were white, and 55% were Catholic). Cigarette smoking and other health behaviors were assessed. A two-item religiosity index asked, "How often do you attend religious services?" and "How religious are you?"; scores were dichotomized into high and low religiousness. Cigarette smoking was significantly lower among the high religious group ($F = 12.7$, $p < .001$, with gender controlled).

Recall Adelekan et al.'s (1993) study of the psychosocial correlates of tobacco and cannabis use among 137 Muslim and 483 Christian undergraduates in Nigeria. While no differences in cigarette smoking or cannabis use were found between Muslims and Christians, those who were "very religious" (regardless of religious group) were less likely than those who were "not religious" to smoke cigarettes (30% vs. 72% lifetime, $p < .001$; 4% vs. 36% current, $p < .001$) or to use cannabis (6% vs. 25% lifetime, $p < .001$). Also recall that Ndom and Adelakan (1996) examined cigarette smoking and religiosity in second- and fourth-year university students (649 subjects in 1988 and 859 subjects in 1993) at Ilorin University, in Nigeria. In both 1988 and 1993, greater self-rated religiosity was associated with a lower lifetime use of cigarettes (for the very religious, 4% and 3%, respectively, vs., for the not religious, 36% and 30%, respectively, both $p < .001$).

Adults. Goldbourt and Medalie (1975) surveyed more than 10,000 men ages 40–65 in Israel to determine the psychosocial characteristics of smokers. Religiousness was measured by three items: religious or secular education, self-definition as orthodox in belief (or traditional or secular), and frequency of synagogue attendance. Smokers were characterized by crowded housing, low education, and little leisure-time activity and were significantly less likely to be categorized as religious. The percentage of current smokers among very orthodox subjects was 39%, compared to 50–53% in secular or agnostic subjects ($p < .001$, uncontrolled).

Koenig, Moberg, & Kvale (1988) evaluated 106 consecutive geriatric clinic outpatients ages 56–94 years (mean age 74) in Springfield, Illinois, examining cigarette smoking, other health behaviors, and religious activities and attitudes. Investigators found a weak inverse relationship between cigarette smoking and organizational religious activity, private religious activity, and intrinsic religiosity; none of these associations, however, reached statistical significance. The relatively low rates of smoking (18.8%) and the small sample size may have contributed to these weak associations.

Brown and Gary (1994) examined the relationship between religious involvement and cigarette smoking among African American men. The sample consisted of 537 persons living in Norfolk, Virginia; 59% of the subjects were under age 45. A 10-item religiosity scale was administered, and information about religious attendance and affiliation (13% claimed no affiliation) was obtained. All of the religious variables were related to smoking status ($p = .001$). Religious attendance, rather than age, income, education, marital status, or employment status, was the strongest predictor of whether a subject was a current smoker in the multivariate model ($p < .001$).

Kendler et al. (1997) examined cigarette smoking and religiousness among 849 white female same-sex twins and 204 single members of twin pairs from the population-based Virginia Twins Registry ($n = 1,902$). Daily cigarette intake was assessed, and measures of personal religious devotion (importance of religious or spiritual beliefs, seeking of religious or spiritual comfort, and frequency of private prayer to God), religious conservatism (belief that God rewards and punishes, literal belief in Bible), and institutional conservatism (judged by the conservativeness of the subjects' religious affiliations) were administered. Using regression modeling, the investigators found that all three religious measures were inversely related to current cigarette smoking ($\beta = -1.59$, $p < .0001$; $\beta = -.04$, $p > .01$; and $\beta = -.058$, $p < .01$, respectively). Personal religious devotion was also inversely related to lifetime nicotine dependence ($\beta = 0.79$, $p < .01$), as were personal devotion and religious conservatism, although to a lesser degree ($\beta = 0.89$ and 0.86, $p < .05$).

Conclusion

In the vast majority of studies reviewed here, whether in adolescents or college students, whether in younger or older adults, whether in Christians, Muslims, or Jews, cigarette smoking is inversely related to personal religiousness and religious practices. Of particular importance are the studies of adolescents and college students. The inverse relationship between cigarette smoking and religious involvement is important because it is during these early years that the habit of cigarette smoking usually be-

gins. Koenig, George, Cohen, et al. (1998b), in their study of almost 4,000 older adults, found that the reason that religiously active elders smoked less than nonreligious elders was that the former were less likely to have ever started smoking (rather than being more likely to quit). If religiousness can help prevent the onset of cigarette smoking during adolescence or young adulthood, people will enjoy the health benefits of avoiding this habit throughout their lifetimes. Recall that 21% of coronary heart disease deaths, 30% of cancer deaths, and almost all deaths from chronic bronchitis and emphysema could be prevented if Americans never started smoking cigarettes (Office on Smoking and Health, 1989). Clearly, the relationship between religious involvement and cigarette smoking has important implications for public health.

SEXUAL BEHAVIORS

We reviewed earlier the physical health and societal consequences of unrestrained sexual activity, including the risk of contracting a variety of sexually transmitted diseases (some of which are lifelong or life-threatening), teen pregnancies, out-of-wedlock births, and families and marriages destroyed by extramarital affairs. We now examine the relationship between religion and sexual behavior.

Religion and Premarital Sex

To what extent does religion influence the decision whether to engage in nonmarital sex among adolescents and teenagers, college students and young adults, and mature adults? We examine, first, *attitudes* toward premarital sex and, second, sexual activity.

Sexually Permissive Attitudes in Adolescents and Teenagers.   Wright and Cox (1971) studied 3,850 teenagers (ages 16–20) from 96 randomly selected schools in England in 1963 ($n = 2,276$) and 1970 ($n = 1,574$). In the 1970 survey, religious beliefs and activities were inversely associated with permissive attitudes toward premarital sex and other delinquent behaviors. However, when the investigators compared the

1963 results with the 1970 results, they found that permissiveness with regard to delinquent behaviors had increased regardless of the subject's expressed religious attitudes in 1963. In other words, both believers and nonbelievers demonstrated greater acceptance. The investigators concluded that, while they are "factually" associated, religious and moral beliefs are not "functionally" related to each other. This interpretation of the results is problematic, since comparing different cohorts and evaluating change within one cohort must be seen in relation to the cultural environment, which in this case became more permissive during those seven years.

Werebe (1983) examined the relationship between religion and attitudes toward sexuality in a survey of 386 French adolescents. The sample included 241 girls and 145 boys ages 16–18, of whom 50 were practicing Catholics, 157 were nonpracticing Catholics, 31 were Jews, 13 were other, and 112 had no religious affiliation. Dependent variables included attitudes toward abortion, homosexuality, masturbation, and premarital sex. Practicing Catholics had more negative views on abortion than did subjects with no religion ($p < .01$, uncontrolled) and more positive views toward marriage (60% of practicing Catholics vs. 6% of "atheists"). The author concluded that religion was associated with more conservative attitudes toward all four topics, including premarital sex.

Brown (1985) examined premarital sexual permissiveness among 702 African American adolescent females ages 15–19 who were participating in the 1976 National Survey of Young Women. Religious commitment was measured by church attendance; the dependent variable was attitude toward premarital sex. Analyses using logistic regression revealed that high religious attendance was related to low sexual permissiveness, independent of the permissiveness of close friends and of income. Brown concluded that "the influence of African American religious institutions on sexual permissiveness may be more important than previously assumed" (p. 385).

Sexually Permissive Attitudes in College Students. Cardwell (1969) examined the relationship between religious commitment and premarital sexual permissiveness in a survey of 187 students at New England State University. A 30-item religious commitment scale measured the five religious dimensions of ritual, knowledge, belief, self-definition, and consequences. Attitudes toward sexual permissiveness were measured with a recognized 24-item scale (Reiss scale). All five religious commitment subscales were inversely related to premarital sexual permissiveness (analyses uncontrolled).

Ruppel (1970) examined religiosity and sexual permissiveness in 437 randomly sampled college students at Northern Illinois University. Religiosity was measured by the eight-item Faulkner-Dejong religiosity scale (which measures primarily religious belief); premarital sexual permissiveness was again measured by the Reiss scale. Religiosity was inversely related to premarital sexual permissiveness ($p < .001$) after the sample was stratified according to sex, academic class, social class, and religious affiliation.

In the study of 444 undergraduates at University College in Cork, Ireland, mentioned earlier, Parfrey (1976) also found that church attendance was positively related (in both men and women) to the feeling that engaging in extramarital sexual intercourse and getting drunk were more serious misdemeanors than was cheating on tests ($p < .001$, uncontrolled).

Davids (1982) examined attitude toward premarital sex and religiosity among 208 Jewish students (139 men, 69 women) who were participating in a computer dating service sponsored by the Jewish Student Federation at York University in Ontario, Canada. Jewish identity, Jewish religiosity (rated on a 0–5 scale), and previous Jewish schooling were the religious variables. Although five out of six students indicated a strong Jewish identity, religiosity was less common; 46% scored a zero on Jewish religiosity, 45% scored 1–3 (some), and 9% scored 4–5 (high). Low religiosity was related to permissive attitudes toward premarital sex; 40% of those with no religiosity had liberal attitudes toward sex, as did 24% of those with "some" religiosity and 11% of those with "high" religiosity ($p < .01$, uncontrolled).

Haerich (1992) surveyed 204 students (61% women, 32% Asian, 30% white, 15% African American) in general psychology classes at La Sierra University in Riverside, California. Religious orientation (the 20-item 1982 adaptation by Batson & Ventis of Allport's scale), religious attendance, and self-rated religiosity were assessed. Premarital sexual permissiveness was again measured by the 12-item Reiss scale. Attitudes were assessed both as they applied to others and as they applied to oneself. Premarital sexual permissiveness was inversely related to church attendance ($r = -.19$ for others, $p < .01$ and $r = -.15$ for self, $p < .05$), self-reported religiosity ($r = -.25$ for others, $p < .01$, and $r = -.22$ for self, $p < .01$), and intrinsic religiosity ($r = -.25$ for others, $p < .01$, and $r = -.20$ for self, $p < .01$). Analyses were not controlled for covariates.

Sexually Permissive Attitudes in Adults. Mol (1970) surveyed a random sample of 1,825 adults in Australia. Subjects' belief in God and their frequency of church attendance were each measured by a three-point scale. Subjects were asked about their attitudes toward sexual relations before marriage. Among those over age 40, men who did not believe in a personal God were less disapproving of sex before marriage than were men who believed in a personal God (37% vs. 78%). For men ages 20–40, the difference was similar (14% vs. 63%). Among women, differences were similar for those ages 20–40 years (28% vs. 77%) but narrowed for those over 40 (69% vs. 87%) ($p < .01$–.001). For infrequent and frequent church attendance, disapproval rates were 50% and 84% for men over 40, 31% and 68% for men under 40, 73% and 92% for women over 40, and 50% and 83% for women under 40. The effects of religious variables on disapproval of premarital sex were equal to or greater than either sex or age effects. Analyses were controlled for gender.

In perhaps the largest study of the relationship between religiousness and attitudes toward premarital sex, Cochran and Beeghley (1991) used data from the NORC General Social Survey, a national probability sample of 14,979 English-speaking persons 18 or older who were

living in the United States, to examine this relationship. The survey assessed religious attendance, strength of religious identification, belief in an afterlife, membership in a religious organization, and religious affiliation. Religious affiliation comprised several categories—highly proscriptive (Protestant fundamentalists and Baptists), moderately proscriptive (Methodists, Lutherans, and Catholics), and least proscriptive (Presbyterians, Episcopalians, and Jews). Subjects were asked three questions about premarital sex; possible responses were "always wrong," "almost always wrong," "wrong only sometimes," or "not wrong at all." Religious affiliation was related to the attitude that premarital sex was "always wrong" (13% for least proscriptive, 25% for moderately proscriptive, and 44% for highly proscriptive). Church attendance, strength of religious beliefs, belief in afterlife, and church membership were all significantly related to permissive attitudes toward premarital sex (correlations were −.22, −.47, −.22, −.18, after researchers controlled for age, race, sex, education, occupation, income marital status, residency, and year of survey). These effects varied considerably by religious denomination; they were strongest among Baptists and nonmainline Protestants and weakest among Jews and those with no religious affiliation.

Reported Sexual Activity in Adolescents and Teenagers. Forliti and Benson (1986) surveyed 8,165 adolescents in grades 5–9 who were involved in religious organizations and 10,467 parents. Adolescents involved in premarital sexual intercourse and other delinquent behaviors tended to place less emphasis on church and religion than did teens who did not engage in these behaviors. Parents' reports of a strong religious emphasis at home was related to lower rates of drug use among their children (no statistical analyses were done).

In some cases, religious involvement may be a double-edged sword. Studer and Thornton (1987) studied 224 18-year-old adolescents in the Detroit metropolitan area, examining the relationship between religious attendance and the likelihood of engaging in premarital sex. Results from logistic regression analyses indicated that while religious attendance was inversely related to participation in premarital sex, attendance was also inversely related to contraceptive usage, even after parental and other variables were controlled. Thus, while frequent church attenders were less likely to engage in premarital sex, they were also less likely to use contraceptives if they became sexually active.

These researchers later reported the results of a prospective study of children in the Detroit area (Thornton & Camburn, 1989); children born in 1961 and their mothers were followed until 1980. In 1980, investigators examined the degree of religious participation and the adolescent sexual behavior and attitudes of the children, who were now age 18. Children who were most likely to have premarital sex, those who had the most partners, and those who had the most permissive attitudes toward sex were those with no religious affiliation, those who never or infrequently attended church, and those who indicated that religion was not important in their lives. These associations largely persisted when the researchers controlled other factors, using structural equation modeling.

DuRant et al. (1990) surveyed a national probability sample (Cycle III of the 1982–1983 National Survey of Family Growth) of 202 unmarried Hispanic adolescent girls ages 15–19. Religious variables included religious affiliation and frequency of church attendance; the dependent variable was sexual intercourse, with nearly 42% of the women being sexually active. Girls with no religious affiliation were significantly more likely to be sexually active than were those with an affiliation (82% vs. 18%, $p < .01$). Sexually active girls also reported significantly less church attendance than did virgins ($p < .001$). In a regression model, factors directly related to sexual activity included lack of religious affiliation ($\beta = .24$), which was the second strongest predictor of sexual activity. Church attendance dropped out as a predictor when race, education, income level, and religious affiliation were added to the model.

Does attending parochial school (rather than public school) affect the likelihood that adolescents will engage in sexual activity? Cullari and

Mikus (1990) surveyed 116 high school students at a Catholic school (50 ninth-grade students and 66 twelfth-grade students) and 92 students from a public school (52 ninth-grade students and 40 twelfth-grade students) in Pennsylvania to examine the correlates of adolescent sexual behavior. Scores on the Sex Knowledge Inventory were significantly higher for Catholic twelfth graders than for public school twelfth graders; no difference in knowledge was found between ninth graders at Catholic and at public schools. Despite their greater sexual knowledge, Catholic students were less likely to have engaged in sexual intercourse than were public school students (24% vs. 48%, $p < .01$). Also, only 10% of Catholic ninth graders and 33% of Catholic twelfth graders were sexually active, compared to 29% of ninth graders and 73% of twelfth graders at the public school. However, when asked how large a role religious beliefs had played in their decisions regarding sexual intercourse, 15% of Catholic students said "none" and 20% said "a large role," whereas 19% of those in public school indicated "none" and 23% said "a large role." The authors concluded that religious beliefs played a relatively small role in influencing the students' attitudes toward sex (at least as far as the students would acknowledge). Nevertheless, the difference in the rate of sexual activity between Catholic and public school students is impressive.

Reported Sexual Activity in College Students and Young Adults. Clayton (1969) examined religious orthodoxy and premarital sexual activity among 887 single undergraduate students at a small, coeducational, liberal arts Baptist college in southern Florida. Of the sample, 52% were female and 31% were Baptist; more than 40% were fraternity or sorority members. Religious orthodoxy was measured by Putney and Middleton's six-item religious orthodoxy scale. The primary dependent variable was premarital sexual intercourse in the past year. Religiously orthodox nonfraternity men were less likely to have had sex than were orthodox fraternity men (21% vs. 55%, $p = .001$), less orthodox fraternity men (21% vs. 62%, $p = .001$), and less orthodox nonfraternity men (21% vs. 39%, $p = .01$). Similarly, religiously orthodox nonsorority women were less likely to have engaged in sex during the past year than were less orthodox nonsorority women (14% vs. 39%, $p = .001$); religiously orthodox sorority women, however, were not less likely than less orthodox sorority women to report having had sexual intercourse during the school year (17.9% vs. 23.9%, $p = $ ns). Clayton concluded that religious orthodoxy was inversely related to experience of premarital sex in nonsorority and nonfraternity undergraduates but not in undergraduates who lived in fraternities or sororities—where, perhaps, peer pressure overwhelmed the effects of religious belief (analyses uncontrolled).

Rohrbaugh and Jessor (1975) surveyed a random sample of 475 high school students and 221 college students from a city in the Rocky Mountain region. Investigators examined the relationship between religiosity and deviance or problem behavior. Religiosity was measured by an eight-item scale that assessed the ritual, consequential, ideological, and experiential dimensions of religiosity. Among high school students, religiosity was significantly and inversely related to premarital sex, marijuana use, and general deviant behavior. For college students, the relationship was significant for premarital sex and marijuana use. The authors concluded that religious youth are characterized by "a relative acceptance of social institutions as worth conserving as they are, a set of values that sustain conformity and eschew self-assertion and autonomy, and a social context that minimizes both opportunity and support for departure from conventional norms" (p. 151).

Gunderson and McCary (1979) interviewed 327 students (135 men, 192 women) enrolled in a course in human sexuality at the University of Houston. Sample participants were mostly white, single, and Protestant. Religious affiliation, religious interest, and frequency of church attendance were assessed, along with sexual attitudes, sexual behaviors, and sexual guilt. Mosher's "G" inventory was used to assess sexual guilt. In both men and women, religious interest and frequent church attendance were significantly related to sexual attitudes, sexual behavior, and sexual guilt. However, when re-

searchers controlled for sexual guilt most of the variance in sexual attitudes and behaviors vanished because of the strong correlation between religious attendance and sexual guilt (although several items on the Mosher inventory are confounded by orthodox religious views) (Mosher & Cross, 1971). The investigators concluded that religiousness predicts sexual guilt, which in turn predicts sexual information obtained, sexual attitudes held, and sexual behaviors expressed. The authors also concluded that sexual guilt "interfered" with students' "sexuality," although they did not specify what this meant. If interfering with students' sexuality means preventing premarital sex, teenage pregnancy, and sexually transmitted diseases, then sexual guilt at this time in life may be an advantage. In the introduction of this article, the investigators conceded that "religion is the single best predictor of sexual attitudes and sexual behavior, especially premarital intercourse" (p. 353).

Mahoney (1980) examined religiosity and sexual behavior in 441 introductory sociology students at Western Washington University in Washington State. Approximately two-thirds of the sample was female, predominantly freshmen or sophomores. Intensity of religious belief was measured by a single item, a 21-point scale ranging from 0 to 20 (not at all intense to very intense). Among men, 13 of 20 sexual behaviors were related to religiosity; among women, seven of 20 sexual behaviors were significantly related to religiosity. Sexual intercourse was more common among students with low religiousness (compared to those with high religiousness) for both men and women (92% vs. 79%, $p < .001$, and 79% vs. 45%, $p < .001$, respectively). In addition, religiousness was inversely related ($p < .05$) to number of sexual partners ($r = -.21$ for men and $r = -.13$ for women), frequency of light and heavy petting ($r = -.19$ for men and $r = -.17$ for women, and $r = -.23$ for men and $r = -.17$ for women), extensiveness of sexual experiences ($r = -.38$ for men and $r = -.25$ for women), thinking about sex ($r = -.25$ for men and $r = -.12$ for women), sexual enjoyment ($r = -.15$ for men only), sexual responsiveness ($r = -.14$ for men only), and ideal frequency of sex per month ($r = -.19$ for men and $r = -.24$ for women). Mahoney concluded that religiosity was negatively correlated with premarital sexual intercourse and with the behaviors and thought processes that lead up to it.

Herold and Goodwin (1981) surveyed 408 college women (87% of whom were freshmen or sophomores) and 106 high school girls in Ontario, Canada (the combined average age of the students was 19). Religiosity was measured by frequency of church attendance. Subjects were asked first whether they had ever had sexual intercourse and second about the likelihood of their doing so in the future (rated on a scale of 1–9). On the basis of these responses, the researchers categorized subjects into "adamant virgins" (32%), "potential nonvirgins" (14%), and "nonvirgins" (48%). Church attendance was strongly related to virginity. Nearly 42% of adamant virgins attended church weekly or more, compared to 17% of potential virgins and 9% of nonvirgins ($p < .001$, uncontrolled). When adamant virgins were asked to name the most important reason they did not engage in sex, half indicated moral or religious beliefs, as did only 2% of potential nonvirgins. Discriminant analysis confirmed that religious attendance was significantly related to virgin status.

Woodruff (1985) surveyed 477 freshman students who attended colleges associated with Churches of Christ to examine the associations between premarital sexual behavior and religious behavior. The sample was all white and single; 60% of the subjects were women, 79% had parents who were Church of Christ members, and 79% attended church three times per week (a very high frequency). An 11-item religious behavior scale and Allport's intrinsic-extrinsic religiosity scale were administered, in addition to a sexual behavior test that comprises five-items: having had sexual intercourse, age at first intercourse, frequency of intercourse, number of current partners, and number of past partners. Students who were intrinsically religious and who scored high in religious behavior had the lowest level of premarital sexual activity: 80% of those who attended religious services three times per week were virgins, compared to 37% of those who attended less than once per week ($p < .0001$). Intrinsic religiosity was inversely related to sexual activity; 86% of intrinsics were virgins, compared to 62% of extrinsics ($p < .0001$). Although regression models were used, the results were essentially uncontrolled, since only a couple of variables were included in the models.

Fox and Young (1989) interviewed 196 first-year college students (60% of whom were female). Religiousness was measured by the Faulkner-Dejong 5-D religiosity scale, which assesses the ideological, ritualistic, intellectual, experiential, and consequential dimensions of religiosity. The variables studied were sexual guilt (again measured by Mosher's scale), history of sexual intercourse, and experience of sexual intercourse within the past 12 months. Women scored higher for sexual guilt and higher for religiosity on all five subscales. Those who had not engaged in sexual intercourse scored higher on sexual guilt and higher religiosity on the ritualistic, experiential, and consequential dimensions ($p < .001$). Recall, however, that Mosher's scale is contaminated by conservative religious attitudes.

Kandel (1990) examined religious involvement and sexual activity in 2,711 people involved in the National Longitudinal Survey of Young Adults, a nationally representative sample of young persons born in 1963 or 1964. Religious affiliation and frequency of attendance were assessed. Regression analysis revealed that the likelihood of initiating sexual intercourse by age 16 was inversely related to religious attendance in men ($\beta = -.09$, $p < .001$) and in women ($\beta = -.13$, $p < .001$). Baptist affiliation was correlated with a greater likelihood of premarital sex among men ($r = .33$, $p < .01$) and women ($r = .28$, $p < .10$), although this result may have been partly due to confounding by race (African Americans are both more likely to be Baptist and more likely to have sex at an early age).

Jensen, Newell, et al. (1990) examined the frequency of sexual intercourse in 423 single men and women ages 17–25 who were enrolled in "family relations" classes at Cameron University, in Lawton, Oklahoma and at the University of Wisconsin at Stout. Belief about and frequency of sexual intercourse were assessed, along with frequency of religious attendance. Students who attended religious services at least weekly had nonpermissive attitudes toward premarital sex and the lowest mean frequency of premarital sexual intercourse. However, those who attended services weekly and had permissive attitudes toward premarital sex had higher rates of intercourse. Jensen and colleagues concluded that religious attendance probably leads to less permissive attitudes toward premarital sex, which leads to less premarital sex. They emphasized that religious belief had to be accepted and internalized by the adolescent before it could affect premarital sexual activity and that going to church by itself was not enough.

Rosenbaum and Kandel (1990) examined the relationship between early onset of adolescent sexual behavior and religious involvement in a random national sample of 2,711 persons ages 19–20. African Americans, Hispanics, and economically disadvantaged white youth were oversampled. Using regression analysis, investigators examined the probability of initiating intercourse by age 16. Frequency of religious attendance was inversely related to having intercourse before age 16 in men (OR = 0.92, $p < .001$) and in women (OR = 0.88, $p < .001$). In other words, for every one-point increase in frequency of religious attendance (rated on a scale from 1–6), the likelihood of initiating sexual intercourse before age 16 dropped by 8% for men and by 12% for women.

Beck et al. (1991) prospectively studied persons ages 14–22 years between 1979 and 1983; the subjects were involved in the National Longitudinal Surveys of Youth, a stratified, random national sample of young persons in the United States. In white women, fundamentalist religious background significantly reduced the likelihood of premarital sex (n for analyses not given). Among African American females, Baptists had higher rates of premarital sex than did mainline Protestants. For both white men and white women, belonging to an "institutionalized sect" (Pentecostals, Jehovah's Witnesses, Mormons) was associated with less premarital sex, independent of control variables. For African American men, there were no significant

differences across affiliation groups. For the white, teen virgin subsample (1,103 women, 969 men), Baptist, fundamentalist, or institutional sect membership significantly predicted abstention from premarital sex in both men and women. Frequency of church attendance was significantly and inversely related to premarital sex in both men and women, an association that persisted ($p < .01$) after other variables were controlled, including denomination, age, marriage before or after age 20, area of country, rural or urban location, education of parents, and presence of both parents in the home.

Nicholas and Durrheim (1995) examined the relationship between religiosity and sexual knowledge, attitudes, beliefs, and practices among 1,817 black South African first-year students at the University of Western Cape. The mean age of the students was 20; 56% were women, and all were black. Religiosity was measured by the eight-item Rohrbaugh and Jessor scale, and scores were divided into quartiles: highly religious, medium religious (middle two quartiles), and low religious. Openness of communication with parents about contraception, attitudes toward homosexuality, attitudes toward AIDS, and sexual and contraceptive behaviors were assessed. Religiosity was not correlated with negative attitudes toward contraception or AIDS. Highly religious students experienced sexual intercourse at an older age than did low religious students (17.5 vs. 15.9 years, $p < .0001$), had fewer sexual partners in high school ($p = .01$), were more likely to intend to remain sexually abstinent during the first year of college ($p < .0001$), but were less likely to use safe sex practices ($p < .0001$) and less likely to use contraceptives ($p < .05$). Note that in the last series of analyses, virgins were excluded, and the researchers compared only those in the top and the bottom quartiles for religiousness. The study concluded that religious commitment was associated with a lower likelihood of engaging in sexual intercourse and a later age of onset. Nevertheless, for those subjects who engaged in sexual activity, safe sexual practices and contraceptive use were practiced less often, just as Studer and Thornton (1987) and Goldscheider and Mosher (1991) found.

Negative Studies. Not all studies find a negative relationship between religiousness and premarital sex. Sack et al. (1984) surveyed 264 male and 255 female undergraduate students at a large mid-Atlantic land-grant university. The frequency of premarital intercourse among one's friends (peer behavior), the feelings of one's friends toward the subject if he or she had sexual intercourse (peer approval), sexual intercourse (coitus), and sex guilt (Mosher index) were assessed. A six-item measure of conventional religious attitudes was also administered. Religiosity was inversely related to peer approval ($r = -.26$), peer behavior ($r = -.22$), and coitus ($r = -.22$) among women and inversely related to peer approval ($r = -.32$), peer behavior ($r = -.05$), and coitus ($r = -.11$) in men. Path analysis showed that in men, religiosity had a weak overall total positive effect on coitus, operating largely through an indirect effect mediated by the sexual behavior of the subject's close friends; religious men were more likely to have close friends who were sexually active, which was strongly correlated with coitus. Among women, conventional religious attitudes had an overall weak total positive effect on coitus. Researchers concluded that the total effect of conventional religiousness on premarital sexual attitudes and behavior was minimal.

From this review it is clear that in almost all studies, whether in adolescents or teenagers, college students, young adults, or mature adults, religious beliefs and practices are associated with less permissive attitudes toward and lower rates of premarital sexual activity. After comprehensively reviewing this research, Donahue and Benson (1995) likewise concluded that religiousness was positively associated with prosocial values and behavior and negatively related to premature sexual involvement.

Extramarital Sexual Affairs

It was Kinsey and colleagues (1953) who provided the first evidence that church activity was inversely related to extramarital coitus. Numerous other studies over the past 50 years have provided further evidence to corroborate this claim. Mol (1970), in a survey of 1,825 adults in Australia, examined the relationship between attitudes toward extramarital affairs and belief in God. Among those over age 40, men who did not believe in a personal God were less disapproving of extramarital sex than were men who believed in a personal God (74% vs. 92%). For men ages 20–40, the difference was similar (66% vs. 88%). Among women, both those who believed in God and those who did not had similar attitudes toward extramarital affairs. Among women ages 20–40 years, 89% of those who believed in God and 90% of those who did not believe disapproved; for those over age 40, the figures were 90% and 95%. Differences were statistically significant only in men.

Bell (1974) examined the sexual behaviors of 2,374 married women (average age 34.9) in the United States and 1,442 married women (average age 35.3) in Australia. Subjects were asked whether they attended religious services (no/yes). The researchers found that extramarital sex was less common among religious attenders than among nonattenders (19% vs. 33% in the United States, 23% vs. 41% in Australia). When asked whether they would engage in extramarital sex in the future, 62% of attenders and 34% of nonattenders in the United States said it would never happen, and 56% of church attenders and 26% of nonattenders in Australia said it would never happen. Bell concluded that religious women are less likely to have extramarital affairs and less likely to expect to have them in the future.

Cochran and Beeghley (1991), in their classic study of 14,979 English-speaking persons age 18 or older in the United States, examined the relationship between extramarital sex and religious attendance, strength of religious identification, belief in afterlife, membership in religious organization, and religious affiliation. Recall that religious affiliation was divided into highly proscriptive (Protestant fundamentalists and Baptists), moderately proscriptive (Methodists, Lutherans, and Catholics), and least proscriptive (Presbyterians, Episcopalians, and Jews) categories. Relating religious affiliation to the attitude that extramarital sex is "always wrong," the researchers found that 50% of those affiliated with the least proscriptive groups, 72% of those affiliated with the moderately proscriptive groups, and 81% of those in the highly proscriptive held this view. Church attendance, strength of religious beliefs, belief in afterlife, and church membership were all inversely related to permissive attitudes toward extramarital sex ($\beta = -.17$ for attendance, $\beta = -.51$ for strength of religious beliefs, and $\beta = -.28$ for belief in afterlife); no significant relationship was found with church membership. Correlations were controlled for subjects' age, race, sex, education, occupation, income, marital status, residency, and year of survey. The effects of these factors varied considerably for different religious denominations, being strongest among Baptists and nonmainline Protestants and weakest among Jews and those with no religious affiliation.

Number of Sexual Partners

Religious persons in general have fewer sexual partners, whether for premarital sex or for extramarital affairs; this factor is particularly important in assessing the likelihood of contracting diseases transmitted by intercourse. Recall that Mahoney (1980) examined religiosity and sexual behavior in 441 introductory sociology students at Western Washington University. Women, most of whom were freshmen or sophomores, made up approximately two-thirds of the sample. Intensity of religious belief was measured by a single item, a 21-point scale ranging from 0 to 20 ("not at all intense" to "very intense"). Mahoney found that religiousness was inversely related to number of sexual partners ($r = -.21$ for men and $r = -.13$ for women, both $p < .05$).

Seidman, Mosher, and Aral (1992) evaluated 7,011 sexually active women ages 15–44 who were surveyed as part of the National Survey of Family Growth Cycle IV conducted by the National Center for Health Statistics. Those with a religious affiliation were less likely than those without to have multiple sexual partners (two or more partners in the past three months) (3.1% vs. 8.7%, $p < .01$). Among white women ($n = 5,354$), lack of religious affiliation independently predicted multiple sexual partners,

whereas among African American women ($n = 2,771$), low or irregular church attendance predicted multiple sexual partners. All analyses were controlled and percentages weighted.

Billy et al. (1993) examined the sexual behavior of men in the United States in a national probability sample of 3,321 men ages 20–39 as part of the 1991 National Survey of Men. Religious affiliation, classified as "conservative Protestant," "other Protestant," "Catholic," and "other or none," was the main religious variable; sexual behavior was the primary dependent variable. Conservative Protestants reported significantly fewer lifetime partners (5.4 vs. 7.3 for the entire sample), a slightly greater likelihood of having had only one partner over the past 18 months (74% vs. 71% overall), and greater frequency of intercourse over the past four weeks (4.6 vs. 3.7). Men with no religious affiliation had the most partners (8.4) and were the least likely to have had a single partner for the past 4 weeks (67%). Men with non-Christian backgrounds or no religious affiliation were somewhat more likely than conservative Protestants to have had anal intercourse (22% vs. 18%, respectively) and with more partners (2.1 vs. 1.4, respectively).

Recall Nicholas and Durrheim's (1995) evaluation of religiosity and sexual behaviors among 1,817 first-year black students at the University of Western Cape, South Africa. Religiosity was measured by an eight-item Rohrbaugh and Jessor scale, and subjects were then divided by score into quartiles: highly religious, medium religious (middle two quartiles), and low religious. Highly religious students had had fewer sexual partners in high school ($p = .01$) and were more likely to intend to remain sexually abstinent during the first year of college ($p < .0001$). In general, then, most studies find that religious affiliation, belief, and activity are associated with having fewer sexual partners.

Religious Activity and Sexually Transmitted Diseases

Despite the high likelihood that a relationship exists, few studies have examined the effects of religious belief and practice on the probability of contracting a sexually transmitted disease.

Recall from chapter 20 the study by Naguib, Lundin, et al. (1966) at the Johns Hopkins School of Public Health, which involved a cytologic screening program for cervical cancer in Washington County, Maryland, in 1963. Among the 3,962 women designated as "Christians," there was an inverse relationship between the frequency of religious service attendance and the rates of abnormal Pap smears or confirmed cases of cervical cancer, an association that persisted after researchers controlled for educational level. Among women who attended services once a week or more, the rate of suspicious or positive smears or confirmed cases was 25/2213, or 1.13%, compared with 15/426 (3.52%) for women who attended services less than twice a year or never. This finding helped establish the relationship between multiple sexual partners and the etiology of cervical cancer (human papillomavirus).

High-Risk Sexual Activity. Folkman, Chesney, Pollack, et al. (1992) examined the relationship between stress, coping, and high-risk sexual behavior (unprotected anal intercourse) in 331 gay and bisexual men involved in the AIDS Behavioral Research Project in San Francisco. Spiritual beliefs and activities were measured by a nine-item scale that we have already described in chapter 5. Discriminant function analysis revealed that unprotected anal intercourse during the previous month was significantly related to having fewer spiritual activities.

OTHER HEALTH BEHAVIORS

Safe Driving and Use of Seat Belts

Recall Oleckno and Blacconiere's (1991) survey of 1,077 college students at Northern Illinois University. Included in the study was a questionnaire that assessed seat-belt use and rate of injuries. The sample was dichotomized on the basis of the results of a two-item religiosity index: "How often do you attend religious services?" and "How religious are you?" Seat belt use was significantly greater among those with high religiosity ($F = 12.3$, $p < .001$). Studies are needed to examine the impact of religion on indicators of unsafe driving (driving above the speed limit, traffic citations, rates of DWI). We hypothesize that unsafe driving practices would be fewer among the more religious (see section on health behaviors in young people).

Risk-Taking Behaviors

From chapters 11 and 12, we know that religiously involved persons tend to avoid behaviors that increase the risk of accidents and injuries. They are also less likely to practice risky sexual behaviors (as noted earlier) and tend to be more conservative in their overall lifestyle. The sociologist David Mechanic (1990) has emphasized that a wide range of religious groups tend to encourage moderation and frown upon "extreme" or risk-taking behaviors, thus contributing to better health among their adherents. Miller and Hoffmann (1995) studied a nationally representative sample of 2,408 high school seniors and found that risk-taking tendency (attraction to risk and to danger) was inversely related to religiosity (attendance at religious services and importance of religion) ($\beta = -.06$, $p < .001$). Indeed, several studies have shown that low risk takers prefer traditional ways (e.g., religion) of handling stress and uncertain situations, whereas high risk takers seek out nontraditional responses (Holloway, 1979; Ferguson & Valenti, 1991).

Regular Sleep Patterns

Almost no research has examined the relationship between religiousness and quality, length, and depth of sleep. One might predict that religious persons would enjoy better sleep patterns, given their greater capacity to deal with stress and to cope with life problems. To our knowledge, only one study has used sleep patterns to examine this question in any depth. Hoch et al. (1987) conducted a case-control study of the nocturnal sleep structure of 10 healthy elderly nuns, comparing them to 10 healthy age-matched female controls. The nuns fell asleep more quickly ($p < .05$ for sleep latency), had less early morning awakening ($p < .05$), spent more time asleep ($p < .05$), and had more REM sleep time ($p < .02$). The researchers concluded that some of the effects of aging on sleep can be offset by attention to good "sleep hygiene," including careful attention to sleep schedule and modest habitual sleep restriction (the nuns on the average slept about 6.5 hours a night, whereas the controls slept 7.5 hours a night). The investigators also acknowledged that greater "security" might have contributed to the nuns' better sleep patterns.

Health Behaviors in Young People

Since health habits learned during adolescence may affect the rest of a young person's life, it is extremely important to study the relationships between religious involvement and behaviors that affect health risk. A recent study by Wallace and Forman (1998) examined these relationships in a random sample of 5,000 students from 135 high schools across the United States (part of the University of Michigan's Monitoring the Future Project). Included among the variables measured were the importance of religion for the subject and attendance at religious services. Outcome variables included behaviors that might unintentionally or intentionally result in injury (carrying a weapon to school, engaging in interpersonal violence, failing to use a seat belt, drinking while driving, riding while drinking), substance use (cigarette smoking, binge drinking, marijuana use), and lifestyle behaviors (poor diet, lack of exercise, and irregular sleep habits).

Religious importance was inversely related to carrying a weapon to school ($p \le = .05$), interpersonal violence ($p \le = .01$), driving while drinking ($p \le = .001$), riding while drinking ($p \le = .001$), and low seat belt use ($p \le = .001$). Similar inverse relationships were noted for cigarette smoking, binge drinking, and marijuana use (all $p \le = .001$). Frequency of religious attendance was even more strongly related to less substance use and fewer intentional and unintentional injury behaviors (except for carrying a weapon to school). Of particular interest is the finding that students who claimed that religion was very important to them or who attended religious services frequently were significantly more likely to have healthier dietary

practices, engage in regular exercise, and have better sleep patterns (all $p \le = .01 - .001$). These relationships persisted after researchers adjusted for demographic variables in multivariate analyses, and time-trend analysis for the years 1976–1996 indicated that these relationships persisted over time.

SUMMARY AND CONCLUSIONS

We examined several health variables and their relationships to the onset and course of physical disease. These variables included diet, serum cholesterol levels, weight, exercise, cigarette smoking, use of alcohol and drugs, sexual practices, seat belt use, risk-taking behaviors, and sleep patterns. We then reviewed studies that have explored the relationships between these health behaviors and religious beliefs and practices. Certain religious groups, particularly Seventh-Day Adventists and Mormons, adhere to healthy diets that are rich in unprocessed grains, fruits, and vegetables and relatively low in fat. These religious groups also tend to have lower serum cholesterol levels and, consequently, lower death rates from coronary artery disease. Studies have generally shown a connection between being overweight and being involved in religious community activity; the focus of such activities around food may encourage overeating. Thus, churches are ideal settings for health programs that promote weight reduction and regular exercise.

There exist considerable data from numerous studies from different areas of the United States and world to show that those who are religious have lower rates of cigarette smoking and alcohol and drug use. Similarly, persons who are very religious are less likely to engage in premarital sex or extramarital affairs or to have multiple sexual partners. They are also more likely to wear seat belts and less likely to engage in risk-taking behaviors. In conclusion, there is ample evidence to demonstrate that religious belief and practice are associated with positive health behaviors. This is likely a major pathway by which religion affects physical health.

25

Understanding Religion's Effects on Physical Health

W E SEEK IN THIS CHAPTER to better understand how religion influences physical health. We do this by first summarizing the research findings and then by developing a hypothetical model that illustrates possible causal mechanisms for religion's apparent effect on health. Again, as we have repeatedly emphasized throughout this book, most of the research done thus far consists of cross-sectional and prospective cohort studies that, while providing evidence that supports a causal relationship, cannot establish such a relationship. Before summarizing the research, we review the criteria for causality as determined by the epidemiologist Hill (1965) and as applied to the religion-health relationship (R-H) by Levin (1994) in table 25.1. Only randomized controlled clinical trials (RCTs) can definitively answer the question "Does religion cause better physical health?" While some RCTs have examined this question, they are few

in number. Bearing this limitation in mind, we freely use such terms as "affects" and "influences" in this chapter as we discuss hypothetical mechanisms.

SUMMARY OF RESEARCH FINDINGS

For more details, the reader should consult the individual chapters on each of the health topics reviewed here. In summarizing the findings, we refer primarily to the studies listed in part VIII of this book under their section headings.

Heart Disease

Our review of religion and heart disease identified 30 quantitative studies, many of which focus on coronary artery disease (CAD) (see part VIII). Of the 16 studies that examined degree of religiousness, 12 (75%) found less heart disease or lower cardiovascular mortality among

TABLE 25.1   Hill criteria for causality applied to the religion-health relationship

Hill Criteria	Levin Application to R-H
Strength of association	Moderate to strong association
Consistency	Repeated observation
Specificity	General effects, not disease specific
Temporality	Evidence present, but not conclusive
Biological gradient	Evidence present, but not conclusive
Coherence	Coherence difficult to assess; complex relations
Experiment	Little evidence (but growing)
Analogy	Yes; other psychosocial influences (e.g., social support) shown to have causal effects
Plausibility	Yes; biologically plausible

those who were more religious than comparison groups; three studies found no association; one study reported mixed findings (but measured parental religious affiliation only). Of the 15 studies that examined the relationship between subjects' religious denomination and CAD, four studies found higher rates of CAD in Jews than in non-Jews. Higher rates were found in secular Jews than in orthodox Jews (who experienced about 20% fewer deaths from CAD than secular Jews) (Medalie, Kahn, Neufeld, et al., 1973b; Friedlander et al., 1986; Goldbourt et al., 1993). Although one study reported more CAD in Catholics than in Protestants or Jews, three other studies found the exact opposite, that is, lower rates of CAD among Catholics than among members of other religious groups, and two studies found no association between CAD and denomination. Finally, two studies found lower rates of CAD in Mormons than in non-Mormons, and three studies found lower CAD mortality in Seventh-Day Adventists than in non-SDAs. Thus, it appears that secular Jews have the highest CAD, followed by Protestants, Catholics, Mormons, and Seventh-Day Adventists.

In the two prospective cohort studies that measured the religiousness of subjects at baseline and examined outcomes over time (Goldbourt et al., 1993; Oxman et al., 1995), both reported that religion had positive effects on CAD mortality. We also identified five clinical trials that included a religious or spiritual component as part of a psychosocial-behavioral intervention (e.g., prayer, yoga, or transcendental meditation) to reduce CAD or improve outcomes. All five reported positive effects.

Cholesterol

Three studies found that Jews had higher serum cholesterol levels than did comparison groups, and four studies found lower serum cholesterol levels in Seventh-Day Adventists than in members of the general population. Effects were explained primarily on the basis of diet. Two clinical trials have also examined the effects of transcendental meditation (TM) on serum cholesterol levels, and both found that TM lowered cholesterol after 6–11 months. Only one study to our knowledge has examined degree of religiousness as a predictor of cholesterol level; it found lower cholesterol levels among the more religious subjects than among those who were less religious (Friedlander et al., 1987).

Hypertension

We identified a total of 34 studies that quantitatively examined the relationship between religious and spiritual practices and blood pressure. Of those 34 studies, 16 examined the association between religiousness and diastolic and/or systolic blood pressure; four studies compared blood pressures in Seventh-Day Adventists with those of members of other religious groups or the general population; one study compared Protestants, Catholics, and

Jews; and 13 studies were clinical trials in which a religious or spiritual intervention (usually meditation) was used to lower blood pressure. Of the 16 studies that examined the relationship between religiousness and blood pressure, 14 studies (88%) reported lower blood pressure among the more religious subjects; diastolic blood pressures, in particular, were lower among highly religious than among less religious subjects.

A single study reported no association between religiousness and blood pressure, and that study did not measure blood pressures but relied on self-reported hypertension (Brown & Gary, 1994). Only one study found that the religious had higher blood pressures. Once again, that study examined self-reported hypertension and correlated it with self-rated religiousness; the researchers found that 30% of those in the "less than very religious" group indicated that they had hypertension, compared to 43% of those in the "very religious" group (Levin & Markides, 1985). In all studies that actually measured the blood pressure of subjects, particularly in the prospective cohort studies, the more religious subjects had lower blood pressures than did other subjects. Of the 13 clinical trials, nine reported a significant effect for the spiritual intervention on lowering blood pressure.

Cerebrovascular Disease

We found six studies that quantitatively examined the relationship between religion and stroke. Five of these studies compared rates of stroke between specific religious groups and, usually, the general population (three were prospective cohort studies). Two studies compared Mormons with non-Mormons; one found a lower rate of stroke in Mormons, and the other found no difference. One study in California found a lower rate of stroke among Seventh-Day Adventists than among non-SDAs.

The last study is the only one to examine the effects of religiousness on rate of stroke (Colantonio et al., 1992). The incidence of stroke among those who attended religious services once a week or more (50/1,055, or 4.7%) was significantly lower than that among those

who attended less frequently (113/1,503, or 7.5%) ($p < <.001$). However, frequency of religious attendance, divided by investigators into two categories, frequent attenders (once or twice a year or more) and infrequent attenders (less than once or twice a year), lost its statistical significance when included in a multiple regression model with other predictors of stroke (e.g., hypertension, myocardial infarction, diabetes, smoking). The weak method of categorizing religious attendance and the statistical controlling of possible mechanisms (e.g., hypertension, smoking) may have caused the loss of statistical significance in the final model.

Immune System Function

To our knowledge, only five studies (three of them published) have examined the relationship between religious involvement and immune system functioning. Four studies are epidemiological, and one study is experimental. Outcomes included interleukin-6 (two studies), CD4+ counts (T-helper-inducer lymphocytes), delayed-type hypersensitivity responses to skin test antigens, NK cell numbers, T-helper cell counts, total lymphocytes (two studies), and salivary IgA. All five studies reported better immune system functioning among the more religious than among the less religious.

Neuroendocrine Function

Eleven studies have examined neuroendocrine function (cortisol, ACTH, catecholamines, growth hormone, prolactin, TSH) and religious involvement. In a study of 30 women who were awaiting breast biopsies for possible cancer (Katz et al., 1970), subjects who employed prayer and faith tended to have lower cortisol levels than other subjects (although no statistical comparison was done). In a study of 112 women with metastatic breast cancer, Schaal et al. (1998) found that overall levels of salivary cortisol were not associated with religious expression, but evening (5 P.M.) cortisol levels were lower among women who reported higher religious expression ($r = .22, p = .01$). The other nine studies examined the effects of transcendental meditation and tai-chi on endocrine function; seven of the nine studies found that these practices significantly lowered cortisol or other stress hormones. Since high serum cortisol levels have been linked with impaired immune system functioning, this pattern is consistent with findings from the epidemiological and experimental studies that examined religious involvement and immunity.

Cancer

We identified 13 studies that quantitatively examined the relationship between religion and the *risk* of developing cancer. Unfortunately, all but three studies were denominational studies; that is, they compared persons from one denomination with those from other denominations. Among the 10 denominational studies, Jews were found to have the highest rates of breast or ovarian cancers (familial types) in three studies but the lowest rates of penile cancer in a fourth study; Seventh-Day Adventists were found to have the lowest rates of lung cancer in two studies (but overall cancer rates were no different in a third study); Mormons were found to have lower rates of cervical cancer than non-Mormons in two studies; and members of the Parsis religious group in India had higher rates of breast cancer than did members of other religious groups in Bombay, India. Of the three studies that examined religiousness, two found lower rates of cervical cancer (or abnormal Pap smears) among the more religious, and one found no difference in cancer risk between religious and less religious subjects.

There are many more studies of cancer-related mortality than of cancer risk. At least 36 studies have examined the relationship between religion and mortality. Unfortunately, most of these are denominational studies ($n = 28$), and the only consistent finding is that Mormons and Seventh-Day Adventists (particularly those who are active in their faith) live longer than persons in the general population. Only seven studies have examined religiousness and cancer mortality, and weak measures of religiousness were used in most of them. Five studies reported that persons with the greatest religious activity and the strongest beliefs were less likely to die of cancer (Gardner & Lyon, 1982a, 1982b; Enstrom, 1989; Dwyer et al., 1990; Ringdal, 1996), and two studies found no association (Yates et al., 1981; LoPrinzi et al., 1994). The last study involved a randomized clinical trial of intercessory prayer involving 18 children with leukemia; 70% of those prayed for were alive at follow-up compared with 25% of those who were not prayed for, but the difference was not statistically significant (Collipp, 1969).

Mortality

Including the cancer studies, we identified a total of 101 studies that quantitatively examined the relationship between religion and mortality or length of survival:

- forty-eight studies explored all-cause mortality only
- thirty-two studied cancer mortality only
- two studied cardiovascular mortality only
- one studied cancer and all-cause mortality
- two studied cancer and cardiovascular mortality
- one studied cancer, cardiovascular, and all-cause mortality
- one studied end-stage renal disease mortality
- one studied accidental mortality
- twelve studied all-cause mortality among clergy
- one studied all-cause mortality and cancer mortality among clergy

Approximately half of the studies ($n = 47$) measured religion as religious affiliation only, the other half ($n = 52$) measured religion in terms of religiousness, and two studies were clinical trials. Of the 52 studies that measured religiousness, the criterion was church attendance ($n = 21$), church membership ($n = 4$), subjective religiousness ($n = 8$), religious belief ($n = 3$), religious coping ($n = 6$), private religious activity ($n = 3$), membership or nonmembership in the clergy ($n = 13$), and other measure of religiousness ($n = 5$).[1] One study examined the effects of transcendental meditation on survival among

---

1. Ns add up to more than 52 because some studies used more than one measure of religiousness.

elderly nursing home patients, and, as noted earlier, one study examined the effects of intercessory prayer in children with cancer. The denominational studies typically found longer survival among the Amish, Seventh-Day Adventists, Mormons, and, to some extent, Jews. The TM study found lower mortality among elderly subjects in the meditation group.

When the religious variable was operationalized as religiousness, 75% ($n = 39$) of the studies found that those who were more religious survived longer, 19% ($n = 10$) found no association, 4% ($n = 2$) reported complex results, and 2% ($n = 1$) found that the more religious survived for a shorter time. The majority of studies, then, find that greater religiousness is associated with longer survival, and studies that examine those who are presumably the most religious of all, the clergy, almost all (12 out of 13) found that clergy lived longer than comparison groups. Frequency of church attendance (an indicator of level of involvement in religious community) seems to be the strongest predictor of survival in the five most recent and best designed studies of the relationship between religion and mortality (Kark et al., 1996b; Strawbridge, Cohen, et al., 1997; Oman & Reed, 1998; Hummer et al., 1999; Koenig, Hays, Larson, et al., 1999).

Functional Disability

We identified 12 studies that directly examined the relationship between physical disability and some indicator of religiousness. Ellen Idler, of Rutgers University, and Stan Kasl, of Yale University, published four of these reports from their investigation of 2,812 persons age 65 or over who participated in the Yale-New Haven EPESE survey. Idler and Kasl have been following this cohort since its initial evaluation in 1982. Their studies, and reports by other investigators, suggest that attendance at religious services is associated with less physical disability when examined cross-sectionally and predicts lower levels of disability in the future when populations are studied over time.

In the best-designed and most thorough study published to date, Idler and Kasl (1997b) reported that religious attendance may delay the onset and progression of physical disability

among older adults. In contrast, subjective measures of religiousness (or religious coping) tend to be either unrelated to physical disability level or positively related to it. One reason for the latter finding is that, as people become more physically ill and disabled, they often turn to religion for support and comfort (Koenig 1994a). In one of her first studies, Idler (1987) found that private religiousness may have a positive effect on perceived level of disability. For any given level of chronic illness, men with high levels of private religiousness reported less disability than did men with lower levels of religiousness (measured by self-rated religiousness and comfort received from religion). In a later study, she went on to show that self-ratings of health represent broad conceptions of self in which physical health and abilities may be de-emphasized and nonphysical characteristics, including religious or spiritual self-identities, emphasized (Idler, 1995).

Pain and Somatic Symptoms

We found 10 studies that quantitatively examined the relationship between religion and pain. The majority of these studies ($n = 6$) looked at the relationship between prayer and pain intensity. Interestingly, all of the four cross-sectional studies found a significant and positive relationship between frequency of prayer and pain intensity (i.e., more prayer was associated with greater pain). This positive relationship could be explained either by an increase in prayer in response to pain or an increase in pain in response to prayer.

The only prospective study among the 10 reviewed reported that "praying and hoping," while positively associated with pain in the cross-sectional analysis, predicted lower pain levels when subjects were assessed over time (Turner & Clancy, 1986). Likewise, the two clinical trials that used a religious intervention both found a reduction in pain level in the treatment group. Kabat-Zinn, Lipworth, et al. (1985) found that prayer or meditation as an intervention for chronic pain resulted in a significant lowering of pain in the meditation group. The other clinical trial examined the effects of a standard intervention by a chaplain on requests for pain medication by orthopedic patients following surgery. Requests for "prn" pain medications by patients who received the chaplain intervention were significantly fewer than those by control patients (Florell, 1973). The single prospective cohort study and these two clinical trials suggest that positive cross-sectional correlations between prayer and pain occur because increasing pain causes people to pray more. Praying, in turn, may ultimately help reduce the pain or at least help people cope better with it.

Among studies have examined the relationship between religiousness and complaints of somatic symptoms, results have been inconsistent. Of the 11 studies located, five compared somatic symptoms across religious denominations, five examined associations with level of religiousness, and one was a clinical trial. Of the five denominational studies, one found more somatic symptoms among Jews than non-Jews, one found more somatic symptoms among Hindus than among Muslims, and two found no association between number of complaints and religious denomination. One study found that children reared in dissimilar neighborhoods in terms of religious affiliation were more likely to manifest somatic symptoms. Of the five studies that examined religiousness, three found fewer somatic symptoms among the more religious, two reported mixed results (i.e., positive correlations with some religious activities and negative correlations with others), and one found a positive correlation between somatic symptoms and certain religious behaviors (glossolalia and possession states) in a small sample of fundamentalists. The only clinical trial that has addressed this topic found a reduction in somatic symptoms with a religious intervention (Carson & Huss, 1979).

Health Behaviors

Health behaviors include drug and alcohol use or abuse, cigarette smoking, weight control, diet, and exercise, sexual behavior, and other health practices (e.g., general safety, regular patterns of sleep and eating). In chapters 11 and 15 we found that the vast majority of studies reported an inverse relationship between greater religiousness and substance use or abuse (particularly among younger persons). A similar pattern was present for cigarette smoking. Of the 25 studies that quantitatively examined the relationship between religiousness and smoking, 24 (96%) reported less smoking by the more religious subjects. The remaining study found no association between smoking status and religious affiliation (any affiliation vs. no affiliation) in Western Scotland (Mullen et al., 1996).

Weight control, on the other hand, seems to be more of a problem among the religious than among the nonreligious. This is particularly true for those who attend religious services frequently. Of the six studies that have examined the relationship between weight and religious activity, all (100%) found a significant positive relationship. On a brighter note, we did identify one study that described a church-based weight control program in Baltimore that was quite successful in helping members lose weight and keep it off (Kumanyika & Charleston, 1992).

Few studies have examined the relationship between diet and religiousness or religious activity. The few that have looked at this are primarily denominational studies that focus on either Jews or Seventh-Day Adventists. Epstein, Carol, et al. (1956) and Epstein, Simpson, et al. (1956) examined the diet of garment factory workers in New York City in the 1950s. The studies found that Jews took in fewer calories than did Italians; unfortunately, those calories were more likely to come from animal fat, resulting in higher serum cholesterol levels in Jews. Phillips (1975), Phillips, Lemon, et al. (1978), and Phillips and Snowdon (1983) published several papers on the dietary habits of Seventh-Day Adventists (focusing on their avoidance of meat) and the impact of this pattern on rates of cancer and cardiovascular disease.

A number of studies have examined the relationship between religion and physical exercise. We identified five such studies. Three showed that religious persons (particularly frequent church attenders) were significantly more likely to exercise than were less religious persons. One study among older adults found no rela-

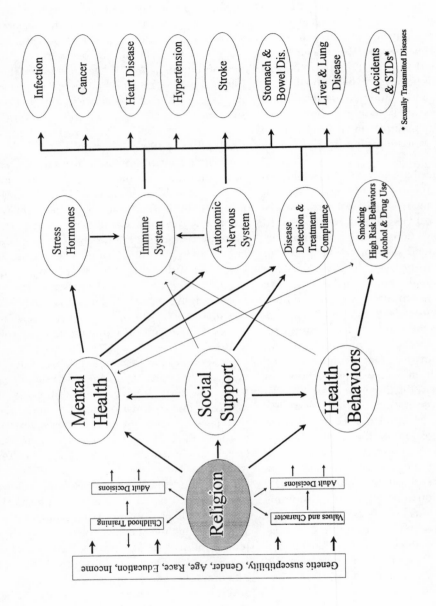

FIGURE 25.1 Theoretical model describing how religion affects physical health. Adapted from Koenig (1999), *The Healing Power of Faith* (New York: Simon & Schuster). Used with permission.

388

tionship between religious attendance and exercise, and one study found a negative relationship between exercise and intrinsic religiosity in college students. The only prospective cohort study (5,286 persons in the Alameda County study) reported that frequent church attenders in 1965 were 38% more likely than less frequent attenders to increase physical exercise during the 28-year follow-up period (Strawbridge, Cohen, et al., 1997).

Studies of sexual behavior suggest that religious involvement is inversely related to favorable attitudes toward nonmarital sex and toward premarital and extramarital sexual activity. Of the 38 quantitative studies we located, 37 (100%) found that religious subjects had more negative attitudes toward nonmarital sex than did the nonreligious subjects and significantly less premarital and extramarital sexual activity. The vast majority of the studies ($n = 32$) were of adolescents or college students. Other studies suggest that religious persons are less likely to engage in risk-taking behavior (e.g., more likely to wear seat belts), and have more structured lifestyles (better sleep patterns and sleep wave architecture) (Hoch et al., 1987; Oleckno & Blacconiere, 1991; Wallace & Forman, 1998) (see chapter 24 for details).

HYPOTHESIZED MECHANISMS FOR RELIGION'S EFFECTS

On the basis of the research we have reviewed, we now develop a theoretical model to illustrate how religious beliefs and practices might impact physical health (see Figure 25.1). This model does not consider "supernatural" or " superempirical" explanations (as defined by Levin, 1994), since such mechanisms (if they exist at all) act outside the laws of science as we know them today. We focus here on known psychological, social, behavioral, and physiological mechanisms by which religion may exert effects on physical health. Such mechanisms must take into account the following:

- Background factors such as genetic susceptibility to disease, socioeconomic status, racial or ethnic influences, and gender effects

- Childhood training as a determinant of values and character that influence decisions affecting later socioeconomic status and physical health
- Psychological and social influences (through psychoneuroimmunological mechanisms) on the development and course of physical disease
- Lifestyle choices and health behaviors that affect the development and course of physical disease
- Health care behaviors that affect health maintenance, disease detection, and treatment compliance
- Interactions among all of these factors.

BACKGROUND FACTORS

Genetic Factors

Genetic susceptibility influences the onset and course of many diseases. Because of inbreeding, specific diseases can arise and become prevalent in certain religious groups. For example, recall from chapter 20 that some groups of Jewish women have higher than expected rates of breast cancer because they carry a mutation in the breast cancer gene BRCA1 (Egan et al., 1996; Toniolo & Kato, 1996). Cardiovascular disease is particularly high among Ashkenazi and non-Mizrahi Sephardi Jews, at least partly because of enhanced genetic susceptibility (Dreyfuss, 1953). Tay-Sachs disease, which results from an inborn error of metabolism that leads to infant death, is 100 times more common in Ashkenazi Jews than in other ethnic groups. Certain genetically transmitted diseases have also been localized in the Old Order Amish community (Egeland et al., 1987).

Religion may interact with genetics to influence health in other ways. Religious involvement and belief may exert a force counter to natural selection, enabling the "less fit" (i.e., the poor, the physically weaker, or those prone to depression, anxiety, substance abuse) to survive. By surrounding these people with a supportive community and providing them with coping behaviors to compensate for their weaknesses, religion may enable them to pass on their defective genes. Thus, one might expect religious people to be less healthy and generally more feeble.

Furthermore, the whole notion of loving, forgiving, showing mercy, or "turning the other cheek" to one's enemies seems to act completely against the primary principle of natural selection (i.e., that survival is enhanced by defeating and annihilating one's enemies). One would think that these types of passive beliefs would lead to extinction, whereas more aggressive beliefs and practices would promote survival. On the other hand, such behaviors may facilitate resolution of conflict and enable disparate communities to bind together and cooperate, rather than destroy each other. This might bring new genetic material into the gene pool, increasing heterogeneity and ultimately enhancing survival (e.g., by reducing homozygote-dependent diseases).

Recent findings suggest that religious tendencies may have a genetic component. Kendler et al. (1997) surveyed 849 white female same-sex twins (496 monozygotic and 353 dizygotic) and 204 single members of twin pairs (total $n = 1,902$) from the population-based Virginia Twin Registry. They found that religious characteristics were more strongly correlated in twin pairs who were monozygotic than in those who were dizygotic. This was true for personal devotion ($r = .52$ vs $r = .40$, respectively) and, to a lesser degree, for personal conservatism ($r = .47$ vs. $r = .43$) and institutional conservatism ($r = .63$ vs. $r = .57$). Using statistical modeling, however, investigators demonstrated that family and other environmental contributions to religious tendencies were more important than genetic influences. Family environment and unknown individual or environmental influences explained twin resemblance in personal devotion (24% family environment and 47% unknown), personal conservatism (45% and 55%), and institutional conservatism (51% and 37%), leaving genetic influences to account for 29% for personal devotion, 0% for personal conservatism, and 12% for institutional conservatism.

Gender, Ethnicity, and Age

For unknown reasons, women tend to be more religious than men, and African Americans tend to be more religious than other racial groups. Women live longer than men and have different susceptibilities to many medical conditions. African Americans are more likely to have hypertension (which is at least partly genetic) and sickle-cell anemia (which is entirely genetic). Older persons tend to be more religious and are also at increased risk for most medical conditions. Gender, race, and age all have strong correlations with religion and with greater or lesser susceptibility to physical disease, thus potentially confounding relationships between religion and other health outcomes.

Socioeconomic Status

Education and income can also influence physical health, especially the quality of medical care that one receives. Education increases knowledge about preventive health behaviors, increases the likelihood that diseases will be detected early, and increases income available to spend on health-related activities. Greater income also increases access to health care resources and to coping resources for adapting to illness and disability. Study after study has shown a powerful connection between socioeconomic status and health (McCally et al., 1998). Because religion tends to be more common among those in the lower socioeconomic classes, who often rely on religion to compensate for lack of other resources, the religious poor may be at greater risk for physical illness and poor medical care.

TRAINING IN CHILDHOOD AND ADOLESCENCE

Devout religious belief and practice may help young persons reach their full adult potential, both economically and physically, partly because of the powerful relationship between socioeconomic status and physical health just noted. Religious training during childhood and adolescence may instill values that promote choices that maintain health and prevent disease in later life. If religious training in childhood prevents drug use, alcohol abuse, and delinquency in adolescence, then disruption of education and career development may be less likely. Likewise, if religious adolescents engage less frequently in premarital sexual activity, then teen pregnancy is less likely to occur and to disrupt the pursuit of higher education and limit later earning capacity. Thus, religion may actually increase the likelihood that persons in later life will have the financial resources to invest in healthy activities and timely medical care.

Recall, however, that low educational level and lack of economic resources (and especially serious physical illness) increase the likelihood that persons will turn to religion for comfort and sustenance—which in cross-sectional studies may party disguise the positive effects of childhood religious training on later socioeconomic and health status.

PSYCHOLOGICAL FACTORS THAT INFLUENCE PHYSICAL HEALTH

As noted in earlier chapters, emotional stress has physiological consequences (Selye, 1936). Enormous progress in psychoneuroimmunology and cardiovascular stress research over the past 10 years has uncovered mechanisms by which psychological factors influence physical health, particularly the onset and spread of cancer (Andersen et al., 1994) and the development of coronary artery disease (McEwen, 1998).

The "fight or flight" response, as described by Walter Cannon in 1941, is activated when the individual experiences external or internal danger. Major life events perceived as threatening to the physical body or to the psychological self (including loss of sources of pleasure or meaning in life) elicit this physiological response. The following is a simple explanation of the fight-flight response. In response to neurological and hormonal signals from the brain, the adrenal medulla releases large amounts of epinephrine and norepinephrine, which cause blood vessels in the hands, feet, and skin to constrict and redirect blood flow to vital organs (the heart and large muscles). In addition, the adrenal cortex releases the steroid hormone cortisol, which helps prepare the body to either confront the threat or flee from it. While in the short run this physiological response is very adaptive in terms of survival, if it continues for hours, days, weeks, or months (as it does in situations of prolonged psychological stress or depression), then these physiological changes damage the body's organs and homeostatic mechanisms.

For example, exposure to endogenous steroids during prolonged stress alters the immune system, weakening the body's primary defense system against infection and foreign invaders. Since the immune system may also be responsible for early detection and destruction of malignant cells and for containment of metastatic spread, this activity may also be impaired (see chapters 19 and 20).

High levels of circulating epinephrine and norepinephrine can likewise increase blood pressure, which may over time lead to coronary and cerebral artery damage, deposits of cholesterol in damaged vessel walls, and consequent plaque formation. These blood vessel changes, together with increased platelet adhesion during stress, can predispose to myocardial infarction or stroke (chapter 16). An impaired immune system can also independently increase the likelihood of coronary and carotid atherosclerosis by another mechanism. There is new evidence that infection with cytomegalovirus, a type of herpes virus, can damage artery walls producing a lesion around which vascular blockages develop (Nieto et al., 1996; Zhou et al., 1996). This may also be true for infection with Chlamydia pneumoniae (Davidson et al., 1998; Hooper, 1999). A healthy immune system may help prevent or control such infections.

Psychological stress may also activate the autonomic nervous system, affecting gastrointestinal function and leading to peptic ulcer disease, irritable bowel disease, and possibly pancreatic dysfunction and diabetes (Engel, 1955; Cobb & Rose, 1973; Hagglof et al., 1991; Lehman et al., 1991).

In addition to suffering these unhealthy physiological consequences of psychological stress, the distressed person may engage in negative health behaviors to cope with the stress. These include cigarette smoking, alcohol or drug use, risky sexual behaviors, and other activities that ultimately add to and compound health problems (see chapter 24). Heatherton and Renin

(1995) have shown that emotional stress can increase the likelihood that persons will reengage in anxiety-reducing behaviors such as smoking or unhealthy eating habits. In fact, this phenomenon occurs so frequently that it has been named the "stress disinhibition effect" (Marlatt, 1985). Thus, the "psychic cost" of stress may lower the person's self-regulatory capacity (Glass et al., 1969). Finally, if stress continues and leads to depressive disorder, then motivation to seek medical care and comply with treatment may be adversely affected (see chapter 27).

If religious beliefs and activities reduce psychological stress, prevent the onset of depression or speed its recovery, and promote greater well-being, life satisfaction, hope, and optimism (chapter 15), then religion may help moderate or prevent the damaging physiological responses to stress we have described. Religion may also prevent stress-related negative health behaviors and counteract the loss of motivation and increased pessimism that interfere with appropriate seeking of health care and compliance with medical treatment. Consequently, one should find lower rates of diseases associated with stress and emotional disorder (and possibly longer survival) among those who are more religious than the general population. In addition to independently and directly reducing psychological stress, religious beliefs and practices may also indirectly affect stress level by increasing social support.

On the other hand, religious beliefs that increase psychological stress by instilling fear or arousing guilt may have the opposite effect, stimulating the fight-flight physiological response and bringing on its long-term negative health consequences. Likewise, religious beliefs that discourage the timely seeking of medical care by substituting religious rituals for traditional treatments are likely to have negative health consequences.

SOCIAL FACTORS THAT INFLUENCE PHYSICAL HEALTH

Social support has been shown to modify the psychological and physiological consequences of stress (Uchino et al., 1996). As noted in chapter 15, emotional support from family and friends buffers stressful life events, reduces the risk of depression, and speeds recovery from depression (Cohen & Wills, 1985; George et al., 1989; George, 1992). Persons who participate in more diversified social networks—those who are married, interact with family and friends, and participate in social groups—have also been shown to live longer (Berkman & Syme, 1979; Vogt et al., 1992; House, Landis, et al., 1988) and may be more resistant to infection because of better immune system functioning (Kiecolt-Glaser, Malarkey, et al., 1994; Cohen et al., 1997). Social support is also associated with less cigarette smoking, less alcohol abuse, healthier diet, more exercise, and better sleep quality (Berkman & Breslow, 1983; Cohen, 1988). In fact, the overall effect of social support on physical health is estimated to equal that of abstention from cigarette smoking (House, Landis, et al., 1988).

Social support may enhance immune function through a number of mechanisms. First, as noted, it may buffer the effects of stressful life events on mental health. If one resists stress better, then the fight-flight response will also be reduced, the production of cortisol and other stress hormones will be lessened, and immunity will be less impaired. Second, social support may have a direct impact on health through mechanisms not yet well defined. As noted in chapter 19, social isolation of primates may adversely affect immune system function and increase susceptibility to disease (Sapolsky, Alberts, et al., 1997). Involvement in a religious community expands one's social network, increases the diversity of one's social contacts, and is associated with greater satisfaction with one's support network (see chapter 15).

By contrast, religious belief systems that isolate persons from their family and the surrounding community may reduce social support from other sources and adversely affect the religion's stress-buffering capacity. Likewise, traditional religious communities can ostracize members who do not "play by the rules," leading to alienation and social isolation.

HEALTH BEHAVIORS AND LIFESTYLE CHOICES

As noted in chapter 24, health behaviors can have an enormous influence on physical health, particularly those behaviors practiced since adolescence or young adulthood. This is particularly true for unhealthy behaviors such as cigarette smoking, alcohol or drug use and abuse, lack of exercise, unhealthy eating habits, and risky sexual behaviors. Many of these behaviors are performed in response to stressful life circumstances and may in turn lead to greater stress and poorer quality of life, plunging the person into a downward spiral.

If religion can help to prevent the development of unhealthy habits or behaviors in youth and early adulthood, it may have an enormous impact on health over the life span of the individual. Religion can reduce negative health behaviors by lessening the mental stress that sometimes precipitates them and by promoting teachings that proscribe behaviors that harm the body or control the mind. As noted, religion may also indirectly reduce negative health behaviors by providing a supportive social network that buffers stress and provides healthier alternatives for coping with stress. On the other hand, if religious beliefs promote unhealthy habits such as neglect of the physical body, overeating, or lack of exercise, then health outcomes will likely suffer. Similarly, being ostracized from a religious community may drive some individuals to return to a lifestyle of addiction and self-neglect.

DISEASE PREVENTION AND DETECTION AND TREATMENT COMPLIANCE

Health care–related behaviors can influence physical health by at least three mechanisms: disease prevention, disease detection, and treatment compliance. People who have regular medical visits for health maintenance are likely to receive education about health practices that may help prevent the development of physical disease. Disease screening procedures, whether in a doctor's office or in a community setting such as a mall or church, may lead to early detection and treatment of diabetes, hypertension, breast cancer, cervical cancer, colon cancer, prostate cancer, and other diseases. Finally, compliance with medical treatments such as taking antihypertensive medications or adhering to a diabetic or low-cholesterol diet may have a substantial impact on health outcomes.

Religion may promote better health care behaviors in a number of ways. First, religious teachings promote respect and care for the body (the "temple of the Holy Spirit"). In early Hebrew times, as noted in chapter 2, Jewish law prohibited Jews from living in towns that did not have a physician. There was great respect for the physician and for his or her profession, and this respect continues in the traditional Jewish community today.

Second, as noted, religious participation increases one's social network and frequency of social contacts. For many, the church becomes an extended family; for some, it may be the *only* family the person has. The social interaction and outreach promoted by religious groups increase the likelihood that physically ill persons will receive monitoring for their medical conditions and be encouraged to seek medical care. For example, if a member of a close-knit religious community does not show up for church one Sunday, he or she is likely to receive a call or a visit from a member of that community expressing concern. Church members may remind the sick person to take her medicine or to follow the doctor's recommendations and may provide her with transportation to the doctor's office for checkups. The medically ill individual who is part of a religious community is less likely to be able to "hide out" and neglect her health than are persons without such support.

Third, religious persons may be more compliant with the treatments offered by their doctors. Accustomed to yielding to authority or because of a sense of responsibility to others, the religious person may be more likely to take medication as prescribed (Koenig, George, Cohen, et al., 1998b) and to show up for medical appointments (Koenig, 1995b). Consequently, medical illnesses receive better treatment and are less likely to advance to a point where they are out of control.

As noted earlier, however, religious beliefs may also prevent the seeking of timely medical care or may promote religious therapies over secular ones, encouraging the patient to stop medications, possibly leading to negative health outcomes (see chapter 4).

INTERACTIVE EFFECTS

Psychological, social, behavioral, genetic, and socioeconomic factors may also interact in their influences on physical health. We already mentioned how depression and stress can lead to maladaptive coping responses and negative health behaviors. Negative health behaviors such as cigarette smoking, alcohol or drug use, and nonmarital sexual activity may themselves lead to decisions and choices that create stress, promote emotional turmoil, and worsen mental health.

Social support may prevent negative health behaviors such as substance abuse or risk-taking behaviors. On the other hand, negative health behaviors may impair social support and reduce number of positive social contacts (i.e., the alcoholic or drug user who loses his job, wife, and family), leading to isolation and associated negative health consequences. Similarly, while social support may buffer negative life events and reduce their mental health consequences, a mental health problem such as depression can itself cause social withdrawal, rejection of social support, and constriction of social network. Finally, failure to seek timely medical care and comply with medical treatments can lead to chronic illness that creates stress, prevents social interactions, and fosters depression. Depression, in turn, may reduce medical compliance and adversely affect motivation for self-care.

Genetic factors likely predispose to introversion and possibly depressive illness, which in turn affects ability to achieve financial and economic success, develop a supportive network of family and friends, and avoid drugs, alcohol, cigarette smoking, and addictive eating patterns. One thing is clear—that the intricate web of causation that is responsible for physical health problems is extremely complex.

Religion, acting either directly through belief, practice, and commitment or indirectly through effects on social support and mental health, can inhibit or promote the vector of causation that moves among psychosocial stress, emotional illness, negative health behaviors, and inadequate medical care.

SUMMARY AND CONCLUSIONS

We began this chapter by summarizing research presented in chapters 16 through 24 on the relationship between religion and physical disease and dysfunction. Our systematic review revealed that the majority of studies indicate that religiousness is associated with less coronary artery disease, hypertension, stroke, immune system dysfunction, cancer, and functional impairment, fewer negative health behaviors (e.g., smoking, drug and alcohol abuse, risky sexual behaviors, and sedentary lifestyle), and lower overall mortality. However, some religious activities are associated with increased weight and inattention to diet.

We then presented a theoretical model of religion's effects on physical health, first describing how genetic, socioeconomic, psychological, social, and behavioral factors lead to disease and then suggesting how religion might influence the links in this intricate web of causation. While both positive and negative effects of religion on health were discussed, we focused primarily on positive influences, given the predominance of research results in that direction. Because most of the research has been conducted among members of established Western religious traditions (largely the Judeo-Christian tradition), this model primarily applies to religious beliefs and practices rooted in those traditions (with the exception of meditation and prayer). Future research, particularly prospective cohort studies and randomized clinical trials, is needed to test the various pathways of this model. Likewise, studies of members of Eastern religious traditions are needed to determine whether this model generalizes to those traditions.

PART V

RELIGION AND USE
OF HEALTH SERVICES

26

Disease Prevention, Disease Detection, and Treatment Compliance

I N THIS CHAPTER, WE EXAMINE how religion influences disease prevention, disease detection, and treatment compliance. In the first section of this chapter we focus on disease prevention, health promotion, and disease detection. Do religious persons live in a way that prevents the development of common diseases and promotes health? Do religious people make more of an effort to identify disease early by getting regular health screenings? Are diseases among the actively religious detected earlier or later? In the second section, we examine treatment compliance. What factors other than religion influence whether persons comply with medical treatments? Are religious individuals more or less likely to take their medications, keep medical appointments, or adhere to medical treatment plans? Why? Is religious belief or commitment (personal faith) or involvement in religious community life (social participation) more im-

portant in terms of maximizing treatment compliance? What about maximizing disease prevention or early detection? While many of these questions have not yet been subject to careful scientific scrutiny, some have, and we review that research here.

NEW EMPHASIS ON HEALTH PROMOTION

There is a growing emphasis in the United States on disease prevention and health promotion. Americans have become more health conscious during the past 25 years. Attention to exercise and diet was less relevant in days past when work was largely physical in nature, taking up most of the waking hours of the day, and food came mostly out of the garden or field. As we have moved from an agricultural country to a largely technological, white-collar society where people are employed in sedentary types of work and eat at fast-food restaurants, work-related exercise and consumption of fresh vegetables, fruits, and whole grains have declined.

As medical knowledge has increased and become disseminated widely through the media, we have also become more aware of the negative effects of sedentary living, high serum cholesterol levels, and obesity. An increase in leisure time has allowed for nonwork-related exercise and for education about the health benefits of a balanced diet, abstinence from cigarette smoking, and temperate use of alcohol. Maintaining youth and health, in fact, has now become a national obsession. *Prevention* magazine, *Health* magazine, *Fitness* magazine, and *Cooking Light* magazine are only a few of several popular journals that focus on disease prevention and health promotion. Many online news programs (*Health News on the Web*), radio programs (*Here's to Your Health, Health Watch*), and even cable television channels (Kaleidoscope's *Health, Wellness, and Ability*) focus on health.

Furthermore, the increasing cost of health care—national health expenditures to skyrocket from $1.1 trillion to $2.1 trillion in less than 10 years—and diminishing resources with which to provide health services have forced Americans to realize that they may not always have unlimited access to health care. This has motivated many to want to stay healthy to reduce their need for health services. In order to obtain affordable health insurance coverage, many Americans have joined managed care or health maintenance organizations (HMOs). Even Medicare patients are now rapidly joining HMOs to reduce their costs and to increase their coverage. In 1998, 6 million older Americans had joined HMOs, and others were joining at a rate of 70,000 a month (Editorial, 1998a). Increasing health care costs, however, have caused HMOs to cut services for many older Americans, forcing many back into the old system, which is expanding rapidly beyond its capacity (Pear, 1999). In order to survive, HMOs must emphasize health promotion, since it is much less expensive to prevent disease than to treat it. Thus, there are growing incentives for both the U.S. populace and the nation's health care system to keep Americans healthy and disease free.

Advances in medical science are helping us in this battle by increasing our knowledge about health and about ways to maintain it. Science has also provided us with screening tools that detect many diseases in their early stages, which will lead to more effective management, increased probability of cure, and, ultimately, lower costs of treatment. Screening now exists for early detection of cancers of the prostate (digital examination, blood screening for prostate-specific antigen), breast (self examination, mammography), colon and rectum (digital examination, sigmoidoscopy, fecal blood test), cervix (Pap smear), lung (chest x-ray, sputum test), oropharynx (examination by dentist or physician), and skin and testes (examination by physician). Screening tests also exist for blood pressure, serum cholesterol, diabetes, and emotional disorders such as depression. Given the rising costs of health care, it is essential to identify and take advantage of whatever resources exist in our communities that might help prevent illness, promote health, and facilitate early detection and timely treatment of disease.

RELIGION AND DISEASE PREVENTION

How might religion influence activities designed to promote health, prevent disease, and facilitate early detection? As we saw in chapter 24, religious persons are more likely to live healthy lifestyles. They are less likely to smoke, abuse alcohol, use illicit drugs, and engage in risky sexual practices or other hazardous behaviors. Some religious groups eat healthier diets, and have lower serum cholesterol levels, and they may even exercise more regularly than the general population. Obesity, however, appears to be a problem in members of most religious groups in the United States, and some religious groups do not emphasize exercise and healthy diets. Is there any other evidence from systematic research that religious persons are at lower risk of contracting physical disease, or are more likely to have disease detected and treated sooner?

Risk of Disease

Are religious persons more or less susceptible to disease? Kuemmerer and Comstock (1967) examined a population-based sample of 7,787 junior and senior high school students in Washington County, Maryland, for tuberculosis (TB). Nearly 4% of students had positive tests; 105 had large reactions, and 197 had small reactions. These students were compared with a random sample of 414 nonreactors from the sample. The frequency of large reactions was greater among children whose parents attended church less than once per month than among those whose parents went to church more often. The researchers did not present any statistics, although the association was apparently significant (but not controlled).

Although many possible explanations exist for this now rather dated finding, it suggests that the likelihood of contracting tuberculosis (as evidenced by "large reactions" to TB skin testing) was higher among students whose families were less involved in religion. Although socioeconomic and racial factors were not controlled, one would expect this bias to further increase the strength of the association, since poor families and African Americans are both more likely to be religious and at higher risk for infectious diseases like TB. Much of the research summarized in chapter 25 indicates that greater religiousness reduces the risk of disease, especially those conditions brought on by psychosocial stress and negative health behaviors.

Knowledge about Health Maintenance

Does religion affect attitudes toward and knowledge about health maintenance activities? Apel (1986) examined attitude toward health and retirement among 246 Lutherans who were living in the midwestern United States. Positive attitudes toward retirement were more common among more frequent church attenders, who also had more positive attitudes about the functional worth and capability of retired persons. Active church members also were significantly more knowledgeable about health maintenance

than were less active church members. Involvement in a religious community is often associated with having more social contacts outside the religious community as well as within it (Strawbridge, Cohen, et al., 1997). Greater social contact with family and nonfamily members increases opportunities for communication of information and knowledge, especially about health-related issues.

Disease Screening

Are religious persons more likely to participate in health screening programs? Naguib, Geiser, et al. (1968) conducted a case control study of 2,612 white women ages 30–45 who were living in rural Washington County. Subjects were mailed self-use pipettes for cervical cancer screening. Women who used and returned the pipettes ($n = 1,970$) were more likely to be members of religious and social organizations than were those who did not use the pipettes ($n = 642$) (45% vs. 30%). Atheists and persons without a religious affiliation were significantly less likely to participate (54% vs. 75% for the overall sample). Among Christians, survey participation was directly related to frequency of church attendance; women who attended church once a week or more had a participation rate of 81%, compared to 60% for women who never attended church. Sociodemographic factors, however, were not controlled in these analyses.

Murray and McMillan (1993) examined the social and behavioral predictors of women's cancer screening practices in Northern Ireland. Surveying a sample of 391 adults, the investigators found that 28% performed breast self-examinations (BSE) regularly, 28% performed them occasionally, and 44% performed them not at all. BSE performance was predicted by several factors, including religious affiliation; women affiliated with the Church of Ireland (Anglicans) were more likely to perform BSE than were other women. To what extent other sociodemographic factors may have confounded this association is again unclear.

Miller and Champion (1993) examined factors that predisposed and enabled women to obtain mammograms. Their subjects were 151 women over age 50 from four urban churches in Indiana. Over 80% reported having had at least one mammogram, and 24% had followed frequency of mammography screening guidelines for the previous three years. Among the factors associated with having had a mammogram and for adherence to the guidelines was religion. Catholic women were nearly six times more likely than Protestants to have followed the recommended mammography guidelines for the past three years ($p = .01$, from logistic regression). Catholics had higher income and education levels than Protestants, although these variables were controlled for in the regression model.

Recall from chapter 4 that Lannin and colleagues (1998) from Eastern Carolina University explored the reasons that African American women have higher breast cancer mortality than white women. Comparing 540 patients with newly diagnosed breast cancer with 414 control women matched by age, race, and area of residence, the investigators found that "cultural beliefs" were a significant predictor of late-stage cancer at diagnosis (stage III or IV). Among these fundamentalist religious beliefs was the belief that "The devil can cause a person to get cancer" and "If a person prays about cancer, God will heal it without medical treatments." Investigators concluded that socioeconomic and cultural beliefs accounted for the delay in diagnosis among African American women. These findings suggest that religious beliefs may actually delay breast cancer diagnosis.

As noted before, however, a careful look at the data raises questions about such a conclusion. While fundamentalist religious beliefs were univariately related to late cancer stage at diagnosis, the investigators did not report whether religious beliefs had an independent effect on stage of diagnosis after race, education, and socioeconomic factors were taken into account. Recall that fundamentalist religious beliefs are much more common among African Americans, the uneducated, and the poor, all of whom are also at greater risk for late-stage diagnosis. While "cultural factors" did independently predict late-stage diagnosis after other variables were taken into account, fundamental-

ist religious beliefs were only two of 24 variables that were combined into a single variable labeled "cultural factors." This study, then, does not tell us what effect fundamentalist religious belief by itself has on stage of diagnosis when other variables, such as race and socioeconomic status, are controlled. Furthermore, other qualitative studies have not found that religious beliefs delay breast cancer diagnosis in African American women (Facione & Giancarlo, 1998; Fox et al., 1998).

For example, Fox et al. (1998) conducted a telephone survey of 1,517 members of 45 Christian churches in Los Angeles County to determine key predictors of whether women seek breast cancer screening. The subjects were women ages 50–80 with low to moderate incomes (or less than a high school education); 31% were African American, 21% were Hispanic, and 43% were white. Most (96%) reported that they attended church at least once a month and 61% were active in church at least once a month. Seventy-nine percent of women who were active in church (once a month or more) followed the guidelines for clinical breast exam compared to 68% of women who were less active in church ($p < .001$); 63% of those active in church adhered to the guidelines for having mammograms (had had a mammogram within the past 24 months and within the 24-month period) compared to 50% for those who were not ($p < .001$). Among subjects who indicated they were very or extremely religious, 76% had regular clinical breast exams and 59% had regular mammograms, compared to 72% and 54%, respectively, of those who were "less religious" ($p < .05$). Multivariate logistic regression was used to control for seven sociodemographic characteristics (age, race, income, education, health status, marital status, depression status) and three physician characteristics (years with same physician, race of physician, enthusiasm of physician about mammography). Controlling for these variables weakened the association between adherence and religious variables to nonsignificance. Some of the control variables, such as depression, however, could have been "explanatory variables" (i.e., helped to explain how religious involvement might increase adherence).

The investigators also compared mammography adherence rates in their church member sample with mammography adherence rates in another community population, a random sample of 510 African American, Hispanic, and white women ages 50–80 who were residing in Los Angeles County (Behavioral Risk Factor System, or BRFS data). In this sample, of 11% of the women were African American, 25% were Hispanic, and 52% were white. Comparing adherence rates between members of the church sample and the BRFS sample for those with incomes below $10,000 per year, the researchers found that mammography adherence for church members was 75%, compared to 60% for the community sample. For those with incomes of more than $10,000 per year, the figures were closer (86% vs. 81%, respectively). Investigators concluded that frequent church attendance, particularly among low-income women, contributes to greater adherence to mammography screening guidelines.

Health Promotion Programs in Churches

In the Fox et al. (1998) study, 72% of church members strongly endorsed the inclusion of health committees within their churches. A number of churches in the United States have developed health promotion programs to increase screening and encourage health behaviors that might prevent disease. A few reports have reviewed these programs in detail. One of the first programs was described by Saunders and Kong (1983), who reported their three-year experience establishing church-based hypertension screening and education programs in 10 medium-size to major U.S. cities. Not long thereafter, Hatch et al. (1984) reported on a project that involved the General Baptist Convention of North Carolina. In their report, they described health promotion clinics that were set up in low-cost, high-access community churches. Such clinics, working with local physicians and medical centers, could have great potential for improving disease detection and long-term treatment compliance in African American and other minority populations.

Saunders and Kong (1983) offer five reasons for the effectiveness of church-based hypertension programs: (1) churches can offer ongoing high blood pressure education and screening to members over time; (2) lay persons with limited education can be effectively trained to measure blood pressure, provide education, refer to medical professionals, and monitor and follow up on treatments initiated; (3) difficult-to-reach members of the population, especially older African American women, often attend church; (4) physicians can accept referrals from church centers and use them to monitor their patients; and (5) persons in the program who are trained to measure and monitor blood pressure can offer services not only in their churches but also to persons in their neighborhoods.

Lasater et al. (1986) described a large-scale research project (an extension of the Pawtucket Heart Health Program) in which church volunteers grouped into task forces helped other church members change their behavior to reduce their cardiovascular risk factors (smoking, elevated blood pressure, elevated serum cholesterol, excess weight, physical inactivity). The task forces were composed of volunteers specifically responsible for the overall management and coordination of the Health and Religion Program (HARP) in their church. Twenty churches were recruited throughout Rhode Island and were randomly assigned to one of five experimental conditions: presence of task forces and high professional involvement, absence of task forces and high professional involvement, presence of task forces and low professional involvement, absence of task forces and low professional involvement, and a no-treatment control group. While Lasater and colleagues described the methodology and implementation of HARP, they presented no results on effectiveness, and we could locate no subsequent published reports.

Davis et al. (1994) examined the efficacy of a church-based model designed to improve access to and participation in a cervical cancer program among underserved minority women in Los Angeles County. Of the 24 churches chosen, 96% ($n = 23$) participated. Approximately 80% of the churches organized support structures to provide child care, buses, and

lunches for families that were attending education and screening sessions. A total of 1,012
women ages 21–89 attended educational classes,
of whom 44% (n = 445) were targeted for
screening since they either hadn't had a Pap
screening over the past two years or had never
been screened. Approximately 85% (372/445)
of these subjects were recruited; most of these
were Hispanic women (who were more than
four times more likely than African Americans
not to have had Pap smear in the past two years).
The investigators concluded that church-based
health screening programs were particularly
useful for serving minority populations, such
as underserved Hispanic women. Scandrett
(1994) discusses further the role of the African
American church as a participant in community
health interventions, particularly the fostering
of health promotion activities and education
programs on nutrition, AIDS, sexuality, drug
use, and mental illness.

Whether or not religiousness is associated
with a greater likelihood of disease screening,
developing health programs in churches may
be an excellent way to provide screening and
education to members of the population who
are particularly hard to reach (e.g., minority
groups, the poor, the elderly).

COMPLIANCE WITH MEDICAL TREATMENTS

In this section, we turn to the topic of compliance. Compliance is defined as the extent to
which a person's behavior coincides with recommended medical care or advice. Noncompliance, then, may be defined as the patient's failure to comply with the regimen prescribed by
his physician. Before we examine the relationship between religion and medical compliance,
we review the seriousness and the incidence
of noncompliance and what psychological and
social factors influence it.

The Problem of Noncompliance

Between 6% and 20% of patients fail to redeem
their prescriptions, and 30–50% delay or drop
doses of medication (Giuffrida & Torgerson,

1997). Noncompliance with long-term medication regimens occurs in about 50% of persons
of different ages, races, and social backgrounds
(Sackett & Snow, 1979). In a study of 220 outpatients age 60 or over, researchers found that 60%
took their medications incorrectly, averaging
2.6 mistakes per patient; 40% of these mistakes
were potentially serious (*Merck Manual of Geriatrics*, 1995, p. 443). Noncompliance takes many
forms, including the failure to take a medication
as prescribed, premature discontinuation of a
medication, use of the medication at the wrong
time, excessive consumption of the medication,
and use of medications not currently prescribed.
Noncompliance involves more than simply not
taking medication as prescribed. It also includes
failure to keep medical appointments, failure to
comply with suggested health-promoting behaviors, and other intentional or unintentional devi-
ances from a prescribed treatment regimen.
Noncompliance with medical appointments, for
example, varies between 19% and 28% (Giuffrida & Torgerson, 1997).

Consequences of Noncompliance

Approximately one-third of persons who do not
comply with medication regimens experience
health problems as a result. At least 10% of
acute hospital admissions and 25% of nursing
home admissions are due to noncompliance
with medication regimens (Berg et al., 1993);
at least one-third of acute hospital admissions
for congestive heart failure (this country's largest
DRG group) is a result of noncompliance with
dietary and medication guidelines (Vinson et
al., 1990). Similarly, only 29% of the 50 million
persons in the United States with hypertension
have their blood pressures controlled to less
than 90/140, largely because they do not comply with medication regimens. In fact, noncompliance costs our health care system more than
$100 billion each year in lost productivity and
in preventable hospital admissions (National
Pharmaceutical Council, 1992).

Factors That Influence Compliance

Compliance is a complex behavior that is influenced by many factors, including the attitudes

and beliefs of the patient, the environment in which the patient lives (especially the social environment), the patient's interaction with health care professionals, and the overall health care system (Miller, Hill, et al., 1997). Factors that increase noncompliance with medication, for example, include being required to take a large number of medications, having visual or cognitive impairment, experiencing side effects from the treatment, having limited income, experiencing poor communication with one's physician, being isolated socially, and lacking motivation to comply.

Beliefs also influence compliance, particularly the beliefs that the disease is serious and that the medication is an effective treatment for the disease (Stewart & Caranosos, 1989). If the patient feels her illness is a medical problem, then she will seek and comply with medical treatments. If, on the other hand, the patient decides her problem is psychological or spiritual, she will seek psychological or spiritual treatments in preference to medical treatments. If the physician is insensitive to the patient's understanding of her problem and prescribes a medical treatment for a problem that the patient has decided is psychological or spiritual, then she is likely not to comply.

Depression.   Just as beliefs can influence motivation to comply, emotional disorders such as depression can likewise affect treatment adherence, particularly if compliance takes a lot of effort (e.g., ingesting multiple medications several times per day, participating in rehabilitation that requires energy and endurance, remembering and getting to multiple doctor visits). Depression causes a loss of interest, a decrease in energy, impairment of concentration, and reduction in motivation to care for oneself. Not surprisingly, then, depression has been shown to adversely affect compliance among patients with many different disorders, including coronary artery disease (Blumenthal, Williams, et al., 1982; Carney, Rich, et al. 1982; Dunbar, 1990; Carney, Freedland, et al., 1995), multiple sclerosis (Mohr et al., 1997), HIV infection (Singh, Squie, et al., 1996), chronic renal failure (Sensky, Leger, et al., 1996), and asthma (Bosley et al., 1995).

For example, Blumenthal, Williams. et al. (1982) prospectively followed 35 consecutive patients to determine the physiological and psychological predictors of compliance with exercise therapy among patients who were recovering from myocardial infarction (MI). Patients underwent comprehensive physical and psychological assessments at entry into the cardiovascular rehabilitation program and were followed for a year. Of the 35 patients, 14 dropped out. The dropouts were found to be more depressed, hypochondriacal, anxious and socially introverted and had lower ego strength than those who remained in the program. Likewise, Carney, Freedland, et al. (1995) found that medication compliance (defined as adherence to a twice-per-day regimen of low-dose aspirin to reduce risk of MI) by 10 patients with major depression was significantly less than that among 45 patients without major depression. Compliance with medication regimens was assessed for three weeks through an electronic monitoring device. Depressed patients adhered to the aspirin regimen on 45% of days, and the nondepressed complied on 69% of days ($p < .02$).

Mohr et al. (1997) found that, among 85 patients with multiple sclerosis who took interferon β-1b, patients who experienced depression were more likely to discontinue the medication than were nondepressed patients. Among patients who reported new or increased depression, 86% of those treated for the depression (with psychotherapy or with antidepressants medication) continued their treatment with interferon β-1b, compared to 38% of depressed patients who were untreated ($p = .003$). It is evident from these and other studies that depression interferes with treatment compliance and that factors that reduce depression (e.g., greater social support, more coping resources) will increase compliance.

Social Support.   When people have concerned relatives or friends who inquire about their medication or treatment regimen or who remind them to adhere to that regimen, the likelihood of compliance increases (Daltroy & Godin, 1989). Research has shown that a simple telephone call to a patient may provide sufficient encouragement to substantially increase compliance (Bond & Monson, 1984; Taylor et al., 1990). Social isolation, on the other hand, is associated with lower rates of compliance for a number of reasons, including both lack of reminders and reduced motivation to comply (because of lack of emotional support) (Blumenthal, Williams, et al., 1982). Many studies have demonstrated a positive association between social support and compliance in a variety of populations and disease conditions.

Burroughs et al. (1997) reviewed 32 studies that examined the relationship between social support and treatment adherence in adolescents with insulin-dependent diabetes and found largely a positive relationship. Crane (1996) reported that nonadherence after abnormal Pap test results was as high as 40%. In a sample of 498 women, he found that adherence was related to numerous measures of social support, including receipt of any social support, receipt of each of three types of social support (informational, emotional, intangible), amount of support received, satisfaction with support, and source of support. Among African American women, emotional support was strongly related to adherence, whereas, among Latino women, tangible support was the strongest predictor of compliance. The investigator concluded that supportive interventions such as provision of medical information, emotional support, child care, and transportation could help decrease noncompliance.

Studying sources of social support, universal self-care, and self-care behaviors, Wang and Fenske (1996) found that noninsulin-dependent diabetics who received support from *friends* in addition to family reported higher universal and self-care health behaviors than did those without such support. Investigators concluded that nonfamily support can be particularly helpful in promoting medical compliance and self-care. On the other hand, Doherty et al. (1983) found that social support from wives was significantly related to medication compliance among 150 middle-aged men ages 40–65 who were participating in the Coronary Primary Prevention Trial at the University of Iowa's Lipid Research Clinic. The researchers assessed spousal support by interviewing patients, spouses, and clinic staff. The sample was divided into thirds, with high and low spousal support groups compared on adherence to medication regimens. Among the high support group ($n = 28$), 96% of the subjects complied; among the low support group ($n = 29$), 70% complied ($t = 3.64$, $p < .001$). Investigators concluded that social support enhances compliance with medication, particularly if that support comes from a spouse.

Kulik and Mahler (1993) studied social support as a predictor of compliance among 85 male patients one, four, and 13 months after coronary artery bypass surgery and found that higher levels of social support significantly and independently predicted higher compliance with behaviors recommended by physicians (ambulating and not smoking). Finally, Garay-Sevilla et al. (1995) examined factors associated with adherence to diet and medication in 200 noninsulin-dependent diabetic patients in Leon, Mexico. Greater social support was associated with greater adherence to dietary restrictions ($p = .007$) and medication ($p = .002$). Regardless of the particular disease condition, then, social support seems to increase the likelihood of compliance with medical advice.

RELIGION AND COMPLIANCE

There are several reasons that religion might influence medical compliance. These include religion's impact on patients' beliefs about the cause of illness, on their ability to cope with illness, on the social support network available to patients, and on patients' attitudes toward compliance in general.

First, religion influences beliefs about the cause of illness. As noted earlier, if patients believe that spiritual factors (e.g., sin, demons) cause illness, they may seek spiritual cures and value them over medical treatments. This may reduce their motivation to comply with medical treatments offered by doctors or cause them to reject the treatments entirely. We saw in chapter 4 some of the negative health consequences that can result from rigid belief systems that favor religious methods over traditional health care. We also saw, however, that most persons in the United States believe in naturalistic mechanisms of disease and use spiritual treatments to complement rather than replace traditional medical therapies.

Second, we have seen in chapters 5, 6, 7, and 9 that religious beliefs and practices help people to cope better with physical disease and disability, particularly when illness is chronic. Chronically ill persons with devout religious commitment are both less likely to become depressed and more likely to recover quicker from depression when it occurs. Religion helps the chronically ill to deal better with suffering and maintain hope, which increases motivation for recovery and helps generate the energy to work toward that goal. Consequently, religious beliefs may counteract the negative effects that discouragement and depression have on compliance.

Third, it is clear that religious persons, particularly those actively involved in a religious community, have larger and more satisfying social support networks than do nonreligious people (see chapter 15). Church members may provide transportation for doctors' visits and encourage compliance with medical treatments. This increased surveillance makes it more difficult for chronically ill church members to neglect themselves. Likewise, religious beliefs and practices may influence marital and family stability (see chapter 13), increasing the likelihood that family members will be available to remind and encourage the person to take her medications and keep her medical appointments. These factors, acting together, can influence compliance in a powerful way.

Fourth, religious persons may be more likely to comply because of their general attitude toward compliance. The religious tend to be low risk takers and are less likely to rebel against authority. They tend to hold more conservative values, follow societal rules (such as keeping appointments), and adhere to the advice of experts or authorities (such as physicians). The Jewish holy man Ben Sira, writing in the third century B.C., remarked that physicians acted according to God's will: "Honor a physician with the honor due to him for the uses which you may have of him, for the Lord created him. . . . The Lord created medicines out of the earth, and he who is wise will not abhor them" (Dorff, 1998).

To what extent have systematic studies demonstrated that religious persons are more compliant with medical treatments? In a review of the compliance literature, Marston (1970), not surprisingly, concluded that "few studies have been concerned with the relationship between religion and (treatment) compliance" (p. 317). While again the research is very limited, we review studies that have addressed this issue.

Religious Belief about Illness Causation and Compliance

Foulks et al. (1986) studied compliance with outpatient treatment among 60 psychiatric patients who received their initial intake evaluation at the University of Pennsylvania Hospital and Clinics. The participants had a mean age of 29; 68% were female, 29% were nonwhite, and 15% were psychotic. Subjects completed the Cause of Illness Inventory, which included 18 medical model items and 17 nonmedical model items, including the following four religious items: "God's will," "having been hexed or given an evil eye," "having committed too many sins," and "being out of grace." Two measures of compliance were collected from the clinical record after the patients ended their care at the clinic. First, investigators assessed the nature of the patient's termination of treatment (abruptly left treatment without discussion with the therapist, discussed termination with the therapist and terminated against advice, or after the therapist and the patient agreed to termination). Second, investigators determined the number of total visits to the clinic before termination occurred. Results showed that the four religious items were among the top seven nonmedical causes given for illness (10% God's will, 4% sins, 3% hex or evil eye, 2% being out of grace).

Multivariate statistical analyses revealed that the strongest predictor of both number of visits made to clinic and type of termination was the number of nonmedical items endorsed ($t = -2.64$, $p < .01$ for visits, and $t = -2.91$, $p < .01$ for termination). Those who endorsed more nonmedical causes for their illness (including religious reasons) were significantly less likely to comply with the therapist's recommendations. Unfortunately, the investigators did not look at the effects of religious beliefs by themselves on compliance. Although religious beliefs were among the top seven nonmedical causes cited, they were still relatively infrequent (2–10%), particularly since the illnesses were psychiatric in nature. One might expect patients with *physical* diseases to be even less likely to attribute their illnesses to religious or spiritual factors. Nevertheless, these findings are notable.

Religious Affiliation and Compliance

Mayer et al. (1965) studied 193 patients who contacted the Peter Bent Brigham Hospital Alcoholism clinic and accepted intake appointments. About 62% kept their appointments, and 38% did not. The researchers examined the characteristics of the persons who did not show up for their appointments. None of the 11 patient characteristics collected during the initial contact predicted who would show up for appointments (including whether the patient was Catholic, Protestant, or Jewish).

O'Brien (1982), who examined the relationship between religiousness and compliance in 126 chronic hemodialysis patients, reported different results. Of the patients in the sample, 75% were African Americans, 69% were Protestant, 20% were Catholic, 6% were Jewish, and 5% reported no affiliation. Persons with no religious affiliation were the least compliant with their hemodialysis treatment regimen, whereas Catholics were the most compliant.

Chang, Uman, et al. (1985) examined the factors that influenced compliance with health care regimens among elderly women ages 56–89. Aspects of care (technical quality, psychosocial issues addressed, and patient participation) were captured by videotaping patients as they visited with a nurse practitioner. Eight videotapes were randomly selected and shown in 26 senior citizen nutrition centers in Los Angeles, California, to 286 elderly women (of whom 46% were Jewish and 51% were Catholic or Protestant). The women were asked how compliant they would have been if they had been the patient in the tape. Intent to adhere was measured by a five-item scale. Education, marital status, importance of examination, social network, patient satisfaction, and religious affiliation were also assessed. Results indicated that technical quality, psychosocial care, and patient participation were not significant predictors of intent to adhere after the effects of the covariates were controlled. Intent to adhere was significantly predicted by marital status (2.8% of explained variance), religious affiliation (1.3%), importance of exam (2%), social network (4.6%), and preexisting satisfaction (1%). Jewish religious affiliation was associated with a significantly greater intent to adhere.

In an earlier study, Archer et al. (1967) also found that Jews were more likely to continue participating in a treatment regimen (i.e., were more compliant) in a study that examined the relationship between diet and coronary artery disease. This 18-month prospective study evaluated 757 men who were enrolled in a coronary heart disease study in New York City. The social characteristics of the 415 dropouts were compared with those of the 342 active participants. No significant relationship was found between religious attendance and participation. Jews were more likely to be active study participants than study dropouts (83.5% active vs. 77.5% inactive) than were Catholics (6.8% active vs. 12.4% inactive) or Protestants (8.5% active vs. 8.6% inactive) ($p < .02$). Investigators noted that "Jews were highly cosmopolitan, a trait associated with a more scientific attitude and with a consequently greater tendency to remain in the study" (p. 30).

Thus, studies of the relationship between compliance and religious affiliation report mixed results; some studies show no difference between religious groups, whereas other studies show higher compliance rates among Catholics and still others find higher compliance rates among Jews.

Religiousness and Compliance

Studies that examine religious affiliation provide little information about how religious involvement affects compliance. Does level of religious participation or religious commitment influence medical compliance? The results here are a bit more consistent.

Compliance with Medical Regimen. In her study of chronic hemodialysis patients, O'Brien (1982) examined the relationship among compliance, religious attendance, and perceptions of the usefulness of religion for coping with end-stage renal disease. Those who attended church infrequently were found to have worse compliance with their hemodialysis treatment regimens than were frequent attenders. Similarly, patients who indicated that religion had no relationship to their adjustment to illness were also the least compliant with their treatment regimen. Recall that Blumenthal, Williams, et al. (1982) found that noncompliance with prescribed exercise therapy regimens among patients who were recovering from myocardial infarction was related to depression, hypochondriasis, anxiety, and social introversion, characteristics that are less common among the religious. On the other hand, Archer et al. (1967) found no relationship between religious attendance and dropout rate in a study of compliance with treatment for coronary artery disease in their largely Jewish sample.

Harris et al. (1995) examined religion's influence on treatment compliance in 40 adult heart transplant patients (80% were male, 80% were white, 55% were Protestant, and 40% were Catholic). Subjects were interviewed two months, seven months, and 12 months after transplant at a university medical center in Pennsylvania. Investigators found that religious factors at baseline predicted outcomes 12 months later. Having strong religious beliefs was related to less physical dysfunction ($r = -.36$, $p < .05$), less anxiety ($r = -.28$), fewer health worries ($r = -.39$, $p < .05$), and less difficulty with the posttransplant medical regimen ($r = -.37$, $p < .05$). Similarly, frequency of prayer and activity in church congregation were both related to reduced difficulty with the posttransplant medical regimen ($r = -.33$, $p < .05$, and $r = -.30$, $p < .10$). The degree to which a person consulted God when making important decisions also predicted better physical functioning and less difficulty with the medical regimen ($r = -.44$, $p < .01$) 12 months postsurgery.

Koenig, George, Cohen, et al. (1998b) examined the relationship between religious activity and compliance with medications taken for high blood pressure in 3,963 randomly selected persons age 65 or over who were participating in the Duke EPESE project. Among subjects who reported that they had been told by a doctor that they had high blood pressure, those who attended religious services at least once per week were significantly more likely to be taking medication for high blood pressure than were persons who attended religious services less frequently (84.9% vs. 79.8%, $p = .01$), a difference that remained significant after researchers adjusted for covariates.

Compliance with Substance Abuse Rehabilitation. Christo and Franey (1995) prospectively studied 101 poly-drug users (mean age 31) who were living in London. At the six-month follow-up, 90% of the sample was reassessed. Spiritual beliefs were measured by a seven-item Spiritual Beliefs Questionnaire that carefully avoided the mention of God, Jesus, or church, assessing instead strength from religious and spiritual beliefs, belief in psychic or spiritual healers, belief in extrasensory perception, belief in the usefulness of prayer, and belief in life after death. Spiritual beliefs significantly predicted location at follow-up (whether or not in treatment) ($F = 4.3$, $p < .007$), which in turn significantly predicted drug use. Similarly, Desmond and Maddux (1981) conducted a prospective study of 248 heroin addicts who were participating in a religious rehabilitation program (87% were Hispanic; the mean age was 26; subjects had used opioid for an average of 8 years). Over a 12-year period, only 11% of the subjects entered religious programs. Among those who did, 45.5% (15/33) remained abstinent for a year or more, markedly exceeding the 5.7% (56/979) who remained in conventional treatment programs.

Thus, although the research database is limited, it appears that a high degree of religiousness and spirituality predicts better compliance with treatment regimens in persons with chronic medical or substance abuse problems. This is what we would expect, given the relationship between religion and known psychosocial predictors of compliance. Despite the substantial public health implications of such research, well-designed studies have not yet specifically examined the relationship between religiousness and medical compliance. Investigations that utilize multidimensional measures of religious activity and intrinsic religious commitment, carefully quantifying "exposure" to the religious variable over the lifetime of the individual and relating this to compliance with medications, outpatient medical visits, and prescribed healthy lifestyle changes, will be particularly useful.

SUMMARY AND CONCLUSIONS

Disease prevention and health promotion have become a high priority in the United States as demographic and economic forces stretch the capacity of our health care system to provide health services. Although greater religiousness is associated with fewer negative health behaviors, disease screening and health promotion have not until recently been much of a priority for churches. Over the past two decades, this has been slowly changing. A number of pilot projects, particularly in minority churches that serve hard-to-reach populations, have been undertaken to see what role the church might play in disease screening, health promotion, and support of medical compliance.

Noncompliance with medical treatment is a major problem in the United States, costing over $100 billion per year and causing much preventable morbidity and mortality. Psychosocial factors that affect compliance include beliefs about illness causation, presence or absence of depressive disorder that impairs motivation, and level of social support provided by family members and friends. Although religious beliefs may in certain populations and illness conditions worsen compliance, this is relatively rare. Religion should increase medical compliance for several reasons: religiousness is associated with lower rates of depression, greater hope, more stable families, and larger nonfamily social support networks, all of which are associated with better compliance. Nevertheless, few studies have directly examined the relationship between religion and compliance. In the limited work done thus far, religious affiliation has not been consistently related to compliance, although there is a tendency for Jews to be more compliant than members of other religious groups. High levels of religiousness or spirituality, regardless of religious affiliation, however, appear to be related to better compliance. The paucity of well-designed research studies that directly examine this relationship, however, weakens our ability to draw any clear conclusions.

27

Use of General Medical and Mental Health Services

A S WE POINTED OUT IN CHAP-
ter 24, the rising cost of health care
is requiring innovative solutions to
meet the need for (and to reduce the
use of) health services in the United States. In
the years ahead, we will not be able to sustain
indefinitely a $100 billion per year increase in
national health expenditures or a $20 billion
per year increase in Medicare expenditures. As
noted in chapter 26, an emphasis on self-care,
disease prevention, and health promotion may
help stem this tide of rising health care costs.
In this chapter, we look at the relationship between religious beliefs and practices and utilization of general medical and mental health services. First, we examine the characteristics of
persons most likely to use general medical services. We then theorize about the ways and the
reasons religion might affect service use and
review research that addresses such questions.
Second, we examine characteristics of persons

most likely to use mental health services and
review research on ways that religious beliefs
and practices affect the use of these services.

TYPES OF GENERAL
MEDICAL SERVICES

General medical services include outpatient
and inpatient services. Outpatient services
include visits to physicians (office, clinic, or
emergency room), visits to nonphysician health
providers (e.g., nurses, physical therapists, occupational therapists, social workers, chiroprac-
tors, podiatrists, dentists), and home health
visits (nurses, rehabilitation therapists, home
health aides). Inpatient services include acute
medical hospitalization, inpatient rehabilitation
services, and nursing home stays. Other medical
costs that may be incurred by inpatients or outpatients are those for therapeutic procedures,

diagnostic tests, medical equipment, assistive devices, and over-the-counter or prescription medications.

Of these services, the most expensive is acute medical hospitalization. Figure 27.1 illustrates the types of expenditures that make up the Medicare budget and allows for comparison of costs incurred from acute medical hospitalization, physician services, and nursing home services. Medicare pays very little of nursing home costs, which fall largely upon the shoulders of patients and family members and, when these resources are exhausted, Medicaid. It is not surprising, then, that great efforts by Medicare, private insurers, and managed care organizations are being made to limit the use of acute hospital services. Indeed, the cost of "high-tech" acute hospitalization dwarfs the costs of all other medical services combined.

FACTORS THAT AFFECT THE USE OF GENERAL MEDICAL SERVICES

While the strongest predictors of service use are type of medical illness, severity of illness, and access to medical services (including pres-

ence of health insurance or ability to pay for services), other biomedical and psychosocial factors also influence the volume of medical services that people use.

Biomedical Factors

Miller, Russell, et al. (1998) examined the influences of cigarette smoking, blood pressure, serum cholesterol levels, and chronic illness on frequency of acute hospital admission during a 12–16-year follow-up of a national U.S. sample of 6,461 adults age 45 or over. Investigators found that current cigarette smoking increased the risk of hospitalization by 17–34%, and high blood pressure did so by 25–28% for those ages 45–64 and 7–15% for persons ages 65 or older. Diabetes, chronic lung conditions, heart attack, peptic ulcer, and arthritis were each associated with an increased risk of acute hospitalization. Interestingly, four of the five chronic conditions noted frequently are at least in part caused by unhealthy habits and/or psychosocial stress.

Functional Disability. While functional disability is strongly correlated with medical illness, psychosocial factors also play a major role in

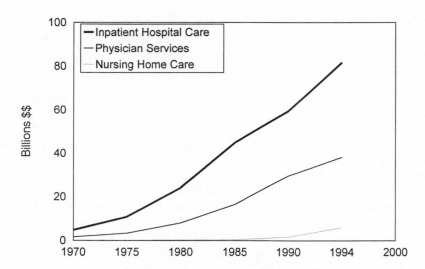

FIGURE 27.1 Medicare expenditures for selected health services in the United States since 1970. Source: *Health: United States 1995*. Department of Health and Human Services, National Center for Health Statistics. DHHS Pub. No. (PHS) 96-1232, Hyattsville, MD, May 1996, p. 263.

determining to what extent physical illness translates into functional disability. For any given level of objective physical illness, disability may range widely depending on how much emotional support the person has and how disabled the person believes he or she is. Meyers et al. (1989) reported that frequency of hospital admissions, length of hospital stays, and frequency of emergency room, outpatient clinic visits, and telephone contacts were all high among 87 independently living adults with spinal cord injury. Level of functional disability was especially predictive of emergency room visits. There is little doubt that *perceived* functional disability strongly predicts use of health services, particularly acute and chronic long-term hospitalization (Asberg, 1986).

Psychosocial Factors

Psychological and social factors also influence health service use. Personality or temperament influences both the perception of illness and behavioral responses to it. The emotionally sensitive, anxious, somatizing individual may readily perceive and worry about physical changes and thus have a low threshold for seeking medical attention. On the other hand, the phlegmatic person who is less emotional and harder to arouse may minimize or deny symptoms, seeking medical attention only when absolutely necessary.

Just as temperament can influence health service use, emotional disorder can likewise influence the threshold for seeking medical care. Persons with anxiety disorder may experience minor physical symptoms or even psychological symptoms as heralding a life-threatening medical condition and readily seek medical attention. Persons with somatization disorder may believe, in the absence of objective physical illness, that they have a physical problem that needs medical attention and repeatedly seek medical services despite reassurance and multiple negative physical examinations and diagnostic tests. Finally, persons with depression may deny or conceal even serious physical symptoms because they either lack motivation to seek services or have self-destructive impulses. Thus, they may delay seeking health care until ill-

nesses are advanced and require more expensive acute inpatient or emergency services, ultimately increasing health care costs beyond the level that would be necessary if the illness had been detected and treated at an early stage.

Anxiety. Souetre and associates (1994) reported that primary care patients with anxiety disorder were more likely to be hospitalized, have laboratory tests, and take medications than were emotionally healthy patients. The costs of acute hospitalization in this study accounted for more than 53% of direct health care costs. In a sample of 327 primary care patients, Simon and colleagues (1995) found that patients with anxiety or depressive disorders had markedly higher baseline costs ($2,390) than those with either subthreshold disorders ($1,098) or no disorder ($1,397). These large cost differences persisted after researchers adjusted for medical morbidity and were attributed to use of general medical services rather than mental health services. Anxiety tends to be energizing and motivating, creating a discomfort that demands relief. Because many of the symptoms of anxiety are similar to those of physical illness, patients often attribute these symptoms to medical causes. Katon and colleagues (1990) also reported that distressed high utilizers of health care frequently had diagnoses of major depression, dysthymic disorder, or generalized anxiety disorder. Patients with generalized anxiety disorder, in particular, may be prone to use general medical services (Carter & Maddock, 1992).

Depression. Studying an older population at high risk for service use, Callahan et al. (1994) followed 1,711 primary care patients (over age 60) for nine months. Patients with CES-D scores of 16 or higher had 38% more outpatient visits and 61% higher outpatient charges. Beekman et al. (1997) examined the effects of major depression on use of medical services by depressed elderly, controlling for potential confounders. Examining 646 persons ages 55–85 years in the Netherlands, these investigators found excess use of medical services among persons with major or minor depression. Greater functional disability among elderly depressed persons helped explain this excess use of health services.

In one of the largest studies to examine the effects of depression on cost of health services, Unutzer et al. (1997) conducted a four-year prospective study of 2,558 Medicare HMO enrollees age 65 or over, assessing depressive symptoms at baseline and two years and four years later. Cost of medical services was determined during the four-year follow-up period. During the year following the baseline survey, depressed patients were more likely to be admitted to the hospital and had more outpatient medical visits, more laboratory tests, more emergency apartment visits, more prescription medications, more ancillary medical visits, and more optometry visits. Subjects with significant depressive symptoms at baseline (CES-D score 16 or above) had a higher median cost of medical services over the four years than nondepressed subjects ($15,423 vs. $10,152) (i.e., a 50% increase in costs). After controlling for relevant factors (e.g., severity of medical illness) in a regression model, investigators found that for every one-point increase on the depression scale (which ranged from 0 to 60), there was a significant 1.9% increase in cost of medical services during the four-year follow-up (95% CI 1.4%–2.3%).

Koenig, Shelp, et al. (1989) compared the length of acute hospital stay in 41 depressed elderly medical inpatients with that for 41 nondepressed controls, matched by age, functional status, severity and type of medical illness, and extent of disease. Average length of hospital stay among depressed patients was 25 days, compared with 14 days for nondepressed patients ($p < .005$). Furthermore, during the five-month follow-up period after hospital discharge, depressed patients spent on average 16 days in the hospital, compared with seven days for nondepressed patients ($p < .05$). Thus, during the index hospitalization and the five-month follow-up period, patients with major depression spent on average 41 days in the hospital compared with 21 days for nondepressed patients with similar medical conditions.

More recently, these investigators examined depression and health service use in 542 patients age 60 or over who were hospitalized

on the medical services of a large university hospital (Koenig & Kuchibhatla, 1998). After controlling for age, sex, race, education, and severity of medical illness, the researchers found that severity of depressive symptoms significantly predicted number of days hospitalized in the past year, total days spent in the hospital or a nursing home, and number of medical outpatient visits in the past three months. Other studies have likewise reported that depressed medical patients (whether young or old) use large amounts of medical services, especially acute hospital services (Mechanic et al., 1982; Fulop et al., 1987; Levenson et al., 1990; Johnson, Weissman, et al., 1992; Verbosky et al., 1993; Simon et al., 1995; Levine et al., 1996).

How does depression cause increased use of health services? Depression may lead to or amplify physical symptoms such as pain, medication-related adverse side effects, or inadequate nutrition, all of which lead to increased use of general medical services. Alternatively, depression may delay diagnosis (because the patient lacks motivation for self-care), which ultimately leads to more expensive medical care, especially acute medical hospitalization. Once admitted to the hospital, these patients may need to stay much longer.

Marital Status. Joung et al. (1995) surveyed a probability sample of 2,662 persons ages 25–74 in the Netherlands, examining the relationship between marital status and utilization of health services. After controlling for multiple sociodemographic and health factors, investigators found that divorced persons were significantly more likely to be hospitalized than were married persons (OR 1.53, CI 1.03–2.22).

Social Support. Social support can reduce overall use of health services by several mechanisms. First, it may increase the likelihood of early detection and timely treatment, preventing diseases from advancing in severity and therefore requiring more expensive and invasive health services. Social contacts likely increase monitoring for health problems, provide support for seeking necessary medical services, and counteract the negative effects of depression on service use. Second, social support may provide an important resource for coping with the psychological stress and anxiety that leads to excessive use of health services.

Meyers et al. (1989) reported that lack of organizational memberships predicted frequent emergency room visits for 87 independently living adults with spinal cord injury. Pini et al. (1995) found that women who seek medical services at a general practice clinic reported more social problems than did women who were not seeking such services. Problems with spouse or partner were far more common among medical service users than among nonusers. Regression analysis demonstrated that problems relating to the spouse or partner doubled the likelihood that a person would seek medical services after physical health factors were taken into account. Likewise, Penning (1995), studying 1,284 noninstitutionalized adults age 60 or over who were living in Manitoba, Canada, reported an association between social support and lower use of medical services. Broadhead et al. (1989) examined the relationship between social support and medical care utilization in 343 family practice patients. Social support (high confidant support and high affective support) was associated with fewer hospital visits per year, lower charges per year, and shorter clinic visits. These findings persisted after researchers controlled for physical health and for seven demographic characteristics. They did find interactions with race, employment status, and gender. The impact of social support was strongest among whites, the unemployed, and women.

On the other hand, Williams et al. (1997) reported an association between low levels of social support and delay in seeking care among HIV-infected mothers. As indicated earlier, persons without strong social support systems are less likely to have persons to encourage them to seek needed health care services.

Psychosocial interventions have been shown to improve both health and cost outcomes (Sobel, 1995). Of particular interest is a clinical trial reported by Cronin et al. (1997) that examined the effects of providing a social support intervention on health care costs among persons with osteoarthritis. A total of 363 HMO members with osteoarthritis were randomly assigned to a social support intervention or to a control group. Health care utilization was assessed on study entry and after one year and two years. A savings of $1,156/participant/year was observed in the experimental group compared to the control group. The authors concluded that social support treatment was a cost-effective intervention. This study is particularly important because it demonstrates that adequate social support can actually reduce the cost of health care in persons with chronic health problems.

RELIGION AND USE OF GENERAL MEDICAL SERVICES

Religion may affect health service use in a number of ways. More than 25 years ago, David Mechanic (1972) pointed out that people's religious background can have a significant impact on their patterns of illness behavior and health service use. According to Donabedian and others, affiliation with certain religious groups may decrease health service use because a socio-organizational "lack of fit" places barriers that block access to services (Morrill & Erickson, 1968; Andersen & Newman, 1973; Donabedian, 1973). For example, certain religious groups may provide members with alternative treatments to medical care (prayer, ritual) and discourage use of traditional medical services.

Members of certain religious groups have an unusually high threshold for seeking traditional medical services. These groups inappropriately underutilize needed health care services, resulting in increased morbidity and mortality. For example, the Christian Science leader Nathan Talbot (1983) wrote in the *New England Journal of Medicine* that Christian Scientists are caring people, but that care includes treating sick children with prayer alone—even for serious conditions like leukemia, club feet, spinal meningitis, bone fracture, and diphtheria. Other examples of underutilization include avoidance of childhood immunizations (e.g., among the Orthodox Dutch Reformed groups in the Netherlands), avoidance of prenatal and obstetrical care (e.g., by the Faith Assembly group in Indiana), and a cessation of medication because one believes that one has been miraculously healed and no longer needs them (see chapter 4 for further discussion). Thus, some groups may use medical services at lower rates because of religious beliefs (1) that advocate religious healing practices and faith over secular medicine and (2) prioritize care of the spirit over care of the physical body. Such underutilization of medical services because of religious beliefs, however, is relatively rare in the United States, where most religious traditions encourage the use of necessary medical services.

Devout religiousness may also enhance physical health so that medical services are simply not needed. Religious groups frequently promote positive health behaviors, such as attention to diet, exercise, regular sleep and waking schedules, safe sexual practices, avoidance of alcohol, drugs, and cigarette smoking, and reduced risk-taking behaviors that lead to accidents (see chapter 24). Partly as a result of these positive health behaviors, religious persons have lower blood pressure, fewer strokes, possibly less coronary artery disease, stronger immune systems, lower rates of cancer, and less disability (see chapter 25).

Religious involvement may also reduce overutilization of expensive services. As indicated, persons who are depressed or anxious use more health services, especially acute hospital services, than do those without emotional problems. If religious beliefs and behaviors either prevent depression or speed its resolution (Pressman et al., 1990; Koenig, Cohen, Blazer, Pieper, et al., 1992; Kennedy, Kelman, et al., 1996; Kendler et al., 1997; Koenig, George, & Peterson, 1998), religion may positively impact the use of medical services (by either increasing use to a more appropriate level or decreasing it if it is inappropriately high). Also, as we saw earlier, greater social support may reduce the use of general medical services by persons with chronic illness (or, again, it may increase it to a more appropriate level). The strong link, repeatedly demonstrated, between religious activities and greater social support (Hatch, 1991; Ellison & George, 1994; Bradley, 1995; Idler & Kasl, 1997a) is another mechanism by which

religious activities may promote a more appropriate level of health service use.

Undoubtedly, mental illness, social support, and religion interact in their effects on health service use. Depressed persons who neglect their medical problems may be helped by regular visits from church members and by participation in church activities. This may counteract a natural tendency for depressed patients to socially isolate themselves, relieve their depression, and reduce the inappropriate use of costly medical services. In the same way, a strong religious faith may foster hope and motivate depressed persons to care for themselves and to reach out to others.

Thus, several plausible mechanisms exist by which religious beliefs and behaviors might influence the use of general medical services, particularly among medical patients who are high utilizers of health care services. Unfortunately, no studies have examined as their primary focus the relationship between religion and use of general medical services. Schiller and Levin (1988) reviewed 200 studies of the relationship between physical disease and religion and found 31 studies that evaluated religion and health care utilization (e.g., physician outpatient services, maternal and child health services, family planning services, pediatric services, psychiatric care, hospital services, and preventive services). In 24 of the 31 studies, a religious variable was significantly related to health service utilization. In all studies, religious variables were peripheral to the primary hypothesis, and the authors offered little explanation for their findings. We review some of these studies, as well as newer studies reported since that update.

RELIGIOUS AFFILIATION AND GENERAL MEDICAL SERVICE USE

Mechanic (1963) examined patterns of illness behavior in two studies that involved a total of 1,300 students at two universities, one a midwestern state university and the other a private university in the western United States. In the first study, he examined students' willingness to consult a physician in three hypothetical illness situations of increasing severity. In the second study, he examined the tendency to visit a physician among male freshmen at the private western university. In the first study, Jews ($n = 34$) were more likely to be in the "high" category for willingness to consult a physician than were Protestants ($n = 398$), those with no religious affiliation ($n = 47$), or Catholics ($n = 59$) (71% vs. 55% vs. 47% vs. 42%, respectively, $p < .05$, uncontrolled). In the second study, he found that Jews ($n = 125$) had a greater tendency to visit a physician than either Protestants ($n = 457$) or Catholics ($n = 159$) (57% vs. 39% vs. 41%, respectively, $p < .01$, uncontrolled). Mechanic concluded, "The 'near-compulsive' concern about health and illness in Jewish culture probably accounts in part for various trends that have been observed" (p. 206).

Wan and Yates (1975) used a multivariate approach to predict dental service utilization in 2,168 randomly selected households surveyed in a five-county area in New York and Pennsylvania. The annual number of dental visits per person per household by religious affiliation was 1.48 for those who chose "no response" ($n = 11$), 1.22 for Protestants ($n = 1,400$), 1.46 for Catholics ($n = 541$), 1.14 for those with "other" affiliations ($n = 202$), and 1.97 for Jews ($n = 14$). A multiple classification analysis adjusted for six covariates (urban-roll residents, residence duration, income, race, dentist/population ratio, social class) revealed that Jewish persons were still more likely to utilize dental services than were persons affiliated with other denominations.

Schiller and Levin (1988) reported findings from an Appalachian Mountain Area study of 909 adults living in an impoverished coal mining region. The authors assessed health care utilization (HSU) by measuring frequency of physician visits, length of time since most recent physician visit, length of time since most recent hospitalization, and length of stay during most recent hospitalization. The religious variables included religious affiliation (Baptist, Methodist, Presbyterian, Roman Catholic, Episcopalians, Mormon, Pentecostal/Holiness, and none). The authors reported no association between affiliation and any of the four HSU variables except length of hospital stay;

Baptists had the longest stay (9.4 days), and nonaffiliates ($n = 10$) had the shortest (3.5 days) ($p < .05$, uncontrolled). When analyses were controlled for age and education, the association lost statistical significance.

RELIGIOUS ACTIVITY AND GENERAL MEDICAL SERVICE USE

Severity of health problems may confound the relationship between religious activities and health service use, and this relationship may vary, depending upon the type of religious activity measured. As noted in previous chapters, frequency of church attendance may be influenced by the physical health of the individual; persons who are very sick and in need of extensive medical services may not be physically able to attend religious services. On the other hand, persons with severe medical illness often turn to religion or prayer as a means of coping with their medical condition (see chapter 5). The frequent use of prayer during illness was underscored in a recent national study published in the *New England Journal of Medicine*. Eisenberg et al. (1993) examined the use of unconventional therapies (UT) for health problems by surveying 1,539 adults of all ages by telephone. The researchers analyzed 16 commonly used health interventions and found that about 83% of participants both used UT and sought treatment from a medical doctor. Nearly 25% used prayer as an UT, which was second only to exercise (26%) in this study.

Thus, prayer and personal religiousness may be associated with more severe illness and greater use of health services, while attendance at religious services may be associated with better health and lower use of health services—influenced by the dynamic issues discussed earlier. Unfortunately, most studies in this area have not considered these complex interactions.

Increased Use of Services

Religious activity may be associated with higher use of medical services. While occasionally a religious person will substitute prayer for seeing a physician, the research suggests that most religious people combine prayer with traditional medicine. Bearon and Koenig (1990) surveyed 40 members drawn from the Duke University Aging Center subject registry (50% female, 53% African American, 100% Protestant), asking them what they thought caused their physical symptoms and illnesses and whether they had prayed about a physical symptom the last time they had it. About 26% agreed that sickness was a test of faith, 15% believed illness was sent as punishment for sin, and 33% believed illness was punishment for disobedience. Nearly 90% reported at least one symptom, with the average number being three, and 53% indicated they had prayed about the symptom. Low education and Baptist affiliation were associated with praying about a symptom. The subjects were more likely to have prayed about a symptom if they had discussed it with a physician or if they were taking medication for it.

In a related study, Trier and Shupe (1991) conducted a telephone survey of a random sample of 325 persons age 18 or older, selected from a metropolitan area in the Great Lakes region. The researchers examined the subjects' tendency to pray for health, their personal relationships, and their financial or material needs. They found that about one-third of the respondents used prayer to maintain their health and to cope with illness. The researchers then measured the subjects' frequency of church attendance, reading the Bible, praying, and watching religious television, as well as their degree of Christian orthodoxy (on the basis of a five-item scale). Frequency of prayer was positively correlated with all religious measures and with consulting a physician ($r = .15$, $p < .05$). Belief that prayer, apart from biomedical care, had helped with healing was also associated with consulting a physician ($r = .13$, $p < .05$), as in the Bearon-Koenig study. While it is likely that subjects prayed for only the more serious health problems (hence the positive association with consulting a physician), there is no indication that prayer or religious activity was substituted for traditional medical care; if anything, the opposite was true (possibly reflecting increased access to care).

In Schiller and Levin's (1988) study, described earlier, church membership, frequency of attendance, and holding a church office ("Are you a church officer?") were assessed along with religious affiliation. Regression analyses controlled for age, sex, race, education, health status, chronic disease status, health locus of control, and the three other indices of health service use. While church membership was unrelated to any of the four HSU variables, church attendance was positively related to number of physician visits (uncontrolled $r = .11$, $p < .01$). When other variables were controlled, however, the association lost its statistical significance ($\beta = .02$, $p = $ ns).

As noted, involvement in religious activities may increase social contacts and friendship networks, thereby increasing one's monitoring of health problems and increasing one's access to and use of health services. There are several ways by which religious organizations may increase access to appropriate and timely medical services. First, congregations can initiate disease screening and health promotion programs. These programs may include screening for cervical cancer, breast cancer, hypertension, hypercholesterolemia, or diabetes (see chapter 27). Second, "prayer chains" may alert members of the congregation that one of their own is having health problems and encourage them to check on the person to ensure that her spiritual and physical health care needs are met. Third, churches are increasingly involving themselves in parish nurse programs. A parish nurse is a member of the congregation (typically a registered nurse) who is employed by the church (sometimes with outside assistance from secular agencies) to provide health screening, education, referral, and follow-up (see chapter 29).

No Association

Levin and Markides (1985) examined the relationship among religious attendance, self-rated religiosity, disability days, and physician visits per year in 1,125 Mexican-Americans, most of whom were Catholic, in San Antonio, Texas. Participants reported the number of days spent in bed during the previous year because of sickness or injury, as well as the number of physician visits they had made that previous year. Overall, investigators found no significant relationship between religious attendance and either days of disability or number of physician visits. Among men ages 65–80 years, however, there was a nonsignificant trend toward fewer disability days and fewer physician visits among frequent church attenders. On the other hand, a significant positive relationship was found between number of disability days and self-rated religiousness among men ages 40–65 years; there was a similar but nonsignificant trend between self-rated religiousness and number of physician visits. Investigators concluded that there was little evidence to support the hypothesis that religious attendance or religiosity reduces use of health services among Mexican-Americans.

In a 14-month prospective study, Koenig (1995b) explored the relationship between religious coping (use of religious beliefs and activities to relieve psychological stress) and acute medical hospitalization in 97 medical inpatients identified as strong religious copers and 165 nonreligious copers. Compared to nonreligious copers, religious copers had a lower number of hospital readmissions per day of follow-up time (average 0.02 vs. 0.05 admissions/day, $p = .01$) and a lower number of hospital days per day of follow-up time (0.19 vs. 0.28 days/day, $p < .05$). These findings, however, were explained by the fact that religious copers were less likely than nonreligious copers to be lost to follow-up after their initial hospitalizations (6% vs. 14%). No independent association was founded between religious coping and use of acute hospital services. As discussed previously, these results may have been confounded by the sickest patients' (and those in need of the most hospital services) turning to religion for comfort and coping, thus nullifying or disguising any long-term positive effects that religious coping may have had on reducing their hospital use.

Decreased Use of Services

Religious activities may decrease use of health services by a number of the mechanisms described earlier (e.g., better health leading to decreased need for services and decreased over-utilization of health services). In Mechanic's study (1963), mentioned earlier, church attendance was inversely related to the tendency to visit a physician among a sample of male freshmen at a private western university. About 38% of persons who attended services every two weeks or more ($n = 425$) had a tendency to visit a physician, compared with 47% of those who attended about once per month ($n = 104$) and 48% of those who attended only a few times a year or less ($n = 225$) ($p < .05$, uncontrolled). When analyses were stratified by religious affiliation, however, the association held true only for Catholics.

Frankel and Hewitt (1994) examined religious involvement and use of health services in two groups of university students at the University of Western Ontario. Of the 299 participants, 172 were members of Christian clubs or faith groups, and 127 were sociology students unaffiliated with any Christian club on campus. The subjects were recruited during club meetings and sociology classes. The religiously affiliated group had fewer emergency room visits ($p < .02$), physician visits ($p = .04$), walk-in clinic visits ($p = .05$), and dentist visits ($p < .02$) and spent fewer days in the hospital ($p < .01$). Compared to nonaffiliated students, religiously affiliated students were slightly older (23 vs. 22 years), were more likely to be employed full time (11% vs. 2%), had lower family incomes ($40,000–60,000 vs. $60,000–75,000), lived closer to home (61% of affiliated students lived within 1 hour vs. 47% of nonaffiliated students), and were more likely to be affiliated with conservative Protestant groups (rather than mainline Protestant). None of these differences explained the observed differences in health service use.

In Schiller and Levin's (1988) study, described earlier, after researchers controlled for other variables, they found that those subjects who held church offices reported longer time lapses since their most recent hospitalization ($\beta = .40$, $p < .01$) and shorter hospital stays ($\beta = -1.92$, $p < .01$). The authors concluded that "perhaps only the sturdiest and most energetic congregants become deacons, elders, ushers, etc." (p. 1375).

Pressman and colleagues (1990) studied rehabilitation progress in 30 hospitalized elderly women with hip fractures. They found that degree of religiousness (measured by church attendance, perceived religiousness, and use of religion as a source of strength and comfort) predicted lower depression scores and ability to walk longer distances at discharge; information on whether there was also an association with length of hospital stay was not reported.

In one of the largest projects to specifically examine the association between religious activity and use of acute inpatient hospital services, Koenig and Larson (1998) studied 542 patients (age 60 or over) consecutively admitted to the Duke University Medical Center's general medicine, cardiology, or neurology inpatient services between September 1993 and July 1996. The investigators examined the subjects' frequency of hospitalization and days hospitalized in the year prior to the index admission, hospital use in the three months prior to index hospitalization, and length of the index hospital stay at Duke. They also examined two religious measures, frequency of church attendance and religious affiliation.

Researchers found that patients who attended religious services once a week or more were 56% less likely to have been hospitalized during the previous year ($p < .0001$). After they controlled for severity of medical illness (assessed by a 12-item physician-rated scale), physical functioning (assessed by questions about ability to perform 20 activities of daily living), social support, depressive symptoms, age, sex, race, and education, frequent attenders were still 43% less likely to be hospitalized ($p < .03$). In terms of actual number of days hospitalized, patients who attended religious services at least several times per month had been hospitalized an average of six days in the previous year; patients who attended services only a few times per year or not at all had been hospitalized for an average of 12 days (Figure 27.2). Length of the index hospital stay at Duke was also significantly shorter for persons who attended religious services more frequently ($p \leq .01$), although this association weakened when covariates were controlled ($p = .09$).

Intrinsic religiosity was also related to number of days hospitalized in the previous year (unpublished data). Scores on the 10-item Hoge scale (range 10–50), which was used to measure intrinsic religiosity, were divided into four quartiles, and the average number of days hospitalized for persons in each quartile was calculated. Higher intrinsic religiosity was associated with fewer days hospitalized; patients in the lowest quartile of intrinsic religiosity were hospitalized an average 9.4 days in the previous year, compared with an average of 5.3 days for those in the highest quartile (Figure 27.3). Intrinsic religiosity as a measure of religious attitude is less likely to be confounded by physical health than is church attendance; intrinsic religiosity is related to religious coping ($r = 0.55$) (Koenig, 1998b), which, if anything, is associated with more severe medical illness, as noted previously (i.e., people turn to religion to cope as they become sicker) (Koenig, 1994a, p. 169).

Most significant, patients not affiliated with any religious denomination were hospitalized an average of 25 days, compared to only 11 days for Catholic, Protestant, or Jewish persons. This large difference in length of stay between affiliated and nonaffiliated patients could not be explained by the severity of the current physical illness, level of physical functioning, social support, psychological state, or demographic characteristics (Koenig & Larson, 1998). In fact, when these other variables were controlled, the strength of the relationship between affiliation status and length of hospital stay became stronger (strength of the association increased from $\beta = -.22$ to $\beta = -.26$, $p < .0001$) (Figure 27.4).

Ongoing Study at Duke University

A group of private foundations, including the John Templeton Foundation, the Arthur Vining Davis Foundation, the Fetzer Foundation, and the Mary Biddle Duke Foundation, has funded a four-year study to examine the effects of religiousness and spirituality on use of medical services by high utilizers of health services. In this project, 600 general medicine patients (age 50 or over) consecutively admitted to the

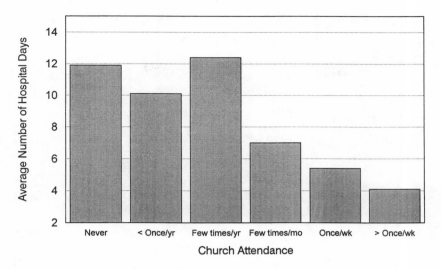

FIGURE 27.2 Days hospitalized in past year by church attendance ($n = 455$).

Duke University Medical Center will be comprehensively assessed during their baseline hospitalization and then carefully followed for one year after discharge. Detailed measures of the subjects' religious and spiritual beliefs and practices will be administered at baseline and at three-month intervals after discharge. Physician visits, acute hospitalizations, inpatient rehabilitation, nursing home stays, home health services, diagnostic and therapeutic procedures, medications, and several other measures of health service use will be carefully tracked during follow-up. Reports from the study are expected in 2002.

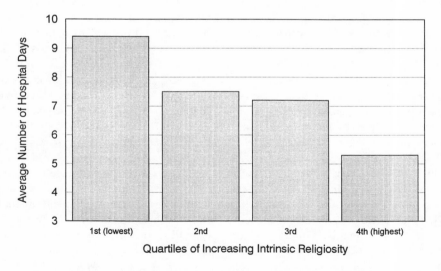

FIGURE 27.3 Average number of days hospitalized in the past year by intrinsic religiosity, assessed by 10-item Hoge scale ($n = 454$).

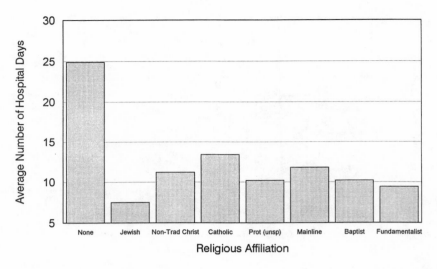

FIGURE 27.4 Length of index hospital stay at Duke by religious affiliation ($n = 363$), from Koenig and Larson (1998). Reprinted with permission from *Southern Medical Journal*.

EFFECT OF CLERGY INTERVENTIONS ON USE OF GENERAL MEDICAL SERVICES

Several epidemiological studies and clinical trials have examined the effects of seeing a clergyperson on volume and cost of medical services.

Recall from chapter 5 Croog and Levine's (1972) 12-month prospective study of 324 men who had suffered their first myocardial infarction (MI). At one-month post-MI, 11% (12% of Catholics, 15% of Protestants, and 2% of Jews) had seen or planned to see a clergyperson for support. Clergy were the second largest group sought for support. At 12 months post-MI, 5.4% of the subjects indicated that they had seen a clergyperson since the interview 11 months earlier. Analyses at 12 months post-MI revealed that a subject's having seen a clergyperson for support was unrelated to the likelihood that he was rehospitalized during the follow-up interval. To what extent the positive effects of seeing a clergyperson (if any) on rehospitalization were canceled out by the tendency of the more seriously ill men to seek clergy assistance, however, is unclear.

Florell (1973) randomized 44 orthopedic injury patients to two groups. One group received daily chaplain visits, and the other received no visits. Chaplain visits, focused on providing support and information, lasted for 15 minutes each day for patients in the intervention group, while patients in the control group received "business as usual." The chaplain intervention reduced patients' length of stay by an average of 20–29% ($p < .05$). Furthermore, patients visited by chaplains needed less "PRN" pain medication, made fewer calls on nursing time, and experienced less pain and stress (all $p < .05$).

McSherry et al. (1986) reviewed the importance of chaplain services for containing costs in hospitals and provided several case examples that show the potential cost savings. McSherry et al. (1987) then reported a study of 43 CABG surgery patients and 37 acute spinal cord injury patients (all middle-aged or older male veterans). Those who rated themselves as moderately or highly religious on admission had post-op lengths of stay 20% shorter than those of patients who had little or no interest in religion ($p < .05$). Later, her research team randomized 331 open-heart surgery patients to either a chaplain intervention ("Modern Chaplain Care") or usual care (Bliss et al., 1995). Patients in the intervention group had post-op hospitalization, that averaged two days shorter than those in the control group, for an overall cost savings of $4,200 per patient.

In summary, the few studies available suggest that chaplain interventions may help reduce use of acute hospital services, particularly following surgery. Unfortunately, none of the studies have been published in major medical journals. Thus, much work remains to be done.

Need for Chaplain Services

Parkum (1985) surveyed 432 patients at six hospitals in Pennsylvania as part of an earlier study that examined patient satisfaction with chaplain services. Significantly more patients felt that pastoral services were helpful (67%) than were helped by visits from social workers (16%), patient representatives (5%), self-help volunteers (7%), or regular volunteers (23%). Patients also indicated that chaplains were more likely (100%) to meet their expressive needs than social workers (37%), patient representatives (78%), self-help volunteers (74%), or regular volunteers (11%). They reported no difference in the extent to which chaplains and other hospital staff met their instrumental needs. Thus, it appears that chaplain services fill an important need that is not addressed by other hospital staff.

Gartner, Lyons, et al. (1990) examined the effects on use of health services that resulted from the elimination of a clinical pastoral education (CPE) program at Northwestern Memorial Hospital in 1985. This action effectively reduced the pastoral care staff from 5.5 full-time chaplains and nine students to 4.5 full-time chaplains and no students. The decision to reduce the chaplaincy staff was in part based on an estimated $90 cost for each hour of direct patient contact with a chaplain. After the program was eliminated, the number of chaplain-initiated or other-initiated referrals for pastoral care dropped from 52 per week to 37 per week. Before the chaplain services were reduced, chaplains had initiated 42 referrals per week, whereas staff had initiated only 10 referrals per week. After the chaplain services were cut, the number of referrals initiated by chaplains dropped to only 17 per week, while the number initiated by hospital staff rose to 21 referrals per week ($p < .01$). The authors concluded that

when pastoral care providers were less available, the demand for their services from nursing and medical staff increased substantially.

RELIGION AND USE OF MENTAL HEALTH SERVICES

Approximately 30% of adults in the United States experience a diagnosable mental illness in any given year (Regier et al., 1993; Kessler et al., 1994). Between 70% and 80% of persons with a recent mental health or addictive disorder receive no treatment for their problem, and, of those who do seek help, fewer than half see a mental health professional. Persons with major depression and anxiety disorder are most likely to seek and receive services for these problems (about one-third do so), and persons with substance abuse problems are least likely (Regier et al., 1993). Persons with low levels of education, the poor, and minorities are least likely to seek help and to receive mental health services. Primary care physicians, psychiatrists, social workers, and psychologists provide 53%, 19%, 15%, and 13%, respectively, of all mental health services (Knesper & Pagnucco, 1987).

Over the past decade the number of persons with depression and other emotional disorders in the population has increased. These emotional disorders are increasingly treated with psychotropic medication, and many persons experience dramatic improvements in their depressive or anxiety symptoms in response to these drugs. Pincus et al. (1998) examined prescribing trends in psychotropic medications between 1985 and 1993, using data from the National Ambulatory Medical Care Surveys. Visits during which a psychotropic drug was prescribed increased from 32.7 million to 45.6 million. The largest category of increase was antidepressant medication. Visits for depression increased from 11.0 million in 1988 to a remarkable 20.4 million in 1993; visits to physicians that included treatment with an antidepressant increased from 5.3 million in 1985 to 12.4 million in 1993. Because of the effectiveness of drugs, there is less and less financial incentive to utilize counseling or psychotherapy in the treatment of these disorders. Nevertheless, many life problems require solutions that drugs cannot provide. Counseling remains an important therapeutic strategy that is necessary to help anxious and depressed persons cope with their problems, make better decisions that create less stress, and improve their interpersonal relationships. Because insurance reimbursement for "talk" therapies is unfortunately rapidly shrinking, pastoral counseling provided by community clergy and chaplains will become increasingly important. In fact, clergy already provide a significant proportion of the mental health services delivered in this country.

Mental Health Services Provided by Clergy

According to calculations performed by Weaver (1995), approximately 312,000 Jewish and Christian clergy serve congregations in the United States (4000 rabbis, 53,000 Catholic priests, 255,000 Protestant ministers). Clergy report that they devote between 10–20% of their average 50-hour work week to counseling. This amounts to 148 million hours of counseling annually, the equivalent of having 77,000 members of the American Psychological Association deliver services at a rate of 38.5 hours per week. Note that this estimate does not include the counseling provided by nearly 100,000 nuns in full-time ministry in the Catholic Church.

A number of epidemiological studies have examined the frequency with which persons seek out clergy for counseling. Gurin et al. (1960) evaluated a national sample of 2,460 adults who spontaneously responded to a question regarding how they handled worries. In this survey, only 16% of respondents mentioned prayer, and 4% indicated that they sought out clergy as their first response. Veroff et al. (1981) reported results from a landmark national study that examined people's patterns of help seeking for personal problems in the United States from 1957 to 1976. Of those who sought help for personal problems in 1957, 43% saw a clergyman, 30% saw a physician, 18% saw a psychiatrist or psychologist, 4% saw a marriage counselor, 10% saw another mental health practitioner, and 3% visited a social services agency.

In 1976, 39% of those who sought help saw a clergyman, 21% saw a primary care physician, 29% saw a psychiatrist or psychologist, 8% saw a marital counselor, and 18% used another mental health source. Among all respondents, a total of 6% saw a clergyman for help in 1957 (similar to Gurin et al.'s figure of 4%), and 10% saw a clergyman in 1976.

For those with mental disorders, the figures are somewhat different. The NIMH Epidemiologic Catchment Area (ECA) Survey assessed mental disorders and use of mental health services by more than 18,000 randomly sampled Americans in 1980–1981. The researchers found that 2.8% of this primarily urban sample sought help from clergy, 12.1% visited mental health specialists, and 2.8% used both resources (Larson, Hohmann, et al., 1988). Interestingly, the types of mental health disorders for which people sought help from clergy were similar to those for which they saw mental health specialists, suggesting that even persons with severe mental health problems often sought help from clergy.

Psychiatrists have had mixed feelings about the role that clergy play in delivering mental health services. For example, Beitman (1982) writes the following in the American Psychiatric Association journal *Hospital and Community Psychiatry*:

> Other nonmedical professionals are also becoming involved in the delivery of mental health services. A large group of *newcomers* [italicized] are ministers and rabbis. . . . There is now one pastoral counseling center for every three mental health centers. . . . Is it the psychiatrist's role to judge the adequacy of care delivered by other professionals? If so, there is much to question about the services offered by ministers and rabbis because their training is highly variable. . . . The pastoral counseling movement may be looked upon as either an ally that reaches a population often untouched by psychiatrists or as a negative force attempting to usurp yet more of what was once psychiatrists' turf. (pp. 486–487)

Whatever information source one uses and regardless of the opinions expressed by mental health professionals, it is clear that clergy see a lot of people with emotional problems and are likely to see a lot more in the days ahead.

FACTORS THAT AFFECT USE OF MENTAL HEALTH SERVICES

In addition to financial considerations, education, and access to services, *psychological* factors (besides the mental disorder itself) and *social* factors also influence the likelihood that persons will seek mental health services.

Psychological Factors

Even more than for use of medical services, beliefs play an important role in decisions about whether to seek formal mental health services for an emotional or psychological problem. Help seeking depends heavily on the extent to which the person or family member believes that the problem is psychological in nature and that mental health professions can help with the problem. For example, if a depressed person believes that her loss of energy and weight loss are caused by a physical problem, she will seek help from a medical doctor, not from a mental health professional. Likewise, a religious person may believe that his problem is spiritual and requires spiritual interventions such as prayer, Bible reading, confession, or exorcism. If the person believes this, he will seek out a religious professional and not a mental health professional for help.

Mental illness or emotional problems also carry with them a stigma that causes embarrassment and shame. Many persons, particularly older adults, deny they have mental health problems and avoid seeing mental health specialists who might confirm their fears ("I'm going crazy"). If people can explain their symptoms in terms of physical or spiritual causes, rather than psychological ones, they are likely to do so and to seek professionals in those areas for help instead.

Social Factors

Social support may increase the appropriate use of mental health services by those with mental disorder in need of treatment, or it may reduce the need for formal treatment of milder emotional disorders by preventing them or by speeding their resolution. In a review of studies of heavy users of psychiatric services, Kent et al. (1995) emphasizes the importance of social issues such as isolation, homelessness, and lack of social support as factors that influence service use. Social support is one of the best predictors of level of functioning in chronically mentally ill patients, which exerts a major influence on their use of mental health services (Meeks et al., 1990). For example, Faccincani et al. (1990) examined psychiatric symptomatology, social functioning, social support, and mental health service use in 41 patients with schizophrenia or other chronic psychoses. They found that social support was negatively correlated with service use; in other words, the greater the patient's social support, the lower his dependency on expensive psychiatric inpatient care.

Social support affects service use not only in the chronically mentally ill but also in community-dwelling adults. Sherbourne (1988) examined the relationship between social support and use of mental health services in a general population of adults age 14 or older who were enrolled in the RAND Health Insurance Experiment (a three to five–year prospective study involving 4,580 person-years of follow-up). Sherbourne found that when social support is defined as social resources, the more support one has, the fewer mental health services one needs. Similarly, Pescosolido et al. (1998) examined social support and use of mental health services by 1,777 low-income Puerto Ricans, and found that persons with larger, more supportive social networks used fewer formal mental health services than did those without such supports. Thus, persons with large support networks use these networks to help them cope with emotional problems that would otherwise require professional assistance.

RELIGION AND USE OF MENTAL HEALTH SERVICES

How might religion influence the use of mental health services? Religion may increase the use of mental health services by chronically mentally ill persons who neglect themselves and shy away from traditional psychiatric care; the increased monitoring and surveillance that occur within the religious community might encourage them to seek such services and even provide access, just as they do for medical services. Timely mental health care, in turn, may ultimately reduce costs by reducing acute hospitalization and by helping the patient maintain functioning and productivity. Religious involvement may also be associated with increased use of mental health services because religious communities may attract persons with chronic mental illness or emotional problems who are seeking relief from these problems in religion. Certain religious groups, such as evangelical Protestants, seek out and evangelize persons with emotional problems (frequently from the lower social classes). These persons may be in particular need of professional mental health services and yet may not seek them until prompted to do so by fellow church members.

Religious persons may use mental health services less frequently than the nonreligious or the weakly religious for many reasons. Perhaps the most likely explanation for the reduced use is that devoutly religious persons who are active in their religious communities simply do not need such services because they are less depressed and less anxious and cope better with life's problems (see chapter 15). By preventing or speeding the resolution of emotional problems, religious involvement decreases the need for secular mental health services. As we have already seen, people with large supportive social networks use fewer mental health services. Church or synagogue involvement appears to increase number of social contacts and the development of high quality supportive relationships (see chapter 15). For many Americans, especially the elderly, church-related social support is the most important source of support outside the family. Such support may prevent the development of emotional problems and replaces formal mental health services for dealing with such problems. Religiously uninvolved and socially isolated people, on the other hand, may be forced to the secular mental health system to meet their psychological and social needs.

Less influential but certainly a factor in reducing service use among some people is the fact that some religious groups discourage the use of mental health services. This is especially the case in small religious sects that advocate using only spiritual methods (prayer, Bible study, confession) for treating mental health problems and see psychology and psychiatry as antireligious. For example, as we noted in chapter 4, Christian writers such as Martin Bobgan, author of *Prophets of Psychoheresy I and II*, and Jay Adams, author of *Competent to Counsel*, condemn all types of psychotherapy, even the religious forms advocated by the Christian mental health professionals Gary Collins, Larry Crabb, and Frank Minirith. Except for the Church of Scientology, these groups are not nearly as vocal against the use of psychotropic medications.

Religious persons themselves may have difficulty deciding whether they have a mental health problem or a spiritual problem, particularly since even mental health professionals at times may have difficulty making this determination. If persons decide or are convinced by others that they have a spiritual problem, then they may seek religious methods of treatment, rather than secular mental health services. Devoutly religious persons may also struggle with whether they should depend upon God for help (as they may feel inclined to do) or on secular health professionals (or the medications they prescribe). Often, it is with great ambivalence and even some guilt that the religious seek out mental health professionals for help with problems that have proved resistant to prayer, Bible study, or help obtained within the church. For these reasons, some devout persons avoid use of mental health services even when they need them.

Access to mental health services can also be a problem for religious persons because they tend to live in rural areas that do not offer such services. In addition, religious beliefs and practices are more prevalent among persons from the lower socioeconomic classes, who may not be able to afford expensive psychotherapy or medication. Thus, religion may affect people's use of mental health services in a number of ways, and the decision to seek help is likely to result from a complex interaction of many influences.

RESEARCH ON RELIGION AND MENTAL HEALTH SERVICE USE

Community Studies

Koenig, George, Meador, Blazer, and Dyck (1994) examined the relationship among religious affiliation, rates of psychiatric disorder, and use of mental health services in a random sample of 2,679 persons ages 18–94 who were participating in the NIMH Epidemiologic Catchment Area survey at its North Carolina site. Of the sample, 30% were mainline Protestants (e.g., Methodists, Presbyterians, Lutherans), 64% were conservative Protestants (primarily Baptists), and 5% were Pentecostals. Rates of psychiatric disorder, especially for the 853 "baby boomers" (those born between 1945 and 1966), were substantially higher among Pentecostals. Despite this finding, Pentecostal baby boomers were no more likely to have seen a mental health professional during the previous six months than were boomers who belonged to other religious groups. Among middle-aged and older participants ($n = 1,826$), fewer Pentecostals and conservative Protestants had made visits to mental health professionals in the previous six months than had mainline Protestants (1.6% vs. 4.0%, $p < .01$); this association persisted after researchers controlled for sex, race, health, and socioeconomic status. Of particular concern was the finding that no Pentecostals of any age who attended church infrequently had seen a mental health professional within the previous six months, even though almost 30% had experienced a recent psychiatric disorder.

When analyses were stratified by occurrence of recent psychiatric disorder, the researchers found that the low rate of use of mental health services among Pentecostal baby boomers could be partially explained by the appropriate absence of mental health visits by those without psychiatric disorder. Although 6% of mainline Protestants without psychiatric disorder had mental health visits, no Pentecostals

without psychiatric disorder did. The same pattern was seen among middle-aged and older adults. When analyses were further stratified by church attendance, the researchers found that Pentecostals with psychiatric disorder and high church attendance were more likely to have made mental health visits than were Pentecostals with mental disorder and low church attendance. These findings suggest that conservative and Pentecostal Protestants are less likely to overuse mental health services than are mainline Protestants; among Pentecostals, increased church attendance is associated with greater and more appropriate use of mental health services.

Psychiatric Patients

A number of studies among psychiatric patients suggest that those who are more religious have less need for inpatient psychiatric care. Chu and Klein (1985) prospectively studied 128 African American schizophrenic patients consecutively admitted to seven hospitals and mental health centers of the Missouri Division of Mental Health. Patients (65 from urban and 63 from rural areas) were interviewed on admission, at discharge, and one year after discharge or on hospital readmission (if this occurred before one year). Urban patients were less likely to be rehospitalized if they said prayers once daily (vs. more often) ($\chi^2 = 8.0$, 3 df, $p < .05$) and if their families encouraged them to continue religious worship while they were in the hospital ($\chi^2 = 12.0$, 1 df, $p < .001$). For the entire sample, fewer rehospitalizations occurred if the patient's family was Catholic; there were more rehospitalizations among those whose families had no religious affiliation ($\chi^2 = 8.7$, 3 df, $p < .025$).

Berg, Reed, et al. (1995) examined length of hospital stay among 37 patients diagnosed with major affective disorder and hospitalized on the St. Cloud, Minnesota, psychiatric inpatient service. Subjects were asked seven questions concerning their spirituality. In response to the statement "God/life has treated you unfairly," respondents were asked to indicate how often they felt this way (1 = never, 2 = sometimes, 3 = often, 4 = very often). For every point increase on this four-point question, researchers found that the patient's length of hospital stay increased by 11.4 days (or $2,252, assuming a cost of $197.38 per hospital day) ($p = .05$). Although this analysis did not control for age, sex, and marital status, those variables were not related to length of stay. Investigators also examined the relationship between frequency of church attendance and length of hospital stay. They compared persons who attended religious services once per week or more (high attenders) with those who attended services less than once per week (low attenders). The average length of stay among 14 low church attenders was 73 days ($14,395), compared with 35 days for the 11 high attenders ($6,944). The statistic of association was not given for this comparison.

As noted, negative attitudes toward mental health treatments among some religious groups may account for the lower use of psychiatric services by members of certain ethnic groups. Postolache et al. (1997) surveyed 41 Hispanic patients (40 of whom were women) who were receiving treatment from the psychiatric outpatient service of Beth Israel Medical Center in New York City. Researchers examined whether certain religious beliefs and practices would predict acceptability of supportive psychotherapy. Some 33 practicing Catholics and 18 exceptionally religious persons were identified. The investigators found three variables that were significant predictors of whether individuals perceived benefits from psychotherapy. Those who believed in a benefit from the sacrament of confession were also likely to believe that psychotherapy had benefit. By contrast, those who went to confession frequently and believed strongly in an afterlife were less likely to believe that psychotherapy had benefits. The authors concluded that knowledge about the patient's religious beliefs may help predict who will and who will not be receptive to psychotherapy.

Members of other religious groups may be more likely to use mental health services than persons in the general population. Flics and Herron (1991) surveyed 152 patients from three psychiatric units at New York City hospitals. Multiple regression analysis was used to identify predictors of patients' prognoses. The researchers found that Jews had better prognoses than did patients affiliated with other religious groups and concluded that this finding was likely a result of Jews' low threshold for seeking mental health services, similar to the findings of other studies (e.g., Sanua, 1989).

SUMMARY AND CONCLUSIONS

In this chapter, we examined the relationship between religious beliefs and practices and use of health services. First, we reviewed factors that affect the use of general medical services, including biomedical factors (cigarette smoking, high blood pressure, functional disability), psychological factors (personality and temperament, anxiety, depression), and social support. We then explored the various ways that religion might influence persons' use of general medical services (e.g., promoting more appropriate use of health services, reducing excess use that is the result of psychological factors, and reducing people's need for health services). The relationship between religious affiliation and use of health services was first examined, and we noted that Jews tend to use more medical services than do members of other religious groups. The relationship between religious activity and use of medical services was also explored. In those studies, we tended to find positive relationships between private religious activities such as prayer and use of medical services *but* a negative relationship between religious community activities such as church attendance and use of services. We also reviewed two studies that found no association between religious variables and health service use. Finally, we explored studies that examined the effects of clergy and chaplain interventions on use and cost of inpatient medical services and found significant effects in terms of length of hospital stay and costs of services in the few studies available.

In the second section of the chapter, we examined the relationship between religion and use of mental health services. First, we acknowledged the huge volume of mental health services provided by clergy in the United States. We found that people seek clergy assistance for all kinds of mental health problems and that these problems are often as severe as those for which they seek psychiatric help. We examined the psychological and social factors that influence use of mental health services, and then linked these factors with religious beliefs and activities. Numerous reasons exist why religion might increase or decrease people's use of formal mental health services. On the one hand, better surveillance and detection of mental health problems among those involved in religious communities may encourage believers to seek help. On the other hand, service use may decrease as people feel less need for professional help because their coping skills improve thanks to the greater social support they receive from the community; service use may also decrease because they are reluctant to seek mental health services. We found that in community and clinical samples, greater religious involvement appears to be associated with more appropriate use of mental health services and less use of acute psychiatric inpatient services.

Although we have reported some positive associations between religious involvement and reduced use of general medical and mental health services, these research findings are preliminary. More studies are clearly needed and are now being designed to more comprehensively measure the religious variable and to study its association with health service use over time in high utilizers. Likewise, intervention studies (e.g., of the effectiveness of prayer-based relaxation techniques or chaplain interventions) are needed to definitively assess the effects of religious beliefs and practices on the use and cost of health services.

28

Understanding Religion's Effects on Health Service Use

I N CHAPTERS 5 THROUGH 15 we explored the effects of religious belief and practice on mental health. In chapters 16 through 25, we saw how religion might impact physical health through psychological, social, and behavioral mechanisms. In chapter 26 we examined how religious involvement can influence disease prevention, disease detection, and compliance with treatment. In chapter 27, we provided evidence for a relationship between religious activities and belief and use of general medical and mental health services. Each of these chapters gives important clues about how religion can impact service use. In this short chapter, we piece together these clues to build a comprehensive and cohesive theoretical model that describes these pathways. Such a model is essential for both research and education as organizations in the public and the private sectors explore ways of reducing the cost of health services. The ultimate goal is to

keep our population as healthy as possible by promoting healthy lifestyles and encouraging self-care and to provide the necessary health services to those who need them in a timely and cost-effective manner. Religion may either help or hinder this process.

DETERMINANTS OF SERVICE USE

As noted in chapter 23, objective disability or physical illness alone explains only about 12–25% of health care use (Berkanovic et al., 1981), and nearly 60% of visits to primary care physicians are due to physical complaints that have no organic basis (Cummings & Follette, 1968; Kroenke & Magelsdorff, 1989). As we saw in the chapter 27, behavioral and psychosocial factors significantly influence the demand for health services (see Fries et al., 1993, for a more extensive review), and interventions that target these factors can reduce service use by 30% or more (Hellman et al., 1990; Caudill, Schnable, et al., 1991; Friedman, Myers, et al., 1995). Although we discussed these points in chapter 27, we now take a careful, more focused look at factors that influence whether people seek health services. These factors, as noted earlier, include:

1. Actual need for services
2. Perceived need for services
3. Perceived benefit from services
4. Access to and availability of services
5. Motivation to seek care

Actual Need for Health Services

Is there true illness present that requires medical or psychiatric services, and, if so, what level of service is needed at this time? For care to be timely and cost-effective, actual need must be matched with the appropriate level of service. For example, a middle-aged, overweight man with high blood pressure needs treatment as soon as possible to prevent a stroke or heart attack that might ultimately cost society much more than the immediate treatment in terms of lost productivity and use of high-technology health services.

Perceived Need for Health Services

Does the patient perceive a need for professional health services, and, if so, does the patient believe the need is for medical or psychiatric services? On the one hand, a person with serious illness may deny that he has a problem and may see no need for health care; on the other hand, a person with no medical illness may believe quite strongly that he has physical illness and may perceive a great need for medical services. In the second case, while physical illness may be absent, a psychiatric illness is present that requires mental health care, not medical treatment. Emotional problems are often perceived as physical problems involving the heart or gastrointestinal system, particularly by persons who are embarrassed about having a psychiatric problem. In other cases, physical disease (e.g., pancreatic cancer or hypothyroidism) may present as an emotional disorder (depression). Diagnosing the correct problem and matching it with the correct health service can be a challenge for even the most skilled clinician.

Gender, ethnic, developmental, and cultural factors also affect the perceived need for health services. Women are more emotionally expressive than men, more in touch with their feelings, and they more readily share these feelings with others, including health professionals. Men, on the other hand, often have a need to maintain a rugged image and wish to appear in control of their own problems; they may deny these problems altogether. Needing to see a doctor may be viewed as a sign of weakness to be avoided whenever possible. Italians and Jews recognize and readily express bodily concerns, whereas the more stoic Irish or English person copes with symptoms by minimizing or denying them. Experiences with parents and siblings during childhood also influence perceived need. Family members provide important role models that influence how we express our concerns later in life and when we seek medical attention. Finally, societal and cultural factors affect how readily people seek health services. Seeing a psychologist or psychiatrist for problems with adjustment was a cause for embarrassment 40 years ago, whereas today it is fashionable to have a therapist for "self-improvement."

Education level heavily influences whether symptoms are recognized as significant enough to require medical treatment and whether they are likely to respond to medical treatment. For example, the uneducated man who experiences pain in his chest, neck, and left arm may interpret the symptoms as indigestion and/or muscle strain and take a minor analgesic for the problem. The educated man, on the other hand, is more likely to recognize these symptoms as heart-related and therefore to seek immediate medical attention. Similarly, the uneducated woman who sees streaks of blood in her stool may interpret the blood as simply coming from hemorrhoids and may not realize that the blood may be a sign of occult colon cancer and that she must therefore see her medical doctor.

Temperament also influences whether people perceive a need for medical treatment. An anxious, hypervigilant, controlling person is more likely than a tranquil, placid individual to be upset by minor physical symptoms and to quickly attribute them to an underlying serious medical condition. Having a need to control every aspect of the situation in order to ward off catastrophe, the high-strung, anxious person rushes to the doctor for reassurance. Many of the anxiety disorders (panic disorder, generalized anxiety disorder, obsessive-compulsive disorder) can foster an inappropriately high level of bodily concern that then fuels a perceived need for health services.

Finally, people usually seek services when a health problem begins to interfere with their ability to function or when they fear this will soon occur. For example, a person with arthritis may simply choose to bear the pain, treating it with over-the-counter pain medication until that pain becomes intolerable or begins to interfere with work or other activity the person values greatly. The pain itself may not be sufficient to motivate the person to seek medical care, but the loss of functioning is. Fear is also a motivating factor for seeking treatment. An older person may forget an old friend's name or get lost in an unfamiliar part of town and may interpret this transient forgetfulness as the first symptoms of Alzheimer's disease. The fear of permanently losing her memory and her ability to function will quickly drive the person to seek medical attention in order to relieve or confirm this fear.

Perceived Benefit from Health Services

People seek health services only if they believe that such services will relieve their problem. That benefit must be seen as outweighing the costs of making an appointment, taking time to keep the appointment, enduring discomfort during the appointment, and bearing the financial burden of the visit. If the person has a lot of faith in the doctor because of prior experience, she will have a lower threshold for seeking care (will more readily see the benefits as outweighing the costs). If, however, the person distrusts doctors or has had bad experiences with them in the past, he may need to perceive a

greater benefit before he will decide to seek medical services.

Lynch (1993) notes that the demand for health care may also be affected by persons who manipulate the system to obtain benefits such as time off from work and workmen's compensation. This goal may be conscious and intentional (as in malingering, where the patient, fully aware of his motivations, produces false or greatly exaggerated physical or psychological symptoms) or unconscious (as in factitious or conversion disorder, in which the patient is not aware that he is producing the symptoms himself).

Access to and Availability of Health Services

If health services are very difficult and costly to acquire, then people will tend to use them less often. Access to health services is determined by a number of factors, including the presence of health insurance, or finances adequate to pay for health care, the availability of transportation and the physical ability to get to health care providers, and the availability of health care providers in the area where the person lives. For example, consider an elderly disabled woman, living on her social security income, who resides in a rural area and who must depend on the good will of neighbors for transportation into town. When she goes to see the busy doctor, she knows that she will have to wait for several hours in a crowded, uncomfortable waiting room. She may expect the doctor to prescribe a medication that will be costly and require her to spend the precious social security income that she needs for other things. It is likely that such a woman will seek medical attention only when it is absolutely necessary—and will probably put off getting help longer than is best for her.

Motivation to Seek Care

Even if the person recognizes the need for health services and the services are readily available, he may not have the energy, interest, or desire to obtain the necessary medical care. Depression and/or social isolation often underlie loss of motivation and lack of interest in self-care. If the disabled elderly woman is also depressed, then she will have even more difficulty perceiving the benefit of medical care (given the effort required for her to overcome the many obstacles she faces in getting care). Depression may also sap her will to live, and she may see an easy way out by letting her medical illnesses take their course. Neglecting physical health by failing to seek timely and appropriate medical care for treatable illness is a form of indirect suicidal behavior (Nelson, 1977).

ROLE OF RELIGION

Religion can affect the determinants of health service use either directly (by promoting beliefs that encourage or discourage service use) or indirectly (by affecting persons' psychosocial resources) and can thereby increase or decrease the volume and cost of services used (see Figure 28.1).

Actual Need for Health Services

As we observed in chapter 25, devout religious involvement may either prevent illness or speed recovery. Additional benefits may be gained from the increased social support that results from religious activity; these may include fewer emotional problems, earlier disease detection, better medical compliance, a stronger immune system, and better overall health. Thus, if religious beliefs and practices help maintain health and prevent disease, religious persons will not need or use medical services as often. Religion may also promote a better matching of actual health need to services sought. For example, Koenig, George, Meador, Blazer, and Dyck (1994) found that use of mental health services was more appropriate among Pentecostal churchgoers who attended services frequently than among mainline Protestants, who appeared to overuse services.

On the other hand, religious beliefs may also prevent people from seeking appropriate medical or psychiatric care when needed (e.g., failure to vaccinate children, obtain prenatal care, ob-

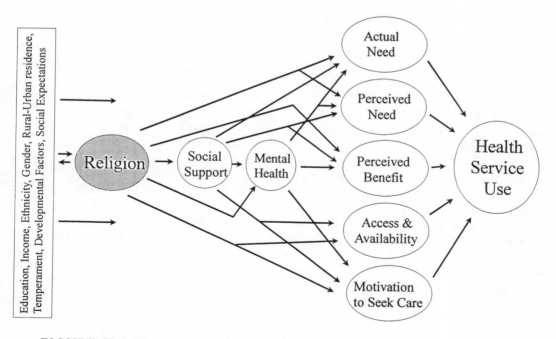

FIGURE 28.1 Theoretical model explaining how religion may influence use of health services.

tain and use necessary medication). In that case, health conditions are likely to worsen and ultimately require more expensive medical care for long-term complications.

Perceived Need for Health Services

Religious involvement may increase the perceived need for treatment by surrounding the ill person with a caring community that encourages timely treatment and thus elevates perception of need to a more appropriate level. Certain religious groups, Jews in particular, may be better educated and wealthier and may have a greater tendency to express their health concerns to medical or psychiatric professionals whom they trust and revere. In contrast, religion may also inappropriately increase the perceived need for medical services by causing the conversion of less acceptable psychological conflicts into physical symptoms, treatment for which carries less or no stigma.

On the other hand, religion may decrease use of health services because it reduces anxiety, somatic preoccupation, and the need for excessive control that drives up perceived need for health services. Religion may calm the anxious person and help her give up control to God, relieving the obsessive concern over minor health problems. Religion may also decrease the perceived need for treatment by providing spiritual explanations for health problems that require spiritual, not medical or psychiatric, care. Some religious people may "claim" their healing, acting as though they no longer have the health condition, entirely denying their illnesses. Of course, such practices may ultimately lead to worse health problems and increase the use of more expensive health services down the road.

Finally, religion can reduce the perceived need for treatment by increasing the level of disability necessary to interfere with valued functioning. Religious persons, because of their spiritual worldview, may value earthly possessions and goals differently than the nonreligious do. In other words, functioning in a certain way may be less important to religious persons who have spiritual hopes and goals that supersede worldly ones. Their sense of value may be less rooted in what they can accomplish or

produce in this life than in spiritual matters, which are less affected by health problems or impaired physical functioning. On the other hand, religious persons may have visions or spiritual goals (i.e., caring for others) that may be impeded by even minor health problems. In such cases, religious beliefs can motivate people to seek medical or psychiatric care to return their health to an optimal level so that they can attain their earthly spiritual goals.

Perceived Benefit from Health Services

Perceived benefit from health services is largely a function of education and knowledge about illnesses and their treatments. Religiousness tends to be associated with lower socioeconomic class, and such medical information may not be as readily available to persons in this class. It is likely, though, that devoutly religious people will view the benefits of medical treatment in a way similar to that of nonreligious persons with similar education and knowledge.

Religious persons might also view health services as less important for healing than would the nonreligious. Religious persons, while understanding that God usually heals through doctors and medications, may believe that God can also heal without them, making medical services less essential for recovery. On rare occasions religious groups may take this view to the extreme, promoting mistrust of medical professionals (particularly psychiatric professionals), who are portrayed as actually causing harm. Such groups may condemn members who seek medical or psychiatric attention as being weak in faith and unable to put their trust in God and may go on to subtly alienate or exclude members who seek such services.

Religious persons may also perceive a lower benefit from health services because they are less likely to manipulate the health care system for secondary gain (in order to avoid work or evade other responsibilities). Devoutly religious people tend to be responsible and to have a strong work ethic, and they may be less likely to complain of somatic symptoms (see chapter 23). Also, because they receive greater social support from the church community, they may be less likely to use the health care system for emotional nurturance and support.

Religion may also increase the perceived benefit of health services. Because most religious beliefs encourage a positive view of life, promote optimism, and instill hope, they may help counteract pessimistic views that see medical treatments as futile and without benefit. This sense of optimism may encourage persons to seek medical care because they have greater hope that God may use these treatments to help them.

Access to and Availability of Health Services

Poor, uneducated, and minority populations, particularly those living in rural locations, may lack both knowledge about health services and the ability to pay for them. These populations also tend to be the most religious (Princeton Religion Research Center, 1996). Thus, the most religious persons may actually have less access than the general population to traditional health services. Involvement in a religious community, however, may increase their exposure to information about available health services and provide them with the emotional, financial, and transportation support to access those services. Some churches may even have a "parish nurse" or other designated health professional whose primary role is to either provide care for ill church members or help them find appropriate medical care in the community (see chapter 29).

Motivation to Seek Care

Because interest in caring for oneself is so strongly influenced by mental health and social support, anything that reduces depression, discouragement, and social isolation or increases hope, optimism, and social support will likely promote more appropriate health care-seeking behaviors. As we saw in chapter 15, devout religious faith, active involvement in religious community, and adaptive use of religion when coping with stress have been associated with a lower risk of depression, faster recovery from depression, and greater well-being, life satisfaction, and hope, particularly in persons with disability

and chronic health problems, the group at highest risk for frequent and costly service use. Likewise, religious teachings promote concern for the physical body as the "temple of the Holy Spirit," to be cared for and maintained.

Spurious Associations

Research studies that examine cross-sectional relationships between religion and health service use may report spurious findings because of a number of factors. As we discussed in chapter 22 and chapter 27, a positive association between prayer or religious coping and increased service use may result when severely ill persons turn to religion or prayer for comfort after they become sick. Second, a negative association between religious involvement and use of health services may result when low education, low income, rural living situation, and minority status are not adequately controlled. All of these factors are positively correlated with both religiousness and inability to gain access to health services (a problem faced by some prospective studies as well).

Finally, a negative association between religious attendance and increased service use may result from inadequate controlling for physical illness or disability that both prevents church attendance and increases service use (again, a problem for some prospective studies also). On the other hand, severe physical illness and disability may be present (and increase the use of health services) because of subjects' lack of religious involvement in the years prior to the study. The ideal study would begin following its subjects when they are young and healthy, assessing their development of illness and their rates of service use over time as a function of their level of religious involvement. Unfortunately, such a project would require many years of follow-up and be very expensive (although it might be worth the cost in the long run).

SUMMARY AND CONCLUSIONS

We saw in chapter 27 that religious activities and commitment are frequently associated with lower use of health services, and occasionally with higher use. In this chapter we try to understand how religion decreases or increases health service use. Religion may decrease health service use by:

- Reducing actual need (promoting better physical and mental health)
- Reducing perceived need (lowering overuse or unnecessary use of services)
- Decreasing perceived benefit (providing alternative methods for healing, and reducing manipulation of health care system for other purposes)
- Increasing timely access to and availability of health services (increasing monitoring for health problems and encouraging better compliance, ultimately reducing use in the long term)
- Increasing motivation to seek care (by reducing depression and other negative mental health states that interfere with early diagnosis and treatment).

On the other hand, religion may increase health service use by:

- Increasing actual need (by promoting beliefs that discourage timely diagnosis and treatment, allowing illnesses to progress unchecked to advanced stages that are more difficult and costly to treat)
- Increasing perceived need (providing a supportive community that encourages appropriate and timely treatment, increasing service use in the short term)
- Increasing perceived benefit (promoting a more optimistic and hopeful attitude toward medical treatments)
- Increasing access to and availability of health services (providing financial assistance, knowledge, and/or transportation that promote greater use of health services in the short term)
- Increasing motivation to seek care (reducing depression and promoting self-care activities, thereby increasing use of health services in the short term)

Thus, religion may affect service use through a number of mechanisms that act either directly on the factors that affect use or indirectly by enhancing social support, improving mental health, and promoting positive health behaviors. Spurious associations are also possible and must be guarded against.

PART VI

CLINICAL APPLICATIONS

29

Health Professionals

IN THE PREVIOUS CHAPTERS OF this book, we focused on reviewing and understanding research that has examined the relationship between religion and health. The question we address in this chapter is, "What does all of this mean for the health care professional?" In many respects, reviewing the research is easy compared to trying to understand the implications for clinical care. This moves our discussion out of the ivory tower of academics and gives it a more practical focus. Addressing religious issues in clinical practice is controversial, and at this time there is very little research to help guide clinicians' behaviors. Because this is a sensitive area for both health professionals and patients, and because of the public and pluralistic nature of the health care setting, we must proceed with the utmost caution when educating professionals how to apply these research findings to patient care.

In this chapter, we review the progress in medical and psychiatric education over the past decade that has attempted to integrate religious and spiritual issues into clinical practice. After briefly overviewing the research and responding to critics, we discuss patient-centered applications relevant to doctors (medical physicians, psychiatrists, and psychologists) and other health professionals (e.g., nurses, social workers, and counselors).

MEDICAL EDUCATION

In 1993, fewer than five medical schools had courses on religion, spirituality and medicine. In 2000, at least 65 of the nation's 126 medical schools were offering such courses, some of which were required, not elective. One reason for this is the medical education grants program sponsored by the John Templeton Foundation, which has offered $25,000 awards (the John

437

Templeton Spirituality and Medicine Curricular Awards) to medical schools each year to initiate courses on spirituality and medicine. The Association of American Medical Colleges (AAMC) initiative, known as the Medical School Objectives Project (MSOP), recently reported that physicians "must seek to understand the meaning of the patients' stories in the context of the patients' beliefs, and family and cultural values" (AAMC, 1998). Dana King, director of the rural family medicine residency program at East Carolina University, has developed a manual for courses on religion, spirituality and medicine to standardize educational content (King, 2000). Course winners during the life of the Templeton awards program are the following:

1995

Johns Hopkins University School of Medicine

Albert Einstein College of Medicine

East Tennessee State University College of Medicine

Ohio State University College of Medicine

Penn State University College of Medicine

1996

University of Pennsylvania School of Medicine

Case Western Reserve University School of Medicine

Bowman Gray School of Medicine

Washington University at St. Louis School of Medicine

West Virginia University School of Medicine

George Washington University School of Medicine

1997

Brown University School of Medicine

Oregon Health Sciences University School of Medicine

Georgetown University School of Medicine

University of Chicago, Pritzker School of Medicine

University of Kentucky, Chandler Medical Center

Morehouse School of Medicine

Loyola University of Chicago Stritch School of Medicine

University of Rochester Medical Center

1998

Harvard University Medical School

Howard University College of Medicine

St. Louis University School of Medicine

Medical University of South Carolina

University of Virginia School of Medicine

Vanderbilt University School of Medicine

University of Texas Medical Branch at Galveston

University of Health Sciences College of Osteopathic Medicine

1999–2000

Southern Illinois University School of Medicine (Carbondale)

State University of New York (SUNY) College of Medicine (Syracuse)

University of California at Los Angeles

University of Florida College of Medicine (Gainesville)

University of Minnesota Medical School (Minneapolis)

Western University of Health Sciences (Pomona, CA)

Kelly et al. (1996) describe the results of a spirituality and medicine course at East Tennessee State University's School of Medicine. Of about 122 students eligible for enrollment, 34 expressed interest in the course, 24 attended the first session, and 16 students completed all course requirements (attendance at didactic presentations, participation in group discussions, and presentation of cases to the group). After taking the elective, medical students reported a higher level of comfort when discussing religious or spiritual issues with patients and showed an improved understanding of what the medical literature indicates about the relationship between religion and health. Bernard et al. (1995) discusses the benefits and liabilities of including courses on religion and medicine in the medical curriculum, again emphasizing the need for a patient-centered approach.

Despite the ethical concerns raised by Sloan et al. (1999), we are not aware of any case reports or systematic studies about physicians having caused harm by addressing patients' religious or spiritual concerns. One would expect to see such reports now that over half of the medical schools in the United States are training physicians to address such issues. This is not to suggest a lackadaisical attitude; if there is one area that needs further research, it is how clinicians can best integrate what we have learned about the religion-health relationship into clinical practice (on which, as noted earlier, there are almost no data).

EDUCATION IN PSYCHIATRY AND PSYCHOLOGY

In 1990, Sansome and colleagues surveyed 276 directors of psychiatric residencies (80% of all program directors in the United States) on whether they taught any aspect of religion to their residents in 1988. Only 12% of programs frequently or always included religion in their training curriculum. This report helped prompt the Accreditation Council on Graduate Medical Education (1994) to mandate in its Special Requirements for Psychiatry Residency Training that all training programs include the following:

- Didactic training in the "presentation of the biological, psychological, socio-cultural, economic, ethnic, gender, religious/spiritual, sexual orientation and family factors that significantly influence physical and psychological development in infancy, childhood, adolescence, and adulthood" (pp. 11–12)
- "Instruction about American culture and subcultures, particularly those found in the patient community associated with the training program. This instruction should include such issues as sex, race, ethnicity, religion/spirituality, and sexual orientation" (p. 18).

To facilitate the inclusion of religion and spirituality into residency education, Larson, Lu, et al. (1997) developed a model curriculum entitled "Integrating Religion and Spirituality

into Clinical Practice." This model curriculum provides three core modules and eight accessory modules that can be incorporated into residency education, depending on the amount of time available. In a short chapter on integrating religion into the education of mental health professionals, Bowman (1998) summarizes this document, succinctly describing "who should be taught . . . what should be taught . . . when should religion/spirituality be taught . . . [and] how can religion/spirituality be taught?"

At the practice level, progress is also being made in the integration of religion and spirituality into patient care. The American Psychiatric Association (1995) notes, in its *Practice Guidelines for the Psychiatric Evaluation of Adults*, that:

- "Important cultural and *religious* influences on the patient's life" should be collected as part of the initial evaluation of the psychiatric patient" (p. 71)
- "Evaluation ought to be performed in a manner that is sensitive to the patient's individuality, identifying issues of development, culture, ethnicity, gender, sexual orientation, familial/genetic patterns, religious/spiritual beliefs, social class, and physical and social environment influencing the patient's symptoms and behavior" (p. 74)
- Assessment must include "information specific to the individual patient that goes beyond what is conveyed by the diagnosis . . . [including] issues related to culture, ethnicity, gender, sexual orientation, and religious/spiritual beliefs" (p. 76).

A model curriculum for residency training programs in primary care is currently being developed at the National Institute for Healthcare Research (NIHR) under the direction of Christina Pulchalski. Thus, it appears that medical education on religion, spirituality and health is advancing forward at many different levels in order to stay abreast of the growing research in this area.

The same changes are occurring in the field of psychology. As noted earlier, Martin E. P. Seligman, a past president of the American Psychological Association, supports including education on religious and spiritual issues in psychology training programs (Seligman, 1998). Allen Bergin has for two decades argued for the integration of spirituality into psychotherapy (Bergin, 1980, 1991). Every psychology training program is now required to ensure that its curriculum "includes exposure to theoretical and empirical knowledge bases relevant to the role of cultural and individual diversity" in science and practice, and religion is included in the definition of "cultural and individual diversity" (American Psychological Association, 1995).

OVERVIEW OF RESEARCH FINDINGS

Religious beliefs and practices arising from established religious traditions are, in general, associated with better health. There is even some basis for suggesting that religion may have positive effects on health. This link is particularly well established for mental health, although there is growing evidence that indicates that physical health benefits accrue as well. We caution, however, that neither mental nor physical health benefits are established beyond doubt; further research is required to expand our knowledge base in this area (Sloan et al., 1999). In particular, we don't know if "prescribing religion" for nonreligious patients will make them any healthier. All we know is that when religious persons are studied (persons who have chosen religion for religion's sake, not in order to be healthy), they appear to be healthier, both mentally and physically. Indeed, becoming religious solely to achieve better health is an extrinsic use of religion, which may actually be associated with worse health outcomes (Batson, 1982; Donahue, 1985).

What is the magnitude of these health "effects"? Sloan et al. (1999) report that it is weak and inconsistent. We disagree. With regard to mental health, we find that recovery from depression occurs 70% faster for every 10-point increase on a 50-point intrinsic religiosity scale, an effect that increases to more than 100% for depressed persons with chronic health problems that are not responding to medical treatment (Koenig, George, & Peterson, 1998). The magnitude of the effect of religious involvement (defined as less than weekly attendance at religious services vs. attendance weekly or

more often) on physical health is equivalent to that of cigarette smoking; high levels of involvement can mean as much as seven years of additional life (Strawbridge, Cohen, et al., 1997; Hummer et al., 1999; Oman & Reed, 1998; Koenig, Hays, Larson, et al., 1999).

What is even more important than the health effects of religion, however, is that many, many people, particularly in the United States, depend heavily on religious beliefs and practices to cope when they are physically ill. More than 40% of medically ill patients in some areas of the country use religion as the first and foremost way of coping with serious health problems (Koenig, 1998b). Regardless of what impact religion has on health or what impact health has on religion, this finding alone makes religious beliefs and practices relevant to health care professionals. If many of our patients cognitively and emotionally deal with their illnesses by relying on religious faith, then health care professionals should be aware of this. Furthermore, if they are not clearly harmful to patients, these beliefs should probably be supported.

How, then, should the clinician make use of this research when treating and caring for patients? We now discuss applications for doctors (medical physicians, psychiatrists, and psychologists) and for other health professionals (e.g., nurses, social workers).

CLINICAL APPLICATIONS FOR DOCTORS

Meeting Patients' Religious and Spiritual Needs

We now describe activities that physicians may wish to perform in order to address the religious or spiritual needs of their patients.

Take a Religious History.   As part of the normal intake or baseline evaluation, physicians may choose to take a religious history—that is, to obtain information about the patient's religious background and whether the patient uses religion to help cope with health problems. At this time, the clinician may communicate to the patient that he or she is open to addressing the religious or spiritual concerns of the patient or will do whatever he or she can to connect the patient with someone who can address these concerns. If the clinician feels unprepared to address a particular religious issue (or any religious issues for that matter), then referral to a chaplain or other religious professional should be made. In any case, the clinician should communicate to the patient that the patient's religious concerns and needs as they relate to health are appropriate topics to address as part of the patient's overall health care. Kuhn (1988) and Matthews and Clark (1998) examine the usefulness of obtaining a spiritual or religious history and provide questions to ask to obtain such a history. Examples of such questions include the following:

- Are religious or spiritual beliefs an important part of your life?
- How do your religious or spiritual beliefs influence the way you take care of yourself?
- Do you rely on your religious or spiritual beliefs to help you cope with health problems?
- Are you part of a religious or spiritual community?
- Are there any religious or spiritual issues that need addressing?
- Who would you like to address religious or spiritual issues should they rise?
- How would you like me to address your spiritual needs?

An American College of Physicians consensus panel, led by Bernard Lo, Timothy Quill, and James Tulsky, has suggested the following questions be asked when taking a spiritual history for patients with severe or terminal illness (Lo et al., 1999).

- Is faith (religion, spirituality) important to you in this illness?
- Has faith (religion, spirituality) been important to you at other times in your life?
- Do you have someone to talk to about religious matters?
- Would you like to explore religious matters with someone?

These questions are general and nonoffensive, yet they open the discussion of this delicate issue between physician and patient.

Certain characteristics of patients may indicate a greater desire or need to discuss religious or spiritual issues. Daaleman and Nease (1994) surveyed 80 patients who were attending the University of Kansas Medical Center family practice outpatient clinic and found that frequency of attendance at religious services (once per month or more often) was a good predictor of whether patients would be receptive to physician-directed inquiry into religious and spiritual issues. In that study, religious attendance also predicted physician referral to clergy for spiritual problems. Surveying 380 family medicine outpatients in North Carolina, Oyama and Koenig (1998) found that greater personal religiousness predicted whether patients knew about the religious beliefs of their physicians and shared their own religious beliefs with their physicians. While it is not particularly surprising, it is notable that patients who frequently attend church or have strong religious beliefs are more receptive to discussing religious or spiritual issues.

Unfortunately, few doctors consistently address religious issues with their patients. In a study of 203 family practice patients in North Carolina and Pennsylvania, King and Bushwick (1994) found that 80% of patients said their physicians rarely if ever addressed spiritual issues (although 77% of these patients believed physicians should). Likewise, in a study of 135 family practice patients and 146 family physicians in Vermont, Maugans and Wadland (1991) found that only 11% of physicians indicated they frequently addressed religious issues with patients. Most of the patients in this study did not recall their physicians ever discussing religious concerns with them, although 40% of patients thought that such discussion should take place. In a random national poll of 1,000 adults, *USA Weekend* confirmed that only about 10% of persons reported that their doctor had talked to them about spiritual faith as a factor in physical health (McNichol, 1996).

Support or Encourage Religious Beliefs. If a patient's religious beliefs and practices appear healthy, then clinicians should feel free to support those that the *patient finds helpful*. According to P. A. Dewald, in *Psychotherapy: A Dynamic*

Approach (1971), providing psychological support is simply part of good clinical care (and good medicine):

> One of the therapist's tasks in supportive treatment is to survey the various defenses available to the patient and determine which of these can most effectively be introduced, strengthened, encouraged or reinforced. . . . He tries to help the patient more effectively use *pre-existing defenses which for him are familiar, rather than introduce new ones the patient is not able to use himself* [our italics]. But when new defenses are to be introduced by the therapist, they are chosen to be compatible with the patient's overall ego structure and already existent major defenses. (pp. 105, 127)

Ensure Access to Religious Resources. Physicians can ensure that hospitalized patients and family members have access to religious resources, including religious Scriptures or inspirational reading material, religious tapes (for the visually impaired), and religious programs on TV or radio and that they have an opportunity to speak with the hospital chaplain, if they so desire.

Respect Visits by Clergy. If community clergy are visiting the patient, physician visits or team rounds should not interrupt these visits, if possible. Clinicians should also make an effort to meet these clergy, since they may be valuable allies in caring for patients and their families after hospital discharge.

View Chaplains as Part of the Health Care Team. Chaplains should be included as members of the health care team, rounding on patients together with the physician, nurse, and other team members. Many clinicians are not aware of the rigorous training required to become a chaplain. After four years of college, the student must usually finish three years of divinity school (to obtain a master's degree in divinity) and then must go on to complete a program in Clinical Pastoral Education (CPE), which typically involves one to four years of additional training in a hospital. After this, chaplains must pass a written and an oral examination before being certified by the Association of Professional Chaplains. Thus, chaplains have as much if not more training than many other health professionals in the hospital. While the physician may not have the interest or expertise to address religious or spiritual issues, the chaplain is the true specialist in this area. In fact, we believe that the procedure for chaplain consultation should be the same as for consultation with any other medical specialty (i.e., that the chaplain should complete a consultation form) so that this information becomes a permanent part of the patient's medical record.

Spiritual needs are also present among psychiatric patients, a group to which chaplains have traditionally had limited access. In many hospitals, until recently, an order had to be written in the chart by the attending physician before a chaplain could visit a psychiatric patient. This is sad, given a recent study that found that 88% of psychiatric inpatients at Chicago's Rush-Presbyterian Medical Center admitted to having three or more current religious needs. More than three-quarters of these patients (76%) had not spoken with a clergyperson during their hospital stay, a figure that contrasted sharply with the 19% of medical inpatients who had not spoken with clergy (Fitchett et al., 1997).

Be Ready to Step in When Clergy Are Unavailable. However, the physician may not be able to delegate all responsibility for spiritual matters to the chaplain or other clergy. For example, a patient may be in extremis, so there is no time to consult a chaplain. The physician may be in the emergency room in the middle of the night facing distraught family members after the death of a loved one. The physician may be seeing patients in an outpatient setting without ready access to chaplains. The patient or family may not want to speak with a chaplain or religious professional because they lack trust in clergy because of previous negative experiences or because they feel overcome by guilt. The physician may be the only person available in these situations. The majority of physicians themselves recognize this fact; almost 70% of primary care doctors agree that physicians should address at least some religious issues with patients (Koenig, Bearon, & Dayringer, 1989).

Use Advanced Spiritual Interventions Cautiously.

The physician may or may not feel comfortable or be competent to perform more advanced spiritual interventions, such as praying with patients, providing specific religious materials to read, or rarely, encouraging religious activities that the patient is not already doing. Such spiritual interventions are not indicated for all patients in all situations. Instead, patients and situations should be carefully selected and the interventions highly individualized to fit the patient's religious background and spiritual need. If the physician chooses to perform any of these interventions, they must be patient centered. In other words, patients should usually initiate such interventions, and physicians should follow their lead. It is also probably necessary that the physician have the same religious background as the patient. "Prescribing" religious activities important for better health is not appropriate.

For example, if a situation calls for prayer, then the patient should do the praying, and the physician may sit quietly and agree with the prayer by saying, "Amen." Patients usually know their own needs better than the physician does, and this practice will help avoid any sense of coercion. If the physician decides to pray, she should obtain explicit consent from the patient beforehand. Remember that about one-third of patients do not wish their physicians to pray with them. Consent should be obtained in a way that the patient is entirely free to refuse. By this we mean that the patient should not be made to fear hurting the doctor's feelings by refusing consent. If the patient agrees, the prayer by the physician should be short and to the point and should focus on God's love and support for the patient.

One study reports that, approximately one-third of randomly sampled primary care physicians had prayed with patients, and the vast majority of these physicians indicated that the prayer was helpful (Koenig, Bearon, & Dayringer, 1989). Olive (1995) questioned 40 religiously devout physicians (defined as "having religious or spiritual beliefs that were an important part of their lives") about praying with patients. These physicians on average prayed privately for 65% of their patients and prayed aloud for 13% of their patients (67% reported having prayed aloud with patients or family members on at least one occasion). The physician initiated the praying aloud 53% of the time. When patients have been asked whether they would like their physician to pray with them, between 46% and 78% indicate that they would (Koenig, Smiley, & Gonzales, 1988; King & Bushwick, 1994; Kaldjian et al., 1998; Oyama & Koenig, 1998). One public opinion poll reported that 64% of Americans think that doctors should join their patients in prayer if the patient so requests (Yankelovich, 1996).

If prayer or any other advanced religious intervention is not patient centered, then it increases the risk that the physician will impose her personal beliefs and agenda on the patient, which we believe is not appropriate in a clinical setting. In situations where religious interventions are considered, it is advisable that the physician and patient be of the same religious background (as noted earlier); alternatively, a clergyperson of the patient's faith can be summoned. Some ethicists go even further, suggesting that no one should be allowed to pray openly with patients without their explicit request and permission and that, whenever possible, prayer should be led by an identified religious leader, rather than a member of the health care team, in order to avoid even the appearance of religious coercion (Dagi, 1995; Post et al., 1999).

Psychiatrists and mental health specialists may need to be even more cautious than medical physicians when addressing spiritual needs of psychiatric patients, particularly if any advanced religious interventions are considered (Meador & Koenig, 2000). There are boundary issues for some psychiatric patients that must be taken into account; these pose less of a problem for medical patients. This is not an excuse to let the spiritual needs of psychiatric patients go unmet, just a suggestion that clinicians proceed more slowly. Koenig and Pritchett (1998) describe ways that psychiatrists, psychologists, and counselors can utilize the religious beliefs of patients to meet therapeutic goals in psychotherapy.

Physicians Who Are
Atheists or Agnostics

What does the atheist or agnostic physician do if a patient who is suffering and in distress asks the clinician to pray with him? There are several views on how to respond. One view suggests that the only honest and appropriate response is for the physician to refuse and to call in someone else to pray with the patient; for the physician to pray with the patient in that situation would be a lie and should never be done.

What if there is no time to get someone else or the patient doesn't want anyone else to pray with him? In the context of the doctor-patient relationship, the physician is obligated, according to the ancient saying, "to cure sometimes, to relieve often, to comfort always." *To comfort always*—the focus is always on the patient, not on the doctor. This leads to a second view of how an atheist or agnostic physician might handle such a situation.

It may be insensitive and is perhaps not good medicine to turn down a request from a suffering patient that may bring the person comfort and hope. Saying "Amen" at the conclusion of a prayer said by the patient for relief of suffering or for healing wouldn't seem to betray the physician's personal convictions or sense of honesty. Indeed, the word "Amen," according to Webster's *New World Dictionary*, does not convey belief in a higher power but is simply the statement "so be it" (Webster's, 1980). Most physicians favor relieving suffering, regardless of their personal beliefs, and therefore might well be able to honestly agree with the patient's request for relief, even if it is made as part of a prayer, whether the request is addressed to God, Jesus, Mohammed, Buddha, the universe, or simply purely random chance or luck.

Certainly there are other views on how to approach this delicate subject. The physician could simply sit by the patient's side, holding his hand while the patient prays. At the conclusion of the prayer, the physician could simply give the patient a warm and reassuring hand squeeze (without saying anything) and then leave the room with a statement such as, "You will be in my thoughts." Cure sometimes, relieve often, *comfort always*.

According to the ethicist Stephen Post and colleagues, "The beneficent physician who is committed to the patient's best interest must consider how to support patient spirituality, if and when the patient deems it relevant; spirituality is also to be respected as an expression of patient autonomy" (Post et al., 2000, p. 579).

Provoking Guilt and a Sense
of Moral Failure

Sloan et al. (1999) express the concern that linking religious activities and better health may be harmful to patients by implying that illness is the result of insufficient faith. We agree that there is a risk that some persons, including health professionals, may conclude that illness is the result of the patient's own moral failure or lack of faith. It could be similarly argued, however, that doctors shouldn't tell patients to quit smoking for fear that patients will blame themselves down the line if emphysema or lung cancer develops because they haven't quit. This problem extends to most of the advice that physicians give patients about any health-related attitude or behavior. Concern over moral failings has long been a problem in stress medicine. If their cancers recur, patients may feel that they haven't dealt adequately with life stressors or practiced relaxation techniques faithfully enough. People who don't or can't lose weight are likely to experience similar feelings. The problem of guilt over becoming sick is not unique to religion.

Health professionals have long had to refrain from "judging" patients for making decisions that do not promote health as they have delved into sensitive, morally dangerous areas. Questions about sexual activity and risk of AIDS, transmission of other STDs, and teenage pregnancy provide some examples. Physicians are not reluctant to encourage patients to use condoms or to refrain from having multiple sexual partners, and it is their duty to educate patients about the risks that unsafe sexual habits pose to their health and to the health of others.

We agree that health care providers should never place on patients an additional burden of guilt for moral failure or inadequate faith simply because their physical health fails. Unfortunately, many patients may already be taking this perspective. Discussing such issues with their physicians will at least get the issue out in the open and allow for referral to chaplains or other clergy who can help the patient deal with such concerns. The patient who believes that God has not healed him because of some moral failing is raising not a medical issue but a theological one. The health care professional should consider involving clergy to handle that issue, since theologians have done a great deal of thoughtful work in this area.

People get sick for many reasons other than those related to religion. These include genetic factors, accidents, and degenerative changes associated with aging. If religion has physical health benefits, then these benefits are likely to accrue over a lifetime. While turning to religion may bring enormous comfort, relieve stress, and help people overcome addictive negative health behaviors, no one is claiming that it immediately reverses all physical health problems or completely prevents such problems from developing in the future.

Importance of Collaboration

Whenever possible, ongoing collaborative relationships should be established among physicians, chaplains in the hospital, and clergy in the community. As we have noted, time spent developing these relationships may pay off in terms of ensuring patient compliance, increasing continuity of care, and facilitating future referrals. Exposure to such collaboration is best begun early in training. Both medical students and CPE (Clinical Pastoral Education) students should take courses together and perform clinical duties together. In this way, both will learn early in their careers the value and the unique contributions of the other.

CLINICAL APPLICATIONS FOR OTHER HEALTH PROFESSIONALS

Other health professionals to whom research on health and religion applies include nurses, social workers, physical therapists, occupational therapists, and miscellaneous health care pro-

viders (e.g., nurses aides, radiology technicians). All of what has been said for physicians and psychologists applies equally to other health professionals, who often work even more closely with patients and address psychological and social needs that heavily overlap with spiritual needs. These health personnel are also especially likely to control the patients' access to religious resources and may be among the first to recognize that such resources are needed. Nursing, in fact, has been far ahead of medicine in addressing spiritual issues, which it has done as a matter of course for decades (Fish & Shelly, 1983; Ross, 1995; Oldnall, 1996).

Both nursing and social work evaluations should include an assessment of spiritual needs, particularly if medical personnel have failed to elicit and record such information. Care must be taken, however, that different health care providers (physicians, nurses, and social workers) do not duplicate the work of one another but rather complement the others' information gathering. The physician may best collect some information as part of a religious history, whereas the nurse might obtain unique information relevant to nursing, and the social worker might acquire spiritual information pertaining to the patient's family. Recall that Fitchett et al. (1997) found that more than three-quarters of medical inpatients had three or more religious needs during their hospitalization. Many of these needs go unaddressed because patients do not volunteer them and health professionals do not ask; unfortunately, this "don't ask, don't tell" policy may be contributing to unnecessary emotional distress and physical morbidity.

Specific Interventions

As noted earlier, supporting the patient's religious beliefs and practices, particularly if they do not conflict with medical treatments, is simply good clinical care. Providing access to religious resources of the patient's choosing is a primary task of nursing and, occasionally, also the task of social workers. As we have noted, religious or spiritual resources include inspirational literature, tapes, radio or television programs, religious services in the hospital chapel, discussions about health care and spiritual concerns, time to pray and, when necessary, someone to pray with (although as stated earlier, this is best done with a religious professional, if possible).

More advanced religious or spiritual interventions should be done cautiously and only by health providers experienced in these techniques. Recall that chaplains have many years of training that have prepared them to meet the spiritual needs of sick patients. Some religious interventions, however, require little training. Often, simply taking the time to listen to patients talk about their religious or spiritual concerns allows the patients to work through these issues themselves. Again, keeping religious interventions patient centered is of utmost importance, and all of the cautions noted for physicians apply to other health professionals as well.

Health care providers can also support patients' spirituality by providing a place and uninterrupted time for patients to pray or meditate. To accomplish this, patient care may need to be interrupted briefly or scheduled around the quiet time. When the patient's community clergy is visiting, nursing staff may delay nonessential duties or work around such visits. Attention must also be paid to the spiritual needs of family members, who, like the patient, may need religious resources for support and someone to talk to about their own spiritual concerns. When doing discharge planning, it is particularly important to have the chaplain (with the patient's permission) communicate with the patient's local clergy about spiritual needs that came up during hospitalization and that require continued help or follow-up after discharge. If there is a parish nurse available in the patient's congregation, then we encourage direct communication between nursing staff and the parish nurse.

PARISH NURSES

Perhaps one of the best ways to promote interaction between health care providers and religious professionals in meeting the spiritual, emotional, and physical needs of patients is to establish a parish nurse program. A parish nurse is usually both a member of the local congregation and a registered nurse. He or she is hired by the church and sometimes receives partial salary support from secular service agencies. The parish nurse assists people within the church and the community to develop healthier lives within the context of their faith tradition by working with members of the congregation or pastoral staff to develop programs and ministries that promote the health of individuals and families.

For example, in the St. Louis, Missouri, metropolitan area alone, there are 70 parish nurses from a variety of Christian faith traditions (Philpot, 1997). As members of the Greater St. Louis Parish Nurse Network, they interact and learn from one another through special educational programs and CME courses. Parish nurses have extensive preparation for their jobs. Typically, a parish nurse must be certified as a registered nurse and receive additional training in parish nursing from a program such as the Parish Nurse Training Institute at the Marquette University School of Nursing, in Milwaukee, Wisconsin. This additional training may last from 2 weeks to as long as one year and involve an internship period during which the nurse receives mentoring on how to set up a parish nurse practice within a congregation. The additional training involves topic areas such as spirituality and health, scriptural foundations for health care, how to give spiritual care within the nursing role, ethics and values, assessment, grief counseling, mental health concepts, how to work with volunteers, how to make referrals, client/family teaching, and legal issues. Duke University's school of nursing and divinity school have collaborated to establish a master's degree program in parish nursing in order to train academic leaders in this field.

The primary activities of the parish nurse involve performing individual consultations (for coping with changes in health status, understanding medications, and so on), visiting patients, teaching small group classes, and conducting volunteer training. Other activities include writing articles on health for the church newsletter and preparing bulletin board displays on specific health topics. The parish nurse may also counsel older persons and their families about how to maintain independent living, or, if that becomes impossible, assist in making decisions on alternative living arrangements. If necessary, the parish nurse can mobilize volunteers from the patient's congregation or from the broader community to help the person remain functionally active at home for as long as possible and delay placement in a nursing home.

When a member of the congregation is hospitalized, the parish nurse often consults with the nursing staff at the hospital and may participate in discharge planning. The parish nurse can also help interpret what the doctor has said to the patient and follow up on the recommendations to ensure that the patient complies with the medical treatment plan. This provides a smoother transition from the hospital back into the community. The parish nurse also works with pastoral staff at the church and with the patient's individual physicians to ensure that the patient's health needs are met. Furthermore, because of the importance of spiritual concerns during times of physical illness, the parish nurse, particularly if she has additional religious training, may pray with clients or encourage them by using Scriptures. Thus, the parish nurse can play a vital role in integrating spirituality into health care and health care into spirituality.

SUMMARY AND CONCLUSIONS

After briefly reviewing the research on religion and health, we explored the implications of this research for doctors (medical physicians, psychiatrists, and psychologists) and for other health professionals (such as nurses, social workers, counselors, and physical and occupational therapists). We focused on how the research findings apply to the everyday work of caring for patients. While the research on clinical application is almost nonexistent, there is sufficient evidence to move ahead cautiously with at least some preliminary recommendations. Medical education at both the doctorate and predoctorate levels is increasingly training physicians to address the religious and spiritual

needs of patients, or at least to consider the religious backgrounds of patients when making decisions about health care.

We encouraged physicians to take a religious history as part of their initial evaluation. Having learned about the religious beliefs and background of the patient, the physician may decide to support healthy religious beliefs and behaviors that the patient finds useful in coping with the stress of medical or psychiatric illness. The physician should also ensure that the patient has access to religious resources, respect the time the patient spends with her clergyperson, and include chaplains as an integral part of the health care team.

Under certain circumstances, physicians may address religious or spiritual issues directly, particularly when a clergyperson is unavailable or not desired. Advanced spiritual interventions such as praying with patients, providing specific religious materials to read, or encouraging religious or spiritual activities should be performed cautiously and only when the physician feels comfortable with and competent to perform such interventions, when the religious background of the physician is the same as the patient's, when circumstances clearly indicate a need for such interventions, and, most of the time, only after the patient initiates such activity. Any intervention must be patient centered, not physician centered, and should be implemented in a sensitive and respectful manner that always follows the patient's lead.

Other health professionals, such as nurses and social workers, may also address religious and spiritual needs of patients in ways similar to those recommended for physicians. Their efforts, however, should be coordinated not only among themselves but also with physicians so that repetition is not a problem. All of the cautions noted earlier for physicians apply equally to other health providers. These health care professionals can support the patient's spirituality in a number of special ways, including by providing a place and an uninterrupted time for the patient to pray or meditate, by attending to the spiritual needs of family members, and by ensuring that the chaplain communicates with the patient's local clergy to inform them about spiritual issues that arose during the hospital stay. One of the best ways to promote interaction between health professionals and religious professionals is to establish a parish nurse program. The parish nurse can serve as a bridge between the medical and the religious communities, promote healthy behaviors and disease screening within congregations, and, when church members become sick, help to improve medical outcomes, quality of life, and spiritual growth.

30

Religious Professionals

MUCH OF THE RESEARCH reviewed in this book supports the work of clergy and religious professionals who have dedicated their lives to meeting the religious and spiritual needs of people. The religious community has long known that devout religious involvement is an effective antidote for spiritual disease. We are now learning, however, that these tools of the clergy's trade—prayer, a trusting faith, inspirational Scripture, powerful ritual, supportive community—may have important influences on mental and physical health, as well. Effective treatment of mental and physical disease, in fact, may require a spiritual dimension of care that health care professionals are not trained to address, an aspect of care that is the primary domain of the religious professional.

As documented in earlier chapters of this book, the vast majority of medical and psychiatric patients have religious or spiritual needs.

Physical or mental illness seems to bring out these needs, particularly when patients perceive their world crumbling around them and their sense of control slipping away. Religion provides answers to questions that secular scientists and medical researchers cannot address, questions that come to the forefront when disease and illness strike and remind us that we are indeed mortal humans—"As for man, his days are like grass, he flourishes like a flower of the field; the wind blows over it and it is gone, and its place remembers it no more" (Psalm 103: 15, NIV). While science can help us understand the "how," only religion can answer the "why." Indeed, it is the "why" question that people most commonly ask when they get sick—particularly after modern medicine has thoroughly investigated and answered the "how" question.

It is the "why" questions, among others, that the clergy must address: Why did God allow me to become sick? Why must I go through this suffering? Why is my illness not responding to treatment? Why doesn't God simply heal me? Why don't I have enough faith? Why continue to struggle for life when I may soon die anyway? Why does God keep me alive when my life has no meaning? Why does my family have to go through all this? There is also a series of "what" questions that clergy must address: What is the purpose of my life now? What will happen to me in the future? What will give my life meaning if I lose my independence? What happened to all my dreams? What will happen to me when I die?

The health professional is likely to have a difficult time answering most of these questions. The religious professional, on the other hand, is better prepared. Armed with faith, hope, spiritual knowledge, spiritual understanding, spiritual power, and, perhaps most important, humility, the religious professional is often the most qualified and sometimes the only person who can meet the underlying spiritual and religious needs that give rise to the patient's questions. Many times, the only answer is not an answer at all but simply a presence. Health professionals have a hard time with this idea because they are accustomed to providing solutions and often become uncomfortable and sometimes irritated when the answers are not there. The religious professional, however, may be more familiar and comfortable with presence—or we would hope so, anyway.

In the pages ahead we examine what the research on religion and health means to chaplains, pastoral counselors, religious educators, community clergy, and congregations and explore how each of these religious professionals can utilize the findings to better meet the spiritual, psychological, social, and physical needs of those they serve. We, the authors, are not religious professionals, nor do we have any religious or spiritual training; thus, our vision and insight are limited by a lack of theological background and experience. Nevertheless, as health care professionals and medical researchers whose lives are devoted to enlightening and facilitating a new reconciliation between religion and medicine, we stand in a position to present at least one view.

CHAPLAINS

Of all religious professionals, the chaplain serves to benefit most from research that documents the health benefits of strong religious faith. Until recently, no one challenged the presence of chaplains on hospital staffs, since it was accepted without proof that their activities were a valuable and necessary part of health care. The spiritual benefits, the inevitable product of chaplain activities, had intrinsic worth, whether or not related to physical health outcomes. Furthermore, these spiritual benefits were thought to be intangible and unmeasurable, and it was considered impossible (and perhaps undesirable) to design research that would link them with mental or physical health.

The Changing Health Care Environment

In many places in the United States today, this view of the chaplain's intrinsic worth is changing. Chaplains now need to justify their presence in modern hospitals, particularly in an era of managed care, when every cost is scrutinized and every benefit carefully assessed. Chaplain services are now expected to demonstrate an impact—speed recovery, improve outcomes, increase patient satisfaction—benefits that can be measured and that will ultimately save the hospital money or increase revenue. The value of chaplains is now being measured by that standard, and it has caught them unprepared. Because chaplains have not in the past had to prove their worth, chaplain programs are largely clinically oriented and seldom train students to conduct research on health outcomes. This lack of a research base by which to justify their existence has recently become the chaplain's Achilles heel, since managed care organizations depend on such data for deciding whether a hospital service is valuable. And many chaplain services in different locations around the country are not passing the test.

Impact on Chaplain Services

On October 31, 1991, chaplains in Georgia's state psychiatric hospitals and prisons received their final paycheck. Because the state budget had fallen $415 million dollars short, legislators decided that one way to make up this deficit was to eliminate all full-time clinical chaplain positions in state-operated facilities (Association of Mental Health Clergy, 1991; Bailey, 1991; Carter, 1991; White, 1991). Chaplains are no longer on the payroll as full-time employees of these facilities. Instead, the needs of patients are served by "volunteer community clergy" or "contract chaplains" (who receive no fringe benefits such as health insurance, retirement, or liability protection). Similar events are taking place in other states. Despite this trend, the directors of most chaplain programs have not been sufficiently motivated to collect outcome data to document the effectiveness of chaplain services. The medical internist and health outcome researcher Elizabeth McSherry (1987) pointed out more than a decade ago that such research is critical for patient care and chaplain department survival in the years ahead.

According to chaplains in Georgia's psychiatric hospital system, Central State Hospital (CSH) in 1991 had nine full-time chaplains and two secretaries. All were released and replaced by contract chaplains paid on an hourly basis with no benefits. Contract chaplains now work about 20 to 30 hours per week at that facility, which houses more than 1,300 patients. In the nearby Georgia War Veterans Home, which has 550 patients, chaplains are hired to work six hours per week. Most chaplain time at these facilities is spent leading worship services. Only a couple of hours per week (30 minutes before and after services) are spent counseling with patients or their families. Are spiritual needs being met? The situation at CSH is actually one of the best in the state as far as chaplains are concerned. In Georgia's nine other state psychiatric hospitals, chaplains are hired for six to 10 hours per week per facility. Interestingly, the situation of part-time contract workers who receive no benefits was the primary issue involved in the 1997 strike by United Parcel Service workers. Remember that chaplains are required to complete four years of college, three years of divinity school, and one to four years of clinical pastoral education and thus have education and

training equivalent to those of many other health care professionals.

Much of the effectiveness of chaplains in the hospital comes from their ministry to hospital staff and the relationships they develop with staff members. Their effectiveness also depends on their involvement as active members of the interdisciplinary care team, being present as important decisions about patient care are made. How is such integrated work possible when the chaplain functions outside the mainstream of the hospital organization? Part of the issue is the need to develop a personal trust that comes from being there when events occur. This is not possible when chaplains are hired as contract laborers for only a few hours per week or when responsibilities are rotated among volunteer pastors from the community.

By mid-1997 the chaplain situation had still not returned to normal at CSH. A half-time chaplain (paid 20 contract hours per week without benefits) was providing chaplain services, along with seven pastors from the community who rotated this chore among them. CSH had no chaplain on staff full time at the hospital and no chaplain who was usually "in house." This arrangement has become the prototype for other human service organizations in the state, including state prisons. In 1991, the Department of Corrections protested vigorously when all full-time chaplains were dismissed, so the state allowed each prison to hire a 40-hour per week contract chaplain (again paid on an hourly basis). However, the Internal Revenue Service cracked down on the department for hiring a full time contract chaplain to avoid creating a permanent position. The Georgia authorities, in order to avoid creating a permanent position, restricted the number of hours for which the chaplain could be hired at a prison facility to a maximum of 29 hours a week, thereby meeting the IRS requirements. Some of these prisons have more than 1,000 inmates.

What about outside Georgia? The situation is not greatly different even in some denomination-run medical center chains. According to chaplains in the Birmingham, Alabama, area, pastoral care services at the two main campuses of the Baptist Medical Center (part of a 13-

hospital chain) have been under enormous pressure to reduce services. A few years ago, their Clinical Pastoral Education (CPE) program had 12 junior residents and four senior residents; all are gone now. The number of full-time chaplains is also being reduced; chaplains are being replaced by part-timers. Some chaplains are covering more than one hospital and are on call 24 hours per day at several hospitals for emergencies. To give these chaplains a break, hospital administration is recruiting volunteer community pastors who come in for training and assist with hospital coverage (as in Georgia). Of course, most community clergy are already overwhelmed by the needs of people in their own congregations and have little spare time for other duties. The hospital administrations at many of these hospitals see chaplains as serving largely a "public relations" function and have made little effort to integrate chaplains as part of the health care team. A message was recently sent to chaplains observing that they are just "icing on the cake" and that "we can't afford that anymore." This is a Baptist hospital system, located in the Bible Belt of the United States! Is this happening elsewhere?

According to chaplains at the University of Tennessee Medical Center in Knoxville, CPE programs have been dramatically cut both at this institution and at others around the country. Efforts are being made to work with the University development office to try to acquire an endowment to salvage chaplain services for the hospital. Medicare has traditionally provided some reimbursement for chaplain services. Recently, however, much of Medicare in the state of Tennessee has been taken over by five large, private management companies (TenCare). Not surprisingly, no or only very limited financial support has been reserved for pastoral services. Again, these moves are setting trends for the rest of the country, since Tennessee is being used by the federal government as a prototype for what may soon occur elsewhere. In addition, MECON, a research group that assesses hospital services at 300 major hospitals and then provides rankings for publication in national magazines, has removed pastoral services as one of the aspects of hospitals care that it measures. The message is clear.

Similar events are occurring in our nation's capital. St. Elizabeth's Hospital in Washington, D.C., formerly associated with the National Institutes of Mental Health, is now being run by the city government. The CPE program here is one of the oldest in the country, having recently celebrated its fiftieth anniversary. According to chaplains in this area, over the past few years the CPE program has been reduced from as many as 11 residency positions to one position in mid-1997. As that institution downsizes, staff chaplain positions are being disproportionately affected. Likewise, chaplains at the University of Virginia Medical Center in Charlottesville are feeling considerable pressure to justify their existence. While the chaplain program has not yet been cut, other departments in the hospital (e.g., social services) have grown about 25% over the past couple of years. Pastoral care, on the other hand, has received no additional funds, despite the increasing number of patients treated (as length of hospital stay drops). Many chaplains are reluctant to talk about these changes for fear that speaking out will jeopardize their positions.

Pressures on chaplain services are occurring in many other areas of the United States, including California and South Carolina. According to the National Association of Catholic Chaplains, as hospitals are taken over by for-profit corporations, these corporations' initial commitments to maintain the chaplain's office have not been upheld; instead, these offices have been subsumed under social work and other departments. Chaplains in California are also under fire, particularly in large managed care organizations like Kaiser Permanente, which are downsizing chaplain departments. If these corporations can get community clergy or lay volunteers to provide care, then why should they pay for trained chaplains? Some of the managed care organizations are asking the churches to pay the salaries of community clergy who come in to perform hospital chaplain duties. Chaplains don't have a union and are often at the mercy of hospital administrators—who base their decisions on data, not tradition.

Need for Chaplain Research

It is important that research on chaplain services be undertaken to show that (1) many hospitalized patients and their families utilize religion as their primary method of coping with serious medical illness; (2) religious and spiritual needs are prevalent among persons with acute and chronic psychiatric and medical conditions; (3) the vast majority of patients want their spiritual needs addressed as part of their medical and psychiatric care; and (4) when such religious or spiritual needs are met, patients get better faster and use fewer costly health care services.

We recommend that chaplain programs be identified around the country that have access to the resources and expertise to conduct research. These chaplain programs should then pool their resources and develop multisite studies to examine the impact they are having on health care costs and health outcomes. Even if chaplain departments don't have chaplains with necessary research expertise, certainly there are persons in local university research departments that would be willing to collaborate. Furthermore, consultants can be brought in from outside institutions to provide expertise on study design, project operation, and data analysis, as well as to help with writing grants to federal and foundation funding agencies to support this research.

Expanded Role for Hospital Chaplains

As noted in chapter 29, we believe that the research already conducted is sufficient to support an expanded role for chaplains in hospital settings. This research clearly demonstrates that many hospitalized patients rely heavily on their religious faith to facilitate coping with medical illness and that at least three-quarters of hospital patients (whether medical or psychiatric) have multiple religious or spiritual needs. There is also evidence that greater religious involvement may prevent depression or speed its recovery and in this way and other ways reduce the need for and the use of acute hospital services.

Chaplain visits have also been associated with shorter lengths of hospital stay (see chapter 27). Thus, we recommend that chaplains:

- Be fully integrated into the multidisciplinary care team
- Participate in morning and afternoon rounds with physicians and nurses
- Be available to provide religious or spiritual support and counseling to patients and families, particularly prior to surgery or other major diagnostic or therapeutic procedures
- Participate in discharge planning, contacting the patient's community clergy to facilitate the patient's transition back into the community and to mobilize congregational support if needed
- Conduct religious services and administer sacraments at bedside
- Possibly conduct routine spiritual histories, assessing religious and spiritual needs of all newly admitted patients
- Be available to provide religious or spiritual support and counseling to hospital staff, including nurses, social workers, nurses aides, and physicians.

Such an expanded role will increase the likelihood that religious and spiritual needs of all patients will be addressed and that spiritual care will be fully integrated into health care activities. The taking of religious histories and meeting of spiritual needs should be coordinated with other spiritual activities performed by the rest of the health care team (e.g., physicians, nurses) to avoid unnecessary overlap and confusion. While the chaplain should be the primary person to conduct these spiritual activities, there should be sufficient flexibility in the system so that health professionals can act independently when necessary and appropriate.

PASTORAL COUNSELORS

Pastoral counselors include any clergyperson who provides individual, family, or group counseling. Such counseling may be either formal (with services billed for like any other professional service) or informal (as may occur between clergy and members of their congregation).

Expanded Need for Services

Rates of emotional disorders in the United States are increasing rapidly, particularly among those facing health problems as they grow older. The baby boom cohort of 76 million persons born between 1945 and 1968, despite living during a time of unprecedented economic growth, widespread employment opportunities, and unlimited health care, are suffering from high rates of depression, anxiety disorder, and substance abuse problems (Koenig, George, & Schneider, 1994). As these persons moved into later life and begin developing health problems, particularly as health services become less and less available (including mental health services), it is likely that a great number will need counseling. Unable or unwilling to obtain such mental health services from traditional secular sources, many will turn to their clergy for such support. Thus, the demand for pastoral services will likely increase substantially in the decades ahead.

Another reason for an increase in demand for pastoral care is the spiritual revival now occurring in the United States. The reasons for this revival are not entirely clear. Nevertheless, many baby boomers are returning to church after years of absence from the pews (Roozen et al., 1990). Likewise, recent Gallup polls suggest that religion's influence in the United States is increasing. Between August 1997 and January 1998, the percentage of Americans who think religion is increasing its influence on American life climbed an amazing 12%, from 36% to 48% (Princeton Religion Research Center, 1998). Michael Novak noted in a *New York Times* article (May 24, 1998) that the twenty-first century will be "the most religious century" in recent times. If these surveys and public opinion polls are correct, then we may see many Americans either return to religion or more seriously pursue spiritual growth. These Americans will need pastoral counseling to help them develop their spiritual lives, as well as cope better with aging and health problems. Several guides are now available to help pastoral counselors address

the mental, physical, and spiritual needs of middle-aged and older adults (Koenig, Lamar, et al., 1997; Koenig & Weaver, 1997, 1998).

Collaboration with Other Mental Health Professionals

Because pastoral counselors will see more and more persons with serious mental illness (as they fall through cracks in the public health system), closer collaboration between pastoral counselors and mental health professionals will be necessary. Patients for whom collaboration is particularly necessary are the severely depressed who are at risk for suicide, those with psychotic symptoms (hallucinations or delusions), and those with disorders that are more clearly biological in nature (obsessive-compulsive disorder, panic disorder, bipolar disorder, Alzheimer's disease). While pastoral counseling is very important for helping these persons cope with their psychiatric illnesses and life circumstances, medications and other biological therapies may be needed in order to treat or control the underlying disease. The psychiatrist of the future will not have a lot of time to talk with patients about what's troubling them but will be very skilled in administering medication and monitoring response to therapy. Pastoral counselors, working with psychiatrists, can provide the spiritual and psychological therapy that patients need in addition to medication. Thus, collaboration is essential if pastoral counselors and mental health specialists wish to obtain the best possible results for their patients.

As mental health professionals become more aware of the research linking religious involvement with mental health and begin inquiring about spiritual needs, they will be more likely to refer patients for pastoral counseling. This, together with the increasing number of persons who will seek help for emotional problems, will provide the pastoral counselor with a large clientele in need of spiritual and emotional assistance. It is essential that pastoral counselors be prepared to meet this increased demand for their services by developing relationships with mental health professionals they can trust and work with. It would be helpful in this regard if there were an overlap in the training of pastoral counselors and mental health professionals so that each could be exposed to the skills of the other and develop positive working relationships early in their professional careers (this idea is similar to that suggested for medical students and CPE students in chapter 29).

Focus of Counseling

As discussed in chapter 3, former APA president Martin Seligman (1998) stressed that our emphasis on trying to build up the self-esteem of our clients has been misplaced. The focus of therapy should be on helping people develop the personality traits and practical skills necessary for acquiring self-esteem, such as building character and promoting personal responsibility. These skills will enhance their ability to make wise choices in their lives and to fulfill their commitments to family, friends, and employers. Making wise choices, in turn, will reduce stressful life events that can precipitate emotional problems and lower quality of life. It will also promote responsibility for self-care, rather than encourage reliance on an already over burdened health care system.

In addition to meeting psychological needs, pastoral counselors are in a unique position to help persons develop their religious and spiritual resources. This can be done in a number of ways, such as emphasizing healthy Scriptural principles, promoting self-discipline (encouraging clients to set aside a time each day to develop their spiritual lives), encouraging personal prayer and prayer with family and friends, supporting regular involvement in religious community life (including participation in small Scripture study or prayer groups), and encouraging volunteer activity where people use their talents to help others in greater need. These activities help reduce loneliness and alienation by developing supportive relationships. Many persons who come in for counseling have lost their sense of vision and are morbidly preoccupied with themselves. They are searching for purpose and meaning and wondering about their roles in this world. Helping patients discover a new spiritual vision for their lives can help fill the void out of which depression,

anxiety, and other emotional symptoms often emerge.

RELIGIOUS EDUCATORS

Religious educators include instructors at seminaries, divinity schools, Bible colleges, and other university and academic settings. Over the years, as secular education has played down and even eliminated religion from its curriculum, secular ways of thinking, behaving, and relating to others have been emphasized. Many religious educators have found their own approach influenced by such trends. Traditional religious teachings are seen as outdated and not relevant to the needs of a modern society. Medical science, however, is beginning to discover that it may be precisely these old religious doctrines and practices that have maintained the mental health and well-being of people through the ages. As the traditional teachings and practices have been stripped from the curriculum, students are finding themselves armed with modern theories and beautifully rational philosophies but otherwise lacking in purpose, direction, and power to lead and inspire congregations. Because research is showing that religious beliefs and practices may be essential for maintaining well-being and quality of life, particularly as people age, lives change, and health deteriorates, religious educators should consider renewing the emphasis on traditional religious teachings, beliefs, and values. At the very least, students should be exposed to the growing body of medical research that demonstrates the mental and physical health benefits of devout religious practice. They should also be made aware of the negative effects that unhealthy religion can have (see chapter 4).

Health Courses and the Curriculum

Because modern clergy will increasingly be responsible for meeting not only the spiritual needs but also the mental and physical health needs of congregations, they will need preparation in seminary and divinity school for this new role. This will probably require that all clergy have a rudimentary knowledge of common health problems that persons face as they grow older. Clergy need to be able to recognize common mental disorders (especially those that increase the risk of suicide), be aware of the available treatments for these disorders, and know when to refer to mental health specialists. Skills in counseling will become more and more necessary for the modern clergyperson attempting to help members of the congregation overcome losses and cope with stressful life events. Knowledge about how to anticipate and handle liability issues associated with counseling will also be useful.

Health Promotion and Disease Prevention

Religious educators should prepare clergy for the important task of helping congregations maintain health and vigor. Since congregations will be looking to clergy in the decades ahead for help in meeting their health needs, a healthy congregation is certainly a goal worth striving for. It is always easier to prevent disease than to treat it. In order to be effective in this area, clergy will need to educate their laity and staff about health maintenance activities (proper diet, weight control, exercise, avoidance of negative health habits) and early disease detection (health screening). Attention to physical health and lifestyle is consistent with most religious teachings but is seldom emphasized in the pulpit. Instead, church members are encouraged to sit and fellowship together at church potlucks and bazaars that often include high-calorie, high-fat, high-cholesterol foods that must be offered and partaken of as a show of hospitality and respect. Perhaps, instead, fruits and vegetables, natural grain breads high in fiber, and low-calorie foods could be provided as a healthy alternative. Likewise, group exercise that includes praying and singing religious hymns can provide both physical and spiritual benefits.

Continuing Education (CE) Courses

Clergy should be required to take CE courses on health-related topics, and such courses should be made available at national denomina-

tional meetings. While there may be little interest today in such topics, interest will pick up in the years ahead as clergy realize that they are unprepared to meet the demands that congregations will soon make of them. These courses should emphasize an integration of spiritual, physical, and mental health, using a spiritual-biopsychosocial model. Indeed, we are learning that it is very difficult to separate the spiritual, the mental, and the physical parts of our nature.

COMMUNITY CLERGY

Emotional Needs of the Congregation

The most rapidly growing churches today are those that are meeting the needs of old and new members in their congregation—needs for fellowship, meaning and purpose in life, hope and optimism, vision, and a common goal for which to strive. Many of these needs are emotional and emerge from a growing dissatisfaction, lack of fulfillment, and sense of isolation that are common in our society today. Many of these emotional needs overlap with spiritual needs, and they are often met when people attend to the spiritual vacuum in their lives. Clergy play a vital role in maintaining the mental health of their congregations. The reason for this is the close link between spiritual and mental health, as the research we have reviewed has demonstrated. Many church members don't recognize the close link between mental and spiritual health and would benefit from such knowledge, knowledge that might encourage them to develop their own spiritual lives. Spiritual development, in turn, may ultimately bring the emotional fulfillment, happiness, and sense of meaning and purpose in life that members are seeking.

Why might information from medical research help guide these educational efforts? While clergy have for many years depended upon authority and tradition for educating and inspiring congregations, modern society operates in a data-driven age where scientific studies often speak with the authority that revelation once had. This research should be particularly exciting for clergy, since it validates what religious traditions have believed and taught for centuries. Also, congregations will benefit from knowing about recent demographic projections and financial projections concerning the cost of health care in the twenty-first century as they plan for a precarious future.

Educational efforts should include an emphasis, in sermons, in adult education classes, and in youth education programs, on the responsibility that church members must assume for one another. Most religious scriptures emphasize this anyway. Since it is the church that will be helping to shoulder the responsibility for caring for the needs of aging baby boomers, it is necessary to start working now on the attitudes of both older and younger church members to prepare them to take on this burden. Having role models in the middle generation who are supporting and providing for the needs of those in the older generation is perhaps the best way of teaching the youth about what their role should be in the years ahead.

Churches can provide a vital role in health promotion and disease prevention, particularly in minority communities (Haugk, 1976; Hatch & Lovelace, 1980; Kong et al., 1982; Saunders & Kong, 1983; Israel, 1985; Lasater et al., 1986; Olson et al., 1988; Davis et al., 1994; Ransdell, 1995; Ford et al., 1996). Because of the increasing responsibility that clergy will have for maintaining the health of congregations, clergy will need to take the lead in developing church health programs and motivating congregants to participate in them. Such programs should:

- Educate youth about (1) the importance of morals and values, (2) the need to avoid alcohol and drugs, premarital sexual activity, and other risky health behaviors, (3) the need to develop healthy eating and exercise habits, (4) the need to participate in activities that require cooperation, team effort, and development of prosocial behaviors, (5) the need to volunteer time to meet the needs of less fortunate people in the community, and (6) the relevance of a strong religious faith in coping with difficult problems in adolescence and young adulthood
- Provide support for elderly church members and their family caregivers, including the formation of support groups for caregivers and

of respite teams to provide caregivers with temporary relief from their duties
- Provide members of the congregation with help overcoming addictions (e.g., alcohol, drugs, sex, smoking, eating, overspending)
- Provide exercise and weight loss programs to help congregants maintain physical fitness; provide healthy cooking classes that teach how to prepare meals and snacks that are nutritious and satisfying but low in fat, cholesterol, and calories
- Provide health programs to identify high blood pressure, diabetes, cervical cancer, breast cancer, and other diseases detectable in their early stages by screening
- Provide or participate in a parish nurse program, as described in chapter 29.

Joining with Other Churches

Because of the increasing needs in our communities (e.g., need for crime control, drug control, mental health services, health care for the poor and elderly), no amount of effort by any single church will be sufficient. Thus, clergy should consider uniting their churches in a cooperative effort to accomplish common health goals. Methodist, Lutheran, Presbyterian, and Baptist congregations in one part of town might decide to join efforts to reduce crime or drug pedaling in their area. Alternatively, they might decide to support a pastoral counseling center or a day-care center to provide respite for weary caregivers of Alzheimer's patients. As a recent example, five churches in Durham, North Carolina (Watts Street Baptist, St. John Baptist, St. James Baptist, Northside Baptist, and Blacknall Presbyterian), two of which are primarily white, and three are African American, joined together to combat violence and crime. Churches in other cities are doing the same. In this way, both racial barriers and denominational barriers are broken down in a cooperative effort to accomplish common goals. An independent organization called Shepherd's Centers of America similarly brings different churches and synagogues together to meet the needs of elderly persons in the community, providing activities, education, respite care, meals, and other services to keep elders at home and avoid nursing home placement (Koenig, Lamar, et al., 1997).

CONGREGATIONS

The increasing evidence from epidemiological research to suggest that social support from the religious community is a powerful way of maintaining health, preventing disease, and improving treatment outcomes has important implications for congregations.

Responsibility for Meeting the Health Needs of Others

If members of the religious community are not willing to help meet the health care needs of their less fortunate neighbors, then much of what is preached in religious institutions around the country has little meaning. It has always been the religious community that met the care needs of the sick and poor when other avenues of support were not available. Recall that the Christian Church's greatest contribution to modern medicine was the care of the sick, not the healing of the sick (see chapter 2). Let us examine what this "caring" might require of the church in the decades ahead.

1. *Monitor Health Status of Members*. We are our brother's keepers. Church members should make an effort to monitor the health status of frail individuals in their congregations. This includes checking up on persons who don't show up for church as usual or who indicate that they have health problems. Such concern will ensure that diseases are detected early, medical care is sought appropriately, and medical treatments are complied with. Ask about when the person last saw her doctor, when her next appointment is scheduled, whether she needs transportation to the appointment or simply wants a companion, whether medications are being taken as prescribed, and so forth. Providing such support in a sensitive and respectful fashion will not only promote positive health behaviors but also convey to the person that she is an important and valued member of the community.

2. *Encourage Healthy Habits*. Church members should be accountable for their own health habits first and then help others maintain healthy lifestyles. This will help to create a healthy congregation that will be physically and emotionally fit to carry out ministry to others in the church and broader community. Encourage others to exercise, maintain an optimal weight, have regular health checkups, drive safely and wear seatbelts, sleep on a regular schedule, balance work and play, and avoid cigarette smoking and other unhealthy habits. For example, a member of the congregation could start up an Overeaters Anonymous group to help obese members in the church achieve and maintain ideal body weight. Alternatively, a member of the congregation might start up a group that takes morning or evening prayer walks, providing fellowship, exercise, and spiritual experiences together. Recall that Kumanyika and Charleston (1992) described a church-based weight control program that enrolled 188 women who each lost an average of six pounds. During a six-month follow-up, 65% of the reassessed women maintained or exceeded the weight loss they had achieved while participating in the program.

3. *Volunteer to Work in Health Programs*. Church members, particularly those with health training, may choose to volunteer time to support the health programs in their church. A nurse, nurse's aide, or other health professional, particularly if retired, might volunteer time to take blood pressures, provide health education, or assist in health screening programs (e.g., cholesterol screening, cervical cancer screening, depression screening). Alternatively, members can volunteer time to sit with a demented elderly person for a couple hours per week, helping the elderly person to remain at home while preventing burnout in the caregiver.

4. *Support Health Programs Financially*. Even those who don't have health skills or who don't have the time to participate in health programs can support these programs financially. Their support provides an opportunity for those who do have the skills and time to use their talents to help maintain the health of the congregation.

5. *Attend Health Programs*. Church members should feel a responsibility both to themselves and to others in the church to regularly participate in health programs, such as going to health education classes, having their blood pressure or cholesterol checked, making an effort to

cook and eat healthy meals, or joining an exercise group. Many such programs do not survive because church members do not participate in them. Again, leadership from the pastor is crucial in motivating participation.

6. *Get to Know Members of Congregation and Their Health Needs.* It is not possible to meet the mental and physical health needs of neighbors unless these needs are made known. Thus, church members should make their needs known and become aware of others' needs. This is different from gossiping. Gossiping involves a desire to be aware of others' problems without any intention of helping with those problems. Many persons are private about their own affairs and don't wish to have them broadcast throughout the church. Perhaps the best way to get to know others' needs is to develop relationships with people in the congregation and build trust so that they will confide their needs. An excellent way of accomplishing this is to create small groups of from five to eight persons who meet regularly in each other's homes, praying together, discussing the sermon together, and developing supportive relationships in which health needs are made known and taken care of in a confidential manner (Koenig, Lamar, et al., 1997).

7. *Ensure That Clergy Take a Leadership Role.* Members of the congregation need to ensure that their clergy take an interest and leadership role in meeting the health needs of the congregation. If they do not, then clergy should be sought who will. The time when churches could be concerned only with the spiritual needs of members is quickly becoming a thing of the past. In the modern church of the twenty-first century, people should expect to have their spiritual, emotional, and, in some cases, physical health needs met (particularly when no other avenues exist for meeting those needs). Both the pastor and church members are responsible for making this happen.

CONCERN BY RELIGIOUS PROFESSIONALS

We would expect all clergy to be overjoyed by scientific reports that indicate a positive relationship between religion and health. This is not so, and there are reasons that it is not so. Many religious professionals feel concerned that people may begin using religion for utilitarian reasons—that is, to achieve better health and longer life—rather than responding to a higher spiritual call to deepen one's faith, regardless of health consequences. An article in *Christian Century*, the voice of mainline Protestant Christianity, drives home this point:

> Perhaps no one is so simple as to start treating church like a nutritional supplement or a leafy green vegetable—something to add to one's life just to be on the safe side. Nevertheless, with their medically authorized praise of religion the scientists subtly confirm their own cultural authority. In our society, it's the scientists not the tellers of sacred stories, that get to define the "value" of the "faith factor." Their reports further inject the dangerous notion that faith is validated by its measurable outcomes. As long as one takes this view of faith, one will never get started on the actual journey of faith. (Faith's Benefits, 1999, p. 77)

We agree that such a use of these research findings would be sad indeed. And yet one wonders whether the urge to respond to a higher spiritual call may not have its origins in the suffering of unfulfilled human need. Let us go back to the sick medical or psychiatric patient who is lying in a hospital bed, struggling with physical or emotional pain, fearful and anxious, feeling isolated and alone, plagued by a vague sense that his life has lost its meaning, purpose, and significance. It is precisely in such circumstances that many of us begin to realize our finiteness and limitations, which then gives rise to spiritual needs and strivings.

For many years, if a doctor or nurse talked with a patient about her religious or spiritual needs, that health professional might lose his job because religion was not felt to be relevant to health care. There was little scientific evidence that religion had anything to do with health; if there was an effect, many health professionals believed that it was a negative one. The chaplain's service was viewed as a fringe benefit, not as an essential part of health care. This view continues today in many different sectors, and in the prevailing atmosphere where cost containment dominates, as we have seen, the chaplain is likely to become the first casualty of a more efficient, streamlined health care system.

Without research from systematic studies that demonstrate a possible link among religious involvement, health maintenance, and use of health services, patients' religious and spiritual needs may easily go unnoticed and unmet. While research on the religion-health relationship may, sadly, be used by some for utilitarian purposes, are not the spiritual strivings of even the loftiest among us to some extent self-serving? One thing is certain—it would be even more sad if the sick were deprived of the spiritual support and comfort on which their hope, health, and well-being may hinge.

SUMMARY AND CONCLUSIONS

The research that demonstrates a link between religious or spiritual factors and health (particularly mental health) has significant implications for clergy. This is especially true for chaplains because of the increasing pressure placed on them by hospital administrators to demonstrate the impact of their work on health outcomes. The research has shown us that the vast majority of patients, both medical and psychiatric, have religious and spiritual needs that likely impact their ability to cope with illnesses and affect the speed at which they recover. Chaplains are uniquely positioned to meet the spiritual needs of patients, and they are the only professional in the health care setting that is trained to do this.

Pastoral counselors (clergy who do not have specific training, and trained counselors) will likely find that more and more persons will turn to them for help in the years ahead. Many of the mental conditions for which pastoral counselors are sought will be as serious as the problems for which people see psychiatrists and psychologists. The simple tools of prayer, Scripture reading, putting one's faith and trust in God, reaching out to help others with worse problems, and becoming more actively involved in

religious community appear to be remarkably effective in helping persons cope with illness, adapt to stress, and recover quickly from depression. They do have their limitations, however, and pastoral counselors must be trained to recognize when referral to mental health specialists for in-depth psychotherapeutic or biological treatment is necessary.

Religious educators will benefit from knowing about recent research on the relationship between religion and health. They should also be aware of changes in population demographics and the increasing problems associated with health care financing. The next generation of clergy must be prepared to lead congregations to mobilize their spiritual resources to help maintain both their own health and the health of others. As noted, the clergy have spiritual tools that are uniquely powerful in addressing the health needs of future congregations, and these should not be too readily traded for a popular psychology whose value remains unproven. Because of the heavy overlap between spiritual and mental health needs, and because of the impact of spiritual factors on mental health, community clergy must be well trained to minister to emotional needs.

Community clergy have a responsibility to educate congregations about the need to care for their physical bodies. This may be accomplished by developing health programs and, in some settings, by participating in a parish nurse program. There is increasing evidence that the church will be largely responsible for caring for the health needs of congregants in the years ahead as government resources are exceeded. That burden of care will be a lot lighter if church members have learned to exercise, maintain ideal body weight, eat healthy diets, have regular medical checkups, participate in disease screening programs, comply with medical treatments, and avoid cigarette smoking and other unhealthy habits. Our youth will bear the burden of caring for millions of aging baby boomers in the decades ahead. Now is also the time for churches to instill in their youth a sense of responsibility toward others, teaching them to volunteer time to learn about the needs of others and help meet those needs.

Finally, members of religious congregations must assume responsibility for their own health behaviors by becoming actively involved in their church's health programs. They must support such programs with their time and their money. In addition, they must look out for the health needs of one another, ensuring that all members have their mental, physical, and spiritual needs met and that their clergy are actively leading this process.

PART VII

PRIORITIES FOR
FUTURE RESEARCH

31

Areas of Research That Need Further Study

B ECAUSE THE FIELD OF RELI- gion and health is so young, there are many areas that require further study. Thus far, we have only scratched the surface in acquiring knowledge about the influences of religion on health, the influences of health on religion, and the mechanisms by which these effects occur. In this chapter we examine specific areas that require further research and should be high-priority areas for future funding. We have divided these areas into eight topics: mental health, substance abuse, neurosciences, physical health, health promotion and disease prevention, use of health services, mechanisms of effect, and application of findings to clinical practice.

MENTAL HEALTH

Chronic Mental Disorders

Future studies are needed to examine the influences of religious belief and practice on the development and course of schizophrenia and other chronic mental disorders. Special attention should be paid to the role of the church in meeting the needs of the chronically mentally ill. This group includes those with severe personality disorders such as borderline and antisocial disorders, people who have not done well within the traditional mental health system. Innovative programs are needed to take advantage of the religious and spiritual resources of patients and of the manpower resources within religious communities to facilitate recovery and to provide the emotional support and understanding these people need. More information is needed also about the relationship between religion, spirituality and the development and course of bipolar disorder and its variants. Positive religious experiences are often heightened during the manic or hypomanic phase of the illness, whereas religious delusions of damnation and guilt may occur in the depressed phase. Again, further research is needed on how religious communities can best support afflicted individuals during both phases of their illness.

Mental Disorders in Children

Studies in children and adolescents are needed to examine the relationship between religious training and depression, anxiety, attention deficit disorder, conduct disorder, and other emotional and mental disorders. It goes without saying that childhood is a critical time in life, and religious factors may have an enormous influence, for better or worse, at this vulnerable stage. We know almost nothing about the relationship between religion and mental health during these early years. Robert Coles (1991) and James Fowler (1981) have begun the dialogue, but much work remains.

While we have considerable data on religion, delinquency, and substance abuse in adolescents, there is almost no research on how religious involvement influences the course of mental disorders in children and adolescents. There is a growing epidemic of depression in this age group that has received almost no attention (Seligman, 1998). To our knowledge, the only research study that examines religion and depression in children is that of Miller, Warner, et al. (1997). Recall that 40% of American families attend religious services weekly or more often and that many of the children in these families participate in religious classes. The potential impact that the church could make in terms of early detection of emotional and mental disorder and in the provision of support to these children and their families is enormous.

Mental Disorders in the Elderly

Although we know more about the relationship between religious beliefs and practices and mental health in the elderly than we do in children, persons in later life may be particularly open and receptive to religion. The elderly population is growing rapidly in the United States and around the world. While the number of persons over age 65 in 1998 was only about 35 million, that number may double in the next 30 years. With improved medical care, persons

with chronic disability are more likely to survive longer. Consequently, the number of severely disabled persons over age 65 in the population is expected to rise from the current number of 2–4 million to more than 12 million during the next few decades. This means that there will be increasing numbers of people with depression related to chronic illness and disability and increased depression among stressed caregivers. Religion as a source of emotional and social support may be a critical factor in meeting the needs of older adults in this new century. Further research is needed to identify how elderly persons can best utilize religious resources and also how we can most effectively mobilize religious communities to provide the care and services that elders need.

Course and Outcome of Mental Disorders

To our knowledge, only three studies have examined the impact of religious beliefs or practices on the course and outcome of major mental disorder. Miller, Warner, et al. (1997) examined religiosity and its association with maternal and offspring depression. These investigators found that (1) a high level of maternal religiosity (degree of religious importance) was protective against maternal depressive disorder, and (2) maternal religiosity and mother-offspring concordance of denomination (e.g., both Protestants or both Catholic) were protective against offspring depression, independent of maternal parental bonding, maternal social functioning, and maternal demographics.

Braam, Beekman, Deeg, et al. (1997) conducted a 12-month prospective study of 177 persons ages 55–89 who were selected from a larger community-based population on the basis of having scored 16 or higher on the CES-D. Religious salience was measured by a single variable. Subjects were asked to choose the three domains of life they considered most important in their present situation. Among the eight domains presented to subjects was "a strong faith"; if the subject chose "strong faith," religion was considered salient (29% of subjects). Absence of religious salience was associated with persistence of depression (OR 5.91, 95% CI 1.48–23.6). Effects were particularly strong among subjects with one or more chronic illnesses, pain, or one or more functional limitations.

Finally, Koenig, George, and Peterson (1998) identified 87 elderly medical inpatients with depressive disorder, using the Diagnostic Interview Schedule. These patients were followed for a median of 47 weeks, as researchers examined baseline predictors of depression remission. Intrinsic religiosity (IR) significantly increased the likelihood of remission; for every 10-point increase on the Hoge IR scale, the speed of remission increased by 70%. Among depressed patients whose physical illnesses were not improving or worsening, the speed at which depression remitted increased by 100% for every 10-point increase on the scale.

These are the only studies that have systematically examined the effects of religion or spirituality on the course or outcome of a mental disorder. We know almost nothing about the impact of religious factors on the outcomes of other mental disorders.

Interactions with Biological, Psychological, and Social Treatments

Another potentially fruitful area of research is the interaction between religion and standard biological, psychological, and social treatments. Traditional therapies for mental disorder may be more or less effective depending upon the religiousness of the patient. Do persons with high intrinsic religiosity respondent faster to antidepressants, antipsychotic medication, or mood stabilizers than do those with low intrinsic religiosity? Do high intrinsics respond more or less quickly to electric shock therapy (ECT)? Is there an interaction between religiousness and psychotherapy? Does the particular type of psychotherapy make a difference in this regard? Is the social support provided by a religious community more helpful to persons with depression or anxiety disorder than the social support offered by nonreligious sources (e.g., bridge club, country club)?

Adaptation and Coping by Families and Caregivers

Because of the increasing number of older and disabled people in the population and the declining resources with which to provide care for these individuals, families in the decades ahead will need to assume more and more responsibility for the care for sick members when they develop dementia, severe arthritis, cancer, or other chronic disabling conditions. Caregiver exhaustion may become a serious public health problem in the years ahead. Once the ill person dies, the suffering does not end, because the family must then cope with the loss of its loved one and the other changes that ensue. This is true whether the sick family member is a child, a spouse, or an elderly parent. Research is needed on the role of religious beliefs, religious practices, and a supportive religious community in the adaptation of families that are caring for sick loved ones or going through bereavement. Preliminary research indicates that religious beliefs and practices may be powerful sources of support for such persons (Rabins, Fitting, Eastham, & Fetting, 1990; Rabin, Fitting, Eastham, & Zabora, 1990; Stolley et al., 1998).

Negative Effects of Religion on Mental Health

Certain religious beliefs and practices may impair recovery from mental disorder. While there have been many claims that this is the case, almost no systematic research has examined how this might occur. While it is likely that religion does negatively influence the course of some mental disorders in certain individuals, how frequently and in what circumstances this occurs has yet to be defined. For example, the obsessive-compulsive individual who prays three to four hours per day and attends religious services daily may be seen by the religious community as very spiritual and be praised for these activities. In this case, religion conceals the disorder and may delay diagnosis and effective treatment. Again, however, this is a hypothetical example, and we do not know how often this actually occurs.

Other questions that need answers include the following: Does the control of anger promoted by religious teachings cause unhealthy repression of aggressive impulses, causing harmful physiological changes (high blood pressure, coronary artery disease, headaches) or resulting in passive-aggressive tendencies that impair functioning and disturb relationships with others? Does devout belief in the supernatural impair a person's ability to deal with reality and cope with problems in the real world? What effect does forcing children to participate in religious practices have on their later development and adult functioning? Does encouraging religious beliefs, practices, and experiences in schizophrenics lead to more delusional activity and destabilize their disease? How does religion affect medication compliance in those with mental disorder?

Effects of Different Religious Belief Systems on Mental Health

Not all religious beliefs and practices may have the same impact on health outcomes. Studies are needed to determine whether different religious beliefs have similar effects on the course and outcome of mental disorders. Does the impact of religion depend on whether one is Jewish, Christian, Muslim, Buddhist, Hindu, atheist, or a New Age believer? Comparison studies are difficult to design but should be possible. Different religious belief systems and practices, because of their differing content, may affect the course of mental disorders in unique ways. No research has yet comprehensively examined this question. Prospective studies are needed that assess and follow persons with different religious beliefs and practices over extended periods of time.

Long-Term Effects of Individual- and Community-Oriented Spirituality

We know that different types of spirituality emphasize religious community to a greater or lesser degree. For example, one type of spirituality relies heavily on individual meditation and

focuses on self and personal control; religious community is not emphasized. Another type of spirituality emphasizes religious participation, group worship and prayer, and involvement in social programs such as visiting the sick, providing food for the hungry, or working to combat drug use and crime in the inner city. What are the short- and long-term mental health effects of individual-centered spirituality compared to spirituality that emphasizes religious community and service?

Effectiveness of Religious Coping

Research is needed to determine what types of religious coping are effective for what types of life stress. Strawbridge et al. (1998) reported data that suggest that religiosity (measured as organizational and nonorganizational religious involvement) buffers the effects of financial and health problems on depression but exacerbates depression among those who are facing family crises. Because of the cross-sectional nature of that study, however, direction of causation could not be determined. What religious coping behaviors in prospective studies predict faster adjustment to health problems, bereavement, or other major losses? What religious coping strategies are effective for dealing with family crises? Which religious behaviors (private religious activities or involvement in religious community) promote more rapid adaptation to acute stress? Which religious activities facilitate adaptation to chronic stress? Are certain religious practices more or less helpful than others in different stages of grief? Does "foxhole" religion (turning to religion only at the time of loss or threatened loss) facilitate adaptation as quickly and as effectively as long-term religious commitment does? Again, longitudinal studies and clinical trials are needed to answer these questions.

Intervention Studies in Mental Health

There have been only a handful of clinical trials that have examined the effects of a religious intervention on the treatment of mental disorder. These studies have involved primarily religious-oriented psychotherapy or prayer. More intervention studies are clearly needed, since only an intervention (experiment or clinical trial) can provide direct evidence of benefit or harm. Intervention studies can also answer the following questions: What effect does involvement in religious community (the intervention) have on the course of a mental disorder? A sample of persons with depression might be recruited and randomized to either a religious community intervention or a control group (perhaps group attendance at a sports event). Similarly, what effect does a chaplain intervention (a series of structured chaplain visits) have on the course of depression or anxiety disorder, compared with traditional therapy? Again, a sample of depressed or anxious persons might be randomly assigned to either the chaplain intervention or to traditional care, with outcomes assessed by raters blinded to group assignment. Other questions can also be asked in such studies. For example, does the effect vary depending on the religiousness of the subject?

Studies are also needed to explore the interactive effects of religious interventions and traditional biological treatments for psychiatric disorder. For example, a study might compare the effects on depressive disorder of (a) antidepressant therapy plus regular participation in a small prayer group and (b) antidepressant therapy alone. Another study might examine religious conversion as an intervention for treating anxiety disorder. The challenge in such research would be to determine a way to induce religious conversion among those randomized to treatment, while at the same time keeping those assigned to the control group from spontaneously converting.

This problem (contamination of the control group) is always present in intervention studies and was most dramatically demonstrated in the Multiple Risk Factor Intervention Trial (MRFIT), which randomly assigned 356,222 subjects to either an intervention (cardiac risk factor reduction program) or a control group (which received standard care). The finding of this multimillion dollar study shocked the scientific community. There was no significant difference in the reduction of cardiac events between the intervention and control groups. Further analy-

sis revealed that the reason for this outcome was that the subjects in the control group, aware that they were in a cardiac risk factor reduction study, began modifying their cardiac risk factors on their own! The end result was that both groups had a similar reduction of cardiac risk factors and consequently a similar reduction in cardiac events (Meaton et al., 1981). Keeping subjects in a control group from engaging in the religious intervention may be a difficult task.

Intervention studies are particularly important in high-risk populations such as children and adolescents, the chronically mentally ill, minority populations, and the medically ill elderly. These populations are often open to religion and may be quite willing to participate in such studies. In addition, secular mental health interventions have had relatively limited success in these populations.

SUBSTANCE ABUSE

Because of widely known religious prohibitions against substance abuse and the effectiveness of spiritually based programs such as Alcoholics Anonymous in helping substance abusers remain abstinent, numerous studies have now examined the relationship between religion and alcohol or drug use (see chapter 11). Many areas, however, have received little or no attention.

Information is needed on the role that religion plays in controlling substance abuse in high-risk populations—those with dual diagnoses (both a mental disorder and a substance abuse disorder), minorities (e.g., African Americans, Mexican Americans, Indians, Asians), adult narcotic abusers (users of heroin, amphetamines, cocaine), and prescription-drug abusers (e.g., users of benzodiazepines, sleeping medications, pain relievers). Both cross-sectional and longitudinal studies are needed in these populations, to be followed by clinical trials.

The effect of religious conversion on the course of substance abuse needs to be more carefully studied. If religious conversion can help some persons become abstinent, information is needed about the characteristics of such persons, the timing of religious conversion in the course of the addiction, and the mechanism by which conversion helps establish abstinence. Likewise, information is needed on how religious alienation or disengagement affects the onset and course of substance abuse. Turning away from religion can make certain individuals more vulnerable to addictive disorders or may worsen prognosis among those who are already addicted.

As with other mental disorders, little information is known about the impact of different religious belief systems on the course of substance abuse. Do certain religious beliefs facilitate the development of addiction? Do certain religious beliefs protect against addiction? Do Western religions, Eastern religions, and New Age spirituality all have the same effect in this regard? Do religious belief systems that emphasize personal religious experience influence substance abuse in the same way that belief systems emphasizing religious community do?

Clinical trials are needed to determine the influence of religious education (e.g., attending religious schools, attending Sunday school classes) on the development and course of substance abuse among adolescents and teenagers. Studies are also needed to determine what effect religious training has on substance abuse and dependence in adulthood. Do the effects of religious education on later substance abuse depend on what age the training is delivered (i.e., is there a certain age at which exposure to such training is more effective)? Are certain types of religious education (with regard to method or content) better than others in preventing substance abuse (for example, is hands-on involvement in helping substance abusers more effective than didactic lectures on the evils of drugs and alcohol)?

These research questions need to be studied in different religious groups, races, and cultures. Social and cultural factors may heavily influence the effects that religious belief and training have on the development or course of substance abuse and dependence.

Interventions for Treating Substance Abuse

In chapter 11 we discussed intervention studies that examined the use of religion and spiritual-

ity in the treatment of addictive disorders. We still don't know whether religious treatment programs are as effective as or more effective than secular treatments. Cost-benefit analyses are needed to identify the most cost-effective treatment for substance abuse, given the low cost of self-help programs such as AA and the high cost of secular inpatient and outpatient programs. Furthermore, not all persons are likely to respond equally well to religious, spiritual, and secular treatment programs. Research is needed to identify the demographic and psychosocial characteristics of those most likely to respond to each approach.

Interventions are needed that involve religious communities in the treatment of substance abuse problems. For example, substance abusers might be randomized to either a group that receives standard inpatient or outpatient treatment or to a group that receives treatment in a monastic-type environment, a religious kibbutz, or a "religious family" environment. Creative ideas are needed on how the resources of religious communities can be best utilized to help those with addictive disorders, ideas that can be incorporated into testable interventions that can be widely applied in church settings. Finally, individual-focused interventions (transcendental meditation and other approaches that focus on personal spirituality) need to be compared with the religious community approaches described earlier. Studies should be designed not only to examine short-term outcomes but also to assess long-term effects that may not be evident until decades later. Such studies are expensive and require long-term commitment both by investigators and by funding agencies.

NEUROSCIENCES

The field of neuroscience is an exciting and growing area that may provide insights into the biological basis for religious experience. The emphasis thus far, however, has been primarily on personal religious experience, with almost no attention given to religious commitment, religious discipline, religious community service, and other religious activities that are not as experience oriented. Nevertheless, trying to understand how religious experiences are rooted in neurological processes is an important area that needs further study.

Neuroanatomical Mediators of Religious Experience

What parts of the brain and central nervous system mediate religious experience? Is this a localized process, occurring in only one specific part of the brain (the temporal lobes, for example)? Is it a whole-brain phenomenon, not restricted to any one part of the brain but a result of interactions between many parts? Is religious experience an epi-phenomenon, related to but not the same as the natural physiological processes that make up thought, emotion, and other brain activity and instead representing "superemperical" processes that have not yet been empirically verified to the satisfaction of mainstream science (Levin, 1996a)?

If natural physiological processes are involved in religious experience, what are they? In other words, what neurotransmitters and neural circuits are responsible for such experiences? Methods such as PET scanning, functional MRI, and use of radio-labeled tracers for identifying specific brain receptors and metabolic processes are becoming increasingly sophisticated, allowing for detailed examination of central nervous system activities during waking and sleeping states.

With this rapidly growing technology, we may soon be able to identify and distinguish physiological and neuroanatomical mediators of different religious and spiritual states. This may allow us to localize the brain areas responsible for traditional Western-type religious experiences and to distinguish these from brain areas responsible for mystical Eastern-type religious experiences, drug-induced experiences, and psychotic religious states. This technology may also help us to distinguish neuroanatomical correlates of solitary and community-oriented religious experiences.

Soon it may be possible to define neuroanatomical correlates of personality types, allowing us to identify personalities that promote or impede religious experience. This technology may eventually help us to predict, on the basis of identifiable and quantifiable structures in the brain, the likelihood that a person will or will not have religious experiences. Such technology, however, will probably give us only one piece of information, which will have to be used in conjunction with psychological, social, and other less quantifiable factors to better understand the human capacity for religious experience.

Prospective Studies

In addition to the largely cross-sectional studies we have described, prospective studies are needed to determine the long-term neuroanatomical and physiological consequences of religious experience. These studies will allow us to determine how religious experience affects the brain, rather than vice versa. For example, one might study a group of persons after their religious conversion (which has occurred naturally) and a group of control subjects, comparing specific areas of brain functioning in the two groups over time. Sudden and gradual conversions could each be studied in this manner. Similarly, one might study the long-term neuroanatomical and physiological consequences of solitary individual religious experience during transcendental meditation and compare these brain changes with those that result from community-oriented religious experiences.

Experimental Studies

Particularly exciting is the potential for intervention and experimental studies. For example, one might attempt to induce religious conversion and then observe short-term and long-term neurophysiological changes in brain, comparing brain functioning over time in converted subjects and in control subjects. Likewise, one might induce religious possession states, fainting ("falling out"), or glossolalia ("speaking in tongues"), observing neurophysiological changes and comparing them to changes in control subjects. Other studies might use drugs to induce religious and spiritual experiences, comparing neurophysiological changes in treated and control subjects. Information from such studies could be used to distinguish drug-induced brain changes from brain changes that occur in persons having natural religious or spiritual experiences.

Theological Implications

If the brain areas responsible for religious experience can be identified, it may become eventually possible to activate these areas of the brain through direct stimulation or by pharmacologic means. Perhaps the benefits of devout religious beliefs and practice could be obtained someday by simply taking a pill, avoiding the responsibilities and encumbrances of religious commitment. Given the far-reaching implications of such work, considerable input from ethicists and theologians will be needed in the design of such studies and the interpretation of results. Also, one would have to clarify how such research would advance human progress and improve society. These questions must be asked before such studies are carried out, not afterward.

PHYSICAL HEALTH

Research on the religion-physical health relationship is far behind that on the religion-mental health relationship. The idea that religion might affect physical health through known social, psychological, and physiological processes capable of being studied and understood by science is a relatively new one. Until recently, it was thought that the effects of religion on physical health were due to supernatural processes beyond our understanding. Since scientists could not study supernatural processes, even if they existed, this subject was placed outside the realm of scientific investigation. With advances in knowledge about how the mind can affect physical health through neuroendocrine and immunological processes (and the role that belief plays in influencing these processes), we are now able to better understand how religion might impact disease susceptibility and outcome through natural mechanisms.

Common Medical Illnesses and Psychosomatic Disorders

Longitudinal studies are needed to determine whether and how different dimensions of religiosity and spirituality influence the development and course of common disabling medical illnesses such as diabetes, heart disease, cancer, stroke, and arthritis. Similar studies are needed to document whether and how religious factors influence psychosomatic illnesses such as chronic fatigue syndrome, fibromyalgia, irritable bowel syndrome, peptic ulcer disease, and asthma. Establishing links between religious practices and these widely prevalent medical conditions could have substantial public health impact.

Outcome Following Surgery

Studies are needed to examine the effects of religious beliefs and activities on outcomes following major surgery (e.g., coronary artery bypass grafting, organ transplantation, cancer surgery, orthopedic surgery). Outcomes that could be assessed include surgical complication rate, need for postop medication, nursing time required, speed of in-hospital recovery, and time to return to work or an active lifestyle. Religious variables could be assessed on both patients and surgeons and their impact on outcomes measured. Randomized trials could examine the effects on surgical outcomes of religious interventions such as prayer before surgery by surgeon, patient, or both, either together or separately. Some patients report that they feel more relaxed if they know their surgeon has prayed before going into the operating room. Numerous studies document the negative effects that anxiety can have on surgical outcomes, need for pain medication, and other outcomes; religious interventions such as prayer or meditation may counteract such anxiety.

Immune System Functioning

We now have data from several studies that suggest that religious activities are in some way related to immune system functioning. More research is needed to explore relationships between different dimensions of religiosity and different components of immune functioning. As noted earlier, we convened a conference at Duke University Medical Center that brought together 13 prominent scientists in the area of psychoneuroimmunology to brainstorm about possible research projects that might explore the link between religion, spirituality and immune functioning. This growing area of research may help to explain how religion affects health and extends survival.

Particularly important are studies that examine the effects of religion on changing immune function over time in persons at high risk for declining immune function, such as the elderly, those experiencing severe chronic stress (caregivers of family members with dementia), HIV-infected persons, and those receiving immunosuppressive drugs or chemotherapy for cancer. The relatively subtle effects of psychosocial factors on immune function may be more easily detected in those with high stress and weakened immune systems that have little reserve strength.

Neuroendocrine Changes

Studies are needed in healthy persons and those with cardiovascular disease to examine the relationship between religious beliefs and practices and autonomic nervous system activity. Such research would measure circulating levels of epinephrine and norepinephrine and assess end-organ responsiveness to these hormones. Studies of this kind may help provide physiological explanations for how different aspects of religion affect blood pressure and influence death rates from coronary heart disease.

Likewise, studies are needed that examine relationship between religious activities and cortisol production by the adrenal glands. Engaging in devout prayer and meditation, reading inspirational religious literature, and attending religious services (group worship, hymn singing, prayer) may affect cortisol levels and other hormones which influence immune function.

Intergenerational Studies

There is a need to examine what effect the religious beliefs and practices of parents has on medical illnesses experienced by their children, both during childhood and later in adult life. Retrospective studies should be conducted first, followed by prospective cohort studies that extend over decades. While intergenerational links between parental religiousness and offspring depression have been identified in one study (Miller, Warner, et al., 1997), these connections have not been studied in a detailed and comprehensive way with depression, other psychiatric disorders, or any medical illness. Psychosomatic diseases (e.g., asthma, peptic ulcer disease, inflammatory bowel disease, hypertension, chronic fatigue syndrome) hold the greatest promise of showing such an influence. Effects from religious influences and personality factors will need to be distinguished.

Faith Healing

Careful follow-up studies are needed of persons who claim miraculous healings at charismatic religious meetings, revivals, and faith healing services. Careful study of those with (and without) persistent healing may yield important insights into the psychological, social, and physiological mechanisms involved. Such research could ultimately identify the psychological and social factors responsible for spontaneous remissions.

Death and Dying

Prospective studies are needed to examine changes in religiousness among persons who are dying (in palliative care) and how these changes affect quality of life (well-being, peace, hope and meaning, cognitive awareness, pain level) and the physiological (cardiovascular, metabolic, immune system, and neurological) processes associated with dying. In addition, further research is needed to examine the relationship between religious beliefs and practices and end-of-life decision making, particularly with regard to advanced directives (e.g., whether to have cardiopulmonary resuscitation, treatment of infections). Research suggests that religious persons are less likely to forgo extraordinary life-saving interventions, perhaps because they have greater hope for recovery.

Intervention Studies

In order to definitively demonstrate that religious beliefs and practices have effects on physical health, intervention studies are needed. As noted earlier, these studies are not easy to design or carry out successfully.

Studies should focus on common, serious, and expensive physical diseases, such as cancer, hypertension, cardiovascular disease, and stroke. Interventions may include structured chaplain or clergy activities, group prayer with and without laying on of hands, practice of regular religious devotion (personal prayer, scripture reading, private worship), involvement in group worship (adoration, prayer, and singing), or participation in religious fellowship. Again, studies are needed to compare the effectiveness of religious practices performed in isolation and those performed in group settings.

Research is needed on the effects of experimentally induced religious conversion on the development or outcome of serious medical illness; use of a wait list control design can ensure that all subjects have an opportunity to experience the intervention. Health effects may be compared between persons converting to different religious faiths (e.g., Christian, Jewish, Muslim). Such studies may or may not be feasible, given the spontaneity that may be required for true conversion to take place. Observational studies that assess and track persons who experience religious conversion in a more natural way will provide important information to assist in the design of experimental studies.

Research is also needed to explore how religious interventions interact with biological treatments in affecting medical illness. For example, a study might compare the effects of group prayer plus chemotherapy and chemotherapy alone for the treatment of cancer. Similar studies could be designed to examine the interactive effects of religious interventions and analgesics for the treatment of chronic pain syndromes or religious interventions and cardiac procedures (CABG or angioplasty) for the treatment of CAD.

HEALTH PROMOTION AND DISEASE PREVENTION

Research on health promotion and disease prevention is strongly encouraged by the National Institutes of Health, which made it a funding priority in the 1990s and plans also to do so in the first decade of the new millennium. Thus, studies that examine the effects of religious beliefs, practices, and community systems on health maintenance and primary prevention may receive special funding consideration. Such studies are essential, given the increasing health needs of an aging U.S. population (and the dwindling financial resources to meet those needs). Keeping people healthy, then, has become a national priority, and the American church stands in a vital position to help with this effort. Consider the following: While people seldom see their doctor more than once or twice a year, almost 70% of Americans are church members, and 43% report having attended religious services in the past seven days (Princeton Religion Research Center, 1996).

Health Programs in Churches and Synagogues

Studies are needed that systematically examine current efforts by religious communities to promote health and detect diseases early in their course. Health promotion programs in churches encourage members to stop smoking, exercise regularly, eat a balanced and healthy diet, or keep their weight under control. Some health programs may persuade members to wear safety belts, drive at or below the speed limit, and maintain a safe home. Churches or synagogues may sponsor screenings for high blood pressure, cancer, or high cholesterol or blood sugar levels. Where such programs are not in place, research is needed to examine the clergy's interest in and openness to developing such programs. In churches that have health programs, studies are needed to examine the level of congregation participation.

Assessing Health Promotion Programs

The effectiveness of health promotion programs must also be studied, and reasons for their effectiveness or lack of effectiveness must be identified. Prospective cohort studies are needed to examine changes in rates of illness and disease outcomes in congregations after health promotion programs have been instituted. Change in health service use and costs should also be assessed. Such naturalistic studies should be performed in congregations that are at high risk for poor health and illness, such as those with a high proportion of elderly and/or minority members.

Intervention studies are needed also to compare the overall health of congregations where such health programs are initiated with that of congregations assigned to a control group without such programs. Several congregations should be included in the intervention and control groups to increase the study's power to detect health differences and increase the generalizability of results. Similarly, studies are needed to examine health outcomes and service use in communities where Shepherd's centers have been started and to compare these communities with control communities that lack Shepherd's centers.

The Shepherd's center concept, in which several local churches, synagogues, and businesses pool their resources to develop programs to assist older adults in the community and keep them out of nursing homes, is rapidly spreading into communities nationwide. These programs are run by elderly persons themselves who volunteer their time and talents to help peers who are less fortunate than they are. Life enrichment and spiritual growth are the goals. These programs keep the healthy elderly healthy by enabling them to use of their talents and feel useful; they also meet the needs of the sick elderly, keeping them at home and reducing health care costs.

Parish Nurse Programs

Parish nurse programs are also spreading rapidly to many areas of the United States. As noted in chapter 29, this innovative program utilizes a registered nurse, ideally, a long-term member of the church congregation, who operates within the congregation. The parish nurse conducts health promotion programs and disease screening for church members. This program had its origins in the Midwest and has quickly spread to the West Coast and to parts of the East Coast. Because the parish nurse is part of the congregation, he is familiar to the members and readily available for consultation, and, if need be, he can refer members to appropriate health professionals.

There is almost no research, however, on how successful parish nurse programs have been. We know very little about what parish nurses actually do or how well they are received or utilized by church members. Furthermore, no studies have examined whether church congregations with parish nurses are any healthier or use any fewer health services than congregations without parish nurses. Consequently, studies are needed to examine the experience of congregations with parish nurses, as well as to gather information about the prevalence of such programs, the activities performed by parish nurses, sources of financial support for parish nurses, and benefits perceived by members of the congregation. Federal agencies may soon help fund parish nurse programs in churches, so such research will be essential.

USE OF HEALTH SERVICES

Given the growing crisis in health care that is resulting from the increased need for services and the decreased resources available to meet the need, research that examines the impact of religious beliefs and practices on decisions to seek health care and on the use of health services is critical. Studies are especially needed to examine relationships between religious factors and service use in populations at high risk for utilization of costly health services.

Religious Influences on Decisions to Seek Health Care

Research is needed to examine the effects of specific religious beliefs and practices on decisions to seek health care, both medical and psychiatric. We know that religion may either decrease or increase the likelihood that persons will seek health services; however, we have almost no information about which religious factors affect these decisions, or when in the natural history of a disease they are likely to do so.

Religious Influences on Service Use

Studies are needed to examine use of health services by members of different religious groups (Jews, Muslims, Catholics, conservative or fundamentalist Protestants, mainline and liberal Protestants) and by intensity of religious belief, practice, and commitment. These studies should be conducted in different racial, socioeconomic, and age groups and should be carefully controlled for confounding factors such as health status, income level, and access to health care services (including type of health insurance).

Service Use over Time

Prospective cohort studies, in particular, are needed to examine use of health services over time by members of different religious groups, by different levels of religious commitment, and by different levels of private and communal religious activity. Priority should be placed on research that examines populations at high risk for using great quantities of expensive health services, such as the medically ill elderly, persons with serious illnesses who are dying (during the last six to 12 months of life), and children or adolescents with chronic diseases (for whom the costs of care will accumulate throughout their lifetime).

Order of Effects

While religious factors may influence use of health services, it is also possible that frequent service use (e.g., acute hospitalization,

outpatient doctor visits) can impact religious activities. Persons who are sick and require many health services may not have the opportunity or the ability to participate in certain religious activities. It is likely, however, that these effects are bidirectional and interact over time. Religious factors may affect health service use at one point in time, and health service use may influence religious activities at another point. At still other times, they may affect each other simultaneously. Carefully designed longitudinal studies are needed to tease out effects of religious variables on service use from effects of service use on religious involvement.

Intervention Studies

Examples of interventions that may directly demonstrate the effects of religion on health service use include the following. A structured chaplain intervention could be administered to patients in a randomized clinical trial. Outcomes might include length of hospital stay, use of PRN medications for pain or anxiety, and demand for nursing time. The chaplain intervention could be administered prior to a major surgical procedure, after admission for a general medical condition, following admission to a rehabilitation unit (for stroke or spinal cord injury), or after admission to a psychiatric unit (for patients with mood or anxiety disorders). Other interventions (e.g., group prayer with laying on of hands, directed congregational prayer during religious services, or private religious activities, such as petitionary prayer, meditation, or scripture study) could likewise be administered, using a clinical trial design in inpatient and outpatient settings in the patient populations described.

Completely unexplored is the impact of the spirituality of the health professional (physician, nurse, or other health care provider) on patient satisfaction and compliance, response to treatment, or use of health services. For example, patients might be randomized to either a religious surgeon who prays or conducts other spiritual rituals (with/without the patient) prior to surgery, or randomized to a nonreligious surgeon who does not perform these spiritual activities. Research could also be conducted on entire health care systems, rather than on individual health practitioners. Patients might be randomized to either a religious hospital that places a strong emphasis on spiritual care from the top administrator to the room cleaning personnel, or randomized to a secular hospital that administers usual care without a spiritual component. In either type of study, investigators could measure and compare requests for pain medication, need for nursing time, length of hospital stay, speed of medical recovery, speed of surgical wound healing, hospital readmission rate, patient and family satisfaction, and so on, between treatment and control groups.

MECHANISMS OF EFFECT

Much work is necessary to more fully elucidate the mechanisms by which religious beliefs and practices affect health and vice versa. While general models are being developed (see chapters 15, 25, 28), these models need further refining and testing. The focus should probably be on known psychosocial-behavioral and biological (neuroendocrine, immunological) processes, rather than on mechanisms that have no plausible scientific basis within nature as we understand it today. The advancement of science depends on investigators' using the building blocks that are available, carefully placing one on top of the other until a solid edifice is constructed.

Epidemiological principles need to be considered when seeking to understand the mechanisms underlying the religion-health relationship (Levin, 1996b). Research is needed to quantify the amount of exposure or "dose" of religious belief or activity necessary to increase or decrease susceptibility to mental or physical illness. Likewise, studies are needed to examine the effects of religious involvement at different ages and at different stages of susceptibility to disease (timing of exposure). Finally, studies are needed to compare the magnitude of the effects of religious variables on health with the effects of other psychosocial, behavioral, heredity/genetic factors. For example, research is needed on how the effects of religiousness on health compare to those of social support, social class, or education level. Similarly, what effect does attending religious services have on survival compared to number of pack-years smoked (i.e., years of smoking one pack of cigarettes per day)? Quantifying the size of an effect by relating it to that of other known psychosocial or behavioral variables will help scientists put into perspective the benefit or risk that religious factors convey.

INTEGRATION OF KNOWLEDGE INTO CLINICAL PRACTICE

While much research is needed to establish and explain the relationships between religion and health, nowhere is work more needed than in integrating what has been learned (and will be learned) into clinical practice. Religiousness and spirituality are personal matters that clinicians must deal with sensitively and carefully. Religiosity is more sensitive than diet or exercise, and is on a level with sexual practices, sexual preference, abortion, extramarital sexual history, decisions about smoking or use of other addictive substances—all of which are very personal areas in people's lives. For many patients, religion and spirituality are indeed a sacred area—holy ground, so to speak—and clinicians must take off their sandals before treading on that ground just as Moses did. Health care providers without training and experience in this area will certainly need to proceed cautiously or risk being the proverbial bull in a china closet.

There exists almost no research and very little discussion on how physicians, nurses, social workers, and other health care providers might address religious issues in a nonoffensive, sensitive manner. For good or for bad, the clinician's own religious beliefs will heavily influence whether and to what extent he addresses the religious or spiritual needs of patients. These personal religious beliefs may cloud the clinician's judgment and impair his sensitivity to where his patients are on their unique spiritual journeys. When people are sick and under stress, their beliefs and values become particularly vulnerable to influence. Systematic research, however, has examined none of these issues. Such research would either validate such concerns or help us dismiss them.

There is need for a random nationwide survey of both health care professionals (e.g., physicians, psychologists, nurses, social workers) and patients to examine their opinions about what religious interventions are appropriate to the clinical setting. There is also a need to examine demographic, social, psychological, and physical health factors that influence patients' opinions about the appropriateness of religious interventions by physicians and other health professionals. Studies are needed to determine how comfortable physicians and other health professionals are with addressing religious and spiritual issues or performing religious interventions. If many clinicians feel uncomfortable about addressing such issues in clinical settings, despite demands by patients that they do so, then educational efforts may be needed to increase this comfort level.

Studies are also needed that ask patients about prior negative experiences with physicians or other health care professionals who have attempted to address religious and spiritual issues in the clinical setting. Such surveys should include questions about patients' fear about having health professionals address these sensitive issues. Similarly, studies are needed to find out how the clinician-patient relationship is affected by different religious interventions (e.g., support of religious practices, prayer with patients, encouragement of religious activities). A significant minority of clinicians already perform these interventions, and yet we know almost nothing about how the therapeutic relationship is altered by such practices, or what type of burden may be placed on the patient because of them.

Finally, studies are needed to determine the most effective time to introduce training about religious or spiritual issues into the education of health professionals and the most effective methods for teaching such material.

SUMMARY AND CONCLUSIONS

While much research that touches on religion and health has already been conducted, most studies have not been designed from the very start to test specific hypotheses about the influence of religious beliefs and practices. A major reason for this has been the lack of funding to support such research. Consequently, many studies have included unrepresentative samples (college students or convenience samples), used only superficial measures of religiousness or spirituality, or reported results based on secondary data analyses performed after the data were collected (and sometimes following the serendipitous discovery of significant results). Because of the growing interest in this area by both federal and private funding sources, support may soon become more readily available to answer specific research questions concerning the religion-health relationship.

In this chapter we discussed eight important areas of research that require further work: mental health, substance abuse, neurosciences, physical health, health promotion/disease prevention, use of health services, mechanisms of effect, and application of findings to clinical practice. We offered specific examples of research questions that need addressing in each of these areas. We hope this discussion will provide ideas for researchers who wishing to advance the field and give funding bodies direction in establishing research needs and priorities.

32

Research Methods

RESEARCH IS THE SYSTEM-atic investigation of a hypothesis, including development, testing, and evaluation, that is designed to contribute to generalizable knowledge. Because of the newness of this field, it is essential that research that examines the religion-health relationship be thoughtfully designed and carefully executed. While journal editors, in general, are not reluctant to publish quality research in the area of religion and health, haphazard research will not pass the stringent peer review process. In addition, because of the heavy competition for grant money in this area, only studies with the best designs are likely to be funded. For these reasons, we briefly review some basic research principles that should be considered when designing research on the religion-health relationship.

STUDY HYPOTHESES

Much of the research on religion and health has been conducted without an a priori hypothesis to guide the design of the study, the analysis of the data, and the interpretation of the findings. Instead, relationships between religion and health outcomes have often been discovered by chance and hypotheses developed only later to explain the associations. In developing a hypothesis, researchers should take these steps:

1. *State the Hypothesis up Front.* Hypotheses or research questions should be developed prior to the beginning of a research project and stated clearly and up front before the study is conducted or the data analyzed. The data analysis plan also should be developed before any data are collected and adhered to throughout the

study. Always be wary of hypotheses developed after analyses are performed. Doing multiple statistical tests in hopes of finding a significant result and then explaining whatever result one obtains by a hypothesis is called a fishing expedition, not research. A primary research question and perhaps two or three secondary questions should always structure and guide the study.

2. *Ground the Hypothesis on Theory and on Prior Research.* The primary hypothesis or research question should be grounded in scientific theory and based on prior work done in the field. For scientific papers or grant applications, the introduction presents the theory on which a hypothesis is based and a review of the prior research that underlies the theory. The statement of the hypothesis usually immediately follows the theory and literature review and ends the introduction section. It will be assumed that this is the order by which the researchers arrived at their idea for the study.

3. *Design the Study to Test the Hypothesis.* The research question or study hypothesis must guide the design of the project. The major criterion for choosing a study design (cross-sectional, longitudinal, or clinical trial) is that it is the best possible and most feasible method for answering the primary research question. The measures used to assess the independent and dependent variables should be sufficiently sensitive, accurate, and valid and should be chosen with the primary research question in mind. The statistical analysis should be focused on and designed to test the primary hypothesis. Typically, power analyses are performed only for testing of the primary hypothesis.

STUDY DESIGNS

Observational Versus Experimental Design

Most epidemiologic research is observational in nature. The researcher observes naturally occurring phenomena without attempting to manipulate the system. In experimental studies, on the other hand, the investigator usually does something to subjects in order to see whether a change can be induced as a result of the intervention.

Observational studies may involve case reports, a case series, case-control studies, cross-sectional studies, or prospective cohort studies. In a case-control study, cases with a particular characteristic are identified and compared with controls that resemble the cases except for lacking the distinguishing characteristic. In a cross-sectional study, the researcher assesses a group of persons at one point in time and correlates certain characteristics with other characteristics of group members. Cross-sectional studies have considerable merit because they are relatively cheap to carry out, since they require no follow-up of the study group over time. Prospective, longitudinal, or cohort studies assess a group of persons at one point in time and follow them over time through periodic reassessments to determine whether an event of interest (e.g., death, recovery, change) has occurred.

Observational studies provide indirect or *circumstantial* evidence that a particular characteristic or experience results in or causes the event of interest. For example, consider a prospective cohort study that examines the effects of being religious on speed of remission of depression. All subjects at the start of the study are depressed, which is the characteristic that defines the cohort. At the beginning of the study, a variety of other characteristics (including religiousness) are measured, especially those that are likely to affect the speed of remission of depression (e.g., age, treatment with antidepressants). Following the baseline assessments, subjects are evaluated periodically to determine which ones remit from depression and how fast they do so. The baseline characteristics are then examined to determine which of them predict the occurrence and speed of remission. Even if religiousness independently predicts faster speed of remission (after taking into account other predictors of remission), we still cannot definitively conclude that religiousness "causes" depression to remit faster; there may have been characteristics of subjects at baseline that the researcher did not measure that may have been related to both religiousness and faster speed of remission. In that case, religiousness would have nothing to do with the speed of depression remission but would simply be related to this other unmeasured factor that affects remission. Thus, one must be careful in concluding that religiousness actually causes faster remission on the basis of the results of a prospective cohort study.

In contrast, experimental studies can provide direct evidence for causation that is unlikely to be confounded by such unmeasured differences. Experimental studies attempt to manipulate the system by some type of intervention. Persons are randomly assigned to either the intervention group or a control group (increasing the likelihood that measured and unmeasured characteristics will be equally distributed between the two groups). Members of the intervention group receive the intervention or treatment, whereas members of the control group do not. If the intervention and the control groups are similar enough at the beginning of the experiment (which should be confirmed by measures of characteristics known to affect outcome), then any differences that arise over time between the two groups can be attributed to the intervention. In other words, the intervention "caused" the differences in outcome. Positive findings from a single intervention study still do not prove that the intervention works, since the scientific community requires that other research groups replicate the results.

For example, suppose 100 patients with congestive heart failure (CHF) are randomly assigned to either an intervention ($n = 50$) or a control group ($n = 50$). Because of random assignment, the intervention group should be similar to the control group at the beginning of the study (especially with regard to characteristics known to affect outcome). Intervention group members then receive a treatment for CHF that control group members do not. If the outcome of interest is severity of CHF, then periodic assessments of heart functioning over time will determine changes in CHF severity for members of both the intervention and the control group. Any improvements in CHF severity among members of the intervention group that exceed those seen in members of

the controls group are assumed to have been caused by the intervention.

Similarly, if the intervention is intercessory off-site prayer, then any differences between the intervention and the control groups on CHF severity could be attributed to the prayer. Ideally, both investigators and subjects should be "blinded" (double-blinded), that is, unaware of who receives the intervention so that they cannot intentionally or unintentionally influence the results. Double-blinding is relatively easy when testing the effectiveness of a drug and a placebo or of intercessory off-site prayer compared to no prayer. Double-blinding is more difficult, however, when testing psychosocial interventions and, for this discussion, religious-based psychosocial interventions.

While randomized clinical trials are important for establishing a causal relationship between religion and health outcomes, these studies are expensive and often require a large number of subjects if they are to achieve sufficient power to detect an effect. Furthermore, clinical trials require a relatively homogeneous patient population, a specific intervention, and a restricted range of outcomes. This creates a relatively narrow focus that often limits generalizability of results that may not be applicable to clinical situations likely to be encountered by health practitioners. Such a lack of generalizability also handicaps the making of policy decisions by government agencies and health insurers. Thus, other research methods (prospective cohort studies, for example) are needed to provide more generalizable data to help inform health care providers, patients, and insurers.

Qualitative versus Quantitative Studies

Qualitative studies involve in-depth interviews with subjects who "tell their story." Questions are typically asked in an open-ended format, and the subject is encouraged to elaborate. For example, the interviewer may ask, "What role does religion play in helping you cope with your physical health problems?" The subject is encouraged to go into as much depth as he can in responding to the question. As another example, subjects may be asked to describe past religious experiences and explain the impact those experiences had in shaping their lives. Subjects' verbatim responses are recorded and analyzed using qualitative methods.

In *quantitative* studies, the investigator attempts to quantify or measure how much of a characteristic the person has. Instead of open-ended questions, the investigator asks closed-ended questions that require that the subject choose among a given set of responses. In a quantitative study of religious coping, for example, the investigator would ask a series of questions to quantify or measure how much subjects rely on religion to help them to cope. A religious coping scale consisting of 10 or 20 questions may be administered; yes responses may be given a score of 1 and no responses a score of 0. Responses are then added up, yielding a score that measures the extent to which the person uses religion to cope. Alternatively, religious coping might be assessed by asking the subject to rate on a 0–10 scale how much she uses religion to cope, where 0 means "not at all" and 10 means "religion is the most important factor that I use to cope." This number/score can then be correlated with other characteristics of the person (well-being, for example) or used to predict changes in that characteristic over time.

Qualitative studies often provide information useful for developing hypotheses that can later be tested by quantitative research. For example, suppose a subject reports in a qualitative study that her religious faith provides peace and relief from depression. The investigator may then design a quantitative study in which he assesses the subjects' religious faith and attempts to correlate it with peace, contentment, or level of depression, first cross-sectionally and then longitudinally. If the studies confirm an association, then a randomized clinical trial may be designed to test the effects of a religious intervention on recovery from depression.

Meta-analytic Studies

According to Leviton and Cook (1981), meta-analysis is "any systematic method that uses statistical analyses for combining data from independent studies to obtain a numerical estimate of the overall effect of a particular procedure or variable on a defined outcome." In other words, an investigator conducts a meta-analysis by compiling several quantitative studies in an effort to determine (a) the average size of an association between two variables or (b) the average effect or change that results from an intervention.

For example, suppose a researcher wishes to know the average increase in survival predicted by weekly religious attendance (i.e., size of the association between attendance and mortality). She would first conduct a literature search to find all the published studies that have examined the association between attendance and survival. She would then calculate an average effect size for the association between attendance and survival for all of the studies found. One study may have reported that weekly attendance reduces the risk of dying during a 10-year period by 25%; another study may have found a decreased risk of 50%; a third study may have reported a reduced risk of only 10%. If these were the only studies published on the topic, then the investigator would average the reduced risks of 25%, 50%, and 10% (called effect sizes). This would result in an average overall reduction of 28%, assuming, for this simplistic example, that each study includes subjects with similar baseline characteristics, employs a similar study design and follow-up period, and uses similar measures for predictor and outcome variables. The statistical significance of this effect size could also be determined using the combined samples from all three studies.

According to Sacks et al. (1987), meta-analyses have four major purposes: (1) to increase the power of an analysis, particularly when the researcher is examining subgroups of a sample that in the original studies were too small to demonstrate a statistically significant effect; (2) to resolve uncertainty when different studies report different or conflicting findings; (3) to improve the estimate of the effect size; and (4) to answer questions not asked in the original studies. Thus, meta-analysis is a legitimate form of research in itself, capable of confirming old hypotheses and testing new ones.

SAMPLNG METHOD

Random or Probability Sample

Most researchers hope that a study's results will apply more widely than just to the subjects studied. In order for the results obtained from subsample A of a larger population B to be generalizable to the larger population B (the reference population), the subjects that make up subsample A must represent a random sample of persons from population B. For example, if we wanted to determine the proportion of persons in New York City who use religion as a coping strategy when dealing with stress, we could question every person in New York City. Alternatively, we could randomly select a small number of persons from New York City and question them about their coping behaviors. It would take a lot less effort and money to survey only this small random sample of New York City residents than to survey the entire population. The method used for identifying a random sample should be stated in the study report. Methods vary and may involve using a random numbers table or some other method of ensuring that each member of the group to be studied is equally likely to be chosen (Rosner, 1986).

The majority of studies that have examined the relationship between religion and health have not utilized random samples; this leads to concern about the generalizability of their results. When random samples have been used, however, the studies are usually large epidemiological surveys in which the religious variable is measured only superficially, which causes concerns regarding the validity of study findings.

Systematic Samples

Another method that approximates random or probability sampling is systematic sampling. Systematic sampling involves the selection of subjects on the basis of a predetermined, systematic, and reproducible method of choosing members representative of a population. For example, one might wish to study hospitalized patients with medical illness. Subjects for the study could be patients consecutively admitted to the hospital during a specified period of time.

Alternatively, one might wish to study patients who visit medical or mental health clinics. Again, one could choose consecutively evaluated patients seen at health clinics in a particular area during a specified period of time. Such a sampling method can be easily reproduced and will capture a fairly unbiased sample of subjects from each of these populations. As with random sampling, the larger the sample, the greater the likelihood that the sample chosen will be representative of the reference population.

Samples of Convenience

Random sampling does not involve haphazard selection of persons who are available for study. Such haphazard methods capture samples of convenience. A sample of convenience is probably not representative of the larger population from which it is taken. Studies that use samples of convenience are easy and inexpensive to carry out. An example of such a study population might be psychology or sociology students who participate in research as part of their educational experience. Students are readily available to professors and eager to please them, and they may even be given course credit for their participation. This introduces a number of biases and self-selection factors that may seriously affect the generalizability of the results. Many studies in the psychology and sociology literature that correlate religious activities with mental health states or personality style involve samples of convenience.

National versus Regional Samples

Because the prevalence and the importance of religious involvement are not the same in all areas of the United States, results from studies conducted in one part of the country (the Bible Belt, for example) may not readily generalize to other parts (the West Coast or the Northeast). For that reason, it is preferable to study relationships between religion and health using national samples. Such studies, however, are expensive to perform and seldom include detailed measures of either religious variables or health outcomes. Studies that examine regional samples, while suffering from the problem of regional bias, are able to assess subjects in much greater depth than are studies that utilize national samples (which are often telephone surveys). Studies that use regional samples are usually better positioned to follow subjects over time and to examine health outcomes on the basis of detailed in-person evaluations. Multi-center studies (in which the same study is performed in several different locations around the country under the direction of a single coordinating center) combine many of the benefits of national and regional sampling in terms of depth of evaluation and quality of tracking.

Different Populations

Studies of religion and health should be performed in different population groups. Studies in middle-aged adults may not reveal the same relationships as studies of children, adolescents, college students, or the elderly. Similarly, studies of healthy community-dwelling adults may not reveal the same relationships as studies of hospitalized medically ill adults or nursing home residents (i.e., clinical samples). Likewise, studies performed in psychiatric patients may not discover the same relationships found in subjects without mental illness.

Studies conducted in different populations not only help to determine the generalizability of results but also help uncover clues to possible mechanisms of effect. For example, a strong relationship may be found between religious behaviors and mental health in persons with severe medical illness or experiencing other psychosocial stressors. Religion may be used very successfully as coping resource among those experiencing certain types of stress. By contrast, among members of nonstressed populations who are generally content and happy with life, there may be no relationship between religion and mental health (because the mechanism of the effect, better coping with stress, is not operative). In psychiatric populations, the relationship between religious beliefs and mental health may actually be negative, particularly if psychiatric patients have religious delusions or preoccupations. A list of different populations that need study would include:

1. Children and adolescents
2. College students
3. Community-dwelling healthy adults
4. Community-dwelling adults with medical or psychiatric illness (outpatients)
5. Acutely hospitalized adults with medical illness
6. Acutely hospitalized adults with psychiatric illness
7. Chronically institutionalized adults with medical illness
8. Chronically institutionalized adults with psychiatric illness
9. Hospitalized children and adolescents (with medical or psychiatric illness)
10. Prisoners
11. Other stressed populations (e.g., caregivers, bereaved persons, disaster victims)
12. Members of different racial groups (e.g., blacks, whites, Hispanics, Native Americans)
13. The elderly, the disabled, the dying
14. Persons with different income and education levels
15. Persons with different payor statuses (Medicare/Medicaid vs. private insurance vs. HMO)

MEASUREMENT

We examine specific measures of religiousness and spirituality in chapter 33. Here we examine issues related to the general topic of measurement. We also make the following recommendations.

1. *Use Quality Measures for Health Outcomes.* To identify relationships between religion and health, scientists must assess the health variable by using a sensitive measure that captures the full range of variability in health seen within the population studied. This is particularly true for community-dwelling populations, where physical and mental functioning are usually pretty high. For example, if a subjective health measure with four possible categories (very good, good, moderate, and poor) is used to assess physical health, approximately 70–80% of community-dwelling adults will place themselves in the very good or good categories. This leaves little variance in health for religious variables to explain. Likewise, purely subjective

measures of physical health, while easy to administer, are often confounded by mental health. Depressed persons may perceive their physical health as worse than it actually is, whereas the optimistic person may do the opposite. Likewise, persons with limited education may not make fine distinctions between physical and mental health, and reports of "feeling bad" may indicate either physical or emotional illness.

Sensitive measures of physical health include the following: number of prescription and over-the-counter medications, ability to perform instrumental activities of daily living (Fillenbaum, 1985), ability to perform vigorous physical activities (Hlatky et al., 1989), and clinician-rated severity of illness scales such as the Cumulative Illness Rating Scale (Conwell et al., 1993). The need to use sensitive measures also applies to assessments of mental health and well-being. For example, the Geriatric Depression Scale (Yesavage et al., 1983) and the Philadelphia Geriatric Center Morale Scale (Lawton, 1975) are multi-item measures that are sensitive to mood state in older populations.

In addition to being sensitive to small changes, measures of physical and mental health must also be reliable, accurate, and valid. *Reliability* is defined as the degree to which a scale or instrument is free of random error; the greater the reliability and accuracy of an instrument, the less likely the results of measurement will change from one administration to another when no actual change has occurred. The most common measures of reliability are the (1) internal consistency of items that make up a multi-item scale (assessed by Cronbach's alpha) and (2) test-retest reliability. Most computer statistical packages have a test for Cronbach's alpha that can be computed from existing data. Test-retest reliability is determined by administering an instrument to subjects at two different time points (but close enough together so that no actual change in the subjects is likely to occur). The same or different interviewers may administer the measure; having different interviewers administer it yields a more stringent test of reliability. If scores involve interval-level or ordinal categories, a correlation of comparison may be calculated between each subject's two scores. If outcomes are categorical

or can be reconstructed as involving two or three categories, then a kappa (κ) of agreement can be calculated between the two administrations.

The *validity* of a measure is perhaps the most important criterion in measure development and assessment (George & Bearon, 1980). It is also perhaps the most difficult to establish. Validity differs from reliability in the following way. A measurement may be perfectly reliable (have no random measurement error) but not measure the intended phenomenon. In other words, someone may very reliably make exactly the same error over and over again. Validity, the extent to which a test actually measures what it purports to measure, may be broken down into a variety of subtypes. These include face validity, convergent validity, discriminant validity, and predictive validity. *Face validity* is the degree to which the questions of the instrument appear on general examination by a sensible person to be measuring the phenomenon of interest. This determination is entirely subjective on the part of the examiner and relies heavily on the examiner's general knowledge of the field and of the construct being measured.

Convergent validity relies on the principle that measures that assess the same variable should correlate highly. For example, two depression scales that claim to assess depression should correlate highly. Likewise, two scales that purport to measure religiosity should correlate highly. Typically, a new scale is compared with an existing scale that has already established validity. A high correlation between the new measure and the established measure is evidence of convergent validity for the new scale.

Discriminant validity is essentially the opposite of convergent validity. Can the new measure discriminate between the phenomenon it is expected to measure and related phenomena? For example, can a new measure of spirituality distinguish this concept from a related concept, such as meaning in life? If the correlation between a new scale for assessing spirituality and an established scale that measures meaning in life is too high (higher than the expected moderate correlation), then the new scale fails the test of discriminant validity (i.e., it cannot discriminate spirituality from meaning in life).

Predictive validity is based upon the concept that if a measure is valid, it should predict other variables in a way that is expected on theoretical grounds. For example, if grades in college are a valid measure of future success and earning power, then one would expect high grades to be a strong predictor of later income. Likewise, if a measure of organizational religiosity is a valid measure of social involvement in religious community, then organizational religiosity should be a strong predictor of number of church friends. While predictive validity can be assessed using cross-sectional data, longitudinal data are preferred.

2. *Use High-Quality Measures of Religion.* Just as measures of health outcome must be sensitive, reliable, accurate, and valid, measures that assess religious variables must likewise have these qualities. If religious and health measures are not sensitive, reliable, and valid, then one should not expect to find a strong correlation between them, even if such a relationship exists, because measurement error will add unexplained variability to the association and weaken the correlation. This is one reason that different studies often report different correlations between religion and health variables or report no association. All studies of religion and health should include some evidence that the measures used are reliable and valid, and the results obtained (whether positive, negative, or indicating no association) should be interpreted in light of this.

3. *Use High-Quality Measures of Covariates.* When assessing the relationship between religion and health, one must be sure that the covariates controlled for in the analysis have been carefully selected and accurately measured. If they are not, this may lead to a false conclusion that a relationship is present (because of failure to control for confounding).

For example, physical disability may confound the relationship between religious attendance and physical health, resulting in a false positive relationship between attendance and better health. This relationship may be entirely a result of the fact that physically ill people are too disabled to attend religious services. In this example, physical disability is related to both physical health and religious attendance and therefore confounds the relationship. Even if physical disability is measured and controlled for, failure to measure disability accurately will result in a spurious relationship between attendance and physical health that does not disappear when disability is controlled.

Likewise, failure to account for social desirability may also affect relationships between religion and health outcomes. Some investigators have argued that religious persons tend to give more socially desirable answers to question concerning marital satisfaction, substance use, and other mental health states (Ellis, 1948; Batson, Naifeh, et al., 1978; Glenn, 1984), although this claim has been challenged by others (Hansen, 1981, 1992; Hunsberger & Ennis, 1982; Hathaway & Pargament, 1990). To be on the safe side, however, one might wish to control for social desirability in such analyses.

Failure to control for or carefully assess covariates may also result in a false conclusion that a relationship is absent (because one has failed to control for confounding that conceals the relationship). For example, failure to control for race in a study of high blood pressure and religiousness might result in failure to find a relationship between religiousness and lower blood pressure. The reason for this is that being African American is associated with both greater religiousness and higher blood pressures; consequently, there will be a spurious positive correlation between religiousness and high blood pressure. The confounding effect of race, then, might cancel out the inverse relationship between religiousness and high blood pressure.

4. *Consider Degree and Duration of Exposure.* If religious beliefs and practices are related to physical or mental health, then one might expect the degree of exposure to the religious variable to determine the strength of the relationship. For example, assuming a linear relationship between exposure to religion and better mental health, one would expect that persons who were raised in the church, who developed a strong intrinsic religiosity early in life, and who maintained a strong faith and active religious life throughout adulthood would have the best mental health as older adults (controlling for confounders, of course).

On the other hand, there may be a window of exposure (in terms of intensity, duration, or timing) that is optimally associated with mental health, and either less or more than this degree of exposure results in poorer mental health. Unfortunately, most measures of religious exposure depend on retrospective self-report, which may not be very accurate; long-term follow-up with repeated measurements is perhaps the most valid method of assessing religious exposure.

5. *Avoid Using Contaminated Measures*. Measures of independent variables are sometimes contaminated by items that are actually assessing the dependent variable. This virtually ensures that the independent variable will correlate with the dependent variable. Such contamination most often occurs when assessing spirituality (rather than religiousness) and relating it to mental health. This results from the broad definition of spirituality that some investigators use. As noted in chapter 1, investigators have included feelings of meaning and purpose in life, peace and contentedness, wholeness and completeness, connectedness, and almost every other positive human emotion under the term "spirituality." If spirituality is defined as a positive emotional state, it will obviously relate positively to better mental health.

For example, a recently developed spirituality measure included the following items: "I feel selfless caring for others"; "I have forgiven those who have hurt or offended me"; "I feel thankful for my blessings"; "I find deep inner peace and harmony"; and "I experience a connection to all of life." Including these positive human emotions in a measure of spirituality virtually ensures a positive relationship with mental health.

The Spiritual Well-Being (SWB) scale of Paloutzian and Ellison (1982) is a widely used measure of spirituality that consists of two subscales: a religious well-being subscale (10 items) and an existential well-being subscale (10 items). The existential well-being subscale is simply a measure of well-being. Consequently, overall scores on the SWB scale will always be related to greater well-being, higher life satisfaction, greater meaning in life, lower depression, and other indicators of positive mental health. The religious well-being

subscale, on the other hand, does not include questions that directly tap well-being. When examining correlations between the SWB scale and mental health, then, only the religious well-being subscale can be used as a valid, uncontaminated predictor.

In conclusion, measures that assess spirituality are often liberally sprinkled with items that assess mental health, making them unsuitable for studies that examine the relationship between spirituality and mental health. This is less of a problem with measures of religiousness. Religious measures are composed primarily of items that inquire about religious beliefs, activities, commitment, orientation, and/or relationship with the transcendent, which are typically not contaminated by items that assess positive emotions.

STATISTICAL ANALYSIS

Researchers should follow these guidelines in designing their statistical analysis.

1. *Develop Analysis Plan before Data Are Collected*. As noted earlier, the analysis plan should be developed and documented prior to collecting any data. Because many research studies published in this century on the religion-health relationship have not resulted from funded research grants designed specifically to examine this relationship, analysis plans have often been developed after data were collected. We hope this will change when research that has as its primary goal the examination of the religion-health relationship is funded (since such grants require a statistical analysis plan up front as part of the grant application). Sometimes, however, large data sets have already been collected and researchers wish to make use of the data, particularly if religious variables have been assessed. In that case, at a minimum, the statistical analysis plan should be developed prior to data analysis. Haphazard analyses not connected with a particular research question or not designed to test a specific hypothesis should not be done.

2. *Choose Appropriate Statistical Tests*. An excellent statistics text for beginners has been written by Freedman et al. (1997); it is very readable and explains the basics. When testing a hypothesis, the investigator typically first ex-

amines the bivariate correlation between the predictor variable (religious factor) and the dependent variable (health). In the second step, the researcher takes into account other variables by including them in a regression model along with the primary predictor variable (religion). The choice of bivariate or multivariate statistic will depend on the type of data that have been collected and whether they are "categorical," "ordinal," or "interval level" (continuous) in nature. Categorical data consist of answers to questions concerning marital status, occupation, sex, or race, which cannot be ordered. Ordinal data involve responses that can be ordered but that do not have specific numerical values; computing means and standard deviations for such data is not meaningful, and they require instead nonparametric statistical methods that can analyze ordered or ranked data. Strictly speaking, only interval-level data can be analyzed using parametric statistics; in practice, however, parametric statistics can be used for ordinal data if an argument can be made that there are multiple response categories that are ordered and separated by equal distances.

Bivariate statistical tests include the chi-square and Mantel-Haenzel tests (for comparing categorical data), student-t test or analysis of variance (for comparing categorical and interval level data), Wilcoxon rank sum test (Mann-Whitney U test) or Spearman rank correlation (for comparing ordinal or ranked data), and Pearson correlation (for comparing interval-level data). A commonly used multivariate method to examine predictors of a categorical dependent variable is logistic regression (if there are only two response categories) or multinomial regression (if more than two categories are present). Linear regression is often used when a multivariate method is needed to examine a dependent variable that involves interval-level data (and sometimes ordered or ranked data, as noted earlier). When time to an event is the dependent variable (e.g., time to remission of depression, time to hospital discharge, or time to death), then proportional hazards regression is useful (it adjusts for covariates and takes into account time to the event and censoring). Structural equation modeling (LISREL) is an advanced form of regression that depends on associations between latent constructs.

3. *Meet Assumptions of Statistical Tests.* All statistical tests have assumptions about the kinds of data they can analyze. One particularly important assumption for parametric statistical tests (correlations, student-t tests, analysis of variance, linear regression) is that variable responses are normally distributed (fall in a bell-shaped curve). Cox proportional hazards regression makes assumptions about predictor variables that can be tested either graphically or with a normal score test of proportionality. If these assumptions are not met, then transformations of the data may be necessary prior to analysis. Failure to transform them may result in an underestimate or overestimate of the association between the variables. Finally, one cannot assume that all relationships between religious and health variables are linear; some relationships may be U-shaped, inverted U-shaped, or logarithmic. Graphically examining the relationship is often the best way to determine its shape.

4. *Perform the Analyses in the Appropriate Order.* When conducting statistical analyses, first perform a bivariate test that examines the relationship between the religious variable and the health state (cross-sectional studies) or health outcome (prospective cohort studies or clinical trials). Next, examine what effect controlling for demographic variables (typically age, sex, race, socioeconomic status) and other *confounders* (e.g., physical functioning) has on the relationship by using multivariate analyses. The result of this analysis will determine whether there is a true relationship between the religious variable and the health outcome. Next, examine variables that might help explain or *mediate* the relationship between the religious variable and the health state or outcome. Mediating variables include social support, mental health, and health behaviors. Note that these variables help to provide information about the mechanism by which religiousness impacts health. If these mediating variables completely explain the relationship between religiousness and health (i.e., the two variables are no longer significantly related), then this does not discount the impor-

tance of the religion-health relationship; it means only that the mechanism for the effect has now been identified and explained by those mediating variables.

5. *Examine Relevant Interactions.* In addition to including all relevant covariates in the analyses, the investigator must be sure to examine all relevant interactions between the primary predictor variable (i.e., religion) and other predictor variables (e.g., sex, race, stress level). By examining such interactions, she can determine whether the religious variable has an especially strong effect in a subgroup of the population. For example, a significant interaction between religiousness and sex (both independent variables) when one is predicting well-being (dependent variable) might suggest that there is a strong relationship between religiousness and well-being in women but not in men. Likewise, a significant interaction between religiousness and stressful life events when one is predicting depression might suggest that there is a strong inverse relationship between religiousness and depression only among those experiencing severe stress but only a weak relationship in those whose lives are less stressful. In this way, clues about mechanism of effect may be discovered.

6. *Avoid Type I Error.* Type I error is the probability of "rejecting the null hypothesis" (i.e., concluding that there is a significant relationship between two variables) given that the null hypothesis is in fact true (i.e., the two variables are not related). The probability of Type I error is commonly referred to as the p value. Type I error can result when the researcher performs too many statistical tests when analyzing a data set. Scientific convention holds that if *the likelihood that the association between two variables occurs by chance alone* is less than 5 in 100 (i.e., $p < .05$), then there is a statistically significant association between the two variables. If one performs 100 statistical tests to examine the association between different variables, however, one can predict that significant associations will occur entirely by chance in at least five instances (even when there is no relationship between the variables). To avoid Type I error, the level of statistical significance (p value) is usually corrected downward. For exam-

ple, if a large number of variables is being examined, the level of statistical significance may be reduced from .05 to .01 or even to .001. In that case, an association will be interpreted as being statistically significant only if the p value is less than .01 or less than .001. For exploratory studies (i.e., those not claiming to answer a research question definitively), these rules are sometimes relaxed.

7. *Avoid Type II Error.* A Type II error is the probability of "accepting the null hypothesis" (i.e., concluding that the two variables are not related) when in fact the alternative hypothesis is true (i.e., the two variables are related). The reason for a Type II error is usually insufficient "power." In other words, there weren't enough subjects in the sample, the subjects weren't followed for long enough, or the variables weren't assessed with sufficient sensitivity. Usually, however, power relates to the number of subjects in the sample. When studies that examine the association between religiousness and health fail to detect a significant difference, it may mean that there were not enough subjects in the sample. When power analyses are performed to estimate the sample size necessary for a successful study, the goal is to identify how many subjects must be recruited so that there will be at least an 80% power to detect a difference of X (usually a clinically significant difference) at a p value $<.05$.

8. *Avoid Multiple Collinearity.* When several religious variables have been measured in a study, investigators often wonder whether it is best to include all religious variables at once in a regression model with covariates. Including several different religious variables in a model as separate variables, however, runs the risk of multiple collinearity. In other words, if several religious variables that strongly correlate with each other (Pearson $r > .40$) are all included in a regression model, they may interfere with each other's ability to predict the dependent variable. Thus, each religious variable (as long as there are not large numbers of these) or each religious dimension (organizational, nonorganizational, subjective, intrinsic) should be examined separately in separate regression models. Religious variables may be combined into a sin-

gle index by summing them, but this method runs the risk that one religious variable will cancel out or conceal the effects of the other (Koenig, Hays, George, et al., 1997). If individual religious variables are summed, they should be combined into categories that follow the religious dimensions noted earlier.

INTERPRETATION OF RESULTS

When interpreting results, researchers should carefully follow these principles.

1. *Distinguish Causation from Association.* If a researcher detects a cross-sectional relationship between a religious variables and a health state, there is absolutely no way of telling whether the religious variable influenced the health state or the health state influenced the religious variable. For example, a positive cross-sectional relationship between frequent church attendance and better physical health might mean that church attendance prevents physical illness or that physical illness prevents church attendance. Likewise, a positive relationship between frequency of religious attendance and absence of depression might mean that either frequent religious attendance prevents depression or that depression prevents people from attending religious services.

Prospective cohort studies provide information on direction of causation, but they still cannot completely eliminate the fact that both better health status and frequent religious involvement may be related to some unknown third variable (perhaps a genetic or personality factor) that has not been measured or controlled in the analysis. Nevertheless, if a religious variable measured at the beginning of a cohort study is able to independently predict a health outcome after other known predictors of the outcome are controlled, this provides at least circumstantial evidence that religion influences the health outcome. Time-lagged analyses can also be used to provide evidence for the direction of causation, but this requires that both religious and health variables be measured a minimum of three times during the course of a prospective study.

As noted earlier, only an intervention study or experiment can definitively demonstrate causation. Such studies are difficult to perform when religion is the intervention. The biggest problem is contamination—keeping the control group from becoming religious. From a practical standpoint this may not be possible, and from an ethical standpoint it may not be desirable. Nevertheless, such studies can be designed, particularly with wait-list control groups, so that everyone eventually receives the intervention. Unfortunately, the follow-up time for intervention studies is limited, usually less than 12 months. This may not be long enough to demonstrate the health effect that a religious intervention is expected to have. In contrast, prospective cohort studies often follow persons anywhere from three months to 30 years or more, allowing for assessment of long-term effects on health. A large intervention study with long multiyear follow-up could provide the benefits of both study methodologies but would be very expensive.

2. *Distinguish Confounding from Mechanism of Effect.* As stressed earlier, investigators must be careful not to confuse the effects of "confounding" with the "mechanism of effect." For example, suppose a prospective cohort study examines the effects of religious attendance at baseline on survival during a 30-year follow-up. If the investigator finds that religious attendance predicts longer survival, then she must include other variables in the model to see whether these covariates can explain the relationship. First, she adds demographic variables to the model. These are true confounders that must be taken into account if a relationship between attendance and survival has any meaning. Similarly, physical health variables (e.g., physical disability, number of medical illnesses) that might have prevented religious attendance at the beginning of the study must be controlled for. These, too, are confounding variables. If demographic variables and physical health can completely explain the relationship between religious attendance and survival, then there is no meaningful independent relationship between these two variables.

If a significant relationship persists after the researcher controls for confounders, however, the investigators must then attempt to explain the effect by controlling for potential mediating variables. Mediating variables might include stressful life events, emotional disorder (i.e., depression or anxiety), social factors (i.e., social support, marital status), health behaviors (i.e., drinking, smoking, sexual practices, exercise, weight, maintaining low blood pressure), and health care practices (i.e., compliance with medical treatment, early recognition of illness, seeking prompt medical attention). Again, these variables are *not confounders*. Rather, they help to explain the *mechanism* by which religious attendance prolongs survival. Even if these variables completely explain the relationship between religious attendance and survival, that relationship remains important; however, we will then know the mechanism by which religion influences survival. If, after the researchers control for these possible mediators of the effect, a significant relationship persists between religious attendance and survival, then unknown factors must exist to explain the relationship and should be the target of future research.

Imprecise measurement of either confounders or mediating variables in this study might account for the unexplained variance in the relationship between attendance and survival. Thus, better measures of the same variables used in the original study might be employed in a second study. Alternatively (or in addition), variables not measured in the original study might be assessed in the second study. Those variables would be chosen on the basis of their likely relationship to both religious attendance and longer survival.

REPLICATION OF RESULTS

Replication by Different Research Teams

A single report of results from a single group of investigators located at a single site cannot be relied upon very confidently. Results need to be replicated by different investigative teams located at different institutions. This not only provides important information with regard to generalizability but also is a check on the validity of the original research. If two or three research teams working separately with different samples report the same findings, then this provides strong evidence that the results are real.

Replication in Different Geographical Areas

Replication of results in different areas of the country is important for generalizing results. In addition, however, the results obtained at different geographical sites may provide helpful clues about mechanisms. For example, if religious variables are related to health in the southern United States (where religious beliefs and practices are part of the dominant culture) but are not related to health in the West or the Northeast (where religious beliefs and practices are less common and, in fact, may be counter to the dominant culture), then one might conclude that social factors play a large role in religion's influence on health.

Replication in Different Populations

Similar or different results found in different races, age groups, and life situations (sick/healthy, stressed/nonstressed) provide further information about the generalizability, the durability, and the mechanism of the effect. (See additional discussion earlier in this chapter in the section on sampling.)

PEER REVIEW PROCESS

Reports of scientific findings have different levels of trustworthiness, depending on what stage in the peer review process the results have passed. In this section we proceed from the highest to the lowest level of credibility assigned by the scientific community to research reports.

Publication in Peer-Reviewed Academic Journals

The way in which the scientific community places its "stamp of approval" on research results is by publishing the results in its scientific journals. Before a scientific paper is accepted for publication, it must go through a rigorous peer review process. First, three or four knowledgeable scientists at different academic institutions carefully read over the report and critique it. They examine the introduction to ensure that the current project is grounded on the most recent research. The reviewers pay attention to whether the hypotheses have been clearly stated in the introduction. They also examine the methods section of the study and look for irregularities or weaknesses in the study design. They then examine the statistical methods and results for validity.

Finally, the reviewers assess the quality of the discussion, focusing on how well the findings are linked to current knowledge in the field, whether the investigators are interpreting results and making implications appropriately, and whether the limitations of the study have been acknowledged. If the paper is felt to have merit, the editor asks the researcher to revise the paper to incorporate the critiques provided by the scientific reviewers. This may involve doing other statistical analyses or even collecting additional data. The paper is then resubmitted and examined by the editor to see if the revisions have been made. The editor may then send out the revised paper a second time to the scientific reviewers for their comments. If the paper is still not satisfactory, then it may be returned to the investigator and further changes requested. Thus, the peer review process is a prolonged and arduous method that is designed to ensure the scientific credibility of results; the entire process often takes up to six months. Until the findings of a study have passed the peer review process and the report has been accepted for publication, results should not be considered reliable.

Abstracts of Papers Presented at Scientific Meetings

Scientific meetings held by national science organizations or associations are designed to provide members of the field with updated information about recent, cutting-edge research. The abstracts of reports presented at these meetings typically must go through a peer-review type process in which members of a scientific committee, made up of knowledgeable scientists in

the field, review and choose which papers should be presented. The abstracts of these papers may be published in the journal of the scientific organization or in the meeting program. Still, until the results are accepted for publication in a scientific journal their credibility remains questionable.

Doctoral Dissertations

In order for a scientist to receive her primary academic credential, a doctor of philosophy (Ph.D.) or similar degree, the scientist must design and carry out a research project, write up the results, and present the findings to a dissertation committee made up of scientists and educators who critically evaluate the work. The abstract of the dissertation may be published in *Dissertation Abstracts* and in that way become available to the wider scientific community. The quality of peer review, however, is usually not as rigorous as that provided by high-quality scientific journals prior to accepting articles for publication.

Nonpeer-Reviewed Academic Book Publications or Book Chapters

The next level of credible results are research findings published in academic books. New research that has not been published in scientific journals may be included in such books. The problem is that usually the research has been neither reviewed nor challenged. The research is then published and circulated, bypassing the critical eye of other scientists.

Solicited Articles for Educational Journals

An editor may make a request to a scientist to write about his research for a popular audience of readers or for educational purposes. Usually, scientists who have published in peer-reviewed journals are asked to write such articles. In such cases, investigators may broaden the implications of their findings to make them more easily understood by a less sophisticated audience. While the journal editor and staff usually perform some checks for accuracy and validity, these reports should not be valued at the same level as the original published research reports.

Popular Nonfiction Books

Popular books are almost never peer reviewed. The publishers urge writers to explain their results and their implications in the simplest terms at a language reading level that an eighth grader can understand. These books are intended primarily to educate the broad public, not speak to a scientific audience. Words such as "causes," "leads to," or "prevents" are often used freely. Indeed, if the writer attempts to explain the limitations of the data, he will likely lose the reader and therefore is discouraged from doing so by editors. Such books contribute to the growth of a field because they translate research findings into a form that average people and political decision makers can understand, which may stimulate financial support for research and career development. From a scientific standpoint, however, information from popular books is usually not dependable.

Newspapers, Popular Magazines, TV, Radio, and Internet

While the popular media often makes substantial attempts to confirm from multiple sources the stories they report (and typically include medical or scientific advisers on their staffs), information from these sources is frequently characterized by overgeneralization and sensationalizing. The popular media have two goals: to report the findings accurately and to sell their product. The latter can often conflict with the former. As with popular books, accuracy is often compromised as writers attempt to translate scientific findings into readable and comprehensible popular language to capture and hold the reader's attention.

PUBLICATION BIAS

Biased Journal Editors and Reviewers

Because of the newness of the field of religion and health, and the understandable uneasiness that the established scientific community has concerning research on this topic, journal editors and scientific reviewers may be biased against publishing research in this area. This problem was more significant in the past, when many journals simply refused to publish this type of research. The scientific atmosphere is changing, though, and is increasingly recognizing the value of such research and its relevance to medicine. Today, most journal editors and reviewers make decisions about manuscripts on the basis of the scientific quality of the work. Nevertheless, some journal editors remain unyielding in their negative attitude toward publishing this research. In fact, negative findings on the religion-health relationship are sometimes more likely to be published than positive findings (regardless of the scientific quality of the work).

The File Drawer Phenomenon

Another bias that affects the publication of research on religion and health is the "file drawer phenomenon." Studies that report no association between religion and health are less likely to be published than are studies that report either significant positive or significant negative findings. Reports that find no association between religion and health are not particularly interesting to a scientific audience that is already skeptical about religion's impact on health. One might expect this bias, however, to lead to the overpublication of both positive and negative studies. The fact that there are so many more published reports of positive than negative findings (even during a time when journal editors and reviewers had largely negative attitudes toward religion) suggests that this bias may be less influential than expected.

SUMMARY AND CONCLUSIONS

In this chapter, we emphasized the need to establish specific hypotheses up front to guide the development of a research study. We explained the different study designs and discussed what inferences each design made possible. We examined sampling methods for recruiting study subjects and discussed the strengths and weaknesses of each method. We emphasized the need to study different populations in different areas of the country to enhance generalizability and to better understand mechanisms of effect. We briefly addressed issues related to measurement and expressed concern about using measures of spirituality that are contaminated by the health outcomes they are attempting to predict. We provided suggestions on how to choose the correct statistical tests and how to subsequently conduct the analysis and interpret the results. We emphasized the importance of having different research teams replicate results at different sites with different populations. Finally, we examined the importance of the peer review process and addressed the issue of publication bias.

Researchers and clinicians need to know basic information about how to design and carry out research studies to examine the relationship between religion and health. Understanding how to conduct such research, from choosing the correct study design to properly analyzing the data and publishing the results, is essential for continued scientific progress in this area.

33

Measurement Tools

AS EMPHASIZED IN CHAPTER 32, it is essential that the religious variable be measured using sensitive and reliable instruments. In this chapter, we present a wide range of scales that can be used to measure religiosity, spirituality, and mysticism. We first examine measures of religiosity and then overview instruments that assess spirituality and mysticism. We do not intend to comprehensively review all existing scales but aim rather to examine and highlight the most commonly used measures. For those who wish a more complete review and critique of such scales, we recommend Peter Hill and Ralph Hood's recent book, *Measures of Religiosity* (1999).

MEASURES OF RELIGIOUSNESS

The following are the dimensions of religiosity that require assessment. These dimensions have been described in chapter 1. We illustrate and discuss measures for assessing each of these dimensions here.

1. Religious belief
   a. Belief vs. nonbelief
   b. Certainty of belief
   c. Orthodoxy of belief
2. Religious affiliation or denomination
3. Organizational religiosity
   a. Membership in church or synagogue or temple
   b. Attendance at religious services
   c. Religious social activity other than attendance
   d. Participating in Scripture study or prayer groups
   e. Holding positions in church (officer, deacon, elder)
   f. Giving financial support to church or temple

g. Receiving the Sacraments or participating in other communal religious
   ritual
4. Nonorganizational religiosity
   a. Engaging in private prayer (at times
      other than meals)
   b. Reading religious Scriptures or inspi-
      rational literature
   c. Watching religious television or lis-
      tening to religious radio
5. Subjective religiosity
   a. Importance of religion
   b. Self-rated religiosity
6. Religious commitment or orientation
   a. Intrinsic religiosity
   b. Extrinsic religiosity
7. Religious "quest" (searching for religious truth)
8. Religious well-being (as part of spiritual well-being)
9. Religious coping (functional)
10. Religious history
11. Religious and spiritual maturity
12. Other religious attitudes and practices

Religious Belief

A question that aims to assess religious belief from a Judeo-Christian or Muslim (and some-times Hindu) religious perspective may simply ask whether one believes in God. This question evokes a "yes," "no," or "unsure" response. As-sessing *certainty* of belief in God is perhaps more useful in the United States, where more than 95% of the population believes in God or a higher power. Measuring certainty of belief pro-vides a wider range of responses and greater variability than simply establishing the presence or absence of belief. Certainty of belief is not the same as *orthodoxy* of belief (conforming to the established, original doctrines of a religious tradition), although the two often overlap in the measures that assess them.

Glock and Stark's (1966) Orthodoxy Index is one of the most commonly used orthodoxy scales. It consists of four items that address beliefs about God, Jesus, miracles, and the devil. For belief in God, the six responses range from "I know God really exists and have no doubts

about it" to "I don't believe in God." For belief in Jesus, the five responses range from "Jesus is the Divine son of God and I have no doubts about it" to "Frankly, I'm not entirely sure there really was such a person as Jesus." Similar state-ments exist for items that tap belief in miracles and belief in the devil. While no evidence of reliability is available, there is some evidence that the index has discriminant validity, in that Unitarians and Congregationalists score low and Southern Baptists score high on the Index.

Related to orthodoxy of belief is *particular-ism*. Particularism is "the Calvinistic doctrine that redemption is possible only for some per-sons, not all" (Guralnik, 1980, p. 1036). Glock and Stark's (1966) Particularism Index consists of three items that concern belief in Jesus and salvation. Other commonly used belief scales are described later. These scales focus primarily on Christian beliefs, and some explicitly state that they should not be used to assess Jewish beliefs. Full versions of these scales can be found in *Measures of Social Psychological Attitudes* (Robinson & Shaver, 1973) or *Measures of Religi-osity* (Hill & Hood, 1999).

One of the first published religious belief scales was Thouless's (1935) Certainty of Beliefs Test, which consists of 40 items, each rated on a scale of 1–6 on the basis of certainty of belief. The scale, however, is heavily contaminated by items that have nothing to do with religion. It consists of 19 items that examine religious be-liefs and 21 items that explore a wide range of other types of beliefs, from "Hornets live in nests under the ground" to "The total national debt of Great Britain is more than a thousand million pounds." Thouless provided no evi-dence of reliability or of validity for the scale, other than face validity for the 19 religious items.

Brown and Lowe (1951) developed a 15-item scale to assess degree of Christian belief. Re-sponses to each item range from 1 to 5 and were based on strength of agreement with the statement. The reliability coefficient for the scale is 0.87 (based on Spearman-Brown for-mula). Concurrent validity was examined by ad-ministering the instrument to Bible college stu-dents and to students at a liberal theological seminary. Bible college students scored much higher than liberal seminary students on the scale.

Martin and Westie (1959) developed a nine-item Religious Fundamentalism scale to assess Christian beliefs about the Bible and Jesus. The five response options for each item range from "strongly agree" to "strongly disagree." No information is given about reliability, although some evidence for discriminant validity is provided.

Brown (1962) modified and expanded the Thouless scale (1935) by deleting most of the nonreligious items, resulting in an orthodoxy scale consisting of 15 items that inquire about subjects' beliefs about God, Jesus, and other elements of Christianity. Brown reported no information on validity, although a test-retest measure of reliability was obtained on 40 subjects over an eight-month period, the two administrations had a correlation coefficient of .85.

Putney and Middleton's (1961) Dimensions of Religious Ideology Scale assesses religious beliefs in terms of orthodoxy, fanaticism, importance, and ambivalence. Each subscale has six items, and each item has a response range from 1 (strong disagreement) to 7 (strong agreement). Except for the religious orthodoxy subscale, this instrument focuses on religion in general without reference to a specific belief system. No measure of reliability or validity is reported, although the investigators indicated that only a small percentage of skeptics (8%) scored high on the orthodoxy subscale, compared with 92% of religious conservatives.

Lenski's (1963) Doctrinal Orthodoxy scale consists of six yes-no items that assess beliefs in God, life after death, God's expectations of humanity, and the Divine nature of Jesus. No information about reliability is given, and validity is primarily in terms of face validity.

Faulkner and DeJong's (1965) Ideological Scale consists of five items that examine belief about God and the Bible. Each item has three to five possible responses. No evidence of validity is provided, although the reliability coefficient (Cronbach α) is reported to be .94 (Robinson & Shaver, 1973).

King and Hunt's (1967) Creedal Assent Scale consists of seven items that examine beliefs in eternal life, God, Christ, and the Bible. Each item is rated on a four-point scale of agreement. The reliability coefficient for the scale is reported to be .91, and evidence for convergent validity is based on the scale's high correlations with several other scales (King & Hunt, 1969).

Religious Affiliation

Denominational affiliation can be assessed in a number of ways. The most common method in Western countries has been to simply ask subjects whether they are Protestant, Catholic, Jewish, none, or other. This method provides little useful information. Other ways of categorizing religious affiliation refine the response categories and provide greater detail. For religious groups in America, the Institute for Social Research (University of Michigan, Ann Arbor) uses the following categories, which are based on degree of institutional conservatism (Kendler et al., 1997) (unfortunately, it categorizes Jews together with the religiously unaffiliated):

Fundamentalist Protestant (e.g., Church of God, Pentecostal, Assembly of God)

Baptist

Catholic

Mainline Protestant (e.g., Episcopalian, Methodist, Presbyterian)

Other or unaffiliated

Roof and McKinney (1987, p. 255) use the categories that follow, which again are based on religious conservatism. Theirs is one of the more commonly used methods today.

Liberal Protestants
   Episcopalians
   United Church of Christ
   Presbyterians

Moderate Protestants
   Methodists
   Lutherans
   Christians (Disciples of Christ)
   Northern Baptists
   Reformed

African American Protestants
  Methodists
  Northern Baptists
  Southern Baptists

Conservative Protestants
  Southern Baptists
  Churches of Christ
  Evangelicals/Fundamentalists
  Nazarenes
  Pentecostals/Holiness
  Assemblies of God
  Churches of God
  Adventists

Catholics

Jews

Others
  Mormons
  Jehovah's Witnesses
  Christian Scientists
  Unitarian-Universalists
  Miscellaneous (Hindus, Buddhists, etc.)

No religious preference

Research studies at Duke University use an even more refined and detailed breakdown of religious groups, although this categorization is weighted heavily toward Protestant Christianity, which is dominant in the southern United States (EPESE, 1984):

General
  None
  Protestant (no denomination given)
  Nondenominational Protestant
  Community church
  Other Protestant not listed

Protestant—Reformation Era
  Presbyterian
  Lutheran
  Congregational
  Reformed, Dutch Reform
  United Church of Christ
  Episcopalian

Protestant—Pietistic
  Methodist
  African Methodist-Episcopal
  Baptist
  Disciples of Christ
  "Christian"

Protestant—Neofundamentalist
  United Missionary

  Church of God
  Nazarene
  Church of God in Christ
  Pentecostal, Holiness
  Church of Christ
  Salvation Army
  Free-Will Baptist
  Seventh-Day Adventist
  Southern Baptist
  Christian Alliance
  Assembly of God

Nontraditional Christian
  Christian Scientist
  Mormon
  Unitarian/Universalist
  Jehovah's Witness
  Other nontraditional Christian

Catholic

Greek Orthodox

Jewish

Buddhist

Hindu

Muslim

Agnostic, atheist

Organizational Religiosity

Organizational religiosity consists of church-related activity and reflects the social dimension of religious practice. Although a number of scales exist that measure this dimension, the most common measure is a simple question about frequency of religious attendance. Glock and Stark (1966) asked the question "How often do you attend Sunday worship services?"; the 10 response options range from "every week" to "never." Likewise, in the five-item Duke Religion Index, Koenig, Meador, and Parkerson (1997) ask the question "How often do you attend church or other religious meetings?"; the six response options range from "more then once per week" to "never."

Hadaway, Marler, and Chaves (1993, 1998), however, reported that responses to general questions about church attendance may be exaggerated. They claim that people overestimate the frequency with which they attend religious services. However, Hout and Greeley (1998) provide more recent evidence that suggests that the magnitude of overreporting of religious attendance is small, closer to a factor of 1.1 rather than 2.0, as suggested by Hadaway, Marler, and Chaves (1998). Smith (1998) indicates that, while questions about church attendance tend to yield modest overreports, subjects typically understand religious attendance in broader terms than simply participation in worship services. Rather, they include participation in prayer groups, Bible studies, and similar social-type religious activities.

George Gallup Jr. has tried to get around this problem by phrasing the question differently. His polls ask, "Did you, yourself, happen to attend church or synagogue in the last seven days, or not?" (Princeton Religion Research Center, 1996). This provides a more specific time frame that can be used as an anchor point by respondents. Differences in rates of religious attendance obtained by the two methods, however, are not great. While religious attendance is a crude measure of religiousness, since people attend religious services for many reasons other than religion, it is a good indicator of level of participation in a religious community.

Other investigators have used multi-item scales to measure organizational religiosity. For example, the Springfield Religiosity Scale (Koenig, Smiley, & Gonzales, 1988) assesses organizational religiosity with three items: frequency of attendance at religious services, participation in other religious group activities (e.g., adult Sunday school classes, Bible study groups, prayer groups), and number among five closest friends who are members of the subject's church congregation.

King and Hunt (1967) use several subscales to assess organizational religious activities. First, a *church attendance* subscale addresses questions about activity within the congregation, frequency of attending church, and frequency of taking Communion. Second, an *organizational activities* subscale inquires about evenings spent at church meetings or in church work, church activities as a source of satisfaction in life, frequency of attendance at Sunday school, extent of being informed about the congregation, enjoyment of activities at church, and the number of offices, special jobs, or com-

mittees in which the subject has been involved. Third, a *church work with friends* subscale asks about close friends who are members of the congregation, self-rating of activity within the congregation, number among five closest friends who are members of the congregation, and frequency of social contacts with members of the congregation other than at church.

Other religious activity, such as giving financial support to the church, may also be included in the organizational dimension. King and Hunt's (1967) Financial Support subscale assesses proportion of income given to church, average monthly contribution, frequency of gifts, and regularity of contributions.

Related to organizational religious involvement is religious support from a congregation. One of the best measures of religious support has recently been developed by Neal Krause (Fetzer Institute, 1999). The measure can be administered in either a long or a shortened scale. The shortened scale consists of eight questions that assess emotional support received from others, emotional support provided to others, negative interactions, and anticipated support if needed.

Nonorganizational Religiosity

Private religious activities are included in the category of *nonorganizational religiosity*. In the Duke Religion Index, Koenig, Meador, and Parkerson (1997) ask the question "How often do you spend time in private religious activities, such as prayer, meditation, or Bible study?" The six response options range from "more then once a day" to "rarely or never." Stark and Glock's (1968) Devotionalism Index consists of two items: frequency of private prayer and importance of prayer in life. Respondents are classified as "high" if they feel prayer is extremely important and if they pray privately once a week or more. The Devotionalism Index developed by Lenski (1963) also consists of two items, frequency of prayer and extent to which one consults God when making everyday decisions. The Springfield Religiosity Scale (Koenig, Smiley, & Gonzales, 1988) includes three items that assess nonorganizational religious behaviors such as engaging in private prayer, reading the Bible or other religious literature, and listening to or watching religious programs on radio or TV.

Some instruments, like that of Faulkner and DeJong (1965), combine both organizational and nonorganizational religious activities into a single scale (ritualistic scale). King and Hunt (1967) combine nonorganizational religious activity with personal religious experience in a subscale that assesses frequency and importance of prayer, impact of religion on decisions, experience of closeness to God, and experience that life has been influenced by God. In general, we advise against such combinations, since each of these dimensions (organizational, nonorganizational, experience) may have different (and sometimes opposite) relationships with health outcomes (Koenig, Hays, George, et al., 1997).

Subjective Religiosity

Subjective religiosity is assessed by asking persons to rate their degree of religiousness or the importance of religion to them. Single items are typically used to assess this dimension. For example, in the Duke NIMH Epidemiologic Catchment Area study, Koenig, George, Meador, Blazer, and Ford (1994) asked, "How important is religion to you?" Response options are "very important," "somewhat important," or "not important." Other investigators ask a question like "How religious do you consider yourself?" Response options are typically "not at all religious," "somewhat religious," "quite religious," and "very religious." Single items with such a limited response range, however, have little variability. A more sensitive alternative is to ask subjects to rate the importance of religion to them using a visual analog scale that ranges from 0 to 10.

Putney and Middleton (1961) have an Importance Scale (with five response options for each item) that assesses importance of religion, influence of religion on views in other areas of life, importance of religion in terms of personal identity, interest in religion, and time spent thinking about religion. Again, having a more sensitive, finely graded measure of this construct will increase the chances of finding a relationship with health (because of the greater variability of responses).

Religious Commitment or Orientation

Religious commitment describes the degree of internal committment a person feels toward his religious beliefs. It also reflects the influence that religious beliefs and teachings have on the person's decisions and lifestyle. Many dimensions of religiosity have been labeled (and perhaps mislabeled) as religious commitment. This is understandable, since all religious dimensions touch upon or reflect religious commitment in one way or another. In our opinion, the best measure of religious commitment is *intrinsic religious orientation*.

As noted in chapter 1, Gordon Allport developed important concepts related to religious orientation in the early 1950s (Allport, 1954). He later led a seminar at Harvard that produced an intrinsic-extrinsic (IE) religiosity scale, which he eventually administered to 309 members of church groups, including Catholics, Lutherans, Nazarenes, Presbyterians, Methodists, and Baptists (Allport & Ross, 1967). The IE scale consists of 20 items; 11 items assess extrinsic religiosity and nine items assess intrinsic religiosity. Agreement with each item is assessed on a 1–4 scale, and intrinsic and extrinsic items are summed separately (see Robinson & Shaver, 1973, pp. 705–708). *Extrinsic* items include statements such as, "One reason for my being a church member is that such membership helps to establish a person in the community," "The church is most important as a place to formulate good social relationships," "A primary reason for my interest in religion is that my church is a congenial social activity," and, "Although I am a religious person, I refuse to let religious considerations influence my everyday affairs." The items that measure *intrinsic* religiosity include statements such as, "I try hard to carry my religion over into all my other dealings in life," "My religious beliefs are what really lie behind my whole approach to life," and "The prayers I say when I am alone carry as much meaning and personal emotion as those said by me during services."

Feagin's (1964) IE scale differs from the Allport-Ross scale by the addition of one extrinsic item ("Religion helps to keep my life balanced and steady in exactly the way as my citizenship, friendships, and other memberships do"). Investigators have sometimes used the six strongest-loading items on the extrinsic factor (Factor I) and the six strongest items on the intrinsic factor (Factor II) reported in Feagin's (1964) study of 286 church members in Texas and in Oklahoma. This is the origin of Feagin's six-item IR and six-item ER scales, and the resulting 12-item Intrinsic/Extrinsic Scale has been recommended over Allport's scale because of its better psychometric properties.

Hoge (1972) developed a 10-item IR scale (based on Allport's scale) that has been used widely to assess the intrinsic dimension. The Hoge scale consists of seven intrinsic items and three extrinsic items (reverse scored). This measure has been related to a number of positive health states, including well-being (Koenig, Kvale, & Ferrel, 1988) and recovery from depression (Koenig, George, & Peterson, 1998).

Gorsuch and McPherson (1989) have developed both 14-item and three-item intrinsic-extrinsic (I-E) scales. These investigators identified two subcategories of "extrinsicness" using factor analysis. They argue that some extrinsic items are concerned with social relationships (Es), while others are concerned with personal benefits (Ep), and they have therefore produced revised I-E scales that contain Es items, Ep items, and intrinsic items that are counterbalanced for "acquiesence." Their three-item scale includes items that tap each of these three major aspects of religious orientation and is attractive because of its brevity. The Gorsuch-McPherson scales, however, have not been used nearly as widely as the Allport-Ross, Feagin, or Hoge measures.

Note that the intrinsic-extrinsic concept has not been without criticism (Hunt & King, 1971; Donahue, 1985; Batson, Oleson, et al., 1989). Hunt and King (1971) had particular problems with the claim that intrinsic and extrinsic religiosity were opposite poles of a continuum. Hunt and King concluded that Allport's I and E scales are not bipolar opposites but rather are separate dimensions made up of several different components. They claimed that Feagin's (1964) six-item Extrinsic Scale (termed "instrumental-selfish") is still the best measure of extrinsic religiousness and suggested that intrinsic religiosity as a single religious dimension be abandoned. Hunt and King based this recommendation on their finding that intrinsic religiousness was made up of several separate factors and that it was hard to distinguish intrinsic religiousness from "indiscriminate proreligiousness." Furthermore, they argued that there were serious problems with the scale's reliability and validity and that terms such as "inner," "real," and "ultimate" were metaphysical, not empirical, constructs.

Religious Quest

According to C. Daniel Batson, two different religious orientations confound Allport's concept of intrinsic religiosity. In addition to the "true believer," he claimed, there are individuals who focus on religion as a *quest*. As noted in chapter 1, "These persons view religion as an endless process of probing and questioning generated by the tensions, contradictions, and tragedies in their own lives and in society" (Batson, 1976, p. 32). Batson assesses the "interactional" or quest dimension of religiosity using a nine-item scale that includes statements such as, "It might be said that I value my religious doubts and uncertainties," "I find my everyday experiences severely test my religious convictions," and "Questions are far more central to my religious experience than are answers" (Batson, 1976, p. 44). Few studies have used Batson's Religious Quest Scale, compared with the number that have utilized IE constructs.

Religious Well-Being

Religious well-being is one of two subscales contained in the 20-item Spiritual Well-Being Scale (SWB) developed by Paloutzian and Ellison (1982). The existential well-being (EWB) subscale assesses well-being unrelated to religion and thus reflects positive mental health; for that reason, finding that SWB is correlated with greater life satisfaction, well-being, or less depression is not surprising, especially when the correlation holds only for the EWB scale. More relevant is whether the religious well-being subscale relates to better mental health. The RWB subscale consists of 10 statements to which agreement or disagreement is indicated on a six-point scale. Examples of statements are, "I believe that God loves me and cares about me," "I have a personally meaningful relationship with God," I feel most fulfilled when I'm in close communion with God," and "I believe that God is concerned about my problems."

While there are other spiritual well-being scales besides the Paloutzian and Ellison scale, the ones that we have examined (Jarel Spiritual Well-Being Scale, Moberg Spiritual Well-Being Scale) are likewise heavily contaminated by items that measure well-being. While these scales are not useful for examining the relationship between spiritual well-being and mental health, their contamination with mental health items is less problematic when one wishes to examine the relationship between spiritual well-being and physical health. One way to avoid the problem entirely, however, is to analyze religious and existential well-being subscales separately.

Religious Coping

Religious coping is defined as the extent to which persons use their religious beliefs and practices to help them to adapt to difficult life situations and stressful events. There has been some discussion on whether religious coping is an "extrinsic" form of religious activity (i.e., using religion as a means of obtaining comfort and relieving stress). Nevertheless, a number of studies have found a stronger relationship between religious coping and intrinsic religiosity than between religious coping and extrinsic religiosity (Bjorck & Cohen, 1993; Pargament, 1997; Koenig, 1998b). Indeed, we would expect persons with strongly internalized religious commitment to readily turn to religion when confronting stressful life problems.

Ken Pargament (1997) provides an in-depth review and discussion of different measures of religious coping. Two different approaches have been used to measure religious coping: a broad general assessment (the extent to which religion is used to cope) and a more detailed assessment of specific religious coping methods (exactly how the person uses religion to cope).

In the first approach, the simplest way of assessing overall degree of religious coping is to ask persons open-ended questions about what enables them to cope with stress. Religion is not even mentioned to the subjects, who must choose whatever method of coping has been most helpful in their experience. While this method has high *specificity* (if the person mentions religion, it is likely to be an important coping behavior), it is not very sensitive. Many persons will not spontaneously mention religion during such a discussion because it is too personal; they may be reluctant to talk about it with strangers, especially skeptical researchers. Another method of assessing religious coping is to directly ask subjects if they use religion to help cope with stress. This strategy, however, suffers the opposite problem from the indirect method. While it is very sensitive in identifying persons who use religion to cope, it has low specificity (many persons may agree only because it is more socially acceptable to answer positively than negatively to such questions).

Koenig, Cohen, Blazer, Pieper, et al. (1992) have developed a three-item Religious Coping Index that combines the indirect and direct methods we have described and adds an interviewer-rated component to increase validity. In the last item, the interviewer rates the patient's religious coping on the basis of an in-depth discussion that delves into how the person uses religion to cope, when she did so, and how frequently she does so. Because of the interviewer component, this measure must be interviewer administered. The Religious Coping Index has a test-retest reliability of 0.81 (when administered on separate occasions by different interviewers with different religious backgrounds) and has been correlated with lower rates of depression both cross-sectionally and longitudinally in hospitalized medically ill patients (Koenig, Cohen, Blazer, Pieper, et al., 1992).

Another method of assessing general religious coping is to provide subjects with a list of different coping behaviors (both religious and nonreligious) and ask them to choose the behaviors they use the most. This checklist method has been particularly useful when studying coping among the medically ill elderly (Conway, 1985; Manfredi & Pickett, 1987).

The second method of assessment involves measuring specific types or styles of religious coping. Ken Pargament (1997) has led the field in the development of such measures. Examples of specific religious coping styles include collaborative religious coping (person and God work together as partners, each doing what is necessary to improve situation), passive religious deferral (person does nothing and relies entirely on God to solve problem), and pleas for direct intercession (person bargains or pleads with God to make things better). Religious coping methods associated with positive and negative mental health states have been identified (Pargament, Kennell, et al., 1988; Pargament, Ensing, et al., 1990; Pargament, Olsen, et al., 1992; Pargament, Ishler, et al., 1994). Most recently, Pargament and Koenig developed a 63-item scale that assesses 21 religious coping methods (the RCOPE). These scales have now been tested in 577 medically ill older patients and 540 healthy college students (Koenig, Pargament, & Nielsen, 1998; Pargament, Koenig, & Perez, 2000).

Pargament, Smith, et al. (1998) have also developed a 14-item brief RCOPE that includes seven items that assess positive religious coping and seven items that measure negative religious coping. Positive religious coping items have generally been related to better mental health, whereas negative religious coping items have been related to both worse mental and worse physical health.

Religious History

While religious activity and involvement are often measured cross-sectionally, we know that persons are often exposed to and participate in religious beliefs and practices throughout their lives. Not infrequently there are "turning points" that initiate a change in direction. A severe stressor or other key experience may cause a person to become much more religious or much less religious. An accurate measure of religious history is essential for determining one's degree of exposure to religious influences across the life span and the reasons for increases or decreases in religiousness; it also helps researchers achieve a greater understanding of the mechanisms by which religion influences health and vice versa. Although no instrument for assessing religious history existed before, now, efforts are now under way at Duke University to develop such a measure (Hays, Meador, et al., 2000; see also the NIA-Fetzer Religiousness/Spirituality measure discussed later in this chapter).

Religious and Spiritual Maturity

Because the influence of religion on health may depend at least in part on the maturity of a person's religious beliefs, measures that assess religious development are of vital importance. Religious maturity involves the extent to which a person has integrated her religious beliefs and practices into daily living. While religious maturity overlaps to some extent with intrinsic religiosity or the degree to which the person has internalized religious motivations (postconventional faith), it is considerably broader. Religious maturity includes consequences of religious faith and nearness to a particular religious goal or ideal.

Religious maturity is best assessed *within* a particular religious tradition. For example, Ellison (1983) has developed the Spiritual Maturity Index, a 30-item measure that assesses spiritual maturity from a Christian perspective. Included in the Index are questions that assess the need for institutional structure to express Christianity (with low need indicating greater maturity), the presence of Christian beliefs and practices as a spontaneous part of everyday life, the absence of need for social support to maintain faith and practice, the degree to which the person is other focused rather than self focused, the person's ability to avoid narrow-minded adherence to laws or rules, the presence of expressions of generosity and love toward others, the closeness of the person's relationship to God, and his acceptance of suffering as part of God's plan. Fowler (1981) and others have attempted to broaden the concept of faith development in order to transcend individual belief systems. This effort has been successful to some degree but has its limitations (Koenig, 1994c). H. Newton Malony, at the Fuller Theological Seminary in Pasadena, California, has also devoted much time to this area of research and coordinated a symposium on this topic at the 1999 meeting of the American Psychological Association.

Other Measures

Numerous other measures of religious beliefs and behavior exist. As noted earlier, these measures can be located by consulting Robinson and Shaver (1973), for some of the older, classic measures, or by obtaining the recently published Hill and Hood (1999) book of measures. We list here a few scales that have not yet been mentioned (by year of publication):

Measures of Religious Belief, Activity, and Commitment

Attitudes toward Church Scale (45-item) (Thurstone & Chave, 1929)

Religion subscale of Chicago Inventory of Activities and Attitudes (Burgess et al., 1948)

Kirkpatrick Religiosity Scale (Kirkpatrick, 1949)

Attitudes toward Religion Scale (Bardis, 1961)

Religious Attitude Scale (Poppleton & Pilkington, 1963)

Glock and Stark's (1966) 5-Dimension Religiosity Scale (originally Glock, 1962)

5-D Religiosity Scale (Faulkner & DeJong, 1966)

Allport-Vernon Scale of Values (Allport et al., 1968)

12-item Wiggins Religiosity Scale (from MMPI) (Wiggins, 1969)

Importance of Religion (single item) (Gorsuch & McFarland, 1972)

King and Hunt Scales (King & Hunt 1967, 1969, 1975; Hunt & King, 1971)

13-item Religiosity Scale (Kenney et al., 1977)

14-item Religious Life Scale (Kauffman, 1979)

5-item Religious Orthodoxy Scale (Shupe & Stacey, 1982; see Trier & Shupe, 1991)

Batson's Orthodoxy Scale (Batson & Ventis, 1982)

Gorsuch-Venable 20-item I-E Scale (Gorsuch & Venable, 1983)

45-item (9 scale) Personal Religiosity Inventory (Lipsmeyer, 1984)

13-item Religious Perspectives Scale (Reed, 1986)

9-item Religious Maturity Scale (Dudley & Cruise, 1990)

10-item Santa Clara Strength of Religious Faith Quest (Plante & Boccaccini, 1997a, 1997b)

Jewish Religiosity Scales

26-item Jewish religiosity Scale (Ben-Meir & Kedem, 1979)

10-item Jewishness Scale (Ressler, 1997)

Jewish Religious Observance Subscale (Katz, 1988)

Hindu Religiosity Scales

36-item Bhushan's Religiosity Scale (India) (Bhushan, 1970)

10-item Hassan Religiosity Scale (Hassan & Khalique, 1981)

Muslim Religiosity Scale

None known

Religiosity Scales used for Muslims

Allport-Vernon Scale of Values (see Shams & Jackson, 1993)

Hoge Intrinsic Religiosity Scale (see Thorson, 1998)

10-item Hassan Religiosity Scale (see Hassan & Khalique, 1981)

Buddhist Belief/Activity Scale

Buddhist Beliefs and Practices Scale (Emavardhana & Tori, 1997)

Religiosity Scale used for Buddhists

20-item Gorsuch-Venable I-E Scale (see Tapanya et al., 1997)

DUREL

The Duke University Religion Index (DUREL) was developed specifically to capture the major dimensions of religiousness that relate to health outcomes. This five-item scale takes less than one minute to administer and taps the three most important religious dimensions: organizational religiousness (one item), nonorganizational religiousness (one item), and intrinsic religiosity (three items) (Koenig, Meador, & Parkerson, 1997). When using this measure, researchers should examine organizational religiousness, nonorganizational religiousness, and intrinsic religiosity separately; the scores should not be combined. Combinations of organizational (ORA) and nonorganizational (NORA) religious activity, however, may be examined (i.e., high ORA-high NORA, high ORA-low NORA, low ORA-high NORA, and low ORA-low NORA). Persons who score high on both ORA and NORA have better health and more positive health behaviors than those who score low on both ORA and NORA (Koenig, George, Cohen, et al., 1998a,b).

MEASURES OF SPIRITUALITY

Researchers may wish to assess spirituality instead of religiosity. As noted in chapter 1, spirituality is a broader, more inclusive term than religiosity. Many measures of spirituality that exist today, however, measure simply religiosity. The label "spirituality" has been given these instruments only because that term is less offensive and more acceptable to academicians than "religiosity." Spirituality and religion frequently become blurred when one is actually trying to measure one or the other. Some researchers may even question the existence of an independent construct called "spirituality" that is distinct from religiousness and other psychological states or traits that already have established labels (meaning in life, forgiveness, awe, beauty, wonder).

Spiritual Well-Being Scale

As discussed earlier, the 20-item Spiritual Well-Being Scale was developed by Paloutzian and Ellison (1982) and consists of a 10-item religious well-being scale and a 10-item existential well-being scale. Religiousness and spirituality are largely synonymous in this instrument.

Index of Spiritual Orientation

Glik (1990a) developed the 19-item Index of Spiritual Orientation, which is based on Sorokin's theory of cultural values and was designed with the intention of capturing "nontraditional religious group orientations." The scale has ideational belief, salience of religion, purpose in life, and mysticism subscales; regular participation in healing groups is used as a proxy for religious practice. There is some concern that this scale may be contaminated by mental health items (for example, purpose in life is often used as an indicator of mental health).

INSPIRIT

Kass et al. (1991) assessed 83 adults with serious medical disorders (musculoskeletal disorders, chronic pain, gastrointestinal disorders, hypertension, and cancer) who were involved in a 10-week study during which they were taught the Relaxation Response. Spiritual experience was measured by using the Index of Core Spiritual Experiences (INSPIRIT), a seven-item scale "measuring the occurrence of experience that convinces a person God exists and evokes feelings of closeness with God, including the perception that God dwells within." Correlation between INSPIRIT and the Intrinsic Religiosity Scale of Allport and Ross's Religious Orientation Inventory is high ($r = .69$, $p < .0001$). Although this scale focuses primarily on God (and thus heavily overlaps with religiousness), it is broad enough to accommodate a wider definition of spirituality than most purely religious measures.

FACIT Spiritual Well-Being Scale (FACIT SpWB)

The FACIT spirituality scale (which is a subscale of the FACIT [Functional Assessment of Chronic Illness Therapy] scale) consists of two parts: a Faith/Assurance subscale and a Meaning/Purpose subscale (Cella, 1996; Cella & Webster, 1997). The Faith/Assurance subscale consists of four items; three of these items are phrased in terms of having found *comfort* in faith and having found *strength* in faith, and one item speaks of feeling connected to God. Again, there is concern that this scale is contaminated by measures of mental health and well-being. If a person admits to finding comfort or strength or connectedness to anything (spiritual things or not), this tells us something about the person's level of well-being (spiritual or nonspiritual). Thus, when one uses the scale to assess the relationship between spiritual beliefs and mental health, tautology becomes a concern. This problem is even greater for the Meaning and Purpose subscale. Examining the 18 items that make up this subscale reveals that this is simply a well-being scale: it measures whether one feels peaceful, has a reason to live, feels that life is productive, has a sense of purpose in life, experiences comfort or harmony, has a sense of connectedness, feels a sense of being loved, experiences love for others, and is hopeful. The definition of spirituality here has become so broad that it includes virtually every positive human experience—love, hope, thankfulness, appreciation, harmony, peace, comfort—whether or not it has any involvement with the transcendent or sacred. There is also a new 24-item version of the scale (Version 4) (FACIT Sp-Ex) (Brady et al., 1999).

Systems of Belief Inventory (SBI-15)

This is a 15-item spiritual beliefs inventory that has been used among patients with severe life-threatening illness (malignant melanoma) (Holland et al., 1998). It consists of two factors, a general factor that consists of 10 items that assess religious beliefs, feelings, and experiences, and a five-item factor that assesses social support received from one's religious community. Most of the research has been done with the longer, 54-item SBI (from which the 15-item scale is derived), which has been correlated with a healthy active-cognitive coping style in patients with malignant melanoma (Holland et al., 1999; Baider et al., 1999). According to unpublished data communicated by Alice Kornblith, a study that used the SBI-15 in a sample of 240 healthy subjects found a significant correlation

between the SBI and the Allport-Ross I-E scale ($r = .60$, $p < .001$) and the Index of Spiritual Experience (INSPIRIT) scale ($r = .74$). These pilot data, however, surprisingly, demonstrated no correlation between measures of psychological distress (Profile of Mood States and Brief Symptom Inventory) and the SBI; this may be a result of the subjective nature of many of the questions and the cross-sectional nature of the data. Spirituality here is largely operationalized in terms of religious beliefs and practices but also attends to broader issues and includes assessment of activity in and support from the religious community.

Fetzer-NIA Measure of Religiousness and Spirituality

The Fetzer-NIA scale arose out of several meetings of a group of prominent social scientists convened by the Fetzer Foundation to discuss issues related to spirituality and measurement (Idler, Ellison, et al., 2000; see Fetzer Institute, 1999, for the expanded instrument). An abbreviated version of this scale was included in the General Social Survey (GSS), a yearly national survey of Americans conducted by the National Opinion Research Center (NORC). The Fetzer-NIA scale taps a broad range of religious and spiritual topics, including denomination (one item), organizational religiousness (two items), private spiritual practices (four items on private religious practices and one item on spiritual meditation), religious social support (four items), religious coping (seven items), religious belief (one item), moral value (one item), religious commitment/intrinsic religiosity (one item), financial contributions to religious causes (one item), time donated on behalf of church or for religious/spiritual reasons (one item), forgiveness (three items), spiritual experience (four religious items and two items that assess peace, harmony, and beauty of creation), spiritual/religious history (three items), and self-ratings of religiousness and spirituality (two items). The only concern with this excellent instrument is that, like the Rush Spiritual Beliefs scale, it includes some items that do not directly measure religiousness or spirituality (i.e., moral value and forgiveness) and is contaminated by items that assess mental health (i.e., feelings of peace and harmony). These items virtually ensure a relationship between spirituality and better mental health should this association be examined.

Spiritual Involvement and Beliefs Scale

Hatch et al. (1998) developed a 26-item scale that they suggest has wide applicability across religious traditions and assesses behaviors as well as beliefs. On the basis of a study of 50 family practice patients and 33 family practice educators, the authors reported that the measure has high internal reliability (Cronbach's α = .92) and strong test-retest reliability (r = .92) and demonstrates convergent validity (a high correlation with Paloutzian and Ellison's Spiritual Well-Being Scale (r = .80). For each of the 26 statements in the scale, there are five response options, ranging from "strongly agree" to "strongly disagree." Many of the items on the scale have little or no relationship to the sacred or transcendent, and there is considerable confounding by questions that assess mental health ("In the future, science will be able to explain everything," "I can find meaning in times of hardship," "I am thankful for all that has happened to me," "My life has a purpose," "When I wrong someone, I make an effort to apologize," "When I am ashamed of something I have done, I tell someone about it"). While these statements may reflect consequences of spirituality (as better mental or physical health may be a consequence of spirituality), they have little to do with the construct of spirituality itself. Many nonspiritual persons might object to definitions that "spiritualize" thankfulness, meaning in life, or the likelihood that one will apologize when one has been wrong.

Pargament's Method

Ken Pargament's research team has developed an interesting method of assessing spirituality that helps to differentiate it from religiousness (Zinnbauer et al., 1998). First, the researchers ask subjects to define for themselves what the terms "spiritual" and "religious" mean to them.

Second, they ask subjects to rate on five-point Likert-type scales how religious and how spiritual they considered themselves. Third, they ask subjects to place themselves into one of four categories: "I am religious but not spiritual," "I am spiritual but not religious," "I am both religious and spiritual," or "I am neither spiritual nor religious." Fourth, the subjects are asked to choose among five sets of statements that describe the way they believe the concepts of religiousness and spirituality are related to each other: Spirituality is a broader concept than religiousness and includes religiousness; religiousness is a broader concept than spirituality and includes spirituality; religiousness and spirituality are different and do not overlap; religiousness and spirituality are the same concept and overlap completely; religiousness and spirituality overlap but are not the same concept. Fifth, participants rate religiousness and spirituality on a 20-item semantic differential scale (a well-established method in social psychology for getting at the qualities of a construct), yielding two scores: evaluation of religiousness and spirituality as positive/negative and evaluation of religiousness and spirituality as potent/impotent. In this way, a qualitative and quantitative picture of the individual's spirituality (as distinct from religiousness) emerges.

In summary, several measures of spirituality exist. Most of these measures actually assess religiousness. In their attempts to expand measures of spirituality beyond religiousness, investigators have included items that tap a wide range of positive human qualities. Qualities such as forgiveness, moral value, thankfulness, purpose and meaning in life, and peace and harmony *already have names that describe these constructs*; there is little reason to include them under the construct "spirituality" (a term that involves relationship to the sacred or the transcendent). If spirituality is itself defined by positive human traits, then it becomes useless and tautological to try to relate it to mental health.

MEASURES OF MYSTICISM

Hood (1975) developed a 32-item Mysticism Scale, using a sample of 300 students at the

University of Tennessee, Chattanooga (most subjects were nominally affiliated with Baptist or Methodist congregations). The scale consists of two subscales: a 20-item general mysticism scale that assesses experiences of unity, temporal and spatial variations, inner subjectivity, ineffability, ego loss, and affect; and a 12-item religious interpretation scale that assesses religious and noetic interpretations, positive affect, and ego loss. Scores on the Mysticism Scale strongly correlate with the Hoge IR scale ($r = .81$), with greater openness to experience in terms of ego permissiveness and with more intense religious experience as measure by Hood's religious experience scale. High scorers on the Mysticism Scale also have somewhat higher scores on the L (lie) scale ($r = .31$, $p < .05$), Hs (hypochondriasis) scale ($r = .38$, $p < .05$), and Hy (hysteria) scale ($r = .47$, $p < .01$) of the MMPI.

Levin (1993) examined 1,481 adults using data from 1988 NORC General Social Survey to assess "psi," or mystical experiences (déja vu, ESP, clairvoyance or visions, contact with dead or spirits, numinous or out-of-body experiences). Only 13.5% of respondents said they had *never* experienced any of the five mystical experiences, although such experiences were clearly not common. Levin constructed a mystical experiences scale that was *inversely* related to organizational religiosity (e.g., church attendance) but was positively related to nonorganizational religious activities and subjective religiosity. Scores on the mysticism scale, particularly the mysticism/psi subscale, were higher among younger than among older participants.

Mathew (1995) developed the Mathew Materialism-Spiritualism Scale, an instrument originally constructed and tested in India. The scale is composed of six subscales: a God scale (belief in God or a power that guides the universe), a Religion scale (examines faith in the value of religion and religious practices), a Mysticism scale (evaluates belief in the genuineness of mystic or transcendental experiences), a Spirits scale (examines belief in the existence of spirits and survival of the soul after death), a Character scale (examines belief in the personal value to the individual of altruism, unselfishness, kind-

ness, and morality), and a Psi scale (examines belief in the genuineness of paranormal phenomena such as extrasensory perception and telepathy). Mathew administered his scale to 62 persons who were recovering from substance abuse, most in 12-step AA or NA programs in North Carolina. These individuals scored significantly higher on character and mysticism than did 61 general controls; however, it is possible that the 12-step program participants exaggerated their spiritual gains or that those with greater than average spirituality chose 12-step programs.

CHOOSING AN INSTRUMENT

When selecting an instrument to assess religiousness, researchers would do well to follow the following guidelines.

1. *Consider Sensitivity, Reliability, and Validity.* As we have repeatedly emphasized, the instrument one chooses must be sensitive enough to capture the full range of religious or spiritual beliefs and practices of the population being studied. It must be sensitive enough to distinguish relatively small differences in religiousness or spirituality among members of the population; this will increase the variability of responses and the likelihood that an association between the religious/spiritual variable and a health outcome will be identified. Using multi-item measures helps to increase the variability and range of responses. For example, suppose an investigator were to use a single item measure of religiosity to assess religiosity and mental health in an elderly group of African American women living in the southern United States. Suppose this single item has five response options that range from low (1) to high (5). It is quite likely that 75% of the sample will indicate either 4 or 5 as their response. This limited variability makes it less likely that the researcher will be able to relate differences in religiosity to a health outcome. The same is true for a measure of the importance of religion, where the response categories are "very," "somewhat," or "not important." In some areas of the United States, 80% of subjects will indicate very important, again providing almost no variability.

If the investigator plans to publish her research in a top-tier journal, the religious measures used must have some established level of reliability (or accuracy). As discussed in chapter 32, measures with low reliability introduce measurement "noise" that reduces the likelihood of identifying a significant relationship. Test-retest reliability is perhaps the best and most stringent indicator of reliability, although it is more difficult to establish than some other indicators. Remember that reliability and accuracy are not the same as *validity*. Measuring religiousness in a valid way is extremely important; few measures, however, attempt to establish this criterion. Since there is no "gold standard" of religiousness or spirituality, validity is difficult to verify. Some investigators have administered their instruments to religious professionals (ministers, priests, rabbis) to establish validity (Hoge, 1972; Koenig, Smiley, et al., 1988).

2. *Assess and Analyze Dimensions of Religiousness Separately.* As noted in chapter 32, researchers should choose measures that clearly assess each of the major dimensions of religiousness separately. In our opinion, the three major dimensions of religiousness are organizational, nonorganizational, and intrinsic or subjective religiousness. Either scales that mix organizational religiousness with nonorganizational religiousness or subjective religiousness should not be used, or each of these dimensions should be analyzed separately when examining relationships to physical or mental health.

3. *Avoid Instruments Contaminated by Health Outcomes.* As we emphasized earlier, items that directly measure mental health should not be included in measures of spirituality or religiousness. The inclusion of items that assess purpose in life, peace, harmony, or satisfaction in these scales virtually ensures a positive correlation with measures of mental health. Discovering a relationship between such scales and life satisfaction or well-being has little meaning. Instruments that include such items should be avoided (or the items should be deleted in the analysis).

4. *Know What You Want to Measure.* Investigators must be clear in their own minds about exactly what they wish to measure. If they desire to measure traditional religiousness, they should use a measure that assesses this construct. If they wish to assess the broader concept of spirituality (relationship to or search for the sacred or transcendent), then they should choose a measure that captures this construct without broadening spirituality to such an extent that it includes virtually every positive human experience. We advise against using a measure that purports to assess spirituality but that actually measures religiousness; this only adds confusion.

Because of the difficulty of defining spirituality, some investigators may decide to allow subjects to provide their own definitions and rate themselves on the basis of those definitions (see Pargament, Zinnbauer et al., 1998). This strategy may unfortunately result in "a mixture of apples and oranges," as different definitions of spirituality are used and rated by participants. One alternative is to have several investigators rate patients' definitions of spirituality according to some "gold standard" definition. This method helps create uniformity in rating that is linked to a specific definition. A second alternative (and the one most often used) is for the investigator to clearly define up front what she means by spirituality and then to ask questions that capture that concept. This, too, is problematic, since investigators have had difficulty agreeing on a common definition, making comparisons between studies almost impossible.

SUMMARY AND CONCLUSIONS

Many, many instruments measure religious beliefs and activities as they are expressed within the Christian religious tradition. We have examined measures that date back to 1929, as well as several new instruments developed in the late 1990s. It is particularly necessary to capture certain dimensions of religiousness, such as organizational religiousness, nonorganizational religiousness, and intrinsic religiosity or level of religious maturity. There are few measures of religiousness that specifically tap Jewish religiosity or religiosity based in other world religions (Hinduism, Buddhism, Islam); it is essential that such instruments be developed to advance research in the field.

In recent years a number of measures have been developed that seek to assess spirituality in a way that transcends any particular religious group. Such worthy attempts have met with only partial success. Further research is needed to develop measures of spirituality that are sensitive, reliable, valid, and distinct from religiousness; that are not contaminated by measures of health outcomes; and that are not so broad that they lose the true meaning of the construct (relationship to the transcendent or sacred).

PART VIII

STUDIES ON
RELIGION AND HEALTH
BY HEALTH OUTCOME

34

The Studies (Earliest to 2000)

Topics Arranged in Order of Chapters in Book

DEFINITION OF ABBREVIATIONS

Investigators: first author plus year of publication are cited. If more than one author is needed to identify the study, the additional authors are given in a footnote to the table page

Type: CS cross-sectional; PC prospective cohort; RS retrospective; CT clinical trial; Exp experimental study; CC case control; D descriptive study; CR case report; CSer case series; Q qualitative; R literature review and/or discussion; SR systematic review; O opinion

Method (Sampling Method): R random, probability, or population-based sample; S systematically identified sampling (e.g., consecutive patients); C convenience/purposive sample

N: number of subjects in sample; in case-control studies, N = cases and Cs = controls

Population: C children; Ad adolescents; HS high school students; CS college students; CDA community-dwelling adults (all ages); E elderly; MP medical patients; PP psychiatric patients; NHP nursing home patients; CM church members; R religious or clergy; F female; M male; B black; W white

Location: city, state, or country

Religious variables: # number of religious questions ("+\>" indicates "or more"); ORA organizational religious activities (e.g., religious attendance, church-related activities, religious giving); NORA (e.g., personal prayer, Scripture study, religious media); SR subjective religiosity (e.g., importance, self-rated religiousness); RCm religious commitment; IR intrinsic religiosity; ER extrinsic religiosity; Q quest; SWB spiritual well-being (RWB religious well-being and EWB existential well-being); RC religious coping; M mysticism; O religious orthodoxy; RB religious belief; RE religious experience; CM church membership; D denomination affiliation; Misc miscellaneous religious variables; SDA Seventh Day Adventist; DIP distant intercessory prayer; DMH distant mental healing

Findings: NA no association with health outcome; P at least one positive association with a better health outcome ($p < .05$); (P) positive association but significance (p value) borderline (trend), effect is indirect, or results are qualitative; NG at least one negative association with a better health outcome ($p < .05$); (NG) negative association but significance (p) borderline, effect is indirect, or results are qualitative; M mixed (both positive and negative associations with better health outcome at $p < .05$); C complex results

Controls: NS no statistical analyses; NONE no controls—analyses not controlled for other covariates (i.e., simple correlation or chi-square analyses); SC some controls (but important other variables not controlled); MC multiple controls (important variables controlled using regression models); DF discriminant function analysis

Rating: 1 to 10 (1 = poor, 10 = excellent) (based on overall study design, sampling method, quality of religious measure, quality of statistical analysis, interpretation of results, and discussion in the context of existing literature).

*indicates that some results from a study have been reported in a previous section
"—" indicates unknown or not applicable

RESEARCH ON RELIGION AND MENTAL HEALTH

Outcome/Investigators	Type	Method	N	Population	Location	Religious Variable	Findings	Controls	Rating
Religious Coping (Ch 5)									
Kidney Disease									
Baldree (1982)	CS	C	35	MP-hemodialysis	Chicago	#1 prayer (RC)	ranked 3rd of 40	–	5
O'Brien (1982)	PC	C	126	MP-hemodialysis	Washington DC	#3+ D,ORA,RC	P	NONE	6
Tix (1997)	PC	S	239	Renal transplant	Minnesota	#11 RC,D	P	MC	9
Diabetes									
Zaldivar (1994)	CS,D	C	104	MP (Hispanic)	New York City	#5+ RC,RB	–	–	6
Cancer (CA)									
Acklin (1983)	CC	C	26 vs. 18 Cs	MP (recurrent CA)	Atlanta, GA	#22 IR/ER,ORA	P	NONE	5
Baider (1999)	CS	S	100	MP (melanoma)	Israel	#54 spiritual beliefs	P (active coping style)		6
Ballard (1997)	CS,D	C	18 with recurrent CA; 20 with new CA	–	#1 depend RC for hope	61% recurrent, 30% new CA			5
Barbarin (1986)	CS	C	74 parents of child with CA	Michigan	#1 RC	NA	SC		6
Carver (1993)	PC	C	59	MP (breast CA)	Miami, FL	#>1 RC	NA	MC	7
Dunkel-Schetter (1992)	CS	C	603	MP (cancer)	Los Angeles	#1 SR,RC	C	MC	6
Ell (1989)	CS	S	369	MP (cancer)	Southern CA	#4 RC	P	NONE	6
Epperly (1983)	O		argues that terminally ill individuals are better able to cope with illness if they have spiritual beliefs							
Fehring (1997)	CS	C	100	MP	Wisconsin	#20+ SWB,IR/ER	P	NONE ?	6
Ferrell (1998)	Q,D	C	21	MP, F	Duarte, CA	describes three SWB domains related to breast CA			5
Ginsburg (1995)	D	S	52	MP (lung CA)	Ontario, Can	#1 RC	44% yes	–	6
Halstead (1994)	CS,D	C	128	Cancer survivors	Baltimore, MD	#1 RC (God & prayer)	68% found helped		6
Highfield (1992)	CS,D	C	23 and 27	MP & nurses	Southwest US	#33 spiritual scale, clergy	–	–	3
Hinton (1975)	CS	C	60	MP (cancer)	London, England	#2 SR,RB	P	NONE	5
Jenkins (1988)	CS	C	62	MP (cancer)	Midwest US	#1 RC	P	SC	6
Jenkins (1995)[a]	R		review of studies examining religious/spiritual coping and cancer							
Johnson SC (1991)	CS,D	C	103	MP (breast CA)	Southwest US	#30+ IR,ER,RC, clergy	85% religion helped		5

514

Study			N / Sample	Population	Location	Religious measure	Finding	Notes	Rating
Kaczorowski (1989)	CS	C	114 (hospice)	MP (cancer)	New York	#10 RWB	P	NONE	6
Kesselring (1986)	D	C	45	MP (cancer)	Switzerland	#1 RC (God & prayer)	38% found helped	—	6
Kurtz (1995)	CS,D	C	191	Cancer survivors	Michigan	#12 "Spiritual outlook"	(P)	—	6
Meyer (1992)	D	C	40	MP (cancer)	Iowa	#20 IR/ER	—	—	4
Mickley (1992)	CS	C	175	MP (breast CA)	Texas	#20+ IR,RWB	C	MC	6
Mickley (1993)	CS	C	50	MP (breast CA)	Texas	#20+ IR,RWB	P	NONE	5
Potts (1996)	Q	C	16	MP, B	New York City	#30+ misc	—	—	4
Raleigh (1992)	CS,D	R	90	MP	Michigan	#2 RC	20% used religion to keep hope		5
Roberts J (1997)	CS,D	C	108	MP,F (cancer)	Ann Arbor, MI	#4+ RC	—	—	6
Salts (1991)	CS,D	C	30	couples,E	Southern US	#1 RC	—	—	4
Sodestrom (1987)	CS,D	C	25	MP (cancer)	Northern CA	#15 RC	prayer most common RC	—	5
Spilka (1983)	D	C	45 parents	MP (cancer)	Denver, CO	experiences with chaplains/home pastors	—	—	6
Spilka (1991)	CS,Q	C	265 relatives of child with CA		Denver, CO	#1+ RC	—	—	6
Heart Disease									
Croog (1972)	PC,D	S	324	MP,M (s/p MI)	Massachusetts	#3+ D,SR,Misc	9% increase/yr	NONE	8
Harris (1995)	PC	C	40	MP (heart transplant)	Pennsylvania	#3+ ORA, NORA,SR	P	NONE	6
Saudia (1991)	CS,D	C	100 pts one day before surgery		Alabama	#2 RC	95% pray, 70% extremely helpful		6
Sears (1994)	CS	S	79 candidates for heart transplant		Mississippi	#15 IR,ER,SR,RC	M	NONE	6
Shapiro (1969)	PC	S	120,000	CDA ages 25–64	New York	#1D (Jews vs. other)	NG	SC-age, sex	6
HIV/AIDS									
Jenkins (1995)	CS	C	422	military	United States	#3 + RC	NG (discontent, pleading)		7
Sexual Dysfunction									
Koenig (1994a)	CS	C	83	MP, M, E	Durham, NC	#2 D,ORA	NG (D)	NONE	6

a. Jenkins and Pargament

Disaster/Crisis

Outcome/Investigators	Type	Method	N	Population	Location	Religious Variable	Findings	Controls	Rating
Cleary (1984)	CS	C	403 (nuclear accident)	CDA	Pennsylvania	#1 ORA	NA	SC	2
Pargament (1994)	PC	C	215 (Gulf war)	CS	Ohio	#18 RC	M	MC	8
Pargament (1995)[a]	CS	C	225 (1993 flood)	CDA	Midwest US	#20+ ORA,SR, RC,IR	P	MC	7
Pargament (1996)	CS	S	310 (OK bomb)	CDA	Oklahoma City	#25+ RC	M	MC	7
Sattler (1994)	CS	–	322 (hurricane)	CDA	Hawaii	#4 RC	NG	–	–
Smith B (1996)	PC	C	131 (flood)	CM	Missouri, Illinois	#2 ORA,SR	M (ORA,SR+)	SC	7
Thompson (1997)	CS	S	150 (family homicide)	CM	Atlanta, GA	#6 RC	M	MC	7
Weinrich (1990)	CS,D	C	61 (hurricane)	CS	S. Carolina	#1 RC	74% used RC	–	4
Zeidner (1992)	CS	C	261 (bombing)	CDA	Israel	#2 RC	NG	MC	7

Caregiving

Outcome/Investigators	Type	Method	N	Population	Location	Religious Variable	Findings	Controls	Rating
Baines (1984)	CS,D	–	–	CGs	–	#1 prayer as primary	74% used it	–	–
Burgener (1994)	CC	C	84 + Cs	CGs for Alz D	Northern New York	#8+ ORA, NORA,RC	P (ORA)	MC	7
Chang (1998)	CS	C?	127	CGs	Bedford, MA	#2+ RB,RC	P (indirect)	–	6
Folkman (1994)	CS	C	82 HIV-pos, 162 HIV-neg	CGs	San Francisco	#10 RB/Misc	P (HIV-positive)	MC	8
Kaye (1994)	R,O	reviews role of spirituality among caregivers							
Keilman (1990)	CS	C	100	CGs for CA pts	Michigan	#? RC	P	NONE	5
Kirschling (1989)	CS	C	70 CGs of terminally ill pts		Northwest US	#20 SWB	NA (RWB)	NONE	6
Millison (1988)	R,O	discusses spirituality as a resource in caregiving							
Picot (1997)	CS	R	391	CGs, E	Ohio	#2+ ORA,RC	(P)	MC	7
Rabins (1990)[b]	CS	C	62 CGs of Alz D & CA pts		Baltimore	#1 RC	P	MC	7
Rabins (1990)[c]	PC	C	62 CGs of Alz D & CA pts		Baltimore	#1 RC	P	MC	8
Richards M (1990,1991)	R,O	meeting the spiritual needs of the cognitively impaired							
Robinson K (1994)	CC	C	17 vs. Cs	CGs for Alz D	Southeast US	#13 scale	NA	NONE	2
Rogers-Dulan (1998)	Q	C	52	CGs, B	Riverside, CA	#2+ RE,ORA	–	–	5
*Salts (1991)	CS,D	C	30	couples,E	Southern US	#1 RC	–	–	4
Segall (1988–89)	D	C	59	CGs, B	–	#2 RC	65% spont mention of RC		–

Study	Type	Design	Sample	N	Location	Religious variable	Findings	Controls	Rating
Whitlatch (1992)	R		reviews the relationship between religion and coping with caregiving in Alzheimer's disease					–	
Wood (1990)	C	CS,D	CGs for Alz D	85	Virginia	#3+ RB,D,SR	P	–	5
Wright (1985)	C	CS	CGs for Alz D	240	Oregon	#1 RC	P	NONE	5
Stress Buffering									
Bjorck (1997)	C	CS	CDA	–	Southern CA	#1 God control beliefs	C	SC	6
Folkman (1997)	C	CS	partners of AIDs	305	Northern CA	#9 spiritual/relig scale	P	NONE/MC	7
Kendler (1997)	C	CS	CDA, twins	1902	Virginia	#11 RB,ORA,NORA,SR	P	MC	9
Koenig (1992)[d]	S	PC	MP, E	850	Durham, NC	#4 D,RC	P	MC	10
Koenig (1998b)	S	PC	MP, E	87	Durham, NC	#12 IR,ORA,NORA	P	MC	10
Lindenthal (1970)	R	CS	CDA	938	New Haven, CT	#3 ORA,NORA,D	M	NONE	7
Maton (1989)	C	CS,PC	bereaved parents/HS	81/68	Maryland	#3 spiritual support	P	MC	7
*Mitchell (1993)	R	CS	CDA,E	868	North Carolina	#7 RB (rlg intervention)	NG	MC	8
Neighbors (1983)	R	CS	CDA,B	2107	National US	#1+ NORA	C (prayer most helpful coping behavior)		7
Williams D (1991)	R	PC	CDA	720	New Haven, CT	#2 D,ORA	P	MC	8
Stress-Related Growth									
Koenig (1998)[e]	S	CS	MP,E	577	Durham, NC	#69 RC,ORA,NORA,SR	P	MC	8
General Religious Coping									
Bjorck (1993)	S	CS	CS	293	Delaware	#7 IR,RC	–		6
Cederblad (1995)	R	CS,D	CDA at risk for mental disorder	148	Sweden	#1 RC	–	1% use RC	6
Compas (1988)	C	CS,D	CS	65	Vermont	#1 RC	–	29% use RC	3
Conway (1985)	C	CS,D	CDA,E,F	65	Kansas City, MO	#4 RC	–	85–91% RC	5
Ebaugh (1984)	C	CS,D	CDA	150	Houston, TX	#1 D (Ca,Bahai, Christian Scientist)	–		5
Ellison CG (1996)	R	CS,D	CDA,B	1344	National US	#1 RC (prayer)	–	80%	8
Ferraro (1994)	R	CS,D	CDA	3417	National US	#1 RC due to stressors	–	greater in South	8
Jalowiec (1981)	C	D	MP	50	Chicago	#1 prayer/trust in God	–	ranked #2 & 10	5

a. Pargament, Smith, & Brant   b. Rabins, Fitting, Eastham, & Fetting   c. Rabins, Fitting, Eastham, & Zabora   d. Koenig, Cohen, Blazer, et al.   e. Koenig, Pargament, & Nielsen

Outcome/Investigators	Type	Method	N	Population	Location	Religious Variable	Findings	Controls	Rating
Koenig (1988)[a]	D	C	100	CDA, E	Durham, NC	#1+ RC (spontaneous)	58%F, 32%M	–	6
Koenig (1989)[b]	CS	C	100	CDA, E	Durham, NC	#1+ RC (spontaneous)	NA	–	6
*Koenig (1998)[c]	CS	S	577	MP, E	Durham, NC	#69 RC,ORA, NORA,SR	M	MC	8
Landis (1996)	CS	C	94	MP (diabetes)	Texas	#10 RWB (SWB)	C	MC	6
Manfredi (1987)	D	C	51	E,CDA	Rhode Island	#1 RC (prayer)	ranked #1	–	6
Mattlin (1990)	D	R	1556	CDA	Detroit	#1 RC	55% some/lot	–	7
McCrae (1986)	CS	C	255, 151	CDA	Baltimore	#1 "faith"	M, ranked #1	NONE	6
Newman (1990)	CS	C	327	CS	Ohio	#81 IR,RC	–	–	5
Nye (1992–93)	Q	C	43	E,CDA,100%B	Southwest VA	#1 RC	–	–	–
*O'Brien (1982)	PC	C	126	MP-hemodialysis	Washington DC	#3+ D,ORA,RC	P	NONE	6
Pargament (1986)	CS	C	124	CS	Ohio	#7+ RC	C	NONE	5
Pargament (1988)	CS	C	197	CDA, CM	Midwest US	#75+ RC,ORA,IR	M	SC	6
Pargament (1990)	CS	C	586	CDA, CM	Midwest US	#45+ RC,SR,IR	M	MC	7
Pargament (1992)	CS	S	538	CM	Midwest US	#30+ IR,ER,Quest	M	SC	8
Pargament (1995)[d]	R	review that examines the many functions of religion including coping, search for meaning, and others								
Pargament (1997)	R	state of the art review of religious coping and mental health outcomes								
Pargament (1998)[e]	CS	C/C/S	196/540/551	CM/CS/MP	OK, OH, NC	#14 "brief RCOPE"	M	NONE	8
Pargament (1998)[f]	CS	C	196/49	CS/CM	Midwest US	#25+ RC	M	NONE	6
Pargament (2000)	CS	S	540/551	CS/MP,E	Ohio & North Carolina	#60+ RC	M	MC	9
Parker (1982)	CS,D	C	108	MP	Australia	#1 RC (prayer)	ranked 7 of 25	–	5
Rehm (1999)	Q	C	25	parents	New Mexico	#6 dimensions of faith	–	–	5
Rutledge (1995)	CS,D	C	102 parents of chronically ill children	couples,E	Virginia	#4 RC	–	–	4
*Salts (1991)	CS,D	C	30	couples,E	Southern US	#1 RC	–	–	4
Shortz (1994)	CS	C	131	CS	Southeast US	#31+ RC	M	SC	4
Stern (1992)	CS, D	S	402	MP-cystic fibrosis	Cleveland, OH	#3 + D,SR,RC	57% religion as non-medical Rx		7
Swanson (1971)	CS,D	R	94	CDA,B	New Orleans	RC	–	–	5
*Thompson (1997)	CS	S	150	family homocide	Atlanta, GA	#6 RC	M	MC	7
Ventura (1982)	CS	C	200	parents	Madison, WI	#1 RC	P	NONE	3
Welford (1947)	CT	C	63	CS (religious)	New Jersey	#1 RC (prayer)	increased with frustration		3

518

Well-Being (Ch 6)

Study			N	Sample	Location	Measure	Result	Control	Rating
Alexander F (1991)	CS	S	156	CDA,E	Southern CA	#5 ORA,NORA	P	NONE	6
Althauser (1990)	CS	C	274	CM (Methodist)	Southern US	#13 IR,ER	P (IR)	SC	4
Anson (1990)[g]	PC	C	639	CDA,E	Israel	#1 observ of rlg rituals	M	MC	6
Anson (1990)[h]	CS	R	105 vs. 125	Kibbutz members	Israel	Relig vs. secular kibbutzim	P (stress buffer)	MC	7
Apel (1986)	CS	C	260	CM,R	Midwest US	#2+ ORA	P	NONE	2
Ayele (1999)	CS	C	100/55	physicians/MP	Richmond, VA	#3+ NORA,IR	P	MC	6
Beckman (1982)	CS	S	719	CDA,E,100%F	Southern CA	#1 SR	P	MC	7
Beutler (1988)	CT	C	120 (40 ea)	CDA	Netherlands	laying on of hands	P	–	9
Bienenfeld (1997)	CS	C	89	R,E,100%F	Ohio	#7 RCm	(P)	MC	6
Blazer (1976)	PC	C	272	CDA,E	N. Carolina	#>10 SR,ORA,NORA	P	NONE	7
Blaine (1995)	CS	C	144	CS	Buffalo, NY	#18 SR,ORA, Misc	P (Blacks)	NONE	6
Bulman (1977)	CS	C	29	MP (paralyzed)	Chicago	#1+ religiousness scale	NA	MC	5
*Burgener (1994)	CC	C	84 vs. Cs	Caregivers	New York	>#8 ORA,NORA	P	NONE	6
Cameron (1973)	CS,D	C	144	Handicapped	Michigan	#1 SR (value of religion)	NA	NONE	5
Carp (1974)	PC,D	C	133	CDA,E	Northern CA	#1 ORA	–	–	6
Chamberlain (1988)	CS	C	188	CDA,100%F	New Zealand	#11 IR-like scales	NA	SC	6
Coke (1992)	CS	C	166	CDA,100%B,E	New York	#2 ORA,SR	P	MC	7
Coleman (1999)	CS/D	C	117	MP,B,AIDS	Los Angeles	#20 SWB	P (EWB)	–	6
Cox (1988)	R			review of research on religion and well-being in elderly					
Cutler (1976)	CS	R	438 and 395	CDA,E	National US	#1 CM	P	MC	7
Decker (1985)	CS	C	100	MP,90%M,A	Northwest US	#1 SR	(P)	NONE	4
Doyle (1984)	CS	R	2306	CDA,E	National US	#1 SR	P	SC	7
Edwards (1973)	CS	R	507	CDA,E	Virginia	#1 ORA	P	MC	8
Ellison CG (1989)	CS	R	1500	CDA	National US	#6 D,ORA,NORA,SR	P	MC	9
Ellison CG (1990)	CS	R	2107	CDA,100%B	National US	#4 D,ORA,NORA,SR	P	MC	9
Ellison CG (1991)	CS	R	997	CDA	National US	#7 D,ORA,NORA,SR	P	MC	9
Emmons (1997)	CS	C	315	CS,CDA	Davis, CA	#>10 spiritual strivings	P	SC	7
Farakhan (1984)	PC	C	30	E,CDA,100%F	Missouri	#2 D,ORA	P	NONE	4
Feigelman (1992)	CS	R	>20,000	CDA	National US	#2 D (dissaffiliates)	NA	MC	8
Francis LF (1997)	CS	C	50	CDA,E	Wales	#2 ORA,NORA	NA	NONE	3

a. Koenig, George, & Siegler b. Koenig, Siegler, & George c. Koenig, Pargament, & Nielsen d. Pargament & Park e. Pargament, Smith, Koenig, et al. f. Pargament, Zimmbauer, et al.
g. Anson, Antonovsky, et al. h. Anson, Carmel, et al.

Outcome/Investigators	Type	Method	N	Population	Location	Religious Variable	Findings	Controls	Rating
Frankel (1994)	CS	C	299	CS	Ontario, Can	#>8 D,RB	P	NONE	6
Gee (1990)	CS	R	6621	CDA	Canada	#2 ORA,D	P	SC	7
Glik (1986,1990a)	CC	C	93/83/137 New Age/Charismatics/MP	(Maryland)	NewA vs. Char vs. MP	P (Char)	MC	7	
Graney (1975)	PC	S	60	E,CDA,100%F	Midwest US	#1 ORA	P	NONE	6
Guy (1982)	CS	S	1170	E,CDA	Memphis, TN	#3 ORA	P	NONE	6
Hadaway (1978)	CS	R	2164	CDA	National US	#3 D,ORA,SR	P	MC	8
Harvey (1987)	CS	R	11071	CDA > 40 y	Canada	#1 SR	P	SC	7
Hater (1984)	CS	S	1174	PP (opioid addicts)	National US	#4 ORA,SR	P (SR)	MC	7
Heisel (1982)	CS	C	122	E,CDA,100%B	New Jersey	>#9 ORA,NORA,E	P	SC	6
Hills (1998)	CS	C	230	CDA	Oxfordshire, England	#? RE	C	NONE	3
Holt (1992)	R	review of research on religion, well-being/morale, and coping behavior in later life							
Hunsberger (1985)	CS	C	85	CDA,E	Ontario, Can	#5 ORA,SR,RB	P	NONE	5
Inglehart (1990)	CS	R	169,776	CDA	14 western nations	#2+ ORA,SR	P	–	7
*Jamal (1993)	CS	S	325	CDA (muslims)	US & Canada	#1 SR	P	SC	6
Kass (1991)	PC	C	83	MP	Boston	#7 INSPIRIT	P	SC	7
Kehn (1995)	CS	C	98	CDA,E	New Jersey	#2 RB,CM	P	NONE	5
Keith (1979)	CS	R	568	CDA	Missouri	#1 ORA	P	NONE	6
Koenig (1988)[a]	CS	C	836	CDA, E	Midwest US	#20+ ORA, NORA,IR	P	MC	7
Krause (1992)	CS	R	448	CDA,E,B	National US	#4 ORA, NORA,SR	P	MC	9
Krause (1993)	CS	R	709	CDA	US and Can	#18 ORA, SR,RB	P	MC	9
Kvale (1989)	CS	C	183	R F,E	Midwest US	#20+ ORA, NORA,IR	C	NONE	4
Lee G (1987)	CS	R	2872	CDA	Washington State	#1 ORA	P (men only)	MC	8
Leonard (1982)	CS	R	320	CDA, E	National US	#1RB (beliefs in after-life)	NA	MC	4
Levin (1988)[b]	CS	R	750	CDA,F,Mex-Am	Texas	#1 ORA	P (women only)	MC	8
Levin (1995)[c]	CS	R	1848	CDA, B	National US	#12 ORA,NORA,SR	P	MC	10
Levin (1996a)	PC	R	624	CDA, Mex-Am	Texas	#1 ORA	P (young)	MC	10
Long J (1990)	Q	C	99	E,CDA	Southeastern US	religion	(P)	–	5

Study			N	Population	Location	Measure			
Magee (1987)	CS	—	150	retired nuns	New York	#10 (Catholic)	NA	SC	5
Marannell (1974)	CS	C	109	CS	Midwest/Southern US	#8 religious dimensions	NG	NONE	4
Markides (1983)	CS,PC	R	338	CDA,70%Mex	Texas	#3 ORA,NORA,SR	P	MC	7
Markides (1987)	PC	R	230	CDA,70%Mex	Texas	#3 ORA,NORA,SR	NA	MC	8
Maton (1987)	PC	C	103	CM	Midwest US	balanced giving & receiving support highest satisfaction			6
McClure (1982)	CS	C	233	CDA,CM	Southwest US	#2+ religious activities & responsibilities	P	NONE	5
McGloshen (1988)	CS	—	226	F,E	Midwest US	#1 ORA	P	MC	7
McNamara (1979)	CS	R	2164	CDA	National US	#8 SR,ORA,D,CM	P	SC	4
Mercer (1995)	CS	C	107	accident victims	–	#4+ SR,ORA,RC	P	NONE	5
Moberg (1953)	CS	C	219	E,NH	Minnesota	#1 CM	NA	MC	6
Moberg (1956)	CS	C	219	E,NH	Minnesota	#11 CM,ORA,NORA	P	MC	7
Moberg (1965)	CS	C	5000	E,CDA	Minnesota, South Dakota, North Dakota, Missouri	#3 CM,ORA	P	MC	7
Moberg (1984)	CS	C	1081	CDA	US & Sweden	#45 SWB scale	P	NONE	6
Moos (1979)	CS	C	122	Alcoholics	Palo Alto,CA	#? moral-religious subscale	P	NONE	5
Morris D (1991)	CS	R	400	E,CDA	Indiana	#2 ORA	P	MC	6
Musick (1996)	PC	R	2623	E,CDA	North Carolina	#2 ORA,NORA	P	MC	9
Myers (1995,1996)	R			comprehensive review of predictors of happiness (including religion)					
O'Connor (1989)	CS	C	176	E,NH	Quebec, Can	#3 IR scale (French)	P	NONE	6
O'Reilly (1957)	CS	R	210	CDA,E,Catholic	Chicago	#2 ORA	P	NONE	5
Ortega (1983)	CS	R	4522	CDA	Northern AL	#2 ORA	P	MC	8
Pfeifer (1995)	CC	C	44 vs. 45 Cs	PP	Switzerland	#35 IR,ER,Misc	P	NONE	5
Pollner (1989)	CS	R	3072	CDA	National US	#7 ORA,NORA,RE	P	MC	8
Poloma (1989)	CS	R	560	CDA	Akron, OH	#3+ NORA,RE	M	MC	7
Poloma (1990)	CS	R	560	CDA	Akron, OH	#7+RE,ORA, NORA,O	M	MC	7
Poloma (1991)	CS	R	560	CDA	Akron, OH	#7+ RE,CM,NORA	M	MC	7
Reyes-Ortiz (1996)	CS	S	55	MP	Richmond, VA	#2+ RC,NORA	P	NONE	6
Rayburn (1991)	CS	C	254	R,F	United States	#2 women religious (Ca,P,J)	P (Ca)	SC	6
Reed K (1991)	GS	R	1473	CDA	National US	#1 strength of affiliation	P	SC	7

a. Koenig, Kvale, & Ferrel   b. Levin & Markides   c. Levin, Chatters, & Taylor

Outcome/Investigators	Type	Method	N	Population	Location	Religious Variable	Findings	Controls	Rating
Reed P (1986)	CC	C	57 vs. Cs	MP (terminal)	Southeast US	#13 scale	P	NONE	6
Reed P (1987)	CC	C	100 vs. Cs	MP (terminal)	Southeast US	#13 scale	P	NONE	7
Riley (1998)	CS	C	216	MP	Ann Arbor, MI	#33 SWB, FACT-SP	P	NONE	5
Ringdal (1995,[a] 1996)	PC	S	253	MP (cancer)	Norway	#2 RB	(P)	SC	8
Rogalski (1987)	CS	C	120	CDA,E	Los Angeles	#1 SR	P	MC	6
Rosen (1982)	CS	C	148	CDA,E	Georgia	#1 RC	P	NONE	5
Schwartz (1997)	CS	S	46	Yale medical students	New Haven, CT	#1 ORA	(P) (no stat)	NONE	4
Shaver (1980)	CS,D	C	2500	F (Redbook)	National US	#4 SR	M	NONE	6
Shuler (1994)	CS	C	50	homeless, F	Los Angeles	#6+ ORA,NORA,RC	P	NONE	5
Singh (1982)	CS	R	1459	CDA,E	National US	#1 ORA	P	MC	9
Spreitzer (1974)	CS	R	1547	CDA	National US	#1 ORA	P (< 65 y)	MC	8
St. George (1984)	CS	R	3362	CDA	National US	#2 ORA,SR	P	MC	8
Steinitz (1980)	CS	R	1493	CDA, E	National US	#4 ORA,SR,RB	P	SC-health	6
Tellis-Nayak (1982)	CS	R	259	CDA,E	New York	#5 D,RB,ORA,RE	NA	MC	6
Thomas (1992)	CS	R	5629	CDA	National US	#2 ORA,SR	P	MC	9
*Tix (1997)	PC	S	239	Renal transplants	Minnesota	#11 RC,D	P	MC	9
Toseland (1979)	CS	R	871	CDA,E	National US	#1 ORA	NA	MC	6
Usui (1985)	CS	R	704	CDA,E	Kentucky	#1 ORA	NA	MC	7
Walls (1991)	CS	R	98	CDA,CM,B	Pennsylvania	#>10 RB,ORA,NORA	NA	MC	6
Weiss (1990)	CS	C	226	Hare Krishna (HK)	United States	#53 HK religiosity	P	NONE	6
Willits (1988)	PC	—	1650	CDA	Pennsylvania	#9 ORA,RB	P	MC	10
Witter (1985)	R	conducted a meta-analysis of religion and well-being relationship							
Zautra (1977)	CS	R	454	CDA	Salt Lake City	#1 religious partici- pation	NA	SC	6

Hope and Optimism (Ch 6)

*Blaine (1995)	CS	C	144	CS	Buffalo, NY	#18 SR,ORA, Misc	P (Blacks)	NONE	6
Bohannon (1991)	CS	C	272	Bereaved parents	Midwest US	#2 D,ORA	P (mothers)	SC	6
Carson (1988)	CS	C	197	Nursing students	Baltimore, MD	#22 EWB,RWB,SR	P	SC	6
Carson (1990)	CS	C	65	MP (HIV+ men)	Baltimore, MD	#20 SWB (EWB,RWB)	P	MC	6
Carver (1993)	PC	C	59	MP breast CA	Miami, FL	#>1 RC	NA	MC	7
Dember (1989)	CS	C	106	CS	–	#1+ RCm	–	NONE	5
Fox (1995)	CS	C	22	MP (Breast CA)	North Ireland	#10 RWB	NA	NONE	4
Herth (1989)	CS	C	120	MP (cancer)	Illinois	#1 SR	P	NONE	5
Idler (1997a)	CS	R	2812	CDA,E	New Haven, CT	#4 ORA,SR	P (disabled)	MC	9

522

*Moberg (1984)	CS	C	1081	CDA	US & Sweden	#45 SWB scale	NA	NONE	6
Plante (1997)	CS	C	102	CS	California	#10 SR,NORA, ORA,RC	P	NONE	4
*Raleigh (1992)	CS, D	R	90 patients with CA or chronic illness	MP (cancer)	Michigan	#2 RC	20% used religion to keep hope (P)	SC	5
*Ringdal (1995,[b] 1996)	PC	S	253		Norway	#2 RB	P	NONE	8
Sanders (1979/80)	CS	S	102 vs. 107 Cs	Bereaved	Florida	#1+ ORA	P		6
Sethi (1993, 1994)	CS	C	623	CM	United States	#4 D,ORA, SR,RB	P	MC	7
Veach (1992)	CS	C	148	CS & health professionals	Nevada	#18 Spiritual Exp	P	NONE	3
Zorn (1997)	CS	C	114	CDA,E, F	Wisconsin	#3+ RWB	P (hope)	SC	5
Purpose/Meaning in Life (Ch 6)									
*Acklin (1983)	CC	C	26 vs. 18 Cs	MP (recurrent CA)	Atlanta, GA	#22 IR/ER,ORA	P	NONE	5
Bolt (1975)	CS	C	52	CS	Michigan	#20 IR,ER	P	NONE	3
Burbank (1992)	CS,D	C	57	E,CDA	Rhode Island	#1 SR	NA	NONE	5
Burns (1991)	CT	C	37 vs. 15 Cs	Alcoholics	Virginia	#1 spiritual awareness	P (pre-post)	–	3
Carroll (1993)	CS	C	100	AA members	Southern CA	#38 (Step 11 spirituality)	P	NONE	6
*Chamberlain (1988)	CS	C	188	CDA,100%F	New Zealand	#11 IR-like scale	P	NONE	6
Crandall (1975)	CS	C	86	CS	Idaho	#20 IR,ER	P (IR)	NONE	5
Ellis J (1991)	CS	C	100	CS	Tennessee	#20 EWB,RWB	P (RWB)	NONE	4
Gifford (1978)	CS	C	38	CDA,E	Palo Alto, CA	#3 D,SR,RB	P	NONE	2
Jackson (1988)	CS	C	98	CM,B	Washington, DC	#13+ IR, RB,ORA	P (RB)	SC	5
Jacobson (1977)	PC	C	57	Alcoholics, PP	DePaul, WI	#20 IR/ER	P	NONE	6
*Kass (1991)	PC	C	83	MP	Boston, MA	#7 INSPIRIT	P	SC	7
Richards D (1990)	CS	C	292	CDA	National US	#8 universal force	P	NONE	3
Richards D (1991)	CS	C	345	CDA	National US	#3+ ORA, NORA,D	P (prayer)	NONE	5
*Tellis-Nayak (1982)	CS	R	259	CDA,E	New York	#5 D,RB, ORA,RE	P	MC	6
VandeCreek (1991)	CS	C	160/150	MP/CDA,F	Columbus, OH	#1 ORA	P (MP only)	SC	6
Self-Esteem (Ch 15)									
Aycock (1985)	CS	C	1466	CS,CDA	Upland, IN	#1 D (evangelicals)	NA	NONE	6
Bahr (1983)	CS	R	500	HS	Middletown, IN	#3 D,ORA,RB	NA	MC	7
Benson P (1973)	CS	C	128	HS, 100%M	Michigan	#12 RB,ORA, NORA	M	MC	5

a. Ringdal 1995; Ringdal, Gotestam, et al. b. Ringdal 1995; Ringdal, Gotestam, et al.

Outcome/Investigators	Type	Method	N	Population	Location	Religious Variable	Findings	Controls	Rating
*Blaine (1995)	CS	C	144	CS	Buffalo, NY	#18 SR,ORA,Misc	P (Blacks)	NONE	6
Commerford (1996)	CS	C	83	NH,E	New York City	#13 ORA,NORA,IR	NA	MC	7
Ellison CG (1993)	CS	R	1933	CDA,100%B	National US	#5 ORA,NORA	P	MC	9
*Ellison CG (1996)	CS	R	1344	CDA,B	National US	#1 RC (prayer)	NG	MC	8
Fehr (1977)	CS	C	120	CS	Cincinnati, OH	#10+ rlg values,O	NA	NONE	4
Flaskerud (1996)	PC	S	491	CDA 100%F	Los Angeles	#1 D (Ca vs. non-Ca)	NA	SC	2
*Gifford (1978)	CS	C	38	CDA,E	Palo Alto, CA	#3 D,SR,RB	NA	NONE	2
Heintzelman (1976)	CS	C	82	CS	Cincinnati, OH	#? relig orthodoxy scale	NA	NONE	4
*Jenkins (1988)	CS	C	62	MP (cancer)	Indiana	#1 RC	P	SC	6
Jensen L (1993)	CS	–	3835	CS	UT,TX,WI,ID	#2 D, "religiosity"	P	SC	6
Krause (1989)	CS	R	2107	CDA, B	National US	#6 ORA,NORA	P	MC	9
*Krause (1992)	CS	R	448	CDA,E,B	National US	#4 ORA,NORA,SR	P	MC	9
Krause (1995)	CS	R	1005	CDA, E	National US	#8 ORA,NORA,RC	P (RC)	MC	9
*Maton (1989)	CS,PC	C	81/68 bereaved parents/HS		Maryland	#3 spiritual support	P	MC	7
Meisenhelder (1986)	CS	R	163	CDA,F,married	Boston	#2 D,SR	P	MC	7
Nelson P (1989)	CS	C	68	E,CDA	Texas	#20 IR/ER scale	P	NONE	5
*O'Connor (1989)	CS	C	176	E,NH	Quebec, Can	#3 IR scale (French)	P	NONE	6
*Plante (1997)	CS	C	102	CS	California	#10 SR,NORA, ORA,RC	NA	NONE	4
Rosenberg M (1962)	CS	R	1021	HS	New York	#1 D (similarity of)	P	NONE	6
Russo (1997)	PC	R	4150	CDA,F	National US	#2 D (affiliation vs. no), ORA	NA	SC-educ, income	8
Ryan (1993)	CS	C	105/151/42/ 342	CS,CM	New York	#72 IR,ER,O,Q,Misc	P (IR)	NONE	3
Sherkat (1992)	CS	C	156	CDA (bereaved)	Southeast US	#3 D,ORA,NORA	P	MC	6
Smith C (1979)	CS	C	1995	Ad (Catholic)	5 countries	#>20 RB,ORA,RE	P	NONE	6
Watson P (1985)	CS	C	127/194	CS	Tennessee	#>20 IR,ER,Q, Misc	P	SC	6
Weltha (1969)	CS	C	565	CS	Iowa	#5+ relig attitude scale	M	NONE	4
Wickstrom (1983)	CS	C	130	CS (Christian)	4 US states	#2 IR,ER	NA	MC	5

Bereavement (Ch 15)

Outcome/Investigators	Type	Method	N	Population	Location	Religious Variable	Findings	Controls	Rating
Azhar (1995a)	CT	C	15 vs. 15 Cs	PP	Malaysia	#1 relig psycho-therapy	P	–	7

Study			Sample	Location	Findings			
Bahr (1979b)	CS	S	44 widows of miners	Idaho	#3 CM,ORA,SR	P	MC	6
Balk (1991)	CS, D	C	42 ad (s/p sibling death)	Midwest US	#3 SR,RC	M	NONE	4
*Bohannon (1991)	CS	C	272 CDA, parents	Midwest US	#2 D,ORA	P	SC	6
Carey (1977)	CS, D	S	119 CDA widows/ers	Illinois	#7+ D,IR	NA	NONE	5
Cook (1983)	CS, D	C	145 parents losing children	Chicago	#3 RB,RC	(P)	—	6
Gass (1987)	CS, D	C	100 widows CDA, F	Midwest US	#1 RC (prayer helpful)	89% yes	—	4
Goodman (1991)	D	C	12 Jewish vs. 17 non-J, CDA	Philadelphia	#1 D (Jewish vs. non-J)	(NG)	—	4
Lasker (1989)	PC	—	138 F having abortion, fetal or neonatal death	Southern US	#2 SR,ORA	P (SR)	NONE (?)	5
Loveland (1968)	CS	C	100 CDA		#3 ORA,NORA,RB	M	increased religiousness	5
Lund (1989)	PC	C	190 CDA, E	Utah	#3+ CM,SR,RB	P	NONE	6
McIntosh (1993)	PC	C	124 CDA (infant death)	Michigan, Illinois	#2 ORA,SR	P	NONE	6
Park (1993)	CS	C	96 CS	Delaware	#56 IR,ER,O	C	MC	5
Purisman (1977)	CS	C	47 Jewish parents losing sons	Israel	#1 "religiosity"	NA	SC-education	5
Richards T (1997)	CS	C	121 bereaved AIDS caregivers	San Francisco	#1 "spiritual responses"	NG	NONE	6
Richards T (1999)	CS	C	70 bereaved AIDS caregivers	San Francisco	#1 "spiritual responses"	NA	NONE	6
Rosik (1989)	CS	C	159 CDA, E	Southern CA	#20 IR,ER	NA	MC	6
*Sanders (1979–80)	CS	S	102 vs. Cs CDA	Tampa, FL	#1 ORA	P	NONE	6
*Sherkat (1992)	CS	C	156 CDA bereaved	Southeast US	#3 D,ORA,NORA	P	MC	6
Siegel (1990)	CS	C	825 CDA, E	Southern CA	#1 CM	P	MC	7
Thearle (1995)	CS	C	258 vs. 249 Cs bereaved parents	Australia	#1 D,ORA	(P)	NS	4
Videka-Sherman (1982)	PC	C	194 bereaved parents	Chicago	#3 ORA,RC	NA	SC	6
Wikan (1988)	R,O	C	discusses how Muslims in Egypt & Bali grieve over dead loved ones					

Social Support (Ch 15)

Study			Sample	Location	Findings			
*Acklin (1983)	CC	C	26 vs. 18 Cs MP (recurrent CA)	Atlanta, GA	#22 IR/ER,ORA	P (ORA)	NONE	5
*Alexander F (1991)	CS	R	156 CDA, retired	Southern CA	relig vs sec retir com	P	NONE	6
Bradley (1995)	CS	R	3597 CDA	National US	#1 ORA	P	MC	8
*Burgener (1994)	CC	C	84 CGs vs. Cs CGs for Alz D	Northern New York	#8+ ORA,NORA,RC	P (ORA)	MC	7
*Commerford (1996)	CS	C	83 NH,E	New York City	#13 ORA,NORA,IR	P (IR)	MC	7
*Cutler (1976)	CS,D	R	438 and 395 CDA,E	National US	#1 CM	(most common voluntary association)	MC	6
Delgado (1981)	R,O		discusses care of aged hispanic elderly by natural support systems (including religion/church)					

Outcome/Investigators	Type	Method	N	Population	Location	Religious Variable	Findings	Controls	Rating
*Ell (1989)	CS	S	369	MP (cancer)	Southern CA	#4 RC	P	NONE	6
Ellison CG (1994a)[a]	CS	R	2956	CDA (ECA)	North Carolina	#1 ORA	P	MC	8
Ellison CG (1994b)	R			includes a review of research on social support and religion					
Ellison CG (1998)	R			comprehensive review on religion and health, but includes excellent discussion on religion-mediated social support					
Hannay (1980)	CS	R	964	CDA	Scotland	#1 ORA	P	SC-age,sex	7
Hatch L (1991)	CS	R	1439	CDA,E,F	National US	#2 ORA	P	MC	9
*Idler (1997a)	CS	R	2812	CDA,E	New Haven, CT	#2 ORA,SR	P (ORA,SR)	MC	9
Kark (1996)[b]	CS	S	437	CDA	Israel	relig vs. secul kibutz	P	SC	8
Koenig (1998a)	CS/PC	C	115	NH,E	Durham, NC	#3 RC	P	MC	6
Koenig (1997a)[c]	CS	R	4000	E,CDA	Durham, NC	#3 ORA,NORA	P	MC	9
McRae (1998)	R,O			examines the role of the Black church as a therapeutic system and source of support					
*Ortega (1983)	CS	R	4522	CDA	Northern AL	#2 ORA	P	MC	8
Scandrett (1994)	R			reviews religion as social support for African Americans & effects on health behaviors					
Steinitz (1981)	Q			examines the local church as a source of support for elderly persons (including interviews and participant-observation)					
Strayhorn (1990)	CS	C	201	parents of Head Start kids	Pittsburgh	#12 ORA,NORA	P	NONE	5
Taylor RJ (1986)	CS,D	R	581	CDA,B,E	National US	#3 ORA,CM,SR	–	MC	7
Taylor RJ (1988)	CS	R	2107	CDA,B	National US	#4 D,ORA,CM,SR	P	MC	8
Thoits (1986)	R			reviews effects of social support on health and relationship between religion and social support					
*Walls (1991)	CS	C	98	CDA,CM,B	Pennsylvania	#>10 RB,ORA,NORA	M	MC	6
Weisner (1991)	CS	C	102	families of retarded children	Los Angeles	#8+ ORA,SR,RC	P	NONE	7
Young (1987)	CS	C	123	CDA,E	El Paso, TX	#15 ORA,NORA, RB,RE	P (NORA)	MC	6
*Zautra (1977)	CS	R	454	CDA	Salt Lake City	#1 relig participation	P	SC	6
Loneliness (Ch 15)									
Bahr (1979a)	CS,D	S	92	widows of mining disaster	Idaho	#5 D,ORA,SR	M	NONE	6
Dufton (1986)	CS	C	232	CS	Winnipeg, Can	#2 RB,RC	NA (RB)	NONE	4
Johnson DP (1989a,b)	CS	C	131	CDA,E	Southern FL	#10 ORA,NORA,SR	P	MC	6
*Lee G (1987)	CS	R	2872	CDA	Washington St	#1 ORA	NA	MC	8
Miller JF (1985)	CS	C	64	rheumatoid arthritis vs. healthy	Wisconsin & Illinois	#10 RWB, #10 EWB	P (RWB,EWB)	NONE	5
*O'Reilly (1957)	CS	R	210	CDA,E,Catholic	Chicago	#2 ORA	NA	NONE	5
Paloutzian (1982)	CS	C	206	CS	Idaho	#10 RWB, #10 EWB	P (RWB,EWB)	NONE	5
Rokach (1996)	CS	C	633	CDA,CS	Ontario, Can	#>12 RC	NG	NONE	5
Schwab (1990)	CS	–	206	CDA	Germany	#3 RC,RB	P	SC	6
Walton (1991)	CS	C	107	CDA,E	Arkansas	#10 RWB, #10 EWB	P/NA (EWB/RWB)		3

Depression (Ch 7)

Study			N		Location	Religious variable	Findings	Controls	Rating
Ai (1997)	CS	S	151	MP (with CABG)	Michigan	#3 SR,ORA,NORA	M	MC	7
Alvarado (1995)	CS	C	200	CS,CDA	Fresno, CA	#8 D,ORA,RB,SR	P	SC	4
Andreasen (1972)	R,O		discusses role of religion in depression						
Azhar (1995b)	CT	C	32 vs. 32 Cs	PP	Malaysia	#1 relig psycho-therapy	P	–	7
Ball (1990)	CS	S	51	PP	London, England	#3 ORA	NA	NONE	7
Bazzoui (1970)	CS	S	98	PP	Iraq	#2 D (Muslim, Ch, J)	–	NONE	1
Belavich (1995)	CS	C	222	CS	Ohio	#6 RC scales	M	SC	6
Bickel (1998)	CS	C	245	CM (Presbyterians)	–	#1+ RC scales	P	NONE (?)	5
*Bienenfeld (1997)	CS	C	89	R,E,100%F	Ohio	#7 RCm	P	MC	6
Bishop (1987)	CC	C	64 vs. Cs	PP	Durham, NC	>#4 D,ORA,other	NA	NONE	4
*Blaine (1995)	CS	C	144	CS	Buffalo, NY	#18 SR,ORA,Misc	P (Blacks)	NONE	6
Blalock (1995)	PC	C	300	MP (arthritis), E	North Carolina	#1 RC	P (neg affect)	MC	8
Blaney (1997)	PC	C	40	HIV+	Miami, FL	#2+ RC	P	MC	7
Braam (1997)[d]	CS	R	2,817	CDA,E	Netherlands	#2 ORA	P	MC	8
Braam (1997)[e]	PC	S	177	CDA,E	Netherlands	#1 SR	P	NONE, but	8
Braam (1998)	CS	R	3020	CDA,E	Netherlands	#3 D, giving up ORA	P	MC	8
Braam (1999)[f]	CS	R	3051	CDA,E	Netherlands	#1 "religious climate"	P	MC	8
Braam (1999)	CS	S	13 nations	CDA,E	Europe	#4 D,ORA,SR,O	P (ORA × Cath)	MC	7
Brant (1995)	CS	–	179	CDA,100%B		#1+ RC scales	M	–	5
Brown D (1987)	CS	R	451	CDA,B	Richmond, VA	#13 scale	NA (stress buf)	SC	6
Brown D (1990)	CS	R	451	CDA,100%B	Richmond, VA	#12 D,ORA,RCm	P	MC	8
Brown D (1992)	CS	R	927	CDA,100%B	Norfolk, VA	#10 RCm	NA	MC	8
Brown D (1994)	CS	R	527	CDA,100%BM	Southeast US	#12 D,ORA,RCm	P (D only)	MC	8
Brown GW (1981)	CS	S	355	CDA,100%F	Scotland	#1 ORA	P	NONE	7
Buckalew (1978)	CS	S	1323	PP	Georgia	#1 D (Pentecostal/Holiness vs.)	Pente/H > others	NONE	5
Caro (1983)	CS,D	C	51	CDA	Spain	#1 RC	–	–	4
Cavenar (1977)	CSer	C	4	PP	Durham, NC	#1 RE (coversion)	–	–	–
*Commerford (1996)	CS	C	83	NH,E	New York City	#13 ORA, NORA,IR	NA	MC	7
Cooklin (1983)	CC	S	64 vs. 722 Cs	PP	London, England	#1 D (Jewish vs. non-J)	Jewish > non-J	NONE	6
Ellison CG (1995)	CS	R	2956	CDA	North Carolina	#3+ D,ORA,NORA	P(ORA),NG(N)	MC	8
Ellison CG (1997)[g]	PC	–	–	CDA,B	National US	#2+ ORA,RB	P	–	–
Ellison CG (1997)[h]	PC	–	–	CDA,B	National US ?	"religious guidance"	P	–	–
*Farakhan (1984)	PC	C	30	CDA,E,100%B	Missouri	#2 D,ORA	NA	NONE	4
Fehring (1987)	CS	C	170	CS	Wisconsin	>#10 RWB,RCm	NA	NONE	4

a. Ellison & George   b. Kark, Carmel, et al.   c. Koenig, Hays, George, et al.   d. Braam, Beekman, van Tilburg, et al.   e. Braam, Beekman, Deeg, et al.   f. Braam, Beekman, van den Eeden, et al.   g. Ellison, Levin, et al.   h. Ellison & Levin

Outcome/Investigators	Type	Method	N	Population	Location	Religious Variable	Findings	Controls	Rating
Fernando (1975,1978)	CC	C	117 vs. Cs	PP	London, England	#2 D,ORA	P	–	8
Ferraro (1998)	CS	R	3497	CDA	National US	#6 D,ORA,NORA,SR,RC	M	MC	9
Figelman (1968)	CS	S/C	65	PP	Boston, MA	#1 D (Jews vs. Blacks)	Jews > Blacks	NONE	5
Flics (1991)	CS	C	152	PP	New York City	#1D (Jews vs. other)	(Jews > other)	NONE	4
Gallemore (1969)	CC	C	62 vs. Cs	PP	Durham, NC	>#4 D,RE, Rlg history	M	NONE	5
Genia (1991,1993)	CS	C	309	CDA	Washington, DC	#21 D,IR,ER	P	–	6
Griffith (1986)	PC	C	16	CM	Barbados	#1 "mourning"	(P)	–	4
Grosse-Holtforth (1996)	CS	C	97	NHP	Durham, NC	#13 IR,RC	NA	SC	6
Hallstrom (1984)	CS	S	800	CDA,100%F	Sweden	#3ORA,NORA,RB	P	MC	8
Hertsgaard (1984)	CS	R	760	CDA,F,farms	North Dakota	#2 ORA,D	P (ORA)	MC	7
Husaini (1998)	CS	R	995	E,CDA	Nashville	#7 ORA,NORA	NA	MC	7
Idler (1987)	CS	R	2811	CDA,E	New Haven, CT	#4 ORA,SR,RC	P	MC	9
Idler (1992)	PC	R	2812	CDA,E	New Haven, CT	#4 ORA,SR,RC	P (men)	MC	10
*Jensen L (1993)	CS	–	3835	CS	UT,TX,WI,ID	#2 D, "religiosity"	P	SC	6
Johnson WB (1992)	CT	C	10	Christians	Indiana	Christian vs. non-C RET	NA	–	5
Johnson WB (1993)	R		reviews Christian psychotherapy outcome studies & presents guidelines						
Johnson WB (1994)	CT	C	32 randomized	Christians	Hawaii	Christian vs. non-C RET	NA (less relapse, though)		6
Jones-Webb (1993)	CS	R	3724	CDA	National US	#1 D (agnostic/none)	P (Blacks)	MC	7
*Kendler (1997)	CS	C	1902	CDA, twins	Virginia	#11 RB,ORA,NORA,SR	P	MC	9
Kennedy (1996)	PC	R	1855	CDA,E	Bronx, NY	#2 ORA,D	P	MC	10
Koenig (1988)[a]	CS	S	106	MP, E	Illinois	#15+ ORA,NORA,IR	P	SC-sex	6
*Koenig (1992)[b]	PC	S	850	MP, E	Durham, NC	#4 D,RC	P	MC	10
Koenig (1994)[b]	CS	R	853 vs. 1826	baby boomers	Durham, NC	#5 D,ORA,SR,NORA	P (ORA)	MC	9
Koenig (1995a)	CS	R	96	prisoners	Butner, NC	#20+ RB,ORA,RC	P (ORA,IR)	NONE	7
Koenig (1995)[c]	CS	S	850	MP, E	Durham, NC	#4 D,RC	P	MC	8
*Koenig (1997)[d]	CS	R	4000	CDA, E	North Carolina	#4 D,ORA,NORA	P (ORA)	MC	9
*Koenig (1998)[e]	CS	C	115	NH, E	Durham, NC	#3 RC	NA	MC	6
*Koenig (1998)[f]	PC	S	87	MP, E	Durham, NC	#12 IR,ORA,NORA	P	MC	10

Study			N	Population/Method	Location	Religious measure	Findings	Controls	Score
*Koenig (1998)[g]	CS	S	577	MP, E	Durham, NC	#69 RC,ORA, NORA,SR	M	MC	8
Kroll (1989)	CS,D	S	52	PP	Minnesota	#26 RB,RE,ORA	(P)	NONE	6
Levav (1997)	CS	R	5772	CDA	New Haven & Los Angeles	#1 Jewish vs. non-J	Jews > non-J	MC	8
Levin (1985)	CS	R	1125	CDA-Mex-Am	Texas	#2 ORA,SR	NA	NONE	6
Lubin (1988)	CS	R	1543	CDA	National US	#1 D (affil vs. none)	P	NONE	6
Malzberg (1973)	CC	S	40,000+	PP	New York	#1 Jewish vs. non-J	Jews > non-J	NONE	6
*Maton (1989)	CS,PC	C	81/68	bereaved parents/HS	Maryland	#3 spiritual support	P	MC	7
McIntosh (1995)	CS	R	1644	CDA, E	National US	#1 Relig volunteering	P	MC	8
Meador (1992)	CS	C	2850	CDA	Durham, NC	#1 D (Pentecostal vs. other)	Pentec > other	MC	7
Miller L (1997)	PC	–	60/151	mothers/children	New York	#4 D,SR	P	MC	8
Mitchell (1993)	CS	R	868	CDA,E	North Carolina	#7 RB (rlg intervention)	M	MC	8
Morris P (1982)	PC	C	24	chronically ill	United Kingdom	Pilgrimage to Lourdes	P	NONE	6
Morse (1987)	CS	C	156	E,CDA	Massachusetts	#3 CM,ORA,RC	P	SC	6
Mosher (1997)	CS	C	461	HS (Catholic)	St. Louis	#45 scale	P	NONE	6
Musick (1998a)	CS	R	586	CDA, B	Detroit	#2 ORA,RC (prayer)	P(ORA),NG(P)	MC	8
Musick (2000)	PC	R	10008	CDA	National US	#4 ORA,RB	M	MC	10
Musick (1998)[h]	PC	R	3007	CDA, E	North Carolina	#3 ORA,NORA	P (blacks only)	MC	10
Neeleman (1994)	CC	S	73 vs. 25 Cs	PP	London, England	#16 ORA, NORA,RB,SR	NG	SC-sex, race	6
Nelson P (1989a,1990)	CS	C	68	E,CDA	Texas	#20 IR-ER scale	P	NONE	5
Nelson P (1989b)	CS	C	26	E,NH	Texas	#1 "religious activity"	P	NONE	5
*O'Connor (1989)	CS	C	176	E,NH	Quebec, Can	#3 IR scale (French)	P	NONE	6
O'Laoire (1997)	CT/PC	C	96/406	CDA	San Francisco	#1 prayer for others	P (those praying)	–	7
Park (1990)	PC	C	83/83	CS (religious)	Delaware	#13 IR,ER,O	M,C	SC	6
Payne (1976)	CS	S	102	MP	Boston	#1 D (Ca vs. other)	Ca > other	NONE	4
Pecheur (1984)	CT	C	21	depressed Christian CS	–	religious CBT	NA	–	6
Plante (1992)	CS	C	86	CS	Santa Clara, CA	#2 SR,D	NA	NONE	5
*Plante (1997)	CS	C	102	CS	California	#10 SR,NORA, ORA,RC	P	NONE	4
Pressman (1990)	CS,PC	C	30	MP, E, F	Chicago	#3 ORA,SR,RC	P	SC	7
Propst (1980)	CT	C	44	mildly depressed Christian CS	Oregon	religious imagery	P	–	7
Propst (1992)	CT	C	59	depressed Christians	Oregon	religious CBT	P	–	10
*Rabins (1990)[i]	CS	C	62	caregivers of Alz D & CA pts	Baltimore	#1 RC	P	MC	7
*Rabins (1990b)[j]	PC	C	62	caregivers of Alz D & CA pts	Baltimore	#1 RC	P	MC	8

a. Koenig, Moberg, & Kvale   b. Koenig, George, Meador, Blazer, & Dyck   c. Koenig, Cohen, Blazer, Kudler, et al.   d. Koenig, Hays, George, et al.   e. Koenig, Weiner, et al.   f. Koenig, George, & Peterson   g. Koenig, Pargament, & Nielsen   h. Musick, Koenig, et al.   i. Rabins, Fitting, Eastham, & Fetting   j. Rabins, Fitting, Eastham, & Zabora

Outcome/Investigators	Type	Method	N	Population	Location	Religious Variable	Findings	Controls	Rating
Razali (1998)	CT	C	203	PP	Malaysia	#1 relig psycho-therapy	P	–	8
*Rosenberg M (1962)	CS	R	1021	HS	New York	#1 D (similarity of neighborhoods)	non-sim > sim	NONE	6
Ross (1990)	CS	R	401	CDA	Illinois	#4 D,SR	P (weak)	MC	7
*Ryan (1993)	CS	C	105/151/42/342	CS,CM	–	#72 IR,ER,O,Q,Misc	P (IR)	NONE	3
Schafer (1997)	CS	C	282	CS	Chico, CA	#8 RB,RC,ORA,NORA	NG	NONE	5
*Sherkat (1992)	CS	C	156	CDA bereaved	Southeast US	#3 D,ORA,NORA	NA	MC	6
*Siegel (1990)	CS	C	825	CDA, E	Southern CA	#1 CM	P	MC	7
*Smith B (1996)	PC	–	131	CDA	Missouri, Illinois	#3+ RC,ORA,SR	P(ORA), NG(SR)		–
Sorenson (1995)	PC	S	261	teenage mothers	S.W. Ontario	#3 D,ORA,SR	NG	SC	6
Spendlove (1984)	CS	R	179	CDA, W, F	Salt Lake City	#12 IR,ORA,CM,D	NA	MC	6
Spiegel (1983)	PC	S	58	MP (breast CA)	California	#2 family ORA, NORA	NG	MC	7
*Strayhorn (1990)	CS	C	201 parents of Head Start kids		Pittsburgh	#12 ORA,NORA	P	NONE	5
Strawbridge (1998)	CS	R	2537	E,CDA	Alameda, CA	#5 ORA,NORA,SR	M	MC	9
Tamburrino (1990)	CS	C	71	F post-abortion dysphoria	Ohio	conversion	P	NONE	5
Toh (1997)	CT	C	46	CDA, religious	Pasadena, CA	lay counselors in church	P	–	8
VandeCreek (1995)	CS	C	150	CDA (relatives)	Ohio	#6 RC	M	SC	6
Varma (1997)	R	review of religious psychotherapy studies for depression							
*Veach (1992)	CS	C	148	CS & health profes-sionals	Nevada	#18 Spiritual Exp, etc.	P	NONE	3
Watson P (1988)	CS	C	314/181	CS	Tennessee	#20 IR,ER	P	SC	6
Watson P (1989)	CS	C	1397	CS	Tennessee	#20 IR,ER	P	NONE	6
Watson P (1990)	CS	C	2435	CS	Tennessee	#>20 IR,ER, Misc	P	NONE	6
Weissman (1978)	PC	C	150	PP	New Haven, CT	#1 (? D)	NA	NONE	1
*Williams D (1991)	PC	R	720	CDA	New Haven, CT	#2 D,ORA	P (stress buffer)	MC	8
Williams R (1997)	CS	R	159	CDA	Glasgow	#1 D (Muslim vs. oth)	Muslim = other	MC	6
Wright (1993)	CS	C	451	HS,Ad	Texas	#3 IR,ORA	P	SC-sex	6
Yeung (1992)	CS	R	3640	CDA	New Haven, CT	#1 Jewish vs. non-J	Jews > non-J	MC	8
Zhang (1996)	CS	C	320/452	CS	China & US	#7 ORA,NORA, SR,RB	P(US),NG (China)	MC	7

530

Suicide (Ch 8)

Bagley (1989)	CS	R	679	CDA	W. Canada	#2+ D,RCm	M	–	7
Bailey (1995)	RS	S	50 states	Suicide rates	National US	#1 D (% Jewish)	Others > Jews	NONE	5
Bainbridge (1981)	RS	S	78 large cities	Suicide rates (1926)	National US	#2 D,CM	P (CM)	SC	6
Bainbridge (1989)	RS	S	75 large cities	Suicide rates (1980)	National US	#1 CM	P to NA	SC	6
Bankston (1983)	RS	S	64 parishes		Louisiana	#1 D (% Catholic)	Cath > others	MC	6
Barry (1997)	R,O		reviews the biblical teachings on suicide						
Bascue (1982)	CS,D	C	49	psychiatric nurse aids	Pennsylvania	recognize suicide lethality	–	–	4
Becker (1987)	CC	S	3503	Suicide attempts	W. Germany	#1+ "religion"	Prot > Others	–	6
Beehr (1995)	CS	S	177 police officers	Suicidal thoughts	Eastern US	#3 RC	NA	MC	5
Beit-Hallahmi (1974)	RS	C	18 countries	Suicide rates	Europe	#1 D (% Ca vs. Prot)	Cath = Prot	NONE	2
Beit-Hallahmi (1975)	RS	S	18 countries	Suicide rates	World	#1 D (of country)	Cath = Prot	NONE	2
Best (1982)	Exp	C	66	CS	–	#1 ministers saw video	Psychol > Minis	–	5
Breault (1982)	RS	S	42 countries	Suicide rates	United Nations	#1 Relig books/newspapers	P	MC	6
Breault (1986)	RS	S	state/county	Suicide rates	National US	#2 D (Ca vs. other), CM	P (CM, Ca)	MC	7
Breier (1984)	CC	S	38 vs. Cs	Suicides	Connecticut	#1 D (Ca vs. others)	Cath > others	NONE	3
Burr (1994)	RS	S	294 SMSAs	Suicide rates	National US	#2 D (Ca vs. other), CM	P (CM, Ca)	MC	7
Burvill (1983)	CC	S	11,806 migrants	Suicides	Australia	#1 D	–	–	1
*Cameron (1973)	CS,D	C	144	Handicapped	Michigan	#1 SR (value of religion)	P	NONE	5
Conrad (1991)	CS	C?	473	HS	–	#1 D	Cath = P = J	–	6
Corder (1974)	CC	S	11 vs. Cs	PP,Ad	Raleigh, NC	#1 stength of rlg affiliation	NA	NONE	2
Danto (1983)	RS	S	Suicide rates	CDA	Oakland Cty, MI	#1 D (Jews vs. non-J)	non-J > J	None ?	5
DeMan (1987)	CS	C	150	CDA	Quebec, Can	#1 SR	P	MC	6
Day (1987)	RS	S	cantons/provinces	Suicide rates	Prussia & Switzerland	#1 D (Ca vs. others)	Ca = others	SC	4
Diespecker (1973)	CC	S	84 suicide attempts		New S. Wales	#1 D (Ca vs. oth, none)	oth/none > Ca	NONE	2
Domino (1985)	CS,D	C	112	clergy	United States	clergy recognition of suicide	poor	–	5
Donahue (1985)	R		review of research on relationship between intrinsic and and extrinsic religiosity and suicide						

Outcome/Investigators	Type	Method	N	Population	Location	Religious Variable	Findings	Controls	Rating
Donahue (1995)	R	review of research on relationship between religion and suicide in adolescents								
Dublin (1933)	RS	–	suicide rate		National US	#1 D (Ca vs. Prot)	Prot > Ca	NONE	–
Durkheim (1897)	R/CS	examines rates of suicide by different religious denominations (Catholics lower suicide rates than Protestants)								
Edland (1973)	CC	S	1418 suicides	CDA	Rochester, NY	#1 D (Jews vs. others)	Jews > others	NONE	6
*Ellis J (1991)	CS	C	100	CS	Tennessee	#10 RWB	P	NONE	4
Ellison CG (1997)[a]	RS	R	296 Standard Metropolitan Statistical Areas	Suicide rates	National US	#1 D homogeneity	P	MC	8
Evans (1967)	RS	S	702 self-poison	hospitalized patients	Oxford, England	#1 D (Ca vs. other)	Ca = Others	NONE	2
Faupel (1987)	RS	S	3108 counties	Suicide rates	National US	#1 D (Ca vs. other)	Others > Ca	MC	7
Feifel (1980)	CS	C	616	PP,prison,oth	Los Angeles	#1 SR	P	MC	7
Fernquist (1995–96)	RS	S	9 countries	Suicide rates	Europe	#1 religious books	P	SC-age,sex	6
Harkavy-Friedman (1987)	CS	S	380	HS	–	#1+ D	–	–	–
Garfinkel (1982)	CC	S	505 vs. Cs	Ad (attempts)	Toronto, Can	#1 D (Ca or Jew vs. Prot)	Prot > Ca/Jew	NONE	3
Gargas (1932)	RS	S	–	Suicide rates	Netherlands	#1 D (Ca vs. Prot vs. Jews)	Jews > Prot > Ca	no stats	4
Ghosh (1994)	R	review of research on suicide (includes religion)								
Gobar (1970)	D	examines suicide in the Moslem country of Afghanistan								
Gold (1965)	CC	S	137	Attempted suicides	NE Tasmania	#1 D (Ca vs. other)	Ca > others	no stats	3
Goss (1971)	CC	S	2975 suicides	CDA,W,>25 yo	New York City	#1 D (Ca vs. other)	Others > Ca	SC-age,sex	6
Gruenewald (1995)	RS	S	532 observ yrs.	Suicide rates	38 US states	#1 D (% Mormon, Baptist)	Others > M/B	MC	6
Hasselback (1991)	RS	S	261 census division	Suicide rates	Canada	#1 D (% none)	P	MC	7
Hoelter (1979)[b]	CS	C	205	CS	Indiana	#5+ ORA,RB,SR,O	P	NONE ?	5
Horton (1973)	CSer	C	3 cases	Ad (schizophrenic)	New Haven, CT	#1 "mystical experience"	(P)	–	–
Iga (1981)	R,O	review of suicide and religion in Japan								
Jasperse (1976)	CC	R	9189 suicides	CDA	Netherlands	#1 D (Ca vs. other)	Ca = others	SC	5
Johnson D (1980)	CS	R	1530	CDA	National US	#3 D,ORA,SR	P	NONE	7
Joubert (1995)	RS	S	50 states	Suicide rates	National US	#1 D (Ca vs. other)	Other > Ca	NONE	5
Kandel D (1991)	CS	R	593	Ad	New York	#1 ORA	P	NONE	6
Kaplan K (1995)	CS	C	117	CS	Detroit, MI	#17+ IR,ER,Q,Misc	P	SC	6
Kehoe (1994)	R	review of suicide and religion								
King S (1996)	CS	C	511	CS	Connecticut	#2 D,ORA	P	NONE	6

Study	Design	Type	N	Outcome	Location	Religious variable	Findings	Controls	Rating
Kirk (1979)	CC	C	20 vs. 20 Cs	PP	Detroit, MI	#2 D,ORA	NA	NONE	3
Kranitz (1968)	CC	C	20 vs. 20 Cs	PP	Los Angeles	#14 Misc	NA	NONE	4
Krull (1994)	RS	S	–	Suicide rates	Quebec, Can	#1 D (% none)	P	MC	8
Krupinski (1966)	CC	S	358	Suicide attempters	Australia	#1 D (Ca vs. other)	Ca > others	NONE	4
Lee D (1987)	CS	C	317	CS	Illinois	#1 SR	P	NONE	5
Lester (1974)	RS	S	244 suicides	PP	Philadelphia, PA	#1 RB (agnostic vs. other)	–	NONE	3
Lester (1987a)	RS	S	49 states	Suicide rates	United States	#1 ORA	P to NA when divorce controlled		5
Lester (1987b)	RS	R	49 states	Suicide rates	United States	#1 D (% Ca/state)	Ca = others	SC–divorce	5
Lester (1988)	RS	R	49 states	Suicide rates	United States	#1 ORA	P	SC–race	6
Lester (1992)	RS	R	13 nations	Suicide rates	crossnational	#2 RB	P	NONE	7
Lester (1993)	CS	C	103	CS	–	#1+ "religiosity"	P to NA when neuroticism controlled		3
Lester (1996a)	RS	S	–	Suicide rates	United States ?	#1 D (Jews vs. non-J)	non-J>J	SC	6
Lester (1996b)	RS	S	18 nations	Suicides	Nations-world	#1 D (% Ca)	Ca = others	SC-GNP	4
Levav (1988)	CS	R	1200	CDA	Israel	#1+ "religiosity"	NA	SC	7
Levav (1989a,b)	RS	S	Israel	Suicide rates	Israel	#1 D (Jews vs. Muslim,Christian)	Jews > Mus,Chr	SC	6
Long D (1991)	CS	C	147 members of MS society	CS	Cincinnati, OH	#3+ RB,SR,O	P (SR)	SC	6
LoPresto (1994)	CS	C	282	CS	Baltimore, MD	#1 SR	P	SC	5
Lukianowicz (1968)	CS,D	C	10	children	North Ireland	#1D (Ca vs. Prots)	Ca = Prots	NONE	1
Marks (1977)	CS	S	98/29/25 vs. Cs	Ad suic attempt	National US	#1 ORA	P	NONE	5
Martin WT (1984)	RS	R	–	Suicide rates	National US	#1 ORA	P	NONE	5
*Minear (1980–81)	CS	C	394	CS	New England	#11 D,ORA,SR,RB	P	NONE	5
Mireault (1996)	CS	C	104	E	Quebec, Can	#1 SR	NA	MC ?	5
Morphew (1968)	D	C	50	Suicide attempts	England	#4 ORA,RB	NA	–	2
Murray (1973)	CS	C	78	CS	E.Europe, US, Can	#1 D	Other > P > Ca	NONE ?	3
Neeleman (1997)	CS	R	23085	CDA (attitude)	National US	#26 D,ORA,RB	P	MC	10
Neeleman (1998)c	CS	R	1729	CDA	National US	#17 ORA,NORA,SR,RB	P	MC	8
Neeleman (1998)	RS	S	11 provinces	Suicide rates	Netherlands	#3+ religiousness	P	MC	8
Neeleman (1999)	RS	S	26 countries	Suicide rates	Europe & America	#25 D,ORA,Misc	P	MC	8
Nelson FL (1977)	CS	R	58	E,NH	Los Angeles	#3 D,SR	–	NONE	4
Nelson FL (1980)	CS	C	99	E,NH	Los Angeles	#2 D,SR	P	NONE	5
Pandey (1968)	R,O		discusses suicide in India						

a. Ellison, Burr, et al.   b. Hoelter & Epley   c. Neeleman, Wessely, et al.

Outcome/Investigators	Type	Method	N	Population	Location	Religious Variable	Findings	Controls	Rating
Paykel (1974)	CS	R	720	CDA	Connecticut	#3 ORA,NORA,CM	P	MC	8
Pescosolido (1986)	RS	S	404 counties	Suicides,accid	National US	#1 D (J,Ca,DOC,B)	NA (suicide)	MC	6
Pescosolido (1989)	RS	S	404 counties	Suicides	National US	#2 D(J,Ca,EP,MP), ORA	P (Ca,EP,ORA)	MC	7
Resnick (1997)	CS	R	12118	Ad	National US	#1 SR	NA	MC	8
Rudestam (1972)	CC	S	50 suicides U.S., 50 suicides Sweden			#1 (Jews vs. P, Ca)	Jews = P,Ca	–	2
Salmons (1984)	D	S	294/149	CS/MP	England	#1 D (relig vs. non-R)	P	NONE	3
Schneider (1989)	CS	C	108	Gay men	Los Angeles	#1 D (no affiliation)	P	NONE	4
Schweitzer (1995)	CS	–	1678	CS	Australia	#2 D,SR	P	NONE	5
Shagle (1995)	CS	S	473	Ad	Tennessee	#2 ORA,SR	P	MC	7
Siegrist (1996)	CS	R	2034	ages 15–30 yo	Germany	#2 D,ORA	P	MC	8
Simpson, M (1989)	RS	S	71 nations	Suicide rates	World	#1 D (%Ca, Prot, Islam)	Ca,Prot > Islam	SC	7
Singh (1986)	CS	R	6521	CDA (attitude)	National US	#? ORA,Misc	P	MC	9
Skog (1995)	RS	S	18 administrative regions	Suicide rates	Portugal	#1% Ca marriages	non-Ca > Ca	SC	6
Stack (1980b)	RS	S	50 states	Suicide rates	National US	#2% Ca,Ca school	non-Ca > Ca	(NA, divorce control)	6
Stack (1981)	RS	S	37 nations	Suicide rates	World	#1% Ca	non-Ca = Ca	MC	6
Stack (1983a)	RS	S	25 nations	Suicide rates	World	#1 relig book production	P (females)	MC	7
Stack (1983b)	RS	S	–	Suicide rates	National US	#1 ORA	P	SC	6
Stack (1983c)	RS	S	nations	Suicide rates	World	#1 relig book production	NA	SC	6
Stack (1985)	RS	S	–	Suicide rate	National US	#1 ORA	P/C	SC	7
Stack (1987)	R		reviews scientific evidence that religiousness is related to lower suicide rates						
Stack (1991)	RS	S	national	Suicide rate	Sweden	#1 relig book production	P (youth suicide)	SC	
Stack (1991)[a]	CS	R	1687	CDA	National US	#2 D,ORA	P (ORA)	SC	7
Stack (1992a)	R		reviews recent research on religion and suicide						
Stack (1992b)	RS	S	–	Suicide rates	Finland	#1 relig book production	P	MC	7
Stack (1992)[b]	CS	R	5726	CDA	National US	#2 D,ORA	P	MC	8
Stack (1994)	CS	R	4946 F, 4475 M	CDA	National US	#1 ORA	P	MC	8
Stack (1995)	CS	R	1197 B, 8204 W	CDA	National US	#1 ORA	P	MC	8

Stack (1998)	CS	R	1500+	CDA		National US	#1+ religiosity	P	MC	8
Stark (1983)	RS	S	214 SMSA			United States	#2 CM, D	P	MC	7
Stein (1989)	CS	S	525	Ad		Israel	#1 SR	P (men)	MC ?	7
Stein (1992)	CS	S	525	Ad		Israel	#1 SR	P	MC	7
Steininger (1978)	CS	C	732	HS,CS		New Jersey	#1 "religion a waste"	P	NONE	4
Stillion (1984)	CS	C	198	HS		Southern US	#1 SR	(P)	NONE	2
Takashasi (1989)	R,O		discusses religion and suicide in Japan							
Templer (1980)	RS	S	50 states	Suicide rates		National US	#1 D (% Ca)	Others > Ca	SC-race	5
Trovato (1986)	RS	S	–	Suicide rates		Canada	#1 D (% Ca)	Ca = Others	MC	4
Trovato (1992)	RS	S	9 provinces	Suicide (young)		Canada	#1 D (none)	P	SC	6
Truett (1992)	CS	C	7620 twins	CDA		Australia	#2 D,ORA	P	SC (factor)	9
Van Egmond (1989)	R		reviews research on factors, including religion, that predict suicidal behavior							
Wagner (1997)	R		reviews research on family risk factors for child and adolescent suicide							
Wandrei (1985)	PC	S	706	F, attempts		San Francisco	#2 D,Misc	P	NONE	6
Wasserman (1993)	RS	S	63 counties	Suicide rates		Louisiana	#1 D (% Catholic)	Ca = other	MC	6
Whitlock (1967)	CC	S	274 vs. Cs	Suicide attempts		Great Britain	#1 D (Ca vs. other)	Ca > other	no statistics	2
Whitt (1972)	RS	S	47 countries	Suicide rates		World	#1 D (Ca,P,non-Christian)	P > Ca,non-Chr	SC	4
Yang (1992)	RS	S	–	Suicide rates		National US	#1 D (Ca membership)	Ca > Others	MC	6
*Zhang (1996)	CS	C	320/452	CS		China & US	#7 ORA,NORA, SR,RB	P (US),NG (China)	MC	7

Assisted Suicide/Euthanasia (Ch. 8)

Doukas (1995)	CS,D	S	154	Oncologists		Michigan	#1 D (any vs. none)	P (against)	–	4
Gilman (1997)	CS	C	240	CDA		Humbolt, CA	#2 D,SR	P (against)	NONE	7
*Johnson D (1980)	CS	R	1530	CDA		National US	#3 D,ORA,SR	P (against)	NONE	7
*Kaplan K (1995)	CS	C	117	CS		Detroit, MI	#17+ IR,ER,Q,Misc	P (against)	SC	6
Koenig (1996)	CS	S	314	MP,PP,families		Durham, NC	spontaneous mention	frequent (against)		7
Monte (1991)	CS	R	1500 ?	CDA		National US	#2 D,ORA	P (against)	MC	7
Ostheimer (1980)	CS	R	–	CDA		National US ?	#1 D	None/J > Prot	–	5
Seiditz (1995)	CS	R	802	CDA,E		National US	#1+ "religiousness"	P (against)	SC	7
Singh (1979)	CS	S	1292	CDA		National US	#3 D,ORA,SR	P (against)	MC	8
Sonnenblick (1993)	CS	S	108	Offspring		Israel	#1 Orthodoxy	P (against)	MC	7
Ward (1980)	CS	R	1530	CDA		National US	#1 SR	P (against)	MC	8

a. Stack & Lester   b. Stack & Wasserman

Anxiety (Ch 9)

Outcome/Investigators	Type	Method	N	Population	Location	Religious Variable	Findings	Controls	Rating
Aday (1984–85)	CS	C	181	CS	Tennessee	#3 D,ORA,RB	P	NONE	5
*Alexander F (1991)	CS	R	156	CDA, retired	Southern CA	relig vs. secular retirement community	P	NONE	6
*Alvarado (1995)	CS	C	200	CS,CDA	Fresno, CA	#8 D,ORA,RB,SR	P	MC	4
Astin (1993)	CS	C	53	battered F	Los Angeles	#3 IR,ER	M	MC	6
Azhar (1994)	CT	C	62	Muslims	Malaysia	religious therapy	P	–	8
Baker (1982)	CS	C	52	CS (?)	Southern CA	#20 IR,ER	P	NONE	4
Beg (1982)	CS	C	200	Muslim CS,CDA	India	>#5 RB scale	NA	NONE	5
Berman (1974)	CS	C	198	CDA with near death experience		#1 "active" vs. "inactive"	NA	NONE	5
Bivens (1994)	CS	C	167	AIDS/HIV MP	Memphis, TN	>#5 O,RB,ORA,IR	P	SC	6
*Bohannon (1991)	CS	C	272	Bereaved parents	Midwest US	#2 D,ORA	P	SC	6
Carlson (1988)	CT	C	36 randomized	CS (Christian)	Chicago	"devotional meditation"	P	–	6
Cooley (1965)	PC	C	72 of 255	Ad, youth camp	Houston, TX	#1 converts, rededicate	P	NONE	4
Dhawan (1986)	Exp	C	40	CS	Northern India	#36 Bhushan relig scale	NA	–	4
*Donahue (1985)	R			reviews research on the relationship between intrinsic/extrinsic religiosity and mental health					
Downey (1984)	CS	C	237	100%M, 40–59	Baltimore, MD	13-item RCm scale	NA (curvilinear)	SC	6
Elkins (1979)	CT	C	42	GM (Baptists)	Tennessee	prayer vs. relax, controls	NA	–	5
Fallon (1990)	CSer	C	10	PP	New York	moral/rlg scrupulosity	Prozac decreased scrupulosity		6
*Fehr (1977)	CS	C	120	CS	Cincinnati, OH	#10+ rlg values,O	NA	NONE	4
Feifel (1974)	CS	C	187	MP,CDA	Los Angeles	#3 RB,SR,ORA	NA	NONE	4
Florian (1983)	CS	C	178	CS	Israel	#20 religious practice	M	NONE	5
Franks (1990–91)	CC	C	51 gay M w AIDS/64 gay without AIDS		San Francisco	#10 ORA,SR,RB,D	NG	NONE	6
Frenz (1989)	CS	C	175	CS	New York	#10+ D,IR,ER	NA	SC	5
Fry (1990)	CS	C	178	homebound, E	Western Canada	#1 prayer	NG	NONE	5
Funk (1956)	CS	C	255	CS	Indiana	>#10 RB,RC	M	NONE	5
Gangdev (1998)	CR	C	1	PP with OCD	Australia	#1 RB	(P)	–	3
Hassan (1981)	CS	R	480	CS (Mus/Hin)	India	#10 religiosity scale	NG	NONE	6
*Heintzelman (1976)	CS	C	82	CS	Cincinnati, OH	#? relig orthodoxy scale	NA	NONE	4

Study	Type		N	Population	Location	Measures	Finding	Controls	Rating
*Hertsgaard (1984)	CS	R	760	CDA,F,farms	North Dakota	#2 ORA,D	P (ORA)	MC	7
Hoelter (1979)	CS	C	375	CS	Indiana	#5+ ORA,RB,SR,O	NA	NONE	5
Iammarino (1975)	CS	C	249	HS (9th grd)	NE Ohio	#1 D (C,P,J vs. N)	NA	NONE	2
Jeffers (1961)[a]	CS	C	260	CDA,E	North Carolina	#6+ORA,NORA, RB,SR	P	NONE	5
Kabat-Zinn (1992)	CT	C	22	PP	Massachusetts	meditation (TM)	P	no controls	6
*Kaczorowski (1989)	CS	C	114 (hospice)	MP (with CA)	New York	#10 RWB	P	NONE	6
Kirkpatrick (1992)	CS	C	213	CDA	Denver, CO	>#25 D,IR,ER,RB	P (x glossolalia)	NONE	5
Koenig (1988)	CS	C	304	CDA, E	Missouri	#3 ORA,RC	P	SC-age, sex	5
*Koenig (1988)[b]	CS	S	106	MP,E	Illinois	#15+ ORA,NORA,IR	P	SC-sex	6
Koenig (1993)[c]	CS	R	1299	CDA, E	North Carolina	#5 ORA,NORA,SR	NA	MC	9
Koenig (1993)[d]	CS	R	2969	CDA	North Carolina	#5 ORA,NORA,SR	P	MC	9
Kraft (1986)	CS	C	107	CS	Louisiana	#10+ IR,ER,SR	P	NONE	4
Kutner (1971)	CS	C	106	CDA,F	California	#2 ORA,D (Ca vs. P)	NA (Ca > P)	NONE	2
Leming (1980)	CS	R	372	CDA	Minnesota	#10 scale	P	SC	7
Levin (1993)[e]	CS	C	266	MP,100%BF	Texas	#1 NORA (prayer)	NG	MC	6
Martin D (1965)	CS	C	58	CM	Tennessee	#5 ORA,NORA,SR	P	NONE	4
McMordie (1981)	CS	C	320	CS	Iowa	#1 SR	C	NONE	5
Miller JJ (1995)	CT,D	C	22	PP	Massachusetts	3-year f/u meditation	(P)	–	4
Minear (1980–81)	CS	C	394	CS	New England	#11 D,ORA,SR,RB	P	NONE	5
*Morris P (1982)	PC	C	24	chronically ill	England	pilgrimage to Lourdes	P	NONE	6
*Morse (1987)	CS	C	156	E,CDA	Massachusetts	#3 CM,ORA,RC	NA	SC	6
Paloutzian (1981)	PC	C	91	CS	Indiana	#1 RE (conversion)	P	SC	5
*Park (1990)	PC	C	83/83	CS (religious)	Delaware	#13 IR,ER,O	M,C	SC	6
*Plante (1992)	CS	C	86	CS	Santa Clara, CA	#2 SR,D	NA	NONE	5
Raphael (1996)	CC	S	49 vs. Cs	PP (OCD)	London, England	#1D (affiliated vs. not)	NG	NONE	4
*Razali (1998)	CT	C	203	PP	Malaysia	#1 relig psycho-therapy	P	–	8
Reid (1978)	CS	R	501	CDA,E	W. Scotland	#3 D,RB,ORA	no stats	NONE	5
Richardson (1983)	CS	R	1428	CDA	National US	#1D (affiliated vs. unaffiliated)	P	SC-age	6
Rokeach (1960)	CS	C	202 and 207	CS	Michigan & NY	#1 D (Ca,P,J vs. N)	NG	NONE	3
*Ryan (1993)	CS	C	105/151/42/342	CS,CM	New York	#72 IR,ER,O,Q,Misc	P (IR)	NONE	3
Schaefer (1991)	CS	C	161	CS (Christian)	Southern CA	#21+ IR,ER,RB,RC	P	SC	6
Shams (1993)	CS	C	140 employed & unemployed Muslims		Great Britain	#15 A-V relig values	P (unemployed)	MC	6
Smith DK (1983–84)	CS	C	20 patients with terminal cancer		Long Beach, CA	#2 ORA,SR	P	NONE	5

a. Jeffers, Nichols, et al.   b. Koenig, Moberg, & Kvale   c. Koenig, George, Blazer, et al.   d. Koenig, Ford, et al.   e. Levin, Lyons, et al.

Outcome/Investigators	Type	Method	N	Population	Location	Religious Variable	Findings	Controls	Rating
Spellman (1971)	CS	C	60	CDA	Texas	#3 SR,ORA,RE	NG (RE)	SC	5
Steketee (1991)	CC	C	33 OCD vs. Cs	PP	Boston	#2 SR,D	NG (SR)	NONE	5
Sturgeon (1979)	CS	C	144	CS (Christian)	Tennessee	#20 IR,ER	P	NONE	6
Tapanya (1997)	CS	C	104	CDA,E	Thailand & Can	#21 I/ER,Buddhist vs. Christian	P	SC-sex	7
*Tellis-Nayak (1982)	CS	R	259	CDA,E	New York	#5 D,RB,ORA,RE	P	MC	6
Templer (1970)	CS	C	213	CS	Kentucky	#8 scale	NA	NONE	5
Templer (1972)	CS	C	267	CM	Midwest, Southern US	#8 scale	P	NONE	5
Thomas (1980)	CS	C	305	CDA	Connecticut	#1 RB	NA	NONE	5
Thorson (1989)	CS	C	103	CDA,E,M	Omaha, NE	#10 IR (Hoge)	NA	NONE	5
Thorson (1990)	CS	C	345	CDA,CS	Omaha, NE	#10 IR (Hoge)	P	NONE	6
Thorson (1991)[a]	CS	C	389	CDA,CS,HS	Omaha, NE	#6 Misc	P	NONE	6
Trenholm (1998)	CS	C	60	PP (anxiety do)	Tennessee	#1+ religious conflict	C	–	5
*Williams D (1991)	PC	R	720	CDA	New Haven, CT	#2 D,ORA	P	MC	8
Williams R (1968)	CS	C	161	CS	Georgia	#5 ORA,NORA	P	NONE	5
Wilson W (1968)	CS	C	100	CS	Alabama	#4+ ORA,RB	NG	NONE	5
Wittkowski (1977)	CS	C	60	E,NHP	Germany	#6 relig dimensions	P	NONE ?	5
Xiao (1998)	CT	C	–	Neurotics	China	#1 Taoistic CBT	(P)	–	6
Young (1980)	CS	R	320	HS	E. Alabama	#1 D (born again vs. not)	P	SC-sex,race	6
Young (1981)	CS	R	320	HS	E. Alabama	#24 scale	M	SC-sex,race	6
*Zeidner (1992)	CS	C	261	CDA	Israel	#2 RC	NG	MC	7

Schizophrenia/Psychosis (Ch 10)

Outcome/Investigators	Type	Method	N	Population	Location	Religious Variable	Findings	Controls	Rating
Armstrong (1962)	CC	C	88 vs. Cs	PP (psychotic)	Illinois	#3+ RB,D	M	NONE	3
Bufford (1989)	R	review and discussion of demonic influence and mental disorders (oriented toward Christian practitioner)							
Carson (1979)	CT	C	20	PP (schizophrenics)	Baltimore, MD	weekly pray/scripture	P	–	3
Cothran (1986)	CC	S	41 vs. Cs	PP	New York	#>5 RB,SR,R delusions	NA	NONE	6
Diduca (1997)	CS	C/S	201	CDA (?)	United Kingdom	#1+ religiosity	NA	–	6
Feldman (1989)	CC	C	31/36 vs. Cs	PP (schizophrenics)	London, England	#2 SR	M	NONE	6
*Flics (1991)	CS,D	S	152	PP (schizo vs. dep)	New York City	#1 D (Jews vs. Ca/Prot)	C (Jews-Dep, P-Schizo)	4

Study	Design	S/R	N	Population	Location	Variable	P	SC	Rating
Francis LJ (1985)	CS	–	132	HS, 15 yo's	England	#110 Relig Attitude Scale	P	SC	5
Francis LJ (1992)	CS	S	50	PP,F (addicts)	Great Britain	#27+ Christian Attitudes	P (psychoticism)	NONE	4
Gaw (1998)	Q/D	C	20	PP, F	China	#1 "possession states"	(P)	–	6
Jones E (1997)	CC	C	20 vs. two Cs	Schizophrenics	London	delusion vs. over-valued idea vs. religious belief			6
Kirov (1998)	CS,D	S	52	PP (psychotic)	United Kingdom	#2+ RC	P	–	6
Lindgren (1995)	CT	C	28	PP	Maryland	spiritual intervention	NA		6
Maltby (1997)	CS	C	216	CDA	Ireland	#3 ORA,NORA,SR	P	SC	6
*Neeleman (1994)	CC	S	73 vs. 25 Cs	PP	London, England	#16 ORA,NORA, RB,SR	NG	SC-race, sex	6
Schofield (1959)	CC	C	158 vs. 150 Cs	PP (schizo)	Minnesota	#2 ORA,RC	NA	NONE	6
Spencer (1975)	CC	S	50 JW with schizophrenia	PP with schizophrenia	Australia	#1 Jehovah Witness vs. other	JW > oth	NONE	5
Sullivan (1993)	Q	C	40 successfully adjusted PP with severe, chronic mental illness in Missouri			48% RC essential to success		5
Trappler (1995,1997)	CC	C	15 vs. Cs	PP	Brooklyn, NY	#1 Jewish conversion	–	NONE	2
Ullman (1988)	CS	C	40	CDA (converts)	Israel	#1 D (J,Ca,Bahai, HK)	B,HK > Ca,J	NONE	5
Verghese (1989)	PC	S	386	PP (schizo)	India	#2 D, relig activites	P	NONE	7
Wahass (1997)	CS,D	C	33 and 37	British & Saudi PP	GB & Saudi Arabia	RC with hallucinations	–	–	6
Wilson WP (1983)	CC	C	72 vs. Cs	PP	Durham, NC	#7 + RB,RE,Misc	P	NONE	5
Wootton (1983)	R,O		reviews research and popular opinion on the relationship between religious conversion and schizophrenic decompensation						

Alcohol Use/Abuse (Ch 11)

Study	Design	S/R	N	Population	Location	Variable	P	SC	Rating
Adelekan (1993)	CS	S/R	636	CS	Nigeria	#2 SR,D (Muslim vs. Christian)	P	NONE	6
Adlaf (1985)	CS	R	2066	Ad	Ontario, Can	#3+ D,ORA,SR	P	SC	7
Alexander (1994)[b]	R		reviews research on transcendental meditation (TM) as a treatment for alcohol, nicotine, and drug abuse						
*Alexander F (1991)	CS	R	156	CDA, retired	Southern CA	#1 relig vs. secular re- tirement com	P	NONE	6
Alford (1991)	PC	C	157	Ad,PP	Nebraska	#1 AA participation	P	NONE	7
Amoateng (1986)	CS	R	17000	HS seniors	National US	#2 ORA,SR	P	MC	9
Bales (1944)	R,O		discussion of therapeutic role of alcoholics anonymous						
Beghley (1990)	CS	R	8652	CDA	National US	#5 ORA,SR,CM,RB	P	MC	9
Benson P (1989)	CS	R	>12000	HS seniors	National US	#2 ORA,SR	P	MC	9
Blacker (1966)	R		review of old studies—low rate in Jews and relig affiliates; increased problems in drinkers of proscriptive relig who drink						
Bliss (1994)	CS	C	143	CS (Catholic)	Ohio	#2 ORA,SR	M	NONE	4
Bock (1987)	CS	R	4289	CDA	National US	#4 D,ORA,SR,CM	P	MC	9

a. Thorson 1991; Thorson & Powell   b. Alexander, Robinson, & Rainforth

Outcome/Investigators	Type	Method	N	Population	Location	Religious Variable	Findings	Controls	Rating
Brizer (1993)	CC	C	65 vs. Cs	PP (alc/drg)	New York	#2+ ORA,NORA	P	NONE	3
*Brown D (1994)	CS	S	537	CDA,B,M	Southeast US	#12 relig scale, ORA,D	P (ORA)	MC	8
Brown H (1991)	PC/D	C	35 and 15	PP (alc)	–	#3+ 12-step spirituality	(P)	–	4
Burkett (1974)	CS	C	855	HS	Pacific NW US	#1 ORA	P	SC-sex	6
Burkett (1977)	CS	S	837	HS	Pacific NW US	#5+ ORA,RB	P (ORA)	SC	7
Burkett (1980)	CS	S	323	HS	Pacific NE US	#4 ORA,SR,RB	P	NONE	6
Burkett (1987)	PC	C	240	HS	Pacific NW US	#6+ ORA,SR,RB	P (indirect)	MC	7
Burkett (1993)	PC	–	–	HS	Pacific NW US	#3 RB; parent SR,RB	P	MC	8
Calahan (1969)	CS	R	2746	CDA	National US	#2 D,ORA	P	SC-sex, age,SES	7
Calahan (1972)	CS	R	1561	CDA,M	National US	#2 D,ORA	P	NONE ?	7
Carlucci (1993)	CS	C	331	CS	New York	#1 D (Ca vs. Prot & J)	Ca > Prot,J	NONE	4
*Carroll (1993)	CS	C	100	AA members	Southern CA	#38 (Step 11 spirituality)	P	NONE	6
Cisin (1968)	CS	R	2746	CDA	National US	#5+ ORA,RC,RB	P	MC ?	9
Cochran (1988)	CS	R	7581	CDA	National US	#4 ORA,RB,SR,CM	P	MC	9
Cochran (1989, '91,[a] '93)	CS	R	3065	Ad	Midwest US	#4 ORA,SR,D	P	MC	8
Cochran (1992)	CS	R	3772	CDA	National US	#3+ R homogamy,SR,D	P	MC	9
Cochran (1994)	CS	C	1600	HS	Oklahoma	#2 ORA,SR	P	MC	6
Coombs (1985)	CS	C	197	Ad,F	Los Angeles	#9 RB,ORA,Misc	P	NONE	5
Corrington (1989)	CS	C	30	AA members	Maryland	#35 spirituality scale	(P) (content-ment)	NS	2
Cronin (1995)	CS	C	216	CS	Maryland	#2 D,SR	P	NONE	3
Dudley R (1987)	CS	R	801	SDA youth	North America	#5+ ORA,NORA,CM	P	SC	6
Edwards (1972)[b]	CS	R	928	CDA	London	#1 D (Ca vs. others)	Ca > others	NONE	4
Edwards (1972)[c]	CS	S	188	prisoners	London	#1 D(Ca vs. others)	Ca > others	NONE	4
Encel (1972)	CS,D	R	820	CDA	Australia	#1 D (vs. none)	–	–	6
Engs (1980)	CS	S	1691	CS	Australia	#2 D,SR	P	NONE	6
Engs (1982)	CS	S	1449	CS	Australia	#3 D,SR,seminarians	P	NONE	6
Engs (1990)	CS	S/R	4911 & 1687	CS	Can & US	#1 D	Ca > P > J	NONE	5
Forster (1993)	CS	R	667	CDA,E	New York	#1 D (none vs. other)	P	MC ?	8
Foshee (1996)	PC	R	2102	Ad & mothers	Southeast US	#4+ ORA,RB,SR,D	P	MC	9
Francis LJ (1994)	CS	C	264	CDA	England	#2 D,ORA	NA	NONE	3

540

Investigators	Type	Meth	N	Population	Location	Rel. variables	Findings	Controls	Rating
Galanter (1982b)	CS,D	R	119 & 227	Sect members	New York	#1 conversion	(P)	–	5
Gelderloos (1991)	CS	S	reviews 24 studies concerning Transcendental Meditation preventing substance abuse				PP > MS		
Goldfarb (1996)	CC	C	101/119	PP/medical students	New York	#12 scale,O	P	NONE	8
Goodwin (1969)	CS	C	98 teetotalers vs. 35 drinkers		St. Louis	#3+ SR,RB	P	NONE	4
Gorsuch (1995)	CS	R	comprehensively reviews relationship between religious factors & substance abuse				P		
Gottlieb (1984)	CS	R	3025	CDA	National US	#1 ORA	P	MC	7
Green (1998)	Q		examines stories of spiritual awakening and its impact on recovery from alcohol abuse						
Guinn (1975)	CS	S/R	1789	HS, Mex-Am	Texas	#1 ORA	P	NONE	6
Hardert (1994)	CS	C	1234	HS,CS	Arizona	#1+"religiosity"	NA (inapp cntl)	MC	7
Hardesty (1995)	CS	C	475	HS,CS (16–19)	Midwest US	#1+"family religiousness"	P	NONE	6
Hasin (1985)	CS	S	835	PP with depress	5 US cities	#1 D (some vs. none)	P	MC	9
Hawks (1992)	CS	R	3591	CDA	Utah	#1 D (LDS/other vs. none)	P	NONE	3
Hays (1986)	CS	R	1121	Ad (13–18)	National US	#5 religiousness scale	P	MC	9
Holman (1993)	CS	C	615	CDA (17–24)	Oklahoma & Wisconsin	#6 RB,ORA	P	SC	5
Hughes (1985)	CS	C	66 teetotalers vs. 60	CM (evangelical)	England	#4+ RB,D	P	NONE	5
Hundleby (1982)	CS	C	231	HS (Catholic)	Ontario, Can	#4 ORA,NORA	NA	NONE	5
Hundleby (1987)	CS	S/R	2048	HS (9th grade)	Ontario, Can	#3 ORA	P	SC	7
*Idler (1997a)	CS	R	2812	CDA,E	New Haven, CT	#2 ORA,SR	P (ORA)	MC	9
Isralowitz (1990)	CS	R	767	CS	Singapore	#1 RB (present vs. absent)	NA	NONE	4
*Jacobson (1977)	PC	C	57	Alcoholics, PP	DePaul, WI	#15 "religious values"	P	NONE	6
Kearney (1970)	Cser	C	5	CDA	Mexico	#1 religious conversion	(P)	–	3
*Kendler (1997)	CS	C	1902	CDA, twins	Virginia	#11 RB,ORA, NORA,SR	P	MC	9
Khavari (1982)	CS	–	4853	CDA	Milwaukee, WI	#2 D,SR	P	NONE	6
Knupfer (1967)	CS	S	1212	CDA	San Francisco Bay Area	#1 D (Jews vs. non-J)	non-J > J	NONE	1
*Koenig (1988)[d]	CS	S	106	MP,E	Illinois	#15+ ORA,NORA,IR	P	SC-sex	6
Koenig (1994)[e]	CS	R	2969	CDA	North Carolina	#5 ORA,NORA,SR	P	MC	9
Krause (1991)	CS	R	1607	CDA, E	National US	#4 ORA,NORA,SR	P	MC	9
Larson DB (1980)	CC	C	81 vs. Cs	PP (alcoholics)	North Carolina	#6+ SR,RE,NORA	P	NONE	5
Lemere (1953)	D	C	500	alcoholics	Seattle, WA	#1 relig conversion	(P)	–	6
*Levav (1997)	CS	R	5772	CDA, New Haven & Los Angeles		#1 D (Jews vs. non-J)	non-J > J	MC	8
Long K (1993)	PC	C	625	grades 3–7	Montana	#2 ORA,NORA	P	MC	7
Lorch (1985)	CS	S/R	13878	HS	Colorado Springs	#6+ CM,ORA,SR	P (SR)	SC-grade, sex	8

a. Cochran & Beeghley   b. Edwards, Chandler, et al.   c. Edwards, Gattoni, et al.   d. Koenig, Moberg, & Kvale   e. Koenig, George, Meador, Blazer, & Ford

Outcome/Investigators	Type	Method	N	Population	Location	Religious Variable	Findings	Controls	Rating
Lorch (1988)	CS, D	S	143	pastors	Colorado Springs	#1 D (conserv vs. lib)	C	—	5
Luna (1992)	CS	R	955	medical, vet, & law students	Spain	#1 SR	P	NONE	6
MacKenzie (1985)	CS	R	3755	CDA	Ireland	#1 D (Ca vs. non-Ca)	Ca > non-Ca	SC	4
Mathew (1995, 1996)	CC	C	62 vs. Cs	PP (alcoholics)	North Carolina	#76 Mathew scale	P	NONE	4
McDowell (1996)	CS	S	101	PP (alcoholics)	New York	#17 IR,ER,ORA,RB	staff underestimated pt's spirituality	NONE	6
Midanik (1995)	CS	R	1603	CDA drinkers	National US	#2 D,SR	P	MC	7
Montgomery (1995)	PC	no relationship between freq of AA attendance & sobriety, but signif assoc between AA "involvement" & abstinence							
Mookherjee (1986)	CS	S	1477	W,M (DWI rehab)	Tennessee	#11 RB scale	NA	NONE	4
Moore M (1995)	CS	C	2366	Ad	Israel	#2 D,SR	P	NONE	5
Moore R (1990)	PC	S	1014	medical students	Baltimore, MD	#1 D (Jews vs. non-J)	non-J >J	MC	7
*Moos (1979)	CS	C	122	alcoholics	Palo Alto, CA	?# moral-relig sub-scale	P	NONE	5
Mullen (1995)	CS	R	1534	HS	Netherlands	#3 D,ORA,RB	P	NONE	6
Mullen (1996)	CS	R	985	CDA > 35 yo	West Scotland	#1 D (vs. none)	P	SC	4
Ndom (1996)	CS	R	1508	CS	Nigeria	#2 D,SR	P	NONE	7
Newcomb (1986)	CS	—	791	Ad	Los Angeles	#1 SR	P	NONE	7
Oleckno (1991)	CS	—	1077	CS	Northern IL	#2 ORA,SR	P	NONE	6
Parfrey (1976)	CS	R	444	CS	Ireland	#3 ORA,RB	P	NONE	5
Park (1998)	CS	R (?)	–	CDA	Korea	#2+ D,RCm	P (women)	–	7
Patock-Peckham (1998)	CS	C	364	CS	Arizona	#22 D,IR/ER	M	SC	6
Peele (1990)	R	reviews studies showing little effectiveness for Alcoholics Annonymous over secular programs							
Perkins (1987)	CS	S	860	CS	New York	#3+ SR,D,misc	P	MC	8
Poulson (1998)	CS	C ?	210	CS	Greenville, NC	#1+ SR	P	SC	5
Query (1985)	PC, D	S	96	PP ages 10–23	North Dakota	#2 ORA,D	(P)	NS	5
*Resnick (1997)	CS	R	12118	Ad	National US	#1 SR	P	MC	8
*Richards D (1990)	CS	C	292	CDA	National US	#8 "universal force"	P	NONE	3
Rosenberg C (1974)	CC	S	22 vs. Cs	alcoholics	Boston	#1 D (Ca)	–	NS	1
Schlegel (1979)	CS	R	842	HS	Ontario, Can	#2 ORA, D(vs. none)	P	NONE	6
Strauss (1953)	CS	S	15747	CS	National US	#2 D,ORA	P	NONE	7
Taub (1994)	CT	C	118	alcoholics	Washington, DC	#1 TM	P	–	6
Taylor J (1990)	CS	R	289 (45% RR)	CDA,B,F	Pittsburgh	#19 IR,NORA,RB	P	MC	6
Thorne (1996)	CS	R	990	CDA,E	Ohio	#3 ORA,D	NA	NONE	7
Tiebout (1944)	R	reviews and discusses effectiveness of Alcoholics Anonymous							

Tuchfeld (1981)	D	C	51 alcoholics (spontaneously remitted)		Southeast US	(results: 13 of 51 did so due to R conversion)	P (affil)	MC	6
Turner (1994)	CS	S	247	HS	Austin, TX	#2 D (affil),ORA	NG	–	5
Waisberg (1994)	CT	C	131	PP	Ontario, Can	#1 spiritual program intervention	P	MC	6
Wallace (1972)	CS	R	4000	CDA	Norway	#4 ORA,NORA	P	MC	9
Wallace, J (1998)	CS	R	5000	HS	National US	#3 D,ORA,SR	P	MC	9
Walters (1957)	CC	C	50 vs. Cs	alcoholics	Topeka, KS	#8 ORA,RE,NORA	(NG)	NS	3
Warfield (1996)	R,O	S	"spirituality: the key to recovery from alcoholism"						
Wechsler (1972)	CS	S	6266	MP	New England	#1 D (Irish Ca vs. others)	Irish Ca > oth	NONE	2
Wechsler (1979)	CS	R	7170	CS	New England	#2 D,ORA	P	NONE	7
Weill (1994)	PC	R	437	Ad (13–18)	France	#1 ORA	P	NONE	7
Williams J (1986)	CS	C	36	alcoholics	New York	#1 alcoholics anonymous	P	NONE	5
Zucker (1987)	PC	C	61	alcoholics	Bronx, NY	#3+ D,SR,ORA	NG	NONE	4

Drug Use/Abuse (Ch 11)

*Adelekan (1993)	CS	S/R	636	CS	Nigeria	#2 SR,D (Muslim vs. Christian)	P	NONE	6
*Adlaf (1985)	CS	R	2066	Ad	Ontario, Can	#3+ D,ORA,SR	P	NONE	6
*Alexander (1994)[a]	R		reviews research showing effectiveness of transcendental meditation on treatment of drug abuse				P		
Amey (1996)	CS	R	11,728	HS	National US	#3 OR,SR,D	P	MC	10
*Amoateng (1986)	CS	R	17000	HS seniors	National US	#2 SR,ORA	P	MC	9
Bell (1997)	CS	R	17952	CS	National US	#2 SR	P	MC	9
*Bliss (1994)	CS	C	143	CS (Catholic)	Ohio	#2 ORA,SR	P	NONE	4
Bowker (1974)	CS	R	948	CS	Ivy College	#2 ORA,D	P (indirect)	NONE ?	5
Brownfield (1991)	CS	R	>800	Ad,W,M	Seattle, WA	#3 D,ORA,SR	P	MC	8
Brunswick (1992)	PC	R	536	Ad,B, 12–17 yo	Harlem, NY	#2 ORA,SR	P	SC	7
*Burkett (1974)	CS	C	855	HS	Pacific NW US	#1 ORA	P	SC-sex	6
*Burkett (1977)	CS	S	837	HS	Pacific NW US	#5+ ORA,RB	P (ORA)	SC	7
*Burkett (1987)	PC	C	240	HS	Pacific NW US	#5+ ORA,SR,RB	P (indirect)	MC	7
Cancellaro (1982)	CC	C	74 vs. Cs (narcotic addicts)		Kentucky	#5+ NORA,RE	P	NONE	4
Christo (1995)	PC	C	101	poly-drug abuse	London	#12 spiritual belief	P	NONE	7
Clark (1992)	CS	R	2036	medical students	Great Britain	#1 D (any vs. none)	P	NONE	6
*Cochran (1989,1991)	CS	R	3065	Ad	Midwest US	#4 ORA,SR,D	P	MC	8
Coleman (1986)	CC	S	50 vs. Cs	Opiate addicts	Philadelphia	#3 ORA,SR	M	MC	6
Cook (1997)	CS	R/S	7666	youth (ages 12–30)	United Kingdom	#1+ RCm	P	–	7

a. Alexander, Robinson, & Rainforth

543

Outcome/Investigators	Type	Method	N	Population	Location	Religious Variable	Findings	Controls	Rating
Desmond (1981)	PC,D	C	248	PP (addicts)	San Antonio,TX	#1 religious rehab program	(P)	NS	7
*Donahue (1995)	R			reviews research on religion and substance abuse					
Dube (1975)	CS	S	566	PP,M	India	#1 D	Hindus > Muslims	NONE	3
*Dudley R (1987)	CS,D	R	801	youth 12–24 y	North America	#5+ ORA,NORA,CM	P	SC	6
*Engs (1980)	CS	S	1691	CS	Australia	#2 D,SR	P	NONE	6
Forliti (1986)	CS,D	C	8165/10,467	Ad/parents,CM	United States	#>15 RB,ORA,SR	(P)	NS	5
Francis LJ (1993)	CS	S	4753	HS	England	#3 ORA,RB	P	NONE	7
*Gelderloos (1991)	R			reviews 24 research studies on transcendental medication and substance abuse					
Gorsuch (1976)	R			reviews relationship between religious factors & initial drug use					
*Gorsuch (1995)	R			reviews relationship between religious factors & substance abuse					
*Guinn (1975)	CS	S/R	1789	HS, Mex-Am	Texas	#1 ORA	P	NONE	6
Hadaway (1984)	CS	R	600	Ad, public HS	Atlanta, GA	#5 ORA,SR,NORA,O	P	SC	6
*Hardert (1994)	CS	C	1234	HS,CS	Arizona	"religiosity"	P	MC	7
*Hardesty (1995)	CS	C	475	HS,CS (16–19)	Midwest US	"family religiousness"	P	NONE	6
*Hasin (1985)	CS	S	835	PP with depress	5 US cities	#1 D (some vs. none)	P	MC	9
*Hater (1984)	CS	S	1174	PP (opioid addicts)	National US	#4 ORA,SR	NA	MC	7
*Hawks (1992)	CS	R	3591	CDA	Utah	#1 D (LDS vs. other vs. none)	P	NONE	3
*Hays (1986)	CS	R	1121	Ad (13–18)	National US	#5 religiousness scale	P	MC	9
Hays (1990)	CS	–	415	HS	–	?# "religious identification"	P	MC	6
*Hundleby (1982)	CS	C	231	HS (Catholic)	Ontario, Can	#4 ORA,NORA	NA	NONE	5
*Hundleby (1987)	CS	S/R	2048	HS (9th grade)	Ontario, Can	#3 ORA	P	SC	7
Jessor (1973)	PC	R	605 and 248	HS and CS	Colorado	#1 ORA	P	NONE	7
Jessor (1977)	PC	R	432 and 205	HS and CS	Colorado	#5 ORA,NORA,SR	P	NONE	7
Jessor (1986)	R			reviews research on marijuana & cocaine use in adolescents & young adults (less attachment to church & lower religious commitment)					
Kandel D (1984)	CS	R	1325	CDA (24–25 yo)	New York	#1 ORA	P	MC	7
*Khavari (1982)	CS	–	4853	CDA	Milwaukee,WI	#2 D,SR	P	NONE	6
*Lorch (1985)	CS	S/R	13878	HS	Colorado Springs	#6+ CM,ORA,SR	P (SR)	SC-grade, sex	8
*Lorch (1988)	CS, D	S	143	pastors	Colorado Springs	#1 D (conserv vs. lib)	(M)	NS	5
Mauss (1959)	CS	S	459	HS	California	#1 D (any vs. none)	P	NONE	4
McIntosh (1981)	CS	R	1358	ages 12–19	Texas	#3 D,ORA,SR	P	MC	8

Delinquency/Crime (Ch 12)

Study			N	Sample	Location	Religion measure	Direction	Controls	Score
McLuckie (1975)	CS	R	27175	grades 7–12	Pennsylvania	#2 D,ORA	P	MC	8
Mohan (1979)	CS	R	3600	CDA	India	#1 D	Sikh > Hindu	NONE	3
*Mullen (1995)	CS	R	1534	HS	Netherlands	#3 D,ORA,RB	P	NONE	6
*Ndom (1996)	CS	R	1508	CS	Nigeria	#2 D,SR	P	NONE	7
*Newcomb (1986)	CS	S ?	791	Ad	Los Angeles	#1 SR	P	NONE	7
Newcomb (1992)	PC	S ?	614	Ad	Los Angeles	#1 SR	P	—	8
Nicholi (1985)	R		review of college students who used drugs; users have fewer religious convictions						
Oetting (1987)	CS	S	415	HS	Western US	#2 SR,ORA	P.	SC	6
*Oleckno (1991)	CS	C ?	1077	CS	Northern IL	#2 ORA, SR	P	NONE	6
*Parfrey (1976)	CS	R	444	CS	Ireland	#3 ORA,RB	P	NONE	5
*Resnick (1997)	CS	R	12118	Ad	National US	#1 SR	P	MC	8
Rohrbaugh (1975)	CS	C	475/221	HS/CS	Colorado	#8 ORA,RB,RE	P	NONE	6
Sarvela (1988)	CS	R	265	7th graders	Northern MI	#1 D (Ca,P,O)	Ca = P = O	MC	5
Tenant-Clark (1989)	CC	C	25 vs. 25 Cs	Ad,PP	Colorado	#1 SR	P	NONE	5
*Veach (1992)	CS	C	148	CS & health professionals	Nevada	#18 Spiritual Exp, etc.	NG	NONE	3
*Wallace, J (1998)	CS	R	5000	HS	National US	#3 D,ORA,SR	P	MC	9
Whitehead (1970)	CS	R	1606	HS	Nova Scotia	#1 D (Ca,P,J,N)	J,N > Ca,P	NONE	3
Delinquency/Crime (Ch 12)									
Avtar (1979)	CS	C	54/59	CS/HS	Ottawa, Can	#1 SR	P	NONE	5
Barrett (1988)	PC	S	326	Mex-Am clients	Texas	#1 ORA	P	MC	7
Benda (1995)	CS	–	>1000	HS	Arkansas & Maryland	#8 Misc	P	SC	7
*Benson P (1989)	CS	R	>12,000	HS	National US	#1 SR	P	MC	9
*Burkett (1974)	CS	C	855	HS	Pacific NW US	#1 ORA	(P)	SC-sex	6
Carr-Saunders (1944)	CC	C	276 vs. 551 Cs	Delinquents	London, England	#1 ORA	(P)	NONE	4
Chadwick (1993)	CS	R	2143	Ad (Mormons)	Eastern US	relig values/practices	P	MC	8
*Cochran (1994)	CS	C	1600	HS	Oklahoma	#2 ORA,SR	NA	MC	6
Cohen (1987)	PC	S	976 mothers/caretakers of 1–10 yo	Ad/ public HS	New York	#1 relig participation	P	MC	8
*Donahue (1995)	R		review of religion and substance abuse in adolescents						
Elifson (1983)	CS	R	600	Ad, public HS	Atlanta, GA	#3 RB,SR,NORA	NA, but inappropriate controls		6
Ellis L (1985)	R		reviews literature on religiosity and criminality (confirming inverse relationship with church attendance)						
Evans (1995)	CS	S	477	CDA,100%W	Midwest US	#12+ OR,SR,RB,D	P	MC	7
Fernquist (1995)	CS	–	180	CS	—	#2+ ORA,NORA	P	–	6
*Forliti (1986)	CS,D	C	8165/10,467	Ad/parents,CM	United States	#15+ RB,ORA,SR	(P)	NS	5

545

Outcome/Investigators	Type	Method	N	Population	Location	Religious Variable	Findings	Controls	Rating
Freeman (1986)	CS	R/R?	2358/4961	Young BM/WM	Boston, Chicago, Philadelphia	#1+ ORA	P	MC	9
Grasmick (1991)	CS	R	304	CDA	Oklahoma City	#6 D,ORA,SR	P/NA	SC	8
*Hater (1984)	CS	S	1174	PP (opioid addicts)	National US	#4 ORA,SR	NA	MC	7
Hersch (1936–37)	CS,D	–	–	Youth	Poland	#1 D	Ca>P>J	NONE ?	–
Higgins (1977)	CS	R	1410	HS (10th grade)	Atlanta, GA	#1 ORA	P	SC-sex,race	7
Hirschi (1969)	CS	R	4077	HS	Northern CA	#1 ORA	NA	NONE	7
Johnson B (1997)	CC	S	201 vs. 201	Prisoners	New York	#2 Prison fellow,ORA	P (ORA)	MC	7
Knudten (1971)	R			reviews literature on delinquency, crime, and religion					
Kvaraceus (1944)	CS	S	>700	Ad	New Jersey	#1 ORA	NA	(NONE)	5
Middleton (1962)	CS	–	554	CS	California, Florida	#3 RB,ORA,SR	P	NONE	6
Montgomery (1996)	CS	–	392	HS (Catholic),F	Great Britain	#1 NORA	P	SC	6
Morris R (1981)	CS	C	134	CS	Tennessee	#20 IR,ER	P	NONE	5
*Parfrey (1976)	CS	R	444	CS	Ireland	#3 ORA,RB	P	NONE	5
Peek (1985)	PC	–	817	HS,M	National US	#1+ religiosity	M	MC	8
Pettersson (1991)	CS	R	118 police districts		Sweden	#1 ORA	P	SC	3
Powell (1997)	CS	S	521	HS high risk, B	Birmingham, AL	#2 ORA,SR	P (SR)	MC	7
*Resnick (1997)	CS	R	12118	Ad	National US	#1 SR	NA (violence)	MC	8
Rhodes (1970)	CS	R	21720	HS	Tennessee	#4 ORA,D,misc	P	MC	9
*Rohrbaugh (1975)	CS	C	475/221	HS/CS	Colorado	#8 ORA,RB,RE	P	NONE	6
Scholl (1964)	CC	C	52 vs. 28 Cs	Ad delinquents	Illinois	#4+ RB,RE	NG	NONE	2
Sloane (1986)	CS	R	1121	HS	National US	#2 ORA,SR	P	MC	9
Smith P (1956)	CS,D	C	50	Inmates	Michigan	#15 CM,ORA,NORA,RB	–	–	1
Stark (1982)	CS	R	1799	white boys	National US	#6 RB,SR,ORA	P	NONE	8
Stark (1996)	CS	R	11955	Ad	National US	#2 D,ORA	P	SC	9
*Wallace, J (1998)	CS	R	5000	HS	National US	#3 D,ORA,SR	P	MC	9
Wattenburg (1950)	CS	S	2137	Delinquent boys	Detroit, MI	#1 ORA	P	NONE (?)	6
*Wickstrom (1983)	CS	C	130	CS (Christian)	4 states	#2 IR,ER	P	MC	5
Wright (1971)	CS	C	3850–1574	CS	England	#3+ RB,ORA,Misc	P	–	6
Zhang (1994)	CS	C	1026	CS in China, Taiwan, & US		#7 SR,NORA,ORA,RE	P	MC	7

Marital Instability (Ch 13)

Study	Design	Method	Population	N	Location	Religious variables	Findings	Controls	Rating
Albrecht (1979)	CS	C	CDA (ever divorced)	500	8 western states	#2 D,ORA, homogamy	P	MC	6
Bahr (1988)	CS	—	CDA	698	Middletown, IN	#2 D,ORA	P	NONE	5
Bell (1974)	CS,D	C	CDA,F,married	2374 and 1442	US & Australia	#1 ORA	P	NONE	7
Booth (1995)	PC	R	CDA married	1008	National US	#4 ORA,NORA,SR	P (divorce)	MC	7
Brutz (1986)	CS	C	Quaker spouses	290	Lake Erie	#4 ORA,SR	M (violence)	NONE	6
Bumpass (1972)	CS	R	CDA,F	5442	National US	#1 D (heterog vs. homogamy)	P(heter > hom)	MC	8
Burchinal (1957)	CS	R	CDA	256 couples	Midwest US	#28 ORA,CM,Misc	P	NONE	6
Butler (1998)	Q	C	relig couples	–	Provo, UT	#1 prayer therapy	(P)	–	6
Call (1997)	CS	R	CDA	4587 couples	National US	#3 D,ORA,RB	P	MC	10
D'Antonio (1982)	SR		review of 76 sociology texts 1951–1980 concerning mention of religion related to marriage and family						
Dudley M (1990)	CS	C	CDA (SDA)	228	IL, IN, MI, WI	#>35 ORA,NORA,IR	P	MC	6
Ellis A (1948)	R,O		claims conventional persons (high religion) are more likely to lie about questions related to marriage						
Ellison CG (1994)[a]	CS	R	CDA,B	1975	National US	#2+ ORA	P	MC	8
Ellison CG (1999)	CS	R	CDA	4662	National US	#3 D,RB,ORA	M (domestic abuse)	MC	9
Filsinger (1984)	CS	C	marital dyads	208	Arizona	#37 scale	P	MC	6
Glenn (1978)	CS	R	CDA	2278	National US	#1 ORA	P	MC	7
Glenn (1982)	CS	R	CDA	1552–5433	National US	#1 D,ORA	P (males)	MC	8
Glenn (1984)	CS	R	CDA	8952	National US	#2 D,ORA	P	MC	8
Gruner (1985)	CS	C	CM,married	416	Los Angeles	#1 RC (prayer,Bible)	P	NONE	6
Hansen (1987)	CS	C	CS,married	220	Kentucky	#3 ORA,SR	P (women)	SC	7
Hansen (1992)	R		reviews research on religiosity and adjustment to marriage (& of marital conventionalization and social desirability argument)						
Heaton (1984)	CS	R	CDA	>1500	National US	#2 D,ORA	P (ORA)	SC	7
Heaton (1990)	CS	R	CDA	12,000	National US	#2+ ORA, R-homogamy	P	SC	8
Hunt (1978)	CS	C	married couples	64	Dallas, TX	#50 + (17 measures of R)	P	SC-sex	6
Johnson M (1973)	CS	—	CS	453	California	#61 ORA,SR,RV	P	NONE	6
Kaslow (1996)	CS,D	C	CDA	57 couples	9 states in US	#1 rlg convictions 3rd most common reason for staying together			5
Kunz (1977)	CS	R	married couples	803	Utah	#1 ORA	P	NONE	7
Larson L (1989)	CS	R	married couples	179	Edmonton, Can	#3 ORA,D,R homogamy	P	MC	8
Lehrer (1993)	CS	R	first marriages	3060	National US	#1 R homogamy	P	MC	8

a. Ellison & George

547

Outcome/Investigators	Type	Method	N	Population	Location	Religious Variable	Findings	Controls	Rating
McCarthy (1979)	CS	R	9797	CDA,F	National US	#2 D,ORA	P	SC	7
Ortega (1988)	CS	S	1070	CDA (Ca & P)	Nebraska	#1 D	NA(heter = hom)	SC	6
*Pollner (1989)	CS	R	3072	CDA	National US	#7 ORA,NORA,RE	P	MC	8
Robinson L (1993,1994)	Q	C	15	couples	Southeast US	explores factors related to enduring marriages			3
Roth (1988)	CS	C	147	couples, CM	Southern CA	#10 RWB	P	NONE	5
Schumm (1982)	CS	R	184	couples	Kansas	#2 SR	P	SC	7
Shehan (1990)	CS	R	1753	CDA	National US	#2 ORA,D	P (esp Catholics)	MC	8
Shrum (1980)	CS	R	7029	CDA	National US	#2 ORA,D	P	MC	9
Sporakowski (1978)	CS, D	C	40 couples, CDA, mean age > 75		Virginia	R most important factor in happy marriage (women)		NONE	5
*Strayhorn (1990)	CS	C	201 parents of Head Start kids		Pittsburgh	#12 ORA,NORA	P (parental practices)	NONE	5
*Truett (1992)	CS	C	7620 twins	CDA	Australia	#2 D,ORA	P	SC (factor)	9
*Weisner (1991)	CS	C	102	fam, MR child	Los Angeles	#8+ ORA,SR,RC	P	NONE	7
Wilson M (1986)	CS	C	190	couples	Southwest US	#37 scale	P	MC	6
Wilson J (1996)	CS	R	5648	CDA	National US	#2+ ORA,D	P	MC	9
Wineberg (1994)	CS	R	506	F,W,CDA	National US	#2 ORA,R homogamy	P	MC	9
*Zautra (1977)	CS	R	454	CDA	Salt Lake City	#1 relig participation	P	SC	6

Personality (Ch 14)

Authoritarianism

Outcome/Investigators	Type	Method	N	Population	Location	Religious Variable	Findings	Controls	Rating
Adorno (1950)	R,D		examines measurement of authoritarianism; includes a description of his widely used scale						
Brown L (1962)	CS	C	203	CS	Australia	#5+ RB	NG	factor analysis	4
Brown L (1966)	CS	C	227	CS	New Zealand	#8+ RB,ORA,D,SR	NA	factor analysis	5
*Fehr (1977)	CS	C	120	CS	Cincinnati, OH	#10+ rlg values,O	NG (O)	NONE	4
Gregory (1957)	CS	C	596	90% CS	California	#? RB,O	NG	NONE	6
*Hassan (1981)	CS	R	480	CS (Mus/Hin)	India	#10 religiosity scale	NG	NONE	6
Jones MB (1958)	CS	C	786	naval cadets	Pensacola, FL	#6+ A-V scale	NG	NONE	4
Kahoe (1974)	CS	C	518	CS (religious)	Midwest US	#20 IR,ER	NG (ER)	NONE	5
Putney (1961)	CS	C	1126	CS	Eastern US	#16 O, RB, SR	NG	NONE	6
Weima (1965)	CS	C	67/101	CM,CS	Utrecht	#17 conservatism scale	NG	NONE	3

Cooperativeness									
*Koenig (1998)[a]	CS	S	577	MP, E	Durham, NC	#69RC,ORA,NORA,SR	P	MC	8
Type A behavior									
Catipovic (1995)	CS	C	1084 employees	CDA	Croatia	#2 ORA,RB	NA	NONE	5
Levin (1988)[b]	PC	C	408	air-traffic controllers, 100%M		#3 ORA,D	M	SC	7
Perfectionism									
Richards P (1993)	CT	C	15	CS (Mormon)	Provo, UT	#1 relig/spiritual intervention	P	(no controls)	4
Hostility									
*Acklin (1983)	CC	C	26 vs. 18 Cs	MP (recurrent CA)	Atlanta, GA	#22 IR/ER,ORA	P	NONE	5
Bateman (1958)	CS	C	51/33	CS	Topeka, KS	#? religious background	C	NONE	4
*Carlson (1988)	CT	C	36 randomized	CS (Christian)	Chicago	"devotional meditation"	P	–	6
*Heinzelman (1976)	CS	C	82	CS	Cincinnati, OH	#? relig orthodoxy scale	P	NONE	4
*Hertsgaard (1984)	CS	R	760	CDA,F,farms	North Dakota	#2 D, ORA	NA	MC	7
*Kark (1996)[c]	CS	S	437	CDA	Israel	relig vs. secular kibbutzim	P	SC	8
*Plante (1992)	CS	C	86	CS	Santa Clara, CA	#2 SR, D	NA	NONE	5
*Strayhorn (1990)	CS	C	201 parents of Head Start kids		Pittsburgh	#12 ORA, NORA	P	NONE	5
Social Order									
Martin-Baro (1990)	R,O					review and discussion of the influence of evangelicals and Catholic charismatics on social order in El Salvador			
Alienation									
Fountain (1986)	CS	C	108	CDA,E	MI, IN, FL	# many, incl ORA,RE	P (ORA)	SC	4

a. Koenig, Pargament, & Nielsen b. Levin, Jenkins, et al. c. Kark, Carmel, et al.

Outcome/Investigators	Type	Method	N	Population	Location	Religious Variable	Findings	Controls	Rating
Guilt (nonsexual)									
*Baker (1982)	CS	C	52	CS (?)	Southern CA	#20 IR,ER	NA	NONE	4
*Bohannon (1991)	CS	C	272	Bereaved parents	Midwest US	#2 D, ORA	P	SC	6
Quiles (1997)	CS	C	101	CS	Boston	#2+ ORA,SR	NG (predispositional guilt)	–	5
Demaria (1988)	–	–	–	–		–	NG	–	
*Lund (1989)	PC	C	190	CDA, E	Utah	#3+ CM, SR, RB	P	NONE	6
*Steketee (1991)	CC	C	33	PP (OCD)	Boston	#2 SR,D	NG (SR)	NONE	5
*Watson P (1989)	CS	C	1397	CS	Tennessee	#20 IR,ER	NG (IR)	NONE	6
Altruism/Humanitarianism									
Annis (1976)	CT	C	71	CS	Mississippi	#>20 RB,ORA,NORA	NA	NONE	6
Batson (1976)	Exp	C	42	CS	Princeton, NJ	#59 IR,ER	P (IR)	NONE	6
Batson 1981	Exp	C	60	CS	Kansas	#20+ IR,ER	NG (IR egoist)	NONE	4
Batson 1989	Exp	C	46 and 60	CS	Kansas	#20+ IR,ER,O,Q,Misc	P (Q only)	NONE	5
Batson 1990	Exp	C	38	CS,F	Kansas	#20+ IR,ER,O,Misc	NG (IR egoist)	NONE	4
Benson P (1980)	CS	C	134	CS	Midwest US	#20+ IR,ORA,SR	P	MC	6
Bernt (1989)	CS	C	178	CS (Catholic)	Pennsylvania	#20+ IR,ER,Q	P (IR)	NONE	5
Cline (1965)	CS	R	155	CDA	Salt Lake, UT	#39 ORA,NORA,RB	NA	NONE	5
Darley (1973)	Exp	C	40	CS	Princeton, NJ	#25 RB,O	NA	–	4
*Fehr (1977)	CS	C	120	CS	Cincinnati,OH	#10+ rlg values,O	P (RV)	NONE	4
Hunsberger (1987)	CS	C	105 and 295	CS	Ontario, Can	#? IR,O scales	P	NONE	5
Leivers (1986)	CS	C	316	NH	W. Australia	#1 relig vs. non-R homes	P	NONE	4
*Moberg (1984)	CS	C	1081	CDA	US & Sweden	#45 SWB scale	P	NONE	6
Nelson LD (1976)	CS	R	663	CDA	Southwest US	#5 ORA,NORA,SR	P	MC	8
Okun (1993)	CS	R	400	CDA, E	Sun City, AZ	#4 ORA, NORA, SR	P	MC	7
Smith R (1975)	Exp	C	402	CS	Washington St	#1 RB	NA	–	5
Watson P (1984)	CS	C	180	CS	Tennessee	#20 IR,ER	P	SC	6
Forgiveness									
Gorsuch (1993)	CS	R	1030	CDA	National US	#15 SR,Misc	P (SR)	SC	7

Study			N		Location				
Cooperativeness									
Ellison CG (1992)	CS	R	2107	CDA,B	National US	#5+ RB,NORA,SR	P	MC	8
*Koenig (1998)[a]	CS	S	577	MP,E	Durham, NC	#69 RC,ORA,NORA,SR	P	MC	8
Prejudice									
Allport (1967)	CS	C	309	CM	Maine, New York, South Carolina, Pennsylvania	#22 D,IR,ORA	M	SC	6
*Batson (1976)	Exp	C	42	CS	Princeton, NJ	#59 IR,ER	P (IR)	NONE	6
Batson (1978)	CS	C	51	CS	Kansas	#30+ IR,ER,O,Q	P (Quest)	SC	6
*Donahue (1985)	R	reviews research on intrinsic/extrinsic religiosity and prejudice							
Hoge (1973)	CS	C	858	CDA,CM	North/South US	#16+ IR,O,NORA, Misc	M	SC	6
Strickland (1971)	CS	C	93	CM & youth	Atlanta, GA	#20 IR,ER	NA (IR)	NONE	4
*Weima (1965)	CS	C	67/101	CM,CS	Utrecht	#? conservatism scale	NG	NONE	3
Dogmatism									
*Donahue (1985)	R	reviews research on intrinsic/extrinsic religiosity and dogmatism							
*Kahoe (1974)	CS	C	518	CS (religious)	Midwest US	#20 IR,ER	NG (ER)	NONE	5
*Strickland (1971)	CS	C	93	CM & youth	Atlanta, GA	#20 IR,ER	NG (IR)	NONE	4
Swindell (1970)	CS	C	135	CS	Georgia	#74 RB,Misc	NG	NONE	4
Locus of Control									
*Benson P (1973)	CS	C	128	HS, 100%M	Michigan	#12 RB,ORA,NORA	P	MC	5
Jackson (1988)	CS	C	98	CM,B	Washington, DC	#13+ IR,RB,ORA	P	SC	5
*Kahoe (1974)	CS	C	518	CS (religious)	Midwest US	#20 IR,ER	P (IR)	NONE	5
Kivett (1979)	CS	C	301	CDA, CM, E	North Carolina	#10 IR	P	MC	7
Levin (1986)[b]	CS	–	909	CDA	Appalachians	#2 D,CM	C	NONE	7
Loewenthal (1993)	CS	C	74	CDA	SE England	#5 ORA,NORA,RB	C	God control—health events only	5
*Richards D (1990)	CS	C	292	CDA	United States	#8 universal force	P	NA	3
Shrauger (1971)	CS	C	465	CS	Buffalo, NY	#2 ORA, D	P (females only)	NONE	5
*Strayhorn (1990)	CS	C	201 parents of Head Start kids	CS (Christian)	Pittsburgh	#12 ORA, NORA	NA	NONE	5
*Sturgeon (1979)	CS	C	144		Tennessee	#20 IR,ER	P	NONE	6
Wolinsky (1996)	CS	S	1051	MP	Indiana	#3+ D,SR,RB	P	MC	9

a. Koenig, Pargament, & Nielsen   b. Levin & Schiller

Outcome/Investigators	Type	Method	N	Population	Location	Religious Variable	Findings	Controls	Rating
Social Desirability									
Batson (1978)	CS	C	51	CS	Kansas	#30+ IR,ER,O	P (IR & O only)	NONE	5
Hunsberger (1982)	CS	C	3 different surveys	CS	Ontario, Can	responses to rlg Q's unrelated to clergy vs. secular administration			6
Stewin (1974)	CS	C	107	HS	Alberta, Can	#22 ORA,IR,ER	P (ER only)	SC (factor analysis)	6
Trimble DE (1997)	R		meta-analysis of correlation between IR/ER and social desirability (minimal correlation)						
General Personality									
Bergin (1987)	CS	C	151	Mormon CS	Utah	#20 IR,ER	P	NONE	4
Bergin (1988)	CS	C	60	Mormon CS	Utah	religious development	P	NONE	4
Bohrnstedt (1968)	CS	R	3700	CS	Wisconsin	#6 conventional relig	P	SC-sex	6
Broen (1955)	CS	C	140	CS	Minnesota	#3+ RB (attitudes)	M	NONE	4
Brown DG (1951)	CS	C	622/58/34	CS	Denver	#16 RB,D	M	NONE	5
*Brown L (1962)	CS	C	203	CS	Australia	#5+ RB	NG	factor analysis	4
*Brown L (1966)	CS	C	227	CS	New Zealand	#8+ RB,ORA,D,SR	NA	factor analysis	5
Costa (1981)	PC	C	557	CDA,M	Baltimore	#7 Misc scale	P (neuroticism)	NONE	7
Dittes (1969)	R		religious experience associated with psychopathology						
*Donahue (1995)	R		reviews research on personality and religion in adolescents						
Dreger (1952)	CS	C	60	CDA	Southern CA	relg conserv vs. liberals	C	NONE	3
Dunn (1965)	R,O		religious persons have dysfunctional personalities						
*Francis LJ (1992)	CS	S	50	PP,F (addicts)	Great Britain	#>27 RB scale	P(psychoticism)	NONE	4
*Hassan (1981)	CS	R	480	CS (Muslims/Hindus)	India	#10 religiosity scale	NG	NONE	6
Hood (1975)	CS	C	300	CS	Tennessee	#32 mysticism scale	NG	NONE	6
Kahoe (1974)	CS	C	518	CS (religious)	Midwest US	#20 IR,ER	P (IR)	NONE	5
*Kaldestad (1995,1996)	CS	C	79/392	PP/CDA	Norway	#26 IR,ER,Q	P (IR), NG (ER,Q)	MC	6
Keene (1967)	CS	C	250	CDA	Tulsa/Chicago	#35 SR,ORA,ORA,IR	NA	NONE	5
Koenig (1990)[a]	PC	C	100	CDA, E	Durham, NC	#1 RC	P	MC	7
Lovekin (1977)	PC	C	51	CM, students	New Mexico	Glossolalia	NA	–	6
Martin C (1962)	CS	C	104	CS, F	Indiana	#96 RB,misc	NG	SC	4
Mayo (1969)	CS	C	166	CS	Texas	#2 SR,D	M	NONE	5

Investigators	Type		N	Population	Location	Religious variable	Findings	Controls	Rating
*Putney (1961)	CS	C	1126	CS	Eastern US	#16 O, RB, SR	C	NONE	6
Pyron (1961)	CS	C	128	unknown	Wisconsin	#>1 D,AV relig subscale	NG	NONE	3
Richek (1970)	CS,D	C	166	CS	Texas	#? MMPI rlg subscale	M	NONE	2
Sanua (1969)	R					reviews research on the relationship between religion and mental health and personality	M	NONE	
Schmidt (1988)	CS	C	191	Ad	Kentucky	Christian students vs. others	P	NONE	4
Strunk O (1959)	CS	C	60 vs. 50	CS	W. Virginia	Divinity vs. business	M	NONE	3
Tennison (1968)	CS	C	299	CS (Protestant)	Ohio	multiple items	NG	NONE	5
Wiebe (1980)	CS	C	158	CS	Canada	#21 IR,ER,D	M	NONE	5
Wilson WP (1972)	CS,D	C	63	CDA (converts)	North Carolina	multiple items	–	–	4
Wilson W (1967)	CS	C	164	CS	Hawaii	#53 ORA,RB, Misc	M	NONE	4

General Mental Health (Ch 15)

Investigators	Type		N	Population	Location	Religious variable	Findings	Controls	Rating
Bergin (1983)	R					reviews results from 24 studies (19 in college students) of religion and mental health (47% of studies with positive findings)			
Carr (1981)	CS	R	219	CDA	Midwestern US	#2 ORA,D	NA	NONE	5
Carson (1992)	CS	C	100	HIV+/AIDS	Baltimore	#20 SWB (EWB, RWB)	P	NONE	6
Carson (1993)	CS	C	100	HIV+/AIDS	Baltimore	#5+ ORA,NORA	P	NONE	6
Crawford (1989)	CS	C	226	CDA	Midwest, SE US	#5 SR	P	NONE	5
Fein (1958)	CS	C	136	CDA,PP,F	Connecticut	#2 RBackground	–	–	4
Epstein (1985)	CS	C	234	HS age 18	Israel	#1 rlg observ vs. secular	NA	NONE	4
Galanter (1978)	CS	C	119	119 Divine Light initiates	United States	#1 conversion	P		5
Galanter (1979)	CS	C	237	237 Unification Church	United States	#1 conversion	(P)	–	5
Galanter (1982b)	R	R				examines effects of charismatic religious sects on mental health			
Galanter (1990)	R	R				compares sect members to self-help groups like AA			
Gartner (1990)	SR	R				religious research in pastoral care journals			
Gartner (1991)	SR	R				religious commitment & mental health			
Griffith (1984)[b]	CS,D	C	13	CM,F,B	Barbados	#1 "mourning"	(P)	–	5
Griffith (1984)[c]	CS,D	C	20	CM,B	Washington, DC	RE in church	(P)	–	5
Handal (1989)	CS	C	114	CDA,B,F	St. Louis, MO	#5 religiosity scale	P	–	4
*Hannay (1980)	CS	R	964	CDA	Scotland	#2 D,ORA	P	SC-age,sex	7
Hathaway (1990)	CS	C	108	CDA,CM	Midwest US	#50+ IR,RC	P	MC	5
Hood (1974)	CS	C	82	CS	Tennessee	#15 RE	P	NONE	5
Katchadourian (1974)	CC	R		psychiatric illness in CDA	Lebanon	Christians vs. Muslims	Christians > Mus	NONE	1
Kelley (1958)	CC	R		women religious	National US	women relig vs. others	P	NONE	6

a. Koenig, Siegler, et al.   b. Griffith, Mahy, et al.   c. Griffith, Young, et al.

Outcome/Investigators	Type	Method	N	Population	Location	Religious Variable	Findings	Controls	Rating
King Mi (1994)	PC	S	300	MP (inpatients)	London, England	#10+ RB,SR,RC	NG (RB)	MC	7
Koenig (1990)	R	reviews research examining the relationship between religion and mental health in later life							
Koenig (1998a)	R	edited book that reviews research on religion and mental health and discusses clinical implications for different world religions							
Larson DB (1986)	SR	systematic review of research in 4 major psychiatric journals between 1978 and 1982							
Larson DB (1989)[a]	R	systematic review that compares the percentages of specific religious affiliations represented in study populations in MH research							
Larson DB (1992)	R	systematic review of religious research published in 2 major psychiatric journals between 1978 and 1989; 72% positive results							
*Lindenthal (1970)	CS	R	938	CDA	New Haven, CT	#3 ORA, NORA, D	M	NONE	7
Lowis (1997)	CT	C	–	E	United Kingdom	#1 sacred vs. secular music	NA (ego integrity) 5		
MacDonald (1983)	CS, D	S	7050	PP (outpatients)	Midwest US	#1 D	C	NONE	6
McAllister (1961)	CC	C	100 vs. lay Cs	PP Catholic R	Baltimore	#1 D	NG	NONE	2
McAllister (1965)	CC	C	200 vs. lay Cs	PP Catholic R	Baltimore	#1 D	NG	NONE	2
McAllister (1969)	R	discusses mental health of clergy based primarily on his 1961 and 1965 studies							
Moore T (1936)	CS	R	600000	Catholic clergy	National US	#1 (clergy vs. non-clergy)	P	NONE	6
Ness (1980)[b]	PC	C	51	Pentecostal CM	Newfoundland	#6 religious activities	P	SC	6
Panton (1979)	CC	C	117 vs. Cs	prisoners	Raleigh, NC	#12 MMPI scale	P	NONE	6
Pargament (1979)	CS	C	133	CDA, CM	Washington, DC	#11 ORA, IR	M	SC	6
Payne (1991)	R	review of literature on religion and well-being, self-esteem, family, substance abuse, suicide, & mental illness							
*Plante (1992)	CS	C	86	CS	Santa Clara, CA	#2 SR, D	NG	NONE	5
Sharkey (1986)	CS	S	440	PP	New York	#1 atheists vs. believers	(P)	NONE	6
Sheehan (1990)	CS, D	S	52	PP	Minnesota	#1 sin as cause of illness	23% yes, 19% need penance	NONE	7
Sherrill (1993)	SR	systematic review of research on religion and mental health in three gerontology journals							
Srole (1962)	CS	R	1660	CDA	Manhattan, NY	#3 D,ORA,RB	P	SC-age,SES	7
Stark (1971)	R	review of the research on religion and mental illness by an outstanding scholar							
Tjeltveit (1996)	CS	C	100	CS	Pennsylvania	#80 ORA,RB,NORA	P	NONE	4
Wright (1959)	CS	C	310	CS	Depauw Univ, Indiana	#50 religious attitudes	M	NONE	5

a. Larson, Donahue, et al. b. Ness & Weintrob

Outcome/Investigators	Type	Method	N	Population	Location	Religious Variable	Findings	Controls	Rating
Heart Disease (Ch 16)									
Alexander (1994)[a]	R		reviews the research concerning transcendental meditation and cardiovascular risk factors						
Brown R (1967)	CC	S	133 vs. Cs	MP w/o hrt dis	Portland, OR	#1 (affiliation vs. none)	NA	NONE	4
Burell (1996)	CT	S	128 vs. Cs	MP-CABG	Sweden	#1 "reflect spiritual issues"	P	–	9
Byrd (1988)	CT	S	393 (randomized)	MP-CCU	San Francisco	"intercessory prayer"	P	–	7
Comstock (1971)	CC	R	189 ASCVD deaths + CS		Maryland	#1 ORA	P	SC	7
Dreyfuss (1953)	CC	S	412	MP-MI	Israel	#1 D	Ashkenazi > Oriental Js		6
Epstein (1955)	CS	R	904	CDA	New York	#1 D (Jews vs. non-J)	Jews > non-J	SC-age,sex	7
Epstein (1957)	CS	R	1275+ (garment)	CDA	New York	#1 D (Jews vs. Italians)	Jews > Italians	SC-age,sex	7
Friedlander (1986)	CC	–	539 vs. Cs	MP (first MI)	Israel	#1 orthodox vs. secular Js	P	MC	8
Friedman (1968)	CS	S	2342	Attorneys	Cleveland/Detroit	#1 D (Jews vs. non-Jews)	Jews > non-J	NONE	6
Goldbourt (1993)	PC	R	10,059	CDA,M	Israel	#3 orthodox vs. secular Js	P (MI death)	MC	10
Gupta (1996)	CS	–	–	CDA	Urban India	#1 prayer & yoga	NA	–	–
Gupta (1997)	CS	R	3148	CDA	Rural India	#1 prayer & yoga	P	MC	9
Jarvis (1977)	CC	R	1169 deaths	CDA, Mormons	Canada	#1 D (Mormon vs. non-M)	non-M > Morm	SC	6
Kaplan B (1976)	R		reviews associations mainly between religious affiliation and CAD						
Kowey (1986)	CR		describes a prayer-meeting cardioversion in a patient (atrial fibrillation to normal sinus rhythm)						
Lasater (1986)	D		describes project in which church volunteers deliver behavior change program for major cardiovascular risk factors						
Lehr I (1973)	PC	C/S	679 industrial employees		San Francisco	#2 parental affiliation	M	MC	7
Lemon (1964)	CC	R	47866	CDA	California	#1 D (SDA vs. non-SDA)	non-SDA > SDA	SC-age,sex	7
Leserman (1989)	CT	C	27 cardiac surgery patients		Boston, MA	Relaxation Response	P	–	6
Lyon (1978)	CC	S	6108	CHD deaths	Utah	#1D (non-Mormon vs. M)	Non-M > Morm	SC	7
Medalie (1973)	PC	S	10000	CDA,100%M	Israel	#3 orthodox vs. secular Js	P	SC	6

a. Alexander, Robinson, Orme-Johnson, et al.

Outcome/Investigators	Type	Method	N	Population	Location	Religious Variable	Findings	Controls	Rating
Oxman (1995)	PC	S	232	MP (open-heart surgery)	New Hampshire	#3 ORA, SR, RC	P (RC)	MC	9
Phillips (1978)	PC	R	24044	CDA	California	#1 D (SDA vs. non-SDA)	non-SDA > SDA	–	6
Phillips (1980)[a]	PC/CC	R	22940 vs. Cs	CDA	California	#1 D (SDA vs. non-SDA)	non-SDA > SDA	SC-age,sex	7
Reyes-Ortiz (1997)	R	reviews some of research concerning religion and cardiovascular disease							
Ross (1965)	CS	S	1272	Parents/medical students	Baltimore, MD	#1 D	J > Ca,P (men)	NONE	6
Skyring (1963)	CC	R	413 deaths	CDA	Baltimore	#1 D (Ca vs. Prot)	Ca = Prot	NONE	2
Thoresen (1990)	CT	–	–	CDA	California	Spiritual intervention	P	–	–
Wardwell (1963)	CC	C	32 vs. Cs	MP	Connecticut	#1 D (Ca vs. Prot)	Prot > Ca	SC-age,sex, race	3
Wardwell (1964)	CC	C	87/16 vs. Cs	MP	Connecticut	#1 D (Ca vs. Prot)	Prot > Ca	SC-age,sex, race	5
Wardwell (1968)	CC	C	87 vs. Cs	MP	Connecticut	#1 D parents (both Ca)	P	SC-age,sex, race	5
Wardwell (1973)	CC	C	114 vs. Cs	MP	Connecticut	#1 D (Ca vs. Prot,J)	Ca > Prot,J	SC-age	5
Watson JS (1991)	CS	S	24 countries	IHD mortality	World	#1 D (% Catholic)	Others > Ca	NONE	5
Winkelstein (1969)	CC	S	123	MP,W,F,E	Buffalo, NY	#1 D (Ca vs. Prot vs. J)	Prot = Ca = J	NONE	2
Yelsma (1990)	CS	C	55	MP & spouses	Michigan	#3+ RC	NA	NONE	4
Zamarra (1996)	CT	C	21	MP with CAD	Buffalo, NY	#1 Transcendental Med	P	–	7
Cholesterol/Hypercholesterolemia									
Barrow (1960)	CS	C	80 and 70	Trappist & Benedictine monks (compared)			–	–	5
Cooper (1978,1979)	CT	C	12 vs. 11 Cs	Hypercholesterolemia		#1 Transcendental Med	P	–	5
Epstein (1956)[b]	CS	C	416 (garment workers)	CDA (chol/cad)	New York City	#1 D (Jew vs. Italian)	Jews > Italians	SC-sex	6
*Epstein (1957)	CS	R	1275+ (garment)	CDA	New York	#1 D (Jews vs. Italians)	Jews > Italians	SC-age,sex	7
Fonnebo (1992b)	CS	C	222 vs. Cs	CDA	Norway	#1 D (SDA vs. non-SDA)	non-SDA > SDA	SC	6
Friedlander (1987)	CS	R	673	Ad	Israel	#7 D,SR	P	MC	8

Study	Design		N	Group	Measure	Location	Hypothesis	Result	Comparison	Control	Score
Glick (1998)	CC	S	223 vs. 12275 Cs	Mennonites	MP	New York			Others > Mennon (men only)		8
Groen (1959)	R	review of religious affiliation effects on diet and cholesterol level; Jews higher cholesterol due to diet									—
Patel (1977)	CT	C	—		MP	—	#1 Transcendental Med	P			—
Schaefer (1953)	CS	S	500		MP	New York	#1 D [Jew vs. non-J]	no statistics	Jew > non-J		4
Torrington (1981)	CC	C	26 vs. Cs		MP	South Africa	#1 D (Dutch Reformed)	—	Dut Ref > Others		6
Walden (1964)	CC	C	145 vs. Cs		CDA	California	#1 D (SDA vs. non-SDA)		Others > SDA	SC	5
Webster (1979)	CC	C	779 vs. Cs		CDA	Australia	#1 D (SDA vs. non-SDA)		non-SDA > SDA	SC-age	7
West (1968)	CC	C	3260 vs. Cs		CDA	Washington, DC	#1 D (SDA vs. non-SDA)		non-SDA > SDA	SC-age	5

Hypertension (Ch 17)

Study	Design		N	Group	Measure	Location	Hypothesis	Result	Comparison	Control	Score
Armstrong (1977)	CC	C	418 vs. Cs		CDA	Australia	#1 (SDA vs. non-SDA)		non-SDA > SDA	MC	7
Alexander (1996)	CT	analysis by gender for Schneider et al (1995) study below					#1 Transcendental Med	P	—	—	10
Benson H (1977)	R	reviews effects of Relaxation Response on blood pressure									—
*Beutler (1988)	CT	C	120 (40 each group)		CDA	Netherlands	laying hands, thought projection	NA	—	—	9
Blackwell (1976)	CT	C	7		MP	—	#1 Transcendental Med	(P)	—	—	—
*Brown D (1994)	CS	S	537		CDA,B,M	Norfolk, VA	#12 relig scale, ORA,D	NA	—	MC	8
Caudill (1987)	R	reviews effects of relaxation therapy (4 studies) & relaxation response (2 studies) on blood pressure									—
*Fonnebo (1992b)	CS	C	222 vs. Cs		CDA	Norway	#1 D (SDA vs. non-SDA)		non-SDA > SDA	SC	6
Graham (1978)	CS	R	355		CDA,W,M	Georgia	#1 ORA	P		MC	7
Hafner (1982)	CT	C	21		MP	—	#1 meditation	NA	—	—	—
Hixson (1998)	CS	C	112		CDA,F	North Carolina	#3+ RC,RE,IR	P		SC	6
Hutchinson (1986)	CS	R	357		CDA	West Indies	#1 ORA	P		SC	6
*Koenig (1988)[c]	CS	S	106		MP,E	Illinois	#15+ ORA,NORA,IR	(P)		SC-sex	6
Koenig (1998a)[d]	PC	R	4000		CDA, E	North Carolina	#4 D, ORA, NORA	P		MC	9
Kong (1982)	D	describes experience of creating high blood pressure control centers in churches									—
Kumanyika (1992)	D/CT	C	188		CM, 100%B,F	Baltimore	church-based wt loss	P		—	7

a. Phillips, Kuzma, et al.   b. Epstein, Simpson, et al.   c. Koenig, Moberg, & Kvale   d. Koenig, George, Cohen, et al.

Outcome/Investigators	Type	Method	N	Population	Location	Religious Variable	Findings	Controls	Rating
Lapane (1997)	CS	R	5145	CDA	Rhode Island	#1 church membership	P	MC	8
Larson DB (1989)[a]	CS	S	401	CDA,M	Georgia	#2 ORA, SR	P	MC	7
*Leserman (1989)	CT	C	27 cardiac surgery patients		Boston	#1 relaxation response	NA	–	7
*Levin (1985)	CS	R	1125	CDA-Mex-Am	Texas	#2 ORA,SR	NG (with SR)	NONE	6
Levin (1989)	R		reviews seven blood pressure studies conducted between 1960 and 1987 that relate to religion						
Livingston (1991)	CS	R	1420	CDA,B	Maryland	#1 church affiliation	P	MC	8
McCullagh (1960)	D	S	44	monks	KY, MA	cholesterol (low) & hypertension (high)		–	2
Merritt (2000)	Exp	C	74	CDA,B,young	Durham, NC	#5 ORA,NORA,IR	P	SC	8
Miller RN (1982)	CT	C	96	MP	–	#1 healing prayers-distant	P	–	6
Patel (1975)	CT	C	34	MP	England	#1 Yoga	P	–	8
Patel (1976)	CT	C	27	MP	England	#1 Yoga (Shavasan)	P	–	7
Pollack (1977)	CT	C	20	MP	New York City	#1 Transcendental Meditation	NA	–	7
*Ross (1965)	CS	S	1272	Parents/medical students	Baltimore, MD	#1 D	J = Ca = P	NONE	6
Rouse (1982)	CS	C	293	CDA	West Australia	#1 D (Mormons vs. SDA)	Morm > SDA	SC	6
Saunders (1983)	D		describes experience of creating high blood pressure control centers in Black churches and why effective						
Schneider (1995)	CT	C	111	CDA,B,E	Oakland, CA	#1 Transcendental Meditation	P	–	10
Scotch (1963)	CS	R	1053	CDA	South Africa	#2 ORA, CM	P	SC	7
Stavig (1984)	CS	R	1757	CDA-Asians	California	#1 (affiliation vs. none)	P	MC	8
Steffen (2000)	CS	–	–	CDA	North Carolina	#1+ RC (from COPE)	P	MC	7
Sudsuang (1991)	CT	C	52	M (ages 20–25)	Thailand	#1 Buddhist meditation	P	–	7
Timio (1988)	PC/CC	S	144 vs. Cs	R (Ca nuns)	Italy	#1 Ca nuns vs. other	P	MC	10
Walsh (1980)	CS	C	75	immigrants	Ohio	#1 ORA	(P)	MC	6
Walsh (1998)	CS	C	137	immigrants	Toledo, OH	#2 ORA,SR	P	MC	7
*Webster (1979)	CC	C	779 vs. Cs	CDA	Australia	#1 SDA vs. non-SDA	non-SDA > SDA	SC-age	7
Wenneberg (1997)	CT	C	39	CDA,M	Iowa City, IA	#1 Transcendental Meditation	P	–	7

Cerebrovascular Disease (Ch 18)

Study					Location	Findings	Result	Controls	Rating
Abu-Zeid (1975)	PC	R	CDA	700,000	Manitoba, Can	#1 D	Jews > Prot/Cath > Mennonites	SC	6
Colantonio (1992)	PC	R	CDA,E	2812	New Haven, CT	#3 ORA,SR,RC	P (no controls) to NA (MC)		9
*Friedman (1968)	CS	S	Attorneys	2342	Michigan, Ohio	#1 D (Jewish vs. non-J)	n-J > J (fam hx)	NONE	5
*Jarvis (1977)	CC	R	CDA, Mormons	1169 deaths	Canada	#1 D (Mormon vs. non-M)	non-M > Morm	SC	6
Lyon (1981)	CC	R	CDA	2521 deaths	Utah	#1 D (Mormon vs. other)	non-M = Morm	SC	6
*Phillips (1980)[b]	PC/CC	R	CDA	22940 vs. Cs	California	#1 D (SDA vs. non-SDA)	non-SDA > SDA	SC-age,sex	7
Wassersug (1989)	CR	C	86 yo s/p stroke	single case	Massachusetts	#1 RE	(P)	–	–

Brain Functioning

Study					Location	Findings	Result	Controls	Rating
Bear (1977)	CC	C	Temp Lobe Epi	27 TLE vs. Cs	Massachusetts	#? religiousness	NG	SC	6
Bear (1982)	CC	C	MP	10 TLE vs. Cs	Massachusetts	#? religiousness	NG	SC-age,sex	6
d'Aquili (1993)	R		reviews studies of the brain and mystical states						
Dewhurst (1970)	CSer	C	6 TLE		England	religious conversion	(NG)	–	2
Fedio (1986)	R		reviews the behavioral characteristics of persons with Temporal Lobe Epilepsy, particularly with regard to religion						
Herzog (1990–91)	D	C	8 subjects		Regional brain glucose metabolism during Yoga meditation (Germany)				4
Mandel (1980)	R,O	R	provides theoretical basis for a psychobiology of religious/spiritual experience						
Newberg (1998)	R		provides a review and recent update on the neuroscience of religious/spiritual experience						
Ogata (1998)	CS	C/S	MP (epileptics)	234	Japan	#2 D, RE	C (seizures)	–	7
Persinger (1984)	CS	C	CS	150 (2 studies)	Ontario, Can	#2 ORA, RE	associated with temporal lobe activation	–	3
Persinger (1987)	R,O		examines the neuropsychological basis for God beliefs						
Ramachandran (1997)	Exp	C	MP	3 TLE vs. Cs	San Diego, CA	religious words	increased galvanic skin response	–	4
Sensky (1984)	CS	S	MP	137 (29 w TLE)	London, England	#? ORA, RB, RE	NA (TLE)	–	7
Surwillo (1978)	Exp	C	6 devout Church of God CDA		Louisville, KY	#1 prayer	no change	–	6
Trimble MR (1997)	R		reviews neuropsychiatric symptoms from temporolimbic lobes						
Tucker (1987)	CC	C	MP	76 TLE vs. Cs	Missouri	#12 scale(RB,ORA,RCm)	NA	NONE	7
Waxman (1975)	R,D	C	MP	3 TLE vs. Cs	Boston, MA	religious tendencies	–	–	2

a. Larson, Koenig, et al.   b. Phillips, Kuzma, et al.

Immune System (Ch 19)

Outcome/Investigators	Type	Method	N	Population	Location	Religious Variable	Findings	Controls	Rating
Koenig (1997)[a]	CS,PC	R	1718	CDA,E	North Carolina	#1 ORA	P	MC	8
Lutgendorf (1997)	CS	S	55	CDA,E	Iowa City, IA	#3+ spiritual support	(P)	SC	7
McClelland (1988)	Exp	C	132	CS	Boston, MA	View Mother Teresa film	P	–	7
Schaal (1998)	CS	C/S	112	MP (breast CA)	Stanford, CA	#2+ ORA, SR	P	SC	8
Woods (1999)	CS	C	106	HIV+ gay M	Florida	#4 ORA,NORA	P	SC	7
Neuroendocrine									
Cooper (1985)	CC	C	10 vs. 9 Cs	–	–	#1 Transcendental Meditation	NA (cortisol, etc.)		6
Infante (1998)	CT	C	18 vs. 9 Cs	CDA	Spain	#1 Transcendental Meditation	P (cortisol/ACTH)		6
Jevning (1978)	CT	C	3 groups	–	–	#1 Transcendental Meditation	P (cortisol)	–	6
Jin (1992)	CT	C	96	–	Australia	#1 Tai Chi meditation	P (cortisol,catecholamines)	–	7
Katz (1970)	D	C	30 breast bx	CDA,100%F	New York	greater prayer/faith, lower cortisol	lower cortisol	no statistics	5
MacLean (1997, 1994)	PC	R	–	–	Iowa	#1 Transcendental Meditation	P (cortisol)	–	6
Michaels (1979)	CC	C	–	–	–	#1 Transcendental Meditation	NA (cortisol)	–	–
*Schaal (1998)	CS	C/S	112	MP (breast CA)	Stanford, CA	#2+ ORA, SR	P	SC	8
*Sudsuang (1991)	CT	C	52	M (ages 20–25)	Thailand	#1 Buddhist meditation	P (lower cortisol)	–	7
Walton (1995)	CS	C	22 vs. 33 Cs	CS	Iowa	#1 Transcendental Meditation	P (lower cortisol)	SC (sex)	6
Werner (1986)	PC	C	11	–	–	#1 TM-Sidhi	P (GH,prolactin, TSH)	–	6

Cancer Risk (Ch 20)

Outcome/Investigators	Type	Method	N	Population	Location	Religious Variable	Findings	Controls	Rating
Egan (1996)	CC	R	6611 vs. Cs	Breast CA risk	National US	#1 D (Jewish vs. non-J)	J > non-J	–	8
Fraser (1991)	PC	R	61 of 34198	Lung CA risk	California	#1 D (SDA vs. non-SDA)	non-SDA > SDA	no controls	5

Gardner (1977)	CC	R	867 cases	Cervical CA risk	Utah	#1 D (Mormon vs. non-M)	non-M > Morm	SC-age,sex	7
Jensen O (1983)	CC	S	781 SDA vs. Cs	Cancer risk	Denmark	#1 D (SDA vs. non-SDA)	SDA = non-SDA	smoking/alc	6
Jussawalla (1977)	CC	S	2130 cases	Breast CA risk	Bombay, India	#1 D (Parsis vs. other)	Parsis > other	NONE	4
Kessler (1974)	CC	R	350 cases	Cervical CA risk	Yugoslavia	#2 D,observ of ritual	P	SC	4
Lyon (1994)	PC,CC	S	49182	CA risk	Utah	#1 D (Mormon vs. non-M)	non-M > Morm	SC	8
Massion (1995)	Exp	R	8 women practicing TM experienced significantly lower urinary metabolite of melatonin than eight controls						4
Mayberry (1982)	R	reviews and discusses risk of cancer in different Christian sects							
Naguib (1966)[b]	CS	R	3962	CDA, F	Maryland	#1 ORA	P (abn PAP)	NONE	7
Phillips (1975)	PC	S	100,000	CA risk	California	#1 D (SDA)	non-SDA > SDA	–	6
Reynolds (1990)	PC	R	6848	CDA	Alameda, CA	#2 ORA, CM	NA	MC	9
Toniolo (1996)	PC	S	10,273	Breast CA risk	New York City	#1 D (Jewish vs. non-J)	J > non-J	MC	6
Troyer (1988)	R	reviews relationship between cancer rates in different religious groups							
Steinberg (1998)	CC	S	471 vs. 4025 Cs	Ovarian Ca risk	National US	#1 D (Jewish vs. non-J)	J > non-J	MC	6
Wolbarst (1932)	CC	R	2484	Penile CA risk	US,India,Java	#1 D (Jewish vs. non-J)	non-J > J	–	6

Mortality (Ch 21)

All-Cause Mortality

Abramson (1982)	PC	S	387	E, 100%M	Israel	#1 + "religiosity"	NA	MC	6
Acheson (1994)	CC	S	6623 births	Perinatal	Ohio	#1 D (Amish vs. non-A)	non-A > Amish	–	8
Alexander (1989)	CT	C	73	E	Massachusetts	#1 Transcendental Meditation	P	–	8
Berkel (1983)	CC	R	522 deaths	CDA	Netherlands	#1 D (SDA vs. non-SDA)	non-SDA > SDA	SC-sex,age	6
Berkman (1979)	PC	R	6928	CDA	Alameda, CA	#1 CM	P	MC	7
Boldman (1933)	CC	R	14047 + Cs	CDA	New York City	#1 D (Jewish vs. non-J)	M	SC-sex,age	6
Bryant (1992)	PC	R	473	CDA,E,B	National US	#1 ORA	P	MC	9
Comstock (1967)	CC	R	234 stillborn babies + Cs		Maryland	#1 ORA	P	SC	7
Comstock (1972)	CC	R	54,848	CDA	Maryland	#1 ORA	P	SC	7
Comstock (1977)	CC	R	47,423	CDA	Maryland	#1 ORA	NA	SC	7
Dysinger (1963)	CC	R	64,256	CDA (SDA)	California	#1 D (SDA vs. non-SDA)	non-SDA > SDA	–	6

a. Koenig, Cohen, George, et al. b. Naguib, Lundin, et al.

Outcome/Investigators	Type	Method	N	Population	Location	Religious Variable	Findings	Controls	Rating
Fonnebo (1992a,1994)	PC	R	7173	CDA (SDA)	Norway	#1 D (SDA vs. non-SDA)	non-SDA > SDA	SC	6
Glass (1999)	PC	R	2761	CDA,E	New Haven, CT	#1 ORA	P	MC	10
Goldman (1995)	PC	R	7500	CDA,E	National US	#1 ORA	P	MC	10
Goldstein (1996)	CC	R	15,520 + Cs	CDA	Rhode Island	#1 D (Jewish vs. non-J)	non-J > Jewish	SC-age, sex	8
Hamman (1981)	CC	R	25,822 (1226)	CDA (Amish)	Indiana, Ohio, Pennsylvania	#1 D (Amish vs. non-A)	M	SC	7
Helm (2000)	PC	R	3851	CDA,E	North Carolina	#1 NORA	P	MC	10
Hogstel (1989)	CS,D	C	302	CDA,E (>85)	Texas	#2 RB,Christian living	(P)	NS	4
House (1982)	PC	R	2754	CDA	Tecumseh	#1 ORA	P	MC	9
Hummer (1999)	PC	R	21,204	CDA	National US	#1 ORA	P	–	10
Idler (1991)	PC	R	2812	CDA,E	New Haven, CT	#4 ORA,NORA	NA	MC	8
*Idler (1992)	PC	R	2812	CDA,E	New Haven, CT	#4 ORA,SR,RC	C	MC	10
Janoff-Bulman (1982)	PC	C	30	NH,E	Massachusetts	#2 SR	NG	SC	6
*Jarvis (1977)	CC	R	1169 deaths	CDA, Mormons	Canada	#1 D (Mormon vs. non-M)	non-M > Morm	SC	6
Kark (1996b)	PC	S	3900	kibbutz members	Israel	#1 relg vs. secular kibbutzim	P	MC	10
Koenig (1995b)	PC	S	262	MP	Durham, NC	#3 RC	NA	MC	6
Koenig (1998)[a]	PC	S	1000	MP	Durham, NC	#3 RC	NA	MC	9
Koenig (1999a)[b]	PC	R	3968	CDA,E	North Carolina	#1 ORA	P	MC	9
Krause (1998a)	PC	R	819	CDA,E	National US	#8 ORA,NORA,RC	P/M	MC	9
Liberson (1956)	CC	R	74079	CDA	New York City	#1 D (Jewish vs. non-J)	non-J > Jewish	NONE	5
Magana (1995)	R,O		examines lower infant mortality in Los Angeles County & relates it to religious beliefs in Mexican American population							
McCullough (1999)	R		meta-analysis of religious involvement and mortality							
Miah (1993)	CS	R	4800+	Perinatal	Bangladesh	#1 D (Muslim vs. Hindu)	Hindu > Muslim	NONE	5
Musick (1999)	PC	R	3617	CDA	National US	#1 ORA	P	MC	9
Needleman (1988)	CC	R	SMR 1920–1971	CDA	Montreal, Can	#1 D (Jewish vs. non-J)	non-J > Jewish	SC-age	5
Oman (1998)	PC	S	1931	CDA, E	Marin, CA	#1 ORA	P	MC	9
Oman (1999)	PC		same cohort as above; found that volunteering associated with lower mortality, but primarily only in the religiously active							9
*Oxman (1995)	PC	S	232	MP (open-heart surgery)	New Hampshire	#3 ORA, SR, RC	P (RC)	MC	9

Study			N	Measure	Finding	Location	Result	Controls	Score
Palmore (1982)[c]	PC	C	252	CDA, E	#6 SR	North Carolina	NA	MC	7
Pargament (2000)[c]	PC	S	595	MP,E	#66 RC,ORA,NORA	Durham, NC	C	MC	8
Rasanen (1996)	PC	R	1624 deaths	CDA,M	#1 D (E. Orthdox, Lutheran)	Finland	EO > Lu	MC	8
Reynolds (1981)	PC	R	193	NH, E	#1 "religious commit"	Los Angeles	(P)	NS	6
Rogers (1996)	PC	R	15,938	CDA,E	#1 ORA	National US	P	MC	9
Saksena (1980)	CS	R	5506 births	Perinatal	#1 D (Hindu vs. Muslim)	India	Muslim > Hindu	NONE	2
Simpson W (1989)	CC	S	5568	CDA	#1 D Christ Sc vs. other)	Illinois	Christ Sc > other	SC-age, sex	8
Schoenbach (1986)	PC	R	2059	CDA	#1 ORA	Georgia	P	MC	10
Seeman (1987)	PC	R	4175	CDA > 38 yo	#1 CM	Alameda, CA	P	MC	10
Seidman (1964)	CC	R	202,851 deaths	CDA	#1 D (Jewish vs. non-J)	New York City	non-J > Jewish	SC-age, sex, SES	5
Smith (1985)	CC	R	–	CDA	#1 D (Morm vs. non-M)	New Zealand	non-M > Morm	–	–
Spence (1984)	CC	R	26,618 Faith Assembly vs. others		#1 D (Faith As vs. other)	Indiana	Faith As > other	SC-age	8
Spence (1987)	CC	R	follow-up study to 1984 report; perinatal mortality declined from 3 to 1.5 rate for Indiana due to laws passed						6
Strawbridge (1997)	PC	R	5286	CDA	#1 ORA	Alameda, CA	P	MC	10
Waaler (1981)	CC	R	–	CDA	#1 D (SDA vs. non-SDA)	Norway	non-SDA > SDA	–	–
*Webster (1979)	CC	C	779 vs. Cs	CDA	#1 D (SDA vs. non-SDA)	Australia	non-SDA > SDA	SC-age	7
Wingard (1982)	PC	R	4725	CDA 30–69 y	#1 CM	Alameda, CA	C	MC	8
Zuckerman (1984)	PC	S	225	CDA,E	#4 D,ORA,SR,RC	New Haven, CT	P	SC-sex, health	7

Clergy Mortality

Study			N	Measure	Finding	Location	Result	Controls	Score
Allison (1999)	RS	S	920	R (Methodists)	#1 Methodist ministers	England	Primitive > Wesleyan		6
De Gouw (1995)	RS	S	1,523	R (monks)	#1 monks vs. others	Netherlands	P	SC	8
Harding le Riche (1985)	CS	C	289	R (clergy)	#1 clergy vs. MDs	Canada	P	NONE	5
Kastenbaum (1990)	CC, D	S	487	Saints	#1 sainthood vs. others	World	P	SC-sex	6
King H (1968)	CC	S	609 deaths	R (Lutheran)	#1 clergy vs. others	US & Canada	P		
King H (1969)	R			review of demographic literature concerning health of the clergy			P	SC-age, sex, race	6

a. Koenig, Larson, et al.   b. Koenig, Hays, Larson, et al.   c. Pargament, Koenig, et al.

Outcome/Investigators	Type	Method	N	Population	Location	Religious Variable	Findings	Controls	Rating
King H (1970)	CC	S	4106 deaths	R (clergy)	US, England	#1 clergy vs. others	P	SC-age,sex	6
King H (1971)	CC	S	1387 deaths	R (Anglican)	US	#1 clergy vs. others	P	SC- age,sex, race	6
King H (1980)	CC	S	5207 deaths	R (Prot,W,M)	US	#1 clergy vs. others	P	SC- age,sex, race	6
Locke (1980)	CC	R	3446 deaths	R (Baptist)	National US	#1 clergy vs. others	P	SC	6
Madigan (1957)	CC	R	6932 deaths	R (Catholic)	National US	#1 clergy vs. others	P	SC-age	6
Madigan (1961)	CC	S	1247 deaths	R (Cath priests)	National US	#1 priests vs. others	P	SC-age	6
Ogata (1984)	CC	S	1396 deaths	R (Zen priests)	Japan	#1 priests vs. others	P	SC-age,sex	7
Taylor RS (1959)	CC	C	2657 deaths	R (Cath nuns)	Massachusetts, New York	#1 nuns vs. others	P	SC-age	6
Versluys (1949)	CC	S	51,124 CA-deaths	R (Catholic)	Netherlands	#1 priests vs. others	NA	NONE (NS)	5
Walker (1990)	RS	S	1038 deaths	R (Catholic)	Brooklyn, NY	#2 deaths not less freq on relg holidays	—	–	4
Cancer Mortality									
Collipp (1969)	CT	C	18 children with leukemia		New York	#1 intercessory prayer	NA (70% vs. 25%)		6
Creagan (1997)	R		reviews relationship between spiritual coping and cancer survival						
Dwyer (1990)	CS	R	3063 counties	CDA	National US	#2 D,CM	P	MC	8
Enstrom (1975)	CC	R	4865 deaths	CDA-Mormons	California	#1 D (Mormon vs. non-M)	non-M > Morm	SC-age,sex	7
Enstrom (1978)	CC	R	55000 vs. Cs	CDA-Mormons	Utah, California	#1 D Act Mor vs. non-M	non-M > Morm	SC-age,sex	8
Enstrom (1980)	CC	R	4 large samples	CDA-Mormons	Utah, California	#1 D Act Mor vs. non-M	non-M > Morm	SC-age,sex	8
Enstrom (1989)	CC	R	9844 vs. 3199 Cs	CDA-Mormons	California	#2 ORA, Mor vs. non-M)	P	SC	9
Gardner (1982a)	CC	S	1819 deaths	M, Mormons	Utah	#2 lay-priesthood level	P	SC-age,sex	7
Gardner (1982b)	CC	S	1354 deaths	F, Mormons	Utah	#2 church activity (ORA)	P	SC-age,sex	7
Greenwald (1975)	CC	S	800 deaths	Russian-born	New York	#1 D (Jews vs. non-J)	M	NONE	6
Herman (1970)	CC	R	572 lung CA deaths	CDA	Pittsburgh	#1 D (Jews vs. non-J)	M	SC-age,sex	5

Hoffman (1932)	CC	R	9405 CA deaths	CDA	Amsterdam, Netherlands	#1 D (Jews vs. non-J)	M	NONE	4
Horowitz (1970)	CC	R	361 lung CA deaths	CDA	Montreal, Can	#1 D (Jews vs. non-J)	M	SC-age,sex	4
*Jarvis (1977)	CC	R	1169 deaths	CDA,Mormons	Canada	#1 D (Mormon vs. non-M)	non-M > Morm	SC	6
King H (1965)	CC	S	1754 deaths	CDA	Baltimore, MD	#1 D (P vs. Ca vs. J)	M	SC-sex	4
Kune (1991,1992)	PC	S	637–705	MP (colon CA)	Australia	#1 D (Jewish vs. non-J)	Jewish = non-J	SC	4
*Lemon (1964)	CC	R	47866	CDA	California	#1 D (SDA vs. non-SDA)	non-SDA > SDA	SC-age,sex	6
Lemon (1966)	PC/CC	R	11071	CDA, 100%M	California	#1 D (SDA vs. non-SDA)	non-SDA > SDA	SC-age	8
Lemon (1969)	CC	R	34271	CDA, >35 yo	California	#1 D (SDA vs. non-SDA)	non-SDA > SDA	SC-age,sex	6
LoPrinzi (1994)	PC	S	1115	MP (advanced CA)	United States	#2 "feelings re relig"	NA	MC	7
Lyon (1976)	CC	R	10641	CDA	Utah	#1 D (Mormon vs. non-M)	non-M > Morm	SC-age,sex	6
Lyon (1977)	CC	R	CA deaths	—	Utah	#1 D (Mormon vs. non-M)	non-M > Morm	NONE	6
MacMahon (1957)	CC	R	1368 leukemia	CDA	New York City	#1 D (Jewish vs. non-J)	Jewish > non-J	NONE	5
MacMahon (1960)	CC	R	14356	CDA	New York City	#1 D (Jewish vs. non-J)	M	NONE	5
Martin AO (1980)	CC	R	53 deaths	CDA	Canada, N Dakota	#1 D (Hutterite vs. non-H)	non-H > Hutt	SC-age ?	6
Newill (1961)	CC	R	83341 deaths	CDA	New York City	#1 D (Jew vs. Ca vs. P)	M	NONE	4
Phillips (1980)[a]	PC/CC	R	22940 vs. Cs	CDA	California	#1 D (SDA vs. non-SDA)	non-SDA > SDA	SC-age,sex	7
Phillips (1983)	CC	R	21295 vs. Cs	CDA	California	#1 D (SDA vs. non-SDA)	non-SDA > SDA	SC-age,sex	7
*Ringdal (1995,[b] 1996)	PC	S	253	MP (cancer)	Norway	#2 RB	(P)	SC	8
Rosenwaike (1984)	RS	R	SMR (lung CA)	CDA	New York City	#1 D (J vs. Ca vs. P)	Ca > P > J	NS	3
Seidman (1966)	CC	R	SMR (lung CA)	CDA	New York City	#1 D (Jewish vs. non-J)	non-J > Jewish	SC-age	5
Seidman (1970,1971)	CC	R	SMR (any CA)	CDA	New York City	#1 D (Jewish vs. non-J)	M	SC-age, sex,SES	5

a. Phillips, Garfinkel, et al.; Phillips, Kuzma, et al.   b. Ringdal, Gotestam, et al.

Outcome/Investigators	Type	Method	N	Population	Location	Religious Variable	Findings	Controls	Rating
Correspondent (1902)	CC	R	113 deaths	CDA	London, England	#1 D (Jewish vs. non-J)	non-J > Jewish	NONE	3
*Versluys (1949)	CC	R	51124	CDA	Netherlands	#1 D (Jewish vs. non-J)	Jewish > non-J	SC-age	6
Wolff (1939)	CC	S	801/947 deaths	CDA	Berlin	#1 D (Jewish vs. non-J)	M	SC-sex,age?	5
Yates (1981)	CS	C	71	MP (adv CA)	Michigan	#7+ RB,RE,SR,ORA	NA	NONE	6
Zollinger (1984)	PC	S	2304	MP (with CA)	California	#1 D (SDA vs. non-SDA)	SDA = non-SDA	MC	8
Cardiovascular Mortality									
*Comstock (1971)	CC	R	189 deaths vs. Cs	CDA	Maryland	#1 ORA	P	SC	7
*Goldbourt (1993)	PC	R	10,059	CDA,M	Isreal	#3 orthodox vs. secular Js	P (MI death)	MC	10
*Jarvis (1977)	CC	R	1169 deaths	CDA,Mormons	Canada	#1 D (Mormon vs. non-M)	non-M > Morm	SC	6
*Lemon (1964)	PC	R	47866	CDA	California	#1 D (SDA vs. non-SDA)	non-SDA > SDA	SC-age,sex	7
*Oxman (1995)	PC	S	232	MP-open-heart	New Hampshire	#3 ORA, SR, RC	P (RC)	MC	9
*Phillips (1978)	PC	R	24044	CDA	California	#1 D (SDA vs. non-SDA)	non-SDA > SDA	–	6
*Phillips (1980)[a]	PC/CC	R	22940 vs. Cs	CDA	California	#1 D (SDA vs. non-SDA)	non-SDA > SDA	SC-age,sex	7
End-Stage Renal Disease									
Devins (1990)	PC	C	97	MP	Alberta, Can	#1 "active vs. inactive"	NA	MC	6
Accidents									
*Pescosolido (1986)	CS	R	404 counties	Suicides,accidents	National US	#1 D (J,Ca,DOC,B)	Others > Ca	MC	6

Functional Disability (Ch 22)

Coping with Disability

Study			N	Population	Location	Findings	Result	Outcome	Score
*Bulman (1977)	CS	C	29	MP (para/quad)	Chicago	#1+ religiousness scale	NA (coping)	MC	5
*Cameron (1973)	CC	C	144/46 vs. Cs	MP (handicapped)	Detroit	#1 SR	disabled value relig more than healthy		6
Dalal (1988)	PC	C	41	MP (acute injured)	India	#1 attribute to God/karma	P (psych recovery)	NONE	5
*Decker (1985)	CS,D	C	100	MP (spinal injury)	Northwest US	#1 SR ?	(P) (coping)	NS	4
Dein (1997)	R			review of whether religion helps with coping with chronic illness					
Kolin (1971)	CS,D	C	13 parents with child with meningomyelocele			#1 RC	(P)	NS	4
Leyser (1994)	PC/CS	C	82 families of disabled children		Israel	#3+ RC	46% prayer	–	5
Rogers-Dulan (1995)	R,O			examine how religion, disability and ethnicity relate to adjustment for families					

Disability Level

Study			N	Population	Location	Findings	Result	Outcome	Score
Adams (1987)	CS	C	412	CDA,E	Rural NC	#2 ORA	P	MC	5
*Idler (1987)	CS	R	2811	CDA,E	New Haven, CT	#4 ORA,SR,D	P (ORA)	MC	9
*Idler (1992)	PC	R	2812	CDA,E	New Haven, CT	#4 ORA,SR,D	M: ORA-p,SR-n	MC	10
Idler (1995)	CS	R	146	MP (rehab clinic)	New Haven, CT	#4 RC,SR,D	NG (RC)	MC	8
*Idler (1997a)	CS	R	2812	CDA,E	New Haven, CT	#4 ORA,SR,D	M: ORA-p,SR-n	MC	9
Idler (1997b)	PC	R	2812	CDA,E	New Haven, CT	#4 ORA,SR,D	P (ORA)	MC	10
Jeffers (1961)[b]	CS	C	251	CDA,E	North Carolina	#2+ORA,RCm (attitude)	NG (RCm)	NONE	5
Krause (1998b)	PC/CS	R	511	CDA,E	National US	#8 ORA,NORA,RC	P (self-rated hlth)	MC	8
*Levin (1985)	CS	R	1125	CDA-Mex-Am	Texas	#2 ORA,SR	M:ORA-p,SR-n	NONE	6
Mackenbach (1993)	CC	S	134	Monks,M	Netherlands	#1 Monks vs. non-Monks	NG	SC-age	6
Musick (1996)	PC	R	2623	CDA,E	North Carolina	#2 ORA,NORA	P (for subj hlth)	MC	9
*Pressman (1990)	CS, PC	C	30	MP, E, F	Chicago	#3 ORA, SR, RC	P	SC	7
Selway (1998)	R			review of the literature examining disability, religion, and health					

a. Phillips, Kuzma, et al.　b. Jeffers & Nichols

Pain and Somatic Symptoms (Ch 23)

Pain

Outcome/Investigators	Type	Method	N	Population	Location	Religious Variable	Findings	Controls	Rating
Abraido-Lanza (1996)	CS,D	C	109	MP (arthritis) F	New York City	#1 prayer	2nd most common coping strategy		6
*Brown GK (1989)	PC	C	287	MP (rheumatology)	Tennessee	#1+ prayer (subsumed under "distraction")	–		2
Cronan (1989)	CS,D	R	382	CDA (MS complaints)	San Diego	#2 (use/helpful)	#1 most common, #2 most helpful		9
Florell (1973)	CT	C	44	MP (orthopedic)	–	#1 chaplain intervention	P (less pain)		6
Foley (1988)	R,O	–	review and discussion of effects of religious coping on pain experience						
*Fry (1990)	CS	C	178	E,MP	Western Canada	#1 prayer	NG	NONE	6
Heiligman (1983)	C	C	single case	MP	Los Angeles	#1 RB (protective angels)	no post-op analgesia	–	–
Kabat-Zinn (1985)	CT	C	90 vs. 20Cs	MP	Massachusetts	#1 Transcendental Meditation	P	–	7
Keefe (1990)	CS	S	62	MP (low back pain)	North Carolina	#1 divert attention & prayer	NG	MC	5
*Koenig (1998)[a]	CS/PC	C	115	E,NH	North Carolina	#3 RC	NA	MC	6
Kotarba (1983)	Q R,O	–	110	CDA	–	#1 relig resources	–	–	6
Low (1997)			examines relationship between religious orientation and pain/suffering						
McBride (1998)	CS	R	442	MP	Georgia	#7 INSPIRIT	C	NONE	7
Rosenstiel (1983)	CS	C	61	MP (low back)	Durham, NC	#1 RC (prayer)	NG	MC	6
Turner (1986)	PC	C	74	MP (low back)	Seattle, WA	#1 "praying or hoping"	P	SC	7
Tuttle (1991)	CS	C	181	MP (chronic pain)	–	#1 "praying or hoping"	NG	–	6
*Yates (1981)	CS	C	71	MP (advanced CA)	Vermont	#7+ RB,RE,SR,ORA	P	NONE	6
Zborowski (1952)	Q	C	103	MP	Bronx, NY	#1 D (Jewish vs. Irish Ca, Italian Ca)	P	–	5

Somatic Symptoms

Outcome/Investigators	Type	Method	N	Population	Location	Religious Variable	Findings	Controls	Rating
Acheson (1960)	CS	R	2329	MP (with GI)	VA hospitals in US	#1 D (Jewish vs. non-J)	Jewish > non-J	NONE	6

Study			N	Measure	Location	Religious variable	Finding	Effect	
*Carson (1979)	CT	C	20 Christian schizophrenics	PP	Maryland	#1 prayer/scripture	(P)	NS	4
Chaturvedi (1989)	CS	S	31		India	#1 D (Hindu vs. Muslim)	Hindu > Muslim	NONE ?	2
De Figueiredo (1978)	CS	R	160	CDA	India	#2 D, ORA,NORA	M:ORA-p,NR-n	NONE	6
Jamal (1993)	CS	C	325	CDA,Muslim	North America	#1 SR	P	SC	6
McIntosh (1990)	CS	C	76	largely CS	Colorado, Georgia	#20+ IR,misc	P	NONE	2
Ness (1980)	CS	C	51/54	CM	Newfoundland	#4 ORA,RE	NG	NONE	4
Polit (1980)	CS	C	167	CDA, F	Boston	#1 D	NA (menopause symps)		2
*Rosenberg M (1962)	CS	R	1021	HS	New York	#1 D (similarity of neighborhood)	P	NONE	6
Rothbaum (1990)	CS	C	121	CDA, F	Pennsylvania	#1 D (J vs. Ca vs. Prot)	NA	NONE	2
*Shaver (1980)	CS,D	C	2500	F (Redbook)	National US	#1 SR	M	NONE	6

Health Behaviors (Ch 24)

Weight

Study			N	Measure	Location	Religious variable	Finding	Effect	
*Ferraro (1998)	CS	R	3497	CDA	National US	#6 ORA,NORA,-SR,RC	NG	MC	9
*Gottlieb (1984)	CS	R	3025	CDA 20–64 y	National US	#1 ORA	NG (women)	MC	7
*Idler (1997a)	CS	R	2812	CDA,E	National US	#2 ORA,SR	NG (SR)	MC	9
*Kumanyika (1992)	D/CT	C	188	CM, 100%B,F	New Haven, CT	church-based wt ctrl	P	–	7
Lapane (1997)	CS	R	5241	CDA	Baltimore	#1 CM	NG	NONE	7
*Oman (1998)	PC	R	1931	CDA,E	Rhode Island	#1 ORA	NG	MC	9
*Strawbridge (1997)	PC	R	5286	CDA	Marin, CA	#1 ORA	NG	MC	10
					Alameda, CA				

Exercise

Study			N	Measure	Location	Religious variable	Finding	Effect	
*Idler (1997a)	CS	R	2438	CDA,E	New Haven, CT	#3 ORA,SR	P	MC	9
*McIntosh (1990)	CS	C	76	largely CS	Colorado, Georgia	#20+ IR,misc	NG	NONE	2
*Oleckno (1991)	CS	–	1077	CS	N. Illinois	#2 ORA, SR	P	NONE	6
*Strawbridge (1997)	PC	R	5286	CDA	Alameda, CA	#1 ORA	P	MC	10
*Thorne (1996)	CS	R	990	CDA,E	Ohio	#3 ORA,D	NA	NONE	7

Diet

Study			N	Measure	Location	Religious variable	Finding	Effect	
Epstein (1956)[b]	CS,D	C	416 (garment workers)	CDA (calories)	New York City	#1 D (Jew vs. Italian)	J fewer calories	–	6

a. Koenig, Weiner, et al. b. Epstein, Carol, et al.

Outcome/Investigators	Type	Method	N	Population	Location	Religious Variable	Findings	Controls	Rating
*Epstein (1956)[a]	CS	C	416 (garment workers)	CDA (chol/cad)	New York City	#1 D (Jew vs. Italian)	J more animal fat	SC-sex	6
*Groen (1959)	R		review of religious affiliation effects on diet and cholesterol level; Jews higher cholesterol due to diet						
Katz (1976)	R		reviews Jewish dietary laws						
*Phillips (1975)	PC	R	100,000 CDA	CA risk	California	#1 D (SDA)	non-SDA > meat	–	6
Phillips (1978)	PC	R	24,044 CDA	CHD mortality	California	#1 D (SDA)	non-SDA > meat	MC	6
Phillips (1983)	CC	R	21295 vs. Cs	CA mortality	California	#1 D (SDA)	non-SDA > meat	SC-age,sex	7
Shatenstein (1998)	R		reviews differences in diet and health behaviors between different religious groups						
*Wallace, J (1998)	CS	R	5000	HS	National US	#3 D,ORA,SR	P	MC	9
*West (1968)	CC	C	3260 vs. Cs	CDA (cholesterol)	Washington, DC	#1 D (SDA)	non-SDA > chol	SC-age	5

Smoking

Outcome/Investigators	Type	Method	N	Population	Location	Religious Variable	Findings	Controls	Rating
*Adelekan (1993)	CS	S/R	636	CS	Nigeria	#2 SR,D (Muslim vs. Christian)	P	NONE	6
Ahmed (1994)	CS	R	266	CDA,B,F	Norfolk, VA	#11 D,ORA, NORA,RB	P (D only)	MC	6
*Brown D (1994)	CS	S	537	CDA,B,M	Norfolk, VA	#12 relig scale,ORA,D	P (ORA)	MC	8
*Engs (1980)	CS	S	1691	CS	Australia	#2 D,SR	P	NONE	6
*Fonnebo (1992b)	CS	C	222 vs. Cs	CDA	Norway	#1 D (SDA vs. non-SDA)	non-SDA > SDA	SC	6
Gmur (1987)	CS	C/S	532 heavy smokers (CDA)		Switzerland	Rx by faith healer, ORA	P (ORA)	NONE	6
Goldbourt (1975)	CS	S	10000	CDA, M	Israel	#3 ORA, SR	P	NONE	8
*Gottlieb (1984)	CS	R	3025	CDA 20–64 y	National US	#1 ORA	P	MC	7
*Hundleby (1982)	CS	C	231	HS (Catholic)	Ontario, Can	#4 ORA,NORA	P	NONE	5
*Hundleby (1987)	CS	S/R	2048	HS (9th grade)	Ontario, Can	#3 ORA	P	SC	7
*Idler (1997a)	CS	R	2812	CDA,E	New Haven, CT	#2 ORA,SR	P (ORA,SR)	MC	9
Kandel C (1981)	CS	R	1108	Ad	France, Israel	#1 ORA or rlg school	(P)	NS	7
*Kendler (1997)	CS	C	1902	CDA, twins	Virginia	#11 RB,ORA, NORA,SR	P	MC	9
*Khavari (1982)	CS	–	4853	CDA	Milwaukee, WI	#2 D,SR	P	NONE	6
*Koenig (1988)[b]	CS	S	106	MP, E	Illinois	#15+ ORA,NORA,IR	(P)	SC-sex	6
Koenig (1998b)[c]	PC	R	4000	CDA, E	North Carolina	#4 ORA, NORA, D	P	MC	10
*Mullen (1996)	CS	R	985	CDA > 35 yo	West Scotland	#1 D (vs. none)	NA	SC	4
*Ndom (1996)	CS	R	1508	CS	Nigeria	#2 D,SR	P	NONE	7

Study	Type	Method	N	Sample	Location	Findings	P	Controls	Rating
*Newcomb (1986)	CS	S?	791	Ad	Los Angeles	#1 SR	P	NONE	7
*Oleckno (1991)	CS	–	1077	CS	N. Illinois	#2 ORA, SR	P	NONE	6
*Parfrey (1976)	CS	R	444	CS	Ireland	#2 ORA, RB	P	NONE	5
*Resnick (1997)	CS	R	12118	Ad	National US	#1 SR	P	MC	8
Spangler (1998)	CS	–	400	Lumbee Indians	North Carolina	#1+ ORA	P	–	6
Torabi (1990)	CS	C	405 Christians	US vs. 406 Muslims Turks (CS)		#1 RB	P	SC	6
*Thorne (1996)	CS	R	990	CDA,E	Ohio	#3 ORA,D	P	NONE	7
*Wallace, J (1998)	CS	R	5000	HS	National US	#3 D,ORA,SR	P	MC	9

Sexual Behavior

Study	Type	Method	N	Sample	Location	Findings	P	Controls	Rating
Beck (1991)	PC	R	several thousand	youth 14–22 y	National US	#2 D,ORA	P	MC	8
Billy (1993)	CS	R	3321	CDA,M,20–39y	National US	#1 D (vs. none)	P	MC	7
Brown S (1985)	CS	R	702	Ad,B,F	National US	#1 ORA	P	MC	8
Cardwell (1969)	CS	C	187	CS	New England	#30 (5 dimensions)	P	NONE	4
Clayton (1969)	CS	S	887	CS	Florida	#6 RB	P	NONE	6
Cochran (1991)	CS	R	14979	CDA	National US	#5 ORA,SR,RB,CM,D	P	MC	10
Cullari (1990)	CS	C	208	HS	Pennsylvania	#2 Ca vs. public school	P	NONE	6
Davids (1982)	CS	C	208	CS,Jewish	Ontario, Can	#2 D,SR	P	NONE	4
*Donahue (1995)	R				reviews research on relationship between religion and sexual behavior in adolescents				
DuRant (1990)	CS	R	202	Ad,F,Hispanic	National US	#2 D,ORA	P	MC	7
*Forliti (1986)	CS,D	C	8165/10,467	Ad/parents,CM	United States	#>15 RB,ORA,SR	(P)	–	5
Fox (1989)	CS	C	196	CS	Southern US	#24 ORA,NORA, RB,RE	P	NONE	5
Goldscheider (1991)	CS	R	8450	CDA,F	National US	#4 ORA,D	P (ORA)	SC	8
Gunderson (1979)	CS	C	327	CS	Houston	#3 ORA,D,SR	P	MC	6
Haerich (1992)	CS	C	204	CS	Riverside, CA	#22 ORA,SR,IR,ER	P	NONE	4
Heltsley (1969)	CS	C	1435	CS	United States	#2+ D, relig scale	P	SC-sex,race	6
Hendricks (1984)	CC	C	48 vs. 50 Cs	Ad,B fathers	Columbus, OH	#5 ORA,NORA	P (ORA)	DF	5
Herold (1981)	CS	C	514	CS,HS	Ontario, Can	#1 ORA	P	SC	6
Jensen L (1990)	CS	C	423	CS, ages 17–25	Oklahoma, Wisconsin	#1 ORA	P	–	6
Kandel D (1990)	CS	R	2711	young adults	National US	#2 ORA,D	P (ORA)	MC	8
Kinsey (1953)	CS	R/S	5940	CDA,F,W	National US	#2+ ORA,SR	P	NONE ?	7
Mahoney (1980)	CS	C	441	CS	Washington St	#1 SR	P	NONE	5
Miller PY (1974)	CS	R	2064	Ad, W	Illinois	#1 SR	P	SC-sex, age	8
Mol (1970)	CS	R	1825	CDA	Australia	# 2 RB, ORA	P	NONE	6

a. Epstein, Simpson, et al. b. Koenig, Moberg, & Kvale c. Koenig, George, Cohen, et al.

Outcome/Investigators	Type	Method	N	Population	Location	Religious Variable	Findings	Controls	Rating
Naguib (1966)[a]	CS	R	5896	CDA,F	Maryland	#2 ORA, D (any vs. none)	P	NONE	7
Nicholas (1995)	CS	S	1817	CS	South Africa	#8 scale	M	NONE	7
*Parfrey (1976)	CS	R	444	CS	Ireland	#3 ORA,RB	P	NONE	5
*Poulson (1998)	CS	C?	210	CS	Greenville, NC	#1+ SR	P (women)	SC	5
*Resnick (1997)	CS	R	12118	Ad	National US	#1 SR	P	MC	8
*Rohrbaugh (1975)	CS	C	475/221	HS/CS	Colorado	#8 ORA, RB, RE	P	NONE	6
Rosenbaum (1990)	CS	R	2711	CDA 19–20 yo	National US	#1 ORA	P	MC	8
Ruppel (1970)	CS	R	437	CS	N. Illinois	#8 RB,Misc	P	MC	6
Sack (1984)	CS	S	519	CS	Eastern US	#6 conventional religiosity	(no p value)	MC	7
Seidman (1992)	CS	R	7011	CDA, F	National US	#2 ORA, D	P	MC	10
Sheeran (1996)	CS	C	682	HS	Scotland	#1 SR	P (females)	NONE	6
Studer (1987)	CS	C	224	Ad (18 yo)	Detroit	#1 ORA	P	SC	6
Thornton (1989)	PC	R	888	Ad (18 yo)	Detroit	#3 D,ORA,SR	P	MC	8
Werebe (1983)	CS	C	386	Ad	France	#2 D, ORA	P	NONE	3
Woodroof (1985)	CS	C	477	CS (Christian)	United States	#31 IR,ER,Misc	P	SC	5
*Wright (1971)	CS	C	3850	CS	England	#5 RB,ORA,Misc	P	NONE	6
General Safety (seat belt use, etc.)									
*Oleckno (1991)	CS	–	1077	CS	N. Illinois	#2 ORA, SR	P	NONE	6
*Wallace, J (1998)	CS	R	5000	HS	National US	#3 D,ORA,SR	P	MC	9
Sleep									
Hoch (1987)	CC	C	10 healthy nuns vs. matched Cs		Pittsburgh, PA	#1 D (nuns vs. other F)	P	–	7
*Wallace, J (1998)	CS	R	5000	HS	National US	#3 D,ORA,SR	P	MC	9
Miscellaneous Health									
Ainlay (1992; also 1984)	CS	R	200	CDA,E	Massachusetts	#13 ORA,NORA,SR	M	MC	7
*Anson (1990)[b]	PC/CS	C	639	CDA,E	Israel	#1 observ of rlg rituals	NG (CS)	MC	6
Benson H (1990)	C	C	3	Buddhist monks	India	meditation	change in metabolism		5
Broyles (1992)	CS	R	3410	CDA,E	Washington	#1 ORA	P (subj hlth)	MC	8

572

Study	CT	C	N	CS	Location	Religious variable	Result	Controls	Score
*Carlson (1988)	CT	C	36 randomized	CS (Christian)	Chicago	"devotional meditation"	M (muscle tension)	NONE	6
Comstock (1970)	CC	R	60,000	TB cases (CDA)	Maryland	#1 ORA	P	NONE	7
Corby (1978)	PC,D	C	3	Meditators,CDA	San Francisco	#1 Tantric Yoga meditation	–	–	4
Courtenay (1992)	CS	–	165	CDA,E	Georgia	#23 RB,ORA,-NORA,RE	NG	NONE	6
Craigie (1988)	SR	found that 1.9–3.5% of 1086 articles in Journal of Family Practice (1976–1986) examined religion							
Craigie (1990)	SR	reviews 64 associations in 52 studies published in JFP 1976–1986 (25 pos, 30 neu, 9 neg)							
Delmonte (1985)	R	review of biochemical changes with meditation (skeptical review)							
Drevenstedt (1998)	CS	R	10,930	CDA	National US	#2 ORA,SR	P (subj hlth)	SC	8
Ferraro (1991)	CS	R	2939	CDA	National US	#7+ RB,ORA,NORA	M	MC	7
*Hannay (1980)	CS	R	964	CDA	Scotland	ORA	P	SC-age,sex	7
Heenan (1972)	R	review of studies on religion, health, and aging							
Jarvis (1987)	R	review of studies on religion and physical morbidity & mortality							
Kesterson (1989)	Exp	C	32 experienced meditators		Iowa	meditation	reduced respiratory exchange ratio		7
King Mi (1994)	PC	S	216	MP	London, England	#8+ Spiritual beliefs	NG	SC ?	7
King Mi (1999)	PC	S	144	MP	London, England	#8 ? Spiritual beliefs	NG	SC	7
Koenig (1994a)	R	review of research on religion, health, and aging							
Koenig (1999)	R	review of the research written for patients and a popular audience of readers							
Levin (1986)[c]	CS	R	1125	CDA, Mex-Am	Texas	#2 ORA, SR	NA (subj hlth)	MC	8
Levin (1987)[d]	R	reviews research evidence that there is a connection between religion and health							
Levin (1987)[e]	R	reviews research evidence that religious attendance is related to health							
Levin (1997)[f]	R	reviews research evidence that there is a connection between religion and health (JAMA)							
Matthews (1998)	R	review of the research written for patients and a popular audience of readers							
*McBride (1998)	CS	R	442	MP	Georgia	#7 INSPIRIT	P	NONE	7
Moberg (1996)	R	review of religion, health, and aging							
Orr (1992)	SR	systematic review of seven major primary care journals; 1% with religious variables							
Osler W (1910)	O	legendary Johns Hopkins professor of medicine discusses "faith" and its healing power							
*Riley (1998)	CS	C	216	MP	Ann Arbor, MI	#33 SWB, FACT-SP	P	NONE	5
Shapira (1998)	CC	R/S	ulcerative colitis in 82,300 CDA		N. Israel	#1 D (Jews vs. Arabs)	Jews > Arabs	SC-age	6
Sijuwade (1994)	CS	C	115	CDA,E	Nigeria	#4 NORA,RE,SR	NA (# illnesses)	MC	5
Simons (1984–85)	CS	C	299	CDA, E	Midwest US	#4 NORA,RE,SR	NA (# illnesses)	MC	5
West (1983)	CS	C	299	CDA,E	Midwest US	#4 NORA,RE,SR	NA (# illnesses)	MC	5

a. Naguib, Lundin, et al. b. Anson, Antonovsky, et al. c. Levin & Markides d. Levin & Schiller e. Levin & Vanderpool f. Levin, Larson, et al.

Outcome/Investigators	Type	Method	N	Population	Location	Religious Variable	Findings	Controls	Rating
Understanding Religion's Health Effects (Ch 25)									
Krause (1997)	R	examines directions for the scientific study of religion, aging, and health							
*Levin (1987)[a]	R	comprehensive review of religion and health							
Levin (1994)	R	provides theoretical foundation for epidemiology of religion							
Levin (1996b)	R	examines how natural history, salutogenesis, and host resistance may explain religion's effects on health							
Levin (1996)[b]	R	reviews literature on religion-health relationship and discusses mechanisms							
Genetics									
Boomsma (1999)	CS	C	1974 twins/families	Netherlands	#5+ ORA,D,SR	?0% genetic	–	8
Bouchard (1999)	CS	C	35 MZ/37 DZ twins	–	#3+ IR,ER	significant	SC	7
Heath (1999)	PC	C?	1687 twins	13–20 yo	–	#3+ RB,ORA	Blacks—yes	SC	8
*Kendler (1997)	CS	C	1902	CDA, twins	Virginia	#11 RB,ORA, NORA,SR	0–29% genetic	MC	9
Kirk (1999)	CS	C?	5670/5614 families	US/Australia	#1 ORA	Significant	SC	8
Landis (1999)	PC	R	357 twins	6–18 yo/mothers	–	#3+ RB,SR,ORA	minor	SC	8
*Truett (1992)	CS	C	7620 twins	CDA	Australia	#2 D, ORA	0–16% genetic	SC	10

a. Levin & Schiller   b. Levin, Chatters, et al.

RESEARCH ON RELIGION AND USE OF HEALTH SERVICES

Outcome/Investigators	Type	Method	N	Population	Location	Religious Variable	Findings	Controls	Rating
Use of General Medical Services (Ch 26)									
Bearon (1990)	CS,D	C	40	CDA,E	Durham, NC	#5+ RB,NORA	NG (prayer)	NONE	4
Bliss (1995)	CT	C	331	MP (open heart surgery)	Massachusetts	#1 chaplain intervention	P	–	–
*Burell (1996)	CT	S	128 vs. Cs	MP (CABG)	Sweden	#1 "reflect spiritual issues"	P	–	9

Reference			N	Variables	Location	Findings	2nd most common	Controls	Q
*Croog (1972)	PC,D	S	324	MP,M (s/p MI)	Massachusetts	#1 consulting clergy	NA (MD visits)	NONE	7
Eisenberg (1993)	CS,D	R	1539	CDA	National US	#1 prayer as unconventional treat	P	–	7
*Florell (1973)	CT	C	44	MP	–	#1 chaplain visits	P	NONE	–
*Frankel (1994)	CS	C	299	CS	Ontario, Can	#10+ D,Belief scale	P	MC	6
*Koenig (1995b)	PC	S	262	MP	Durham, NC	#3 RC	NA	MC	6
Koenig (1998)[a]	CS,PC	S	542	MP, E	Durham, NC	#2 ORA,D	P	NONE	9
*Levin (1985)	CS	S	1125	CDA (MexAm)	San Antonio, TX	#2 ORA,SR	NG (with SR)	NONE	7
McSherry (1986)[b]	R,O			reviews effects that chaplains may have on cost and use of health services					
McSherry (1987)	PC	C	80	MP	Massachusetts	#1 SR	P	NONE	6
Mechanic (1963)	CS	C	1300	CS	West, Midwest US	#2 D,ORA	P	NONE	6
Mechanic (1990)	R			notes that a wide range of religious groups tend to encourage moderation and to frown upon "extreme" or risk-taking behaviors					
*Pressman (1990)	CS	C	30	MP,E	Chicago	#3 ORA,SR,RC	P	NONE	6
Schiller (1988)	R,CS	–	909	CDA	Appalachia	#4 CM,ORA	P	MC	7
Trier (1991)	CS	R	325	CDA	Michigan	#9 RB,ORA,NORA	NG (prayer)	NONE	6
Wan (1975)	CS	R	2168	CDA	New York, Pennsylvania	#1 D	Jews > others	MC	3
*Yeung (1992)	CS	R	3640	CDA	New Haven, CT	#1 Jewish vs. non-J	Jews > Non-J	MC	8

Use of Mental Health Services (Ch 26)

Reference			N	Variables	Location	Findings	2nd most common	Controls	Q
Chu (1985)	PC	S	128	PP (Schizophrenics,B)	Missouri	#3+ D,ORA,NORA	M	NONE	6
Berg (1995)	PC	C	37	PP	Minnesota	#7 ORA,RB,E	P	NONE	6
Gurin (1960)	CS,D	R	2460	CDA	National US	#3 ORA,RC,clergy	–	–	6
*Kennedy (1996)	PC	R	1855	CDA,E	Bronx, NY	#1 Jews vs. others	Jews > others	SC	10
*Koenig (1994)[c]	CS	R	853 vs. 1826	baby boomers	Durham, NC	#5 D,ORA,SR,NORA	C (D)	MC	9
Kulka (1979)	D	R	4724	CDA	National US	#1 sought clergy help	43%	–	7
Larson DB (1988)	CS, D	R	18000+	CDA	5 US cities	#1 seeking clergy for psychiatric problems (often)	–		9
Murstein (1993)	D	C	90	PP	Connecticut	#1 clergy 3rd-4th most preferred MH provider			3
Postolache (1997)	CS	C	41	PP (Hispanic)	New York City	#3 RB,D,NORA	M	MC	6
Regier (1978)	CS	R	–	CDA	National US	#1 saw relig counselors			6
*Srole (1962)	CS	R	1660	CDA	Manhattan, NY	#1 D	Jews > others	SC-age,SES	7
*Yeung (1992)	CS	R	3640	CDA	New Haven, CT	#1 Jewish vs. non-J	Jews > Non-J	MC	8

Disease Prevention (Ch 27)

(">" indicates less prevention activity in this section)

Reference			N	Variables	Location	Findings	2nd most common	Controls	Q
*Apel (1986)	CS	C	260	CM,R	Midwest US	#2+ ORA	P	NONE	2

a. Koenig & Larson b. McSherry 1986; McSherry, Kratz, et al. c. Koenig, George, Meador, Blazer, & Dyck

Outcome/Investigators	Type	Method	N	Population	Location	Religious Variable	Findings	Controls	Rating
*Goldscheider (1991)	CS	R	8450	CDA,F	National US	#4 ORA,D	NG (D-conserv)	MC	8
Kuemmerer (1967)	C	R	7787	HS (TB screen)	Maryland	#1 parents ORA	P	NONE	5
Loue (1999)	R,O			discusses how Buddhist religious beliefs may be utilized to reduce spread of HIV infection in Pacific Islanders					
Miller SL (1980)	CS	C	260	MP, F (SBE)	San Diego, CA	#1 D	Ca > P,J	NONE	5
Miller AM (1993)	CS	C	161	CDA,F (mammography)	Indiana	#1 D (Ca vs. P)	Ca > P	MC	6
Murray M (1993)	CS	S	391	CDA,F (SBE)	North Ireland	#1 D (Anglican vs. others)	Others > Anglican	MC	7
*Lasater (1986)	D			describes project in which church volunteers deliver behavior change programming for major cardiovascular risk factors					

SBE = self breast examination

Health Responsibility

*Oleckno (1991)	CS	–	1077	CS	N. Illinois	#2 ORA, SR	P	NONE	6
Miller AS (1995)	CS	R	2408	HS	National US	#2 ORA, SR	P	SC	7

Compliance with Treatment

Archer (1967)	PC	S	757	Anti-coronary club	New York City	#2 D,ORA	P (J > Ca)	NONE	6
Blumenthal (1982)	PC	S	35	MP (recent MI)	Durham, NC	#1 (social isolation)	(P)	–	7
Chang (1985)	CS	C	286	CDA,E,F	Los Angeles	#1 D (Jews vs. other)	J > other	MC	7
*Christo (1995)	PC	C	101	poly-drug abusers	London, England	#10 spiritual belief	P (Narcotics Anonymous participation)	NONE	7
DeVellis (1988)	CS	C	72	CM	Chapel Hill, NC	#1 RB (affects health care decisions)	–	–	3
Foulks (1986)	CS	C	60	PP	Pennsylvania	#4 RB (R cause of ill)	NG	MC	6
Fox (1998)	CS	C	1517	CM	Los Angeles	#3 ORA,SR	P	SC	7
*Harris (1995)	PC	C	40	MP (heart transplant)	Pennsylvania	#3+ ORA,NORA,SR	P	NONE	6
*Kirov (1998)	CS/D	S	52	PP (psychotic)	United Kingdom	#2+ RC	(P)	–	6
Mayer (1965)	CS	S	193	PP (alcoholics)	Boston	#1 D (P vs. Ca vs. J)	NA	NONE	2
Naguib (1968)	CS	R	2612	CDA, F	Maryland	#2 ORA,D (any)	P	NONE	7
*O'Brien (1982)	PC	C	126	MP (hemodialysis)	Washington, DC	#3+ D,ORA,RC	P	NONE	6

CLINICAL IMPLICATIONS AND APPLICATIONS

Health Professionals (Ch 29)

Medical Practice

Outcome/Investigators	Type	Method	N	Population	Location	Religious Variable	Findings	Controls	Rating
Barnard (1995)	R,O			examines medical education and incorporation of relligious studies in medical curriculum					
Cornish (1998)	R,O			overviews religious beliefs and issues in care of Mormon patients					
Daaleman (1994)	CS	C	80	MP	Kansas		ORA predicts receptivity to religious inquiry		5
Daaleman (1998,1999)	CS	S	438	physicians-FPs	National US	#5 ORA,NORA,RE	–	–	7
Ellis M (1999)	CS	C	170	physicians-FPs	Missouri	#20+ SWB, Misc	–	–	6
Hamilton (1998)	R,O			discusses the importance of physicians acknowledging potential role of spirituality in health and affirming patients' beliefs					
Hiatt (1986)	Q		–	general practice	–	spiritual care	–	–	–
Kelly MJ (1996)	D			describes results of a course on religion and health at E. Tennessee State University					
Koenig (1989)[a]	CS,D	R	160	physicians	Illinois	#20+ misc	–	–	8
Koenig (1991)	CS,D	C	130	physicians	Durham, NC	#3+ RB, RC,ORA	–	–	6
Kuhn (1988)	R,O			provides useful information for obtaining a spiritual or religious history, including questions					
Larson DB (1995)	R			reviews whether religion and spirituality are clinically relevant to health care					
Lo (1999)	O			American College of Physicians panel suggestions concerning religious/spiritual history in seriously ill patients					
Malak (1998)	R,O			overviews religious beliefs and issues involved in treating Jehovah's Witnesses					
Magaletta (1997)	R,O			discusses the issue of physicians praying with patients					
Maugans (1991)	CS,D	S	115/135	physicians/pts	Vermont	#15 misc	–	–	6
Maugans (1996)	R,O			discusses physician spiritual history taking with The SPIRITual History method					
McKee (1992)	R			review and discussion of the role of spirituality in practice of family medicine					
Mohiuddin (1998)	R			overview of Sufi healing practices					
Olive (1995)	CS	C	26	physicians	Tennessee		practices with patients described		5
Orr (1997)	R,O			discusses medical ethics involved in physicians' responses to "inappropriate" requests from patients based on their religious beliefs					
Orr (1998)	R,O			responds to assertion that medicine, ethics and atheism are objective, rational and true, while religion is irrational and false					
Oyama (1998)	CS,D	C	380/31	pts/physicians	North Carolina		religious practices of patients and physicians described		6
Post (2000)	O			discusses ethical issues concerning use of prayer and other religious intervention in medical practice					
Puchalski (1998)	R,O			discusses the development of curricula in medical schools concerning spirituality and medicine					
Sansome (1990)	CS	S	276	directors of psychiatric training programs; 12 percent of programs have a course on religion					8
Sinha (1998)	R,O			overviews religious beliefs and issues in care of Hindu patients					
Tate (1998)	R,O			overviews religious beliefs and issues in care of Jewish patients					
Tauxe (1998)	R,O			overviews religious beliefs and issues in care of Unitarian-Universalist patients					
Walter (1997)	R,O			discusses three approaches to organizing spiritual care in hospices					

a. Koenig, Bearon, & Dayringer

Outcome/Investigators	Type	Method	N	Population	Location	Religious Variable	Findings	Controls	Rating
Nursing Practice									
Bauer (1995)	CS	C	50	E	Omaha, Neb	spiritual care preferences	–	–	6
Bay (1997)	R,O			examines relationship between oncology nurse and parish nurse					
Boland (1998)	R,O			discusses the role of the parish nurse in promoting health in the elderly					
Carson (1997)	R,O			examines nurses giving spiritual care to family caregivers of cancer patients					
Clark (1997)	R,O			examines the spiritual needs of orthopedic patients					
Hart (1997)[a]	R,O			examines spiritual care of children with cancer					
Highfield (1997)	R,O			examines spiritual assessment of cancer patients by nurses					
Magilvy (1997)	R,O			examines parish nursing as an advanced practice model for stimulating health care reform					
Mickley (1995)	R			reviews the major empirical data on religion and mental health pertinent to nursing					
Newshan (1998)	R,O			examines spiritual interventions for treating pain in patients with HIV or cancer					
Oldnall (1996)	R,O			explores possibilities for nurses meeting spiritual needs in context of British National Health Service					
O'Neill (1998)	R,O			comprehensive overview of spirituality and strategies to support the spiritual dimensions of nursing care for those with chronic illness					
Penner (1997)	R,O			discusses the role of parish nursing in community health					
Roberson (1987)	Q			examines folk health beliefs of health professionals, nurses in particular (120 health professionals)					
Ross (1995)	R,O			reviews the nurse's role in spiritual care					
Ross (1997)	R,O			discusses spiritual needs and care in elderly patients					
Van Loon (1998)	R,O			reviews parish nurse program (faith community nursing program) development in Australia					
VandeCreek (1997)	R,O			examines collaboration between nurses and chaplains in caring for cancer patients					
Weinrich (1998)	R			examines African-American churches as an outlet for prostate cancer education					
Weis (1997)	R/CS			major review and evaluation of the parish nurse model, including interventions used by 11 parish nurses over one-year					
Wright (1998)	R,O			examines the nurse's professional, ethical, and legal responsibility to provide spiritual care					
Psychiatric Practice									
Abernethy (1998)	R,O			examines religious transference and counter-transference when examining religious themes					
Ball (1991)	CS,D	S	174 and 30	Chr therapists	California	therapy techniques	–	–	5
Bergin (1980)	R,O			discusses whether or not to consider patient's religious values in psychotherapy					
Bergin (1991)[b]	R,O			review of how to incorporate spirituality in psychotherapy					
Cary (1997)	O			Archbishop of Canterbury discusses need to integrate religion and psychiatrict practice					
Fitchett (1997)	CC,D	C	51 PP, 50 MP	PP and MP	Chicago	spiritual needs of pts	–	–	6
Gartner (1986)	Exp	C	356 MP	psychology graduate programs	National US	evangelical/integrationalist applicant		–	7
Jones S (1992)	CS/D	S	8639	alumni of Christian graduate training programs of professional psychology–clinical interventions					7
Jones S (1994)	R,O			examines the relationship between religion and the science and profession of psychology					

Larson DB (1993)	D					found that 22.2% of case examples of pathology in DSM-III-R glossary had substantial religious content			6
Larson DB (1997)	R					provides model curriculum for training of psychiatry residents in religious/spiritual issues			
Lehr E (1989)	D					compares handling of religion in psychology textbooks in 1950s and 1970s with 1980s			
Lukoff (1992)	R					explores nomenclature barriers that prevent accurate diagnosis and management of psycho-spiritual and religious problems			
Marcus (1995)	R,O								
Martinez (1991)	PC/D	C	30	PP	Midwest US	discusses role of religion as support in extreme situations (self-psychology of Kohut)	#1 religious vs. non-R	—	
Morgan (1994)	R,O					review & discussion of growing interest in spirituality among North American psychiatrists			
Neeleman (1995)	R					review of implications of research between religion and mental health to psychiatrists			
Pattison (1966)	R,O					early discussion of social and psychological aspects of religion in psychotherapy			
*Pfeifer (1995)	CC	C	44 vs. 45 Cs	PP	Switzerland		#35 IR,ER,Misc	NONE / NA	5
Pichot (1973)	CS	C	3952	PP	France		#1 RB	NONE / M	5
Roberts D (1997)	R,O					discusses transcending barriers between religion and psychiatry			
Runions (1974)	R,O					early discussion of religion and psychiatric practice			
Saucer (1992)	R,O					review of a psychotherapeutic technique called evangelical renewal therapy			
Sivan (1996)	CC,D	51 PP, 50 MP		PP and MP	Chicago		#1 spoke with clergy	MP > PP	6
Taubes (1998)	D					discusses first form of psychiatric care in America—moral treatment—with its strong religious component			
Tillman (1998)	R,O					discusses whether or not therapists should self-disclose their religious beliefs to patients			
Turbott (1996)	R,O					reviews implications of research between religion and mental health for psychiatrists			
Turner (1995)	R					discusses new DSM category for spiritual problems			
Waldfogel (1993)	Cser	—	—	cases	Philadelphia		relig considerations in C-L psychiatry	—	—
Waldfogel (1996)	Cser	—	—	cases	Philadelphia		relig considerations in capacity evaluations	—	—
Worthington (1991)	R					review of psychotherapy & religious values			
Worthington (1996)	R					review of research on religious psychotherapy			

Social Work Practice

Babler (1997)	CS	C/S		hospice nurses, social workers, etc	National US		"spiritual care" differences	—	6
*Bergin (1990)	CS	S	425	therapists	National US		#23 D,ORA,RB	(fewest agnostics/atheists among social workers)	—
Hart (1997)[c]	R,O					describes an educational program where hospital chaplains collaborate with social workers in meeting patient needs			

Religious Professionals (Ch 30)

Anderson (1993)	D	S	152	MP	Baltimore, MD		R/S needs	—	6
Arnold (1979)	R					reviews research on counseling by clergy			
Beitman (1982)	O					discusses the challenge that pastoral counseling presents to community mental health centers			
Blasi (1998)	D	S	51	R	Nashville		Services	—	
Chalfant (1990)	CS,D	R	530	CDA	El Paso, TX		clergy sought for help	41%	6 / 7

a. Hart & Schneider   b. Bergin 1991; Bergin & Payne   c. Hart & Matorin

Outcome/Investigators	Type	Method	N	Population	Location	Religious Variable	Findings	Controls	Rating
Chatters (1998)	R				examines public health and health education in faith communities				
Davis (1994)	D	C	24 churches	minority gps	Los Angeles	cervical CA screening	–	–	5
Emblen (1993)	CS,D	C	19	MP	Illinois	meeting spiritual needs	–	–	3
Eng (1980)	D				describes church-based interventions to disseminate a wide range of health information and services				
Ford (1996)	D				describes church-based asthma education program for African-Americans				
Haber (1984)	D				describes 12-hour caregiving program at 8 church sites				
Hatch J (1980)	R,O				reviews disease prevention programs in Black churches				
Haugk (1976)	R,O				examines contribution of churches and clergy to mental health effort				
Holmes (1980)	Exp	C	180	groups of professionals (physicians, clergy, etc.)			clergy recognize suicide poorly	–	7
Jones (1992)	D	S	639	psychologists	National US	Christian college alumni	–	–	7
Kaseman (1977)	Q	C	18	R	Illinois, Minnesota	discusses clergy involvement in community mental health programs (based on qualitative study)			–
Kloos (1995)	Q					discusses collaboration with mental health professionals			
Koenig (1997)[a]	R				review and discussion to help clergy identify and treat mental disorders in older adults				
Koenig (1998)[b]	R				review and discussion of geriatric mental and medical problems relevant to clergy				
*Kumanyika (1992)	D/CT	C	188	CM, 100%B,F	Baltimore	church-based wt ctrl	P		7
*Larson DB (1988)	CS, D	R	18000+	CDA	5 US cities	#1 seeking clergy for psychiatric problems (often)	–	–	9
*Lasater (1986)	D				describes project in which church volunteers deliver behavior change programming for major cardiovascular risk factors				
Levin (1984)	R				discusses role of Black church in community medicine				
Maton (1995)	R				reviews role of religious community (through volunteering) in maintaining health of congregations, others				
Mollica (1986)	D	S	214	R	Connecticut	pastoral counseling activities	–	–	9
Neighbors (1998)	CS, D	R	2107	CDA, B	National US	#1 sought clergy help	–		7
Olson (1988)	D	C	176 Black church pastors		Chicago	interviews to assess church-based social & health programs	–	–	6
Parkum (1985)	CS/D	C	432	MP	Pennsylvania	chaplains	–	–	7
Pieper (1992)	CS/D	C	160	R	Midwest US	pastors	NG	–	6
Ransdell (1995)	R,O				discusses church-based health promotion for women age 65 or over				
*Rayburn (1991)	CS	C	254	R,F	United States	women relig (Ca,P,J)	P (Ca)	SC	6
*Saunders (1983)	D				describes three-years of experience establishing and running a church-based hypertension program				
Shifrin (1998)	R				examines role of faith community as a supportive network for persons with mental illness				
*Spilka (1983)	CS,D	C	101 pts/45 parents of children with cancer		Denver, CO	experiences with chaplains and home pastors		–	6
Thomas (1994)	CS	C	635	Black churches	Northern US	health outreach prgms		–	8

Uhlman (1984)	CS/D	C	120	NH,E	National US	pastoral visitation	—	—	7
VandeCreek (1996)	CS	S	471	R	Ohio	pastoral visit made	—	—	8
*VandeCreek (1997)	R,O	examines collaboration between nurses and chaplains in caring for cancer patients							
Weaver A (1993a)	R	discusses what clergy need to know about depression							
Weaver A (1993b)	R	discusses what clergy need to know about psychological trauma							
Weaver A (1997)c	SR	systematic review of 8 APA journals—need for collaboration between psychologists and clergy							
Weaver A (1997)d	SR	systematic review of marriage and family journals—need for collaboration between M & F therapists and clergy							
Weaver A (1998)e	SR	systematic review of 4 psychiatric journals—need for collaboration between psychiatrists and clergy							
Weaver A (1998b)f	SR	systematic review of major mental health nursing journals—need for collaboration between nurses and clergy							
Worthington (1986)	R	reviews outcome research on religious counseling							

a. Koenig & Weaver   b. Koenig & Weaver   c. Weaver, Samford, Kline, et al.   d. Weaver, Koenig, et al.   e. Weaver, Samford, Larson, et al.   f. Weaver, Flannelly, et al.

PRIORITIES FOR FUTURE RESEARCH

Outcome/Investigators	Type	Method	N	Population	Location	Religious Variable	Findings	Controls	Rating
Measurement (Ch 33)									
*Allport (1967)	CS	C	309	CM	Maine, New York, Tennessee	#20 IR-ER	—	—	7
Ben-Meir (1979)	CS,D	—	—	CDA	Israel	#26 Jewish beliefs & activities scale	—	—	7
Dudley R (1990)	CS	C	491	CS (religious)	Michigan	#58 IR,ER 11-item maturity index	—	—	6
Duke (1984)	CS	R	1384	CDA Mormons	National US	#12+ ORA,NORA,RB	—	—	4
Fetzer Institute (1999)	Q	development of multi-dimensional religious/spiritual scale at Fetzer Institute (CS & PC studies in progress)							
*Genia (1993)	CS	C	309	CDA	Washington, DC	#21 D,IR,ER	—	—	6
Glock (1966)	R	review, development, and testing of the renowned Glock & Stark religiosity scales							
Gorsuch (1972)	CS	C	84	CS	Kentucky, Tennessee	#40 + RB, IR/ER (compared single vs multiple-item scales)	—	—	6
Gorsuch (1984)	R	reviews ways of measuring religiousness							
Gorsuch (1989)	CS	C	768	CS (?)	Pasadena, CA	#3 & #14 IR-Es-Ep	—	—	7
Hadaway (1993)	CS	R	604	CDA	Ohio	ORA (compares rates of reported with actual attend)	—	—	7
Hall (1996)	CS	C	470	CS	Arizona	#40 item spirituality	—	—	6
Hatch R (1998)	CS	C	50/33	MP/physicians	Florida	#26 item spirituality	—	—	6
Himmelfarb (1975)	CS	C	1278	CDA (Jews)	Chicago	#66 Jewish beliefs & activities scale	—	—	7
Hoge (1972)	CS	C	93	CDA	New Jersey	#10 IR scale	—	—	7

Outcome/Investigators	Type	Method	N	Population	Location	Religious Variable	Findings	Controls	Rating
*Hood (1975)	CS	C	300	CS	Tennessee	#32 mysticism scale	–	–	6
Hunt (1971)	R	review and critique of Allport's IE scales							
Idler (2000)	R	review and development of a 38-item Fetzer Institute spirituality measure (see Fetzer Institute, 1999, above)							
*Kass (1991)	PC	C	83	MP	Boston	#7 INSPIRIT	–	–	7
Kirkpatrick (1990)[a]	R	review & discussion of intrinsic and extrinsic religiosity scales							
King MB (1972)	CS	S	1356	CM	Texas	#59 scale development	–	–	8
King MB (1975)	CS	R	1990	CM (Presbyt)	United States	#98 scale development	–	–	8
King Mi (1995)	CS	C	305	MP,staff, etc.	London, England	#15+ scale development	–	–	7
King Mi (1998)	R	discusses the inclusion and measurement of the spiritual variable in psychiatric research							
Koenig (1988)[b]	CS	C	906	CDA,E,R	Illinois/Iowa	#34 (long), #21 (short) versions of Springfield Religiosity Schedule	–	–	
Koenig (1997)[c]	CS,PC	S	7000/86	CDA/MP	North Carolina	#5 ORA,NORA,IR	–	–	7
*Krause (1993)	CS	R	709	CDA	US and Can	#18 ORA,SR,RB	–	–	9
Krause (1996)	Q	report on development of measures of religion for studies on health : The SWAN project							
Levin (1995)[d]	CS	R	1978	CDA, B	National US	#12 ORA,NORA,SR	–	–	8
Mindel (1978)	CS	C	106	CDA,E	Missouri	#7 ORA,NORA (measuring religiousness in older adults)	–	–	5
*Moberg (1984)	CS	C	1081	CDA	US & Sweden	#45 SWB scale	–	–	7
*Palloutzian (1982)	CS	C	206	CS	Idaho	#10 RWB	–	–	7
*Pargament (1998, 2000)[e]	CS	S	540/551	CS/MP,E	Ohio & NC	#63 RC	–	–	9
*Plante (1997)	CS	C	102	CS	California	#10 SR,NORA, ORA,RC	–	–	5
Schaefer (1993)	CS	C	137	CM, Christian CS	S. California	#>20 RC, D	–	–	4
Schaler (1996)	CS	C	295	Addiction Rx providers	S. California	#8 spiritual beliefs scale (measures AA spiritual philosophy)	–	–	7
*Strayhorn (1990)	CS	C	201	parents of Head Start kids	Pittsburgh	#12 ORA, NORA	–	–	5
Underwood (1999)	Q	development of 15-item daily spiritual experiences scale at Fetzer Intitute (several CS & PC studies in progress)							
*Veach (1992)	CS	C	148	CS & health professionals	Nevada	#18 Spiritual Exp, etc.	–	–	3
Wilson J (1978)	R	review of measurement of religion							

a. Kirkpatrick & Hood   b. Koenig, Smiley, & Gonzales   c. Koenig, Meador, & Parkerson   d. Levin, Taylor, & Chatters   e. Pargament, Smith, Koenig, et al.; Pargament, Koenig, & Perez

MISCELLANEOUS TOPICS CONCERNING RELIGION AND HEALTH

Outcome/Investigators	Type	Method	N	Population	Location	Religious Variable	Findings	Controls	Rating
Religious Beliefs/Behaviors									
Medical Patients									
*Ai (1997)	PC	S	151	MP (with CABG)	Michigan	#3 SR,ORA,NORA	–	–	7
Ehman (1999)	CS	S	177	MP	Philadelphia	#5+ (patient attitudes toward MD addressing religious issues)	–	–	8
Ide (1992)	CS,D	C	50	MP,F, Saudi	Saudia Arabia	#1 RB (God causes)	–	–	4
King D (1994)	CS,D	S	203	MP (inpatients)	North Carolina, Pennsylvania	#8+ RB,ORA, NORA,O	–	–	7
*Koenig (1988)[a]	CS	S	106	MP, E	Illinois	#15+ ORA,NORA,IR	–	–	7
*Koenig (1991)	CS,D	C	130	MP, families	Durham, NC	#3+ RB, RC,ORA	–	–	6
Koenig (1998b)	CS,D	S	542	MP, E	Durham, NC	#12 ORA,NORA, IR	–	–	7
*Oyama (1998)	CS,D	C	380/31	pts/physicians	North Carolina	#33 ORA,IR,RE,RB	–	–	6
Psychiatric Patients									
*Fitchett (1997)	CC,D	C	51 PP, 50 MP	PP and MP	Chicago	spiritual needs of pts	–	–	6
*Lindgren (1995)	D	C	28	PP	Maryland	#5+ RB, RC, NORA	–	–	6
Lyles (1983)	CC,D	C	21 + Cs	PP	North Carolina	#5+ RB,RE,ORA	–	–	3
*Pichot (1973)	CS,D	C	3952	PP	France	#1 RB	–	–	5
Roberts B (1954)	CS,D	S	1963	PP	New Haven, CT	#1 D (CA,J,P)	–	–	4
Sexually Abused									
Johnsen (1996)	CC	C	491 vs. 51 Cs	CS,F	New England	#2 D, SR	NA	NONE	5
Community-Dwelling Adults									
Barna (1991)	CS	R	1000+	CDA	National US	Many	–	–	8
Barron (1958)	CS,D	–	1206	CDA,E, M	National US	#3 ORA,NORA	–	–	5
*Bearon (1990)	CS,D	C	40	CDA,E	Durham, NC	multiple (NORA,RB)	–	–	4
Campbell (1994)	CS	R	28764	CDA	22 countries	#12 ORA,SR,RB	effects of secularization	–	8
Chavis (1989)	CS	R	10655	CDA	National US	#1 ORA	–	–	7
Glamser (1987)	PC,D	C	51 industrial workers (CDA)		Pennsylvania	#3 D,ORA,RB	rlg activity increase in retirement	–	7
Levin (1993)[b]	CS	R	2107	CDA, 100%B	National US	#12 ORA,NORA,SR	–	–	8

a. Koenig, Moberg, & Kvale   b. Levin & Taylor

Outcome/Investigators	Type	Method	N	Population	Location	Religious Variable	Findings	Controls	Rating
Levin (1993)	CS	R	1481	CDA	National US	#10+ ORA,NORA,Mystical experiences	—	—	8
Levin (1994)[a]	CS	R	1209/2797/ 1669/551	CDA	National US	#4/#4/#7/#6 ORA, NORA,SR	—	—	9
Levin (1997)[b]	CS	R	1481	CDA	National US	#1 NORA (prayer)	—	—	8
Orbach (1961)	CS,D	R	6911	CDA	Detroit	#1 ORA	—	—	4
Petrowsky (1976)	CS	R	273	CDA,E	Florida	# 1 ORA	—	—	6
PRRC (1939–96)	CS	R	1000's	CDA	National US	Many	—	—	9
Roozen (1990)	CS	R	1015/1130	CDA	National US	#1 ORA	—	—	7
Shebani (1986)	CS	C	215	CDA,E vs. CS	Libya	#2 ORA,RB	—	—	4
Stark (1968)	CS,D	R	2871	CDA	National US	#>20 D,ORA,RCm,NORA	—	—	6
*Taylor RJ (1986)	CS,D	R	581	CDA,E,B	National US	#3 ORA,CM,SR	—	—	7
Taylor RJ (1991)	CS	R	581	CDA,E,B	National US	#4 NORA	—	—	8
Zinnbauer (1997)	CS	C	346	CDA,CS,CM	Pennsylvania, Ohio	#>50 RB (spiritual vs. religious)	—	—	7

Physicians/Nurses

Outcome/Investigators	Type	Method	N	Population	Location	Religious Variable	Findings	Controls	Rating
*Daaleman (1998,1999)	CS	S	438	physicians-FPs	National US	#5 ORA,NORA,RE	—	—	7
*Ellis M (1999)	CS	C	170	physicians-FPs	Missouri	#20+ SWB, Misc	—	—	6
Hall (1993)	CS,D	C	303	Christian nurses	North America	#10+ ORA,RB,Misc	—	—	5
*Koenig (1991)	CS,D	C	130	physicians	Durham, NC	#3+ RB, RC,ORA	—	—	6
Manusov (1995)	Q	C	59	FP residents	4 major US cities	religion noted as contributer to well-being	—	—	5
*Maugans (1991)	CS,D	S	115/135	physicians/pts	Vermont	#15 misc	—	—	6
*Olive (1995)	CS	C	26	physicians	Tennessee		practices with patients described	—	5
*Oyama (1998)	CS,D	C	31	physicians	North Carolina	#33 ORA,IR,RE,RB	—	—	6
*Roberson (1987)	CS,D	C	97/23	Nurses/MDs	Southern US	#9 RB,NORA	—	—	4
Schwartz (1971)	CS,D	C	46	medical students	New Haven, CT	#2 D,ORA	(P) (ORA)	NS	4

Mental Health Professionals

Outcome/Investigators	Type	Method	N	Population	Location	Religious Variable	Findings	Controls	Rating
Bergin (1990)	CS,D	S	425	Psychotherapists	National US	#23 D,ORA,RB	—	—	7
Galanter (1991)	CS,D	S	193	Christian psychiatrists	National US	characteristics & practices of	—	—	7
Ganje-Fling (1991)	CS,D	C	50 therapists/68	spiritual healers	Midwestern US	characteristics & practices of	—	—	4
Jensen J (1988)	CS	S	425	MH professionals	National US	#4+ D,RB (religious values)	—	—	7

Study			N	Population	Location	Measures	Findings	
Marx (1969)	CS,D	S	3990	MH professionals	New York, Louisiana, Chicago	#3+ D,misc	—	7
Neeleman (1993)	CS,D	C	231	psychiatrists	England	#32 RB,misc	—	7
Ragan (1980)	CS,D	R	555	psychologists	National US	$3+ RB,ORA	—	7
Shafranske (1990b)	CS, D	S	409	psychologists	National US	#10+ RB,RE,ORA,D	—	7
Shafranske (1990a)	CS,D	R	47	psychologists	California	#20+ RB,Q,ORA,D	—	6

Religious/Faith Development

Study			N	Population	Location	Measures	Findings	
Barns (1989)	CS	S	277 and 301	theologians,CM	Dayton, OH	Fowler's faith stages, RB	—	6
Fowler (1981)	CS	C	356	CDA in & around academic communities		(describes widely known theory of faith development)		7
Glover (1986)	CS	C	147	Ad, young	Arkansas	#4+ four rlg factors	differences between age groups	4
Hertel (1995)	CS	–	3400 triads	father-mo-child	National US	(parenting styles predicted images of God)		7
Kirkpatrick (1990)[c]	CS	C	213	CDA	Denver, CO	#25+ IR,ER,ORA	assoc w maternal attachment styles	5
*Kirkpatrick (1992)	CS	C	213	CDA	Denver, CO	#5+ D,IR,ER,RB	God as compensatory	5
Koenig (1994c)	R,O		discusses theory of religious faith development in later life					5
Masters (1991)	PC	C	60	CS (Mormon)	Utah	#20-IR, others (continuous vs. discontinuous religious development)		5
Shulik (1988)	CS,D	C	40	CDA,E		descriptive attempt to validate Fowler's faith stages in older adults		5
Worthington (1989)	R		theories of religious development are reviewed, from childhood to adolescence and beyond					

Religious Conversion

Study			N	Population	Location	Measures	Findings	
Bragan (1977)	CR		discusses case report of conversion and need for psychotherapy to integrate experience					
*Cavenar (1977)	Cser		reviews four cases of depressive disorder and religious conversion					
Christensen (1963)	R,O		discusses the psychology of religious conversion					
*Galanter (1979)	CS,D	C	237	CDA-Moonies	New York City	#10 D, religiosity scale (describes expriences of converts)		7
Gritzmacher (1988)	R,O		examines psychodynamics of Pentecostalism					
Heirich (1977)	CC	C	152 recently coverted Catholic Pentacostals vs. 158 controls					7
James (1902)	R,D		examines extreme cases of religious conversion					
Koenig (1994)[d]	CS	S	276	MP, <40,>65		examines frequency and mental health effects of religious conversion		7
*Kirkpatrick (1990)	CS	C	213	CDA	Denver, CO	#25+ IR,ER,ORA (with maternal attachment styles)		7
Pattison (1980)	Cser	C	11 white homosexual males reporting profound changes in sexual orientation following conversion					5
Salzman (1953)	R,O		discusses the psychology of religious and ideological conversion					
*Ullman (1988)	CS	C	40	CDA (converts)	Jerusalem	#2 D (J,Ca,Bahai, HK), RE	—	5

a. Levin, Taylor, et al.   b. Levin & Taylor   c. Kirkpatrick & Shaver   d. Koenig & Herman

Outcome/Investigators	Type	Method	N	Population	Location	Religious Variable	Findings	Controls	Rating
*Wilson WP (1972)	CS,D	C	63	CDA	Durham, NC	#10+ RE	—	—	5
Wiztum (1990)	CS,D	S	561	PP	Jerusalem	#2 D,RE (coversion to Judaism)	—	—	5
*Wootton (1983)	R,O	reviews effects of religious conversion on mental health							

Spiritual/Faith Healing

Outcome/Investigators	Type	Method	N	Population	Location	Religious Variable	Findings	Controls	Rating
Am Acad Peds (1997)	R,O	position statement regarding religious healing and concerns over child safety							
Fitzgerald (1970)	CS,D	C	66	CDA (blind)	London, England	seeking faith healing	>1/3	—	6
*Glik (1986,1990a)	CC	C	93/83/137	New Age/Charismatics/MP	(Maryland)	NewA. vs. Char vs. MP	P (Char)	MC	7
Glik (1988)	PC,Q	C	250–300	CDA	Baltimore, MD	healings in New Age and Charismatic healing groups	—	—	4
Glik (1990b)	PC	C	160 members of healing groups		Baltimore, MD	outcome of healings	NA (with objective outcomes)	—	6
Johnson DM (1986)	CS,D	C	586	CDA	Richmond, VA	faith healing experiences	—	—	7
King D (1988)	CS/D	C	203	MP	Gatesville, NC	faith healing experiences	6% healed by faith healer	—	6
King D (1992)	CS/D	R	594	Physicians	North Carolina, New York, Florida, Illinois	faith healing experiences & opinions	—	—	7
*King D (1994)	CS	S	203	MP	North Carolina, Pennsylvania	faith healing & prayer	—	—	7
Koss (1987)	CS	C	96/100	Therapists/PP	Puerto Rico	compares treatment in community MHC with treatment by spiritist	—	—	6
Levin (1986)[a]	R	reviews and discusses "New Age" healing practices in the United States							
Paulsen (1926)	R	early review of religious groups and beliefs about faith healing							
Pattison (1973)	D	C	43 pentacostals/fundamentalists		Seattle, WA	faith healing experiences and MMPI scores	—	—	5
Uyanga (1979)	CS,D	C	18/472	Spiritual healers/MP	Nigeria	compares pts of spiritual healing homes & traditional doctors	—	—	6
Wirth (1995)	PC,D	C	48	MP	Marin, CA	spiritual healing ("magnetic laying on of hands")	NA	—	4

Prayer Studies (DIP distant intercessory prayer; DMH distant mental healing)

Outcome/Investigators	Type	Method	N	Population	Location	Religious Variable	Findings	Controls	Rating
Benor (1992)	R	reviews studies of distant mental effects/healing, including studies involving bacteria and non-human subjects							
Benson H (in progress)	CT	S	1800	MP (CABG)	Multisite	DIP	pending	—	10
*Beutler (1988)	CT	C	120	CDA	Netherlands	DIP,DMH	NA	—	8

*Byrd (1988)	CT	S	393	MP (CCU)	San Francisco	DIP	P	—	7
*Collipp (1969)	CT	C	18 children with leukemia		New York	DIP	NA	—	6
Dossey (1993)	R		discusses effects of intercessory prayer and distant mental effects in this popular book						
Duckro (1994)	R		review and critique of research concerning effects of prayer upon physical health						
Finney (1985a)	R		review of prayer studies and mental health outcomes						
Finney (1985b)	CT/PC	C	9 outpatients seeking therapy		Pasadena, CA	"contemplative prayer"	P (before vs. after) (no ctrls)		4
Galton (1872)	CC		members of royal house, missionaries, praying classes			DIP	NA	—	3
Harris (1999)	CT	R	466 vs. 524 Cs	MP	Kansas City	DIP	P	—	7
Horrigan/Krucoff (1999)	CT	C	120	MP-angioplasty	Durham, NC	DIP,DMH	NA	—	7
Joyce (1965)	CT	C	48	PP,MP	London, England	DIP	NA	—	6
Levin (1996a)	R		describes various theoretical models of how prayer heals						
Matthews (1999)	CT	C	40	MP (Rheumatoid arthritis)	Florida	DIP, hands on prayer	NA (DIP)/P (hands on prayer)	—	7
McCullough (1995)	R		review of studies examining the effects of prayer on health (including clinical trials)						
*Miller RN (1982)	CT	C	96	MP (hypertension)		DMH	P	—	6
*O'Laoire (1997)	CT	C	406	CDA	San Francisco	DIP	NA	—	7
Parker W. (1957)	CT	C	45	CDA	Southern CA	2 prayer groups vs. secular controls	(P) (prayer therapy group)		5
Sicher, Targ (1998)	CT	C	40	PP (AIDS)	San Francisco	DMH	P	—	7
Targ (1997)	R		defines and reviews research concerning "distant healing" and "psychic healing"						
Walker (1997)	CT	C	40	Alcoholics	New Mexico	DIP	NA	—	7

Death and Dying

*Babler (1997)	CS	C/S		hospice nurses, social workers, etc	National US	"spiritual care" differences	–	SC	6
Carey (1974)	CS	C	84	MP (terminal)	Illinois	#10+ RB,IR,ER,D	P	SC	6
Faunce (1958)	D	C	104	Ad	Michigan	#1 D	–	–	5
Gibbs (1978)	CS	C	16	MP (cancer)	Dallas, TX	#28 IR,RB,O	P	NONE	4
Kaldjian (1998)	CS	S	90	MP (HIV+)	New Haven, CT	#8+ RB,ORA, NORA,D	P	NONE	7
Pace (1997)	CS	C	55	MP (AIDS,CA)	Atlanta, GA	#5+ SWB	P (loneliness, social support)		6
*Reed P (1986)	CC	C	57 vs. Cs	MP (terminal)	Southeast US	#13 scale	P	NONE	6
*Reed P (1987)	CC	C	100 vs. Cs	MP, terminal	Southeast US	#13 scale	P	NONE	7
Silber (1985)	CS	S	114	severely ill Ad ages 11–19	Washington, DC	#9 spiritual concerns scale	C	NONE	7
*Smith DK (1983–84)	CS	C	20 patients with terminal cancer		Long Beach,CA	#2 ORA, SR	P	NONE	5
Spilka (1977)	CS	C	167	CM (most CS)	Colorado, Indiana, Georgia	#20+ IR,SR	P	NONE	4

a. Levin & Coriel

Religious Harm

Outcome/Investigators	Type	Method	N	Population	Location	Religious Variable	Findings	Controls	Rating
*Am Acad Peds (1997)	R,O	PC	official statement by American Academy of Pediatrics concerning medical neglect of children based on faith healing						
Anonymous (1991)	CS	R	400 cases of rubella in 9 outbreaks in Amish communities due to lack of vaccination of children						
Asser (1998)	R	C	reports on 172 cases of child death possibly due to medical neglect secondary to faith healing						
Bottoms (1995)	R		reviews child abuse by clergy						
Bowker (1988)	CS	C	144 and 854	battered wives	Wisconsin, US	#3 ORA,D,clergy help	—	—	5
Bullis (1991)	R		examines spiritual healing "defense" in crimes against children						
Capps (1992)	R,O		discusses religion and child abuse with anecdotal case reports; makes few references to systematic research						
CDC (1991)	CC	S	documents significantly higher death rates among Christian Scientists						
Clark (1981)	CR		describes a case of self-mutilation based on religious delusions						
Coakley (1986)	CR		describes case of person discontinuing medical treatment due to faith healing (with negative results)						
Conyn-van S. (1996)	CS	R	2400 children	poliovirus	Netherlands	#1 Orthodox Reformed	NG	—	8
*Ellis A (1980)	O		examines negative effects of religion on mental health						
Ellis A (1983)	O		examines negative effects of religion on mental health						
Ellis A (1987)	O		examines negative effects of religion on mental health						
Ellis A (1988)	O		examines negative effects of religion on mental health						
Etkind (1992)	CS	S	examines pertussis outbreaks in groups claiming religious exemptions to vaccinations						
Freud (1907)	CR		describes and discusses how religious practices are similar to obsessive acts						
Freud (1913)	O		discusses negative effects of religion on mental health						
Freud (1919)	O		discusses psychoanalytic origins of religious practices						
Freud (1927)	O		discusses religion and neurosis						
Freud (1928)	O		discusses case of religious experience						
Freud (1933a)	O		discusses negative mental health effects of religion						
Freud (1933b)	O		discusses negative mental health effects of religion						
Freud (1939)	O		discusses negative mental health effects of religion						
Hughes (1990)	R,O		discusses psychological perspectives on infanticide in a faith healing sect						
Kaunitz (1984)	CC		examines perinatal and maternal mortality in a religious group avoiding obstetric care (see Spence 1984, 1987 below)						
Lannin (1998)	CC	S	540	women with breast CA		examines religious beliefs and delay of breast CA diagnosis			7

Reference			Description						
MMWR (1991)	CC	S	outbreaks of rubella among the Amish due to failure to vaccinate children						
Novotny (1988)	CC	S	measles outbreak in religious groups exempt from immunization laws						
Purcell (1998)	R,O		discusses the definition of spiritual abuse and spiritual terrorism, with examples						
Pruyser (1977)	O		discusses the "seamy side" of religious beliefs						
Rodgers (1993)	CC	S	measles outbreak in groups with religious exemption to vaccination						
Salzman (1965)	O		discusses healthy and unhealthy religion from a psychodynamic perspective						
Sajwaj (1973)	CR		discusses negative effects of forcing prayer on an oppositional retarded boy						
*Simpson W (1989)	CC	S	5568	CDA	Illinois	#1 D Christian Scientists vs. other)	Christ Sc > other	SC-age, sex	8
Skolnick (1990)	R		discusses religious exemptions to child neglect						
Sloan (1999)	R		presents skeptical review of research on religion, spirituality, and medicine						
Smith DM (1986)	CR		describes case of person discontinuing medical treatment due to faith healing (with negative results)						
*Sorenson (1995)	PC	S	261	teenage mothers	S.W. Ontario	#3 D,ORA,SR	NG	SC	6
*Spence (1984)	CC	R	26,618	Faith Assembly vs. others	Indiana	#1 D (Faith As vs. other)	Faith As > other	SC-age	8
*Spence (1987)	CC	R	follow-up study to 1984 report; perinatal mortality declined from 3 to 1.5 rate for Indiana due to laws passed						6
Swan (1983)	R,O		discusses faith healing, Christian Science, and the medical care of children						
Swan (1997)	R,O		discusses faith healing, Christian Science, and the medical care of children						
Trew (1971)	O		opinion piece about religion and psychopathology						
Watters (1992)	R,O		reviews negative effects of Christianity on physical and mental health						
Wilson GE (1965)	CC		higher death rate among Christian Scientists compared with others in general population						

Print Media

Arthritis Today (3/96)
USA Weekend (4/96)
Time (5/96)
Newsweek (3/97)
Reader's Digest (10/98)
Prevention Magazine (12/98)
McCalls Magazine (12/98)
New York Times (6/99)
Readers Digest (10/99)
USA Today (6/00, 7/00)

Conclusions

THE TWIN HEALING TRADItions of religion and medicine have slowly split apart over the past 500 years. Within the past decade, however, there are signs that the deep rift between these two traditions may be closing. Research has shown that medical patients have religious and spiritual needs that are intimately related to their physical health conditions and that religious beliefs and practices can often be important for emotional healing. The fields of psychoneuroimmunology and psychosomatic medicine have shed light on the physiological mechanisms by which psychological, social, and behavioral factors can affect physical health. These mechanisms provide us with rational and highly plausible explanations of why and how religion may impact *physical* health, quite apart from supernatural influences that are likely beyond scientific investigation.

The twenty-first century will be a rich one for research on religion and health. Of the more than 1,200 research studies reviewed in this book, few were initially designed to examine the effects of religious involvement on health. Only a handful of these studies were intervention studies capable of truly testing the hypothesis that religion influences health, positively or negatively. Nevertheless, in the vast majority of the cross-sectional studies and prospective cohort studies we identified, religious beliefs and practices rooted within established religious traditions were found to be consistently associated with better health and predicted better health over time; in a few clinical trials, groups that received spiritual interventions experienced superior clinical outcomes compared with controls. This is not to say that religious influences *always* convey health benefits, which they clearly do not; sometimes the exact opposite occurs.

Much work remains in order to develop

and mature the scientific base upon which this field rests. Improvements are needed in the way that religious involvement and commitment are measured and lifetime exposure is quantified. Prospective cohort studies are needed to help identify the time order of effects, particularly for those religious variables that cannot be tested using clinical trial methodology. For religious variables that can be tested according to the principles of experimental design, randomized clinical trials are sorely needed to definitively demonstrate cause-effect relationships. Studies in persons with different religious backgrounds are also needed to determine whether the content of religious belief makes a difference in the observed health effects. We hope this review, discussion, and synthesis of the research conducted during the twentieth century will stimulate research in the new century that will further our understanding of what appears to be an intimate relationship between religion and health.

Returning now to definitions: What is health? What is religion? What is healing? The American Heritage Dictionary (1995) defines "health" as "1. The *overall condition* of an organism at a given time. 2. *Soundness*, especially of body or mind. . . . 3. The condition of *optimal well-being* . . . [our italics]." The word "healing" comes from the Greek word *heilen*, which means "to become whole," "to set right," or "to restore." "Religion" comes from the Latin word *religare*, which is composed of two roots, *re* and *ligare*. *Re* means "back," and *ligare* means "to bind, bind together." Thus, the word "religion" literally means "to bind back together." When our patients become physically ill or mentally out of balance, they need to be bound back together. Thus, the word "religion" itself involves a description of healing. Health, religion, and healing all have the common theme and task of making the person whole, sound, transforming him into a state of optimal well-being—restoring the person, both mind and body, to order and balance.

We would agree that when mind, body, and spirit are balanced and in order, this is *true health*—and it is around this common goal that medicine and religion may someday join hands once again—this time on equal footing, each understanding, valuing, and utilizing the healing power the other has to offer.

References

AAMC (1998). *Report I: Learning Objectives for Medical School Education: Guidelines for Medical Schools*. Washington, D.C.: Association of American Medical Colleges.

Aanson, O. (1988). Living arrangements and women's health. *Social Science and Medicine*, 26, 201–208.

Abernethy, A. D., & Lancia, J. J. (1998). Religion and the psychotherapeutic relationship. Transferenial and counter-transferential dimensions. *Journal of Psychotherapy Practice and Research*, 7, 281–289.

Abraido-Lanza, A. F., Guier, C., & Revenson, T. A. (1996). Coping and social support resources among Latinas with arthritis. *Arthritis Care and Research*, 9(6), 501–508.

Abramson, J. H., Gofin, R., & Peritz, E. (1982). Risk markers for mortality among elderly men—a community study in Jerusalem. *Journal of Chronic Disease*, 35, 565–572.

Abu-Zeid, H. A. H., Choi, N. W., Maini, K. K., & Nelson, N. A. (1975). Incidence and epidemiologic features of cerebrovascular disease (stroke) in Manitoba, Canada. *Preventive Medicine*, 4, 567–578.

Accreditation Council on Graduate Medical Education (1994). *Special Requirements for Residency Training in Psychiatry*. Chicago: Accreditation Council on Graduate Medical Education.

Acheson, E. D. (1960). The distribution of ulcerative colitis and regional enteritis in United States veterans with particular reference to the Jewish religion. *Gut*, 1, 291–293.

Acheson, L. S. (1994). Perinatal, infant, and child death rates among the Old Order Amish. *American Journal of Epidemiology*, 139, 173–183.

Acklin, M. W., Brown, E. C., & Mauger, P. A. (1983). The role of religious values and coping with cancer. *Journal of Religion and Health*, 22, 322–333.

Adams, R. G., & Brittain, J. L. (1987). Functional status and church participation of the elderly: Theoretical and practical implications. *Journal of Religion and Aging*, 3(3/4), 35–48.

Aday, R. H. (1984–1985). Belief in afterlife and death anxiety: Correlates and comparisons. *Omega*, 15, 67–75.

Adelekan, M. L., Abiodun, O. A., Imouoklhome-Obayan, A. O., Oni, G. A., & Ogunremi, O. O. (1993). Psychosocial correlates of alcohol, tobacco and cannabis use: Findings from a Nigerian university. *Drug and Alcohol Dependence*, 33, 247–256.

Ader, R. (1981). *Psychoneuroimmunology*. New York: Academic Press.

Adlaf, E. M., & Smart, R. G. (1985). Drug use and religious affiliation, feelings, and behavior. *British Journal of Addiction*, 80, 163–171.

Adler, N. E., Boyce, W. T., Chesney, M. A., Folkman, S., & Syme, S. L. (1993). Socioeconomic inequalities in health. *Journal of the American Medical Association*, 268, 3140–3145.

Adorno, T. W., Frenkel-Brunswick, E., Levinseson, D. J., & Sanford, R. N. (1950). *The Authoritarian Personality*. New York: Harper & Row.

Advisory Committee to the Surgeon General of the Public Health Service (1964). *Smoking and Health*. Publication 1103. Washington, D.C.: U.S. Department of Health, Education and Welfare.

Advisory Council on Church and Society (1986). *Alcohol Use and Abuse: The Social and Health Effects*. New York: Pilgrim Agency, Presbyterian Church.

Agrawal, M., & Dalal, A. K. (1993). Beliefs about the world and recovery from myocardial infarction. *Journal of Social Psychology*, 133, 385–394.

Ahern, D. K., Gorkin, L., Anderson, J. L, Tierney, C., Hallstrom, A., & Ewart, C. (1990). Biobehavioral variables and mortality or cardiac arrest in the Cardiac Arrhythmias Pilot Study (CAPS). *American Journal of Cardiology*, 66, 59–62.

Ahmed, F., Brown, D. R., Gary, L. E., & Saadatmand, F. (1994). Religious predictors of cigarette smoking: Findings for African American women of childbearing age. *Behavioral Medicine*, 20, 34–43.

Ai, A. L., Dunkle, R. E., Peterson, C., & Bolling, S. F. (1998). The role of private prayer in psychological recovery among midlife and aged patients following cardiac surgery (CABG). *Gerontologist*, 38, 591–601.

Ainlay, S. C., & Smith, D. R. (1984). Aging and religious participation. *Journal of Gerontology*, 39, 357–363.

Ainlay, S. C., Singleton, R., & Swigert, V. L. (1992). Aging and religious participation: Reconsider-

ing the effects of health. *Journal for the Scientific Study of Religion*, 31, 175–188.

Akabaliev, V., & Dimitrov, I. (1997). Attitudes towards alcohol use among Bulgarians-Christians and Turks-Muslims. *Folia Med (Plovdiv)*, 39(1), 7–12.

Akimoto, M., Nakajima, Y., Tan, M., Ishii, H., Iwasaki, H., & Abe, R. (1986). Assessment of host immune response in breast cancer patients. *Cancer Detection and Prevention*, 9, 311–317.

Albrecht, S. L. (1979). Correlates of marital happiness among the re-married. *Journal of Marriage and the Family*, 41, 857–867.

Albrecht, S. L., Bahr, H. M., & Goodman, K. L. (1983). *Divorce and Remarriage: Problems, Adaptations, and Adjusments*. Westport, Conn.: Greenwood.

Alcohol Effects on the Immune System (1993). Alcohol effects on the immune system: Third Annual Meeting of the Alcohol and Drug Abuse Immunology Symposium, Vail, Colorado, March 25–29 (abstracts). *Alcohol*, 10, 335–342.

Alcoholics Anonymous (1976). *Alcoholics Anonymous*, 3rd ed. New York: Alcoholics Anonymous World Services.

Alexander, C. N., Langer, E. J., Newman, R. I., Chandler, H. M., & Davies, J. L. (1989). Transcendental meditation, mindfulness, and longevity: An experimental study with the elderly. *Journal of Personality and Social Psychology*, 57, 950–964.

Alexander, C. N., Robinson, P., Orme-Johnson, D. W., Schneider, R. H., & Walton, K. G. (1994). Effects of transcendental meditation compared to other methods of relaxation and meditation in reducing risk factors, morbidity and mortality. *Homeostasis*, 35, 243–264.

Alexander, C. N., Robinson, P., & Rainforth, M. (1994). Treating and preventing alcohol, nicotine, and drug abuse through transcendental meditation: A review and meta-analysis. *Alcoholism Treatment Quarterly*, 11(1/2), 13–87.

Alexander, C. N., Schneider, R. H., Staggers, F., Sheppard, W., Clayborne, B. M., Rainforth, M., Salerno, J., Kondwani, K., Smith, S., Walton, K. G., & Egan, B. (1996). Trial of stress reduction for hypertension in older African Americans: II. Sex and risk subgroup analysis. *Hypertension*, 28(2), 228–237.

Alexander, F., & Duff, R. W. (1991). Influence of religiosity and alcohol use on personal well-being. *Journal of Religious Gerontology*, 8, 11–19.

Alexander, F. G. (1966). Contributions of the ancients: The Hebrews. In F. G. Alexander & S. T.

Selesnick, *The History of Psychiatry: An Evaluation of Psychiatric Thought and Practice from Prehistoric Times to the Present*. New York: New American Library.

Alexander, F. G., & Selesnick, A. S. T. (1966). *The History of Psychiatry: An Evaluation of Psychiatric Thought and Practice from Prehistoric Times to the Present*. New York: New American Library.

Alexander, R. W., Schlant, R. C., Fuster, V., Alexander, W., & Sonnenblick, E. H. (1998). *The Heart, Arteries and Veins*, 9th ed. New York: McGraw-Hill.

Alford, G. S., Koehler, R. A., & Leonard, J. (1991). Alcoholics anonymous–narcotics anonymous model inpatient treatment of chemically dependent adolescents: A 2-year outcome study. *Journal of Studies on Alcohol*, 52, 118–126.

Allen-Hagen, B. (1991). *Public Juvenile Facilities: Children in Custody 1989*. OJJDP Update on Statistics. Juvenile Justice Bulletin. Washington, D.C.: Office of Juvenile Justice and Delinquency Prevention, U.S. Department of Justice.

Allison, T., & St. Leger, S. (1999). The life span of Methodist ministers: An example of the use of obituaries in epidemiology. *Journal of Epidemiology and Community Health*, 53, 253–254.

Allport, G. W. (1950). *The Individual and His Religion: A Psychological Interpretation*. New York: Macmillan.

Allport, G. W. (1954). *The Nature of Prejudice*. New York: Addison-Wesley.

Allport, G. W., & Ross, J. M. (1967). Personal religious orientation and prejudice. *Journal of Personality and Social Psychology*, 5, 432–443.

Allport, G. W., Vernon, P. E., & Linzey, G. (1968). *Study of Values*, 3rd ed. Boston: Houghton Mifflin.

Althauser, R. P. (1990). Paradox in popular religion: The limits of instrumental faith. *Social Forces*, 69, 585–602.

Alvarado, K. A., Templer, D. I., Bresler, C., & Thomas-Dobson, S. (1995). The relationship of religious variables to death depression and death anxiety. *Journal of Clinical Psychology*, 51, 202–204.

Amato, P. R. (1988). Parental divorce and attitudes toward marriage and family. *Journal of Marriage and the Family*, 50, 453–461.

Amato, P. R., & Keith, B. (1991). Parental divorce and well-being of children: A meta-analysis. *Psychological Bulletin*, 110, 26–46.

American Academy of Pediatrics (1997). Religious objections to medical care. *Pediatrics*, 99, 279–281.

Americana Healthcare Corporation (1980–1981). *Aging in America: Trials and Triumphs*. Westport, Conn.: U.S.-Research and Forecasts Survey Sampling Corporation.

American Cancer Society (1994). *Cancer Facts and Figures 1993*. New York: American Cancer Society.

American Cancer Society (1998). *Cancer Facts and Figures 1998: Basic Cancer Facts*. Atlanta: National Center for Health Statistics, Centers for Disease Control and Prevention.

American Cancer Society (1999). *Cancer Facts and Figures 1999: Basic Cancer Facts, Statistics, and Selected Cancers*. Atlanta: National Center for Health Statistics, Centers for Disease Control and Prevention (www.cancer.org/statistics).

American Heart Association (1998). Data from National Heart, Lung, and Blood Institute ARIC, CHS, and Framingham Heart studies. American Heart Association (www.americanheart.org).

American Heart Association (1999a). Stroke statistics; stroke risk factors. *1999 Heart and Stroke Statistical Update*. Dallas, Texas: American Heart Association (www.americanheart.org).

American Heart Association (1999b). *1999 Heart and Stroke Statistical Update*. Dallas, Texas: American Heart Association (www.americanheart. org).

American Heart Association (1999c). National Health and Nutrition Examination Survey III (NHANES III), 1988–94, CDC/NCHS and the American Heart Association. *1999 Heart and Stroke Statistical Update*. Dallas, Texas: American Heart Association (www.americanheart.org).

American Heart Association (1999d). Coronary heart disease and angina pectoris. *1999 Heart and Stroke Statistical Update*. Dallas, Texas: American Heart Association (www.americanheart. org).

American Heritage Dictionary (1995). 3rd ed. Microsoft Bookshelf CD ROM. Seattle, Wash.: Microsoft.

American Psychiatric Association (1994). *Diagnostic Manual of Mental Disorders*, 4th ed. Washington, D.C.: American Psychological Association.

American Psychiatric Association (1995). American Psychiatric Association practice guidelines for psychiatric evaluation of adults. *American Journal of Psychiatry* supplement, 152(11), 64–80.

American Psychological Association (1995). Guidelines and principles for accreditation of programs in professional psychology (pp. 5, Iw-27). In *American Psychological Association Committee on Accreditation Site Visitor Handbook*. Washington, D.C.: American Psychological Association.

Amey, C. H., Albrecht, S. L., & Miller, M. K. (1996). Racial differences in adolescent drug use: The impact of religion. *Substance Use and Misuse*, 31, 1311–1332.

Amoateng, A.Y., & Bahr, S. J. (1986). Religion, family, and adolescent drug use. *Sociological Perspectives*, 29, 53–76.

Amundsen, D. W. (1978). Medieval canon law on medical and surgical practice by the clergy. *Bulletin of the History of Medicine*, 52, 22–44.

Amundsen, D. W. (1982). Medicine and faith in early Christianity. *Bulletin of the History of Medicine*, 56, 326–350.

Amundsen, D. W. (1998). The medieval Catholic tradition. In R. L. Numbers & D. W. Amundsen (eds.), *Caring and Curing: Health and Medicine in the Western Religious Traditions* (pp. 65–107). Baltimore: Johns Hopkins University Press.

Anda, R., Williamson, D., Jones, D., Macera, C., Eaker, E., & Glassman, A. (1993). Depressed affect, hopelessness, and risk of ischemic heart disease in a cohort of U.S. adults. *Epidemiology*, 4, 285–294.

Andersen, B. L., Farrar, W. B., Golden-Kreutz, D., Kutz, L. A., MacCallum, R., Courtney, J. E., & Glaser, R. (1998). Stress and immune responses after surgical treatment for regional breast cancer. *Journal of the National Cancer Institute*, 90, 30–38.

Andersen, B. L., Kiecolt-Glaser, J. K., & Glaser, R. (1994). A biobehavioral model of cancer stress and disease course. *American Psychologist*, 49, 389–404.

Andersen, R., & Newman, J. (1973). Societal and individual determinants of medical care utilization. *Milbank Memorial Fund Quarterly*, 51, 95–124.

Anderson, D., Deshaies, J., & Jobin, J. (1996). Social support, social networks and coronary artery disease rehabilitation: A review. *Canadian Journal of Cardiology*, 12, 739–744.

Anderson, J. M., Anderson, L. J., & Felsenthal, G. (1993). Pastoral needs and support within an inpatient rehabilitation unit. *Archives of Physical Medicine and Rehabilitation*, 74, 574–578.

Andreasen, N. J. C. (1972). The role of religion in depression. *Journal of Religion and Health*, 11, 153–166.

Andrews, F. M., & Withey, S. B. (1976). *Social Indicators of Well-Being: America's Perception of Life Quality*. New York: Plenum.

Angell, M., & Kassirer, J. P. (1999). Alternative medicine: The risks of untested and unregulated remedies. *Skeptical Inquirer* (January/February), 58–60.

Angell, R. C. (1951). The moral integration of American cities. *American Journal of Sociology*, 57, entire monograph.

Annis, L. V. (1976). Emergency helping and religious behavior. *Psychological Reports*, 39, 151–158.

Anson, O., Antonovsky, A., & Sagy, S. (1990). Religiosity and well-being among retirees: A question of causality. *Behavior, Health, and Aging*, 1, 85–97.

Anson, O., Carmel, S., Bonneh, D.Y., Levenson, A., & Maoz, B. (1990). Recent life events, religiosity, and health: An individual or collective effect. *Human Relations* 43, 1051–1066.

Antonovsky, A. (1979). *Health, Stress and Coping*. San Francisco: Jossey-Bass.

Apel, M. D. (1986). The attitude and knowledge of church members and pastors related to older adults and retirement. *Journal of Religion and Aging*, no. 293, 31–43.

Archer, M., Rinzler, S., & Christakis, G. (1967). Social factors affecting participation in a study of diet and coronary heart disease. *Journal of Health and Social Behavior*, 8, 22–31.

Armstrong, B., Van Merwyk, A. J., & Coates, H. (1977). Blood pressure in Seventh-Day Adventist vegetarians. *American Journal of Epidemiology*, 105, 444–449.

Armstrong, R. G., Larsen, G. L., & Mourer, S. A. (1962). Religious attitudes and emotional adjustment. *Journal of Psychological Studies*, 13, 35–47.

Arnold, D., & Schick, C. (1979). Counseling by clergy: A review of empirical research. *Journal of Pastoral Counseling*, 14, 76–101.

Aromaa, A., Raitasalo, R., Reunanen, A., Impivaara, O., Heliovaara, M., & Knekt, P. (1994). Depression and cardiovascular diseases. *Acta Psychiatrica Scandinavica*, supplement 377, 77–82.

Asberg, K. H. (1986). Assessment of ADL in homecare for the elderly: Change in ADL and use of short-term hospital care. *Scandinavian Journal of Social Medicine*, 14, 105–111.

Aspinwall, L. G., & Taylor, S. E. (1992). Modeling cognitive adaptation: A longitudinal investigation of the impact of individual differences and coping on college adjustment and performance. *Journal of Personality and Social Psychology*, 63, 989–1003.

Asser, S. M., & Swan, R. (1998). Child fatalities from religion-motivated medical neglect. *Pediatrics*, 101, 625–629.

Associated Press (1996). Doctors find attending church good for the body. February 12.

Association of Mental Health Clergy (1991). Here we are again! Crisis in Georgia. *AMHC Newsletter*, 3(10), 1.

Astin, M. C., Lawrence, K. J., & Foy, D. W. (1993). Posttraumatic stress disorder among battered women: Risk and resiliency factors. *Violence and Victims*, 8, 17–28.

Augustyn, M., & Simons-Morton, B. G.. (1995). Adolescent drinking and driving: Etiology and interpretation. *Journal of Drug Education*, 25(1), 41–59.

Austin, J. T., & Vancouver, J. B. (1996). Goal constructs in psychology: Structure, process, and content. *Psychological Bulletin*, 120, 338–375.

Avtar, S. (1979). Religious involvement and antisocial behavior. *Perceptual and Motor Skills*, 48, 1157–1158.

Aycock, D. W., & Noaker, S. (1985). A comparison of the self-esteem levels in evangelical Christian and general populations. *Journal of Psychology and Theology*, 13, 199–208.

Ayele, H., Mulligan, T., Gheorghiu, S., & Reyes-Ortiz, C. (1999). Religious activity improves life satisfaction for some physicians and older patients. *Journal of the American Geriatrics Society*, 47, 453–455.

Azhar, M. Z., & Varma, S. L. (1995a). Religious psychotherapy as management of bereavement. *Acta Psychiatrica Scandinavica*, 91, 233–235.

Azhar, M. Z., & Varma, S. L. (1995b). Religious psychotherapy in depressive patients. *Psychotherapy and Psychosomatics*, 63, 165–168.

Azhar, M. Z., Varma, S. L., & Dharap, A. S. (1994). Religious psychotherapy in anxiety disorder patients. *Acta Psychiatrica Scandinavica*, 90, 1–3.

Babler, J. E. (1997). A comparison of spiritual care provided by hospice social workers, nurses, and spiritual care professionals. *Hospice Journal*, 12(4), 15–27.

Bagley, C., & Ramsay, R. (1989). Attitudes toward suicide, religious values, and suicidal behavior. In R. F. W. Diekstra, R. Maris, S. Platt, A. Schmidtke, & G. Sonneck (eds.), *Suicide and Its Prevention* (pp. 78–90). Leiden: Brill.

Bahr, H. M. (1981). Religious intermarriage and divorce in Utah and the mountain states. *Journal for the Scientific Study of Religion* 20, 251–261.

Bahr, H. M., & Chadwick, B. A. (1988). Religion and family in Middletown, U.S.A. In T. L. Darwin (ed.), *The Religion and Family Connection: Social Science Perspectives* (pp. 51–65). Provo, Ut.: Brigham Young University.

Bahr, H. M., & Harvey, C. D. (1979a). Correlates of loneliness among widows bereaved in a mining disaster. *Psychological Reports*, 44, 367–385.

Bahr, H. M., & Harvey, C. D. (1979b). Widowhood and perceptions of change in quality of life: Evidence from the Sunshine Mine Widows. *Journal of Comparative Family Studies*, 10, 411–428.

Bahr, H. M., & Martin, T. K. (1983). "And thy neighbor as thyself": Self-esteem and faith in people as correlates of religiosity and family solidarity among Middletown high school students. *Journal for the Scientific Study of Religion*, 22, 132–144.

Baider, L, Russak, S. M., Perry, S., Kash, K. M., Gronert, M. K., Fox, B., Holland, J. C., & Kaplan-Denour, A. (1999). The role of religious and spiritual beliefs in coping with malignant melanoma: An Israeli sample. *Psycho-oncology*, 8, 27–35.

Bailey J. (1991). Legislature approves budget cuts: Cuts also endanger Central State chaplaincy program. *Union-Recorder* (Milledgeville, Ga.), 173(174) (August 29), p. 1.

Bailey, W. T., & Stein, L. B. (1995). Jewish affiliation in relation to suicide rates. *Psychological Reports*, 76(2), 561–562.

Bainbridge, W., & Stark, R. (1981). Suicide, homicide, and religion. *Annual Review of the Social Sciences of Religion*, 5, 33–56.

Bainbridge, W. S. (1989). The religious ecology of deviance. *American Sociological Review*, 54, 288–295.

Baines, E. (1984). Caregiver stress in the older adult. *Journal of Community Health Nursing*, 1, 257–263.

Baker, M., & Gorsuch, R. (1982). Trait anxiety and intrinsic-extrinsic religiousness. *Journal for the Scientific Study of Religion*, 21, 119–122.

Baldree, K. S., Murphy, S. P., & Powers, M. J. (1982). Stress identification and coping patterns in patients on hemodialysis. *Nursing Research*, 31, 107–112.

Bales, R. F. (1944). The therapeutic role of alcoholics anonymous as seen by a sociologist. *Quarterly Journal of Studies on Alcohol*, 5, 267–278.

Bales, R. F. (1946). Cultural differences in rates of alcoholism. *Quarterly Journal of Studies on Alcohol*, 6, 480–499.

Balk, D. E. (1991). Sibling death, adolescent bereavement, and religion. *Death Studies*, 15, 1–20.

Ball, R. A., & Clare, A. W. (1990). Symptoms and social adjustment in Jewish depressives. *British Journal of Psychiatry*, 156, 379–383.

Ball, R. A., & Goodyear, R. K. (1991). Self-reported professional practices of Christian psychotherapists. *Journal of Psychology and Christianity*, 10, 144–153.

Ballard, A., Green, T., McCaa, A., & Logsdon, M. C. (1997). A comparison of the level of hope in patients with newly diagnosed and recurrent cancer. *Oncology Nursing Forum*, 24, 899–904.

Bankston, W. B., Allen, H. D., & Cunningham, D. S. (1983). Religion and suicide: A research note on sociology's "one law." *Social Forces*, 62, 521–528.

Barbarin, O. A., & Chesler, M. (1986). The medical context of parental coping with childhood cancer. *American Journal of Community Psychology*, 14, 221–235.

Bardis, P. D. (1961). A religion scale. *Social Science*, 36, 120–123.

Barefoot, J. C., & Schroll, M. (1996). Symptoms of depression, acute myocardial infarction, and total mortality in a community sample. *Circulation*, 93, 1976–1980.

Barefoot, J. C., Dahlstrom, D. W. G., & Williams, R. B., Jr. (1983). Hostility, CHD incidence and total mortality: A 25-year follow-up study of 255 physicians. *Psychosomatic Medicine*, 45(45), 59–63.

Barefoot, J. C., Helms, M. J., Mark, D. B., Blumenthal, J. A., Califf, R. M., & Haney, T. L. (1996). Depression and long-term mortality risk in patients with coronary artery disease. *American Journal of Cardiology*, 78, 613–617.

Barna, G. (1991). *The Barna Report: What Americans Believe*. Ventura, Calif.: Regal Books.

Barnard, D., Dayringer, R., & Cassel, C. K. (1995). Toward a person-centered medicine: Religious studies in the medical curriculum. *Academic Medicine*, 70, 806–813.

Barnes, V., Schneider, R., Alexander, C., & Staggers, F. (1997). Stress, stress reduction, and hypertension in African-Americans: in updated review. *Journal of the National Medical Association*, 89, 464–476.

Barns, M., Doyle, D., & Johnson, B. (1989). The formulation of a Fowler scale: An empirical assessment among Catholics. *Review of Religious Research*, 30, 412–420.

Baron, R. S., Cutrona, C. E., Hicklin, D., Russel, D. W., & Lubaroff, D. M. (1990). Social support and immune function among spouses of cancer patients. *Journal of Personality and Social Psychology*, 59, 344–352.

Barrett, M. E., Simpson, D. D., & Lehman, W. E. K. (1988). Behavioral changes of adolescents in drug abuse intervention programs. *Journal of Clinical Psychology*, 44, 461–473.

Barrett-Connor, E. L. (1985). OECD, atherosclerosis, and coronary artery disease. *Annals of Internal Medicine*, 103, 1010–1019.

Barron, M. L. (1958). The role of religion and religious institutions in creating the milieu of older people. In *Organized Religion and the Older Person*. Report from the Eighth Annual Southern Conference on Gerontology, April 10–11. Gainesville: University of Florida, Institute of Gerontology.

Barrow, J. G., Quinlan, C. B., Cooper, G. R., Whitner, V. S., & Goodloe, M. H. R. (1960). Studies in atherosclerosis: III. An epidemiologic study of atherosclerosis in Trappist and Benedictine monks: A preliminary report. *Annals of Internal Medicine*, 42, 368–377.

Barry, J., Mead, K., Nabel, E. G., Rocco, M. B., Campbell, S., Fenton, T., Mudge, G. H., & Selwyn, A. P. (1989). Effect of smoking on the activity of Ischemic Heart Disease. *Journal of the American Medical Association*, 261, 398–402.

Barry, R. (1997). The biblical teachings on suicide. *Issues in Law and Medicine*, 13(2), 83–99.

Bart, P. (1968). Depression in middle-aged women: Some sociocultural factors. Ph.D. diss., University of California, Los Angeles.

Bartrop, R. W., Lazarus, L., Luckhurst, E., Kiloh, L. G., & Penny, R. (1977). Depressed lymphocyte function after bereavement. *Lancet*, April 16, 834–836.

Bascue, L. O., Inman, D. J., & Kahn, W. J. (1982). Recognition of suicide lethality factors by psychiatric nursing assistants. *Psychological Reports*, 51(1), 197–198.

Bateman, M. M., & Jensen, J. S. (1958). The effect of religious background on modes of handling anger. *Journal of Social Psychology*, 47, 133–141.

Batson, C. D. (1976). Religion as prosocial: Agent or double agent? *Journal for the Scientific Study of Religion*, 15(1), 29–45.

Batson, C. D. (1987). Prosocial motivation: Is it ever truly altruistic? In L. Berkowitz (ed.), *Advances in Experimental Social Psychology*, Vol. 20. (pp. 65–122) San Diego, Calif.: Academic Press.

Batson, C. D., & Flory, J. D. (1990). Goal-relevant cognitions associated with helping by individuals high on intrinsic, end religion. *Journal for the Scientific Study of Religion*, 29, 346–360.

Batson, C. D., & Gray, R. A. (1981). Religious orientation and helping behavior: Responding to one's own or to the victim's needs? *Journal of Personality and Social Psychology*, 40, 511–520.

Batson, C. D., & Ventis, W. L. (1982). *The Religious Experience: A Social Psychological Perspective*. New York: Oxford University Press.

Batson, C. D., Naifeh, S. J., & Pate, S. (1978). Social desirability, religious orientation, and racial prejudice. *Journal for the Scientific Study of Religion*, 17, 31-41.

Batson, C. D., Oleson, K. C., Weeks, J. L., Healy, S., Reeves, P. J., Jennings, P., & Brown, T. (1989). Religious prosocial motivation: Is it altruistic or egoistic? *Journal of Personality and Social Psychology*, 57, 873-884.

Bauer, T., & Barror, C. R. (1995). Nursing interventions for spiritual care: Preferences of the community-based elderly. *Journal of Holistic Nursing*, 13(3), 268-279.

Bay, M. J. (1997). Healing partners: The oncology nurse and the parish nurse. *Seminars in Oncology Nursing*, 13, 275-278.

Baydar, N. (1988). Effects of parental separation and reentry into union on the emotional well-being of children. *Journal of Marriage and the Family*, 50, 967-981.

Bazzoui, W. (1970). Affective disorders in Iraq. *British Journal of Psychiatry*, 117, 195-203.

Bear, D., Levin, K., Blumer, D., Chetham, D., & Ryder, J. (1982). Interictal behavior in hospitalized temporal lobe epileptics: Relationship to idiopathic psychiatric syndromes. *Journal of Neurology, Neurosurgery, and Psychiatry*, 45, 481-488.

Bear, D. M., & Fedio, P. (1977). Quantitative analysis of interictal behavior in temporal lobe epilepsy. *Archives of Neurology*, 34, 454-467.

Bearon, L. B., & Koenig, H. G. (1990). Religious cognitions and use of prayer in health and illness. *Gerontologist*, 30, 249-253.

Beck, A. T. (1976). *Cognitive Therapy and Emotional Disorders*. New York: International Universities Press.

Beck, S. H., Cole, B. S., & Hammond, J. A. (1991). Religious heritage and premarital sex: Evidence from a national sample of young adults. *Journal for the Scientific Study of Religion*, 30, 173-180.

Becker, U., Bohme, K., Breitmaier, J., Drisch, D., Schaefer, D., Kulessa, C., & Wahl, P. (1987). Self-poisoning in Heidelberg, 1974-1980. *Crisis*, 8(2), 103-111.

Beckman, L. J., & Houser, B. B. (1982). The consequences of childlessness on the social-psychological well-being of older women. *Journal of Gerontology*, 37, 243-250.

Bedell, K. B. (ed.) (1997). *Yearbook of American and Canadian Churches 1997*. Nashville: Abingdon Press.

Beecher, H. K. (1961). Surgery as a placebo. *Journal of the American Medical Association*, 176, 1102.

Beeghley, L., Bock, E. W., & Cochran, J. K. (1990). Religious change and alcohol use: An application of reference group and socialization theory. *Sociological Forum*, 5, 261-278.

Beehr, T. A., Johnson, L. B., & Nieva, R. (1995). Occupational stress: Coping of police and their spouses. *Journal of Organizational Behavior*, 16(1), 3-25.

Beekman, A. T. F., Deeg, D. J. H., Braam, A. W., Smit, J. H., & Van Tilburg, W. (1997). *Psychological Medicine*, 27, 1397-1409.

Beg, M. A., & Zilli, A. S. (1982). A study of the relationship of death anxiety and religious faith to age differentials. *Psychologia*, 25, 121-125.

Beit-Hallahmi, B. (1974). Psychology of religion 1880-1930: The rise and fall of a psychological movement. *Journal of the History of the Behavioral Sciences*, 10, 84-90.

Beit-Hallahmi, B. (1975). Religion and suicidal behavior. *Psychological Reports*, 37, 1303-1306.

Beitman, B. D. (1982). Pastoral counseling centers: A challenge to community mental health centers. *Hospital and Community Psychiatry*, 33, 486-487.

Belavich, T. G., & Pargament, K. I. (1995). The role of religion in coping with daily hassles. Paper presented at the Annual Meeting of the American Psychological Association, New York City.

Bell, R., Wechsler, H., & Johnston, L. D. (1997). Correlates of college student marijuana use: Results of a U.S. national survey. *Addiction*, 92, 571-581.

Bell, R. R. (1974). Religious involvement and marital sex in Australia and the United States. *Journal of Comparative Family Studies*, 5(2), 109-116.

Benassi, V. A., Sweeney, P. D., & Dufour, C. L. (1988). Is there a relationship between locus of control orientation and depression? *Journal of Abnormal Psychology*, 97, 357-367.

Benda, B. B. (1995). The effect of religion on adolescent delinquency revisited. *Journal of Research in Crime and Delinquency*, 32(4), 446-466.

Ben-Eliyahu, S., Yirmirya, R., Liebeskind, J. C., Taylor, A. N., & Gale, R. P. (1991). Stress increases metastatic spread of a mammary tumor in rats: Evidence for mediation by the immune system. *Brain, Behavior, and Immunity*, 5, 193-205.

Benfante, R., & Reed, D. (1990). Is elevated serum cholesterol level a risk factor for coronary heart disease in the elderly? *Journal of the American Medical Association*, 263, 393–396.

Ben-Meir, Y., & Kedem, P. (1979). Index of religiosity of the Jewish population of Israel. *Megamot*, 24, 353–362. Translated from Hebrew into English by Rabbi Dayle A. Friedman, chaplain at the Philadelphia Geriatric Center.

Benner, D. G. (1992). *Strategic Pastoral Counseling*. Grand Rapids, Mich.: Baker.

Bennett, W. J. (1998). Neuroscience and the human spirit. *National Review* (December 31), 32–35.

Benor, D. J. (1992). *Healing Research: Holistic Energy, Medicine, and Spirituality*: Vol. 1. *Research in Health*. Munich: Helix.

Benson, H. (1975). *The Relaxation Response*. New York: William Morrow.

Benson, H. (1977). Systemic hypertension and the relaxation response. *New England Journal of Medicine*, 296(20), 1152–1156.

Benson, H. (1984). *Beyond the Relaxation Response*. New York: Times Books.

Benson, H. (1996). *Timeless Healing: The Power and Biology of Belief*. New York: Scribners.

Benson, H. (In progress). Study of the therapeutic effects of intercessory prayer. Grant funded by John Templeton Foundation. Results to be available in early 2002.

Benson, H., & Stuart, E. M. (1993). *The Wellness Book: A Comprehensive Guide to Maintaining Health and Treating Stress-Related Illness*. New York: Fireside.

Benson, H., Alexander, S., & Feldman, C. L. (1975). Decreased premature venture tool or contractions through use of the relaxation response in patients with stable ischemic heart-disease. *Lancet*, 2, 380–382.

Benson, H., Malhotra, M. S., Goldman, R. F., Jacobs, G. D., & Hopkins, P. J. (1990). Three case reports of the metabolic and electroencephalographic changes during advanced Buddhist meditation techniques. *Behavioral Medicine* (Summer), 90–95.

Benson, H., Shapiro, D., Bursky, B., & Schwartz, G. (1971). Decreased systolic blood pressure through opera on conditioning techniques in patients with essential hypertension. *Science*, 173, 740–742.

Benson, P. L., & Donahue, M. J. (1989). Ten-year trends in at-risk behaviors: A national study of black adolescents. *Journal of Adolescent Research*, 4, 125–139.

Benson, P. L., & Spilka, B. P. (1973). God image as a function of self-esteem and locus of control. *Journal for the Scientific Study of Religion*, 12, 297–310.

Benson, P. L., Dehority, J., Garman, L., Hanson, E., Hochschwender, M., Lebold, C., Rohr, R., & Sullivan, J. (1980). Intrapersonal correlates of nonspontaneous helping behavior. *Journal of Social Psychology*, 110, 87–95.

Berdoe, E. (1893). *The Origin and Growth of the Healing Art: A Popular History of Medicine in All Ages and Countries*. London: Sonnenschein.

Berg, G., Reed, A., Fonss, N., & VandeCreek, L. (1995). The of religious faith and practice on patients suffering from a major affective disorder: A cost. *Journal of Pastoral Care*, 49, 359–363.

Berg, J. S., Dischler, J., Wagner, D. J, Raia, J. J., & Palmer-Shevlin, N. (1993). Medication compliance: a health care problem. *Annals of Pharmacotherapy*, 27 (supplement), S5–S24.

Bergin, A. E. (1980). Psychotherapy and religious values. *Journal of Consulting and Clinical Psychology*, 48, 95–105.

Bergin, A. E. (1983). Religiosity and mental health: A critical reevaluation and meta-analysis. *Professional Psychology: Research and Practice*, 14, 170–184.

Bergin, A. E. (1991). Values and religious issues in psychotherapy and mental health. *American Psychologist*, 46, 394–403.

Bergin, A. E., & Jensen, J. P. (1990). Religiosity and psychotherapists: A national survey. *Psychotherapy*, 27, 3–7.

Bergin, A. E., & Payne, I. R. (1991). Proposed agenda for a spiritual strategy in personality and psychotherapy. *Journal of Psychology and Christianity*, 10, 197–210.

Bergin, A. E., Masters, K. S., & Richards, P. S. (1987). Religiousness and mental health reconsidered: A study of an intrinsically religious sample. *Journal of Counseling Psychology*, 34, 197–204.

Bergin, A. E., Stinchfield, R. D., Gaskin, R. A., Masters, K. S., & Sullivan, C. E. (1988). Religious life styles and mental health: An exploratory study. *Journal of Counseling Psychology*, 35, 197–204.

Berglund, M., & Ojehagen, A. (1998). The influence of alcohol drinking and alcohol use disorders on psychiatric disorders and suicidal behavior. *Alcohol Clinical and Experimental Research*, 22(7 Suppl.), 333S–345S.

Berk, M. L., & Taylor, A. K. (1984). Women and divorce: Health insurance coverage, utilization, and health care expenditures. *Public Health Briefs*, 74(11), 1276–1278.

Berkanovic, E., Telesky, C., & Reeder, S. (1981). Structural and social psychological factors in the decision to seek medical care for symptoms. *Medical Care*, 21, 693–709.

Berkel, J. (1979). *Clean Life*. Amsterdam: Drukkerij Insulinde.

Berkel, J., & deWaard, F. (1983). Morality pattern and life expectancy of Seventh-Day Adventists in the Netherlands. *International Journal of Epidemiology*, 12, 455–459.

Berkman, L. F., & Breslow, L. (1983). *Health and Ways of Living: The Alameda County Study*. New York: Oxford University Press.

Berkman, L. F., & Syme, S. L. (1979). Social networks, host resistance, and mortality: A nine-year follow-up study of Alameda County residents. *American Journal of Epidemiology*, 109, 186–204.

Berkman, L. F., Leo-Summers, L., & Horwitz, R. I. (1992). Emotional support and survival after myocardial infarction. *Annals of Internal Medicine*, 117, 1003–1009.

Berman, A. L. (1974). Belief in afterlife, religion, religiosity and life-threatening experiences. *Omega*, 5, 127–135.

Bernard, D., Dayringer, R., & Cassel, C. K. (1995). Toward a person-centered medicine: Religious studies in the medical curriculum. *Academic Medicine*, 70, 806–813.

Bernt, F. M. (1989). Being religious and being altruistic: A study of college service volunteers. *Personality and Individual Differences*, 10, 663–669.

Best, J. B., & Kirk, W. G. (1982). Religiosity and self destruction. *Psychological Record*, 32, 35–39.

Beutler, J. J., Attevelt, J. T. M., Schouten, S. A., Faber, J. A. J., Mees, E. J. D., & Giejskes, G. G. (1988). Paranormal healing and hypertension. *British Medical Journal*, 296, 1491–1494.

Bhushan, L. I. (1970). Religiosity scale. *Indian Journal of Psychology*, 45, 335–342.

Bianchi, M., Sacerdote, P., & Locatelli, L. (1991). Corticotropin releasing hormone, interleukin-1 alpha, and tumor necrosis factor share characteristics of stress mediators. *Brain Research*, 546,139–142.

Bickel, C. O., Ciarrocchi, J. W., Sheers, N. J., Estadt, B. K., Powell, D. A., & Pargament, K. I. (1998). Perceived stress, religious coping styles, and depressive affect. *Journal of Psychology and Christianity*, 17(1), 33–42.

Bienenfeld, D., Koenig, H. G., Sherill, K. A., & Larson, D. B. (1997). Psychosocial predictors of mental health in a population of elderly women: Test of a simple model. *American Journal of Geriatric Psychiatry*, 5, 43–53.

Billings, J. S. (1891). Vital statistics of the Jews. *North American Review*, 153, 70–84.

Billy, J. O. G., Tanfer, K., Grady, W. R., & Klepinger, D. H. (1993). The sexual behavior of men in the United States. *Family Planning Perspectives*, 25(2), 52–60.

Bilu, Y., & Witztum, E. (1997). The mental health of Jews outside and inside Israel. In I. Al-Issa and A. M. Tousignant (eds.), *Ethnicity, Immigration, and Psychopathology*. New York: Plenum.

Bishop, L. C., Larson, D. B., & Wilson, W. P. (1987). Religious life of individuals with affective disorders. *Southern Medical Journal*, 80, 1083–1086.

Bivens, A. J., Neumeyer, R. A., Kirchberg, T. M., & Moore, M. K. (1994–1995). Death concern and religious beliefs among gays and bisexuals of variable proximity to AIDS. *Omega*, 30, 105–120.

Bjorck, J. P., & Cohen, L. H. (1993). Coping with threats, losses, and challenges. *Journal of Social and Clinical Psychology*, 12, 36–72.

Bjorck, J. P., Lee, Y. S., & Cohen, L. H. (1997). Control beliefs and faith as stress moderators for Korean American vs. Caucasian American Protestants. *American Journal of Community Psychology*, 25, 61–72.

Blackburn, H., & Jacobs, D. R. (1988). Physical activity and the risk of coronary heart disease. *New England Journal of Medicine*, 319, 1217–1219.

Blacker, E. (1966). Sociocultural factors in alcoholism. *International Psychiatry Clinics*, 3(2), 51–80.

Blackwell, B., Bloomfield, S., Gartside, P., Robinson, A., Hanenson, I., Magenheim, H., Nidich, S., & Zigler, R. (1976). Transcendental meditation in hypertension: Individual response patterns. *Lancet* 1(7953), 223–226.

Blaine, B., & Crocker, J. (1995). Religiousness, race, psychological well-being—exploring social-psychological mediators. *Personality and Social Psychology Bulletin*, 21, 1031–1041.

Blalock, S. J., DeVellis, B. M., & Giorgino, K. B. (1995). The relationship between coping and psychological well-being among people with osteoarthritis—a problem-specific approach. *Annals of Behavioral Medicine*, 17, 107–115.

Blaney, N. T., Goodkin, K., Feaster, D., Morgan, R., Millon, C., Szapocznik, J., & Eisdorfer, C. (1997). A psychosocial model of distress over time in early HIV-1 infection: The role of life stressors, social support and coping. *Psychology and Health*, 12, 633–653.

Blasi, A. J., Hussaini, B. A., & Drumwright, D. A. (In press). Seniors' mental health and pastoral practices in African American churches: An exploratory study in a Southern city. *Review of Religious Research*.

Blay, J. Y., Farcet, J. P., Lavaud, A., Radoux, D., & Chouaib, S. (1994). Serum concentrations of cytokines in patients with Hodgkin's disease. *European Journal of Cancer*, 39A, 321–324.

Blazer, D. (1998). *Freud vs. God: How Psychiatry Lost Its Soul and Christianity Lost Its Mind*. Downers Grove, Ill.: Inter-Varsity Press.

Blazer, D. G., & Palmore, E. (1976). Religion and aging in a longitudinal panel. *Gerontologist*, 16, 82–85.

Bliss, J. R., McSherry, E., & Fassett, J. (1995). Chaplain intervention reduces costs in major DRGs: An experimental study. In H. Heffernan, E. McSherry, & R. Fitzgerald (eds.), *Proceedings of the NIH Clinical Center Conference on Spirituality and Health Care Outcomes*, March 21, 1995. Bethesda, Md.: National Institute of Health.

Bliss, S. K., & Crown, C. L. (1994). Concern for appropriateness, religiosity, and gender as predictors of alcohol and marijuana use. *Social Behavior and Personality*, 22, 227–238.

Bloom, B. L., Hodges, W. F., Stern, M. B., & McFadden, S. C. (1985). A preventive intervention program for the newly separated: Final evaluations. *American Journal of Orthopsychiatry*, 55, 9–26.

Blum, S. B., & Mann, J. H. (1960). The effect of religious membership on rleigious prejudice. *Journal of Social Psychology*, 42, 97–101.

Blumenthal, J. A., Burg, M. M., Barefoot, J., Williams, R. B., Haney, T., & Zimet, G. (1987). Social support, type A behavior, and coronary artery disease. *Psychosomatic Medicine*, 49, 331–340.

Blumenthal, J. A., Williams, R. B., & Wallace, A. G. (1982). Physiological and psychological variables predict compliance to prescribed exercise therapy in patients recovering from myocardial infarction. *Psychosomatic Medicine*, 44, 519–527.

Bobgan, M., & Bobgan, D. (1989). *Prophets of Psychoheresy I*. Santa Barbara, Calif.: EastGate Publishers.

Bobgan, M., & Bobgan, D. (1990). *Prophets of Psychoheresy II*. Santa Barbara, Calif.: EastGate Publishers.

Bock, E. W., Cochran, J. K., & Beehgley, L. (1987). Moral messages: The relative influence of de-nomination on the religiosity-alcohol relationship. *Sociological Quarterly*, 28, 89–103.

Bohannon, J. R. (1991). Religiosity related to grief levels of bereaved mothers and fathers. *Omega*, 23, 153–159.

Bohrnstedt, G. W., Borgatta, E. F., & Evans, R. R. (1968). Religious affiliation, religiosity, and MMPI scores. *Journal for the Scientific Study of Religion*, 7, 255–258.

Boland, C. S. (1998). Parish nursing: Addressing the significance of social support and spirituality for sustained health-promoting behaviors in the elderly. *Journal of Holistic Nursing*, 16, 355–368.

Bolduan, C., & Weiner, L. (1933). Causes of death among Jews in New York City. *New England Journal of Medicine*, 208, 407–416.

Bolt, M. (1975). Purpose in life and religious orientation. *Journal of Psychology and Theology*, 3, 116–118.

Bomalaski, J. S., & Phair, J. P. (1982). Alcohol, immunosuppression, and the lung. *Archives of Internal Medicine*, 142, 2073–2074.

Bond, C. A., & Monson, R. (1984). Sustained improvement in drug documentation, compliance, and disease control: A four-year analysis of an ambulatory care model. *Archives of Internal Medicine*, 144, 1159–1162.

Boomsma, D. I., de Geus, E. J., Van Baal, G. C., & Koopmans, J. R. (1999). A religious upbringing reduces the influence of genetic factors on disinhibition: Evidence for interaction between genotype and environment on personality. *Twin Research*, 2, 115–125.

Booth, A., Johnson, D. R., Branaman, A., & Sica, A. (1995). Belief and behavior: Does religion matter in today's marriage? *Journal of Marriage and the Family*, 57(3), 661–671.

Bosley, C. M., Fosbury, J. A., & Cochrane, G. M. (1995). The psychological factors associated with poor compliance with treatment in asthma. *European Respiratory Journal*, 8, 899–904.

Bottoms, B. L., Shaver, P. R., Goodman, F. S., & Qin, J. (1995). In the name of God: A profile of religion-related child abuse. *Journal of Social Issues*, 51, 85–112.

Bouchard, T. J., McGue, Lykken, D., Tellegen, A. (1999). Intrinsic and extrinsic religiousness: genetic and environmental influences and personality correlates. *Twin Research*, 2, 88–98.

Bourin, M., Baker, G.B., & Bradwejn, J. (1998). Neurobiology of panic disorder. *Journal of Psychosomatic Research*, 44(1): 163–180.

Boutelle, F. C., Epstein, S., & Ruddy, M. C. (1987). The relation of essential hypertension to feelings of anxiety, and depression, and anger. *Psychiatry*, 50, 206–217.

Bovbjerg, D. H. (1991). Psychoneuroimmunology implications for oncology? *Cancer*, 67, 828–832.

Bowker, D. (1978). Pain and suffering–Religious perspective. In W. T. Reich (ed.), *Encyclopedia of Bioethics*, vol. 4 (pp. 1185–1189). New York: Free Press.

Bowker, L. H. (1974). Student drug use and the perceived peer drug environment. *International Journal of the Addictions*, 9, 851–861.

Bowker, L. H. (1988). Religious victims and their religious leaders: Services delivered to one thousand battered women by the clergy. In A. L. Horton & J. A. Williamson (eds.), *Abuse and Religion: When Praying Isn't Enough* (pp. 229–234). Lexington, Ky.: Lexington Books.

Bowman, E. S. (1998). Integrating religion into the education of mental health professionals. In H. G. Koenig (ed.), *Handbook of Religion and Mental Health* (pp. 367–378). San Diego: Academic Press.

Braam, A. (1999). Religion and depression in later life: An empirical approach. Doctoral diss., Vrije University. Amsterdam: Thela Thesis.

Braam, A. W., Beekman, A. T. F., Deeg, D. J. H., Smith, J. H., & van Tilburg, W. (1997). Religiosity as a protective or prognostic factor of depression in later life: Results from the community survey in the Netherlands. *Acta Psychiatrica Scandinavia*, 96, 199–205.

Braam, A. W., Beekman, A. T., van den Eeden, P., Deeg, D. J., Knipscheer, K. P., & van Tilburg, W. (1998). Religious denomination and depression in the older Dutch citizens. *Journal of Aging and Health*, 10, 483–503.

Braam, A. W., Beekman, A. T., van den Eeden, P., Deeg, D. J., Knipscheer, K. P., & van Tilburg, W. (1999). Religious climate and geographical distribution of depressive symptoms in older Dutch citizens. *Journal of Affective Disorders*, 54(1–2), 149–159.

Braam, A. W., Beekman, A. T. F., van Tilburg, T. G., Deeg, D. J. H., & van Tilburg, W. (1997). Religious involvement and depression in older Dutch citizens. *Social Psychiatry and Psychiatric Epidemiology*, 32, 284–291.

Braceland, F. J., & Stock, M. (1963). *Modern Psychiatry*. Garden City, N.Y.: Doubleday.

Bradburn, N. M. (1969). *The Structure of Psychological Well-Being*. Chicago: Aldine.

Bradford, D., & Spero, M. (eds.) (1990). Psychotherapy and religion (Special Issue). *Psychotherapy*, 15, 432–440.

Bradley, D. E. (1995). Religious involvement and social resources: Evidence from the data set "Americans' Changing Lives." *Journal for the Scientific Study of Religion*, 34, 259–267.

Bradley, L. A., Young, L. D., Anderson, K. O., McDaniel, L. K., Turner, R. A., & Agudelo, C. A. (1984). Psychological approaches to the management of arthritis pain. *Social Science and Medicine*, 19, 1353–1360.

Bradley, L. A., Young, L. D., Anderson, K. O., Turner, R. A., Agudelo, C. A., McDaniel, L. K., Pisko, E. J., Semble, E. L., & Morgan, T. M. (1987). Effects of psychological therapy on pain behavior of rheumatoid arthritis patients: Treatment outcome and six-month follow-up. *Arthritis and Rheumatism*, 30, 1105–1114.

Brady, M. J., Peterman, A. H., Fitchett, G., & Cella, D. (1999). The expanded version of the functional assessment of chronic illless therapy-spiritual well-being scale (FACIT Sp-Ex): Initial report of psychometric properties. Paper presented at the 20th annual meeting of the Society of Behavioral Medicine, San Francisco, March.

Bragan, K. (1977). The psychological gains and losses of religious conversion. *British Journal of Medical Psychology*, 50, 177–180.

Branden, N. (1994). *The Six Pillars of Self-Esteem*. New York: Bantam.

Brandsma, J. M., Maultsby, M. C., & Welsh, R. J. (1980). *The Outpatient Treatment of Alcoholism*. Baltimore: University Park Press.

Brant, C. R., & Pargament, K. I. (1995). Religious coping with racist and other negative life events among African-Americans. Paper presented at the meeting of the American Psychological Association, New York, August.

Bravender, T., & Knight, J. R. (1998). Recent patterns of use and associated risks of illicit drug use in adolescents. *Current Opinions in Pediatrics*, 10(4), 344–349.

Breault, K. D. (1986). Suicide in America: A test of Durkheim's theory of religious and family integration 1933–1980. *American Journal of Sociology*, 92, 628–656.

Breault, K. D., & Barkey, K. (1982). A comparative analysis of Durkheim's theory of egoistic suicide. *Sociological Quarterly*, 23, 321–331.

Breed, W. (1966). Suicide, migration, and race: A study of new cases in New Orleans. *Journal of Social Issues*, 22, 30–43.

Breier, A., & Astrachan, B. M. (1984). Characterization of schizophrenic patients who commit suicide. *American Journal of Psychiatry*, 141, 206–209.

Breier, A., Albus, M., Pickar, D., Zahn, T. P., Wolkowitz, O. M., & Paul, S. M. (1987). Controllable and uncontrollable stress in humans: Alterations in mood and neuroendocrine and psychophysiological function. *American Journal of Psychiatry*, 144, 1419–1425.

Bridges, K. W., & Goldberg, D. P. (1985). Somatic presentation of DSM-III psychiatric disorders in primary care. *Journal of Psychosomatic Research*, 29, 563–569.

Brizer, D. A. (1993). Religiosity and drug abuse among psychiatric inpatients. *American Journal of Drug and Alcohol Abuse*, 19, 337–345.

Broadhead, W. E., Gehlbach, S. H., deGruy, F. V., & Kaplan, B. H. (1989). Functional vs. structural social support and health-care utilization in a family medicine outpatient practice. *Medical Care*, 27, 221–233.

Brody, D. S. (1980). Psychological distress and hypertension control. *Journal of Human Stress*, (March), 2–6.

Broen, W. E. (1955). Personality correlates of certain religious attitudes. *Journal of Consulting Psychology*, 19, 23.

Bromet, E. J., Dew, M. A., & Eaton, W. (1995). Epidemiology of psychosis with special reference to schizophrenia. In M. T. Tusang, M. Tohen, & G. E. P. Zahner (eds.), *Textbook in Psychiatric Epidemiology*. New York: Wiley.

Brooks, N. A., & Matson, R. R. (1982). Social-psychological adjustment to multiple sclerosis. *Social Science and Medicine*, 16, 2129–2135.

Brown, D. G., & Lowe, W. L. (1951). Religious beliefs and personality characteristics of college students. *Journal of Social Psychology*, 33, 103–129.

Brown, D. R., & Gary, L. E. (1987). Stressful life events, social support networks, and the physical and mental health of urban African-American adults. *Journal of Human Stress*, Winter, 165–174.

Brown, D. R., & Gary, L. E. (1988). Unemployment and psychological distress among Black African-American women. *Sociological Focus*, 21, 209–222.

Brown, D. R., & Gary, L. E. (1994). Religious involvement and health status among African-American males. *Journal of the National Medical Association*, 86, 825–831.

Brown, D. R., Gary, L. E., Greene, A. D., & Mulburn, N. G. (1992). Patterns of social affiliation as predictors of depressive symptoms among urban Blacks. *Journal of Health and Social Behavior*, 33, 242–253.

Brown, D. R., Ndubuisi, S. C., & Gary, L. E. (1990). Religiosity and psychological distress among Blacks. *Journal of Religion and Health*, 29(1), 55–68.

Brown, G. K., Nicassio, P. M., & Wallston, K. A. (1989). Pain coping strategies and depression in rheumatoid arthritis. *Journal of Consulting and Clinical Psychology*, 57, 652–657.

Brown, G. W., & Prudo, R. (1981). Psychiatric disorder in a rural and an urban population: 1. Aetiology of depression. *Psychological Medicine*, 11, 581–599.

Brown, H. P., & Peterson, J. H. (1991). Assessing spirituality in addiction treatment and follow-up: Development of the Brown-Peterson Recovery Progress Inventory (BPRI). *Alcohol Treatment Quarterly*, 8(2), 21–50.

Brown, L. B. (1962). A study of religious belief. *British Journal of Psychology*, 53, 259–272.

Brown, L. B. (1966). The structure of religious belief. *Journal for the Scientific Study of Religion*, 5, 259–272.

Brown, R. C., & Ritzmann, L. (1967). Some factors associated with absence of coronary heart disease in persons aged 65 or older. *Journal of the American Geriatrics Society*, 15, 239–250.

Brown, S. V. (1985). Premarital sexual permissiveness among black adolescent females. *Social Psychology Quarterly*, 48, 381–387.

Brownfield, D., & Sorenson, A. M. (1991). Religion and drug use among adolescents: A social support conceptualization and interpretation. *Deviant Behavior*, 12, 259–276.

Broyles, P. A., & Drenovsky, C. K. (1992). Religious attendance and the subjective health of the elderly. *Review of Religious Research*, 34, 152–160.

Brozan, N. (1998). Breaking down the barriers between religion and medicine. *New York Times* (July 18), B1, B4.

Bruce, M. L., & Kim, K. M. (1992). Differences in the effects of divorce on major depression in men and women. *American Journal of Psychiatry*, 149(7), 914–917.

Bruns, C., & Geist, C. S. (1984). Stressful life events and drug use among adolescents. *Journal of Human Stress*, 10(3), 135–139.

Brunswick, A. F., Messeri, P. A., & Titus, S. P. (1992). Predictive factors in adult substance abuse: A prospective study of African American adolescents. In M. Glantz & R. Pickens (eds.), *Vulnerability to Drug Abuse* (pp. 419–472). Washington, D.C.: American Psychological Association.

Brutz, J. L., & Allen, C. M. (1986). Religious commitment, peace, activism, and marital violence in Quaker families. *Journal of Marriage and the Family*, 48, 491–502.

Bryant, S., & Rakowski, W. (1992). Predictors of mortality among elderly African Americans. *Research on Aging*, 14, 50–67.

Buckalew, L.W. (1978). A descriptive study of denominational concomitants in psychiatric diagnosis. *Social Behavior and Personality*, 6, 239–242.

Budd, R. J., Eiser, J., Morgan, M., & Gammage, P. (1985). The personal characteristics and lifestyle of the young drinker: The results of a survey of British adolescents. *Drug and Alcohol Dependence*, 16, 145–157.

Bufford, R. K. (1989). Demonic influence and mental disorders. *Journal of Psychology and Christianity*, 8, 35–48.

Bull, C. N., & Aucoin, J. B. (1975). Voluntary association participation and life satisfaction: A replication note. *Journal of Gerontology*, 30, 73–76.

Bullis, R. K. (1991). The spiritual healing "defense" in criminal prosecutions for crimes against children. *Child Welfare*, 30, 541–555.

Bulman, J., & Wortman, C. (1977). Attributions of blame and coping in the "real world": Severe accident victims react to their lot. *Journal of Personality and Social Psychology*, 35, 351–363.

Bumpass, L. L., & Sweet, J. A. (1972). Differentials in marital instability: 1972. *American Sociological Review*, 37, 754–767.

Burbank, P. M. (1992). An exploratory study: Assessing the meaning in life among older adult clients. *Journal of Gerontological Nursing*, 18, 19–28.

Burchinal, L. G. (1957). Marital satisfaction and religious behavior. *American Sociological Review*, 22, 306–310.

Bureau of the Census (date unknown). *Projections of the Numbers of Households and Families: 1986 to 2000*. Washington, D.C.: U.S. Department of Commerce.

Burell, G. (1996). Group psychotherapy in Project New Life: Treatment of coronary-prone behaviors for patients who have had coronary artery bypass graft surgery. In R. Allan & S. Scheidt (eds.), *Heart and Mind: The Practice of Cardiac Psychology* (pp. 291–310). Washington, D.C.: American Psychological Association.

Burgener, S. C. (1994). Caregiver religiosity and well-being in dealing with Alzheimer's dementia. *Journal of Religion and Health*, 33, 175–189.

Burgess, E. W., Cavan, R. S., & Havighurst, R. J. (1948). *Your Attitudes and Activities*. Chicago: Science Research Associates.

Burkett, S. R. (1977). Religion, parental influence, and adolescent alcohol and marijuana use. *Journal of Drug Issues*, 7, 263–273.

Burkett, S. R. (1980). Religiosity, beliefs, normative standards and adolescent drinking. *Journal of Studies on Alcohol* 41, 662–671.

Burkett, S. R. (1993). Perceived parents' religiosity, friends' drinking, and hellfire: A panel study of adolescent drinking. *Review of Religious Research*, 35, 134–153.

Burkett, S. R., & Warren, B. O. (1987). Religiosity, peer associations, and adolescent marijuana use: A panel study of underlying causal structures. *Criminology* 25(1), 109–131.

Burkett, S. R., & White, M. (1974). Hellfire and delinquency: Another look. *Journal for the Scientific Study of Religion*, 13D, 455–462.

Burnet, F. M. (1970). The concept of immunological surveillance. *Progress in Experimental Tumor Research*, 13, 1–27.

Burns, C. M., & Smith, L. L. (1991). Evaluating spiritual well-being among drug and alcohol dependent patients: A pilot study examining the effects of supportive/educative nursing interventions. *Addictions Nursing Network*, 3 (3), 89–94.

Burnside, M., Baer, P., McLaughlin, R., & Pokorny, A. (1986). Alcohol use by adolescents in disrupted families. *Alcoholism: Clinical and Experimental Research* 10, 274–278.

Burr, J. A., McCall, P. L., & Powell-Griner, E. (1994). Catholic religion and suicide–the mediating effect of divorce. *Social Science Quarterly*, 75, 300–318.

Burroughs, T. E., Harris, M. A., Pontious, S. L., & Santiago, J. V. (1997). Research on social support in adolescents with IDDM: A critical review. *Diabetes Educator*, 23, 438–448.

Burvill, P. W., McCall, M. G., Woodings, T., & Stenhouse, N. S. (1983). Comparison of suicide rates and methods in English, Scots and Irish migrants in Australia. *Social Science and Medicine*, 17, 705–708.

Buscaglia, L. (1975). *The Disabled and Their Parents*. Thorofare, N.J.: Charles B. Slack.

Buss, A. H., & Durkee, A. (1957). An inventory for assessing different kinds of hostility. *Journal of Clinical Psychology*, 21, 343–349.

Butler, M. H., Gardner, B. C., & Bird, M. H. (1998). Not just a time-out: Change dynamics of prayer for religious couples in conflict situations. *Family Process*, 37, 451–478.

Byrd, R. C. (1988). Positive therapeutic effects of intercessory prayer in a coronary care unit population. *Southern Medical Journal*, 81, 826–829.

Byrne, D. G., Byrne, A. East, & Reinhart, M. I. (1995). Personality, stress and the decision to commence cigarette smoking in adolescence. *Journal of Psychosomatic Research*, 39, 53–62.

Cacioppo, J. T., Malarkey, W. B., Kiecolt-Glaser, J. K., Uchino, B. N., Sgoutas-Emch, S. A., Sheridan, J. F., Berntson, G. G., & Glaser, R. (1995). Heterogeneity in neuroendocrine and immune responses to brief psychological stressors as a function of autonomic cardiac activation. *Psychosomatic Medicine*, 57, 154–164.

Caffrey, B. (1969). Behavior patterns and personality characteristics related to prevalence rates of coronary heart disease in American monks. *Journal of Chronic Diseases*, 22(2), 93–103.

Cahalan, D., & Room, R. (1972). Problem drinking among American men aged 21–59. *American Journal of Public Health*, 62, 1473–1482.

Cairns, D. M., Adkins, R. H., & Scott, M. D. (1996). Pain and depression in acute traumatic spinal cord injury: origins of chronic problematic pain? *Archives of Physical Medicine and Rehabilitation*, 77, 329–335.

Calabrese, J. R., King, M. A., & Gold, P. W. (1987). Alterations in immunocompetence during stress, bereavement, and depression: Focus on neuroendocrine regulation. *American Journal of Psychiatry*, 144, 1123–1134.

Calahan, D., Cisin, I. H., & Crossley, H. M. (1969). *American Drinking Practices*. New York: United Printing Services.

Call, V. R. A., & Heaton, T. B. (1997). Religious influence on marital stability. *Journal for the Scientific Study of Religion*, 36(3), 382–392.

Callahan, C. M., Hui, S. L., Nienaber, N. A., Musick, B. S., & Tierney, W. M. (1994). Longitudinal study of depression and health services use among elderly primary care patients. *Journal of the American Geriatric Society*, 42, 833–838.

Cameron, P., Titus, D. G., Kostin, J., & Kostin, M. (1973). The life satisfaction of nonnormal persons. *Journal of Consulting and Clinical Psychology*, 41(2), 207–214.

Campbell, A. (1981). *The Sense of Well-Being in America: Recent Patterns and Trends*. New York: McGraw-Hill.

Campbell, A., Converse, P., & Rogers, W. L. (1976). *The Quality of American Life*. New York: Russell Sage Foundation.

Campbell, R. A., & Curtis, J. E. (1994). Religious involvement across societies: Analysis for alternative measures in national surveys. *Journal for the Scientific Study of Religion*, 33(3), 219–229.

Cancellaro, L. A., Larson, D. B., & Wilson, W. P. (1982). Religious life of narcotic addicts. *Southern Medical Journal*, 75, 1166–1168.

Cannon, W. B. (1941). The emergency function of the adrenal medulla in pain and the major emotions. *American Journal of Physiology*, 33, 356.

Capps, D. E., Ransohoff, P., & Rambo, L. (1976). Publication trends in the psychology of religion to 1974. *Journal for the Scientific Study of Religion*, 15, 15–28.

Cardwell, J. D. (1969). The relationship between religious commitment and premarital sexual permissiveness: A five-dimensional analysis. *Sociological Analysis*, 30, 72–80.

Caren, L. D., Leveque, J. A., & Mandel, A. D. (1983). Effect of ethanol on the immune system in mice. *Developments in Toxicology and Environmental Science*, 11, 435–438.

Carey, R. G. (1974). Emotional adjustment in terminal patients: A quantitative approach. *Journal of Counseling Psychology*, 21, 433–439.

Carey, R. G. (1977). The widowed: A year later. *Journal of Counseling Psychology*, 24, 125–131.

Carlens, E. (1976). Smoking and the immune response in the air passages. *Broncho-Pneumologie*, 26, 322–323.

Carlson, C. R., Bacaseta, P. E., & Simanton, D. A. (1988). A controlled evaluation of devotional meditation and progressive relaxation. *Journal of Psychology and Theology*, 16, 362–368.

Carlson, G. A., & Cantwell, D. P. (1982). Suicidal behavior and depression in children and adolescents. *American Academy of Child Psychiatry* 21, 361–368.

Carlucci, K., Genova, J., Rubackin, F., & Rubackin, R. (1993). Effects of sex, religion, and amount of alcohol consumption on self-reported drinking-related problem behaviors. *Psychological Reports*, 72(3, pt. 1), 983–987.

Carnegie, D. (1936). *How to Win Friends and Influence People*. New York: Pocket Books.

Carney, R. M. (1998). Psychological risk factors for cardiac events: could there be just one? *Circulation*, 97, 128–129.

Carney, R. M., Freedland, K. E., Eisen, S. A., Rich, M. W., & Jaffe, A. S. (1995). Major depression and medication adherence in elderly patients with coronary artery disease. *Health Psychology,* 14, 88–90.

Carney, R. M., Rich, M. W., Freedland, K. E., Saini, J., te Velde, A., Simeone, C., & Clark, K. (1988). Major depressive disorder predicts cardiac events in patients with coronary artery disease. *Psychosomatic Medicine,* 50, 627–633.

Carney, R. M., Saunders, R. D., Freedland, K. E., Stein, P., Rich, M. W., & Jaffe, A. S. (1995). Association of depression with reduced heart rate variability in coronary artery disease. *American Journal of Cardiology,* 76, 562–564.

Caro, I., Miralles, A., & Rippere, V. (1983). What's the thing to do when you're feeling depressed? A cross-cultural replication. *Behavior, Research, and Therapy,* 21, 477–483.

Carp, F. M. (1974). Short-term and long-term prediction of adjustment to a new environment. *Journal of Gerontology,* 29, 444–453.

Carr, L. G., & Hauser, W. J. (1981). Class, religious participation, and psychiatric symptomatology. *International Journal of Social Psychiatry,* 27, 133–142.

Carroll, S. (1993). Spirituality and purpose in life in alcoholism recovery. *Journal of Studies on Alcohol,* 54, 297–301.

Carr-Saunders, A. M., Mannheim, H., & Rhodes, E. C. (1944). *Young Offenders.* New York: Macmillan.

Carson, V., & Huss, K. (1979). Prayer: An effective therapeutic and teaching tool. *Journal of Psychiatric Nursing and Mental Health Services,* 17, 34–37.

Carson, V., Soeken, K. L., & Grimm, P. M. (1988). Hope and its relationship to spiritual well-being. *Journal of Psychology and Theology,* 16(2), 159–167.

Carson, V., Soeken, K. L., Shanty, J., & Terry, L. (1990). Hope and spiritual well-being: Essentials for living with AIDS. *Perspectives in Psychiatric Care,* 26, 28–34.

Carson, V. B. (1993). Prayer, meditation, exercise, and special diets: Behaviors of the hardy person with HIV/AIDS. *Journal of the Association of Nurses in AIDS Care,* 4(3), 18–28.

Carson, V. B. (1997). Spiritual care: The needs of the caregiver. *Seminars in Oncology Nursing,* 13, 271–274.

Carson, V. B., & Green, H. (1992). Spiritual well-being: A predictor of hardiness in patients with AIDS. *Journal of Professional Nursing,* 8, 209–220.

Carter, C. S., & Maddock, R. J. (1992). Chest pain in generalized anxiety disorder. *International Journal of Psychiatry in Medicine,* 22, 291–298.

Carter, H. G. (1991). Save prison, mental hospital chaplains. *Atlanta Constitution* (September 12), p. A14.

Carver, C. S., & Gaines, J. G. (1987). Optimism, pessimism, and postpartum depression. *Cognitive Therapy and Research,* 11, 449–462.

Carver, C. S., Pozo, C., Harris, S. D., Noriega, V., Scheier, M. F., Robinson, D. S., Ketcham, A. S., Moffat, F. L., & Clark, K. C. (1993). How coping mediates the effect of optimism on distress: A study of women with early stage breast cancer. *Journal of Personality and Social Psychology,* 65, 375–390.

Carver, C. S., Scheier, M. F., & Weintraub, J. K. (1989). Assessing coping strategies: A theoretically based approach. *Journal of Personality and Social Psychology,* 56, 267–283.

Cary, G. (1997). Towards wholeness: Transcending the barriers between religion and psychiatry. *British Journal of Psychiatry,* 170, 396–397.

Caspersen, C. J., Christenson, G. M., & Pollard, R. A. (1986). Status of the 1990 physical fitness and exercise objectives—evidence from NHIS-1985. *Public Health Reports,* 101, 587–592.

Cassileth, B. R., Lusk, E. J., Miller, D. S., Brown, L. L., & Miller, C. (1985). Psychosocial correlates of survival in advanced malignant disease? *New England Journal of Medicine,* 312, 1551–1555.

Casten, R. J., Parmelee, P. A., Kleban, M. H., Lawton, M. P., & Katz, I. R. (1995). The relationships among anxiety, depression, and pain in a geriatric institutionalized sample. *Pain,* 61, 271–276.

Catipovic-Veselica, K., Buric, D., Ilakovac, V., Amidzic, V., Kozmar, D., Durjancek, J., Skrinjaric, S., & Catipovic, B. (1995). Association of scores for Type A behavior with age, sex, occupation, education, life needs satisfaction, smoking, and religion in 1084 employees. *Psychological Reports,* 77, 131–138.

Caudill, M., Schnable, R., Zuttermeister, P., Benson, H., & Friedman, R. (1991). Decreased clinic use by chronic pain patients: response to behavioral medicine intervention. *Clinical Journal of Pain,* 7, 305–310.

Caudill, M. A., Friedman, R., & Benson, H. (1987). Relaxation therapy in the control of blood pressure. *Biblioteca Cardiologica,* 41, 106–119.

Cavenar, J. O., & Spaulding, J. G. (1977). Depressive disorders and religious conversions. *Journal of Nervous and Mental Disease,* 165, 209–212.

Cederblad, M., Dahlin, L., Hagnell, O., et al. (1995). Coping with life span crises in a group at risk of mental and behavioral disorders: From the Lundby study. *Acta Psychiatrica Scandinavia*, 91, 322–330.

Cella, D. (1996). Quality of life outcomes: measurement and validation. *Oncology*, 10(11, Suppl.), 233–246.

Cella, D., & Webster, K. (1997). Linking outcomes management to quality-of-life measurement. *Oncology*, 11(11A), 232–235.

Centers for Disease Control (1990). Infant mortality by marital status of mother–United States, 1983. *Morbidity and Mortality Weekly Report*, 39, 521–522.

Centers for Disease Control (1991). Comparative mortality of two college groups. *CDC Mortality and Morbidity Weekly Report*, 40, 579–582.

Centers for Disease Control and Prevention (1993). Public health focus: Physical activity in the prevention of coronary heart disease. *Journal of the American Medical Association*, 270, 1529–1530.

Centers for Disease Control and Prevention (1997). *Physical Activity and Health: A Report of the Surgeon General*. Washington, D.C.: U.S. Department of Health and Human Services.

Cesana, G., Ferario, M., & Sega, R. (1996). Job strain in the ambulatory blood pressure levels in a population-based employed sample of men from northern Italy. *Scandinavian Journal of Work, Environment, and Health*, 22, 294–305.

Chadwick, B. A., & Top, B. L. (1993). Religiosity and delinquency among LDS adolescents. *Journal for the Scientific Study of Religion*, 32, 51–67.

Chalfant, H. P., Heller, P. L., Roberts, A., Vriones, D., Aquirre-Hochbaum, S., & Farr, W. (1990). The clergy as a resource for those encountering psychological distress. *Review of Religious Research*, 31, 306–313.

Chamberlain, K., & Zika, S. (1988). Religiosity, life meaning and well-being: Some relationships in a sample of women. *Journal for the Scientific Study of Religion*, 27, 411–420.

Chan, L. Y., & Heaton, T. B. (1989). Demographic determinants of delayed divorce. *Journal of Divorce*, 13(1), 97–112.

Chan, R. S., Huey, E. D., Maecker, H. L., Cortopassi, K. M., Howard, S. A., Iyer, A. M., Mcintosh, L. J., Ajilore, O. A., Brooke, S. M., & Sapolsky, R. M. (1996). Endocrine modulators of necrotic neuron death. *Brain Pathology*, 6, 481–491.

Chandra, R. K., & Newberne, P. M. (1977). *Nutrition, Immunity, and Infection: Mechanisms of Interactions*. New York: Plenum.

Chang, B. H., Noonan, A. E., & Tennstedt, S. L. (1998). Role of religion/spirituality and in coping with caregiving for disabled elders. *Gerontologist*, 38, 463–470.

Chang, B. L., Uman, G. C., Linn, L. S., Ware, J. E., & Kane, R. L. (1985). Adherence to health care regimens among elderly women. *Nursing Research*, 34, 27–31.

Chase-Lansdale, P. L., Cherlin, A. J., & Kiernan, K. E. (1995). The long-term effects of parental divorce on the mental health of young adults: A developmental perspective. *Child Development*, 66, 1614–1634.

Chatters, L. M., Levin, J. S., & Ellison, C. G. (1998). Public health and health education in faith communities. *Health Education and Behavior*, 25, 689–699.

Chaturvedi, S. K., & Bhandari, S. (1989). Somatization and illness behavior. *Journal of Psychosomatic Research*, 33, 147–153.

Chavis, M. (1989). Secularization and religious revival: Evidence from U.S. church attendance rates 1972–1986. *Journal for the Scientific Study of Religion*, 28, 464–477.

Cherpitel, C. J. (1997). Alcohol and violence-related injuries in the emergency room. *Recent Developments in Alcohol*, 13, 105–118.

Chesney, M. A., Hecker, M. H., & Black, G. W. (1988). Coronary-prone components of Type A behavior in the WCGS: A new methodology. In B. K. Houston & C. Snyder (eds.), *Type A Behavior Pattern: Research, Theory, and Intervention* (pp. 168–188). New York: Wiley.

Chick, J., & Erickson, C. K. (1996). Conference summary: Consensus Conference on Alcohol Dependence and the Role of Pharmacotherapy in Its Treatment. *Alcohol Clinical and Experimental Research*, 20(2), 391–402.

Cho, P. Y. (1987). *The Fourth Dimension*. New York: Logos Associates.

Christensen, C. W. (1963). Religious conversion. *Archives of General Psychiatry*, 9, 207–216.

Christo, G., & Franey, C. (1995). Drug users' spiritual beliefs, locus of control and the disease concept in relation to Narcotics Anonymous attendance and six-month outcomes. *Drug and Alcohol Dependence*, 38, 51–56.

Chu, C. C., & Klein, H. E. (1985). Psychosocial and environmental variables in outcome of black schizophrenics. *Journal of the National Medical Association*, 77, 793–796.

Cigarette Smoking among U.S. Adults (1996). Cigarette smoking among adults—United States,

1994. *Mortality and Morbidity Weekly Reports*, 45, 588–590.

Cisin, I. H., & Cahalan, D. (1968). Comparison of abstainers and heavy drinkers in a national survey. *Psychiatric Research Reports*, 24, 10–21.

Clark, C. C. (1997). Recognizing spiritual needs of orthopedic patients. *Orthopedic Nursing*, 16 (6), 27–32.

Clark, D. C., Daughterty, S. R., Baldwin, D. C., & Hughes, P. H. (1992). Assessment of drug involvement: Applications to a sample of physicians in training. *British Journal of Addiction*, 87, 1649–1662.

Clark, R. A. (1980). Religious delusions among Jews. *American Journal of Psychotherapy*, 34, 62–71.

Clark, R. A. (1981). Self-mutilization accompanying religious delusions—a case report and review. *Journal of Clinical Psychiatry*, 42, 243–245.

Clayton, R. R. (1969). Religious orthodoxy and premarital sex. *Social Forces*, 47, 469–474.

Cleary, P. D., & Houts, P. S. (1984). The psychological impact of the Three Mile Island incident. *Journal of Human Stress*, Spring, 28–34.

Cline, V. B., & Richards, J. M. (1965). A factor analytic study of religious belief and behavior. *Journal of Personality and Social Psychology*, 1, 569–578.

Cloninger, C. R. (1987). A systematic method for clinical description and classification of personality. *Archives of General Psychiatry*, 44, 573–588.

Coakley, D. V., & McKenna, G. W. (1986). Safety of faith healing. *Lancet*, February 22, 444.

Cobb, S., & Rose, R. M. (1973). Hypertension, peptic ulcer, and diabetes in air traffic controllers. *Journal of the American Medical Association*, 224, 489–492.

Cochran, J. K. (1993). The variable effects of religiosity and denomination on adolescent self-reported alcohol use by beverage type. *Journal of Drug Issues*, 23, 479–491.

Cochran, J. K., & Akers, R. L. (1989). Beyond hellfire: An exploration of the variable effects of religiosity on adolescent marijuana and alcohol use. *Journal of Research in Crime and Delinquency*, 26, 198–225.

Cochran, J. K., & Beeghley, L. (1991). The influence of religion on attitudes toward nonmarital sexuality: A preliminary assessment of reference group theory. *Journal for the Scientific Study of Religion*, 30, 45–62.

Cochran, J. K., Beeghley, L., & Bock, E. W. (1988). Religiosity and alcohol behavior: An explora-tion of reference group theory. *Sociological Forum*, 3, 256–276.

Cochran, J. K., Beeghley, L., & Bock, E. W. (1992). The influence of religious stability and homogamy on the relationship between religiosity and alcohol use among Protestants. *Journal for the Scientific Study of Religion*, 31, 441–456.

Cochran, J. K., Wood, P. B., & Arneklev, B. J. (1994). Is the religiosity-delinquency relationship spurious? Social control theories. *Journal of Research in Crime and Delinquency*, 31, 92–123.

Cohen, H. J., Pieper, C. F., Harris, T., Rao, K. M., & Currie, M. S. (1997). The association of plasma IL-6 levels with functional disability in community-dwelling elderly. *Journals of Gerontology*, Series A, Medical Sciences, 52, M201–208.

Cohen, M. A. (1998). The monetary value of saving a high-risk youth. *Journal of Quantitative Criminology* 14(1), 5–33.

Cohen, P., & Brook, J. (1987). Family factors related to the persistence of psychopathology in childhood and adolescence. *Psychiatry*, 50, 332–345.

Cohen, S. (1988). Psychosocial models of the role of social support in the etiology of physical disease. *Health Psychology*, 7, 269–297.

Cohen, S., & Willis, T. A. (1985). Stress, social support, and the buffering hypothesis. *Psychological Bulletin*, 98, 310–357.

Cohen, S., Doyle, W. J., Skoner, D. P., Rabin, B. S., & Gwaltney, J. M. (1997). Social ties and susceptibility to the common cold. *Journal of the American Medical Association*, 277, 1940–1944.

Cohen, S., Tyrell, D. A. J., & Smith, A. P. (1991). Psychological stress and susceptibility to the common cold. *New England Journal of Medicine*, 325, 606–612.

Cohen-Mansfield, J., & Marx, M. S. (1993). Pain and depression in the nursing home: Corroborating results. *Journal of Gerontology*, 48, 96–97.

Coke, M. M. (1992). Correlates of life satisfaction among elderly African Americans. *Journal of Gerontology*, 47, 316–320.

Colantonio, A., Kasl, S. V., & Ostfeld, A. M. (1992). Depressive symptoms and other psychosocial factors as predictors of stroke in the elderly. *American Journal of Epidemiology*, 136, 884–894.

Colby, J. P. Jr., Linsky, A. S., & Straus, M. A. (1994). Social stress and state-to-state differences in smoking and smoking-related mortality in the United States. *Social Science and Medicine*, 38, 373–381.

Coleman, C. L., & Holzemer, W. L. (1999). Spirituality, psychological well-being, and HIV symptoms for African-Americans living with HIV disease. *Journal of the Association of Nurses in the AIDS Care*, 10, 42–50.

Coleman, S. B., Kaplan, J. D. & Downing, R. W. (1986). Life cycle and loss: The spiritual vacuum of heroin addiction. *Family Process*, 25, 5–23.

Coles, R. (1991). *Spiritual Life of Children*. New York: Houghton Mifflin.

Collins, G. R. (1988). *Christian Counseling: A Comprehensive Guide* (rev. ed.). New York: Word Books.

Collipp, P. J. (1969). The efficacy of prayer: A triple-blind study. *Medical Times*, 97, 201–204.

Commerford, M. C., & Reznikoff, M. (1996). Relationship of religion and perceived social support to self-esteem and depression in nursing home residents. *Journal of Psychology*, 130, 35–50.

Committee on Trauma Research (1988). Commission on Life Sciences, National Research Council, and Institute of Medicine. *Injury in America: A Continuing Public Health Problem*. Washington, D.C.: National Academy Press.

Committee on Ways and Means, U.S. House of Representatives (1993). *The Green Book: Overview of Entitlement Programs*. Washington, D.C.: U.S. Government Printing Office.

Compas, B. E., Forsythe, C. J., & Wagner, B. M. (1988). Consistency and variability in causal attributions and coping with stress. *Cognitive Therapy and Research*, 12, 305–320.

Comstock, G., & Partridge, K. (1972). Church attendance and health. *Journal of Chronic Disease*, 25, 665–672.

Comstock, G. W. (1971). Fatal arteriosclerotic heart disease, water hardness at home, and socioeconomic characteristics. *American Journal of Epidemiology*, 94, 1–10.

Comstock, G. W., & Lundin, F. E. (1967). Parental smoking and perinatal mortality. *American Journal of Obstetrics and Gynecology*, 98, 708–718.

Comstock, G. W., & Partridge, K. B. (1972). Church attendance and health. *Journal of Chronic Disease*, 25, 665–672.

Comstock, G. W., & Tonascia, J. A. (1977). Education and mortality in Washington County, Maryland. *Journal of Health and Social Behavior*, 18, 54–61.

Comstock, G. W., Abbey, H., & Lundin, F. E. (1970). The nonofficial census as a basic tool for epidemiologic observations in Washington County, Maryland. In I. I. Kessler & M. L. Levin (eds.), *The Community as an Epidemiologic Laboratory: A Casebook of Community Studies* (pp. 73–97). Baltimore: Johns Hopkins University Press.

Conrad, N. (1991). Where do they turn? Social support systems of suicidal high school adolescents. *Journal of Psychosocial Nursing and Mental Health Services*, 29(3), 14–20.

Conway, K. (1985). Coping with the stress of medical problems among black and white elderly. *International Journal of Aging and Human Development*, 21, 39–48.

Conwell, Y., Forbes, N. T., Cox, C., & Caine, E. D. (1993). Validation of a measure of physical illness burden at autopsy: The Cumulative Illness Rating Scale. *Journal of the American Geriatrics Society*, 41, 38–41.

Conyn-van Spaendonck, M. A., Oostvogel, P. M., van Loon, A. M., van Wijgaarden, J. K., & Kromhout, D. (1996). Circulation of poliovirus during the poliomyelitis outbreak in the Netherlands, in 1992–1993. *American Journal of Epidemiology*, 143, 929–935.

Cook, A. J. (1998). Cognitive-behavioral pain management for elderly nursing home residents. *Journal of Gerontology*, 53, 51–59.

Cook, C. C., Goddard, D., & Westall, R. (1997). Knowledge and experience of drug use amongst church-affiliated young people. *Drug and Alcohol Dependence*, 46(1–2), 9–17.

Cook, J. A., & Wimberley, D. W. (1983). "If I should die before I wake": Religious commitment and adjustment to the death of a child. *Journal for the Scientific Study of Religion*, 22, 222–238.

Cook, W., & Medley, D. (1954). Proposed hostility and pharisaic-virtue scales for the MMPI. *Journal of Applied Psychology*, 38, 414–418.

Cooklin, R. S., Ravindran, A., & Carney, M. W. P. (1983). The patterns of mental disorder in Jewish and non-Jewish admissions to a district general hospital psychiatric unit: Is manic-depressive illness a typically Jewish disorder? *Psychological Medicine*, 13, 209–212.

Cooley, C. E., & Hutton, J. B. (1965). Adolescent response to religious appeal as related to IPAT anxiety. *Journal of Social Psychology*, 56, 325–327.

Coombs, R. H., Wellisch, D. K., & Fawzy, F. I. (1985). Drinking patterns and problems among female children and adolescents: A comparison of abstainers, past users, and current users. *American Journal of Drug and Alcohol Abuse*, 11, 315–348.

Cooper, H. M. (1984). *The Integrated Research Review: A Systematic Approach*, vol. 2 (pp. 66–71). Beverly Hills: Sage.

Cooper, M., & Aygen, M. (1978). Effect of meditation on blood cholesterol and blood pressure. *Journal of the Israel Medical Association*, 95, 1–10.

Cooper, M., & Aygen, M. (1979). A relaxation technique in the management of hypercholesterolemia. *Journal of Human Stress*, 5, 24–27.

Cooper, R., Joffe, B. I., Lamprey, J. M., Botha, K., Shires, L. R., Baker, S. G., & Seftel, H. C. (1985). Hormonal and biochemical responses to transcendental meditation. *Postgraduate Medical Journal*, 61, 301–304.

Coordinating Council on Juvenile Justice and Delinquency Prevention (1996). *Combating Violence and Delinquency: The National Juvenile Justice Action Plan*. Washington, D.C.: Office of Juvenile Justice and Delinquency Prevention, U.S. Department of Justice.

Copeland, K. (1996). *Healing Promises*. Fort Worth, Tex.: Kenneth Copeland.

Corby, J. C., Orth, W. T., Carcone, V. P., & Kopell, B. S. (1978). Psychophysiological correlates of the practice of Tantric Yoga meditation. *Archives of General Psychiatry*, 35, 571–577.

Corder, B., Shorr, W., & Corder, R. (1974). A study of social and psychological characteristics of adolescent suicide attempters in an urban, disadvantaged area. *Adolescence*, 9(33), 1–6.

Cornish, J. D. (1998). Mormons and health: Impact of Latter-Day Saints' scriptures on health and health practices. *Journal of the Medical Association of Georgia*, 87, 303–304.

Correspondent (1902). Cancer among Jews. *British Medical Journal* (March 15), 681–682.

Corrington, J. E. (1989). Spirituality and recovery: Relationships between levels of spirituality, contentment, and stress during recovery from alcoholism in AA. *Alcoholism Treatment Quarterly*, 6 (3/4), 151–165.

Corti, M. C., Guralnik, J. M., Salive, M. E., Harris, T., Ferrucci, L., Glynn, R. J., & Havlik, R. J. (1997). Clarifying the direct relation between total cholesterol levels and death from coronary heart disease in older persons. *Annals of Internal Medicine*, 126, 753–760.

Costa, P. T., McCrae, R. R., & Norris, A. H (1981). Personal adjustment to aging: Longitudinal prediction from neuroticism and extraversion. *Journal of Gerontology*, 36, 78–85.

Cothran, M. M., & Harvey, P. D. (1986). Delusional thinking in psychotics: Correlates of religious content. *Psychological Reports*, 58, 191–199.

Cotton, S. P., Levine, E. G., Fitzpatrick, C. M., & Dold, K. H. (1998). Spirituality, quality of life and psychological adjustment in women with breast cancer. Paper presented at the Annual Conference of the American Psychological Association, San Francisco, August.

Courtenay, B. C., Poon, L. W., Martin, P., Clayton, G. M., & Johnson, M. A. (1992). Religiosity and adaptation in the oldest-old. *International Journal of Aging and Human Development*, 34, 47–56.

Covinsky, K. E., Kahana, E., Chin, M. H., Palmer, R., Fortinsky, R. H., & Landefield, C. S. (1999). Depressive symptoms and three-year mortality in older hospitalized medical patients. *Annals of Internal Medicine*, 130, 563–569.

Coward, H. (1986). Intolerance in the world's religions. *Studies in Religion*, 15, 419–431.

Cowen, E. L. (1954). The negative concept as a personality measure. *Journal of Consulting Psychology*, 18, 138–142.

Cox, H., & Hammonds, A. (1988). Religiosity, aging, and life satisfaction. *Journal of Religion and Aging*, 5, 1–21.

Craigie, F. C., Liu, I. Y., Larson, D. B., & Lyons, J. S. (1988). A systematic analysis of religious variables in the *Journal of Family Practice*, 1976–1986. *Journal of Family Practice*, 27, 509–513.

Crandall, J. E., & Rasmussen, R. D. (1975). Purpose in life as related to specific values. *Journal of Clinical Psychology*, 31, 483–485.

Crane, L. A. (1996). Social support and adherence behavior among women with abnormal Pap smears. *Journal of Cancer Education*, 11, 164–173.

Crawford, M. E., Handal, P. J., & Wiener, R. L. (1989). The relationship between religion and mental health/distress. *Review of Religious Research*, 31, 16–22.

Creagan, E. T. (1997). Attitude and disposition: Do they make a difference in cancer survival? *Mayo Clinic Proceedings*, 72, 160–164.

Cronan, T. A., Kaplan, R. M., Posner, L., Lumberg, E., & Kozin, F. (1989). Prevalence of the use of unconventional remedies for arthritis in a metropolitan community. *Arthritis and Rheumatism*, 32, 1604–1607.

Cronin, C. (1995). Religiosity, religious affiliation, and alcohol and drug use among American college students living in Germany. *International Journal of Addictions*, 30, 231–238.

Cronin, T. A., Groessl, T. E., & Kaplan, R. M. (1997). The effects of social support and education interventions on health-care costs. *Arthritis Care and Research*, 10, 99–110.

Croog, S. H., & Levine, S. (1972). Religious identity and response to serious illness: A report on heart patients. *Social Science and Medicine*, 6, 17–32.

Crumley, E. E. (1979). Adolescent suicide attempts. *Journal of the American Medical Association* 241, 2404–2407.

Cullari, S., & Mikus, R. (1990). Correlates of adolescent sexual behavior. *Psychological Reports*, 1179–1184.

Cummings, N. A., & Follette, W. T. (1968). Psychiatric services and medical utilization in a prepaid health plans setting: Part II. *Medical Care*, 6, 31–41.

Cutler, S. J. (1976). Membership in different types of voluntary associations and psychological well-being. *Gerontologist*, 16, 335–339.

Daaleman, T. P., & Frey, B. (1999). Spiritual and religious beliefs and practices of family physicians: A national survey. *Journal of Family Practice*, 48, 98–104.

Daaleman, T. P., & Nease, D. E. (1994). Patient attitudes regarding physician inquiry into spiritual and religious issues. *Journal of Family Practice*, 39, 564–568.

Dagi, T. F. (1995). Prayer, piety, and professional propriety: Limits on religious expression in hospitals. *Journal of Clinical Ethics*, 6, 275–279.

Dalal, A. K., & Pande, N. (1988). Psychological recovery of accident victims with temporary and permanent disability. *International Journal of Psychology*, 23, 25–40.

Daltroy, L. H., & Godin, G. (1989). The influence of spousal approval and patient perception of spousal approval on cardiac participation in exercise programs. *Journal of Cadiopulmonary Rehabilitation*, 9, 363–367.

Danto, B. L., & Danto, J. M. (1983). Jewish and non-Jewish suicide in Oakland County, Michigan. *Crisis*, 4, 33–60.

D'Antonio, W. V., Newman, W. M., & Wright, S. A. (1982). Religion and family life: How social scientists view the relationships. *Journal for the Scientific Study of Religion*, 21, 218–225.

D'Aquili, E. G., & Newberg, A. B. (1993). Religious and mystical states: A neuropsychological model. *Zygon*, 28, 177–200.

Darley, J. M., & Batson, C. D. (1973). From Jerusalem to Jericho: A study of situational and dispositional variables in helping behavior. *Journal of Personality and Social Psychology*, 27, 100–108.

Davids, L. (1982). Ethnic identity, religiosity, and youthful deviance: The Toronto computer dating project-1979. *Adolescence*, 17(67), 673–684.

Davidson, M., Kuo, C. C., Middaugh, J. B., Campbell, L. A., Wang, S. P., Newman, W. P., Finley, J. C., & Grayston, J. T. (1998). Confirmed previous infection with Chlamydia pneumonia (TWAR) and its presence in early coronary atherosclerosis. *Circulation*, 98, 628–633.

Davies, P. (1995). *Are We Alone?* New York: Harper-Collins.

Davis, D. T., Bustamante, A., Brown, C. P., Wolde-Psadik, G., Savage, E. W., Cheng, X., & Howland, L. (1994). The urban church and cancer control: A source of social influence in minority communities. *Public Health Reports*, 109, 500–506.

Davis, K. (1948). *Human Society*. New York: Macmillan.

Dawson, D. A. (1991). Family structure and children's health and well-being: Data from the 1988 National Survey of Child Health. *Journal of Marriage and the Family*, 53, 573–584.

Day, L. (1987). Durkheim on religion and suicide: A demographic critique. *Sociology*, 21, 449–461.

Decker, S. D., & Schulz, R. (1985). Correlates of life satisfaction and depression in middle-aged and elderly spinal cord-injured persons. *American Journal of Occupational Therapy*, 39, 740–745.

De Figueiredo, J. M., & Lemkau, P. V. (1978). The prevalence of psychosomatic symptoms in a rapidly changing bilingual culture: An exploratory study. *Social Psychiatry*, 13, 125–133.

De Gouw, H. W. F. M., Westendorp, R. G. J., Kunst, A. E., Mackenbach, J. P., & Vandenbroucke, J. P. (1995). Decreased mortality among contemplative monks in the Netherlands. *American Journal of Epidemiology*, 141, 771–775.

Dein, S. Z., & Stygall, J. (1997). Does being religious help or hinder coping with chronic illness? A critical literature review. *Palliative Medicine*, 11, 291–298.

Delgado, M. (1981). Ethnic and cultural variations in the care of the aged hispanic elderly and natural support systems: a special focus on Puerto Ricans. *Journal of Geriatric Psychiatry*, 239–251.

Delmonte, M. M. (1985). Biochemical indices associated with meditation practice: A literature review. *Neuroscience and Biobehavioral Review*, 9(4), 557–561.

DeMan, A. F., Balkou, S., & Iglesias, R. I. (1987). Social support and suicidal ideation in French Canadians. *Canadian Journal of Behavioural Science*, 19(3), 342–346.

Demaria, T., & Kassinove, H. (1988). Predicting guilt from irrational beliefs, religious affiliation, and religiosity. *Journal of Rational-Emotive and Cognitive-Behavioral Therapy,* 6, 259–272.

Dember, W. N., & Brooks, J. (1989). A new instrument for measuring optimism and pessimism: Test-retest reliability and relations with happiness and religious commitment. *Bulletin of the Psychonomic Society,* 27(4), 365–366.

Denier, E. (1984). Subjective well-being. *Psychological Bulletin,* 95, 542–575.

Denison, H., Berkowicz, A., Oden, A., & Wendestam, C. (1997). The significance of coronary death for the excess mortality in alcohol-depended men. *Alcohol and Alcoholism,* 32, 517–526.

Desmond, D. P., & Maddux, J. F. (1981). Religious programs and careers of chronic heroin users. *American Journal of Drug and Alcohol Abuse,* 8, 71–83.

Deutscher, S., Rockette, H. E., & Krishnaswami, V. (1984). Evaluation of habitual excessive alcohol consumption on myocardial infarction risk in coronary disease patients. *American Heart Journal,* 108, 988–995.

DeVellis, B. M., DeVellis, R. F., & Spilsbury, J. C. (1988). Parental actions when children are sick: The role of belief in divine influence. *Basic and Applied Social Psychology,* 9, 185–196.

Devins, G. M., Mann, J., Mandin, H., Paul, L. C., Hons, R. B., Burgess, E. D., Taub, K., Schorr, S., Letourneau, P. K., & Buckle, S. (1990). Psychosocial predictors of survival in end-stage renal disease. *Journal of Nervous and Mental Disease,* 178, 127–133.

Dewald, P. A. (1971). *Psychotherapy: A Dynamic Approach.* New York: Basic Books.

Dewhurst, K., & Beard, A. W. (1970). Sudden religious conversions in temporal lobe epilepsy. *British Journal of Psychiatry,* 117, 497–507.

Dhabhar, F. S., & McEwen, B. S. (1996). Moderate stress enhances and chronic stress suppresses cell-mediated immunity in vivo. *Society of Neurosciences,* 22, 1350.

Dhawan, N., & Sripat, K. (1986). Fear of death and religiosity as related to need for affiliation. *Psychological Studies,* 31, 35–38.

Diagnostic and Statistical Manual of Mental Disorders, 4th ed. (1994). Washington, D.C.: American Psychiatric Press.

Diamond, E. L. (1982). The role of anger in essential hypertension and coronary heart disease. *Psychological Bulletin,* 92, 410–433.

Dickey, B., Normand, S. L., Norton, E. C., Azeni, H., Fisher, W., & Altaffer, F. (1996). Managing the care of schizophrenia: Lessons from a 4-year Massachusetts Medicaid study. *Archives of General Psychiatry,* 53, 945–952.

Diduca, D., & Joseph, S. (1997). Schizotypal traits and dimensions of religiosity. *British Journal of Clinical Psychology,* 36(part 4), 635–638.

Diekstra, R., & Kerkhof, A. (1989). Attitudes toward suicide: The development of a suicide-attitude questionnaire. In R. F. W. Diekstra, R. Maris, S. Platt, A. Schmidtke, & G. Sonneck (eds.), *Suicide and Its Prevention* (pp. 91–107). Leiden: Brill.

Diener, E. (1984). Subjective well-being. *Psychological Bulletin,* 95, 542–575.

Diespecker, D. D. (1973). Some characteristics of attempted suicide. *Medical Journal of Australia,* 2, 121–125.

Dietary Guidelines (1995). U.S. Department of Agriculture and U.S. Department of Health and Human Services. Nutrition and Your Health: Dietary Guidelines for Americans, 4th ed. (Home and Garden Bull 232). Washington, D.C.: Government Printing Office.

Dilulio, J. J. (1994). America's ticking crime bomb and how to diffuse it. *Wisconsin Interest,* 3(1),16–17.

Ditman, K. S., Crawford, G. G, Forgy, E. W., Moskowitz, H., & MacAndrew, C. (1967). A controlled experiment on the use of court probation for drunk arrests. *American Journal of Psychiatry,* 124, 160–163.

Dittes, J. E. (1969). Psychology and religion. In G. Lindzey & E. Aronson (eds.), *The Handbook of Social Psychology,* 2nd ed., Vol. 5 (pp. 602–659). Reading, Mass.: Addison Wesley.

Dittes, J. E. (1971). Two issues in measuring religion. In M. P. Stronmen (ed.), *Research on Religious Development: A Comprehensive Handbook.* New York: Hawthorne.

Dobson, J. (1970). *Dare to Discipline.* Wheaton, Ill.: Tyndale House.

Dodd, D. K., & Mills, L. L. (1985). FADIS: A measure of the fear of accidental death and injury. *The Psychological Record,* 35: 269–275.

Doherty, W. J., Schrott, H. G., & Metcalf, L. (1983). Effect of spouse support and health beliefs on medication adherence. *Journal of Family Practice,* 17, 837–841.

Domino, G. (1985). Clergy's attitudes toward suicide and recognition of suicide lethality. *Death Studies,* 9, 187–199.

Donabedian, A. (1973) *Aspects of Medical Care Administration.* Cambridge, Mass.: Harvard University Press.

Donahue, M. J. (1985). Intrinsic and extrinsic religiousness: Review and meta-analysis. *Journal of Personality and Social Psychology*, 48, 400–419.

Donahue, M. J., & Benson, P. L. (1995). Religion and the well-being of adolescents. *Journal of Social Issues*, 51, 145–160.

Dorff, E. N. (1998). The Jewish tradition. In R. L. Numbers & D. W. Amundsen (eds.), *Caring and Curing: Health and Medicine in the Western Religious Traditions* (pp. 5–40). Baltimore: Johns Hopkins University Press.

Doria, G., Biozzi, G., Mouton, D., & Covelli, V. (1997). Genetic control of immune responsiveness, aging and tumor incidence. *Mechanisms of Aging and Development*, 96, 1–13.

Dorian, B. J., & Garfinkel, P. E. (1987). Stress, immunity, and illness—A review. *Psychological Medicine*, 17, 393–407.

Dossey, L. (1995). *Healing Words: The Power of Prayer and The Practice of Medicine*. New York: HarperCollins.

Doukas, D. J., Waterhouse, D., Gorenflo, D. W., & Seid, J. (1995). Attitudes and behaviors on physician-assisted death: A study of Michigan oncologists. *Journal of Clinical Oncology*, 13, 1055–1061.

Dovey, K., & Graham, J. (1987). *The Experience of Disability: Social Construction and Imposed Limitation*. Burwood, Victoria: Victoria College Press.

Dowley, T. (ed.) (1982). *Handbook to the History of Christianity*. Grand Rapids, Mich.: Eerdmans.

Downey, A. M. (1984). Relationship of religiosity to death anxiety of middle-aged males. *Psychological Reports*, 54, 811–822.

Doyle, D., & Forehand, M. J. (1984). Life satisfaction and old age. *Research on Aging*, 6, 432–448.

Dreger, R. M. (1952). Some personality correlates of religious attitudes as determined by projective techniques. *Psychological Monographs*, 66, 335.

Drevenstedt, G. T. (1998). Race and ethnic differences in the effects of religious attendance on subjective health. *Review of Religious Research*, 39, 245–263.

Dreyfuss, F. (1953). The incidence of myocardial infarctions in various communities in Israel. *American Heart Journal*, 45, 749–755.

Dube, K. C., Jain, S. C., Basu, A. K., & Kumar, N. (1975). Patterns of the drug habit (cannabis) in hospitalized psychiatric patients. *Bulletin on Narcotics*, 27(2), 1–10.

Dublin, L. I. (1933). *To Be or Not to Be*. New York: Smith & Haas.

Duckro, P. N., & Magaletta, P. R. (1994). The effect of prayer on physical health—experimental evidence. *Journal of Religion and Health*, 33, 211–219.

Dudley, M. G., & Kosinski, F. A. (1990). Religiosity and marital satisfaction: A research note. *Review of Religious Research*, 32, 78–86.

Dudley, R. L., & Cruise, R. J. (1990). Measuring religious maturity: A proposed scale. *Review of Religious Research*, 32, 97–109.

Dudley, R. L., Mutch, P. B., & Cruise, R. J. (1987). Religious factors and drug usage among Seventh-day Adventist Youth in North America. *Journal for the Scientific Study of Religion*, 26, 218–233.

Dufton, B. D., & Perlman, D (1986). Loneliness and religiosity: In the world but not of it. *Journal of Psychology and Theology*, 14, 135–145.

Duke, J. T., & Johnson, B. L. (1984). Spiritual well-being and the consequential dimension of religiosity. *Review of Religious Research*, 26, 59–72.

Dunbar, J. (1990). Predictors of patient adherence: Patient characteristics. In S. A. Shumaker, E. B. Schron, & J. K. Ockene (eds.), *The Handbook of Health Behavior Change* (pp. 348–360). New York: Springer.

Duncan, D. F. (1978). Family stress and the initiation of adolescent drug abuse: A retrospective study. *Corrective and Social Psychiatry*, 24, 111–114.

Dunkel-Schetter, C., Fernstein, L. G., Taylor, S. E., & Falke, R. L. (1992). Patterns of coping with cancer. *Health Psychology*, 11, 79–87.

Dunn, D. S. (1996). Well-being following amputation: Salutary effects of positive meaning, optimism, and control. *Rehabilitation Psychology*, 41(4), 285–302.

Dunn, R. F. (1965). Personality patterns among religious personnel. *Review of Catholic Psychological Records*, 3, 125–137.

DuPont, R. L., Rice, D. P., Miller, L. S., Shiraki, S. S., Rowland, C. R., & Harwood, H. J. (1996). Economic costs of anxiety disorders. *Anxiety*, 2(4): 167–172.

DuRant, R. H., Pendergrast, R., & Seymore, C. (1990). Sexual behavior among Hispanic female adolescents in the United States. *Pediatrics*, 85, 1051–1058.

Durkheim, E. (1951). *Suicide*. Trans. J. A. Spaulding & G. Simpson. New York: Free Press. Original edition: *Le Suicide* (Paris: Felix Alcan, 1897). Original English edition: *Suicide* (London: Routledge & Kegan Paul).

Durkheim, E. (1995). *The Elementary Forms of Religious Life*. New York: Free Press. Original edition: 1912.

Dwyer, J. W., Clarke, L. L., & Miller, M. K. (1990). The effect of religious concentration and affiliation on county cancer mortality rates. *Journal of Health and Social Behavior*, 31, 185–202.

Dysinger, P. W., Lemon, F. R., Crenshaw, G. L., & Walden, R. T. (1963). Pulmonary emphysema in a non-smoking population. *Diseases of the Chest*, 43, 17–25.

Ebaugh, H. R. F., Richman, K., & Chafetz, J. S. (1984). Life crises among the religiously committed: Do sectarian differences matter? *Journal for the Scientific Study of Religion*, 23, 19–31.

Editorial (1998a). HMOs lured elderly into fold, now abandon them to uncertainty. *USA Today* (December 24), 9A.

Editorial (1998b). Spirit of the age: Malignant sadness is the world's great hidden burden. *Economist* (December 19), 113–117.

Edland, J. F., & Duncan, C. E. (1973). Suicide notes in Monroe County: A 23-year look (1950–1972). *Journal of Forensic Sciences*, 18, 364–369.

Edmonds, V. H. (1967). Marital conventionalization: Definition and measurement. *Journal of Marriage and the Family*, 29, 681–688.

Edmonds, V. H., Withers, G., & Dibattista, B. (1972). Adjustment, conservatism, and conventionalism. *Journal of Marriage and the Family*, 34, 96–103.

Edwards, G., Chandler, J., & Hensman, C. (1972). Drinking in a London suburb: Correlates of normal drinking. *Quarterly Journal of Studies on Alcohol*, Suppl. 6, 69–93.

Edwards, G., Gattoni, F., & Hensman, C. (1972). Correlates of alcohol-dependence scores in a prison population. *Quarterly Journal of Studies on Alcohol*, 33, 417–429.

Edwards, G., Kyle, E., & Nicholls, P. (1974). Alcoholics admitted to four hospitals in England. *Quarterly Journal of Studies on Alcohol*, 35, 499–522.

Edwards, J. N., & Klemmack, D. L. (1973). Correlates of life satisfaction: A re-examination. *Journal of Gerontology*, 28, 497–502.

Egan, K. M., Newcomb, P. A., Longnecker, M. P., Trentham-Dietz, A., Baron J. A., Trichopoulos, D., Stampfer, M. J., & Willett, W. C. (1996). Jewish religion and risk of breast cancer. *Lancet*, 347 (9016), 1645–1646.

Egeland, J. A., Gerhard, D. S., Paula, D. L., & Sussex, J. N. (1987). Bipolar affective disorder linked to DNA markers on chromosome 11. *Nature*, 325, 783–787.

Ehman, J., Ott B., Short, T., Ciampa R., Hansen-Flaschen, J. (1999). Do patients want physicians to inquire about their spiritual or religious beliefs if they become gravely ill? *Archives of Internal Medicine*, 159, 1803–1806.

Einstein, A. (1941). *Science, Philosophy and Religion: A Symposium*. In A. Partington (ed.), *The Oxford Dictionary of Quotations* (p. 268), 4th ed. New York: Oxford University Press.

Eiseman, R., & Cole, S. N. (1964). Prejudice and conservatism in denominational college students. *Psychological Reports*, 14, 644.

Eisenberg, D. M., Davis, R. B., Ettner, S. L., Appel, S., Wilkey, S., Rompay, M. V., & Kessler, R. C. (1998). Trends in alternative medicine use in the United States, 1990–1997. *Journal of the American Medical Association*, 280, 1569–1575.

Eisenberg, D. M., Kessler, R. C., Foster, C., Norlock, F. E., Calkins, D. R., & Delbanco, T. L. (1993). Unconventional medicine in the United States. *New England Journal of Medicine*, 328, 246–252.

Elifson, K. W., Petersen, D. M., & Hadaway, C. K. (1983). Religiosity and delinquency. *Criminology*, 21, 505–527.

Elkins, D., Anchor, K. N., & Sandler, H. M. (1979). Relaxation training and prayer behavior as tension reduction techniques. *Behavioral Engineering*, 5, 81–87.

Ell, K. O., Mantell, J. E., Hamovitch, M. B., & Nishimoto, R. H. (1989). Social support, sense of control, and coping among patients with breast, lung, or colorectal cancer. *Journal of Psychosocial Oncology*, 7, 63–89.

Ellis, A. (1948). The value of marriage prediction tests. *American Sociological Review*, 13, 710–718.

Ellis, A. (1962). *Reason and Emotion in Psychotherapy*. Secaucus, N. J.: Lyle Stuart.

Ellis, A. (1980). Psychotherapy and atheistic values: A response to A. E. Bergin's "Psychotherapy and religious values." *Journal of Consulting and Clinical Psychology*, 48, 635–639.

Ellis, A. (1983). *The Case against Religiosity*. New York: Institute for Rational-Emotive Therapy.

Ellis, A. (1987). Religiosity and emotional disturbance: A reply to Sharkey and Malony. *Psychotherapy*, 24, 826–827.

Ellis, A. (1988). Is religiosity pathological? *Free Inquiry*, 18, 27–32.

Ellis, J. B., & Smith, P. C. (1991). Spiritual well-being, social desirability and reasons for living:

Is there a connection? *International Journal of Social Psychiatry, 37,* 57–63.

Ellis, L. (1985). Religiosity and criminality: Evidence and explanations of complex relationships. *Sociological Perspectives, 28,* 501–520.

Ellis, M. R., Vinson, D. C., & Ewigman, B. (1999). Addressing spiritual concerns up patients: family physicians' attitudes and practices. *Journal of Family Practice, 48,* 105–109.

Ellison, C. G. (1991). Religious involvement and subjective well-being. *Journal of Health and Social Behavior, 32,* 80–99.

Ellison, C. G. (1992). Are religious people nice people? Evidence from the National Survey of Black Americans. *Social Forces, 71,* 411–430.

Ellison, C. G. (1993). Religious involvement and self-perception among Black Americans. *Social Forces, 71,* 1027–1055.

Ellison, C. G. (1994a). Religion, the life stress paradigm, and the study of depression. In J. S. Levin (ed.), *Religion in Aging and Health: Theoretical Foundations and Methodological Frontiers* (pp. 78–121). Thousand Oaks, Calif.: Sage.

Ellison, C. G. (1994b). Religious involvement and subjective quality of family life among African Americans. In R. J. Taylor, J. S. Jackson, & L. M. Chatters (eds.), *Family Life in Black America.* Thousand Oaks, Calif.: Sage.

Ellison, C. G. (1995). Race, religious involvement, and depressive symptomatology in a southeastern U.S. community. *Social Science and Medicine, 40,* 1561–1572.

Ellison, C. G. (1996). Conservative Protestantism and the parental use of corporal punishment. *Social Forces, 75,* 1003–1028.

Ellison, C. G., & Gay, D. A. (1990). Region, religious commitment, and life satisfaction among black Americans. *Sociological Quarterly, 31,* 123–147.

Ellison, C. G., & George, L. K. (1994). Religious involvement, social ties, and social support in a southeastern community. *Journal for the Scientific Study of Religion, 33,* 46–61.

Ellison, C. G., & Levin, J. S. (1997). Religious guidance and major depression. Paper presented at the annual meeting of the Society for the Scientific Study of Religion, San Diego, November 7–9.

Ellison, C. G., & Levin, J. S. (1998). The religion-health connection: Evidence, theory, and future directions. *Health Education and Behavior, 25,* 700–720.

Ellison, C. G., & Taylor, R. J. (1996). Turning to prayer: Social and situational antecedents of religious coping among African Americans. *Review of Religious Research, 38,* 111–131.

Ellison, C. G., Bartkowski, J. P., & Anderson, K. L. (1999). Are there religious variations in domestic violence? *Journal of Family Issues, 20,* 87–113.

Ellison, C. G., Burr, J. A., & McCall, P. L. (1997). Religious homogeneity and metropolitan suicide rates. *Social Forces, 76,* 273–299.

Ellison, C. G., Gay, D. A., & Glass, T. A. (1989). Does religious commitment contribute to individual life satisfaction? *Social Forces, 68,* 100–123.

Ellison, C. G., Levin, J. S., & Taylor, R. J. (1997). Religious involvement and psychological distress in a national panel study of African Americans. Paper presented at the joint meetings of the Society for the Scientific Study of Religion and the Religious Research Association, San Diego, November 7–9.

Ellison, C. W. (1983). Spiritual Maturity Index. Unpublished manuscript. Contact Craig W. Ellison (Alliance Theological Seminary, Nyack, New York) for copy of index.

Emavardhana, T., & Tori, C. D. (1997). Changes in self concept, ego defense mechanisms, and religiosity following seven-day Vipassana meditation retreats. *Journal for the Scientific Study of Religion, 36,* 194–206.

Emblen, J. D., & Halstead, L. (1993). Spiritual needs and interventions: Comparing the views of patients, nurses, and chaplains. *Clinical Nurse Specialist, 7*(4), 175–182.

Emmons, R. A. (1999). *The Psychology of Ultimate Concerns: Motivation and Spirituality in Personality.* New York: Guilford.

Emmons, R. A., Cheung, C., & Tehrani, K. (1998). Assessing spirituality through personal goals: Implications for research on religion and subjective well-being. *Social Indicators Research, 45,* 391–422.

Emrick, C. D., Tonigan, J. S., Montgomery, H., & Little, L. (1993). Alcoholics Anonymous: What is currently known? In B. S. McCrady & W. R. Miller (eds.), *Research on Alcoholics Anonymous: Opportunities and Alternatives* (pp. 41–76). New Brunswick, N.J.: Rutgers Center of Alcohol Studies.

Encarta Encyclopedia (1999). *Microsoft Encarta Encyclopedia 99.* Redmond, Wash.: Microsoft Corporation.

Encel, S., Kotowicz, K. C., & Resler, H. E. (1972). Drinking patterns in Sydney, Australia. *Quarterly Journal of Studies on Alcohol,* Suppl. 6, 1–27.

Eng, E., Hatch, J., & Callan, A. (1985). Institutionalizing social support through the church and into the community. *Health Education Quarterly*, 12, 81–92.

Engel, G. (1955). Studies of ulcerative colitis: III. The nature of the psychological processes. *American Journal of Medicine*, 19, 231–256.

Engs, R. C. (1980). The drug-use patterns of helping-profession students in Brisbane, Australia. *Drug and Alcohol Dependence*, 6, 231–246.

Engs, R. C. (1982). Drinking patterns and attitudes toward alcoholism of Australian human-service students. *Journal of Studies on Alcohol*, 43, 517–531.

Engs, R. C., Hanson, D. J., Gliksman, L., & Smythe, C. (1990). Influence of religion and culture on drinking behaviors: A test of hypotheses between Canada and the USA. *British Journal of Addiction*, 85, 1475–1482.

Enstrom, J. E. (1975). Cancer mortality among Mormons. *Cancer*, 36, 825–841.

Enstrom, J. E. (1978). Cancer and total mortality among active Mormons. *Cancer*, 42, 1943–1951.

Enstrom, J. E. (1979). Cancer mortality among low-risk populations. *Ca.: A Cancer Journal for Clinicians*, 29, 352–361.

Enstrom, J. E. (1980). Cancer mortality among Mormons in California during 1968–75. *Journal of the National Cancer Institute*, 65, 1073–1082.

Enstrom, J. E. (1989). Health practices and cancer mortality among active California Mormons. *Journal of the National Cancer Institute*, 81, 1807–1814.

EPESE (1984). *NIA Established Population for Epidemiologic Studies in the Elderly*. Durham, N.C.: Center for the Study of Aging and Human Development, Duke University Medical Center.

Epperly, J. (1983). The cell and the celestial: Spiritual needs of cancer patients. *Journal of the Medical Asocciation of Georgia*, 72, 374–376.

Epstein, F. H., & Boas, E. P. (1955). The prevalence of manifest atherosclerosis among randomly chosen Italian and Jewish garment workers: A preliminary report. *Journal of Gerontology*, 10, 331–337.

Epstein, F. H., Arbor, A., Simpson, R., & Boas, E. P. (1957). The epidemiology of atherosclerosis among a random sample of clothing workers or different ethnic origins in New York City. *Journal of Chronic Disease*, 5, 300–341.

Epstein, F. H., Carol, R., & Simpson, R. (1956). Estimation of caloric intake from dietary histories among population groups. *American Journal of Clinical Nutrition*, 4(1), 1–10.

Epstein, F. H., Simpson, R., Boas, E. P. (1956). Relations between diet and atherosclerosis among a working population of different ethnic origins. *American Journal of Clinical Nutrition*, 4(1), 10–19.

Epstein, L., Tamir, A., & Natan, T. (1985). Emotional health state of adolescents. *International Journal of Adolescent Medicine and Health*, 1, 14–22.

Erikson, K. T. (1966). *Wayward Puritans: A Study in the Sociology of Deviance*. New York: Wiley.

Ershler, W. B. (1993). Interleukin-6: A cytokine for gerontologists. *Journal of the American Geriatric Society*, 41, 176–181.

Ershler, W. B., Sun, W. H., & Binkley, N. (1994). The role of interleukin-6 in certain age-related diseases. *Drugs and Aging*, 5, 358–365.

Esquirol, J. E. D. (1838). *Des maladies mentales*. Paris: Bailliere.

Esterling, B. A., Kiecolt-Glaser, J. K., Bodnar, J. C., & Glaser, R. (1994). Chronic stress, social support, and persistent alterations in the natural killer cell response to cytokines in older adults. *Health Psychology*, 13, 291–298.

Esterling, B. A., Kiecolt-Glaser, J. K., & Glaser, R. (1996). Psychosocial modulation of cytokine-induced natural killer cell activity in older adults. *Psychosomatic Medicine*, 58, 264–272.

Etkind, P., Lett, S. M., MacDonald, P. D., Silva, E., & Peppe, J. (1992). Pertussis outbreaks in groups claiming religious exemptions to vaccinations. *American Journal of Diseases of Children*, 146, 173–176.

Evans, D. L., Leserman, J., Perkins, D. O., Stern, R. A., Murphy, C., Zheng, B., Gettes, D., Longmate, J. A., Silva, S. G., van der Horst, C. M., Hall, C. D., Folds, J. D., Golden, R. N., & Petitto, J. M. (1997). Severe life stress as a predictor of early disease progression in HIV infection. *American Journal of Psychiatry*, 154, 630–634.

Evans, J. G. (1967). Deliberate self-poisoning in the Oxford area. *British Journal of Preventative and Social Medicine*, 21, 97–107.

Evans, M. B. (1985). Emotional stress and diabetic control: A postulated model for the effect of emotional distress upon intermediary metabolism in the diabetic. *Biofeedback and Self-Regulation*, 10, 241–254.

Evans, T. D., Cullen, F. T., Dunaway, R. G., & Burton, V. S. (1995). Religion and crime re-examined: The impact of religion, secular controls, and social ecology on adult criminality. *Criminology*, 33, 195–217.

Everett, C., & Everett, S. V. (1994). *The Health Divorce*. San Franscisco: Jossey-Bass.

Everson, S. A., Goldberg, D. E., & Kaplan, G. A. (1996). Hopelessness and risk of mortality and incidence of myocardial infarction and cancer. *Psychosomatic Medicine, 58,* 113–121.

Everson, S. A., Kaplan, G. A., Goldberg, D. E., Salonen, R., & Salonene, J. T. (1997). Hopelessness and 4-year progression of carotid artherosclerosis: The Kuopio Ischemic Heart Disease Risk Factor Study. *Artherosclerosis, Thrombosis, and Vascular Biology, 17*(8), 1490–1495.

Everson, S. A., Roberts, R. T., Goldberg, D. E., & Kaplan, G. A. (1998). Depressive symptoms and increased risk of stroke mortality over a 29-year period. *Archives of Internal Medicine, 158,* 1133–1138.

Faccincani, C., Mignolli, G., & Platt, S. (1990). Service utilization, social support and psychiatric status in a cohort of patients with schizophrenic psychoses: A 7-year follow-up study. *Schizophrenia Research, 3,* 139–146.

Facione, N. C., & Giancarlo, C. A. (1998). Narratives of breast symptom discovery and cancer diagnosis: Psychologic risk for advanced cancer at diagnosis. *Cancer Nursing, 21,* 430–440.

Fadaei-Tehrani, R. (1990). Crime, unemployment, and poverty. *Mankind Quarterly* 31(1–2), 109–127.

Faith's Benefits (1999). *Christian Century,* January 27, p. 77.

Fallon, B. A., Liebowitz, M. R., Hollander, E., Schneier, F. R., Campeas, R. B., Fairbanks, J., Papp, L. A., Hatterer, J. A., & Sandberg, D. (1990). The pharmacotherapy of moral or religious scrupulosity. *Journal of Clinical Psychiatry, 51,* 517–521.

Farakhan, A., Lubin, B., & O'Connor, W. A. (1984). Life satisfaction and depression among retired black persons. *Psychological Reports, 55,* 452–454.

Farrington, D. P. (1990). Implications of criminal career research for the prevention of offending. *Journal of Adolescence, 13,* 93–113.

Farrington, D. P., Morley, L., St. Ledger, R. J., & West, D. J. (1988). Are there successful men from criminologic backgrounds? *Psychiatry, 51,* 116–130.

Faucett, J. A. (1994). Depression in painful chronic disorders: The role of pain and conflict about pain. *Journal of Pain and Symptomatic, 9,* 520–526.

Fauci, A. S., Braunwald, E., Isselbacher, K. J., Wilson, J. D., Martin, J. B., Kasper, D. L., Hauser, S. L., & Longo, D. L. (eds.) (1998). *Harrison's Principles of Internal Medicine,* 14th ed. New York: McGraw-Hill.

Faulkner, J. E., & DeJong, G. F. (1966). Religiosity in 5-D: An empirical analysis. *Social Forces, 45,* 246–254.

Faunce, W. A., & Fulton, R. L. (1958). The sociology of death: A neglected area of research. *Social Forces, 3,* 205–209.

Faupel, C. E., Kowalski, G. S., & Starr, P. D. (1987). Sociology's one law: Religion and suicide in the urban context. *Journal for the Scientific Study of Religion, 26*(4), 523–534.

Fawzy, F. I., Cousins, N., Fawzy, N. W., Kemeny, M. E., Elashoff, R., & Morton, D. (1990). A structured psychiatric intervention for cancer patients: I. Changes over time and methods of coping and affective disturbance. *Archives of General Psychiatry, 47,* 720–725.

Fawzy, F. L., Fawzy, N. W., Arndt, L. A., & Pasnau, R. O. (1995). Critical review of psychosocial interventions in cancer care. *Archives of General Psychiatry, 52,* 100–113.

Fawzy, F. L., Fawzy, N. W., Hyun, C., Elashoff, R., Guthrie, D., Fahey, J. L. & Morton, D. L. (1993). Malignant melanoma: Effects of an earlier structured psychiatric intervention, coping, and affective state on recurrence and survival six years later. *Archives of General Psychiatry, 50,* 681–689.

Fawzy, F. I., Kemeny, M. E., Fawzy, N. W., Elashoff, R., Morton, D., Cousins, N., & Fahey, J. L. (1990). A structured psychiatric intervention for cancer patients: II. Changes over time in immunological measures. *Archives of General Psychiatry, 47,* 729–735.

Feagin, J. R. (1964). Prejudice and religious types: A focused study of Southern fundamentalists. *Journal for the Scientific Study of Religion, 4,* 3–13.

Federal Bureau of Investigation (1994). *Crime in the United States, 1993: Uniform Crime Reports.* Washington, D.C.: U.S. Department of Justice.

Fedio, P. (1986). Behavioral characteristics of patients with temporal lobe epilepsy. *Psychiatric Clinics of North America, 9,* 267–281.

Fehr, L. A., & Heintzelman, M. E. (1977). Personality and attitude correlates of religiosity: A source of controversy. *Journal of Psychology, 95,* 63–66.

Fehring, R. J., Brennan, P. F., & Keller, M. L. (1987). Psychological and spiritual well-being in college students. *Research in Nursing and Health, 10,* 391–398.

Fehring, R. J., Miller, J. F., & Shaw, C. (1997). Spiritual well-being, religiosity, hope, depression, and other mood states in elderly people coping with cancer. *Oncology Nursing Forum*, 24, 663–671.

Feifel, H. (1974). Religious conviction and fear of death among the healthy and the terminally ill. *Journal for the Scientific Study of Religion*, 13, 353–360.

Feifel, H., & Schag, D. (1980–1981). Death outlook and social issues. *Omega: Journal of Death and Dying*, 11(3), 201–215.

Feigelman, W., Gorman, B. S., & Varacalli, J. A. (1992). Americans who give up religion. *Journal for the Scientific Study of Religion*, 76(3), 138–144.

Feigenson, J. (1979). Stroke rehabilitation: Effectiveness, benefits, and cost—some practical considerations (editorial). *Stroke*, 10,1–4.

Fein, L. G. (1958). Religious observance and mental health: A note. *Journal of Pastoral Care*, 12, 99–101.

Feldman, J., & Rust, J. (1989). Religiosity, schizotypal thinking, and schizophrenia. *Psychological Reports*, 65, 587–593.

Felten, D. L., & Felten, S. Y. (1991). Innervation of lymphoid tissue. In R. Ader, D. L. Felten, & N. Cohen (eds.), *Psychoneuroimmunology* (pp. 87–101). San Diego: Academic Press.

Felten, D. L., Felten, S. Y., Bellinger, D. L., Carlson, S. L., Ackerman, K., Madden, K. S., Olschowski, J. A., & Livnat, S. (1987). Noradrenergic sympathetic neural interactions with the immune system: Structure and function. *Immunological Reviews*, 100, 225–260.

Ferdinand, K. C. (1997). Lessons learned from the Healthy Heart Community Prevention Project in reaching the African American population. *Journal of Health Care for the Poor and Underserved* 8(3), 366–371; discussion 371–372.

Ferguson, M. A., & Valenti, J. (1991). Communicating with environmental and health risk takers: An individual differences perspective. *Health Education Quarterly*, 18, 303–318.

Fernando, S. J. M. (1975). A cross-cultural study of some familial and social factors in depressive illness. *British Journal of Psychiatry*, 127, 46–53.

Fernando, S. J. M. (1978). Aspects of depression in a Jewish minority group. *Psychiatrica Clinica*, 11, 22–33.

Ferngren, G. B. (1992). Early Christianity as a religion of healing. *Bulletin of the History of Medicine*, 66, 1–15.

Fernquist, R. M. (1995). A research note on the association between religion and delinquency. *Deviant Behavior*, 16, 169–175.

Fernquist, R. M. (1995–1996). Elderly suicide in western Europe 1975–1989: A different approach to Durkheim's theory of political integration. *Omega: Journal of Death and Dying*, 32(1), 39–48.

Ferrada-Noli, M., & Sundbom, E. (1996). Cultural bias in suicidal behavior among refugees with post-traumatic stress-disorder. *Nordic Journal of Psychiatry*, 50, 185–191.

Ferraro, K. F. (1998). Firm believers? Religion, body weight, and well-being. *Review of Religious Research*, 39(3), 224–244.

Ferraro, K. F., & Albrecht-Jensen, C. M. (1991). Does religion influence adult health? *Journal for the Scientific Study of Religion*, 30, 193–202.

Ferraro, K. F., & Koch, J. R. (1994). Religion and health among black and white adults: Examining social support and consolation. *Journal for the Scientific Study of Religion*, 33, 362–375.

Ferrell, B. A., Ferrell, B. R., & Osterweil, D. (1990). Pain in the nursing home. *Journal of the American Geriatrics Society*, 38, 409–414.

Ferrell, B. R., Grant, M., Funk, B., Otis-Green, S., & Garcia, N. (1998). Quality of life in breast cancer: Part II. Psychological and spiritual well-being. *Cancer Nursing*, 21, 1–9.

Fetzer Institute (1999). *Multidimensional Measurement of Religiousness/Spirituality for Use in Health Research*. Kalamazoo: John E. Fetzer Institute.

Figelman, M. A. (1968). A comparison of affective and paranoid disorders in Negroes and Jews. *International Journal of Social Psychiatry*, 14, 277–281.

Fillenbaum, G. (1985). Screening the elderly: A brief instrumental activities of daily living measure. *Journal of the American Geriatrics Society*, 33, 698–705.

Filsinger, E. F., & Wilson, M. R. (1984). Religiosity, socioeconomic rewards, and family development: Predictors of marital adjustment. *Journal of Marriage and the Family*, 46, 663–670.

Fimian, M. J., Zacherman, J., & McHardy, R. J. (1985) . Substance abuse and teacher stress. *Journal of Drug Education*, 15(2), 139–155.

Finney, J. R., & Malony, H. N. (1985a). Empirical studies of Christian prayer: A review of the literature. *Journal of Psychology and Theology*, 13, 104–115.

Finney, J. R., & Malony, H. N. (1985b). An empirical study of contemplative prayer as an adjunct to psychotherapy. *Journal of Psychology and Theology*, 13, 172–181.

Fish, S., & Shelly, J. A. (1983). *Spiritual Care: The Nurse's Role*. Downers Grove, Ill.: InterVarsity Press.

Fitchett, G., Burton, L. A., & Sivan, A. B. (1997). The religious needs and resources of psychiatric patients. *Journal of Nervous and Mental Disease*, 185, 320–326.

Fitzgerald, R. G. (1970). Reactions to blindness: An exploratory study of adults with recent loss of sight. *Archives of General Psychiatry*, 22, 370–379.

Fitzpatrick, J. P. (1967). The role of religion in programs for the prevention and correction of crime and delinquency. In *Task Force Report: Juvenile Delinquency and Youth Crime*. Washington, D.C.: Government Printing Office.

Flaskerud, J. H., & Uman, G. (1996). Acculturation and its effects on self-esteem among immigrant Latina women. *Behavioral Medicine*, 22, 123–133.

Flics, D. H., & Herron, W. G. (1991). Activity-withdrawal, diagnosis, and demographics as predictors of premorbid adjustment. *Journal of Clinical Psychology*, 47, 189–196.

Florell, J. L. (1973). Crisis-intervention in orthopedic surgery: Empirical evidence of the effectiveness of a chaplain working with surgery patients. *Bulletin of the American Protestant Hospital Association*, 37(2), 29–36.

Florian, V., & Kravetz, S. (1983). Fear of personal death: attribution, structure, and relation to religious belief. *Journal of Personality and Social Psychology*, 44, 600–607.

Florian, V., Kravetz, S., & Frankel, J. (1984). Aspects of fear and personal death, levels of awareness, and religious commitment. *Journal of Research in Personality*, 18: 289–304.

Foley, D. P. (1988). Eleven interpretations of personal suffering. *Journal of Religion and Health*, 27, 321–328.

Foley, K. M. (1987). Pain syndromes in patients with cancer. *Medical Clinics of North America*, 71, 169–184.

Folkman, S. (1997). Positive psychological states and coping with severe stress. *Social Science and Medicine*, 45, 1207–1221.

Folkman, S., Bernstein, L., & Lazarus, R. S. (1987). Stress processes and the misuse of drugs in older adults. *Psychology & Aging*, 2(4), 366–374.

Folkman, S., Chesney, M. A., Cooke, M., Boccellari, A., & Collette, L. (1994). Caregiver burden in HIV-positive and HIV-negative parners of men with AIDS. *Journal of Consulting and Clinical Psychology*, 62, 746–756.

Folkman, S., Chesney, M. A., Pollack, L., & Phillips, C. (1992). Stress, coping, and high-risk sexual behavior. *Health Psychology*, 11, 218–222.

Fones, C. S., Manfro, G. G., & Pollack, M. H. (1998). Social phobia: An update. *Harvard Review of Psychiatry*, 5(5): 247–259.

Fonnebo, V. (1992a). Coronary risk factors in Norwegian 7th Day Adventists: A study of 247 SDA's and matched controls—the cardiovascular disease studies in Norway. *American Journal of Epidemiology*, 135, 504–508.

Fonnebo, V. (1992b). Mortality in Norwegian SDA's 1962–1986. *Journal of Clinical Epidemiology*, 45, 157–167.

Fonnebo, V. (1994). The healthy Seventh Day Adventist lifestyle: What is the Norwegian experience? *American Journal of Clinical Nutrition*, 59, S1124–S1129 (suppl).

Fontaine, K. R., & Jones, L. C. (1997). Self-esteem, optimism, and postpartum depression. *Journal of Clinical Psychology*, 53(1), 59–63.

Ford, D. E., Mead, L. A., Chang, P. P., Cooper-Patrick, L., Wang, N. Y., & Klag, M. J. (1998). Depression is the risk factor or coronary artery disease in man. *Archives of Internal Medicine*, 158, 1422–1426.

Ford, M. E., Edwards, G., Rodriguez, J. L., Gibson, R. C., & Tilley, B. C. (1996). An empowerment-centered, church-based asthma education program for African American adults. *Health and Social Work*, 21, 71–75.

Fordyce, M. W. (1983). A program to increase happiness: Further studies. *Journal of Counseling Psychology*, 30, 483–498.

Forehand, R., Wierson, M., Thomas, A. M., Armistead, L., Kempton, T., & Neighbors, B. (1991). The role of family stressors and parent relationships in adolescent functioning. *Journal of the American Academy of Child and Adolescent Psychiatry*, 30, 316–322.

Forliti, J. E., & Benson, P. L. (1986). Young adolescents: A national study. *Religious Education*, 81, 199–224.

Forster, L. E., Pollow, R., & Stoller, E. P. (1993). Alcohol use and potential risk for alcohol-related adverse drug reactions among community-based elderly. *Journal of Community Health*, 18, 225–239.

Foshee, V. A., & Hollinger, B. R. (1996). Maternal religiosity, adolescent social bonding, and adolescent alcohol use. *Journal of Early Adolescence*, 16, 451–468.

Foulks, E. F., Persons, J. B., & Merkel, R. L. (1986). The effect of patients' beliefs about their illnesses on compliance in psychotherapy. *American Journal of Psychiatry*, 143, 340–344.

Fountain, D. E. (1986). How to assimilate the elderly into your parish: The effects of alienation on church attendance. *Journal of Religion and Aging*, 2(3), 45–55.

Fowler, J. W. (1981). *Stages of Faith*. San Francisco: Harper & Row.

Fox, E., & Young, M. (1989). Religiosity, sex guilt and sexual behavior among college students. *Health Values*, 13(2), 32–37.

Fox, S. A., Pitkin, K., Paul, C., Carson, S., & Duan, N. (1998). Breast cancer screening adherence: Does church attendance matter? *Health Education and Behavior*, 26, 742–758.

Fox, W. P., & Odling-Smee, G. W. (1995). Spiritual well-being, hope and psychological morbidity in breast cancer patients. *Psycho-Oncology*, 4, 87.

Francis, L. F., & Bolger, J. (1997). Religion and psychological well-being in later life. *Psychological Reports*, 80, 1050.

Francis, L. J. (1994). Denominational identity, church attendance and drinking behavior among adults in England. *Journal of Alcohol and Drug Education*, 39(3), 27–33.

Francis, L. J., & Bennett, G. A. (1992). Personality and religion among female drug misusers. *Drug and Alcohol Dependence*, 30, 27–31.

Francis, L. J., & Mullen, K. (1993). Religiosity and attitudes towards drug use among 13–15 year-olds in England. *Addiction*, 88, 665–672.

Francis, L. J., & Pearson, P. R. (1985). Psychoticism and religiosity among 15-year-olds. *Personality and Individual Differences*, 6, 397–398.

Frank, J. D. (1975). The faith that heals. *Johns Hopkins Medical Journal*, 137, 127–131.

Frankel, B. G., & Hewitt, W. E. (1994). Religion and well-being among Canadian university students. *Journal for the Scientific Study of Religion*, 33, 62–73.

Frankl, V. (1959). *Man's Search for Meaning*. New York: Simon & Schuster.

Franks, K., Templer, D. L., Cappelletty, G. G., & Kauffman, I. (1990–1991). Exploration of death anxiety as a function of religious variables in gay men with and without AIDS. *OMEGA*, 22(1), 43–50.

Fraser, G. E., Beeson, W. L., & Phillips, R. L. (1991). Diet and lung cancer in California Seventh-Day Adventists. *American Journal of Epidemiology*, 133, 683–693.

Frasure-Smith, N. (1991). In-hospital symptoms of psychological stress as predictors of long-term outcome after acute myocardial infarction in men. *American Journal of Cardiology*, 67, 121–127.

Frasure-Smith, N., & Prince, R. (1989). Long-term follow-up of the Ischemic Heart Disease Life Stress Monitoring Program. *Psychosomatic Medicine*, 51, 485–513.

Frasure-Smith, N., Lesperance, F., & Talajic, M. (1993). Depression following myocardial infarction: Impact on 6-month survival. *Journal of the American Medical Association*, 270, 1819–1825.

Frasure-Smith, N., Lesperance, F., & Talajic, M. (1995). Depression and 18-month prognosis after myocardial infarction. *Circulation*, 91, 999–1005.

Frazer, G. E., Strahan, T. M., Sabate, J., Beeson, W. L., & Kissinger, D. (1992). Effects of traditional coronary risk factors on rates of incident coronary events in a low-risk population: The Adventist Health Study. *Circulation*, 86, 406–413.

Freedman, D., Pisani, R., & Purves, R. (1997). *Statistics*, 3rd ed. New York: Norton.

Freeman, R. B. (1986). Who escapes? The relation of churchgoing and other background factors to the socioeconomic performance of black male youths from inner-city tracts. In R. B. Freeman & H. J. Holzer (eds.), *The Black Youth Employment Crisis*. Chicago: University of Chicago Press.

Frenz, A. W., & Carey, M. P. (1989). Relationship between religiousness and trait anxiety: Fact or artifact? *Psychological Reports*, 65, 827–834.

Freud, S. ([1907] 1962). *Obsessive Acts and Religious Practices*. In J. Strachey (ed. and trans.), *Standard Edition of the Complete Psychological Works of Sigmund Freud*. London: Hogarth Press.

Freud, S. ([1913] 1962). *Totem and Taboo: Some Points of Agreement between the Mental Lives of Savages and Neurotics*. In J. Strachey (ed. and trans.), *Standard Edition of the Complete Psychological Works of Sigmund Freud*. London: Hogarth Press.

Freud, S. ([1919] 1962). *Psychoanalysis and Religious Origins*. In J. Strachey (ed. and trans.), *Standard Edition of the Complete Psychological Works of Sigmund Freud*. London: Hogarth Press.

Freud, S. ([1927] 1962). *Future of an Illusion*. In J. Strachey (ed. and trans.), *Standard Edition of the Complete Psychological Works of Sigmund Freud*. London: Hogarth Press.

Freud, S. ([1928] 1962). *A Religious Experience*. In J. Strachey (ed. and trans.), *Standard Edition of the Complete Psychological Works of Sigmund Freud*. London: Hogarth Press.

Freud, S. ([1930] 1962). *Civilization and Its Discontents*. In J. Strachey (ed. and trans.), *Standard*

Edition of the Complete Psychological Works of Sigmund Freud. London: Hogarth Press. Quote from p. 25.

Freud, S. ([1933a] 1962). *New Introductory Lectures.* In J. Strachey (ed. and trans.), *Standard Edition of the Complete Psychological Works of Sigmund Freud.* London: Hogarth Press.

Freud, S. ([1933b] 1962). *Why War?* In J. Strachey (ed. and trans.), *Standard Edition of the Complete Psychological Works of Sigmund Freud.* London: Hogarth Press.

Freud, S. ([1939] 1962). *Moses and Monotheism.* In J. Strachey (ed. and trans.), *Standard Edition of the Complete Psychological Works of Sigmund Freud.* London: Hogarth Press.

Friedberg, B. A., & Friedberg, R. D. (1985). Locus of control and religiosity in college students. *Psychological Reports,* 56(3), 757–758.

Friedlander, Y., Kark, J. D., & Stein, Y. (1986). Religious orthodoxy and myocardial infarction in Jerusalem: A case-control study. *International Journal of Cardiology,* 10, 33–41.

Friedlander, Y., Kark, J. D., & Stein, Y. (1987). Religious observance and plasma lipids and lipoproteins among 17-year-old Jewish residents of Jerusalem. *Preventive Medicine,* 16, 70–79.

Friedman, E. H., & Hellerstein, H. K. (1968). Occupational stress, law school hierarchy, and coronary artery disease in Cleveland attorneys. *Psychosomatic Medicine,* 30(1), 72–86.

Friedman, H. (1986). Marijuana effects on immunity: Suppression of human natural killer cell activity of delta-9-tetrahydrocannabinol. *International Journal of Immunopharmacology,* 8, 741–745.

Friedman, H., Klein, T., & Specter, S. (1991). Immunosupression by marijuana and components. In R. Ader, D. L. Felten, & N. Cohen (eds.), *Psychoneuroimmunology* (pp. 66–85). San Diego: Academic Press.

Friedman, H. S., Tucker, J. S., Schwartz, J. E., Martin, L. R., Wingard, D. L., & Criqui, M. H. (1995). Psychosocial and behavioral predictors of longevity: The aging and death of the "Termites." *American Psychologist,* 50(2), 69–78.

Friedman, M. (1976). Emotional factors and heart disease. *Journal of the American Medical Association,* 235, 2081.

Friedman, R., Myers, P., Sobel, D., Caudil, M., & Benson, H. (1995). Behavioral medicine, clinical health psychology, and cost offset. *Health Psychology,* 14, 509–518.

Friedrich, W. N., Cohen, D. S., & Wilturner, L. T. (1988). Specific beliefs as moderator variables in maternal coping with mental retardation. *Children's Health Care,* 17, 40–44.

Fries, J. F., Koop, C. E., Beadle, C. E., Cooper, P. P., England, M. J., Greaves, R. F., Sokolov, J. J., & Wright, D. (1993). Reducing health care costs by reducing the need in demand for mental services. *New England Journal of Medicine,* 329, 321–325.

Fritzsche, S. (1988). Über die Einheit von Physischem und Psychischem bei Alkohol- und Arzneimittelabhängigkeit. *Psychiatrica Neurologika Medicina und Psychologia* (Leipzig), 40(3), 129–135.

Fry, P. S. (1990). A factor analytic investigation of homebound elderly individuals' concerns about death and dying, and their coping responses. *Journal of Clinical Psychology,* 46, 737–748.

Fulop, G., Strain, J. J., Vita, J., Lyons, J. S., & Hammer, J. S. (1987). Impact of psychiatric comorbidity on length of hospital stay for medical/surgical patients: a preliminary report. *American Journal of Psychiatry,* 144, 878–882.

Funk, R. A. (1956). Religious attitudes and manifest anxiety in a college population (abstract). *American Psychologist,* 11, 375.

Furhnam, A. F. (1982). Locus of control and theological beliefs. *Journal of Psychology and Theology,* 10, 130–136.

Galanter, M. (1982a). Altered use of social intoxicants after religious conversion. In J. Solomon (ed.), *Alcoholism and Clinical Psychiatry* (pp. 49–55). New York: Plenum.

Galanter, M. (1982b). Charismatic religious sects and psychiatry: An overview. *American Journal of Psychiatry,* 139, 1539–1548.

Galanter, M. (1990). Cults and zealous self-help movements: A psychiatric perspective. *American Journal of Psychiatry,* 147, 543–551.

Galanter, M., & Buckley, P. (1978). Evangelical religion and meditation: Psychotherapeutic effects. *Journal of Nervous and Mental Disease,* 166, 685–691.

Galanter, M., Larson, D., & Rubenstone, E. (1991). Christian psychiatry: The impact of evangelical belief on clinical practice. *American Journal of Psychiatry,* 148, 90–95.

Galanter, M., Rabkin, R., Brabkin, J., & Deutsch, A. (1979). The "moonies": A psychological study of conversion and membership in a contemporary religious sect. *American Journal of Psychiatry,* 136, 165–170.

Gallagher, W. (1999). Seeking help for the body in the well-being of the soul. *New York Times,* June 13, Women's Health section.

Gallemore, J. L., Wilson, W. P., & Rhoads, J. M. (1969). The religious life of patients with affective disorders. *Diseases of the Nervous System*, 30, 483–486.

Gallo, O., Gori, A. M., & Atanasio, M. (1993). Interleukin-1 beta and interleukin-6 released by peripheral blood monocytes in head and neck cancer. *British Journal of Cancer*, 68, 465–468.

Galton, F. (1872). Statistical inquiries into the efficacy of prayer. *Fortnightly Review*, 12, 125–135.

Gamwell, L., & Tomes, N. (1995). *Madness in America: Cultural and Medical Perceptions of Mental Illness before 1914*. Binghamton and Ithaca: State University of New York at Binghamton and Cornell University Press.

Gangdev, P. S. (1998). Faith-assisted cognitive therapy of obsessive-compulsive disorder. *Australian and New Zealand Journal of Psychiatry*, 32, 575–578.

Ganje-Fling, M. A., & McCarthy, P. R. (1991). A comparative analysis of spiritual direction and psychotherapy. *Journal of Psychology and Theology*, 19, 103–117.

Garay-Sevilla, M. E., Nava, L. E., Malacara, J. M., Huerta, R., Diaz de Leon, J., Mena, A., & Fajardo, M. E. (1995). Adherence to treatment and social support in patients with non-insulin-dependent *Diabetes mellitus*. *Journal of Diabetes and Its Complications*, 9, 81–86.

Gardner, J. W., & Lyon, J. L. (1977). Low incidence of cervical cancer in Utah. *Gynecologic Oncology*, 5, 68–80.

Gardner, J. W., & Lyon, J. L. (1982a). Cancer in Utah Mormon men by lay priesthood level. *American Journal of Epidemiology*, 116, 243–257.

Gardner, J. W., & Lyon, J. L. (1982b). Cancer in Utah Mormon women by church activity level. *American Journal of Epidemiology*, 116, 258–265.

Garfinkel, B., Froese, A., & Hood, J. (1982). Suicide attempts in children and adolescents. *American Journal of Psychiatry*, 139, 1257–1261.

Gargas, S. (1932). Suicide in the Netherlands. *American Journal of Sociology*, 37, 697–713.

Garland, A. F., & Zigler, E. (1993). Adolescent suicide prevention: Current research and social policy implications. *American Psychologist*, 48, 169–182.

Gartner, J. D. (1986). Antireligious prejudice in admissions to doctoral programs in clinical psychology. *Professional Psychology, Research, and Practice*, 17, 473–475.

Gartner, J. G., Lyons, J. S., Larson, D. B., Serkland, J., & Peyrot, M. (1990). Supplier induced demand for pastoral care services in the general hospital: A natural experience. *Journal of Pastoral Care*, 44, 266–270.

Gartner, J. W., Larson, D. B., & Allen, G. D. (1991). Religious commitment and mental health: a review of the empirical literature. *Journal of Psychology and Theology*, 19, 6–25.

Gartner, J. W., Larson, D. B., & Vachar-Mayberry, C. D. (1990). A systematic review of the quantity and quality of empirical research published in four pastoral counseling journals: 1975–1984. *Journal of Pastoral Care*, 44, 115–123.

Gass, K. A. (1987). The health of conjugally bereaved older widows: The role of appraisal. *Research in Nursing and Health*, 10, 39–47.

Gatz, M., & Smyer, M. A. (1992). The mental health system and older adults in the 1990's. *American Psychologist*, 47, 741–751.

Gaudette, L. A., Holmes, T. M., Laing, L. M., Morgan, K., & Grace, M. G. A. (1978). Cancer incidence in a religious isolate of Alberta, Canada, 1953–1974. *Journal of the National Cancer Institute*, 60, 1233–1238.

Gaw, A. C., Ding, Q., Levine, R. E., & Gaw, H. (1998). The clinical characteristics of possession disorder among 20 Chinese patients in the Hebrei province of China. *Psychiatric Services*, 49, 360–365.

Gee, E. M., & Veevers, J. E. (1990). Religious involvement and life satisfaction in Canada. *Sociological Analysis*, 51, 387–394.

Geist, C. R., & Daheim, C. M. (1984). Religious affiliation and manifest hostility. *Psychological Reports*, 55(2), 493–494.

Gelato, M. C. (1996). Aging and immune function: A possible role for growth hormone. *Hormone Research*, 45, 46–49.

Gelderloos, P., Walton, K. G., Orme-Johnson, D. W., & Alexander, C. N. (1991). Effectiveness of the transcendental meditation program in preventing and treating substance misuse: A Review. *International Journal of the Addictions*, 26, 293–325.

Gelfand, T. (1993). The history of the medical profession. In W. F. Bynum & R. Porter (eds.), *Companion Encyclopedia of the History of Medicine*. New York: Routledge, Chapman, & Hall.

Genia, V. (1993). A psychometric evaluation of the Allport-Ross I/E Scales in a religiously heterogeneous sample. *Journal for the Scientific Study of Religion*, 32, 284–290.

Genia, V., & Shaw, D. G. (1991). Religion, intrinsic-extrinsic orientation, and depression. *Review of Religious Research*, 32, 274–283.

George, L. K. (1992). Social factors and the onset and outcome of depression. In K. W. Schaie, D. Blazer, & J. S. House (eds.), *Aging, Health Behaviors, and Health Outcomes* (pp. 137–159). Hillsdale, N.J.: Lawrence Erlbaum Associates.

George, L. K., & Bearon, L. B. (1980). *Quality of Life in Older Persons: Meaning and Measurement.* New York: Human Sciences Press.

George, L. K., Blazer, D. G., Hughes, D. C., & Fowler, N. (1989). Social support and the outcome of major depression. *British Journal of Psychiatry,* 154, 478–485.

Georgemiller, R. J., & Getsinger, S. H. (1987). Reminiscence therapy: Effects on more and less religious elderly. *Journal of Religion and Aging,* 4, 47–58.

Ghosh, T. B., & Victor, B. S. (1994). Suicide. In R. E. Hales, S. C. Yudofsky, & J. A. Talbott (eds.), *Textbook of Psychiatry* (pp. 1251–1271). Washington, D.C.: American Psychiatric Association.

Gibbs, H. W., & Achterberg-Lawlis, J. (1978). Spiritual values and death anxiety: Implications for counseling with terminal cancer patients. *Journal of Counseling Psychology,* 25, 563–569.

Gibbs, J. (1961). Suicide. In R. Merton (ed.), *Contemporary Social Problems* (pp. 281–321). New York: Harcourt, Brace, and World.

Gifford, A., & Golde, P. (1978). Self-esteem in an aging population. *Journal of Gerontological Social Work,* 1, 69–80.

Gil, K. M., Keefe, F. J., Crisson, J. E., & Van Dalfsen, P. J. (1987). Social support and pain behavior. *Pain,* 29, 209–217.

Gilliland, B. C. (1980). Introduction to clinical immunology. In K. J. Isselbacher, R. D. Adams, E. Braunwald, R. G. Petersdorf, & J. D. Wilson (eds), *Harrison's Principles of Internal Medicine,* 9th ed. (pp. 315–325). New York: McGraw-Hill.

Gilman, P. A., Merrill, L. L., & Reid, J. L. (1997). Attitudes toward euthanasia. *Perceptual and Motor Skills,* 84, 317–318.

Ginsburg, M. L., Quirt, C., Ginsburg, A. D., & MacKillop, W. J. (1995). Psychiatric illness and psychosocial concerns of patients with newly diagnosed lung cancer. *Canadian Medical Association Journal,* 152, 701–708.

Gitlow, S. E., Dziedzic, L. B., & Dziedzic, S. W. (1986). Alcohol and hypertension: Implications from research for clinical practice. *Journal of Substance Abuse Treatment,* 3, 121–129.

Giuffrida, A., & Torgerson, D. J. (1997). Should we pay the patient? Review of financial incentives to enhance patient compliance. *British Medical Journal,* 315, 703–707.

Glamser, F. D. (1987). The impact of retirement upon religiosity. *Journal of Religion and Aging,* 4, 27–37.

Glaser, R., & Kiecolt-Glaser, J. K. (1994). Stress-associated immune modulation and its implications for reactivation of latent herpesviruses. In R. Glaser & J. Jones (eds.), *Human Herpesvirus Infections* (pp. 245–270). New York: Marcel Dekker.

Glaser, R., Rabin, B., Chesney, M., Cohen, S., & Natelson, B. (1999). Stress-induced immunomodulation: Are there implications for infectious diseases? *Journal of the American Medical Association,* 281, 2268–2270.

Glaser, R., Rice, J., & Sheridan, J. (1987). Stress-related immune suppression: Health implication. *Brain, Behavior, and Immunity,* 1, 7–20.

Glass, D. C., Singer, J. E., & Friedman, L. (1969). Psyche cost of adaptation to an environmental stressor. *Journal of Personality and Social Psychology,* 12, 200–210.

Glass, T. A., Mendes de Leon, C., Marottoli, M. A., & Berkman, L. F. (1999). Population based study of social and productive activities as predictors of survival among elderly Americans. *British Medical Journal,* 319, 478–485.

Glassman, A. H., & Shapiro, P. A. (1998). Depression and the course of coronary artery disease. *American Journal of Psychiatry,* 155, 4–11.

Glenn, N. D. (1982). Interreligious marriage in the United States: Patterns and recent trends. *Journal of Marriage and the Family,* 44, 555–566.

Glenn, N. D. (1984). Social and demographic correlates of divorce and separation in the United States: An update and reconsideration. *Journal of Marriage and the Family,* 46, 563–576.

Glenn, N. D., & Supancic, M. (1984). The social and demographic correlates of divorce and separation in the United States: An update and reconsideration. *Journal of Marriage and the Family,* 46, 563–576.

Glenn, N. D., & Weaver, C. N. (1978). A multivariate, multisurvey study of marital happiness. *Journal of Marriage and the Family,* 40, 269–282.

Glenn, N. D., & Weaver, C. N. (1979). A note on family situation and global happiness. *Social Forces,* 57, 960–967.

Glick, M., Michel, A. C., Dorn, J., Horwitz, M., Rosenthal, T., & Trevisan, M. (1998). Dietary cardiovascular risk factors and serum cholesterol in an Old Order Mennonite community. *American Journal of Public Health,* 88, 1202–1205.

Glicksman, A. (1991). *The New Jewish Elderly*. New York: American Jewish Committee.

Glik, D. C. (1986). Psychosocial wellness among spiritual healing participants. *Social Science and Medicine*, 22, 579–586.

Glik, D. C. (1988). Symbolic, ritual and social dynamics of spiritual healing. *Social Science and Medicine*, 27, 1197–1206.

Glik, D. C. (1990a). Participation in spiritual healing, religiosity, and mental health. *Sociological Inquiry*, 60, 158–176.

Glik, D. C. (1990b). The redefinition of the situation: The social construction of spiritual healing experiences. *Sociology of Health and Illness*, 12, 151–168.

Glock, C. Y. (1962). On the study of religious commitment. *Religious Education* (research supplement), 42 (July–August), 98–110.

Glock, C. Y., & Stark, R. (1965). *Religion and Society in Tension*. Chicago: Rand McNally.

Glock, C. Y., & Stark, R. (1966). *Christian Beliefs and Anti-Semitism*. San Francisco: Harper & Row.

Glover, R. J. (1996). Religiosity in adolescence and young adulthood: Implications for identity formation. *Psychological Reports*, 78, 427–431.

Glueck, S., & Glueck, E. (1950). *Unraveling Juvenile Delinquency*. Cambridge: Harvard University Press.

Gmur, M., & Tschopp, A. (1987). Factors determining the success of nicotine withdrawal: 12-year follow-up of 532 smokers after suggestion therapy (by a faith healer). *International Journal of the Addictions*, 22, 1189–1200.

Gobar, A. H. (1970). Suicide in Afghanistan. *British Journal of Psychiatry*, 116, 493–496.

Gold, N. (1965). Suicide and attempted suicide in North-Eastern Tasmania. *Medical Journal of Australia*, August 28, 361–364.

Goldbourt, U., & Medalie, J. H. (1975). Characteristics of smokers, nonsmokers and ex-smokers among 10,000 adult males in Israel: I. Distribution of selected sociodemographic and behavioral variables and the prevalence of disease. *Israel Journal of Medical Sciences*, 11, 1079–1101.

Goldbourt, U., Yaari, S., & Medalie, J. H. (1993). Factors predictive of long-term coronary heart disease mortality among 10,059 male Israeli civil servants and municipal employees. *Cardiology*, 82, 100–121.

Goldfarb, L. M., Galanter, M., McDowell, D., Lifshutz, H., & Dermatis, H. (1996). Medical student and patient attitudes toward religion and spirituality in the recovery process. *American Journal of Drug and Alcohol Abuse*, 22, 549–561.

Goldman, N., Korenman, S., & Weinstein, R. (1995). Marital status and health among the elderly. *Social Science and Medicine*, 40, 1717–1730.

Goldscheider, C., & Mosher, W. C. (1991). Patterns of contraceptive use in the United States: The importance of religious factors. *Studies in Family Planning*, 22(2), 102–115.

Goldstein, S. (1996). Changes in Jewish mortality and survival, 1963–1987. *Social Biology*, 43, 72–97.

Goodman, M., Rubinstein, R. L., Alexander, B. B., & Lubersky, M. (1991). Cultural differences among elderly women in coping with the death of an adult child. *Journal of Gerontology* (social sciences), 6, 321–329.

Goodwin, D. W., Johnson, J., Maher, C., Rappaport, A., & Guze, S. B. (1969). Why people do not drink: A study of teetotalers. *Comprehensive Psychiatry*, 10, 209–214.

Goodwin, J. S., Hunt, W. C., & Samet J. M. (1991). A population-based study of functional status and social support networks of elderly patients newly diagnosed with cancer. *Archives of Internal Medicine*, 151, 366–370.

Gopinath, N., Chada, S. L., Jain, P., Shekhawat, S., & Tandon, R. (1995). An epidemiological study of coronary heart disease in different ethnic groups in a Delhi urban population. *Journal of the Association of Physicians of India*, 43, 30–33.

Gorsuch, R. L. (1984). The boon and bane of investigating religion. *American Psychologist*, 39, 228–236.

Gorsuch, R. L. (1995). Religious aspects of substance abuse and recovery. *Journal of Social Issues*, 51(2), 65–83.

Gorsuch, R. L., & Butler, M. (1976). Initial drug abuse: A review of predisposing social psychological factors. *Psychological Bulletin*, 83, 120–137.

Gorsuch, R. L., & Hao, J. Y. (1993). Forgiveness: An exploratory factor analysis and its relationship to religious variables. *Review of Religious Research*, 34(4), 333–347.

Gorsuch, R. L., & McFarland, S. (1972). Single vs. multiple-item scales for measuring religious values. In H. N. Malony, *Current Perspectives in the Psychology of Religion*. Grand Rapids, Mich.: Eerdmans., 1977. Originally published in 1972.

Gorsuch, R. L., & McPherson, S. E. (1989). Intrinsic/extrinsic measurement: I/E-revised and single-item scales. *Journal for the Scientific Study of Religion*, 28, 348–354.

Gorsuch, R. L., & Venable, G. D. (1983). Development of an "Age Universal" I-E scale. *Journal for the Scientific Study of Religion*, 22, 181–187.

Gorwood, P. H. (1998). Is anxiety hereditary? *Encephale*, 24(3): 252–255.

Goss, M. E. W., & Reed, J. I. (1971). Suicide and religion: A study of white adults in New York City, 1963–67. *Life-Threatening Behavior*, 1, 163–177.

Gottlieb, N. H., & Green, L. W. (1984). Life events, social network, life-style, and health: An analysis of the 1979 National Survey of Personal Health Practices and Consequences. *Health Education Quarterly*, 11, 91–105.

Gould, K. L., Ornish, D., Kirkeeide, R., Brown, S., Stuart, Y., Buchi, M., Billings, J., Armstrong, W., Ports T., & Scherwitz, L. (1992). Improved stenosis geometry by quantitative coronary arteriography after vigorous risk factor modification. *American Journal of Cardiology*, 69, 845–853.

Graham, T. W., Kaplan, B. H., Cornoni-Huntley, J. C., James, S. A., Becker, C., Hames, C. G., & Heyden, S. (1978). Frequency of church attendance and blood pressure elevation. *Journal of Behavioral Medicine*, 1, 37–43.

Graney, M. J. (1975). Happiness and social participation in aging. *Journal of Gerontology*, 30, 701–706.

Granshaw, L. (1993). The hospital. In W. F. Bynum & R. Porter (eds.), *Companion Encyclopedia of the History of Medicine*. New York: Routledge, Chapman, & Hall.

Green, L. L., Fullilove, M. T., & Fullilove, R E. (1998). Stories of spiritual awakening: The nature of spirituality in recovery. *Journal of Substance Abuse Treatment*, 15, 325–331.

Greenberg, D., Witztum, E., & Buchbinder, J. T. (1992). Mysticism and psychosis: The fate of Ben Zoma. *British Journal of Medical Psychology*, 65, 223–235.

Greenberg, I., Spitz, M., Weltz, S., Spitz, C., & Bizzozero, O. J., Jr. (1975). Factors of adjustment in chronic hemodialysis patients. *Psychosomatics*, 16, 178–184.

Greenwald, P., Korns, R. F., Nasca, P. C., & Wolfgang, P. E. (1975). Cancer in United States Jews. *Cancer Research*, 35, 3507–3512.

Greenwood, D. C., Muir, K. R., Packham, C. J., & Madley, R. J. (1996). Coronary heart disease: A review of the role of psychosocial stress and social support. *Journal of Public Health Medicine*, 18, 221–231.

Gregory, W. E. (1957). The orthodoxy of the authoritarian personality. *Journal of Social Psychology*, 45, 217–232.

Griffith, E. E. H., Mahy, G. E., & Young, J. L. (1984). Psychological benefits of Spiritual Baptist "mourning": II. An empirical assessment. *American Journal of Psychiatry*, 143, 226–229.

Griffith, E. E. H., Young, J. L., & Smith, D. L. (1984). An analysis of the therapeutic elements in a black church service. *Hospital and Community Psychiatry*, 35, 464–469.

Gritzmacher, S. A., Bolton, B., & Dana, R. H. (1988). Psychological characteristics of Pentecostals: A literature review and psychodynamic synthesis. *Journal of Psychology and Theology*, 16, 233–245.

Groen, J., & Van Der Heide, R. M. (1959). Atherosclerosis and coronary thrombosis. *Medicine*, 38, 1–23.

Groen, J. J., Tijong, K. B., Koster, M., Willebrands, A. F., Verdonck, G., & Pierloot, M. (1962). The influence of nutrition and ways of life on blood cholesterol and the prevalence of hypertension and coronary heart disease among Trappist and Benedictine monks. *American Journal of Clinical Nutrition*, 10, 456–470.

Gross, L. (1982). *The Last Jews in Berlin*. New York: Simon & Schuster.

Grosse-Holtforth, M., Pathak, A., Koenig, H. G., Cohen, H. J., Pieper, C. F., & VanHook, L. G. (1996). Medical illness, religion, health control and depression of institutionalized medically ill veterans in long-term care. *International Journal of Geriatric Psychiatry*, 11, 613–620.

Gruenewald, P. J., Ponicki, W. R., & Mitchell, P. R. (1995). Suicide rates and alcohol consumption in the United States, 1970–1989. *Addiction*, 90(8), 1063–1075.

Gruner, L. (1985). The correlation of private, religious devotional practices and marital adjustment. *Journal of Comparative Family Studies*, 16, 47–59.

Guagliardo, M. F., Huang, Z., Hicks, J., & D'Angelo, L. (1998). Increased drug use among old-for-grade and dropout urban adolescents. *American Journal of Preventive Medicine*, 15(1), 42–48.

Guggenheim, F. G. (1981). Approach to the patient with obesity. In A. H. Goroll, L. A. May, & A. G. Mulley (eds.), *Primary Care Medicine*. Philadelphia: Lippincott.

Guinn, R. (1975). Characteristics of drug use among Mexican-American students. *Journal of Drug Education*, 5(3), 235–241.

Gunderson, M. P., & McCary, J. L. (1979). Sexual guilt and religion. *Family Coordinator*, July, 353–357.

Gupta, R. (1996). Lifestyle risk factors and coronary heart disease prevalence in Indian men. *Journal of the Association of Physicians of India*, 44, 689–693.

Gupta, R., Prakash, H., Gupta, V. P., & Gupta, K. D. (1997). Prevalence and determinants of coronary heart disease in a rural population of India. *Journal of Clinical Epidemiology*, 50, 203–209.

Gupta, S., & Camm, A. J. (1997). Chlamydia pneumoniae and coronary heart disease (editorial). *British Medical Journal* (clinical research edition), 314 (7097), 1778–1779.

Guralnik, D. B. (ed.) (1980). *Webster's New World Dictionary of the American Language*. New York: Simon & Schuster.

Gurin, G., Veroff, J., & Feld, S. (1960). *Americans View Their Mental Health*. New York: Basic Books.

Guy, R. F. (1982). Religion, physical disabilities, and life satisfaction in older age cohorts. *International Journal of Aging and Human Development*, 15, 225–232.

Guyton, A. C. (1971). *Textbook of Medical Physiology*, 4th ed. Philadelphia: Saunders.

Haber, D. (1984). Church-based programs for black care-givers of non-institutionalized elders. *Gerontological Social Work in Home Health Care*, 7(4), 43–55.

Hadaway, C. K., & Roof, W. C. (1978). Religious commitment and the quality of life in American society. *Review of Religious Research*, 19, 295–307.

Hadaway, C. K., Elifson, K. W., & Peterson, D. M. (1984). Religious involvement and drug use among urban adolescents. *Journal for the Scientific Study of Religion*, 23, 109–128.

Hadaway, C. K., Marler, P., & Chaves, M. (1993). What the polls don't show: A closer look at U.S. church attendance. *American Sociological Review*, 58, 741–752.

Hadaway, C. K., Marler, P., & Chaves, M. (1998). Over-reporting church attendance in America: Evidence that demands the same verdict. *American Sociological Review*, 63, 122–130.

Haerich, P. (1992). Premarital sexual permissiveness and religious orientation: A preliminary investigation. *Journal for the Scientific Study of Religion*, 31, 361–365.

Hafner, R. J. (1982). Psychological treatment of essential hypertension: A controlled comparison of meditation and meditation plus biofeedback. *Biofeedback and Self Regulation*, 7(3), 305–316.

Hagglof, B., Blom, L., Dahlquist, G., Lonnberg, G., & Sahlin, B. (1991). The Swedish childhood diabetes study: Indications of severe psychological stress as a risk factor for type I (insulin-dependent) diabetes mellitus in childhood. *Diabetologia*, 34, 579–583.

Hagin, K. (1982). *Must Christians Suffer?* Falls Church, Va.: Kenneth Hagin Ministries.

Hall, C., & Lanig, H. (1993). Spiritual caring behaviors as reported by Christian nurses. *Western Journal of Nursing Research*, 15(6), 730–741.

Hall, S. M., Havassy, B. E., & Wasserman, D. A. (1991). Effect of commitment to abstinence, positive moods, stress, and coping on relapse to cocaine use. *Journal of Consulting and Clinical Psychology*, 59, 526–532.

Hall, T. W., & Edwards, K. J. (1996). The initial development and factor analysis of the Spiritual Assessment Inventory. *Journal of Psychology and Theology*, 24, 233–246.

Hallstrom, T., & Persson, G. (1984). The relationship of social setting to major depression. *Acta Psychiatrica Scandinavica*, 70, 327–336.

Halstead, M. T., & Fernsler, J. I. (1994). Coping stratgies of long-term cancer survivors. *Cancer Nursing*, 17(2), 94–100.

Hamilton, D. G. (1998). Believing in patients' beliefs: Physician attunement to the spiritual dimension as a positive factor in patient healing and health. *American Journal of Hospice and Palliative Care*, 15, 276–279.

Hamman, R. F., Barancik, J. I., & Lilienfeld, A. M. (1981). Patterns of mortality in the old order Amish: I. Background and major causes of death. *American Journal of Epidemiology*, 114, 845–861.

Handal, P. J., Black-Lopez, W., & Moergen, S. (1989). Preliminary investigation of the relationship between religion and psychological distress in black women. *Psychological Reports*, 65, 971–975.

Hanna, E. Z., Chou, S. P., & Grant, B. F. (1997). The relationship between drinking and heart disease morbidity in the United States: Results from the National Health Interview Survey. *Alcoholism, Clinical and Experimental Research*, 21, 111–118.

Hannay, D. R. (1980). Religion and health. *Social Science and Medicine*, 14, 683–685.

Hansen, G. L. (1981) Marital adjustment and conventionalization: A reexamination. *Journal of Marriage and the Family* (November), 855–863.

Hansen, G. L. (1982). Religion and marital adjustment. In J. F. Schumaker (ed.), *Religion and Mental Health* (pp. 189-198). New York: Oxford University Press.

Hansen, G. L. (1987). The effect of religiosity on factors predicting marital adjustment. *Social Psychology Quarterly*, 50, 264-269.

Hansen, G. L. (1992). Religion and marital adjustment. In J. F. Schumaker (ed.), *Religion and Mental Health* (pp. 189-198). New York: Oxford University Press.

Hanson, D. J., & Engs, R. C. (1987). Religion and collegiate drinking problems over time. *Psychology*, 24, 10-12.

Hardert, R. A., & Dowd, T. J. (1994). Alcohol and marijuana use among high school and college students in Phoenix, Arizona: A test of Kandel's socialization theory. *International Journal of Addictions*, 29, 887-912.

Hardesty, P. H., & Kirby, K. M. (1995). Relation between family religiousness and drug use within adolescent peer groups. *Journal of Social Behavior and Personality*, 10, 421-430.

Harding le Riche, W. (1985). Age at death: Physicians and ministers of religion. *Canadian Medical Association Journal*, 133, 107.

Harkavy-Friedman, J. M., Asnis, G. M., Boeck, M., & DiFiori, J. (1987). Prevalence of specific suicidal behaviors in a high school sample. *American Journal of Psychiatry*, 144, 1203-1206.

Haroun, A. (ed.) (1997). Psychiatric aspects of wickedness. *Psychiatric Annals*, 27, 613-641.

Harris, R. C., Dew, M. A., Lee, A., Amaya, M., Buches, L., Reetz, D., & Coleman, G. (1995). The role of religion in heart transplant recipients' health and well-being. *Journal of Religion and Health*, 34(1), 17-32.

Harris, W. S., Bowda, M., Kolb, J. W., Strychacz, C. P., Vacek, J. L., Jones P. G., Forker, A., O'Keefe, J. H., McCallister, B. D. (1999). The randomized, controlled trial of the effects of remote, intercessory prayer on outcomes in patients admitted to the coronary care unit. *Archives of Internal Medicine*, 159, 2273-2278.

Hart, C. W., & Matorin, S. (1997). Collaboration between hospital social work and pastoral care to help families cope with serious illness and grief. *Psychiatric Services*, 48, 1549-1552.

Hart, D., & Schneider, D. (1997). Spiritual care for children with cancer. *Seminars in Oncology Nursing*, 13, 263-270.

Harvey, C. D. H., Barnes, G. E., & Greenwood, L. (1987). Correlates of morale among Canadian widowed persons. *Social Psychiatry*, 22, 65-72.

Harwood, H., Fountain, D., & Livermore, G. (1998). *The Economic Costs of Alcohol and Drug Abuse in the United States, 1992*. Bethesda, Md.: National Institute for Drug Abuse.

Hasdai, D., Garratt, K. N., Grill, D. E., Lerman, A., & Holmes, D. R. (1997). Effect of smoking status on the long-term outcome after successful percutaneous coronary revascularization. *New England Journal of Medicine*, 336, 755-761.

Hasin, D., Endicott, J., & Collins, L. (1985). Alcohol and drug abuse in patients with affective syndromes. *Comprehensive Psychiatry*, 26, 283-295.

Hassan, M. K., & Khalique, A. (1981). Religiosity and its correlates in college students. *Journal of Psychological Researches*, 25 (3), 129-136

Hasselback, P., Lee, K. I., Mao, Y., Nichol, R., & Wigle, D. T. (1991). The relationship of suicide rates to sociodemographic factors in Canadian census divisions. *Canadian Journal of Psychiatry*, 36(9), 655-659.

Hatch, J. W., & Lovelace, K. A. (1980). Involving the Southern rural church and students of the health professions in health education. *Public Health Reports*, 95, 23-25.

Hatch, J. W., et al. (1984). General Baptist Convention of North Carolina: HHS Project. *Contact*, 77, 1-6.

Hatch, L. R. (1991). Informal support patterns of older African-American and White women. *Research on Aging*, 13, 144-170.

Hatch, R. L., Burg, M. A., Naberhasu, D. S., & Hellmich, L. K. (1998). The Spiritual Involvement and Beliefs Scale: Development and testing of a new instrument. *Journal of Family Practice*, 46, 476-486.

Hater, J. J., Singh, I., & Simpson, D. D. (1984). Influence of family and rleigion on long-term outcomes among opioid addicts. *Advances in Alcohol and Substance Abuse*, 4(1), 29-40.

Hathaway, W. L., & Pargament, K. I. (1990). Intrinsic religiousness, religious coping, and psychosocial competence: a covariance structure analysis. *Journal for the Scientific Study of Religion*, 29, 423-441.

Haugk, K. C. (1976). Urban contributions of churches and clergy to community mental health. *Community Mental Health Journal*, 12, 20-28.

Hawkins, J. D., & Catalano, R. F., Jr. (1992). *Communities That Care: Action for Drug Abuse Prevention*. San Francisco: Jossey-Bass.

Hawks, R. D., & Bahr, S. H. (1992). Religion and drug use. *Journal of Drug Education*, 22, 1-8.

Haynes, B. F., & Fauci, A. S. (1998). Introduction to the immune system. In A. S. Fauci, E. Braunwald, K. J. Isselbacher, J. D. Wilson, J. B. Martin, D. L. Kasper, S. L. Hauser, & D. L. Longo, (eds.), *Harrison's Principles of Internal Medicine*, 14th ed. (pp. 1753–1776). New York: McGraw-Hill.

Hays, J. C., Meador, K. G., & George, L. K. (2000). Developing a major of religious history. Durham, N.C.: Center for Aging and Human Development, Duke University Medical Center.

Hays, R. D., & Revetto, J. P. (1990). Peer cluster theory and adolescent drug use: A reanalysis. *Journal of Drug Education*, 20, 191–198.

Hays, R. D., Stacy A. W., Widaman, D. M. R., & Downey, R. (1986). Multistage path models of adolescent alcohol and drug use: A reanalysis. *Journal of Drug Issues*, 16, 357–369.

Healthy People 2000: National Health Promotion and Disease Prevention Objectives (1991). DHHS publication no. (PHS) 91–50212. Washington, D.C.: Department of Health and Human Services, Public Health Service.

Heath, A. C., Madden, P. A., Grant, J. D., McLaughlin, T. L., Todorov, A. A., Bucholz, K. K. (1999). Resiliency factors protecting against teenage alcohol use and smoking: influences of religion, religious involvement and values, and ethnicity in the Missouri Adolescent Female Twin Study. *Twin Research*, 2, 145–155.

Heather, N. (1998). A conceptual framework for explaining drug addiction. *Journal of Psychopharmacology*, 12(1), 3–7.

Heatherton, T. F., & Renin, R. J. (1995). Stress and the disinhibition of behavior. *Mind/Body Medicine*, 1, 72–81.

Heaton, R. B., & Pratt, E. L. (1990). The effects of religious homogamy on marital satisfaction and stability. *Journal of Family Issues*, 11, 191–207.

Heaton, T. B. (1984). Religious homogamy and marital satisfaction reconsidered. *Journal of Marriage and the Family*, 46, 729–733.

Heenan, E. (1972). Sociology of religion and the aged: The empirical lacunae. *Journal for the Scientific Study of Religion*, 2, 171–176.

Heiligman, R. M., Lee, L. R., & Kramer, D. (1983). Pain relief associated with a religious visitation: A case report. *Journal of Family Practice*, 16, 299–302.

Heinemann, A. W., & Kim, J. (1998). Spirituality in the lives of persons with disabilities: Qualitative methods. Paper presented at the 106th annual convention of the American Psychological Association, San Francisco.

Heintzelman, M. E., & Fehr, L. A. (1976). Relationship between religious orthodoxy and three personality variables. *Psychological Reports*, 38, 756–758.

Heirich, M. (1977). Change of heart: A test of some widely held theories about religious conversion. *American Journal of Sociology*, 83, 653–680.

Heisel, M. A., & Faulkner, A. O. (1982). Religiosity in an older Black population. *Gerontologist*, 22, 354–358.

Hellman, C. J. C., Budd, M., Borysenko, J., McCleland, D. C., & Benson, H. (1990). A study of the effectiveness of two group behavioral medicine intervention's four patients with psychosomatic complaints. *Behavioral Medicine*, Winter, 165–173.

Helm, H., Hays, J. C., Flint, E., Koenig, H. G., & Blazer, D. G. (2000). Does private religious activity prolong survival? A six-year follow-up study of 3,851 older adults. *Journal of Gerontology* (Medical Sciences), 55A, M400–M405.

Heltsley, M. E., & Broderick, C. (1969). Religiosity and premarital sexual permissiveness: Reexamination of Reiss's traditionalism proposition. *Journal of Marriage and the Family*, 31, 441–443.

Hendricks, L. E., Robinson-Brown, D. P., & Gary, L. E. (1984). Religiosity and unmarried Black adolescent fatherhood. *Adolescence*, 19(74), 417–424.

Herberman, R. B. (1981). Natural killer cells: Their roles in defenses against disease. *Science*, 214, 24–30.

Herberman, R. B. (1991). Principles of tumor immunology. In A. I. Holleb, D. J. Fink, & G. P. Murphy (eds.), *Textbook of Clinical Oncology* (pp. 69–79). Atlanta: American Cancer Society.

Herman, B., & Enterline, P. E. (1970). Lung cancer among the Jews and non-Jews of Pittsburgh, Pennsylvania, 1953–1967: Mortality rates and cigarette smoking behavior. *American Journal of Epidemiology*, 91, 355–367.

Herold, E. S., & Goodwin, M. S. (1981). Adamant virgins, potential nonvirgins and nonvirgins. *Journal of Sex Research*, 17(2), 97–113.

Hersch, L. (1936). Delinquency among Jews. *Journal of Criminal Law and Criminology*, 27, 515–516.

Hersch, L. (1936–1937). Complementary data on Jewish delinquency in Poland. *Journal of Criminal Law and Criminology*, 27, 857–873.

Hertel, R. B., & Donahue, M. J. (1995). Parental influences on God images among children: Testing Durkheim's metaphoric parallelism. *Journal for the Scientific Study of Religion*, 34, 186–199.

Herth, K. (1989). The relationship between level of hope and level of coping response and other variables in patients with cancer. *Oncology Nursing Forum*, 16, 67–72.

Hertsgaard, D., & Light, H. (1984). Anxiety, depression, and hostility in rural women. *Psychological Reports*, 55, 673–674.

Herzog, H., Lele, V. R., Kuwert, T., Langen, K. J., Kops, E. R., & Feinendegen, L. E. (1990–1991). Changed pattern of regional glucose metabolism during Yoga meditative relaxation. *Neuropsychobiology*, 23, 182–187.

Hess, C. B. (1977). A seven-year follow-up study of 186 males in a religious therapeutic community. In A. Schecter, H. Alksne, & E. Kaufman (eds.), *Critical Concerns in the Field of Drug Abuse*. New York: Marcel Dekker.

Hewitt, D. J., & Foley, K. M. (1997). Pain and pain management. In C. K. Cassel, H. J. Cohen, E. B. Larson, D. E. Meier, N. M. Resnick, L. Z. Rubinstein, & L. B. Sorensen (eds.), *Geriatric Medicine*, 3rd ed. (pp. 865–881). New York: Springer.

Hiatt, J. F. (1986). Spirituality, medicine and healing. *Southern Medical Journal*, 79, 736–743.

Higgins, P. C., & Albrecht, G. L. (1977). Hellfire and delinquency revisited. *Social Forces*, 55, 952–958.

Highfield, M. F. (1992). Spiritual health of oncology patients: Nurse and patient perspectives. *Cancer Nursing*, 15, 1–8.

Highfield, M. F. (1997). Spiritual assessment across the cancer trajectory: Methods and reflections. *Seminars in Oncology Nursing*, 13, 237–241.

Hill, A. B. (1965). The environment and disease: Association or causation? *Proceedings of the Royal Society of Medicine*, 58, 1217–1219.

Hill, P. C., & Hood, R. (1999). *Measures of Religiosity*. Birmingham, Ala.: Religious Education Press.

Hills, P., & Argyle, M. (1998). Musical and religious experiences and their relationship to happiness. *Personality and Individual Differences*, 25, 91–102.

Himmelfarb, H. S. (1975). Measuring religious involvement. *Social Forces*, 53, 606–618.

Hinn, B. (1997). *The Anointing*. Nashville: Thomas Nelson.

Hinton, J. (1975). The influence of previous personality on reactions to having terminal cancer. *Omega*, 6, 95–111.

Hirschfeld, R. M., & Cross, C. K. (1982). Epidemiology of affective disorders. *Archives of General Psychiatry*, 39, 35–46.

Hirschfeld, R. M. J. (1996). Panic disorder: Diagnosis, epidemiology, and clinical course. *Clinical Psychiatry*, 57(Suppl.), 3–8.

Hirshi, T., & Stark, R. (1969). Hellfire and delinquency. *Social Problems*, 17(2), 202–213.

Hixson, K. A., Gruchow, H. W., & Morgan, D. W. (1998). The relation between religiosity, selected health behaviors, and blood pressure among adult females. *Preventive Medicine*, 27, 545–552.

Hlatky, M. A., Boineau, R. E, Higginbotham, M. B., Lee, K. L., Mark, D. B., Califf, R. M., Cobb, F. R., & Pryor, D. B. (1989). A brief self-administered questionnaire to determine functional capacity (the Duke activity status index). *American Journal of Cardiology*, 64, 651–654.

Hoch, C. C., Reynolds, C. F., Kupfer, D. J., Houck, P. R., Berman, S. R., & Stack, J. A. (1987). The superior sleep of healthy elderly nuns. *International Journal of Aging and Human Development*, 25, 1–9.

Hoelter, J. W. (1979). Religiosity, fear of death and suicide acceptability. *Suicide and Life-Threatening Behavior*, 9, 163–172.

Hoelter, J. W., & Epley, R. J. (1979). Religious correlates of fear of death. *Journal for the Scientific Study of Religion*, 18, 404–411.

Hoffman, F. L. (1932). The cancer mortality of Amsterdam, Holland, by religious sects. *American Journal of Cancer*, 17, 142–153.

Hoge, D. R. (1972). A validated intrinsic religious motivation scale. *Journal for the Scientific Study of Religion*, 11, 369–376.

Hoge, D. R., & Carroll, J. W. (1973). Religiosity and prejudice in Northern and Southern churches. *Journal for the Scientific Study of Religion*, 12, 181–197.

Hogstel, M. O., & Kashka, M. (1989). Staying healthy after 85. *Geriatric Nursing*, January/February, 16–18.

Holland, J. C., Passik, S., Kash, K. M., Russak, S. M., Gronert, M. K., Sison, A, Lederberg, M., Fox, B., & Baider, L. (1999). The role of religious and spiritual beliefs in coping with malignant melanoma. *Psycho-oncology*, 8, 14–26.

Holloway, C. A. (1979). *Decision-making under Uncertainty: Models and Choices*. Englewood Cliffs, N.J.: Prentice Hall.

Holman, T. B., Jensen, L., Capell, M., & Woodard, F. (1993). Predicting alcohol use among young adults. *Addictive Behaviors*, 18, 41–49.

Holmes, C. B., & Howard, M. E. (1980). Recognition of suicide lethality factors by physicians, mental health professionals, ministers, and college students. *Journal of Consulting and Clinical Psychology*, 48, 383–387.

Holt, M. K., & Dellmann-Jenkins, M. (1992). Research and implications for practice: Religion, well-being/morale, and coping behavior in later life. *Journal of Applied Gerontology*, 11, 101–110.

Holt, P. G. (1987). Immune and inflammatory function in cigarette smokers. *Thorax*, 42, 241–249.

Holt, P. G., & Keast, D. (1977). Environmentally induced changes in immunological function: Acute and chronic effects of inhalation of tobacco smoke and other atmospheric contaminants in man and experimental animals. *Bacterialogical Reviews*, 41, 205–216.

Hood, R. W. (1974). Psychological strength and the report of intense religious experience. *Journal for the Scientific Study of Religion*, 13, 65–71.

Hood, R. W. (1975). The construction and preliminary validation of a measure of reported mystical experience. *Journal for the Scientific Study of Religion*, 14, 29–41.

Hooper, J. (1999). A new germ theory. *Atlantic Monthly* (February), 41–53.

Hoover, J. E. (1948). The youth problem today. *Chicago Schools Journal*, 30, 33–35.

Hope, S., Power, C., & Rogers, B. (1998). The relationship between parental separation in childhood and problem drinking in adulthood. *Addiction*, 93, 505–514.

Horowitz, I., & Enterline, P. E. (1970). Lung cancer among the Jews. *American Journal of Public Health*, 60, 275–282.

Horrigan, B. (1999). Mitchell W. Krucoff, M.D.: The Mantra Study Project. *Alternative Therapies*, 5(3), 75–82.

Horton, P. C. (1973). The mystical experience as a suicide preventive. *American Journal of Psychiatry*, 130, 294–296.

House, A., Dennis, M., Mogridge, L., Hawton, K., & Warlow, C (1990). Life events and difficulties preceding stroke. *Journal of Neurology, Neurosurgery and Psychiatry*, 53, 1024–1028.

House, J. S., Landis, K. R., & Umberson, D. (1988). Social relationships and health. *Science*, 241, 540–545.

House, J. S., Robbins, C., & Metzner, H. L. (1982). The association of social relationships and activities with mortality: Prospective evidence from the Tecumseh Community Health Study. *American Journal of Epidemiology*, 116, 123–140.

Hout, M., & Greeley, A. (1998). What church officials' reports don't show: Another look at church attendance data. *American Sociological Review*, 63, 113–119.

Hu, Y., & Goldman, N. (1990). Mortality differentials by marital status: An international comparison. *Demography*, 27(2), 233–250.

Hughes J., Stewart, M., & Barraclough, B. (1985). Why teetotallers abstain. *British Journal of Psychiatry*, 146, 204–208.

Hughes, R. A. (1990). Psychological perspectives on infanticide in a faith healing sect. *Psychotherapy*, 27, 107–115.

Huizinga, D. (1994). *Urban Delinquency and Substance Abuse: Research Summary*. Washington, D.C.: Office of Juvenile Justice and Delinquency Prevention, Department of Justice.

Huizinga, D., & Menard, B. (1989). *Multiple Problem Youth: Delinquency Substance Abuse, and Mental Health Problems*. New York: Springer-Verlag.

Hull, D. (1997). Dieters putting their faith in sustenance of the spirit. *Washington Post* (May 17), p. C6.

Hummer, R., Rogers, R., Nam, C., & Ellison, C. G. (1999). Religious involvement and U.S. adult mortality. *Demography*, 36, 273–285.

Hundleby, J. D. (1987). Adolescent drug use in a behavioral matrix: A confirmation and comparison of the sexes. *Addictive Behaviors*, 12, 103–112.

Hundleby, J. D., Carpenter, R. A., Ross, R. A. J., & Mercer, G. W. (1982). Adolescent drug use and other behaviors. *Journal of Child Psychology and Psychiatry*, 23, 61–68.

Hunsberger, B. (1985). Religion, age, life satisfaction, and perceived sources of religiousness: A study of older persons. *Journal of Gerontology*, 40, 615–620.

Hunsberger, B., & Ennis, J. (1982). Experimenter effects in studies of religious attitudes. *Journal for the Scientific Study of Religion*, 21, 131–137.

Hunsberger, B., & Platonow, E. (1987). Religion and helping charitable causes. *Journal of Psychology*, 120(6), 517–528.

Hunt, I. E., Murphy, N. J., & Henderson, C. (1988). Food and nutrient intake of Seventh-Day Adventist women. *American Journal of Clinical Nutrition*, 48, 850–851.

Hunt, R. A., & King, M. B. (1971). The intrinsic-extrinsic concept: A review and evaluation. *Journal for the Scientific Study of Religion*, 10, 339–356.

Hunt, R. A., & King, M. B. (1978). Religiosity and marriage. *Journal for the Scientific Study of Religion*, 17, 399–406.

Hunter, J. E., & Schmidt, F. L. (1990). *Methods of Meta-analysis*. Newbury Park, Calif.: Sage.

Husaini, B. A., Blasi, A. J., & Miller, O. (1999). Does public and private religiosity have a moderating effect on depression? A biracial study of elders in the American south. *International Journal of Aging and Human Development*, 48(1), 63–72.

Hutchinson, J. (1986). Association between stress and blood pressure variation in a Caribbean population. *American Journal of Physical Anthropology*, 71, 69–79.

Iammarino, N. K. (1975). Relationship between death anxiety and demographic variables. *Psychological Reports*, 37, 262.

IASP (1979). International Association for the Study of Pain Subcommittee on Taxonomy of Pain Terms: A list with definitions and notes on usage. *Pain*, 6, 249.

Ide, B. A., & Sanli, T. (1992). Health beliefs and behaviors of Saudi women. *Women and Health*, 19, 97–113.

Idler, E. L. (1987). Religious involvement and the health of the elderly: some hypotheses and an initial test. *Social Forces*, 66, 226–238.

Idler, E. L. (1994). *Cohesiveness and Coherence: Religion and the Health of the Elderly*. New York: Garland.

Idler, E. L. (1995). Religion, health, and nonphysical senses of self. *Social Forces*, 74, 683–704.

Idler, E., & Kasl, S. (1991). Health perceptions and survival: Do global evaluations of health status really predict mortality? *Journal of Gerontology* (social sciences), 46, 55–65.

Idler, E., & Kasl, S. (1992). Religion, disability, depression, and the timing of death. *American Journal of Sociology*, 97, 1052–1079.

Idler, E. L., & Kasl, S. V. (1997a). Religion among disabled and nondisabled persons: I. Cross-sectional patterns in health practices, social activities, and well-being. *Journal of Gerontology*, 52B(6), 294–305.

Idler, E. L., & Kasl, S. V. (1997b). Religion among disabled and nondisabled persons: II. Attendance at religious services as a predictor of the course of disability. *Journal of Gerontology*, 52B(6), 306–316.

Idler, E. L., Ellison, C. G., George, L. K., Krause, N., Levin, J. S., Ory, M., Pargament, K. I., Powell, L. H., Williams, D. R., & Underwood-Gordon, L. (2000). Brief measure of religiousness and spirituality: Conceptual development. *Research on Aging*.

Iga, M. (1981). Suicide of Japanese youth. *Suicide and Life-Threatening Behavior*, 11(1), 17–30.

Imamura, H., Tanaka, K., Hirae, C., Futagami, T., & Yoshimura, Y. (1996). Relationship of cigarette smoking to blood pressure and serum lipids and lipoproteins in men. *Clinical and Experimental Pharmacology and Physiology*, 23, 397–402.

Infante, J. R., Peran, F., Martinez, M., Roldan, A, Poyatos, R., Ruiz, C., Samaniego, F., & Garrido, F. (1998). ACTH and beta-endorphin in transcendental medication. *Physiology and Behavior*, 64, 311–315.

Inglehart, R. (1990). *Culture Shift in Advanced Industrial Society*. Princeton, N.J.: Princeton University Press.

Inui, A., Kitaoka, H., Majima, M, Takamiya, S., Uemoto, M., Yonenaga, C., Honda, M., Shirakawa, K., Ueno, N., Amano, K., Morita, S., Kawara, A., Yokono, K., Kasuaga, M., & Taniguchi, H. (1998). Effect of the Kobe earthquake on stress and a glycemic control in patients with diabetes mellitus. *Archives of Internal Medicine*, 158, 274–278.

Ironson, G., LaPerrier, A., Antoni, M., O'Hearn, P., Schneiderman, N., Klimas, N., & Fletcher, M. A. (1990). Changes in immune and psychological measures as a function of anticipation and reaction to news of HIV-A antibody status. *Psychosomatic Medicine*, 52, 247–270.

Irwin, M., Britton, K. T., & Vale, W. (1987). Central corticotropin releasing factor suppresses natural killer cell activity. *Brain, Behavior, and Immunity*, 1, 81–87.

Irwin, M., Daniels, M., & Risch, S. C. (1988). Plasma cortisol and natural killer cell activity during bereavement. *Biological Psychiatry*, 24, 173–178.

Irwin, M., Patterson, T., Smith, T. L., Caldwell, C., Brown, S. A., Gilin, C., & Grant, I. (1990). Reduction of immune function in life stress and depression. *Biological Psychiatry*, 27, 22–30.

Irwin, M., Smith, T. L., & Gillin, J. C. (1987). Low natural killer cytotoxicity in major depression. *Life Science*, 41, 2127–2133.

Irwin, M., Smith, T. L., & Gillin, J. C. (1992). EEG sleep and natural killer activity in depressed patients and control subjects. *Psychosomatic Medicine*, 54, 10–21.

Israel, B. A. (1985). Social networks and social support: Implications for natural helper and community level interventions. *Health Education Quarterly*, 12, 65–80.

Isralowitz, R. E., & Ong, T. H. (1990). Religious values and beliefs and place of residence as predictors of alcohol use among Chinese college students in Singapore. *International Journal of Addictions, 25,* 515–529.

Jabaaij, P. M., Grosheide, R. A., & Heijtink, R. A., (1993). Influence of perceived psychological stress and distress of antibody response to low dose rDNA Hepatitis B vaccine. *Journal of Psychosomatic Research, 37,* 361–369.

Jackson, L. E., & Coursey, R. D. (1988). The relationship of God control and internal locus of control to intrinsic religious motivation, coping and purpose in life. *Journal for the Scientific Study of Religion, 27,* 399–410.

Jacob, R. G., Kramer, H. C., & Agras, W. S. (1977). Relaxation therapy in the treatment of hypertension. *Archives of General Psychiatry, 34,* 1417–1427.

Jacobson, G. R., Ritter, D. P., & Mueller, L. (1977). Purpose in life and personal values among adult alcoholics. *Journal of Clinical Psychology, 33,* 314–316.

Jaffe, J. H. (1980). Drug addiction and drug abuse. In A. G. Gilman & L. S. Goodman (eds.), *The Pharmacological Basis of Therapeutics,* 6th ed. (pp. 150–175). New York: Macmillan.

Jalowiec, A., & Powers, M. J. (1981). Stress and coping in hypertensive and emergency room patients. *Nursing Research, 30,* 10–15.

Jamal, M., & Badawi, J. (1993). Job stress among Muslim immigrants in North America: Moderating effects of religiosity. *Stress Medicine, 9,* 145–151.

James, W. (1890). *The Principles of Psychology.* New York: Holt.

James, W. (1902). *The Varieties of Religious Experience.* New York: New American Library.

Jamison, R. N., & Virts, K. L. (1990). The influence of family support on chronic pain. *Behavior Research and Therapy, 28,* 283–287.

Janoff-Bulman, R., & Marshall, G. (1982). Mortality, well-being, and control: A study of a population of institutionalized aged. *Personality and Social Psychology Bulletin, 8,* 691–698.

Jarvis, G. K. (1977). Mormon mortality rates in Canada. *Social Biology, 24,* 294–302.

Jarvis, G. K., & Northcott, H. C. (1987). Religion and differences in morbidity and mortality. *Social Science and Medicine, 25,* 813–824.

Jasperse, C. W. G. (1976). Self-destruction and religion. *Mental Health and Society, 3,* 154–168.

Jeffers, F. C., & Nichols, C. R. (1961). The relationship of activities and attitudes to physical well-being in older people. *Journal of Gerontology, 16,* 67–70.

Jeffers, F. C., Nichols, C. R., & Eisdorfer, C. (1961). Attitudes of older persons toward death. *Journal of Gerontology, 16,* 53–56.

Jenkins, R. A. (1995). Religion and HIV: Implications for research and intervention. *Journal of Social Issues, 51,* 131–144.

Jenkins, R. A., & Pargament, K. I. (1988). Cognitive appraisals in cancer patients. *Social Science and Medicine, 26,* 625–633.

Jenkins, R. A., & Pargament, K. I. (1995). Religion and spirituality as resources for coping with cancer. *Journal of Psychosocial Oncology, 13,* 51–74.

Jensen, J. P., & Bergin, A. E. (1988). Mental health values of professional therapists: A national interdisciplinary study. *Professional Psychology: Research and Practice, 19,* 290–297.

Jensen, L., Newell, R. J., & Holman T. (1990). Sexual behavior, church attendance, and permissive beliefs among unmarried young men and women. *Journal for the Scientific Study of Religion, 29,* 113–117.

Jensen, L. C., Jensen, J., & Wiederhold, T. (1993). Religiosity, denomination, and mental health among young men and women. *Psychological Reports, 72,* 1157–1158.

Jensen, O. M. (1983). Cancer risk among Danish male Seventh-Day Adventists and other temperance society members. *Journal of the National Cancer Institute, 70,* 1011–1014.

Jessor, R., & Jessor, S. L. (1977). *Problem Behavior and Psychosocial Development: A Longitudinal Study of Youth.* New York: Academic Press.

Jessor, R., Donovan, J. E., & Costa, F. (1986). Psychosocial correlates of marijuana use in adolescence and the young adult: The past as prologue. International Symposium on Marijuana, Cocaine and Traffic Safety. *Alcohol, Drugs, and Driving Abstracts and Reviews, 2(3–4),* 31–49.

Jessor, R., Jessor, S. L., & Finney, J. (1973). A social psychology of marijuana use: Longitudinal studies of high school and college youth. *Journal of Personality and Social Psychology, 26,* 1–15.

Jevning, R., Wilson, A. F., & Davidson, J. M. (1978). Adrenocortical activity during meditation. *Hormones and Behavior, 10(1),* 54–60.

Jex, S. M., Hughs, P., Storr, C., Conard, S., Baldwin, D. C., & Sheehan, D. V. (1992). Relations among stressors, strains, and substance use among residents physicians. *International Journal of the Addictions, 27,* 979–994.

Jilek, W. G. (1974). *Salish Indian Mental Health and Culture Change.* Toronto: Holt, Rinehart, & Winston.

Jin, P. (1992). Efficacy of Tai Chi, brisk walking, meditation, and reading in reducing mental and emotional stress. *Journal of Psychosomatic Research*, 36, 361–370.

John, O. P. (1990). The "Big Five" factor taxonomy: Dimensions of personality in the natural language and in questionnaires. In L. A. Pervin (ed.), *Handbook of Personality: Theory and Research* (pp. 66–100). New York: Guilford.

Johnsen, L. W., & Harlow, L. L. (1996). Childhood sexual abuse linked with adult substance use, victimization, and AIDS risk. *AIDS Education and Prevention*, 8, 44–57.

Johnson, B., Larson, D. B., & Pitts, T. C. (1997). Religious programs, institutional adjustment, and recidivism among former inmates in prison fellowship programs. *Justice Quarterly*, 14(1), 145–166.

Johnson, B., Spencer, D. L., Larson, D. B., & McCullough, M. (1997). A systematic review of the religiosity and delinquency literature. Paper presented at the American Society of Criminology, San Diego.

Johnson, D., Fitch, S. D., Alston, J. P., & McIntosh, W. A. (1980). Acceptance of conditional suicide and euthanasia among adult Americans. *Suicide and Life Threatening Behavior*, 10, 157–166.

Johnson, D. M., Williams, J. S., & Bromley, D. G. (1986). Religion, health, and healing: Findings from a southern city. *Sociological Analysis*, 47, 66–73.

Johnson, D. P., & Mullins, L. C. (1989a). Religiosity and loneliness among the elderly. *Journal of Applied Gerontology*, 8, 110–131.

Johnson, D. P., & Mullins, L. C. (1989b). Subjective and social dimensions of religiosity and loneliness among the well elderly. *Review of Religious Research*, 31, 4–15.

Johnson, J., Weissman, M. M., & Klerman, G. L. (1992). Service utilization and social morbidity associated with depressive symptoms in the community. *Journal of the American Medical Association*, 267, 1478–1483.

Johnson, L. D., & O'Malley, P. M. (1998). *Monitoring the Future*. Ann Arbor: University of Michigan Survey Research Center.

Johnson, M. A. (1973). Family life and religious commitment. *Review of Religious Research*, 14, 144–150.

Johnson, S. C., & Spilka, B. (1991). Coping with breast cancer: The roles of clergy and faith. *Journal of Religion and Health*, 30, 21–33.

Johnson, W. B. (1993). Outcome research and religious psychotherapies: Where are we and where are we going? *Journal of Psychology and Theology*, 21, 297–308.

Johnson, W. B., & Ridley, C. R. (1992). Brief Christian and non-Christian rational-emotive therapy with depressed Christian clients: An exploratory study. *Counseling and Values*, 36, 220–229.

Johnson, W. B., DeVries, R., Ridley, C. R., Pettorini, D., & Peterson, D. R. (1994). The comparative efficacy of Christian and secular rational-emotive therapy with Christian clients. *Journal of Psychology and Theology*, 22, 130–140.

Johnston, L., O'Malley, P., & Bachman, J. (1996). National survey results on drug use from the Monitoring the Future Study, 1975–1994. Rockville, Md.: National Institute on Drug Abuse.

Jonas, B. S., Franks, P., & Ingram, D. D. (1997). Are symptoms of anxiety and depression risk factors for hypertension? Longitudinal evidence from the National Health and Nutrition Examination Survey I epidemiologic follow-up study. *Archives of Family Medicine*, 6, 43–49.

Jones, E., & Watson, J. P. (1997). Delusion, the overvalued idea and religious beliefs: A comparative analysis of their characteristics. *British Journal of Psychiatry*, 170, 381–386.

Jones, M. B. (1958). Religious values and authoritarian tendency. *Journal of Social Psychology*, 48, 83–89.

Jones, S. (1994). A constructive relationship for religion with the science and profession of pscyhology. *American Psychologist*, 49, 184–199.

Jones, S. L., Watson, E. J., & Wolfram, T. J. (1992). Results of the Rech Conference Survey on religious faith and professional psychology. *Journal of Psychology and Theology*, 20, 147–158.

Jones-Webb, R. J., & Snowden, L. R. (1993). Symptoms of depression among blacks and whites. *American Journal of Public Health*, 83, 240–244.

Jorm, A. F., van Duijn, C. M., Chandra, V., Fratiglioni, L., Graves, A. B., Heyman, A., Kokmen, E., Kondo, K., Mortimer, J. A., & Rocca, W. A. (1991). Psychiatric history and related exposures as risk factors for Alzheimer's disease: A collaborative re-analysis of case-control studies. EURODEM Risk Factors Research Group. *International Journal of Epidemiology*, 20 (Suppl. 2), S43–S47.

Joubert, C. E. (1995). Catholicism and indices of social pathology in the states. *Psychological Reports*, 76(2), 573–574.

Joung, I. M. A., Van der Meer, J. B. W., & Mackenbach, J. P. (1995). Marital status and health care utilization. *International Journal of Epidemiology*, 24, 569–575.

Joyce, C. R. B., & Welldon, R. M. C. (1965). The objective efficacy of prayer, a double-blind clinical trial. *Journal of Chronic Disease*, 18, 367–377.

Jung, C. (1933). *Modern Man in Search of Soul*. New York: Harcourt Brace Jovanovich.

Jussawalla, D. J., & Jain, D. K. (1977). Breast cancer and religion in greater Bombay women: An epidemiological study of 2,130 women over a 9-year period. *British Journal of Cancer*, 36, 634–638.

Kabat-Zinn, J., Lipworth, L., & Burney, R. (1985). The clinical use of mindfulness meditation for the self-regulation of chronic pain. *Journal of Behavioral Medicine*, 8, 163–190.

Kabat-Zinn, J., Massion, A. O., Kristeller, J., Peterson, L. G., Fletcher, K. E., Pbert, L., Lenderking, W. R., & Santorelli, S. F. (1992). Effectiveness of a meditation-based stress reduction program in the treatment of anxiety disorders. *American Journal of Psychiatry*, 149, 936–943.

Kaczorowski, J. M. (1989). Spiritual well-being and anxiety in adults diagnosed with cancer. *Hospice Journal*, 5, 105–116.

Kahoe, R. D. (1974). Personality and achievement correlates of intrinsic and extrinsic religious orientations. *Journal of Personality and Social Psychology*, 29, 812–818.

Kaldestad, E. (1995). The empirical relationships of the religious orientations to personality. *Scandinavian Journal of Psychology*, 36, 95–108.

Kaldestad, E. (1996). The empirical relationships between standardized measures of religiosity and personality mental health. *Scandinavian Journal of Psychology*, 37, 205–220.

Kaldjian, L.C., Jekel, J. F., & Friedland, G. (1998). End-of-life decisions in HIV-positive patients: The role of spiritual beliefs. *AIDS*, 12(1), 103–107.

Kandel, C. B., Adler, I., & Sudit, M. (1981). The epidemiology of adolescent drug use in France and Israel. *American Journal of Public Health*, 71, 256–265.

Kandel, D. B. (1984). Marijuana users in young adulthood. *Archives of General Psychiatry*, 41, 200–209.

Kandel, D. B. (1990). Early onset of adolescent sexual behavior and drug involvement. *Journal of Marriage and the Family*, 42, 783–798.

Kandel, D. B., Raveis, V. H., & Davies, M. (1991). Suicidal ideation in adolescence: Depression, substance use, and other risk factors. *Journal of Youth and Adolescence*, 20, 289–301.

Kane, R. L., Ouslander, J. G., & Abrass, I. B. (1984). *Essentials of Clinical Geriatrics*. New York: McGraw-Hill.

Kang, S. H., & Bloom, J. R. (1993). Social support and cancer screening among older black Americans. *Journal of the National Cancer Institute*, 85, 737–742.

Kaplan, B. H. (1976). A note on religious beliefs and coronary heart disease. *Journal of the South Carolina Medical Association*, 72 (Suppl.), 60–64.

Kaplan, H. I., & Sadock, B. J. (1988a). Normal sleep and sleep disorders. In *Synopsis of Psychiatry*, 5th ed. (pp. 381–395). Baltimore: Williams & Wilkins.

Kaplan, H. I., & Sadock, B. J. (1988b). *Synopsis of Psychiatry*, 5th ed. Baltimore: Williams & Wilkins.

Kaplan, K., & Ross, L. (1995). Life ownership orientation and attitude toward abortion, suicide, and captial punishment. *Journal of Psychology and Judasim*, 19(2), 177–193.

Kark, J. D., Carmel, S., Sinnreich, R., Goldberger, N., & Friedlander, Y. (1996). Psychosocial factors among members of religious and secular kibbutzim. *Israel Journal of Medical Science*, 32, 185–194.

Kark, J. D., Shemi, G., Friedlander, Y., Martin, O., Manor, O., & Blondheim, S. H. (1996). Does religious observance promote health? Mortality in secular vs. religious kibbutzim in Israel. *American Journal of Public Health*, 86(3), 341–346.

Kaseman, C. M., & Anderson, R. G. (1977). Clergy consultation as a community mental health program. *Community Mental Health Journal*, 13, 84–91.

Kasl, S. V., Evans, A. S., & Niederman, J. C. (1979). Psychosocial risk factors in the development of infectious mononucleosis. *Psychosomatic Medicine*, 41, 445–466.

Kaslow, F., & Robinson, J. A. (1996). Long-term satisfying marriages: Perceptions of contributing factors. *American Journal of Family Therapy*, 24, 154–170.

Kass, J. D., Friedman, R., Leserman, J., Zuttermeister, P. C., & Benson, H. (1991). Health outcomes and a new index of spiritual experience (INSPIRIT). *Journal for the Scientific Study of Religion*, 30, 203–211.

Kastenbaum, R. (1990). The age of saints and the saintliness of age. *International Journal of Aging and Human Development*, 30, 95–118.

Katchadourian, H. (1974). A comparative study of mental illness among the Christians and Moslems of Lebanon. *International Journal of Social Psychiatry*, 20(1–2), 56–67.

Katerndahl, D. A. J. (1996). Panic attacks and panic disorder. *Family Practice*, 43(3): 275–282.

Katkin, S., Zimmerman, V., Rosenthal, J., & Ginsburg, M. (1975). Using volunteer therapists to reduce hospital readmissions. *Hospital and Community Psychiatry*, 26, 151–153.

Katon, W., Von Korff, M., Lin, E., & Lipscomb, P. (1990). Distressed high utilizers of medical care: DSM-III-R diagnoses and treatment needs. *General Hospital Psychiatry* 12, 355–362.

Katz, J., Weiner, H., Gallagher, T., & Hellman, L. (1970). Stress, distress, and ego defenses. *Archives of General Psychiatry*, 23, 131–142.

Katz, M. (1976). Jewish dietary laws. *Southern Australian Medical Journal* (November 20), 2004–2005.

Katz, Y. J. (1988). A validation of the Social-Religious-Political Scale. *Educational and Psychological Measurement*, 48, 1025–1028.

Katzel, L. I., Bleecker, E. R., & Colman, E. G. (1995). Effects of weight loss versus aerobic exercise training on risk factors for coronary disease in healthy, obese, middle aged and older men: A randomized controlled trial. *Journal of the American Medical Association*, 274, 1915–1921.

Kauffman, C. (1976). *Tamers of Death: The History of the Alexian Brothers from 1300 to 1789.* New York: Seabury Press.

Kauffman, C. (1978). *The Ministry of Healing: Vol. 2 of the History of the Alexian Brothers.* New York: Seabury Press.

Kauffman, J. H. (1979). Social correlates of spiritual maturity among North American Mennonites. In D. Moberg (ed.), *Spiritual Well-Being: Sociological Perspectives* (pp. 237–254). Washington, D.C.: University Press of America.

Kaufman, D. M. (1990). *Clinical Neurology for Psychiatrists*, 3rd ed. Philadelphia: Saunders.

Kaunitz, A. M., Spence, C., Danielson, T. S., Rochat, R. W., & Grimes, D. A. (1984). Perinatal and maternal mortality in a religious group avoiding obstetric care. *American Journal of Obstetrics and Gynecology*, 150, 826–831.

Kaye, J., & Robinson, K. M. (1994). Spirituality among caregivers. *IMAGE: Journal of Nursing Scholarship*, 26, 218–221.

Kearney, M. (1970). Drunkenness and religious conversion in a Mexican village. *Quarterly Journal of Studies on Alcohol*, 31, 132–152.

Keefe, F. J., & Williams, D. A. (1990). A comparison of coping strategies in chronic pain patients in different age groups. *Journal of Gerontology*, 45, 161–165.

Keefe, F. J., Crisson, J., Urban, B. J., & Williams, D. A. (1990). Analyzing chronic low back pain: The relative contribution of pain coping strategies. *Pain*, 40, 293–301.

Keene, J. J. (1967). Religious behavior and neuroticism, spontaneity, and worldmindedness. *Sociometry*, 30, 137–157.

Kehn, D. J. (1995). Predictors of elderly happiness. *Activities, Adaptation, and Aging*, 19(3), 11–29.

Kehoe, N. C., & Gutheil, T. G. (1994). Neglect of religious issues in scale-based assessment of suicidal patients. *Hospital and Community Psychiatry*, 45, 366–369.

Keilman, L. J., & Given, B. A. (1990). Spirituality: an untapped resource for hope and coping in family caregivers of individuals with cancer. *Oncology Nursing Forum*, 17, 159.

Keith, P. M. (1979). Life changes and perceptions of life and death among older men and women. *Journal of Gerontology*, 34, 870–878.

Kelley, M. W. (1958). The incidence of hospitalized mental illness among religious sisters in the U.S. *American Journal of Psychiatry*, 115, 72–75.

Kelly, M. J., Olive, K. E., Harvill, L. M., & Maddry, H. A. (1996). Spiritual and religious issues in clinical care: An elective course for medical students. *Annals of Behavioral Science and Medical Education*, 3(2), 1–7.

Kelsen, D. P., Portenoy, R. K., Thaler, H. T., Niedzwiecki, D., Passik, S. D., Tao, Y., Banks, W., Brennan, M. F., & Foley, K. M. (1995). Pain and depression in patients with newly diagnosed pancreas cancer. *Journal of Clinical Oncology*, 13, 748–755.

Kendler, K. S. (1988). The genetics of schizophrenia. In M. T. Tsuang & J. C. Simpson (eds.), *Handbook of Schizophrenia: Vol. 3. Nosology, Epidemiology and Genetics.* Amsterdam: Elsevier Science.

Kendler, K. S., Gardner, C. O., & Prescott, C. A. (1997). Religion, psychopathology, and substance use and abuse: A multimeasure, genetic-epidemiologic study. *American Journal of Psychiatry*, 154, 322–329.

Kennedy, G. F., Hofer, M. A., Cohen, D., Shindledecker, R., & Fisher, J. D. (1987). Significance of depression and cognitive impairment in patients undergoing programmed stimulation of cardiac arrhythmias. *Psychosomatic Medicine*, 49, 410–421.

Kennedy, G. J. (1998). Religion and depression. In H. G. Koenig (ed.), *Handbook of Religion and Mental Health* (pp. 129–145). San Diego: Academic Press.

Kennedy, G. J., Kelman, H. R., Thomas, C., & Chen, J. (1996). The relation of religious preference and practice to depressive symptoms among 1,855 older adults. *Journal of Gerontology,* 51B, P301–308.

Kennedy, S., Kiecolt-Glaser, J., & Glaser, R. (1988). Immunological consequences of acute and chronic stressors: Mediating role of interpersonal relationships. *British Journal of Medical Psychology,* 61, 77–85.

Kenney, B. P., Cromwell, R. E., & Vaughan, C. E. (1977). Identifying the socio-contextual forms of religiosity among urban ethnic minority group members. *Journal for the Scientific Study of Religion,* 16, 237–244.

Kent, S., Fogarty, M., & Yellowlees, P. (1995). The review of studies of heavy users of psychiatric services. *Psychiatric Services,* 46, 1247–1253.

Kesselring, A., Dodd, M. J., Lindsey, A. M., & Strauss, A. L. (1986). Attitudes of patients living in Switzerland about cancer and its treatment. *Cancer Nursing,* 9, 77–85.

Kessler, I. I., Kulcar, Z., Zimolo, A., Grgurevic, M., Strnad, M., & Goodwin, B. (1974). Cervical cancer in Yugoslavia: II. Epidemiologic factors of possible etiologic significance. *Journal of the National Cancer Institute,* 53, 51–60.

Kessler, R. C., McGonagle, K. A., Zhao, S., Nelson, C. B., Hughes, M., & Eshleman, S. (1994). Lifetime and 12-month prevalence of DSM-III-R psychiatric disorders in the United States: Results from the National Co-Morbidity Survey. *Archives of General Psychiatry,* 51, 8–19.

Kesterson, J., & Clinch, N. F. (1989). Metabolic rate, respiratory exchange ratio, and apneas during meditation. *American Journal of Physiology,* 256, 632–638.

Keys, A., Aravanis, C., Blackburn, H., & Van Buchem, F. S. (1972). Coronary heart disease: Overweight and obesity as risk factors. *Annals of Internal Medicine,* 77, 15–27.

Khavari, K. A., & Harmon, T. M. (1982). The relationship between the degree of professed religious belief and use of drugs. *International Journal of the Addictions,* 17, 847–857.

Kiecolt-Glaser, J. K., & Glaser, R. (1988). Psychological influences on immunity: Implications for AIDS. *American Psychologist,* 43(11), 892–898.

Kiecolt-Glaser, J. K., & Glaser, R. (1994). Caregivers, mental health, and immune function. In E. Light, G. Niederehe, & B. D. Lebowitz (eds.), *Stress Effects on Family Caregivers of Alzheimer's Patients: Research and Intervention* (pp. 64–75). New York: Springer.

Kiecolt-Glaser, J. K., & Glaser, R. (1995). Psychoneuroimmunology and health consequences: Data and shared mechanisms. *Psychosomatic Medicine,* 57, 269–274.

Kiecolt-Glaser, J. K., Dura, J. R., Speicher, C. E., Trask, O. J., & Glaser, R. (1991). Spousal caregivers of dementia victims: Longitudinal changes in immunity and health. *Psychosomatic Medicine,* 53, 345–362.

Kiecolt-Glaser, J. K., Fisher, L., Ogrocki, P., Stout, J. C., Spelcher, C. E., & Glaser, R. (1987). Marital quality, marital disruption and immune function. *Psychomatic Medicine,* 49, 13–34.

Kiecolt-Glaser, J. K., Garner, W., & Spelcher, C. (1984). Psychosocial modifiers of immunocompetence in medical students. *Psychosomatic Medicine,* 46, 7–14.

Kiecolt-Glaser, J. K., Glaser, R., Cacioppo, J. T., MacCallum, R. C., Snydersmith, M., Kim. C., & Malarkey, W. B. (1997). Marital conflict in older adults: Endocrinological and immunological correlates. *Psychosomatic Medicine,* 49, 339–349.

Kiecolt-Glaser, J. K., Glaser, R., Gravenstein, S., Malarkey, W. B., & Sheridan, J. (1996). Chronic stress alters the immune response to influenza virus vaccine in older adults. *Proceedings of the National Academy of Sciences of the United States of America,* 93, 3043–3047.

Kiecolt-Glaser, J. K., Malarkey, W. B., Cacioppo, J. T, & Glaser, R. (1994). Stressful personal relationships: Immune and endocrine function. In R. Glaser & J. Kiecolt-Glaser (eds.), *Handbook of Human Stress and Immunity* (pp. 321–339). San Diego: Academic Press.

Kiecolt-Glaser, J. K., Malarkey, W. B., Chee, M., Newton, T., Cacioppo, J. T., Mao, H. Y., & Glaser, R. (1993). Negative behavior during marital conflict is associated with immunological downregulation. *Psychosomatic Medicine,* 55, 395–409.

Kiecolt-Glaser, J. K., Marucha, P. T., Malarkey, W. B., Mercado, A. M., & Glaser, R. (1996). Slowing of wound healing by psychological stress. *Lancet,* 346(8984), 1194–1196.

Kiecolt-Glaser, J. K., Newton, T., Cacioppo, J. T., MacCallum, R. C., Glaser, R., & Malarkey, W. B. (1996). Marital conflict and endocrine function: Are men really more physiologically affected than women? *Journal of Consulting and Clinical Psychology,* 64, 324–332.

Kiecolt-Glaser, J. K., Ricker, D., & George, J. (1984). Urinary cortisol levels, cellular immunocompetence, and loneliness in psychiatric inpatients. *Psychosomatic Medicine,* 46, 15–23.

Kim, J., & Heinemann, A. W. (1998). Spirituality, quality of life, and functional recovery following medical rehabilitation. Paper presented at the

106th annual convention of the American Psychological Association, San Francisco.

King, C. A., Radpour, L., Naylor, M. W., Segal, H. G., & Jouriles, E. N. (1995). Parents' marital functioning and adolescent psychopathology. *Journal of Consulting and Clinical Psychology*, 63(5), 749–753.

King, D. (2000). *Faith, Spirituality, and Medicine: Towards the Making of the Healing Practitioner*. Binghamton, N.Y.: Haworth Press.

King, D. E., & Bushwick, B. (1994). Beliefs and attitudes of hospital inpatients about faith healing and prayer. *Journal of Family Practice*, 39, 349–352.

King, D. E., Sobal, J., & DeForge, B. R. (1988). Family practice patients' experiences and beliefs in faith healing. *Journal of Family Practice*, 27, 505–508.

King, D. E., Sobal, J., Haggerty, J., Dent, M., & Patton, D. (1992). Experiences and attitudes about faith healing among family physicians. *Journal of Family Practice*, 35, 158–162.

King, H., & Locke, F. B. (1980). American white Protestant clergy as a low-risk population for mortality research. *Journal of the National Cancer Institute*, 65, 1115–1124.

King, H., Zafros, G., & Hass, R. (1975). Further inquiry into Protestant clerical mortality patterns. *Journal of Biosocial Science*, 7, 243–254.

King, H. G. (1970). Health in the medical and other learned professions. *Journal of Chronic Disease*, 23, 257–281.

King, H. G. (1971). Clerical mortality patterns of the Anglican communion. *Social Biology*, 18, 164–177.

King, H. G., & Bailar, J. C. (1968). Mortality among Lutheran clergymen. *Milbank Memorial Fund Quarterly*, 46, 527–548.

King, H. G., & Bailar, J. C. (1969). The health of the clergy: A review of demographic literature. *Demography*, 6, 27–43.

King, H. G., Diamond, E., & Bailar, J. C. (1965). Cancer mortality and religious preference. *Milbank Memorial Fund Quarterly*, 43, 349–357.

King, K. B. (1997). Psychological and social aspects of cardiovascular disease. *Annals of Behavioral Medicine*, 19, 264–270.

King, M., & Hunt, R. (1967). Dimensions of religiosity in "measuring the religious variable." *Journal for the Scientific Study of Religion*, 6, 173–190.

King, M., & Hunt, R. (1969). Measuring the religious variable: Amended findings. *Journal for the Scientific Study of Religion*, 8, 321–323.

King, Michael B., & Dein, S. (1998). The spiritual variable in psychiatric research. *Psychological Medicine*, 28, 1259–1262.

King, Michael B., Speck, P., & Thomas, A. (1994). Spiritual and religious beliefs in acute illness: Is this a feasible area of study? *Social Science and Medicine*, 38, 631–635.

King, Michael B., Speck, P., & Thomas, A. (1995). The Royal Free Interview for Religious and Spiritual Beliefs: Development and standardization. *Psychological Medicine*, 25, 1125–1134.

King, Michael B., Speck, P., & Thomas, A. (1999). The effect of spiritual beliefs on outcome from illness. *Social Science and Medicine*, 48, 1291–1299.

King, Morton B., & Hunt, R. A. (1972). Measuring the religious variable: Replication. *Journal for the Scientific Study of Religion*, 11, 240–251.

King, Morton B., & Hunt, R. A. (1975). Measuring the religious variable: National replication. *Journal for the Scientific Study of Religion*, 14, 13–22.

King, S. R., Hampton, W. R., Bernstein, B., & Schichor, A. (1996). College students' views on suicide. *Journal of American College of Health*, 44, 283–287.

Kinosian, B., Glick, H., & Garland, G. (1994). Cholesterol and coronary heart disease: Predicting risks by levels and ratios. *Annals of Internal Medicine*, 121, 641–647.

Kinsey, A. C., Pomeroy, W. B., & Martin, C. E. (1953). *Sexual Behavior in the Human Female*. Philadelphia: Saunders.

Kirk, A., & Zucker, R. (1979). Some sociological factrors in attempted suicide among urban black males. *Suicide and Life-Threatening Behavior*, 9(2), 76–86.

Kirk, K. M., Maes, H. H., Neale, M. C., Heath, A. C., Martin, N. G., Eaves, L. J. (1999). Frequency of church attendance in Australia and the United States: models of family resemblance. *Twin Research*, 2, 99–107.

Kirkpatrick, C. (1949). Religion and humanitarianism: A study of institutional implications. *Psychological Monographs*, 63 (4, Whole No. 304).

Kirkpatrick, L. A., & Hood, R. W. (1990). Intrinsic-extrinsic religious orientation: The boon or bane of contemporary psychology of religion. *Journal for the Scientific Study of Religion*, 29, 442–462.

Kirkpatrick, L. A., & Shaver, P. R. (1990). Attachment theory and religion: Childhood attachments, religious beliefs, and conversion. *Journal for the Scientific Study of Religion*, 29, 315–334.

Kirkpatrick, L. A., & Shaver, P. R. (1992). An attachment-theoretical approach to romantic love and religious belief. *Personality and Social Psychology Bulletin*, 18, 266–275.

Kirmayer, L. J., Robbins, J. M., Dworkind, M., & Yaffe, M. J. (1993). Societies and the recognition of depression and anxiety in primary care. *American Journal of Psychiatry*, 150, 734–741.

Kirov, G., Kemp, R., Kirov, K., & David, A. S. (1998). Religious faith after psychotic illness. *Psychopathology*, 31, 234–245.

Kirschling, J. M., & Pittman, J. F. (1989). Measurement of spiritual well-being: A hospice caregiver sample. *Hospice Journal*, 5, 1–11.

Kitagawa, J. M. (1989). Buddhist medical history. In L. E. Sullivan (ed.), *Healing and Restoring: Health and Medicine in the World's Religious Traditions*. New York: Macmillan.

Kitson, G. C., & Sussman, M. (1982). Marital complaints, demographic characteristics, and symptoms of mental distress in divorce. *Journal of Marriage and the Family*, 44, 87–101.

Kivett, V. R. (1979). Religious motivation in middle age: Correlates and implications. *Journal of Gerontology*, 34, 106–115.

Kivett, V. R., Watson, J. A., & Busch, J. C. (1977). The relative importance of physical, psychological, and social variables to locus of control orientation in middle age. *Journal of Gerontology*, 32, 203–210.

Klein, B., Lu, Z. Y., Gallard, J. P., Harousseau, J. L., & Bataille, L. R. (1992). Inhibiting IL-6 in human multiple myeloma. *Current Topics in Micro-Immunology*, 182, 237–243.

Kloos, B., Horneffer, K., & Moore, T. (1995). Before the beginning: Religious leaders perceptions of the possibility for mutual beneficial collaboration with psychologists. *Journal of Community Psychology*, 23, 275–291.

Knapp, M., & Kavanagh, S. (1997). Economic outcomes and costs in the treatment of schizophrenia. *Clinical Therapeutics*, 19, 128–138.

Knekt, P., Raitasaio, R., & Heliovaara, M. (1996). Elevated lung cancer risk among persons with depressed mood. *American Journal of Epidemiology*, 144, 1096–1103.

Knesper, D. J., & Pagnucco, D. J. (1987). Estimated distribution of effort by providers of mental health services to U.S. adults in 1982 and 1983. *American Journal of Psychiatry*, 144, 883–888.

Knudten, R. D., & Knudten, M. S. (1971). Juvenile delinquency, crime, and religion. *Review of Religious Research*, 12, 130–152.

Knupfer, G., & Room, R. (1967). Drinking patterns and attitudes of Irish, Jewish, and white Protestant American men. *Quarterly Journal of Studies on Alcohol*, 28, 676–699.

Koenig, H. G. (1988). Religion and death anxiety in later life. *Hospice Journal*, 4(1), 3–24.

Koenig, H. G. (1990). Research on religion and mental health in later life: A review and commentary. *Journal of Geriatric Psychiatry*, 23, 23–53.

Koenig, H. G. (1994a). *Aging and God: Spiritual Paths to Mental Health in Midlife and Later Years*. Binghamton, N.Y.: Haworth.

Koenig, H. G. (1994b). Religious conversion. In H. G. Koenig, *Aging and God* (pp. 419–438). Binghamton, N.Y.: Haworth.

Koenig, H. G. (1994c). A theory of religious faith development. In H. G. Koenig, *Aging and God* (pp. 105–135). Binghamton, N.Y.: Haworth.

Koenig, H. G. (1995a). Religion and older men in prison. *International Journal of Geriatric Psychiatry*, 10, 219–230.

Koenig, H. G. (1995b). Use of acute hospital services and mortality among religious and non-religious copers with medical illness. *Journal of Religious Gerontology*, 9(3), 1–22.

Koenig, H. G. (1998a). *Handbook of Religion and Mental Health*. San Diego: Academic Press.

Koenig, H. G. (1998b). Religious beliefs and practices of hospitalized medically ill older adults. *International Journal of Geriatric Psychiatry*, 13, 213–224.

Koenig, H. G. (1999). *The Healing Power of Faith*. New York: Simon & Schuster.

Koenig, H. G., & George, L. K. (1998). Depression and physical disability outcomes in depressed medically ill hospitalized older adults. *American Journal of Geriatric Psychiatry*, 6, 230–247.

Koenig, H. G., & Herman, S. (1994). Religion and coping with sexual impotence in later life. *Journal of Religious Gerontology*, 9(1), 73–87.

Koenig, H. G., & Kuchibhatla, M. (1998). Use of health services by hospitalized medically ill depressed elderly patients. *American Journal of Psychiatry*, 155, 871–877.

Koenig, H. G., & Larson, D. B. (1998). Use of hospital services, church attendance, and religious affiliation. *Southern Medical Journal*, 91, 925–932.

Koenig, H. G., & Pritchett, J. (1998). Religion and psychotherapy. In H. G. Koenig (ed.), *Handbook of Religion and Mental Health* (pp. 324–335). San Diego: Academic Press.

Koenig, H. G., & Weaver, A. J. (1997). *Counseling Troubled Older Adults: A Handbook for Pastors and Religious Caregivers*. Nashville: Abingdon.

Koenig, H. G., & Weaver, A. J. (1998): *Pastoral Care of Older Adults*. Minneapolis: Augsburg-Fortress.

Koenig, H. G., Bearon, L., & Dayringer, R. (1989). Physician perspectives on the role of religion in the physician-older patient relationship. *Journal of Family Practice*, 28, 441–448.

Koenig, H. G., George, L. K., & Peterson, B. L. (1998). Religiosity and remission from depression in medically ill older patients. *American Journal of Psychiatry*, 155, 536–542.

Koenig, H. G., George, L. K., & Schneider, R. (1994). Mental health care for older adults in the year 2020: A dangerous and avoided topic. *Gerontologist*, 34, 674–679.

Koenig, H. G., George, L. K., & Siegler, I. (1988). The use of religion and other emotion-regulating coping strategies among older adults. *Gerontologist*, 28, 303–310.

Koenig, H. G., Kvale, J. N., & Ferrel, C. (1988). Religion and well-being in later life. *Gerontologist*, 28, 18–28.

Koenig, H. G., Lamar, T., & Lamar, B. (1997). *A Gospel for the Mature Years: Finding Fulfillment by Knowing and Using Your Gift*. Binghamton, N.Y.: Haworth.

Koenig, H. G., Meador, K. G., & Parkerson, G. (1997). Religion index for psychiatric research. *American Journal of Psychiatry*, 154, 885–886.

Koenig, H. G., Moberg, D. O., & Kvale, J. N. (1988). Religious activities and attitudes of older adults in a geriatric assessment clinic. *Journal of the American Geriatrics Society*, 36, 362–374.

Koenig, H. G., Pargament, K. I., & Nielsen, J. (1998). Religious coping and health status in medically ill hospitalized older adults. *Journal of Nervous and Mental Disease*, 186, 513–521.

Koenig, H. G., Siegler, I. C., & George, L. K. (1989). Religious and non-religious coping: Impact on adaptation in later life. *Journal of Religion and Aging*, 5(4), 73–94.

Koenig, H. G., Smiley, M., & Gonzales, J. (1988). *Religion, Health, and Aging*. Westport, Conn.: Greenwood Press.

Koenig, H. G., Wildman-Hanlon, D., & Schmader, K. (1996). Attitudes of elderly patients and their families toward physician-assisted suicide. *Archives of Internal Medicine*, 156, 2240–2248.

Koenig, H. G., Cohen, H. J., Blazer, D. G., Kudler, H. S., Krishnan, K. R. R., & Sibert, T. E. (1995). Cognitive symptoms of depression and religious coping in elderly medical patients. *Psychosomatics*, 36, 369–375.

Koenig, H. G., Cohen, H. J., Blazer, D. G., Pieper, C., Meador, K. G., Shelp, F., Goli, V., & DiPasquale, R. (1992). Religious coping and depression in elderly hospitalized medically ill men. *American Journal of Psychiatry*, 149, 1693–1700.

Koenig, H. G., Cohen, H. J., George, L. K., Hays, J. C., Larson, D. B., & Blazer, D. G. (1997). Attendance at religious services, interleukin-6, and other biological indicators of immune function in older adults. *International Journal of Psychiatry in Medicine*, 27, 233–250.

Koenig, H. G., Ford, S., George, L. K., Blazer, D. G., & Meador, K. G. (1993). Religion and anxiety disorder: An examination and comparison of associations in young, middle-aged, and elderly adults. *Journal of Anxiety Disorders*, 7, 321–342.

Koenig, H. G., George, L. K., Blazer, D. G., Pritchett, J., & Meador, K. G. (1993). The relationship between religion and anxiety in a sample of community-dwelling older adults. *Journal of Geriatric Psychiatry*, 26(1), 65–93.

Koenig, H. G., George, L. K., Cohen, H. J., Hays, J. C., Blazer, D. G., & Larson, D. B. (1998a). The relationship between religious activities and blood pressure in older adults. *International Journal of Psychiatry in Medicine*, 28, 189–213.

Koenig, H. G., George, L. K., Cohen, H. J., Hays, J. C., Blazer, D. G., & Larson, D. B. (1998b). The relationship between religious activities and cigarette smoking in older adults. *Journal of Gerontology* (medical sciences), 53A, 426–434.

Koenig, H. G., George, L. K., Meador, K. G., Blazer, D. G., & Dyck, P. B. (1994). Religious affiliation and psychiatric disorder in Protestant baby boomers. *Hospital and Community Psychiatry*, 45, 586–596.

Koenig, H. G., George, L. K., Meador, K. G., Blazer, D. G., & Ford, S. M. (1994). The relationship between religion and alcoholism in a sample of community-dwelling adults. *Hospital and Community Psychiatry*, 45, 225–231.

Koenig, H. G., Hays, J. C., George, L. K., Blazer, D. G., Larson, D. B., & Landerman, L. R. (1997). Modeling the cross-sectional relationships between religion, physical health, social support, and depressive symptoms. *American Journal of Geriatric Psychiatry*, 5, 131–143.

Koenig, H. G., Hays, J. C., Larson, D. B., George, L. K., Cohen, H. J., McCullough, M., Meador, K., & Blazer, D. G. (1999). Does religious attendance prolong survival?: A six-year follow-up study of 3,968 older adults. *Journal of Gerontology* (medical sciences) 54A: M370–377.

Koenig, H. G., Hover, M., Bearon, L. B., & Travis, J. L. (1991). Religious perspectives of doctors, nurses, patients and families: Some interesting differences. *Journal of Pastoral Care*, 45, 254–267.

Koenig, H. G., Idler, E., Kasl, S., Hays, J. C., George, L. K., Musick, M., Larson, D. B., Collins, T. B., & Benson, H. (1999). Religion, spirituality, and medicine: A rebuttal to skeptics. *International Journal of Psychiatry in Medicine*, 29, 123–131.

Koenig, H. G., Larson, D. B., Hays, J. C., McCullough, M. E., George, L. K., Branch, P. S., Meador, K. G., & Kuchibhatla, M. (1998). Religion and survival of 1010 male veterans hospitalized with medical illness. *Journal of Religion and Health*, 37, 15–29.

Koenig, H. G., Shelp, F., Goli, V., Cohen, H. J., & Blazer, D. G. (1989). Survival and health-care utilization in elderly medical inpatients with major depression. *Journal of the American Geriatrics Society*, 37, 599–606.

Koenig, H. G., Siegler, I. C., Meador, K. G., & George, L. K. (1990). Religious coping and personality in later life. *International Journal of Geriatric Psychiatry*, 5(2), 123–131.

Koenig, H. G., Weiner, D. K., Peterson, B. L., Meador, K. G., & Keefe F. J. (1998). Religious coping in institutionalized elderly patients. *International Journal of Psychiatry in Medicine*, 27, 365–376.

Kolin, I. S., Scherzer, A. L., New, B., & Garfield, M. (1971). Studies of the school-age child with meningomyelocele: Social and emotional adaptation. *Journal of Pediatrics*, 78, 1013–1019.

Kong, B. W., Miller, J. M., & Smoot, R. T. (1982). Churches as high blood pressure control centers. *Journal of the National Medical Association*, 74, 920–923.

Koopman, C., Hermanson, K., Diamond, S., Angell, K., & Spiegel, D. (1998). Social support, life stress, pain and emotional adjustment to advanced breast cancer. *Psycho-Oncology*, 7, 101–111.

Koos, J. D. (1977). Social process, healing, and self-defeat among Puerto Rican spiritists. *American Ethnology*, 4, 453–460.

Kosmin, B. A., & Lachman, S. P. (1993). *One Nation under God*. New York: Harmony.

Koss, J. D. (1987). Expectations and outcomes for patients given mental health care or spiritist healing in Puerto Rico. *American Journal of Psychiatry*, 144, 56–61.

Kosten, T. R., Markou, A., & Koob, G. F. (1998). Depression and stimulant dependence: neurobiology and pharmacotherapy. *Journal of Nervous and Mental Disease*, 186(12), 737–745.

Kotarba, J. A. (1983). Perceptions of death, belief systems and the process of coping with chronic pain. *Social Science and Medicine*, 17, 681–689.

Kowey, P. R., Friehling, T. D., & Marinchak, R. A. (1986). Prayer-meeting cardioversion. *Annals of Internal Medicine*, 104, 727–728.

Kozma, A., & Stones, M. J. (1978). Some research issues and findings in the study of psychological well-being in the aging. *Canadian Psychological Review*, 19, 241–249.

Kraeplin, E. (1899). Studirende und Ärtzte. In *Psychiatrie: Ein Lehrbuch für Studirende und Ärtze*, Vol. 1. Leipzig: Von Johann Ambrosius Barth.

Kraft, W. A., Litwin, W. J., & Barber, S. E. (1986). Religious orientation and assertiveness: Relationship to death anxiety. *Journal of Social Psychology*, 127, 93–95.

Kranitz, L., Abrahams, J., Spiegel, D., & Keith-Spiegel, P. (1968). Religious beliefs of suicidal patients. *Psychological Reports*, 22, 936.

Krause, N. (1991). Stress, religiosity, and abstinence from alcohol. *Psychology and Aging*, 6, 134–144.

Krause, N. (1992). Stress, religiosity, and psychological well-being among older blacks. *Journal of Aging and Health*, 4, 412–439.

Krause, N. (1993). Measuring religiosity in later life. *Research on Aging*, 15, 170–197.

Krause, N. (1995). Religiosity and self-esteem among older adults. *Journal of Gerontology*, 50, P236–P246.

Krause, N. (1996). Embedding measures of religion in later studies on health: The SWAN project as a case study. Paper presented at the Fetzer Institute and National Institute on Aging, July 22–23, Kalamazoo, Michigan.

Krause, N. (1997). Religion, aging, and health: Current status and future prospects. *Journal of Gerontology*, 52B, S291–S293.

Krause, N. (1998a). Neighborhood deterioration, religious coping, and changes in health during late life. *Gerontologist*, 38, 653–664.

Krause, N. (1998b). Stressors in highly valued roles, religious coping, and mortality. *Psychology and Aging*, 13, 242–255.

Krause, N., & Van Tran, T. (1989). Stress and religious involvement among older Blacks. *Journal of Gerontology*, 44, S4–S13.

Krause, N., Herzog, A. R., & Baker, E. (1992). Providing support to others in well-being in later life. *Journal of Gerontology*, 47, P300–P311.

Krause, S. J., Wiener, R. L., & Tait, R. C. (1994). Depression and pain behavior in patients with chronic pain. *Clinical Journal of Pain*, 10, 122–127.

Krieger, D. (1975). The imprimatur of nursing. *American Journal of Nursing*, 5, 784–787.

Kroenke, K., & Mangelsdorff, A. D. (1989). Common symptoms in ambulatory care: Incidence, evaluation, therapy, and outcome. *American Journal of Medicine*, 86, 262–266.

Kroll, J. (1973). A reappraisal of psychiatry in the middle ages. *Archives of General Psychiatry*, 29, 276–283.

Kroll, J., & Bachrach, B. (1984). Sin and mental illness in the Middle Ages. *Psychological Medicine*, 14, 507–514.

Kroll, J., & Sheehan, W. (1989). Religious beliefs and practices among 52 psychiatric inpatients in Minnesota. *American Journal of Psychiatry*, 146, 67–72.

Kronfol, Z., Silva, J., & Greden, J. (1983). Impaired lymphocyte function in depressive illness. *Life Science*, 33, 241–247.

Krull, C., & Trovato, F. (1994). The quiet revolution and the sex differential in Quebec's suicide rates: 1931–1986. *Social Forces*, 72(4), 1121–1147.

Krupinski, J. (1966). Attempted suicides admitted to the mental health department, Victoria, Australia: A socio-epidemiological study. *International Journal of Social Psychiatry*, 13, 5–13.

Kuemmerer, J. M., & Comstock, G. W. (1967). Sociologic concomitants of tuberculin sensitivity. *American Review of Respiratory Diseases*, 96, 885–892.

Kuhlman, K. (1962). *I Believe in Miracles*. Englewood Cliffs, N.J.: Prentice Hall.

Kuhn, C. C. (1988). A spiritual inventory of the medically ill patient. *Psychiatric Medicine*, 6, 87–100.

Kulik, J. A., & Mahler, H. I (1993). Emotional support as a moderator of adjustment and compliance after coronary artery bypass surgery: a longitudinal study. *Journal of Behavioral Medicine*, 16, 45–63.

Kulka, R. A., Veroff, J., & Douvan, E. (1979). Social class and the use of professional help for personal problems: 1957 and 1976. *Journal of Health and Social Behavior*, 20, 2–17.

Kulkarni, S., O'Farrell, I., Erasi, M., & Kochar, M. S. (1998). Stress and hypertension. *Wisconsin Medical Journal*, 97(11), 34–38.

Kumanyika, S. K., & Charleston, J. B. (1992). Lose weight and win: A church-based weight loss program for blood pressure control among Black women. *Patient Education and Counseling*, 19, 19–32.

Kumpfer, K. L., Molgaard, V., & Spoth, R. (1996). The strengthening families program for the prevention of delinquency and drug use. In R. Peters & R. J. McMahon (eds.), *Preventing Childhood Disorders, Substance Abuse, and Delinquency*. Banff International Behavioral Science Series, Vol. 3 (pp. 241–267). Thousand Oaks, Calif.: Sage.

Kune, C. A., Kune, S., & Watson, L. F. (1992). The effect of family history of cancer, religion, parity and migrant status on survival in colo-rectal cancer. *European Journal of Cancer*, 28A, 1484–1487.

Kune, C. A., Kune, S., Watson, L. F., & Bahnson, C. B. (1991). Personality as risk factor in large-bowel cancer. *Psychological Medicine*, 21, 29–41.

Kunkel, S. R., & Applebaum, R. A. (1992). Estimating the prevalence of long-term disability for an aging society. *Journal of Gerontology* (social sciences), 47, S253–S260.

Kunz, P. R., & Albrecht, S. L. (1977). Religion, marital happiness, and divorce. *International Journal of Sociology of the Family*, 7, 227–232.

Kunzendorff, R. (1985). Repressed fear of inexistence and its hypnotic recovery in religious students. *Omega Journal of Death and Dying*, 16: 23–33.

Kurtz, M. E., Wyatt, G., & Kurtz, J. C. (1995). Psychological and spiritual well-being, philosophical/spiritual views, and health habits of long-term cancer survivors. *Health Care for Women International*, 16, 253–262.

Kushner, M. G., Sher, K. J., & Beitman, B. D. (1990) The relation between alcohol problems and the anxiety disorders [see comments]. *American Journal of Psychiatry*, 147(6): 685–695.

Kutner, S. J. (1971). A survey of fear of pregnancy and depression. *Journal of Psychology*, 79, 263–272.

Kvale, J. N., Koenig, H. G., & Ferrel, C. (1989). Life satisfaction of the aging woman religious. *Journal of Religion and Aging*, 5(4), 68–72.

Kvaraceus, W. (1944). Delinquent behavior and church attendance. *Sociology and Social Research*, 28, 284–289.

Ladwig, K. H., Kieser, M., Konig, M., Breithardt, G., & Borggrefe, M. (1991). Affective disorders and survival after acute myocardial infarction: Results from the post-infarction late-potential study. *European Heart Journal*, 12, 959–964.

LaHaye, T. (1974). *How to Win over Depression*. Grand Rapids, Mich.: Zondervan.

Lamison-White, L. (1992). Income, poverty, and wealth in the United States: A chart book. *Current Population Reports*. U.S. Bureau of Census, Series P-60, No. 179. Washington, D.C.: U.S. Government Printing Office.

Landis, B. J. (1996). Uncertainty, spiritual well-being, and psychosocial adjustment to chronic illness. *Issues in Mental Health Nursing*, 17, 217–231.

Landis, J. L., Maes, H. H. (1999). Adolescent religiousness and its influence on substance use: preliminary findings from the Mid-Atlantic School-age Twin study. *Twin Research*, 2, 156–168.

Landis, J. R., & Koch, G. G. (1977). The measurement of observer agreement for categorical data. *Biometrics*, 33, 159–174.

Landsbergis, P. A., Schnall, P. L., & Warren, K. (1994). Association between ambulatory blood pressure and alternative formulations of job stress. *Scandinavian Journal of Work, Environment, and Health*, 20, 349–363.

Lannert, J. L. (1991). Resistance and countertransference issues with spiritual and religious clients. *Journal of Humanistic Psychology*, 31, 68–76.

Lannin, D. R., Mathews, H. F., Mitchell, J., Swanson, M. S., Swanson, F. H., & Edwards, M. S. (1998). Influences of socioeconomic and cultural factors on racial differences in late-stage presentation of breast cancer. *Journal of the American Medical Association*, 279, 1801–1807.

Lapane, K. L., Lasater, T. M., Allan, C., & Carleton, R. A. (1997). Religion and cardiovascular disease risk. *Journal of Religion and Health*, 36(2), 155–163.

Larson, B. (1968). *Living on the Growing Edge*. Grand Rapids, Mich.: Zondervan.

Larson, D. B., & Greenwold, M. A. (1995). Are religion and spirituality clinically relevant in health care? *Mind/Body Medicine*, 1(3), 147–157.

Larson, D. B., & Wilson, W. P. (1980). Religious life of alcoholics. *Southern Medical Journal*, 73, 723–727.

Larson, D. B., Donahue, M. J., Lyons, J. S., Benson, P. L., Pattison, M., Worthington, E. L., & Blazer, D. G. (1989). Religious affiliations in mental health research samples as compared with national samples. *Journal of Nervous and Mental Disease*, 177, 109–111.

Larson, D. B., Hohmann, A. A., Kessler, L. G., Meador, K. G., Boyd, J. H., & McSherry, E. (1988). The couch and the cloth: The need for linkage. *Hospital and Community Psychiatry*, 39, 1064–1069.

Larson, D. B., Koenig, H. G., Kaplan, B. H., Greenberg, R. S., Logue, E., & Tyroler, H. A. (1989). The impact of religion on men's blood pressure. *Journal of Religion and Health*, 28, 265–278.

Larson, D. B., Lu, F. G., & Swyers, J. P. (1997). *Model curriculum for psychiatric residency training programs: Religion and spirituality in clinical practice, a course outline*. Rockville, Md.: National Institute for Healthcare Research.

Larson, D. B., Pattison, E. M., Blazer, D. G., Omran, A. R., & Kaplan, B. H. (1986). Systematic analysis of research on religious variables in four major psychiatric journals, 1978–1982. *American Journal of Psychiatry*, 143, 329–334.

Larson, D. B., Sherrill, K. A., Lyons, J. S., Craige, F. C., Thielman, S. B., Greenwold, M. A., & Larson, S. S. (1992). Dimensions and valences of measures of religious commitment found in the *American Journal of Psychiatry and the Archives of General Psychiatry*, 1978–1989. *American Journal of Psychiatry*, 149, 557–559.

Larson, D. B., Swyers, J. P., & Larson, S. (1995). *The Costly Consequences of Divorce*. Rockville, Md.: National Institute for Healthcare Research.

Larson, D. B., Swyers, J. P., & McCullough, M. E. (1997). *Scientific Research on Spirituality and Health: A Consensus Report*. Rockville, Md.: National Institute for Healthcare Research.

Larson, D. B., Thielman, S. B., Greenwold, M. A., Lyons, J. S., Post, S. G., Sherrill, K. A., Wood, G. G., & Larson, S. S. (1993). Religious content in the DSM-III-R glossary of technical terms. *American Journal of Psychiatry*, 150, 1884–1885.

Larson, E. J., & Witham, L. (1997). Scientists are still keeping the faith. *Nature*, April 3, 435–436.

Larson, L. E., & Goltz, J. W. (1989). Religious participation and marital commitment. *Review of Religious Research*, 30, 387–400.

Lasater, T. M., Wells, B. L., Carleton, R. A., & Elder, J. P. (1986). The role of churches in disease prevention research studies. *Public Health Reports*, 101, 125–131.

Lasker, J. N., Lohmann, J., & Toedter, L. (1989). The role of religion in bereavement: The case of pregnancy loss. Paper presented at the Society for the Scientific Study of Religion, Salt Lake City, Utah.

Lawton, M. P. (1975). The Philadelphia Geriatric Center Morale Scale: A revision. *Journal of Gerontology*, 30, 85–89.

Lee, D. E. (1987). The self-deception of the self-destructive. *Perceptual and Motor Skills*, 65(3), 975–989.

Lee, G. R., & Ishii-Kuntz, M. (1987). Social interaction, loneliness, and emotional well-being among the elderly. *Research on Aging*, 9, 359–482.

Lefcourt, H. M., & Davidson-Katz, K. (1991). Locus of control and health. In C. R. S. D. R. Forsyth (ed.), *Handbook of Social and Clinical Psychology* (pp. 246–266). New York: Pergamon.

Lefcourt, H. M., Sordoni, C., & Sordoni, C. (1974). Locus of control, field dependence, and the expression of humor. *Journal of Personality*, 42, 130–143.

Lehman, C., Rodin, J., McEwen, B. S., & Brinton, R. (1991). Impact of environmental stress on the expression of insulin-dependent diabetes mellitus. *Behavioral Neurosciences*, 105, 241–245.

Lehr, E., & Spilka, B. (1989). Religion in the introductory psychology textbook: A comparison of three decades. *Journal for the Scientific Study of Religion*, 28, 366–371.

Lehr, I., Messinger, H. B., & Rosenman, R. H. (1973). A sociobiological approach to the study of coronary heart disease. *Journal of Chronic Disease*, 26, 13–30.

Lehrer, E. L., & Chiswick, C. U. (1993). Religion as a determinant of marital stability. *Demography*, 30, 385–404.

Leivers, S., Serra, P. I., & Watson, J. S. (1986). Religion and visiting hospitalized old people: Sex differences. *Psychological Reports*, 58, 705–706.

Leland, J. (1998). God vs. gangs. What's the hottest idea in crime fighting? The power of religion. *Newsweek* (June 1), 20–25.

Lemere, F. (1953). What happens to alcoholics. *American Journal of Psychiatry*, 109, 674–676.

Leming, M. R. (1980). Religion and death: A test of Homans' thesis. *Omega: Journal of Death and Dying*, 10, 347–359.

Lemon, F. R., & Kuzma, J. W. (1969). A biologic cost of smoking: Decreased life expectancy. *Archives of Environmental Health*, 18, 950–955.

Lemon, F. R., & Walden, R. T. (1966). Death from respiratory system disease among Seventh-Day Adventist men. *Journal of the American Medical Association*, 198, 137–146.

Lemon, F. R., Walden, R. T., & Woods, R. W. (1964). Cancer of the lung and mouth in Seventh-Day Adventists. *Cancer*, 17 (April), 486–497.

Lenski, G. (1963). *The Religious Factor*. Garden City, N.Y.: Doubleday

Leonard, W. M. (1982). Successful aging: An elaboration of social and psychological factors. *International Journal of Aging and Human Development*, 14, 223–232.

Leserman, J., Stuart, E. M., Mamish, M. E., & Benson, H. (1989). The efficacy of the relaxation response in preparing for cardiac surgery. *Behavioral Medicine*, 15(3), 111–117.

Lester, D. (1987a). Religion, suicide, and homicide. *Social Psychiatry*, 22(2), 99–101.

Lester, D. (1987b). Religiosity and personal violence: A regional analysis of suicide and homicide rates. *Journal of Social Psychology*, 127(6), 685–686.

Lester, D. (1988). Religion and personal violence (homicide and suicide) in the USA. *Psychological Reports*, 62, 618.

Lester, D. (1992). Religiosity, suicide, and homicide: A cross-national examination. *Psychological Reports*, 71, 1282.

Lester, D. (1996a). Comment on "Jewish affiliation in relation to suicide rates." *Psychological Reports*, 78(3, pt. 1), 834.

Lester, D. (1996b). Religiosity and suicide. *Psychological Reports*, 78, 1090.

Lester, D., & Beck, A. T. (1974). Suicide in the spring: A test of Durkheim's explanation. *Psychological Reports*, 35, 893–394.

Lester, D., & Francis, L. J. (1993). Is religiosity related to suicidal ideation after personality and mood are taken into account? *Personality and Individual Differences*, 15(5), 591–592.

Leuba, J. H. (1896). A study in the psychology of religious phenomena. *American Journal of Psychology*, 5, 309–385.

Leuba, J. H. (1912). *A Psychological Study of Religion*. New York: Macmillan.

Levav, I., & Aisenberg, E. (1989a). The epidemiology of suicide in Israel: International and intranational comparisons. *Suicide and Life-Threatening Behavior*, 19(2), 184–200.

Levav, I., & Aisenberg, E. (1989b). Suicide in Israel: Crossnational comparisons. *Acta Psychiatrica Scandinavia*, 79(5), 468–473.

Levav, I., Kohn, R., Dohrenwend, B. P., Shrout, P. E., Skodol, A. E., Schwartz, S., Link, B. G., & Naveh, G. (1993). An epidemiological study of mental disorders in a 10-year cohort of young adults in Israel. *Psychological Medicine*, 23, 691–707.

Levav, I., Kohn, R., Golding, J. M., & Weissman, M. M. (1997). Vulnerability of Jews to affective disorders. *American Journal of Psychiatry*, 154, 941–947.

Levav, I., Magnes, J., Aisenberg, E., Rosenblum, I., & Gil, R. (1988). Sociodemographic correlates of suicidal ideation and reported attempts: A brief report on a community survey. *Israel Journal of Psychiatry and Related Sciences*, 25(1), 38–45.

Levenson, J. L., Hamer, R. M., & Rossiter, L. F. (1990). Relation of psychopathology in general medical inpatients to use and cost of services. *American Journal of Psychiatry*, 147, 1498–1503.

Levin, J. S. (1984). The role of the Black church in community medicine. *Journal of the National Medical Association*, 76, 477–483.

Levin, J. S. (1993). Age differences in mystical experience. *Gerontologist*, 33, 507–513.

Levin, J. S. (1994). Religion and health: Is there an association, is it valid, and is it causal? *Social Science and Medicine*, 38, 1475–1482.

Levin, J. S. (1996a). How prayer heals: A theoretical model. *Alternative Therapies*, 2(1), 66–73.

Levin, J. S. (1996b). How religion influences morbidity and health: Reflections on natural history, salutogenesis and host resistance. *Social Sciences and Medicine*, 43, 849–864.

Levin, J. S., & Coriel, J. (1986). "New Age" healing in the U.S. *Social Science and Medicine*, 23, 889–897.

Levin, J. S., & Markides, K. S. (1985). Religion and health in Mexican Americans. *Journal of Religion and Health*, 24, 60–69.

Levin, J. S., & Markides, K. S. (1986). Religious attendance and subjective health. *Journal for the Scientific Study of Religion*, 25, 31–40.

Levin, J. S., & Markides, K. S. (1988). Religious attendance and psychological well-being in middle-aged and older Mexican Americans. *Sociological Analysis*, 49, 66–72.

Levin, J. S., & Schiller, P. L. (1986). Religion and the multidimensional health locus of control scales. *Psychological Reports*, 69, 26.

Levin, J. S., & Schiller, P. L. (1987). Is there a religious factor in health? *Journal of Religion and Health*, 26, 9–36.

Levin, J. S., & Taylor, R. J. (1993). Gender and age differences in religiosity among black Americans. *Gerontologist*, 33, 16–23.

Levin, J. S., & Taylor, R. J. (1997). Age differences in patterns and correlates of the frequency of prayer. *Gerontologist*, 37, 75–88.

Levin, J. S., & Vanderpool, H. Y. (1987). Is frequent religious attendance *really* conducive to better health? Toward an epidemiology of religion. *Social Science and Medicine*, 24, 589–600.

Levin, J. S., & Vanderpool, H. Y. (1989). Is religion therapeutically significant for hypertension? *Social Science and Medicine*, 29, 69–78.

Levin, J. S., Chatters, L. M., Ellison, C. G., & Taylor, R. J. (1996). Religious involvement, health outcomes, and public health practice. *Current Issues in Public Health*, 2, 220–225.

Levin, J. S., Chatters, L. M., & Taylor, R. J. (1995). Religious effects on health status and life satisfaction among black Americans. *Journal of Gerontology* (social sciences), 50B, S154–S163.

Levin, J. S., Jenkins, C. D., & Rose, R. M. (1988). Religion, type A behavior, and health. *Journal of Religion and Health*, 27, 267–278.

Levin, J. S., Larson, D. B., & Puchalski, C. M. (1997). Religion and spirituality in medicine: Research and education. *Journal of the American Medical Association*, 178, 792–793.

Levin, J. S., Lyons, J. S., & Larson, D. B. (1993). Prayer and health during pregnancy: Findings from the Galveston Low Birthweight Survey. *Southern Medical Journal*, 86, 1022–1027.

Levin, J. S., Markides, K. S., & Ray, L. A. (1996). Religious attendance and psychological well-being in Mexican Americans: A panel analysis of three-generations data. *Gerontologist*, 36, 454–463.

Levin, J. S., Taylor, R. J., & Chatters, L. M. (1994). Race and gender differences in religiosity among older adults: Findings from four national surveys. *Journal of Gerontology: Social Sciences*, 49, S137–S145.

Levin, J. S., Taylor, R. J., & Chatters, L. M. (1995). A multidimensional measure of religious involvement for African Americans. *Sociological Quarterly*, 36, 157–173.

Levin, J. S., Wickramasekera, I. E., & Hirschberg, C. (1998). Is religiousness a correlate of absorption? Implications for psychophysiology, coping, and morbidity. *Alternative Therapies in Health and Medicine*, 4 (6), 72–77.

Levine, J. B., Covino, N. A., Slack, W. V., Safran, C., Safran, D. B., Boro, J. E., Davis, R. B., Buchanan, G. M., & Gervino, E. V. (1996). Psychological predictors of subsequent medical care among patients hospitalized with cardiac disease. *Journal of Cardiopulmonary Rehabilitation*, 16, 109–116.

Levinson, R. M., Fuchs, J. A., Stoddard, R. R., Jones, D. H., & Mullet, M. (1989). Behavioral risk factors in an Amish community. *American Journal of Preventive Medicine*, 5, 150–156.

Levinton, L. C., & Cook, T. D. (1981). What differentiates meta-analysis from other forms of review? *Journal of Personality*, 49, 231–236.

Levy, S., Herberman, R. B., Lee, J., Whiteside, I., Kirkwood, J., & McFeeley, S. (1990). Estrogen receptor concentration and social factors as predictors of natural killer cell activity in early-stage breast cancer patients. *Natural Immunity and Cell Growth Regulation*, 9, 313–324.

Levy, S., Lee, J., Bagley, C., & Lippman, Gamma (1988). Survival hazards analysis in first recurrent breast cancer patients: The seven-year follow-up. *Psychosomatic Medicine*, 50, 520–528.

Levy, S., Lippman, M., & d'Angelo, T. (1987). Correlation of stress factors with sustained suppression of natural killer cell activity and predictive prognosis in patients with breast cancer. *Journal of Clinical Oncology*, 5, 348–353.

Lewis, C., & Whalin, W. T. (1998). *First Place: The Original Spiritually Based Weight Loss Plan for Whole Person Fitness*. Nashville: Broadman & Holdman.

Leyser, Y. (1994). Stress and adaptation in orthodox Jewish families with a disabled child. *American Journal of Orthopsychiatry*, 31, 376–385.

Liberson, D. M. (1956). Causes of death among Jews in New York City in 1953. *Jewish Social Studies*, 18, 83–117.

Lilienfeld, A. M., Levin, M. L., & Kessler, I. I. (1972). Mortality and marital status. In A. M. Lilienfeld, M. L. Levin, & I. I. Kessler (eds.), *Cancer in the United States*. Cambridge, Mass.: Harvard University Press.

Linden, W., & Feuerstein, M. (1981). Essential hypertension and social coping behavior. *Journal of Human Stress*, March, 28–34.

Lindenthal, J. J., Myers, J. K., Pepper, M. P., & Stern, M. S. (1970). Mental status and religious behavior. *Journal for the Scientific Study of Religion*, 9, 143–149.

Lindgren, K. N., & Coursey, R. D. (1995). Spirituality and serious mental illness: A two-part study. *Psychosocial Rehabilitation Journal*, 18(3), 93–111.

Lipid Research Clinics Coronary Primary Prevention Trial (1984). The Lipid Research Clinics coronary primary prevention trial results: I. Reduction in incidence of coronary heart disease. *Journal of the American Medical Association*, 251, 351–364.

Lipsmeyer, M. E. (1984). The measurement of religiosity and its relationship to mental health impairment. *Dissertation Abstracts International*, 45, 1918–1919.

Livingston, I. L., Levine, D. M., & Moore, R. D. (1991). Social integration and black intraracial variation in blood pressure. *Ethnicity and Disease*, 1(2), 135–149.

Lloyd, C. E., Robinson, N., Stevens, L. K., & Fuller, J. H. (1991). The relationship between stress and the development of diabetic complications. *Diabetic Medicine*, 8,146–150.

Lo, B., Quill, T., & Tulsky, J. (1999). Discussing palliative care with patients. *Annals of Internal Medicine*, 130, 744–749.

Locke, F. B., & King, H. (1980). Mortality among Baptist clergymen. *Journal of Chronic Disease*, 33, 581–590.

Loewenthal, K. N., & Cornwall, N. (1993). Religiosity and perceived control of life events. *International Journal for the Psychology of Religion*, 3, 39–45.

Long, D. D., & Miller, B. J. (1991). Suicidal tendency and multiple sclerosis. *Health and Social Work*, 16, 104–109.

Long, J. D., Anderson, J., & Williams, R. L. (1990). Life reflections by older kinsmen about critical life issues. *Educational Gerontology*, 16, 61–71.

Long, J. V. F., & Scherl, D. J. (1984). Developmental antecedents of compulsive drug use: A report on the literature. *Journal of Psychoactive Drugs*, 16, 169–182.

Long, K. A., & Boik, R. J. (1993). Predicting alcohol use in rural children: A longitudinal study. *Nursing Research*, 42, 79–86.

LoPresto, C. T., Sherman, M. F., & DiCarlo, M. A. (1994–1995). Factors affecting the unacceptability of suicide and the effects of evaluator depression and religiosity. *Omega: Journal of Death and Dying*, 30(3), 205–221.

Loprinzi, C. L., Laurie, J. A., Wieand, H. S., Krook, J. E., Novotny, P. J., Kugler, J. W., Bartel, J., Law, M., Bateman, M., & Klatt, N. E. (1994). Prospective evaluation of prognostic variables from patient-completed questionnaires. *Journal of Clinical Oncology*, 12, 601–607.

Lorch, B. R., & Hughes, R. H. (1985). Religion and youth substance use. *Journal of Religion and Health*, 24, 197–208.

Lorch, B. R., & Hughes, R. H. (1988). Church, youth, alcohol and drug education programs and youth substance use. *Journal of Alcohol and Drug Education*, 33, 14–26.

Loue, S., Lane, S. D., Lloyd, L. S., & Loh, L. (1999). Integrating Buddhism and HIV prevention in US southeast Asian communities. *Journal of Health Care for the Poor and Underserved*, 10, 100–121.

Lourdes (1999). Our Lady of Lourdes. All 64 cures pronounced "miraculous" by the Church—briefly described by Dr. Magiapan, President of the Medical Bureau of Lourdes. (http://abbey.

apana.org.au/Bvm/LOURDES/Homepage. htm).

Lovekin, A., & Malony, H. N. (1977). Religious glossolalia: A longitudinal study of personality changes. *Journal for the Scientific Study of Religion*, 16, 383–393.

Loveland, G. G. (1968). The effects of bereavement on certain religious attitudes and behaviors. *Sociological Syposium*, 1, 17–27.

Low, J. F. (1997). Religious orientation and pain management. *American Journal of Occupational Therapy*, 51, 215–219.

Lowis, M. J., & Hughes, J. (1997). The comparison of the effects of sacred and secular music on elderly people. *Journal of Psychology*, 13, 45–55.

Lown, B., Verrier, R. L., & Rabinowtiz, S. H. (1977). Neural and psychologic mechanisms and the problem of sudden cardiac death. *American Journal of Cardiology*, 39, 890–902.

Lu, Z. Y., Brailly, H., Wijdenes, J., Bataille, R., Rosse, J. F., & Klein, B. (1995). Measurement of whole blood interleukin-6 (IL-6) production: Prediction of the efficacy of anti-IL-6 treatments. *Blood*, 86, 3123–3131.

Lubin, B., Zuckerman, M., Breytspraak, L. M., Bull, N. C., Gumbhir, A. K., & Rinck, C. M. (1988). Affects, demographic variables, and health. *Journal of Clinical Psychology*, 44, 131–141.

Lukianowicz, N. (1968). Attempted suicide in children. *Acta Psychiatrica Scandinavia*, 44, 415–435.

Lukl, P. (1971). Stress and heart disease. *Cardiovascular Clinics*, 2, 143–149.

Lukoff, D., Lu, F., & Turner, R. (1992). Toward a more culturally sensitive DSM-IV: Psychoreligious and psychospiritual problems. *Journal of Nervous and Mental Disease*, 180, 673–682.

Luna, A., Osuna, E., Zurera, L., Gracia-Pastor, M. V., & Castillo del Toro, L. (1992). The relationship between perception of alcohol and drug harmfulness and alcohol consumption by university students. *Medicine and Law*, 11, 3–10.

Lund, D. A., Caserta, M. S., & Dimond, M. F. (1989). A comparison of bereavement adjustments between Mormon and non-Mormon older adults. *Journal of Religion and Aging*, 5(1/2), 75–92.

Lundy, J., Raaf, J. H., Deakins, S., Wanebo, H. J., Jacobs, D. A., Lee, T., Jacobowitz, D., Spear, C., & Oettgen, H. F. (1975). The acute and chronic effects of alcohol on the human immune system. *Surgery, Gynecology and Obstetrics*, 141, 212–218.

Lupien, S., Lecours, A. R., & Lussier, I. (1994). Basil cortisol levels and cognitive deficits in human aging. *Journal of Neurosciences*, 14, 2893–2903.

Lutgendorf, S. (1997). IL-6 level, stress, and spiritual support in older adults. Psychology Department, University of Iowa and Iowa City. Personal communcation, May 1997.

Lyles, M. R., Wilson, W. P., & Larson, D. B. (1983). Mental health and discipleship. *Journal of Psychology and Christianity*, 2, 62–66.

Lynch, J. J. (1977). *The Medical Consequences of Loneliness.* New York: Basic Books.

Lynch, W. D. (1993). The potential impact of health promotion on health care utilization: An introduction to demand management. *Association for Worksite Health Promotion Practitioners' Forum*, 8, 87–92.

Lynskey, M. T. (1998). The comorbidity of alcohol dependence and affective disorders: treatment implications. *Drug & Alcohol Dependence*, 52, 201–209.

Lyon, J. L., Bishop, C. T., & Nielsen, N. S. (1981). Cerebrovascular disease in Utah, 1968–1971. *Stroke*, 12, 564–566.

Lyon, J. L., Gardner, J. W., Klauber, M. R., & Smart, C. R. (1977). Low cancer incidence and morality in Utah. *Cancer*, 39, 2608–2618.

Lyon, J. L., Klauber, M. R., Gardner, J. W., & Smart, C. R. (1976). Cancer incidence in Mormons and non-Morons in Utah, 1966–1970. *New England Journal of Medicine*, 294, 129–133.

Lyon, J. L., Wetzler, H. P., Gardner, J. W., Klauber, M. R., & Williams, R. R. (1978). Cardiovascular mortality in Mormons and non-Mormons in Utah, 1969–1971. *American Journal of Epidemiology*, 108(5), 357–366.

MacDonald, C. B., & Luckett, J. B. (1983). Religious affiliation and psychiatric diagnoses. *Journal for the Scientific Study of Religion*, 22, 15–37.

MacDonald, D. I. 1984. *Drugs, Drinking, and Adolescents.* Chicago: Year Book Medical.

Macdonald, S. (1996). Faith is good medicine, family physicians agree. *Seattle Times* (December 28).

MacGregor, R. R. (1986) Alcohol and immune defense. *Journal of the American Medical Association*, 256, 1474–1479.

Mackenbach, J. P., Kunst, A. E., Devrij, J. H., & VanMeel, D. (1993). Self-reported morbidity and disability among Trappist and Benedictine monks. *American Journal of Epidemiology*, 138, 569–573.

MacKenzie, G., & Blaney, R. (1985). Further correlates of problem drinking in Northern Ireland from a population study. *International Journal of Epidemiology*, 14(3), 410–414.

MacLean, C. R., Walton, K. G., Wenneberg, S. R., Levitsky, D. K., Mandarino, J. V., Waziri, R., Hillis, S. L., & Schneider, R. H. (1997). Effects of the transcendental meditation program on adaptive mechanisms: Changes in hormone levels and responses to stress after four months of practice. *Psychoneuroendocrinology*, 22, 277–295.

MacLean, C. R., Walton, K. G., Wenneberg, S. R., Levitsky, D. K., Mandarino, J. V., Waziri, R., & Schneider, R. H. (1994). Altered responses of cortisol, GH, TSH and testosterone to acute stress after four months' practice of transcendental meditation (TM). *Annals of the New York Academy of Sciences*, 746, 381–384.

MacMahon, B. (1960). The ethnic distribution of cancer mortality in New York City, 1955. *Acta Unio Internationale Contra Cancrum*, 16, 1716–1724.

MacMahon, B., & Koller, E. K. (1957). Ethnic differences in the incidence of leukemia. *Blood*, 12, 1–10.

Maddi, S. R. (1989). *Personality Theories: A Comparative Analysis*, 5th ed. Homewood, Ill.: Dorsey.

Maddox, G. L. (1963). Activity and morale: A longitudinal study of selected elderly subjects. *Social Forces*, 42, 195–204.

Maddox, W. R. (1998). Bawling alone: An epidemic of clinical depression in the midst of material prosperity can be related to the breakdown of family and the decline of civic virtue. *Policy Review*, September-October, 40–42.

Madigan, F. C. (1957). Are sex mortality differentials biologically caused? *Milbank Memorial Fund Quarterly*, 35, 202–223.

Madigan, F. C. (1961). Role satisfactions and length of life in a closed population Catholic priests. *American Journal of Sociology*, 67, 640–649.

Magaletta, P. R., Duckro, P. N., & Staten, S. F. (1997). Prayer in office practice: On the theshold of integration. *Journal of Family Practice*, 44, 254–256.

Magana, A., & Clark, N. M. (1995). Examining a paradox: Does religiosity contribute to positive birth outcomes in Mexican American populations? *Health Education Quarterly*, 22, 96–109.

Magee, J. J. (1987). Determining the predictors of life satisfaction among retired nuns: Report from a pilot project. *Journal of Religion and Aging*, 4(1), 39–49.

Magilvy, J. K., & Brown, N. J. (1997). Parish nursing: Advancing practice nursing. Model for healthier communities. *Advanced Practice Nursing Quarterly*, 2(4), 67–72.

Magni, G., Moreschi, C., Rigatti-Luchini, S., & Merskey, H. (1994). Prospective steady on the relationship between depressive symptoms and chronic musculoskeletal pain. *Pain*, 56, 289–297.

Mahabeer, M., & Bhana, K. (1984). The relationship between religion, religiosity, and death anxiety among Indian adolescents. *South African Journal of Psychology*, 14, 7–9.

Maheswaran, R., Potter, J. F., & Beavers, D. G. (1986). The role of alcohol in hypertension. *Journal of Clinical Hypertension*, 2, 172–178.

Mahoney, E. R. (1980). Religiosity and sexual bahavior among heterosexual college students. *Journal of Sex Research*, 16, 97–113.

Malak, J. (1998). Jehovah's Witnesses and medicine: An overview of beliefs and issues in their care. *Journal of the Medical Association of Georgia*, 87, 322–327.

Maltby, J. (1997). Personality correlates of religiosity among adults in the Republic of Ireland. *Psychological Reports*, 81 (3, Part 1), 827–831.

Malzberg, B. (1973). Mental disease among Jews in New York State, 1960–1961. *Acta Psychiatrica Scandinavica*, 49, 479–518.

Mancini, J. A., & Orthner, D. J. (1980). Situational influences on leisure satisfaction and morality and old age. *Journal of the American Geriatrics Society*, 28, 466–471.

Mandel, A. J. (1980). Toward a psychobiology of transcendence: God in the brain. In R. J. Davidson & J. M. Davidson (eds.), *The Psychobiology of Consciousness* (pp. 379–479). New York: Plenum.

Manfredi, C., & Pickett, M. (1987). Perceived stressful situations and coping strategies utilized by the elderly. *Journal of Community Health Nursing*, 4, 99–110.

Manicourt, D. H., Triki, R., Fukuda, K., Devogelaer, J. P., Nagant de Deuxchaisnes, C., & Thonar, E. J. (1993). Levels of circulating tumor necrosis factor alpha and interleukin-6 in patients with rheumatoid arthritis: Relationship to serum levels of hyaluronan and antigenic keratan sulfate. *Arthritis and Rheumatism*, 36, 490–499.

Mann, S. J., James, G. D., Wang, R. S., & Pickering, T. G. (1991). Elevation of ambulatory systolic blood pressure in hypertensive smokers: A case control study. *Journal of the American Medical Association*, 265, 2226–2228.

Manson, J. E., Colditz, G. A., Stampfer, M. J., Willett, W. C., Rosner, B., Monson, R. R., Speizer,

F. E., & Hennekens, C. H. (1990). A prospective study of obesity and risk of coronary heart disease in women. *New England Journal of Medicine*, 322, 882–889.

Manusov, E. G., Carr. R. J., Rowane, M., Beatty, L. A., & Nadeau, M. T. (1995). Dimensions of happiness: A qualitative study of family practice residents. *Journal of the American Board of Family Practice*, 8, 367–375.

Maranell, G. M. (1967). An examination of some religious and plitical attitude correlates of bigotry. *Social Forces*, 45, 356–362.

Maranell, G. M. (1974). *Responses to Religion*. Lawrence: University Press of Kansas.

Marcus, P., & Rosenberg, A. (1995). The value of religion in sustaining the self in extreme situations. *Psychoanalytic Review*, 82, 81–105.

Marcus, S. C., Olfson, M., Pincus, H. A., Shear, M. K., & Zarin, D. A. (1997). Self-reported anxiety, general medical conditions, and disability bed days. *American Journal of Psychiatry*, 154, 1766–1768.

Margolis, R. D., & Elifson, K. W. (1983). Validation of a typology of religious experience and its relation to the psychotic experience. *Journal of Psychology and Theology*, 11, 135–141.

Maris, R. (1985). The adolescent suicide problem. *Suicide and Life-Threatening Behaviors*, 15, 91–109.

Markides, K. S. (1983). Aging, religiosity, and adjustment: A longitudinal analysis. *Journal of Gerontology*, 38, 621–625.

Markides, K. S., Levin, J. S., & Ray, L. A. (1987). Religion, aging, and life satisfaction: An eight-year, three-wave longitudinal study. *Gerontologist*, 27, 660–665.

Marks, P., & Haller, D. (1977). Now I lay me down for keeps: A study of adolescent suicide. *Journal of Clinical Psychology*, 33, 390–400.

Marks, R. U. (1967). Socioenvironmental stress and cardiovascular disease: A review of empirical findings. *Milbank Memorial Fund Quarterly*, 45, 51–108.

Marland, H., & Pelling, M. (eds.) (1996). *The Task of Healing: Medicine, Religion, and Gender in England and the Netherlands, 1450–1800*. Rotterdam: Erasmus.

Marlatt, G. A. (1985). Relapse prevention: Theoretical rationale and overview of the model. In G. A. Marlatt & J. R. Gordon (eds.), *Relapse Prevention* (pp. 3–70). New York: Gillford.

Marston, M. V. (1970). Compliance with medical regimens: a review of the literature. *Nursing Research*, 19, 312–322.

Martin, A. O., Dunn, J. K., Simpson, J. L., Olsen, C. L., Kemel, S., Grace, M., Elias, S., Sarto, G. E., Smalley, B., & Steinberg, A.G. (1980). Cancer mortality in a human isolate. *Journal of the National Cancer Institute*, 65, 1109–1113.

Martin, C., & Nichols, R. C. (1962). Personality and religious belief. *Journal of Social Psychology*, 56, 3–8.

Martin, D., & Wrightsman, L. S. (1965). The relationship between religious behavior and concern about death. *Journal of Social Psychology*, 65, 317–323.

Martin, J., & Westie, F. (1959). Religious fundamentalism scale in "the tolerant personality." *American Sociological Review*, 24, 521–528.

Martin, W. T. (1984). Religiosity and United States suicide rates, 1972–1978. *Journal of Clinical Psychology*, 40, 1166–1169.

Martin-Baro, I. (1990). Religion as an instrument of psychological warfare. *Journal of Social Issues*, 46, 93–107.

Martinez, F. I. (1991). Therapist-client convergence and similarity of religious values: Their effect on client improvement. *Journal of Psychology and Christianity*, 10, 137–143.

Marx, J. H., & Spray, S. L. (1969). Religious biographies and professional characteristics of psychotherapists. *Journal of Health and Social Behavior*, 10, 275–288.

Massion, A. O., Teas, J., Hebert, J. R., Wertheimer, M. D., & Kabat-Zinn, J. (1995). Meditation, melatonin and breast/prostate cancer: Hypothesis and preliminary data. *Medical Hypothesis*, 44, 39–46.

Masters, K. S., Bergin, A. E., Reynolds, E. M., & Sullivan, C. E. (1991). Religious life-styles and mental health: A follow-up study. *Counseling and Values*, 35, 211–224.

Mathew, R. J. (1995). Measurement of materialism and spiritualism in substance abuse research. *Journal of Studies on Alcohol*, 56, 470–475.

Mathew, R. J., Georgi, J., Wilson, W. H., & Mathew, V. G. (1996). A retrospective study of the concept of spirituality as understood by recovering individuals. *Journal of Substance Abuse Treatment*, 13, 67–73.

Maton, K. I. (1987). Patterns and psychological correlates of material support within a religious setting: The bidirectional support hypothesis. *American Journal of Community Psychology*, 15, 185–208.

Maton, K. I. (1989). The stress-buffering role of spiritual support: Cross-sectional and prospective investigations. *Journal for the Scientific Study of Religion, 28,* 310–323.

Maton, K. I., & Wells, E. A. (1995). Religion as a community resource for well-being: Prevention, healing, and empowerment pathways. *Journal of Social Issues, 51,* 177–193.

Matthews, D. A., & Clark, C. (1998). *The Faith Factor: Proof of the Healing Power of Prayer.* New York: Viking (Penguin-Putnam).

Matthews, D. A., Marlowe, S. M., & MacNutt, F. S. (1999). Effects of intercessory prayer ministry on patients with rheumatoid arthritis (abstract). *Journal of General Internal Medicine, 13*(4, Suppl. 1), 17.

Mattlin, J. A., Wethington, E., & Kessler, R. C. (1990). Situational determinants of coping and coping effectiveness. *Journal of Health and Social Behavior, 31,* 103–122.

Maugans, T. A. (1996). The SPIRITual history. *Archives of Family Medicine, 5,* 11–16.

Maugans, T. A., & Wadland, W. C. (1991). Religion and family medicine: A survey of physicians and patients. *Journal of Family Practice, 32,* 210–213.

Mauldon, J. (1990). The effect of marital disruption on children's health. *Demography, 27,* 431–436.

Mauss, A. L. (1959). Anticipatory socialization toward college as a factor in adolescent marijuana use. *Social Problems, 16,* 357–364.

Mayberry, J. F. (1982). Epidemiological studies of gastrointestinal cancer in Christian sects. *Journal of Clinical Gastroenterology, 4,* 115–121.

Mayer, J., Merril, A., & Myerson, D. J. (1965). Contact and initial attendance at an alcoholism clinic. *Quarterly Journal of Studies on Alcohol, 26,* 480–485.

Mayo, C. C., Puryear, H. B., & Richek, H. G. (1969). MMPI correlates of religiousness in late adolescent college students. *Journal of Nervous and Mental Disease, 149,* 381–385.

McAdams, D. P. (1995). What do we know when we know a person? *Journal of Personality, 63,* 365–396.

McAdams, D. P. (1996). Personality, modernity, and the storied self: A contemporary framework for studying persons. *Psychological Inquiry, 7,* 295–321.

McAdams, D. P., Diamond, A., de St. Aubin, E., & Mansfield, E. (1997). Stories of commitment: The psychosocial construction of generative

lives. *Journal of Personality and Social Psychology, 72,* 678–694.

McAll, R. K. (1982). *Healing the Family Tree.* London: Sheldon.

McAllister, R. J. (1969). The mental health of members of religious communities. *International Psychiatric Clinics,* 211–222.

McAllister, R. J., & Vander Veldt, A. (1961). Factors in mental illness among hospitalized clergy. *Journal of Nervous and Mental Disease, 132,* 80–88.

McAllister, R. J., & Vander Veldt, A. J. (1965). Psychiatric illness in hospitalized Catholic religious. *American Journal of Psychiatry, 121,* 881–884.

McBride, J. L., Arthur, G., Brooks, R., & Pilkington, L. (1998). The relationship between eight patients spirituality and health experiences. *Family Medicine, 30*(2), 122–126.

McCall, P. L., & Land, K. C. (1994). Trends in white male adolescent, young adult, and elderly suicide: Are there common structural factors? *Social Science Research, 23,* 57–81.

McCally, M., Haines, A., Fein, O., Addington, W., Lawrence, R. S., & Cassel, C. K. (1998). Poverty and ill health: Physicians can and should make a difference. *Annals of Internal Medicine, 129,* 726–733.

McCarthy, J. (1979). Religious commitment, affiliation, and marriage dissolution. In R. Wuthnow (ed.), *The Religious Dimension: New Directions in Quantitative Research* (pp. 179–197). New York: Academic Press.

McClelland, D. C. (1988). The effect of motivational arousal through films on salivary immunoglobulin A. *Psychology and Health, 2,* 31–52.

McClelland, J. W., Demark-Wahnefried, W., Musttian, R. D., Cowan, A. T., & Campbell, M. K. (1998). Fruit and vegetable consumption of rural African-Americans: Baseline survey results of the Black Churches United for Better Health 5-A-Day Project. *Nutrition and Cancer, 30,* 148–157.

McClure, R. F., & Loden, M. (1982). Religious activity, denomination membership and life satisfaction. *Psychological Quarterly Journal of Human Behavior, 19,* 12–17.

McConnell, M. (1998). Faith can help you heal. *Reader's Digest* (October), 108–113.

McCracken, L. M., Gross, R. T., Aikens, J., & Carnrike, C. L. (1996). The assessment of anxiety and fear in persons with chronic pain: A comparison of instruments. *Behavior Research in Therapy*, 34, 927–933.

McCrae, R. R., & Costa, P. T. (1986). Personality, coping and coping effectiveness in an adult sample. *Journal of Personality*, 54, 385–405.

McCrae, R. R., & Costa, P. T. (1990). *Personality in Adulthood*. New York: Guilford.

McCullagh, E. P., & Lewis, L. A. (1960). A study of diet, blood lipis and vascular disease in trappist monks. *New England Journal of Medicine*, 263, 569–573.

McCullough, M. E. (1995). Prayer and health: Conceptual issues, research review, and research agenda. *Journal of Psychology and Theology*, 23, 15–29.

McCullough, M. E. (1999). Research on religion-accommodation counseling: Review and meta-analysis. *Journal of Counseling Psychology*, 46, 92–98.

McCullough, M. E., Hoyt, W. T., Larson, D. B., Koenig, H. G., & Thoresen, C. E. (2000). Religious involvement and mortality: A meta-analytic review. *Health Psychology*, 19, 211–222.

McCullough, M. E., Larson, D. B., Koenig, H. G., & Lerner, R. (1999). The mismeasurement of religion: A systematic review of mortality research. *Mortality*, 4, 183–194.

McDowell, D., Galanter, M., Goldfarb, L., & Lifshutz, H. (1996). Spirituality and the treatment of the dually diagnosed: An investigation of patient and staff attitudes. *Journal of Addictive Diseases*, 15(2), 55–68.

McEwen, B. S. (1998). Protective and damaging effects of stress mediators. *New England Journal of Medicine*, 338, 171–179.

McEwen, B. S., & Magarinos, A. M. (1997). Stress effects on morphology and function of the hippocampus. *Annals of the New York Academy of Science*, 821, 271–284.

McEwen, B. S., & Stellar, E. (1993). Stress and the individual mechanisms leading to disease. *Archives of Internal Medicine*, 153, 2093–2101.

McEwen, B. S., Albeck, D., & Cameron, H. (1995). Stress and the brain: A paradoxical role for adrenal steroids. *Vitamins and Hormones*, 51, 371–402.

McEwen, B. S., Biron, C. A., & Brunson, T. W. (1997). The role of adrenocorticoids as modulators of immune function in health and disease: Neural, endocrine, and immune interactions. *Brain Research and Brain Research Reviews*, 23, 79–113.

McGloshen, T. H., & O'Bryant, S. L. (1988). The psychological well-being of older, recent widows. *Psychology of Women Quarterly*, 12, 99–116.

McIntosh, B. R., & Danigelis, N. L. (1995). Race, gender, and the relevance of productive activity for elders' affect. *Journal of Gerontology* (social sciences), 50B, S229–S239.

McIntosh, D., & Spilka, B. (1990). Religion and physical health: The role of personal faith and control beliefs. *Research in the Social Scientific Study of Religion*, 2, 167–194.

McIntosh, D. N., Silver, R. C., & Wortman, C. B. (1993). Religion's role in adjustment to a negative life event: Coping with the loss of a child. *Journal of Personality and Social Psychology*, 65, 812–821.

McIntosh, W. A., Fitch, S. D., Wilson, J. B., & Nyberg, K. L. (1981). The effects of mainstream religious social controls on adolescent drug use in rural areas. *Review of Religious Research*, 23, 54–75.

McKee, D. D., & Chappel, J. N. (1992). Spirituality and medical practice. *Journal of Family Practice*, 35, 201–208.

McLuckie, B. F., Zahn, M., & Wilson, A. (1975). Religious correlates of teenage drug use. *Journal of Drug Issues*, 5(2), 129–139.

McMordie, W. R. (1981). Religiosity and fear of death: Strength of belief system. *Psychological Reports*, 49, 921–922.

McNamara, P. H., & St. George, A. (1979). Measures of religiosity and the quality of life. In D. O. Moberg (ed.), *Spiritual Well-Being: Sociological Perspectives* (pp. 229–236). Washington, D.C.: University Press of America.

McNeill, J. M. (1997). *Americans with disabilities: 1994–95*. Current Population Report C3.186: P-70/2/61. Washington, D.C.: U.S. Department of Commerce.

McNichol, T. (1996). The new faith in medicine. *USA Weekend* (April 5–7), 4–5.

McRae, M. B., Carey, P. M., & Anderson-Scott, R. (1998). Black churches as therapeutic systems: A group process perspective. *Health Education and Behavior*, 25, 778–789.

McSherry, E. (1986). Critical role of VA policymakers in modernizing chaplaincy for major gains in quality of care and economics. *National VA Endorsers Bulletin (NAVAC)*, Winter 1986.

McSherry, E. (1987). The need and appropriateness of measurement and research in chaplaincy: Its criticalness for patient care and chaplain department survival post-1987. *Journal of Health Care Chaplaincy*, 1, 3–41.

McSherry, E., Ciulla, M., Salisbury, S., & Tsuang, D. (1987). Spiritual resources in older hospitalized men. *Social Compass*, 35, 515–537.

McSherry, E., Kratz, D., & Nelson, W. A. (1986). Pastoral care departments: More necessary in the DRG era? *Health Care Management Research*, 11, 47–59.

Meador, K. G., & Koenig, H. G. (2000). Spirituality and religion in psychiatric practice: Parameters and implications. *Psychiatric Annals*, September–October.

Meador, K. G., Koenig, H. G., Turnbull, J., Blazer, D. G., George, L. K., & Hughes, D. (1992). Religious affiliation and major depression. *Hospital and Community Psychiatry*, 43, 1204–1208.

Meaton, J. D., Broste, S., Cohen, L., Fishmen, E. L., Kjelsberg, M. O., & Schoenberger, J. (1981). The multiple risk factor intervention trial (MRFIT): VII. A comparison of risk factor changes between the two study groups. *Preventive Medicine*, 10, 519–543.

Mechanic, D. (1963). Religion, religiosity, and illness behavior: The special case of the Jews. *Human Organization*, 22, 202–208.

Mechanic, D. (1972). *Public Expectations and Health Care: Essays on the Changing Organization of Health Services* (pp. 206–208). New York: Wiley.

Mechanic, D. (1990). Promoting health. *Society*, January/February, 16–22.

Mechanic, D., Clearly, P. D., & Greenly, J. R. (1982). Distress syndromes, illness behavior, access to care, and medical utilization in a defined population. *Medical Care*, 20, 361–372.

Medalie, J. H., Kahn, H. A., Neufeld, H. N., Riss, E., Goldbourt, U., Perlstein, T., & Oron, D. (1973a). Myocardial infarction over a five-year period: I. Prevalence, incidence and mortality experience. *Journal of Chronic Disease*, 26, 63–84.

Medalie, J. H., Kahn, H. A., Neufeld, H. N., Riss, E., & Goldbourt, U. (1973b). Five-year myocardial infarction incidence: II. Association of single variables to age and birthplace. *Journal of Chronic Disease*, 26, 325–349.

Meeks, S., Carstensen, L. L., Stafford, P. B., Brenner, L. L.,Weathers, F., Welch, R., & Oltmanns, T. F. (1990). Mental health needs of the chronically mentally yield elderly. *Psychology and Aging*, 5, 163–171.

Meisenhelder, J. B. (1986). Self-esteem in women: The influence of employment and perception of husbands' appraisals. *Image: Journal of Nursing Scholarship*, 18, 8–14.

Meliska, C. J., Strunkard, M. E., Gilbert, D. J., Jensen, R. A., & Martinko, J. M. (1995). Immune function in cigarette smokers who quit smoking for 31 days. *Journal of Allergy and Clinical Immunology*, 95, 901–910.

Melzack, R. (1982). Recent concepts of pain. *Journal of Medicine*, 13, 147–160.

Melzack, R. (1993). Pain: Past, present and future. *Canadian Journal of Experimental Psychology*, 47, 615–629.

Meneghan, E. G., & Lieberman, M. A. (1986). Changes in depression following divorce. *Journal of Family Issues*, 6, 295–306.

Mercer, D., Lorden, R., & Falkenberg, S. (1995). Mediating effects of religiousness on recovery from victimization. Paper presented at the Annual Meeting of the American Psychological Association, New York City.

Merck Manual of Geriatrics (1995). White House Station, N.J.: Merck & Co.

Merikangas, K. R., Prusoff, B. A., Kupfer, D. J., & Frank, E. (1985). Marital adjustment and major depression. *Journal of Affective Disorders*, 9(1), 5–11.

Merritt, M. M., Bennett, G. G., Williams, R. B. (1999). Low religiosity enhances cardiovascular reactivity among black males with low education. Presented at Annual Meeting of the American Psychosomatic Society, Savannah, Georgia, March 2000.

Meyer, M. S., Altmaier, E. M., & Burns, C. P. (1992). Religious orientation and coping with cancer. *Journal of Religion and Health*, 31, 274–249.

Meyers, A. R., Branch, L. G., Cupples, L. A., Lederman, R. I, Feltin, M., & Master, R. J. (1989). Predictors of medical care utilization by independently living adults with spinal cord injuries. *Archives of Physical Medicine and Rehabilitation*, 70, 471–476.

Miah, M. M. R. (1993). Factors influencing infant/child mortality in Bangladesh: Implication for family planning programs and policies. *International Journal of Sociology of the Family*, 23 (Autumn), 21–34.

Michaels, R. R., Parra, J., McCann, D. S., & Vander, A. J. (1979). Renin, cortisol, and aldosterone during transcendental meditation. *Psychosomatic Medicine*, 41(1), 50–54.

Michaud, E. (1998). Unlock the secret healer within. *Prevention* (December), 106–113.

Michelson, D., Stratakis, C., & Hill, L. (1996). Bone mineral density in women with depression. *New England Journal of Medicine*, 335, 1176–1181.

Mickley, J. R., & Soeken, K. (1993). Religiousness and hope in Hispanic- and Anglo-American women with breast cancer. *Oncology Nursing Forum,* 20, 1171–1177.

Mickley, J. R., Carson, V., & Soeken, K. L. (1995). Religion and adult mental health: State of the science in nursing. *Issues in Mental Health Nursing,* 16, 345–360.

Mickley, J. R., Soeken, K., & Belcher, A. (1992). Spiritual well-being, religiousness, and hope among women with breast cancer. *IMAGE: Journal of Nursing Scholarship,* 24(4), 267–272.

Midanik, L. T., & Clark, W. B. (1995). Drinking-related problems in United States: Description and trends, 1984–1990. *Journal of Studies on Alcohol,* 56, 395–402.

Middleton, W. C., & Putney, S. (1962). Religious, normative standards and behavior. *Sociometry,* 25, 141–152.

Miller, A. M., & Champion, V. L. (1993). Mammography in women greater than or equal to 50 years of age: Predisposing and enabling characteristics. *Cancer Nursing,* 16, 260–269.

Miller, A. S., & Hoffmann, J. P. (1995). Risk and religion: An explanation of gender differences in religiosity. *Journal for the Scientific Study of Religion,* 34, 63–75.

Miller, J. E., Russell, L. B., Davis, D. M., Milan, E., Carson, J. L., & Taylor, W. C. (1998). Biomedical risk factors for acute admission in older adults. *Medical Care,* 36, 411–421.

Miller, J. F. (1985). Assessment of loneliness and spiritual well-being in chronically ill and healthy adults. *Journal of Professional Nursing,* 1, 79–85.

Miller, J. J., Fletcher, K., & Kabat-Zinn, J. (1995). Three-year follow-up and clinical implications of mindfulness meditation-based stress reduction intervention in the treatment of anxiety disorders. *General Hospital Psychiatry,* 17, 192–200.

Miller, L. (1979). Culture and psychopathology of Jews in Israel. *Psychiatric Journal of the University of Ottawa,* 4, 302–306.

Miller, L., Warner, V., Wickramaratne, P., & Weissman, M. (1997). Religiosity and depression: Ten-year follow-up of depressed mothers and offspring. *Journal of the American Academy of Child and Adolescent Psychiatry,* 36, 1416–1425.

Miller, N. H., Hill, M., Kottke, T., & Ockene, I. S. (1997). The multi-level compliance challenge: Recommendations for a call to action—a statement of health-care professionals. *Circulation,* 95, 1085–1090.

Miller, P. Y., & Simon, W. (1974). Adolescent sexual behavior: Context and change. *Social Problems,* 22, 58–76.

Miller, R. N. (1982). Study on the effectiveness of remote mental healing. *Medical Hypotheses,* 8(5), 481–490.

Miller, S. L., Norcross, W. A., & Bass, R. A. (1980). Breast self-examination in the primary care setting. *Journal of Family Practice,* 10, 811–815.

Miller, T. Q., Smith, T. W., Turner, C. W., Guijarro, M. L., & Hallet, A. J. (1996). A meta-analytic review of research on hostility and physical health. *Psychological Bulletin,* 119(2), 322–348.

Miller, T. R., Cohen, M. A., & Wiersema, B. (1996). *Victim Costs and Consequences: A new Look.* Washington, D.C.: National Institute of Justice, U.S. Department of Justice.

Miller, W. R. (1995). Toward a biblical view of drug use. *Journal of Ministry in Addiction and Recovery,* 2, 77–86.

Miller, W. R. (1998). Researching the spiritual dimension of alcohol and other drug problems. *Addiction,* 93(7), 979–990.

Millison, M. B. (1988). Spirituality and the caregiver: Developing and underutilized facet of care. *American Journal of Hospice Care,* 5, 37–44.

Mindel, C. H., & Vaughan, C. E. (1978). A multidimensional approach to religiosity and disengagement. *Journal of Gerontology,* 33, 103–108.

Minear, J. D., & Brush, L. R. (1980–1981). The correlations of attitudes toward suicide with death anxiety, religiosity, and personal closeness. *Omega: Journal of Death and Dying,* 11, 317–324.

Minirth, F. B., Meier, P., & Tournier, P. D. (1994). *Happiness Is a Choice: The Symptoms, Causes, and Cures of Depression.* New York: Baker.

Mireault, M., & deMan, A. (1996). Suicidal ideation among the elderly: Personal variables, stress, and social support. *Social Behavior and Personality,* 24(4), 385–392.

Mitchell, J., Mathews, H. F., & Yesavage, J. A. (1993). A multidimensional examination of depression among the elderly. *Research on Aging,* 15, 198–219.

MMWR (1991). Outbreaks of rubella among the Amish: United States, 1991. *Morbidity and Mortality Weekly Report,* 40 (16), 264–265.

Moberg, D. O. (1953). Church membership and personal adjustment in old age. *Journal of Gerontology,* 8, 207–211.

Moberg, D. O. (1956). Religious activities and personal adjustment in old age. *Journal of Social Psychology,* 43, 261–267.

Moberg, D. O. (1984). Subjective measures of spiritual well-being. *Review of Religious Research,* 25, 351–364.

Moberg, D. O. (1996). Religion in gerontology: From benign neglect to belated respect. *Gerontologist*, 36, 264–267.

Moberg, D. O., & Taves, M. J. (1965). Church participation and adjustment in old age. In A. M. Rose & W. A. Peterson (eds.), *Older People and Their Social World*. Philadelphia: F. A. Davis.

Mohan, D., Sharma, K., & Sundaram, R. (1979). Patterns and prevalence of opium use in rural Punjab (India). *Bulletin on Narcotics*, 31, 45–56.

Mohiuddin, A. (1998). Sufi healing practices. *Journal of the Medical Association of Georgia*, 87, 319–320.

Mohr, D. C., Goodkin, D. E., Likosky, W., Gatto, N., Baumann, K. A., & Rudnick, R. A. (1997). Treatment of depression improves adherence to interferon beta-1b therapy for multiple sclerosis. *Archives of Neurology*, 54, 531–533.

Mol, H. (1970). Religion and sex in Australia. *Australian Journal of Psychology*, 22(2), 105–114.

Mollica, R. F., Streets, F. J., Boscarino, J., & Redlich, F. C. (1986). A community study of formal pastoral counseling activities of the clergy. *American Journal of Psychiatry*, 143, 323–328.

Monk, M., Lilienfield, A., & Mendeloff, A. (1962). Preliminary report of an epidemiologic study of cancers of the colon and rectum. Paper presented at meeting of the epidemiology section, American Public Health Association.

Monte, P. (1991). Attitudes toward the voluntary taking of life: An updated analysis of euthanasia correlates. *Sociological Spectrum*, 11(3), 265–277.

Montgomery, A., & Francis, L. J. (1996). Relationship between personal prayer and school-related attitudes among 11–16-year-old girls. *Psychological Reports*, 78, 787–793.

Montgomery, H. A., Miller, W. R., & Tonigan, S. (1995). Does Alcoholics Anonymous involvement predict treatment outcome? *Journal of Substance Abuse Treatment*, 12, 241–246.

Mookherjee, H. N. (1986). Comparison of some personality characteristics of male problem drinkers in rural Tennessee. *Journal of Alcohol and Drug Education*, 31, 23–28.

Moore, M., & Weiss, S. (1995). Reasons for nondrinking among Israeli adolescents of four religions. *Drug and Alcohol Dependence*, 38, 45–50.

Moore, R. D., Mead, L., & Pearson, T. A. (1990). Youthful precursors of alcohol abuse in physicians. *American Journal of Medicine*, 88, 332–336.

Moore, T. V. (1936). Insanity in priests and religious. *American Ecclesiastical Review*, 95, 485–498, 601–613.

Moos, R. H., Bromet, E., Tsu, V., & Moose, B. (1979). Family characteristics and the outcome of treatment for alcoholism. *Journal of Studies on Alcohol*, 40, 78–88.

Morgan, P. P. (1994). Spirituality slowly gaining recognition among North American psychiatrists. *Canadian Medical Association Journal*, 150, 582–585.

Morphew, J. A. (1968). Religion and attempted suicide. *International Journal of Social Psychiatry*, 14, 188–192.

Morrill, R. L., & Erickson, R. (1968). Hospital service areas, Parts I–IV. Working papers I.3, I.4, I.5, I.6, and I.17. Chicago: Chicago Regional Hospital.

Morris, D. C. (1991). Church attendance, religious activities, and the life satisfaction of older adults in Middletown, U.S.A. *Journal of Religious Gerontology*, 8, 83–96.

Morris, J., Mor, V., & Goldberg, R. (1986). The effect of treatment setting and patient characteristics on pain in terminal cancer patients: the report from the National Hospice Study. *Journal of Chronic Disease*, 39, 27–35.

Morris, J., Suissa, S., & Sherwood, S. (1986). Last days: A steady of the quality of life of terminally ill cancer patients. *Journal of Chronic Disease*, 39, 47–62.

Morris, P. A. (1982). The effect of pilgrimage on anxiety, depression, and religious attitude. *Psychological Medicine*, 12, 291–294.

Morris, P. L. P., Robinson, R. G., Andrzejewski, P., Samuels, J., & Price, T. R. (1993). Association of depression with 10-year post-stroke mortality. *American Journal of Psychiatry*, 150, 124–129.

Morris, R. J., & Hood, R. W. (1981). The generalizability and specificity of intrinsic/extrinsic orientation. *Review of Religious Research*, 22, 245–254.

Morrow, D. J. (1998). Lusting after Prozac. *New York Times* (October 11), section 3, 1, 8.

Morse, C. K., & Wisocki, P. A. (1987). Importance of religiosity to elderly adjustment. *Journal of Religion and Aging*, 4, 15–25.

Mosher, D., & Cross, H. (1971). Sex guilt in premarital sexual experiences of college students. *Journal of Consulting and Clinical Psychology*, 36, 22–32.

Mosher, J. P., & Handal, P. J. (1997). The relationship between religion and psychological distress in adolescents. *Journal of Psychology and Theology*, 25, 449–457.

Moss, M. S., Lawton, M. P., & Glicksman, A. (1991). The role of pain in the last year of life of older persons. *Journal of Gerontology*, 46, 51–57.

Moszczynski, P. (1992). Effect of smoking on the indicators of immunity and the acute-phase reaction in persons professionally exposed to solvents. *Wiadomosci Lekarskie*, 45(5–6), 180–184.

Muchnik, B., & Rosenheim, E. (1982). Fear of death, defense style, and religiosity among Israeli Jews. *Israeli Journal of Psychiatry and Related Services*, 19, 157–164.

Muffler, J., Langrod, J. G., & Larson, D. (1992). There is a balm in Gilead: Religion and substance abuse treatment. In J. H. Lowenson, P. Ruiz, R. B. Millman, & J. G. Langrod (eds.), *Substance Abuse: A Comprehensive Textbook* (pp. 584–595). Baltimore: Williams & Wilkins.

Muhlhauser, I. (1994). Cigarette smoking and diabetes: An update. *Diabetic Medicine*, 11, 336–343.

Mullen, K., & Francis, L. J. (1995). Religiosity and attitudes towards drug use among Dutch school children. *Journal of Alcohol and Drug Education*, 41, 16–25.

Mullen, K., Williams, R., & Hunt, K. (1996). Irish descent, religion, and alcohol and tobacco use. *Addiction*, 91, 243–254.

Mundy, L. (1997). *The Complete Guide to Prayer Walking: A Simple Path to Body-&-Soul Fitness.* New York: Abbey Press.

Murray, D. C. (1973). Suicidal and depressive feelings among college students. *Psychological Reports*, 33(1), 175–181.

Murray, M., & McMillan, C. (1993). Social and behavioral predictors of women's cancer screening practices in Northern Ireland. *Journal of Public Health Medicine*, 15, 147–153.

Murstein, B. I., & Fontaine, P. A. (1993). The public's knowledge about psychologists and other mental health professionals. *American Psychologist*, 48, 839–845.

Musick, M. A. (1996). Religion and subjective health among black and white elders. *Journal of Health and Social Behavior*, 37, 221–237.

Musick, M. A., & Strulowitz, S. (2000). Public religious activity and depressive symptomatology: A comparison of religious groups in the United States. *Social Science and Medicine.*

Musick, M. A., House, J. S., & Williams, D. R. (1999). Attendance at religious services and mortality in a national sample. Paper presented at the Annual Meeting of the American Sociological Association, August 6, Chicago.

Musick, M. A., Koenig, H. G., Hays, J. C., & Cohen, H. J. (1998). Religious activity and depression among community-dwelling elderly persons with cancer: The moderating effect of race. *Journal of Gerontology*, 53B, S218–S227.

Musick, M. A., Williams, D. R., & Jackson, J. S. (1998). Race-related stress, religion and mental health among African American adults. Paper presented at the Seventh International Conference on Social Stress Research, Budapest, Hungary.

Musselman, D. L., Evans, D. L., & Nemeroff, C. B. (1998). The relationship of depression to cardiovascular disease: Epidemiology, biology, and treatment. *Archives of General Psychiatry*, 55, 580–592.

Musselman, D. L., Tomer, A., Manatunga, A. K., Knight, B. T., Porter, M. R., & Kasey, S. (1996). Exaggerated platelet reactivity in major depression. *American Journal of Psychiatry*, 153, 1313–1317.

Myers, D. G. (1993). *The Pursuit of Happiness: Who Is Happy–and Why*. London: Aquarian Press (HarperCollins).

Myers, D. G., & Diener, E. (1995). Who is happy? *Psychological Sciences*, 6, 10–19.

Myers, D. G., & Diener, E. (1996). The pursuit of happiness: New research uncovers some anti-intuitive insights into how many people are happy–and why. *Scientific American*, 274(5), 54–56.

Naguib, S. M., Comstock, G. W., & Davis, H. J. (1966). Epidemiologic study of trichomoniasis in normal women. *Obstetrics and Gynecology*, 27, 607–616.

Naguib, S. M., Geiser, P. B., & Comstock, G. W. (1968). Responses to a program of screening for cervical cancer. *Public Health Reports*, 83, 990–998.

Naguib, S. M., Lundin, F. E., & Davis, H. D. (1966). Relation of various epidemiologic factors to cervical cancer as determinants of a screening program. *Obstetrics and Gynecology*, 28, 451–459.

Naitoh, Y., Fukata, J., & Tominaga, T. E. (1988). Interleukin-6 stimulates the secretion of adrenocorticotrophic hormone in conscious, freely-moving rats. *Biochemistry and Biophysics Research Communications*, 155, 1459–1463.

NARSAD (1998). National Alliance for Research in Schizophrenia and Depression: Frequently asked questions (http://www.mhsource.com/advocacy/narsad/narsadfaqs.html).

National Center for Health Statistics. (1989). *Monthly Vital Statistics Report of Final Mortality Standards 1987*, 38, No. 5 (Suppl.)

National Center for Health Statistics. (1996). *Health, United States, 1995.* No. PHS-96-1232. Hyattsville, Md.: U.S. Department of Health and Human Services.

National Committee for Adoption (1985). *Adoption Fact Book: United States Data, Issues, Regulations, and Resources.* Washington, D.C.: National Committe for Adoption.

National Heart, Lung, and Blood Institute. (1997). *Sixth Report of the Joint National Committee on Prevention, Detection, Evaluation, and Treatment of High Blood Pressure.* Bethesda, Md.: National Insitutes of Health.

National Institute for Drug Abuse (1997). *National Household Survey of Drug Abuse, 1997.* Bethesda, Md.: National Institute for Alcohol Abuse and Alcoholism.

National Institute for Drug Abuse. (1998). *Understanding Drug Abuse and Addiction.* Washington, D.C.: U.S. Government Printing Office.

National Institute for Mental Health. (1997). *Anxiety Disorders.* No. NIH-94-3879. Washington, D.C.: Government Printing Office.

National Institute on Alcohol Abuse and Alcoholism. (1997). *Ninth Special Report to Congress on Alcohol and Health.* Washington, D.C.: U.S. Government Printing Office.

National Pharmaceutical Council (1992). *Emerging Issues in Pharmaceutical Cost Containment,* vol. 2 (pp. 1–16). Reston, Va.: National Pharmaceutical Council.

Ndom, R. J. E., & Adelekan, M. L. (1996). Psychosocial correlates of substance use among undergraduates in Ilorin University, Nigeria. *East African Medical Journal,* 73, 541–547.

Needleman, L. (1988). Fifty years of Canadian Jewish mortality. *Social Biology,* 35, 110–122.

Neeleman, J. (1998). Regional suicide rates in the Netherlands: Does religion still play a role? *International Journal of Epidemiology,* 27, 466–472.

Neeleman, J., & King, M. B. (1993). Psychiatrists' religious attitudes in relation to their clinical practice: A survey of 231 psychiatrists. *Acta Psychiatrica Scandinavia,* 88, 420–424.

Neeleman, J., & Lewis, G. (1994). Religious identity and comfort beliefs in three groups of psychiatric patients and a group of medical controls. *International Journal of Social Psychiatry,* 40(2), 124–134.

Neeleman, J., & Lewis, G. (1999). Suicide, religion, and socioeconomic conditions. An ecological study in 26 countries, 1990. *Journal of Epidemiology and Community Health,* 53, 204–210.

Neeleman, J., & Persaud, R. (1995). Why do psychiatrists neglect religion? *British Journal of Medical Psychology,* 68 (part 2), 169–178.

Neeleman, J., Halpern, D., Leon, D., & Lewis, G. (1997). Tolerance of suicide, religion, and suicide rates: An ecological and individual study in 19 Western countries. *Psychological Medicine,* 27(5), 1165–1171.

Neeleman, J., Wessely, S., & Lewis, G. (1998). Suicide acceptability in African- and white Americans: The role of religion. *Journal of Nervous and Mental Disease,* 186, 12–16.

Neher, L. S., & Short, J. L. (1998). Risk and protective factors for children's substance use and antisocial behavior following parental divorce. *American Journal of Orthopsychiatry,* 68, 154–161.

Neighbors, H., Musick, M., & Williams, D. R. (1998). The African American minister as a source of health for serious personal crises. *Health Education and Behavior,* 25, 759–777.

Neighbors, H. W., Jackson, J. S., Bowman, P. J., & Gurin, G. (1983). Stress, coping, and Black mental health: Preliminary findings from a national study. *Prevention in Human Services,* 2, 5–29.

Nelson, A. A., & Wilson, W. P. (1984). The ethics of sharing religious faith in psychotherapy. *Journal of Psychology and Theology,* 12, 15–23.

Nelson, F., & Farberow, N. (1980). Indirect self-destructive behavior in the elderly nursing home patient. *Journal of Gerontology,* 35(6), 949–957.

Nelson, F. L. (1977). Religiosity and self-destructive crises in the institutionalized elderly. *Suicide and Life-Threatening Behavior,* 7(2), 67–74.

Nelson, L. D., & Cantrell, C. H. (1980). Religiosity and death anxiety: A multi-dimensional analysis. *Review of Religious Research,* 21, 148–157.

Nelson, L. D., & Dynes, R. R. (1976). The impact of devotionalism and attendance on ordinary and emergency helping behavior. *Journal for the Scientific Study of Religion,* 15, 47–59.

Nelson, P. B. (1989a). Ethnic differences in intrinsic/extrinsic religious orientation and depression in the elderly. *Archives of Psychiatric Nursing,* 3, 199–204.

Nelson, P. B. (1989b). Social support, self-esteem, and depression in the institutionalized elderly. *Issues in Mental Health Nursing,* 10, 55–68.

Nelson, P. B. (1990). Intrinsic/extrinsic religious orientation of the elderly: relationship to depression and self-esteem. *Journal of Gerontological Nursing,* 16, 29–35.

Nelson, S. (1997). Pastoral care and moral government: Early 19th-century nursing and solutions to the Irish question. *Journal of Advanced Nursing*, 26, 6–14.

Ness, R. C. (1980). The impact of indigenous healing activity: An empirical study of two fundamentalist churches. *Social Science and Medicine*, 14B, 167–180.

Ness, R. C., & Wintrob, R. M. (1980). The emotional impact of fundamentalist religious participation: An empirical study of intragroup variation. *American Journal of Orthopsychiatry*, 50, 302–315.

New International Version of the Holy Bible (1984). East Brunswick, N.J.: International Bible Society.

Newberg, A. B., & D'Aquili, E. G. (1998). The neuropsychology of spiritual experience. In H. G. Koenig (ed.), *Handbook of Religion and Mental Health* (pp. 76–91). San Diego: Academic Press.

Newcomb, M. D. (1992). Understanding the multidimensional nature of drug use and abuse: The role of consumption, risk factors, and protective factors. In M. Glantz & R. Pickens (eds.), *Vulnerability to Drug Abuse* (pp. 255–298). Washington, D.C.: American Psychological Association.

Newcomb, M. D., Maddahian, E., & Bentler, P. M. (1986). Risk factors for drug use among adolescents: Concurrent and longitudinal analyses. *American Journal of Public Health*, 76, 525–531.

Newill, V. A. (1961). Distribution of cancer mortality among ethnic subgroups of the White population of New York City, 1953–1958. *Journal of the National Cancer Institute*, 26, 405–417.

Newman, J. S., & Pargament, K. I. (1990). The role of religion in the problem-solving process. *Review of Religious Research*, 31, 390–404.

Newshan, G. (1998). Transcending the physical: Spiritual aspects of pain in patients with HIV and/or cancer. *Journal of Advanced Nursing*, 28, 1236–1241.

Nias, D. K. B. (1973). Measurement in structure of children's attitudes. In G. E. Wilson (ed.), *The Psychology of Conservatism*. London: Academic Press.

Nicholas, L., & Durrheim, K. (1995). Religiosity, AIDS, and sexuality knowledge, attitudes, beliefs, and practices of black South African first-year university students. *Psychological Reports*, 77, 1328–1330.

Nicholi, A. M. (1985). Characteristics of college students who use psychoactive drugs for nonmedical reasons. *College Health*, 33, 189–192.

Nieto, F. J., Adam, E., Sorlie, P., Farzadegan, H., Melnick, J. L., Comstock, G. W., & Szklo, M. (1996). Coronary heart disease/atherosclerosis/ myocardial infarction: Cohort study of cytoegalovirus infection as a risk factor for carotid intimal-medial thickening, a measure of subclinical atherosclerosis. *Circulation*, 94, 922–927.

Nock, S. L. (1987). *The Sociology of the Family*. Englewood Cliffs, N.J.: Prentice Hall.

Nolen, W. (1974). *Healing: A Doctor in Search of the Miracle*. New York: Random House.

Norman, W. T. (1963). Toward an adequate taxonomy of personality attributes: Replicated factor structure in peer nomination personality ratings. *Journal of Abnormal and Social Psychology*, 66, 574–583.

Novak, M. (1998). The most religious century. *New York Times* (Op-Ed, Sunday, May 24).

Novak, M. (1999). With liberty and prayer for all. *New York Times* (June 18), OP-ED section.

Novotny, T. E., Jennings, C. E., & Doran, M.. (1988). Measles outbreaks in religious groups exempt from immunization laws. *Public Health Reports*, 103, 49–54.

Numbers, R. L., & Amundsen, D. W. (eds.) (1998). *Caring and Curing: Health and Medicine in the Western Religious Traditions*. Baltimore: Johns Hopkins University Press.

Nunn, J. F. (1996). *Ancient Egyptian Medicine*. Norman: University of Oklahoma Press.

Nutt, D.J., Bell, C.J., & Malizia, A. L. (1998). Brain mechanisms of social anxiety disorder. *Journal of Clinical Psychiatry*, 59(Suppl. 17), 4–11.

Nye, W. P. (1992–93). Amazing grace: Religion and identity among elderly black individuals. *International Journal of Aging and Human Development*, 36, 103–114.

O'Brien, M. E. (1982). Religious faith and adjustment to long-term hemodialysis. *Journal of Religion and Health*, 21, 68–80.

O'Connell, M. R. (1998). The Roman Catholic tradition since 1545. In R. L. Numbers & D. W. Amundsen (eds.), *Caring and Curing: Health and Medicine in the Western Religious Traditions* (pp. 108–145). Baltimore: Johns Hopkins University Press.

O'Connor, B. P., & Vallerand, R. J. (1990). Religious motivation in the elderly: A French-Canadian replication and an extension. *Journal of Social Psychology*, 130, 53–59.

O'Donnell, J., Hawkins, J. D., & Abbott, R. D. (1995). Predicting serious delinquency and substance abuse among agressive boys. *Journal of Consulting and Clinical Psychology*, 63(4), 529–537.

Oetting, E. R., & Beauvais, F. (1987). Peer cluster theory, socialization characteristics, and adolescent drug use: A path analysis. *Journal of Counseling Psychology, 34,* 205–213.

Office on Smoking and Health (1989). *Reducing the health consequences of smoking: 25 years of progress. A report of the surgeon general.* DHHS publication no. (CDC) 89–8411. Washington, D.C.: U.S. Department of Health and Human Services.

Ogata, A., & Miyakawa, T. (1998). Religious experiences in epileptics patients with a focus on ictus-related episodes. *Psychiatry and Clinical Neurosciences, 52,* 321–325.

Ogata, M., Ikeda, M., & Kuratsune, M. (1984). Mortality among Japanese Zen priests. *Journal of Epidemiology and Community Health, 38,* 161–166.

Okun, M. A. (1993). Predictors of volunteer status in a retirement community. *International Journal of Aging and Human Development, 36,* 57–74.

Okun, M. A., Stock, W. A., Haring, M J., & Witter, R. A. (1984). The social activity/subjective well-being relation: a quantitative synthesis. *Research on Aging, 6,* 45–65.

O'Laoire, S. (1997). An experimental study of the effects of distant, intercessory prayer on self-esteem, anxiety, and depression. *Alternative Therapies in Health and Medicine, 3*(6), 38–53.

Oldnall, A. (1996). A critical analysis of nursing: Meeting the spiritual needs of patients. *Journal of Advanced Nursing, 23,* 138–144.

Oleckno, W. A., & Blacconiere, M. J. (1991). Relationship of religiosity to wellness and other health-related behaviors and outcomes. *Psychological Reports, 68,* 819–826.

Olfson, M., Broadhead, E. W., Weissman, M. M., Leon, C. L., Farber, L., Hoven, C., & Kathol, R. (1996). Subthreshold psychiatric symptoms in a primary care group practice. *Archives of General Psychiatry, 53,* 880–886.

Olive, K. E. (1995). Physician religious beliefs and the physician-patient relationship: A study of devout physicians. *Southern Medical Journal, 88,* 1249–1255.

Olson, L. M., Reis, J., Murphy, L., & Gehm, J. H. (1988). The religious community as a partner in health care. *Journal of Community Health, 13,* 249–257.

Oman, D., & Reed, D. (1998). Religion and mortality among the community-dwelling elderly. *American Journal of Public Health, 88,* 1469–1475.

Oman, D., Thoresen, C., & McMahon, K. (1999). Volunteerism and mortality among the community-dwelling elderly. *Journal of Health Psychology, 4,* 301–316.

O'Neill, D. P., & Kenny, E. K. (1998). Spirituality and chronic illness. *Image: The Journal of Nursing Scholarship, 30,* 275–280.

Opler, M. E. (1936). Some points of comparison and contrast between the treatment of functional disorrders by Apache shamans and modern psychiatric practice. *American Journal of Psychiatry, 92,* 1371.

Orbach, H. L. (1961). Aging and religion. *Geriatrics, 16,* 530–540.

O'Reilly, C. T. (1957). Religious practice and personal adjustment of older people. *Sociology and Social Research, 41,* 119–121.

Ornish, D., Brown, S. E., Scherwitz, L. W., Billings, J. H., Armstrong, W. T., Ports, T. A., McLanahan, S. M., Kirkeeide, R. L., Brand, R. J., & Gould, K. L. (1990). Can lifestyle changes reverse coronary heart disease? The Lifestyle Heart Trial. *Lancet, 336* (8708), 129–133.

Orr, R. D., & Genesen, L. B. (1997). Requests for "inappropriate" treatment based on religious beliefs. *Journal of Medical Ethics, 23* (3), 142–147.

Orr, R. D., & Genesen, L. B. (1998). Medicine, ethics and religion: rational or irrational? *Journal of Medical Ethics, 24,* 385–387.

Orr, R. D., & Isaac, G. (1992). Religious variables are infrequently reported in clinical research. *Family Medicine, 24,* 602–606.

Ortega, S. T., Crutchfield, R. D., & Rushing, W. A. (1983). Race differences in elderly personal well-being. *Research on Aging, 5,* 101–118.

Ortega, S. T., Whitt, H. P., & William, J. A. (1988). Religious homogamy and marital happiness. *Journal of Family Issues, 9,* 224–239.

Orth-Gomer, K., & Unden, A. L. (1990). Type A behavior, social support, and coronary risk: Interaction and significance or mortality in cardiac patients. *Psychosomatic Medicine, 52,* 59–72.

Orth-Gomer, K., Rosengren, A., & Wilhelmsen, L. (1993). Lack of social support and incidence of coronary heart disease in middle-aged Swedish men. *Psychosomatic Medicine, 55,* 37–43.

Osler, W. (1910). The faith that heals. *British Medical Journal,* 1470–1472.

Ostheimer, J. (1980). The polls: Changing attitudes toward euthanasia, revisited. *Social Biology, 28*(Spring/Summer), 145–148.

Outbreaks of rubella among the Amish: United States, 1991. (1991). *Mortality and Morbidity Weekly Reports, 40,* 264–265.

Outler, A. (1954). *Psychotherapy and the Christian Message.* New York: Harper & Row.

Oxman, T. E., Freeman, D. H., & Manheimer, E. D. (1995). Lack of social participation or religious strength and comfort as risk factors for death after cardiac surgery in the elderly. *Psychosomatic Medicine, 57,* 5–15.

Oyama, O., & Koenig, H. G. (1998). Religious beliefs and practices in family medicine. *Archives of Family Medicine*, 7, 431–435.

Pace, J. C., & Stables, J. L. (1997). Correlates of spiritual well-being in terminally ill care persons with AIDS and terminally ill persons with cancer. *Journal of the Association of Nurses in AIDS Care*, 8(6), 31–42.

Packer, S. (1998). Jewish mystical movements and the European ergot epidemics. *Israel Journal of Psychiatry and Related Sciences*, 35, 227–239.

Palmore, E. B. (1982). Predictor of the longevity difference: A 25-year follow-up. *Gerontologist*, 22, 513–518.

Paloutzian, R. F. (1981). Purpose in life and value changes following conversion. *Journal of Personality and Social Psychology*, 41, 1153–1160.

Paloutzian, R. F., & Ellison, C. W. (1982). Loneliness, spiritual well-being and quality of life. In L. A. Peplau & D. Perlman (eds.), *Loneliness: A Sourcebook of Current Theory, Research and Therapy* (pp. 224–237). New York: Wiley.

Pan, W. H., Chin, C. I, Sheu, C. T., & Lee, M. H. (1993). Hemostatic factors and blood lipids in young Buddhist vegetarians and omnivores. *American Journal of Clinical Nutrition*, 58, 354–359.

Pandey, R. E. (1968). The suicide problem in India. *International Journal of Social Psychiatry*, 14, 193–200.

Panton, J. H. (1979). An MMPI item content scale to measure religious identification within a state prison population. *Journal of Clinical Psychology*, 35, 588–591.

Parfrey, P. S. (1976). The effect of religious factors on intoxicant use. *Scandinavian Journal of Social Medicine*, 4, 135–140.

Pargament, K. I. (1997). *The Psychology of Religion and Coping: Theory, Research, and Practice*. New York: Guilford.

Pargament, K. I., & Brant, C. R. (1998). Religion and coping. In H. G. Koenig (ed.), *Handbook of Religion and Mental Health* (pp. 111–128). San Diego: Academic Press.

Pargament, K. I., & Hahn, J. (1986). God and the just world: Causal and coping attributions to God in health situations. *Journal for the Scientific Study of Religion*, 25, 193–207.

Pargament, K. I., & Park, C. L. (1995). Merely a defense: The variety of religious means and ends. *Journal of Social Issues*, 51, 13–32.

Pargament, K. I., Ensing, D. S., Falgout, K., Olsen, H., Reilly, B., Van Haitsma, K., & Warren, R. (1990). God help me: I. Religious coping efforts as predictors of the outcomes to significant life events. *American Journal of Community Psychology*, 18, 793–824.

Pargament, K. I., Ishler, K., Dubow, E., Stanik, P., Rouiller, R., Crowe, P., Cullman, E., Albert, M., & Royster, B. J. (1994). Methods of religious coping with the Gulf War: Cross-sectional and longitudinal analyses. *Journal for the Scientific Study of Religion*, 33, 347–361.

Pargament, K. I., Kennell, J., Hathaway, W., Grevengoed, N., Newman, J., & Jones, W. (1988). Religion and the problem-solving process: Three styles of coping. *Journal for the Scientific Study of Religion*, 27, 90–104.

Pargament, K. I., Koenig, H. G., et al. (2000). Measuring religious coping in hospitalized medically ill older patients: The impact of specific religious coping methods on health outcomes two years later. File report submitted to the Retirement Research Foundation, 1/1/2000.

Pargament K. I., Koenig, H. G., & Perez, L. M. (2000). A comprehensive measure of religious coping: Development and initial validation of the RCOPE. *Journal of Clinical Psychology*.

Pargament, K. I., Olsen, H., Reilly, B., Falgout, K., & Ensing, D. S. (1992). God help me: II. The relationship of religious orientations to religious coping with negative life events. *Journal for the Scientific Study of Religion*, 31, 504–513.

Pargament, K. I., Smith, B., & Brant C. (1995). Religious and nonreligious coping methods with the 1993 Midwest flood. Paper presented at the Annual Meeting of the Society for the Scientific Study of Religion, St. Louis, Mo.

Pargament, K. I., Smith, B. W., & Koenig, H. G. (1996). Religious coping with the Oklahoma City bombing: The brief RCOPE. Paper presented at the Annual Meeting of the American Psychological Association, Toronto.

Pargament, K. I., Smith, B. W., Koenig, H. G., & Perez, L. (1998). Patterns of positive and negative religious coping with major life stressors. *Journal for the Scientific Study of Religion* 37(4), 710–724.

Pargament, K. I., Steele, R. E., & Tyler, F. B. (1979). Religious participation, religious motivation and individual psychosocial competence. *Journal for the Scientific Study of Religion*, 18, 412–419.

Pargament, K. I., Zinnbauer, B. J., Scott, A. B., Butter, E. M., Zerowin, J., & Stanik, P. (1998). Red flags and religious coping: Identifying some religious warning signs among people in crisis. *Journal of Clinical Psychology*, 54, 77–89.

Park, C. L., & Cohen, L. H. (1993). Religious and nonreligious coping with the death of a friend. *Cognitive Therapy and Research,* 17, 561–577.

Park, C. L., Cohen, L. H., & Herb, L. (1990). Intrinsic religiousness and religious coping as life stress moderators for Catholics versus Protestants. *Journal of Personality and Social Psychology,* 59, 562–574.

Park, J. Y., Danko, G. P., Wong, S. Y., Weatherspoon, A. J., & Johnson, R. C. (1998). Religious affiliation, religious involvement, and alcohol use in Korea. *Cultural Diversity and Mental Health,* 4, 291–296.

Parker, G. B., & Brown, L. B. (1982). Coping behaviors that mediate between life events and depression. *Archives of General Psychiatry,* 39, 1386–1391.

Parker, W. R., & St. Johns, E. (1957). *Prayer Can Change Your Life.* Carmel, N.Y.: Guideposts.

Parkum, K. H. (1985). The impact of chaplaincy services in selected hospitals in the eastern United States. *Journal of Pastoral Care,* 39, 262–269.

Patel, C., & Carruthers, M. (1977). Coronary risk factor reduction through biofeedback-aided relaxation and meditation. *Journal of the Royal College of Genteral Practice,* 27, 401–405.

Patel, C., & Datey, K. K. (1976). Relaxation and biofeedback techniques in the management of hypertension. *Angiology,* 27(2),106–113.

Patel, C., & North, W. R. (1975). Randomised controlled trial of yoga and bio-feedback in management of hypertension. *Lancet* 2(7925), 93–95.

Patlock-Peckham, J. A., Hutchinson, G. T., Cheong, J., & Nagoshi, C. T. (1998). Effect of religion and religiosity on alcohol use in a college student sample. *Drug and Alcohol Dependence,* 49(2), 81–88.

Pattison, E. M. (1966). Social and psychological aspects of religion in psychotherapy. *Journal of Nervous and Mental Disease,* 141, 586–597.

Pattison, E. M., & Pattison, M. L. (1980). "Ex-Gays": Religiously mediated change in homosexuals. *American Journal of Psychiatry,* 137, 1553–1562.

Pattison, E. M., Lapins, N. A., & Doerr, H. A. (1973). Faith healing: A study of personality and function. *Journal of Nervous and Mental Disease,* 157, 397–399.

Paulsen, A. E. (1926). Religious healing. *Journal of the American Medical Association,* 86, 1519–1524, 1617–1623, 1692–1697.

Paykel, E. S., Myers, J. K., Lindenthal, J. J., & Tanner, J. (1974). Suicidal feelings in the general population: A prevalence study. *British Journal of Psychiatry,* 124, 460–469.

Payne, E. C., Kravitz, A. R., Notman, M. T., & Anderson, J. V. (1976). Outcome following therapeutic abortion. *Archives of General Psychiatry,* 33, 725–733.

Payne, I. R., Bergin, A. E., Bielema, K. A., & Jenkins, P. H. (1991). Review of religion and mental health: Prevention and the enhancement of psychosocial functioning. *Prevention in Human Services,* 11–40.

Peale, N. V. (1952). *The Power of Positive Thinking.* Englewood Cliffs, N.J.: Prentice Hall.

Pear, R. (1999). HMOs to up Medicare charge or cut service: Trade association predicts 250,000 members will be forced from their current plans. *New York Times* (July 2).

Pearl, R. (1938). Tobacco smoking and longevity. *Science* 8, March 4, 216–217.

Pearlin, L. I., & Johnson, J. S. (1977). Marital status, life strains, and depression. *American Sociological Review,* 42, 704–715.

Pecheur, D. R., & Edwards, K. J. (1984). A comparison of secular and religious versions of cognitive therapy with depressed Christian college students. *Journal of Psychology and Theology,* 12, 45–54.

Peck, M. S. (1983). *People of the Lie: The Hope for Healing Human Evil.* New York: Simon & Schuster.

Peek, C. W., Curry, E. W., & Chalfant, H. P. (1985). Religiosity and delinquency over time: Deviance deterrence and deviance amplification. *Social Science Quarterly,* 66, 120–131.

Peele, S. (1990). Resarch issues in assessing addiction treatment effiacy: How cost effective are Alcoholics Anonymous and private treatment centers? *Drug and Alcohol Dependence,* 25, 179–182.

Penner, S. J., & Galloway-Lee, B (1997). Parish nursing:. Opportunities in community health. *Home Care Provider,* 2(5), 244–249.

Penning, M. J. (1995). Health, social support, and the utilization of health services among older adults. *Journals of Gerontology: Psychological Sciences and Social Sciences,* 50, S330–S339.

Perkins, H. W. (1987). Parental religion and alcohol use problems as intergenerational predictors. *Journal for the Scientific Study of Religion,* 26, 340–357.

Perkins, K. A., & Gorbe, J. E. (1992). Increased desire to smoke during acute stress. *British Journal of Addictions,* 87, 1037–1040.

Perrine, M., Peck, R., & Fell, J. (1989). Epidemiologic perspectives on drunken driving. In *Sur-*

geon General's Workshop on Drunk Driving: Background Papers. Washington, D.C.: U.S. Department of Health and Human Services.

Persinger, M. A. (1984). People who report religious experiences may also display enhanced temporal lobe signs. *Perceptual and Motor Skills,* 58, 963–975.

Persinger, M. A. (1987). *Neuropsychological Bases of God Beliefs.* New York: Praeger.

Pescosolido, B., & Georgianna, S. (1989). Durkheim, suicide, and religion: Toward a network theory of suicide. *American Sociological Review,* 54, 33–48.

Pescosolido, B. A., & Mendelsohn, R. (1986). Social causation or social construction of suicide? An investigation into the social organization of official rates. *American Sociological Review,* 51, 80–101.

Pescosolido, B. A., Wright, E. R., Alegria, M., & Vera, M. (1998). Social networks and patterns of use among the poor with mental health problems in Puerto Rico. *Medical Care,* 36, 1057–1072.

Petersen, B. H., Lemberger, L., Graham, J., & Dalton, B. (1975). Alterations in the cellular-mediated immune responsiveness of chronic marijuana smokers. *Psychopharmacology Communications,* 1, 67–74.

Peterson, C., Seligman, M. E. P., & Vaillant, G. E. (1988). Pessimistic explanatory style is a risk factor for physical illness: A thirty-five-year longitudinal study. *Journal of Personality and Social Psychology,* 55, 23–27.

Peterson, C., Seligman, M. E. P., Yurko, K. H., Martin, L. R., & Friedman, H. S. (1998). Catastrophizing and untimely death. *Psychological Science,* 9(2), 127–130.

Petraitis, J., Flay, B. R., Miller, T. Q., Torpy, E. J., & Greiner, B. (1998) Illicit substance use among adolescents: A matrix of prospective predictors. *Substance Use and Misuse,* 33(13), 2561–2604.

Petrowsky, M. (1976). Marital status, sex, and the social networks of the elderly. *Journal of Marriage and the Family,* 5, 749–756.

Pettersson, T. (1991). Religion and criminality: Structural relationships between church involvement and crime rates in contemporary Sweden. *Journal for the Scientific Study of Religion,* 30, 279–291.

Peveler, R., Kilkenny, L., & Kinmonth, A. L. (1997). Medically unexplained physical symptoms in primary care: A comparison of self-report screening questionnaires and clinical opin-

ion. *Journal of Psychosomatic Research,* 42, 245–252.

Peyrot, M. F., & McMurry, J. F., Jr. (1992). Stress buffering and glycemic control: The role of coping styles. *Diabetes Care,* 15, 842–846.

Pfeifer, S., & Waelty, U. (1995). Psychopathology and religious commitment: A controlled study. *Psychopathology,* 28, 70–77.

Phillips, R. L. (1975). Role of life-style and dietary habits in risk of cancer among Seventh-Day Adventists. *Cancer Research,* 35, 3513–3522.

Phillips, R. L., & Snowdon, D. A. (1983). Association of meat and coffee use with cancers of the large bowel, breast, and prostate among Seventh-Day Adventists: Preliminary results. *Cancer Research,* 43, 2403s–2408s.

Phillips, R. L., Garfinkel, L., Kuzma, J. W., Beeson, W. L., Lotz, T., & Brin, B. (1980). Mortality among California Seventh-Day Adventists for selected cancer sites. *Journal of the National Cancer Institute,* 65, 1097–1107.

Phillips, R. L., Kuzma, J. W., Beeson, W. L., & Lotz, T. (1980). Influence of selection versus lifestyle on risk of fatal cancer and cardiovascular disease among Seventh-Day Adventists. *American Journal of Epidemiology,* 112, 296–314.

Phillips, R. L., Lemon, F. R., Beeson, W. L., & Kuzma, J. W. (1978). Coronary heart disease mortality among Seventh-Day Adventists with differing dietary habits: A preliminary report. *American Journal of Clinical Nutrition,* 31, S191–S198.

Philpot, C. D. (1997). Parish nursing. *Missouri Gateway Geriatric Education Center* (Saint Louis University) *Newsletter,* 7, 10–11.

Pichot, P., & Overall, J. E. (1973). The significance of background variables for psychopathology in France. *International Pharmacopsychiatry,* 8, 1–26.

Pickens, R. W., & Johanson, C. E. (1992). Craving: Consensus of status and agenda for future research. *Drug and Alcohol Dependence,* 30(2), 127–131.

Picot, S. J., Debanne, S. M., Namazi, K. H., & Wykle, M. (1997). Religiosity and perceived rewards of black and white caregivers. *Gerontologist,* 37, 89–101.

Pieper, H. G., & Garrison, T. (1992). Knowledge of social aspects of aging among pastors. *Journal of Religious Gerontology,* 8, 89–101.

Pincus, H. A., Tanielian, T. L., Marcus, S. C., Olfson, M., Zarin, D. A., Thompson, J., & Magno Zito, J. (1998). Prescribing trends in psychotropic medications: Primary care, psychiatry, and other medical specialties. *Journal of the American Medical Association*, 279, 526–531.

Pini, S., Piccinelli, M., & Zimmerman-Tansella, C. (1995). Social problems as factors affecting medical consultation: A comparison between general practice attenders and community probands with emotional distress. *Psychological Medicine*, 25, 33–42.

Plante, T. G., & Boccaccini, M. T. (1997a). The Santa Clara strength of religious faith questionnaire. *Pastoral Psychology*, 45, 375–387.

Plante, T. G., & Boccaccini, M. T. (1997b). Reliability and validity of the Santa Clara strength of religious faith questionnaire. *Pastoral Psychology*, 45, 429–437.

Plante, T. G., & Manuel, G. M. (1992). The Persian Gulf War: Civilian war related stress and influence of age, religious faith, and war attitudes. *Journal of Clinical Psychology*, 48, 178–182.

Polit, D. F., & LaRocco, S. A. (1980). Social and psychological correlates of menopausal symptoms. *Psychosomatic Medicine*, 42, 335–345.

Pollack, A. A., Case, D. B., Weber, M. A., & Laragh, J. H. (1977). Limitations of transcendental meditation in the treatment of essential hypertension. *Lancet* 1(8002), 71–73.

Pollak, K. (1963). *The Healers: The Doctor, Then and Now*. Camden, N. J.: Thomas Nelson and Sons.

Pollner, M. (1989). Divine relations, social relations, and well-being. *Journal of Health and Social Behavior*, 30, 92–104.

Poloma, M. M., & Pendleton, B. F. (1989). Exploring types of prayer and quality of life: A research note. *Review of Religious Research*, 31, 46–53.

Poloma, M. M., & Pendleton, B. F. (1990). Religious domains and general well-being. *Social Indicators Research*, 22, 255–276.

Poloma, M. M., & Pendleton, B. F. (1991). The effects of prayer and prayer experiences on measures of general well-being. *Journal of Psychology and Theology*, 19, 71–83.

Pomerleau, O. F., & Pomerleau, C. S. (1991). Research on stress and smoking: Progress and problems. *British Journal of Addictions*, 86, 599–603.

Pope, W. (1976). *Durkheim's Suicide: A Classic Reanalyzed*. Chicago: University of Chicago Press.

Poppleton, P. K., & Pilkington, G. W. (1963). The measurement of religious attitudes in a university population. *British Journal of the Society of Clinical Psychology*, 2, 20–36.

Porter, B., & O'Leary, K. D. (1980). Marital discord and childhood behavior problems. *Journal of Abnormal Child Psychology*, 8, 287–295.

Porter, R. (1993). Religion and medicine. In W. F. Bynum & R. Porter (eds.), *Companion Encyclopedia of the History of Medicine*. New York: Routledge, Chapman, & Hall.

Post, S. G., Puchalski, C. M., & Larson, D. B. (2000). Physicians and patient spirituality: Professional boundaries, competency, and ethics. *Annals of Internal Medicine*, 132, 578–583.

Postolache, T., Londono, J., Pinsker, H., Luccerini, S., Augustin, L., & Muran, J. C. (1997). A study of religion and psychotherapy (letter). *Psychiatric Services*, 48, 1592.

Potts, R. G. (1996). Spirituality and the experience of cancer in an African-American community: Implications for psychosocial oncology. *Journal of Psychosocial Oncology*, 14(1), 1–19.

Poulson, R. L., Eppler, M. A., Satterwhite, T. N., Wuensch, K. L., & Bass, L. A. (1998). Alcohol consumption, strength of religious beliefs, and risky sexual behavior in college students. *Journal of American College Health*, 46, 227–232.

Powell, G. E., & Stewart, R. A. (1978). The relationship of age, sex and personality to social attitudes in children aged 8–15 years. *British Journal of Social and Clinical Psychology*, 17, 307–317.

Powell, K. B. (1997). Correlates of violent and nonviolent behavior among vulnerable inner-city youths. *Family and Community Health*, 20(2), 38–47.

Powell, K. E., Thompson, P. D., Caspersen, C. J., & Kendrick, J. S. (1987). Physical activity and the incidence of coronary heart disease. *Annual Review of Public Health*, 8, 253–287.

Pratt, L. A., Ford, D. E., & Crum, R. M. (1996). Depression, psychotropic medication, and risk of myocardial infarction. *Circulation*, 94, 3123–3129.

Pressman, P., Lyons, J. S., Larson, D. B., & Gartner, J. (1992). Religion, anxiety, and fear of death. In J. F. Schumaker (ed.), *Religion and Mental Health* (pp. 98–109). New York: Oxford University Press.

Pressman, P., Lyons, J. S., Larson, D. B., & Strain, J. J. (1990). Religious belief, depression, and ambulation status in elderly women with broken hips. *American Journal of Psychiatry*, 147, 758–760.

Prigerson, H. G., Bierhals, A. J., Kasl, S. V., Reynolds, C. F., Shear, M. K., Day, N., Beery, L. C., Newsom, J. T., & Jacobs, S. (1997). Traumatic grief as a risk factor for mental and physical morbidity. *American Journal of Psychiatry*, 154, 616–623.

Prince, R. (1964). Indigenous Yoruba psychiatry. In A. Kiev (ed.), *Magic, Faith, and Healing*. New York: Free Press.

Princeton Religion Research Center (1939–1998). *Religion in America*. Princeton, N.J.: Gallup Poll.

Princeton Religion Research Center (1982). Religion in America: Who are the "truly devout" among us? Princeton, N.J.: Gallup Poll.

Princeton Religion Research Center (1996). Religion in America: Will the vitality of the church be the surprise of the 21st century? Princeton, N.J.: Gallup Poll.

Princeton Religion Research Center (1998). Dramatic rise seen in those who say religion increasing influence. *Emerging Trends*, 19(4), 1.

Princeton Religion Research Center (1999). Index of leading religious indicators at highest point in 13 years. *Emerging Trends*, 21(February), 1.

Prioreschi, P. (1995). *A History of Medicine*. Omaha: Horatius.

Propst, L. R. (1980). The comparative efficacy of religious and nonreligious imagery for the treatment of mild depression in religious individuals. *Cognitive Therapy and Research*, 4, 167–178.

Propst, L. R. (1996). Cognitive-behavioral therapy and the religious person. In E. P. Shafranske (ed.), *Religion in the Clinical Practice of Psychology* (pp. 391–408). Washington, D.C.: American Psychological Association.

Propst, L. R., Ostrom, R., Watkins, P., Dean, T., & Mashburn, D. (1992). Comparative efficacy of religious and nonreligious cognitive-behavior therapy for the treatment of clinical depression in religious individuals. *Journal of Consulting and Clinical Psychology*, 60, 94–103.

Pruyser, P. W. (1977). The seamy side of current religious beliefs. *Bulletin of the Menninger Clinic*, 41, 329–348.

Puchalski, C. M., & Larson, D. B. (1998). Developing curricula in spirituality and medicine. *Academic Medicine*, 73, 970–974.

Pugh, T. J. (1951). A comparative study of the values of a group of ministers and two groups of laymen. *Journal of Social Psychology*, 33, 223–235.

Purcell, B. C. (1998). Spiritual abuse. *American Journal of Hospice and Palliative Care*, 15, 227–231.

Purisman, R., & Maoz, B. (1977). Adjustment and war bereavement: Some considerations. *British Journal of Medical Psychology*, 50, 1–9.

Putney, S., & Middleton, R. (1961). Dimensions and correlates of religious ideologies. *Social Forces*, 39, 285–290.

Pyron, B. (1961). Belief, Q-Sort, Allport-Vernon Study of Values and Religion. *Psychological Reports*, 8, 399–400.

Query, J. M. N. (1985). Comparative admission and follow-up study of American Indians and whites in a youth chemical dependency unit on the North Central Plains. *International Journal of the Addictions*, 20, 489–502.

Quiles, Z. N., & Bybee, J. (1997). Chronic and predispositional guilt: Relation to mental health, prosocial behavior, and religiosity. *Journal of Personality Assessment*, 69, 104–126.

Raab, W. (1972). Cardiotoxic effects of emotional, socioeconomic, and environmental stresses. *Recent Advances in Studies on Cardiac Structure and Metabolism*, 1, 707–713.

Rabin, B. S. (1999). *Stress, Immune Function, and Health: The Connection*. New York: Wiley-Liss.

Rabins, P. V., Fitting, M. D., Eastham, J., & Fetting, J. (1990). The emotional impact of caring for the chronically ill. *Psychosomatics*, 31, 331–336.

Rabins, P. V., Fitting, M. D., Eastham, J., & Zabora, J. (1990). Emotional adaptation over time in care-givers for chronically ill elderly people. *Age and Ageing*, 19, 185–190.

Rabkin, J. G., & Streuning, E. L. (1976). Life events, stress, and illness. *Science*, 194, 1013–1020.

Ragan, C., Malony, H. N., & Beit-Hallahmi, B. (1980). Psychologists and religion: Professional factors and personal beliefs. *Review of Religious Research*, 21, 208–217.

Rahav, M., Goodman, A. B., Popper, M., & Lin, S. P. (1986). Distribution of treated mental illness in the neighborhoods of Jerusalem. *American Journal of Psychiatry*, 143, 1249–1254.

Rahman, F. (1989). Islam and health/medicine: A historical perspective. In L. E. Sullivan (ed.), *Healing and Restoring: Health and Medicine in the World's Religious Traditions*. New York: Macmillan.

Raikkonen, K., Hautanen, A., & Keltikangas-Jarvinen, L. (1996). Feelings of exhaustion, emotional distress, and pituitary adrenocortical hormones in borderline hypertension. *Journal of Hypertension*, 14, 713–718.

Raikkonen, K., Keltikangas-Jarvinen, L., Adlercreutz, H., & Hautenen, A. (1996). Psychosocial stress and the insulin resistance syndrome. *Metabolism*, 45, 1533–1538.

Raleigh, E. D. H. (1992). Sources of hope in chronic illness. *Oncology Nursing Forum*, 19, 443–448.

Ramachandran, V. S., Hirstein, W. S., Armel, K. C., Tecoma, F., & Iragui, V. (1997). The neural basis of religious experience. Poster presented at the Annual Meeting of the Society of Neurosciences, New Orleans, October 27 (Abstract #519.1, Vol. 23).

Ransdell, L. B. (1995). Church-based health promotion: An untapped resource for women 65 and older. *American Journal of Health Promotion*, 9, 333–336.

Raphael, F. J., Rani, S., Bale, R., & Drummond, L. M. (1996). Religion, ethnicity and obsessive-compulsive disorder. *International Journal of Social Psychiatry*, 42, 38–44.

Rasanen, J., Kauhanen, J., Lakka, T. A., Kaplan, G. A., & Salonen, J. T. (1996). Religious affiliation and all-cause mortality: A prospective population study in middle-aged men in eastern Finland. *International Journal of Epidemiology*, 26, 1244–1249.

Rasmussen, P. K., & Ferraro, K. J. (1979). The divorce process. *Alternative Lifestyles*, 2, 443–460.

Rassnick, S., Sved, A. F., & Rabin, B. S. (1994). Locus coeruleus stimulation by corticotropin-releasing hormone suppresses in-vitro cellular immune responses. *Journal of Neuroscience*, 14, 6033–6040.

Rayburn, C. A. (1991). Counseling depressed female religious professionals: nuns and clergywomen. *Counseling and Values*, 35, 136–148.

Razali, S. M., Hasanah, C. I., Aminah, K., & Subramaniam, M. (1998). Religious-sociocultural psychotherapy in patients with anxiety and depression. *Australian and New Zealand Journal of Psychiatry*, 32, 867–872.

Rednick, R. W., & Johnson, C. (1974). *Marital Status, Living Arrangements, and Family Characteristics of Admissions to State and County Mental Hospitals and Outpatient Psychiatric Clinics, United States*. Statistical Note 100. National Institute for Mental Health, Washington, D.C.: U.S. Government Printing Office.

Reed, K. (1991). Strength of religious affiliation and life satisfaction. *Sociological Analysis*, 52, 205–210.

Reed, P. G. (1986). Religiousness among terminally ill and healthy adults. *Research in Nursing and Health*, 9, 35–41.

Reed, P. G. (1987). Spirituality and well-being in terminally ill hospitalized adults. *Research in Nursing and Health*, 10, 335–344.

Regier, D. A., Goldberg, I. D., & Taube, C. A. (1978). The de facto U.S. mental health services system. *Archives of General Psychiatry*, 35, 685–693.

Regier, D. A., Narrow, W. E., Rae, D. S., Manderscheid, R. W., Locke, B. Z., & Goodwin, F. K. (1993). The de-facto U.S. mental and addictive disorders service system: Epidemiologic catchment. A prospective one-year prevalence rate of disorders and services. *Archives of General Psychiatry*, 50, 85–94.

Rehm, R. S. (1999). Religious faith in Mexican-American families dealing with chronic childhood illness. *Image: The Journal of Nursing Scholarship*, 31, 33–38.

Reid, D. W., & Ziegler, M. (1981). The desired control measure and adjustment among the elderly. In H. M. Lefcourt (ed.), *Research with the Locus of Control Construct* (pp. 127–159). New York: Academic Press.

Reid, W. S., Gilmore, A. J. J., Andrews, G. R., & Caird, F. I. (1978). A study of religious attitudes of the elderly. *Age and Ageing*, 7, 40–45.

Relman, A. S. (1998). The trip to stonesville: Andrew Weil, the boom in alternative medicine, and the retreat from science. *New Republic* (December 14), 28–37.

Rene, J., Weinberger, M., Mazzuca, S. A., Brandt, K. D., & Katz, B. P. (1992). Reduction of joint pain in patients with knee osteoarthritis who have received monthly telephone calls from late personnel and whose medical treatment regimens have remained stable. *Arthritis and Rheumatism*, 35, 511–515.

Rennison, C. M. (1998). *National Crime 1998: Changes 1997–1998 with Trends 1993–1998*. Bureau of Justice Statistics, National Crime Victimization Survey. Washington, D.C.: U.S. Department of Justice, Office of Justice Programs.

Resnick, M. D., Bearman, P. S., Blum, R. W., Baumann, K. E., Harris, K. M., Jones, J., Tabor, J., & Beuhring, T. (1997). Protecting adolescents from harm: Findings from the National Longitudinal Study of Adolescent Health. *Journal of the American Medical Association*, 278, 823–832.

Ressler, W. H. (1997). Jewishness and well-being: Specific identification and general psychological adjustment. *Psychological Reports*, 81, 515–518.

Restak, R. M. (1989). The brain, depression, and the immune system. *Journal of Clinical Psychiatry*, 50(5, Suppl.), 23–25.

Reyes-Ortiz, C. A. (1997). Psychosocial and spiritual supports in coronary disease. *Journal of the American Geriatrics Society* (letter), 45, 1412–1413.

Reyes-Ortiz, C. A., Ayele, H., & Mulligan, T. (1996). Religious activity improves quality of life for ill older adults. *Journal of the American Geriatrics Society*, 44, 1139.

Reynolds, D. K., & Nelson, F. L. (1981). Personality, life situation, and life expectancy. *Suicide and Life-Threatening Behavior*, 11, 99–110.

Reynolds, P., & Kaplan, G. (1990). Social connections and risk for cancer: Prospective evidence from the Alameda County Study. *Behavioral Medicine*, Fall, 101–110.

Rhodes, A. L., & Reiss, A. J. (1970). The "religious factor" and delinquent behavior. *Journal of Research in Crime and Delinquency*, 7, 83–98.

Rice, D. P., & MacKenzie, E. J. (1989). *Cost of Injury in The United States: A Report to Congress, 1989*. San Francisco: University of California at San Francisco Injury Prevention Center.

Richards, D. G. (1990). A "Universal Forces" dimension of locus of control in a population of spiritual seekers. *Psychological Reports*, 67, 847–850.

Richards, D. G. (1991). The phenomenology and verbal correlates of prayer. *Journal of Psychology and Theology*, 19, 354–363.

Richards, M. (1990). Meeting the spiritual needs of the cognitively impaired. *Generations: Aging and the Human Spirit*, 63–64.

Richards, M., & Seicol, S. (1991). The challenge of maintaining spiritual connectedness for persons institutionalized with dementia. *Journal of Religious Gerontology*, 7, 27–40.

Richards, P. S., Owen, L., & Stein, S. (1993). A religiously oriented group counseling intervention for self-defeating perfectionism: A pilot study. *Counseling and Values*, 37, 96–104.

Richards, T. A. & Folkman, S. (1997). Spiritual aspects of loss at the time of a partner's death from AIDS. *Death Studies*, 21, 527–552.

Richards, T. A., Acree, M., & Folkman, S. (1999). Spiritual aspects of loss among partners of men with AIDS: Postbereavement follow-up. *Deaths Studies*, 23, 105–127.

Richardson, V., Berman, S., & Piwowarski, M. (1983). Projective assessment of the relationships between the salience of death, religion, and age among adults in America. *Journal of General Psychology*, 109, 149–156.

Richek, H. G., Mayo, C. D., & Puryear, H. B. (1970). Dogmatism, religiosity and mental health in college students. *Mental Hygiene*, 54, 572–574.

Rigby, R. M., Ryan, S., & King, K. (1993). Two types of religious internalization and their relations to religious orientations and mental health. *Journal of Personality and Social Psychology*, 65, 586–596.

Riley, B. B., Perna, R., Tate, D. G., Forchheimer, M., Anderson, C., & Luera, G. (1998). Types of spiritual well-being among persons with chronic illness: Their relation to various forms of quality of life. *Archives of Physical Medicine and Rehabilitation*, 79, 258–264.

Ringdal, G. I. (1995). Correlates of hopelessness in cancer patients. *Journal of Psychosocial Oncology*, 13(3), 47–66.

Ringdal, G. I. (1996). Religiosity, quality of life, and survival in cancer patients. *Social Indicators Research*, 38, 193–211.

Ringdal, G., Gotestam, K., Kaasa, S., Kvinnslaud, S., & Ringdal, K. (1995). Prognostic factors and survival in a heterogeneous sample of cancer patients. *British Journal of Cancer*, 73, 1594–1599.

Roberson, M. H. B. (1987). Folk health beliefs of health professionals. *Western Journal of Nursing Research*, 9, 257–263.

Roberts, B. H., & Myers, J. K. (1954). Religion, national origin, immigration, and mental illness. *American Journal of Psychiatry*, 110, 759–764.

Roberts, D. (1997). Transcending barriers between religion and psychiatry. *British Journal of Psychiatry*, 171, 188.

Roberts, D., Andersen, B. L., & Lubaroff, A. (1994). Stress and immunity at cancer diagnosis. Unpublished manuscript cited in Andersen et al. (1994).

Roberts, J. A., Brown, D., Elkins, T., & Larson, D. B. (1997). Factors influencing views of patients with gynecologic cancer about end-of-life decisions. *American Journal of Obstetrics and Gynecology*, 176, 166–172.

Roberts, O. (1995). *Expect a Miracle: My Life and Ministry*. Nashville: Thomas Nelson.

Robinson, J. P., & Shaver, P. R. (1973). *Measures of Social Psychological Attitudes*, rev. ed. Ann Arbor, Mich.: Surveyed Research Center, Institute for Social Research.

Robinson, K. M., & Kaye, J. (1994). The relationship between spiritual perspective, social support, and depression in caregiving and noncaregiving wives. *Scholarly Inquiry for Nursing Practice*, 8, 375–389.

Robinson, L. C. (1994). Religious orientation in enduring marriages: An exploratory study. *Review of Religious Research*, 35(3), 207–218.

Robinson, L. C., & Blanton, P. W. (1993). Marital strengths in enduring marriages. *Family Relations*, 42, 38–45.

Robinson-Whelen, S., Kim, C., MacCallum, R. C., & Kiecolt-Glaser, J. K. (1997). Distinguishing optimism from pessimism in older adults: Is it more important to be optimistic or not to be pessimistic? *Journal of Personality and Social Psychology*, 73(6), 1345–1353.

Robison, S. (1960). *Juvenile Delinquency: Its Nature and Control*. New York: Holt, Rinehart, and Winston.

Rodgers, D. V., Gindler, J. S., Atkinson, W. L., & Markowitz, L. E. (1993). High attack rates and case fatality during a measles outbreak in groups with religious exemption to vaccination. *Pediatric Infectious Disease Journal*, 12, 288–292.

Rogalski, S., & Paisey, T. (1987). Neuroticism versus demographic variables as correlates of self-reported life satisfaction in a sample of older adults. *Personality and Individual Differences*, 8, 397–401.

Rogers, R. G. (1996). The effects of family composition, health, and social support linkages on mortality. *Journal of Health and Social Behavior*, 37, 326–338.

Rogers-Dulan, J. (1998). Religious connectedness among urban African-American families who have a child with disabilities. *Mental Retardation*, 36, 91–103.

Rogers-Dulan, J., & Blacher, J. (1995). African American families, religion, and disability: A conceptual framework. *Mental Retardation*, 33, 226–238.

Rohrbaugh, J., & Jessor, R. (1975). Religiosity in youth: A control against deviant behavior. *Journal of Personality*, 43, 136–155.

Rokach, A. (1996). The subjectivity of loneliness and coping with it. *Psychological Reports*, 79, 475–481.

Rokeach, M. (1960). *The Open and Closed Mind*. New York: Basic Books.

Roof, W. C., & McKinney, W. M. (1987). *American Mainline Religion*. New Brunswick, N.J.: Rutgers University Press.

Roozen, D. A., McKinney, W., & Thompson, W. (1990). The "Big Chill" generation warms to worship: A research note. *Review of Religious Research*, 31, 314–323.

Rose, L. (1971). *Faith Healing*. Baltimore: Penguin.

Rosen, C. E. (1982). Ethnic differences among impoverished rural elderly in use of religion as a coping mechanism. *Journal of Rural Community Psychology*, 3, 27–34.

Rosenbaum, E., & Kandel, D. B. (1990). Early onset of adolescent sexual behavior and drug involvement. *Journal of Marriage and the Family*, 52, 783–798.

Rosenberg, C. M., & Amodeo, M. (1974). Long-term patients seen in an alcoholism clinic. *Quarterly Journal of Studies on Alcohol*, 35, 660–666.

Rosenberg, M. (1962). The dissonant religious context and emotional disturbance. *American Journal of Sociology*, 68, 1–10.

Rosenbloom, A. L. (1959). Ethnic prejudice as related to social class and religiosity. *Sociological and Social Research*, 43, 272–275.

Rosengren, A., Tibblin, G., & Wilhelmsen, L. (1991). Self-perceived psychological stress and incidence of coronary artery disease in middle-aged men. *American Journal of Cardiology*, 68, 1171–1175.

Rosengren, A., Wilhelmsen, L., Pennert, K., Berglund, G., & Elmfeldt, D. (1987). Alcoholic intemperance, coronary heart disease and mortality in middle-aged Swedish men. *Acta Medica Scandinavica*, 222, 201–213.

Rosenheim, E., & Muchnik, B. (1984). Death concerns in differential levels of consciousness as functions of defense strategy and religious belief. *Omega Journal of Death and Dying*, 15, 15–24.

Rosenstiel, A. K., & Keefe, F. J. (1983). The use of coping strategies in chronic low back pain patients: Relationship to patient characteristics and current adjustment. *Pain*, 17, 33–44.

Rosenwaike, I. (1984). Changing patterns of lung cancer among socio-cultural groups in New York City. *American Journal of Public Health*, 74, 839–840.

Rosik, C. H. (1989). The impact of religious orientation in conjugal bereavement among older adults. *International Journal of Aging and Human Development*, 28, 251–260.

Rosner, B. (1986). *Fundamentals of Biostatistics*, 2nd ed. Boston: Duxbury.

Ross, C. E. (1990). Religion and psychological distress. *Journal for the Scientific Study of Religion*, 29, 236–245.

Ross, D. C., & Thomas, C. B. (1965). Precursors of hypertension and coronary disease among health medical students: Discriminant funcion analysis III. *Bulletin of the Johns Hopkins Hospital*, 117, 37–57.

Ross, L. A. (1995). The spiritual dimension: Its importance to patients' health, well-being, and quality of life and its implications for nursing practice. *International Journal of Nursing Studies*, 32(5), 457–468.

Ross, L. A. (1997). Elderly patients' perceptions of their spiritual needs and care: A pilot study. *Journal of Advanced Nursing*, 26, 710–715.

Rossow, I. (1993). Suicide, alcohol, and divorce: Aspects of gender and family integration. *Addiction*, 88, 1659–1665.

Roth, P. D. (1988). Spiritual well-being and marital adjustment. *Journal of Psychology and Theology,* 16, 153–158.

Rothbaum, B. O., & Jackson, J. (1990). Religious influence on menstrual attitudes and symptoms. *Women and Health,* 16, 63–78.

Rotter, J. B. (1966). Generalized expectancies for internal versus external control of reinforcement. *Psychological Monographs,* 80, 1–28.

Rouse, L., Armstrong, B. K., & Beilin, L. J. (1982). Vegetarian diet, lifestyle and blood pressure in two religious populations. *Clinical and Experimental Pharmacology and Physiology,* 9(3), 327–330.

Rudestam, K. E. (1972). Demographic factors in suicide, in Sweden and the United States. *International Journal of Social Psychiatry,* 79–90.

Runions, J. E. (1974). Religion and psychiatric practice. *Canadian Psychiatric Association Journal,* 19, 79–85.

Ruoff, G. E. (1996). Depression in the patient with chronic pain. *Journal of Family Practice,* 43, S25–S33.

Ruppel, H. J. (1970). Religiosity and premarital sexual permissiveness: A response to the Reiss-Heltsley and Broderick debate. *Journal of Marriage and the Family,* 32, 647–655.

Russo, N. R., & Dabul, A. J. (1997). The relationship of abortion to well-being. Do race and religion make a difference? *Professional Psychology: Research and Practice,* 28, 23–31.

Rutledge, C. R., Levin, J. S., Larson, D. B., & Lyons, J. S. (1995). The importance of religion for parents coping with a chronically ill child. *Journal of Psychology and Christianity,* 14, 50–57.

Rutledge, J., & Spilka, B. (1993). Coping with intimacy: A problem for the single adult Mormon. Paper presented at the meeting of the American Psychological Association, Toronto, Ontario.

Ryan, R. M., Rigby, S., & King, K. (1993). Two types of religious internalization and their relations to religious orientations and mental health. *Journal of Personality and Social Psychology,* 65, 586–596.

Sack, A. R., Keller, J. F., & Hinkle, D. E. (1984). Premarital sexual intercourse: A test of the effects of peer group, religiosity, and sexual guilt. *Journal of Sex Research,* 20, 168–185.

Sackett, D. L., & Snow, J. C. (1979). The magnitude of compliance and noncompliance. In R. B. Haynes, D. W. Taylor, & D. L. Sackett (eds.), *Compliance in Health Care* (pp. 11–12). Baltimore: Johns Hopkins University Press.

Sacks, H. S., Berrier, J., Reitman, D., & Ancona-Berk, V. A. (1987). Meta-analyses of randomized controlled trials. *New England Journal of Medicine,* 316, 450–455.

Sajwaj, T., & Hedges, D. (1973). A note on the effects of saying grace on the behavior of an oppositional retarded boy. *Journal of Applied Behavior Analysis,* 6, 711–712.

Saksena, D. N., & Srivastava, J. N. (1980). Biosocial correlates of perinatal mortality: Experiences of an Indian hospital. *Journal of Biosocial Science,* 12, 69–81.

Salmons, P. H., & Harrington, R. (1984). Suicidal ideation in university students and other groups. *International Journal of Psychiatry,* 30, 201–205.

Salts, C. J., Denham, T. E., & Smith, T. A. (1991). Relationship patterns and role of religion in elderly couples with chronic illness. *Journal of Religious Gerontology,* 7, 41–54.

Saluter, A. F. (1992). Marital status and living arrangements. *U.S. Bureau of Census Current Population Reports,* Series P20–486, Washington, D.C.: U.S. Government Printing Office.

Salzman, L. (1953). The psychology of religious and ideological conversion. *Psychiatry,* 16, 177–187.

Salzman, L. (1965). Healthy and unhealthy patterns of religion. *Journal of Religion and Health,* 4, 322–326.

Sanders, C.M. (1979–1980). A comparison of adult bereavement in the death of a spouse, child, and parent. *Omega,* 10, 303–322.

Sansome, R. A., Khatain, K., & Rodenhauser, P. (1990). The role of religion in psychiatric education: A national survey. *Academic Psychiatry,* 14, 34–38.

Sanua, V. D. (1969). Religion, mental health, and personality: A review of empirical studies. *American Journal of Psychiatry,* 125, 1203–1213.

Sanua, V. D. (1989). Studies in mental illness and other psychiatric deviance among contemporary Jewry: Favorite view of the literature. *Israel Journal of Psychiatry and Related Sciences,* 26, 187–211.

Sanua, V. D. (1992). Mental illness and other forms of psychiatric deviance among contemporary Jewry. *Transcultural Psychiatric Research Review,* 29, 197–233.

Sapolsky, R. M. (1992). *Stress, the Aging Brain, and the Mechanisms of Neuron Death.* Cambridge, Mass.: MIT Press.

Sapolsky, R. M. (1996). Why stress is bad for your brain. *Science,* 273, 749–750.

Sapolsky, R. M., Alberts, S. C., & Altman, J. (1997). Hypercortisolism associated with social subordinance or social isolation among wild baboons. *Archives of General Psychiatry*, 54, 1137–1143.

Sapolsky, R. M., Krey, L. C., & McEwen, B. S. (1985). Prolonged glucocorticoid exposure reduces hippocampal neuron number: Implications for aging. *Journal of Neurosciences*, 5, 1221–1226.

Sarton, G. (1931). *Introduction to the History of Science*. 2 vols. Baltimore: Williams & Wilkins.

Sarvela, P. D., & McClendon, E. J. (1988). Indicators of rural youth drug use. *Journal of Youth and Adolescence*, 17, 335–347.

Sattler, D. N., Hamby, B. A., Winkler, J. M., & Kaiser, C. (1994). Hurricane Iniki: Psychological functioning following disaster. Paper presented at the Annual Meeting of the American Psychological Association, Los Angeles.

Saucer, P. R. (1992). Evangelical renewal therapy: A proposal for integration of religious values into psychotherapy. *Psychological Reports*, 69, 1099–1106.

Saudia, T. L., Kinney, M. R., Brown, K. C., & Young-Ward, L. (1991). Health locus of control and helpfulness of prayer. *Heart and Lung*, 20, 60–65.

Saunders, E., & Kong, B. W. (1983). A role for churches in hypertension management. *Urban Health*, 12, 49–51, 55.

Saver, J. L., & Rabin, J. (1997). The neural substrates of religious experience. *Journal of Neuropsychiatry*, 9, 498–510.

Sawicki, P. T., Muhlhauser, I., Bender, R., Pethke, W., Heinemann, L., & Berger, M. (1996). Effects of smoking on blood pressure and proteinuria in patients with diabetic nephropathy. *Journal of Internal Medicine*, 239, 345–352.

Scandrett, A. (1994a). The Black church as a participant in community health interventions. *Journal of Health Education*, 25, 183–185.

Scandrett, A. (1994b). Religion as a support component in the health behavior of Black Americans. *Journal of Religion and Health*, 33, 123–129.

Schaal, M. D., Sephton, S. E., Thoreson, C., Koopman, C., & Spiegel, D. (1998). Religious expression and immune competence in women with advanced cancer. Paper presented at the Meeting of the American Psychological Association, San Francisco, August.

Schaefer, C. A., & Gorsuch, R. L. (1991). Psychological adjustment and religiousness: The multivariate belief-motivation theory of religiousness. *Journal for the Scientific Study of Religion*, 30, 448–461.

Schaefer, C. A., & Gorsuch, R. L. (1993). Situational and personal variations in religious coping. *Journal for the Scientific Study of Religion*, 32, 136–147.

Schaefer, L. E., Drachman, S. R., Steinberg, A. G., & Adlersberg, D. (1953). Genetic studies on hypercholesteremia: Frequency in hospital population and in families of hypercholesteremic index patients. *American Heart Journal*, 46, 99–116.

Schafer, W. E. (1997). Religiosity, spirituality, and personal distress among college students. *Journal of College Student Development*, 38, 633–644.

Schaler, J. A. (1996). Spiritual thinking in addiction-treatment providers: The Spiritual Belief Scale (SBS). *Alcoholism Treatment Quarterly*, 14(3), 7–33.

Schatzberg, A. F. (1991). Overview of anxiety disorders: Prevalence, biology, course, and treatment. *Journal of Clinical Psychiatry*, 52(Suppl.): 5–9.

Scheier, M. F., & Carver, C. S. (1993). On the power of positive thinking: The benefits of being optimistic. *Psychological Science*, 2(1), 26–30.

Scheier, M. F., Matthews, K. A., Owens, J. F., Magovern, G. J., Sr., Lefebvre, R., Abbott, R. C., & Carver, C. S. (1989). Dispositional optimism and recovery from coronary artery bypass surgery: The beneficial effects of optimism on physical and psychological well-being. *Journal of Personality and Social Psychology*, 57, 1024–1040.

Schiller, P. L., & Levin, J. S. (1988). Is there a religious factor in health care utilization? A review. *Social Science and Medicine*, 27, 1369–1379.

Schinke, S. P., Moncher, M. S., Palleja, J., & Zayas, L. H. (1988). Hispanic youth, substance abuse, and stress: Implications for prevention research. *International Journal of the Addictions*, 23, 809–826.

Schlegel, R. P., & Sanborn, M. D. (1979). Religious affiliation and adolescent drinking. *Journal of Studies on Alcohol*, 40, 693–703.

Schleifer, S. J., Keller, S. E., & Bond, R. N. (1989). Major depressive disorder and immunity. *Archives of General Psychiatry*, 46, 81–87.

Schleifer, S. J., Keller, S. E., Camerino, M., Thornton, J. C., & Stein, M. (1983). Supression of lymphocyte stimulation following bereavement. *Journal of the American Medical Association*, 250, 274–277.

Schleifer, S. J., Keller, S. E., & Myerson, A. T. (1984). Lymphocyte function in major depressive disorder. *Archives of General Psychiatry, 41,* 484–486.

Schleifer, S. J., Keller, S. E., & Siris, S. G. (1985). Depression and immunity. *Archives of General Psychiatry, 42,* 129–133.

Schmader, K. (1996). Herpes zoster. In C. K. Cassel (ed.), *Geriatric Medicine,* 3rd ed. (pp. 841–854). New York: Springer.

Schmelzer, W. (1994). Religion and health in the elderly. *National Public Radio,* September 6.

Schmidt, F. L., & Hunter, J. E. (1996). Measurement error in psychological research: Lessons from 26 research scenarios. *Psychological Methods, 1,* 199–223.

Schmidt, P. F. (1988). Moral values of adolescents: Public versus Christian schools. *Journal of Psychology and Christianity, 7,* 50–54.

Schnall, P. L., Landsbergis, P. A., & Peiper, C. F. (1992). The impact of anticipation of job loss on psychological distress and work site blood pressure. *American Journal of Indian Medicine, 21,* 417–432.

Schneck, M. J. (1997). Is psychological stress a risk factor for cerebrovascular disease? *Neuroepidemiology, 16,* 174–179.

Schneider, E. L. (1999). Aging in the third millennium. *Science, 283,* 796–797.

Schneider, R. H., Staggers, F., Alexander, C., Sheppard, W., Rainforth, M., Kondwani, K., Smith, S., & King, C. G. (1995). A randomized controlled trial of stress reduction for hypertension in older African Americans. *Hypertension, 26,* 820–829.

Schneider, S. G., Farberow, N. L., & Kruks, G. N. (1989). Suicidal behavior in adolescent and young gay men. *Suicide and Life-Threatening Behavior, 19*(4), 381–394.

Schoenbach, V. J., Kaplan, B. H., Fredman, L., & Kleinbaum, D. G. (1986). Social ties and mortality in Evans County, Georgia. *American Journal of Epidemiology, 123,* 577–591.

Schoenborn, C. A., & Morano, M. (1987). Current estimates from the National Health Interview Survey. *Series Reports,* Series 10, No. 166 (PHS-88-1594, PB-89-140669, PCA-1MFA03). Hyattsville, Md.: National Center for Health Statistics.

Schofield, W., & Balian, L. (1959). A comparative study of the personal histories of schizophrenics and non-psychiatric patients. *Journal of Abnormal and Social Psychology, 59,* 216–225.

Scholl, M. E., & Beker, J. (1964). A comparison of religious beliefs of delinquent and non-delinquent Protestant adolescent boys. *Religious Education, 59,* 250–253.

Schuckit, M. A., Smith, T. L., Daeppen, J. B., Eng, M., Li, T. K., Hesselbrock, V. M., Nurnberger, J. I. Jr, & Bucholz, K. K. (1998). Clinical relevance of the distinction between alcohol dependence with and without a physiological component. *American Journal of Psychiatry, 155*(6), 733–740.

Schuller, R. (1983). *Tough Times Never Last, but Tough People Do!* Nashville: Thomas Nelson.

Schulz, R., Bookwala, J., Knapp, J. E., Scheier, M., & Williamson, G. M. (1996). Pessimism, age, and cancer mortality. *Psychology and Aging, 11,* 304–309.

Schumm, W. R., Bollman, S. R., & Jurich, A. P. (1982). The "marital conventionalization" argument: Implications for the study of religiosity and marital satisfaction. *Journal of Psychology and Theology, 10,* 236–241.

Schwab, R., & Petersen, K. U. (1990). Religiousness: Its relation to loneliness, neuroticism, and subjective well-being. *Journal for the Scientific Study of Religion, 29,* 335–345.

Schwartz, A. H., & Slaby, A. E. (1971). Adjustment and fantasy in medical students. *American Journal of Psychiatry, 128,* 117–122.

Schwartz, J. E., Pickering, T. G., & Landsbergis, P. A. (1996). Work-related stress and blood pressure: Current theoretical models and considerations from a behavioral medicine perspective. *Journal of Occupational Health and Psychology, 1,* 287–310.

Schwartz, M. A., Wiggins, O. P., & Spitzer, M. (1997). Psychotic experience and disordered thinking: A reappraisal from new perspectives. *Journal of Nervous and Mental Disease, 185,* 176–187.

Schweitzer, R., Klayich, M., & McLean, J. (1995). Suicidal ideation and behaviours among university students in Australia. *Australia and New Zealand Journal of Psychiatry, 29*(3), 473–479.

Scioli, A., Chamberlin, C. M., Samor, C. M., LaPointe, A. B., Campbell, T. L., & MacLeod, A. R. (1997). A prospective study of hope, optimism, and health. *Psychological Reports, 81,* 723–733.

Scotch, N. (1963). Sociocultural factors in the epidemiology of Zulu hypertension. *American Journal of Public Health, 53,* 1205–1213.

Scott, A. W. (1993). Masters of the ordinary: Integrating personal experience and vernacular knowledge in Alcoholics Anonymous. Ph.D. diss. Ann Arbor: Michigan Microfilms.

Seamands, D. (1983). *Healing for Damaged Emotions.* Wheaton, Ill.: Victor.

Sears, S. F., & Greene, A. F. (1994). Religious coping and the threat of heart disease. *Journal of Religion and Health*, 33, 221–229.

Seat Belt Safety (1997). Health education: Fast facts (www.bahsc.org/seatbelt.html).

Seeman, T. (1991). Personal control and coronary artery disease: How generalized expectancies about control may influence disease risk. *Journal of Psychosomatic Medicine*, 35, 661–669.

Seeman, T., & Syme, S. L. (1987). Social networks and coronary artery disease: A comparison of the structure and function of social relations as predictors of disease. *Psychosomatic Medicine*, 49, 341–354.

Seeman, T. E., Kaplan, G. A., Knudsen, L., Cohen, R., & Guralnik, J. (1987). Social network ties and mortality among the elderly in the Alameda County study. *American Journal of Epidemiology*, 126, 714–723.

Segall, M., & Wykle, M. (1988–1989). The black family's experience with dementia. *Journal of Applied Social Sciences*, 13, 170–191.

Segerstrom, S. C., Taylor, S. E., Kemeny, M. E., & Fahey, J. L. (1998). Optimism is associated with mood, coping, and immune change in response to stress. *Journal of Personality and Social Psychology*, 74(6), 1646–1655.

Seidlitz, L., Duberstein, P., Cox, C., & Conwell, Y. (1995). Attitudes of older people toward suicide and assisted suicide: An analysis of Gallup poll findings. *Journal of the American Geriatrics Society*, 43(9), 993–998.

Seidman, H. (1966). Lung cancer among Jewish, Catholic, and Protestant males in New York City. *Cancer*, 19, 185–190.

Seidman, H. (1970). Cancer death rates by site and sex for religious and socioeconomic groups in New York City. *Environmental Research*, 3, 234–250.

Seidman, H. (1971). Cancer mortality in New York City for country-of-birth, religious, and socioeconomic groups. *Environmental Research*, 4, 390–429.

Seidman, H., Garfinkel, L., & Craig, L. (1964). Death rates in New York city by socio-economic class and religious group and by country of birth, 1949–1951. *Jewish Journal of Sociology*, 4, 254–273.

Seidman, S. N., Mosher, W. D., & Aral, S. O. (1992). Women with multiple sexual partners: United States, 1988. *American Journal of Public Health*, 82, 1388–1394.

Seidman, S. N., Mosher, W. D., & Aral, S. O. (1994). Predictors of high-risk behavior in unmarried women: Adolescent environment as a risk factor. *Journal of Adolescent Health*, 15, 126–132.

Seligman, M. E. P. (1998). Optimism, hope, and ending the epidemic of depression. Address given at the John Templeton Foundation Board of Advisors Meeting, Philadelphia, February 10.

Selway, D., & Ashman, A. F. (1998). Disability, religion and health: A literature review in search of the spiritual dimensions of disability. *Disability and Society*, 13(3), 429–439.

Selye, H. (1936). A syndrome produced by diverse noxious agents. *Nature*, 138, 32.

Sensky, T., Leger, C., & Gilmour, S. (1996). Psychosocial and cognitive factors associated with adherence to dietary and food restriction regimens by people on chronic hemodialysis. *Psychotherapy and Psychosomatics*, 65, 36–42.

Sensky, T., Wilson, A. Petty, R., Fenwick, P. B. C., & Rose, F. C. (1984). The interictal personality traits of temporal lobe epileptics: Religious belief and its association with reported mystical experiences. In R. J. Porter, et al. (eds.), *Advances in Epileptology: 15th Epilepsy International Symposium* (pp. 545–549). New York: Raven Press.

Sethi, S., & Seligman, M. E. P. (1993). Optimism and fundamentalism. *Psychological Science*, 4, 256–259.

Sethi, S., & Seligman, M. E. P. (1994). The hope of fundamentalists. *Psychological Science*, 5, 58.

Seventeenth Annual Report of the Officers of the Retreat for the Insane at Hartford (1841). Hartford, Conn.: Case, Tiffany & Burnham, Printers.

Shaffer, J. A. (1978). Pain and suffering: Philosophical perspectives. In W. T. Reich (ed.), *Encyclopedia of Bioethics*, Vol. 4 (pp. 1181–1185). New York: Free Press.

Shafranske, E. P., & Malony, H. N. (1990a). California psychologists' religiosity and psychotherapy. *Journal of Religion and Health*, 29, 219–231.

Shafranske, E. P., & Malony, H. N. (1990b). Clinical psychologists' religious and spiritual orientations and their practice of psychotherapy. *Psychotherapy*, 27, 72–78.

Shagle, S. C., & Barber, B. K. (1995). A socio-ecological analysis of adolescent suicidal ideation. *American Journal of Orthopsychiatry*, 65(1), 114–124.

Shams, M., & Jackson, P. R. (1993). Religiosity as a predictor of well-being and moderator of the psychological impact of unemployment. *Journal of Medical Psychology*, 66, 341–352.

Shapira, M., & Tamir, A. (1998). Ulcerative colitis in the Kinneret subdistrict, Israel 1965–1994:

Incidence and prevalence in different sub-groups. *Journal of Clinical Gastroenterology, 27,* 134–137.

Shapiro, D. H., Schwartz, C. E., & Astin, J. A. (1996). Controlling ourselves, controlling our world. *American Psychologist, 51,* 1213–1230.

Shapiro, S., Weinblatt, E., Frank, C. W., & Sager, R. V. (1969). Incidence of coronary heart disease in a population insured for medical care (HIP): Myocardial infarction, angina pectoris, and possible myocardial infarction. *American Journal of Public Health, 59,* 1–100.

Sharkey, P. W., & Malony, H. N. (1986). Religiosity and emotional disturbance: A test of Ellis's thesis in his own counseling center. *Psychotherapy, 23,* 640–641.

Shatenstein, B., & Ghadirian, P. (1988). Influences on diet, health behaviors and their outcome in select ethnocultural and religious groups. *Nutrition, 14*(2), 223–230.

Shaver, P., Lenauer, M., & Sadd, S. (1980). Religiousness, conversion, and subjective well-being: The "healthy-minded" religion of modern American women. *American Journal of Psychiatry, 137,* 1563–1568.

Shebani, B. L., Wass, H., & Guertin, W. H. (1986). Correlates of life satisfaction for old Libyans compared with the judgments of Libyan youth. *International Journal of Aging and Human Development, 24,* 19–28.

Sheehan, W., & Kroll, J. (1990). Psychiatric patients' belief in general health factors and sin as causes of illness. *American Journal of Psychiatry, 147,* 112–113.

Sheeran, P., Spears, R., Abraham, S. C. S., & Abrams, D. (1996). Religiosity, gender, and the double standard. *Journal of Psychology, 130,* 23–33.

Shehan, C. L., Bock. E. W., & Lee, G. R. (1990). Religious heterogamy, religiosity, and marital happiness: The case of Catholics. *Journal of Marriage and the Family, 52,* 73–79.

Shekelle, R. B., Raynor, W. J., Ostfeld, A. M., Garron, D. C., Bieliauskas, L. A., Liu, S. C., Maliza, C., & Oglesby, P. (1981). Psychological depression and 17-year risk of death from cancer. *Psychosomatic Medicine, 43,* 117–125.

Shekelle, R. B., Shryock, A. M., Paul, O., Lepper, M., Stamler, J., Liu, S., & Raynor, W. J. (1981). Diet, serum cholesterol, and death from coronary heart disease: The Western Electric study. *New England Journal of Medicine, 304,* 65–70.

Sher, L. (1998). The role of the endogenous opioid system in the pathogenesis of anxiety disorders. *Medical Hypotheses, 50*(6), 473–474.

Sherbourne, C. D. (1988). The role of social support and life stress events in use of mental health services. *Social Science and Medicine, 27,* 1393–1400.

Sherkat, D. E., & Reed, M. D. (1992). The effects of religion and social support on self-esteem and depression among the suddenly bereaved. *Social Indicators Research, 26,* 259–275.

Sherrill, K. A., Larson, D. B., & Greenwold, M. (1993). Is religion taboo in gerontology? A systematic review of research on religion in three major gerontology journals, 1985–1991. *American Journal of Geriatric Psychiatry, 1,* 109–117.

Shifrin, J. (1998). The faith community as a support for people with mental illness. *New Directions for Mental Health Services, 80,* 69–80.

Shortz, J. L., & Worthington, E. L. (1994). Young adults' recall of religiosity, attributions, and coping in parental divorce. *Journal for the Scientific Study of Religion, 33,* 172–179.

Shrauger, J. S., & Silverman, R. E. (1971). The relationship of religious background and participation to locus of control. *Journal for the Scientific Study of Religion, 10,* 11–16.

Shrum, W. (1980). Religion and marital instability: Change in the 1970's? *Review of Religious Research, 21,* 135–147.

Shu, S., Plautz, G. E., Krause, J. C., & Chang, A. E. (1997). Tumor immunology. *Journal of the American Medical Association, 278,* 1972–1981.

Shuler, P. A., Gelberg, L., & Brown, M. (1994). The effects of spiritual/religious practices on psychological well-being among inner city homeless women. *Nurse Practitioner Forum, 5*(2), 106–113.

Shulik, R. N. (1988). Faith development in older adults. *Educational Gerontology, 14,* 291–301.

Shupe, A., & Stacey, W. A. (1982). *Born Again Politics and the Moral Majority: What Social Surveys Really Show.* Lewiston, N.Y.: Edwin Mellen.

Sicher, F., Targ, E., Moore, D., & Smith, H. S. (1998). A randomized double-blind study of the effect of distant healing in a population with advanced AIDS. *Western Journal of Medicine, 169,* 356–363.

Siegel, B. S. (1986). *Love, Medicine and Miracles.* New York: Harper & Row.

Siegel, J. M., & Kuykendall, D. H. (1990). Loss, widowhood, and psychological distress among the elderly. *Journal of Consulting and Clinical Psychology, 58,* 519–524.

Siegrist, J., Peter, R., Motz, W., & Strauer, B. E. (1992). The role of hypertension, left ventricular hypertrophy and psychosocial risks in cardiovascular disease: Prospective evidence from blue-collar men. *European Heart Journal,* 13(Suppl. D), 89–95.

Siegrist, M. (1996). Church attendance, denomination, and suicide ideology. *Journal of Social Psychology,* 136(5), 559–566.

Sijuwade, P. O. (1994). Sex differences in stress, illness and coping resources among Nigerian elderly. *Social Behavior and Personality,* 22, 239–260.

Silber, T. J., & Reilly, M. (1985). Spiritual and religious concerns of the hospitalized adolescent. *Adolescence,* 20 (77), 217–224.

Simon, G. E., Ormel, J., VonKorff, M., & Barlow, W. (1995). Health care costs associated with depressive and anxiety disorders in primary care. *American Journal of Psychiatry,* 152, 352–357.

Simons, R. L., & West, G. E. (1984–85). Life changes, coping resources, and health among the elderly. *International Journal of Aging and Human Development,* 20, 173–187.

Simonton, D. K. (1997). Achievement domain and life expectancies in Japanese civilization. *International Journal of Aging and Human Development,* 44, 103–114.

Simpson, M. E., & Conklin, G. H. (1989). Socioeconomic development, suicide, and religion: A test of Durkheim's theory of religion and suicide. *Social Forces,* 67(4), 945–964.

Simpson, W. F. (1989). Comparative longevity in a college cohort of Christian scientists. *Journal of the American Medical Association,* 262, 1657–1658.

Singh, B. K. (1979). Correlates of attitudes toward euthanasia. *Social Biology,* 26, 247–254.

Singh, B. K., & Williams, J. S. (1982). Satisfaction with health and physical condition among the elderly. *Journal of Psychiatric Treatment and Evaluation,* 4, 403–408.

Singh, B. K., Williams, J. S., & Ryther, B. J. (1986). Public approval of suicide: A situational analysis. *Suicide and Life-Threatening Behavior,* 16(4), 409–418.

Singh, N., Squier, C., Sivek, C., Wagener, M., Nguyen, M. H., & Yu, V. L. (1996). Determinants of compliance with antiretroviral therapy in patients with human immunodeficiency virus: Prospective assessment with implications for enhancing compliance. *AIDS Care,* 8, 261–269.

Single, E., Robson, L., Rehm, J., & Xi, X. (1999). Morbidity and mortality attributable to alcohol, tobacco, and illicit drug use in Canada. *American Journal of Public Health,* 89(3), 385–390.

Sinha, P. K. (1998). Hinduism and medical practice. *Journal of the Medical Association of Georgia,* 87, 312–314.

Sivan, A. B., Fitchett, G. A., & Burton, L. A. (1996). Hospitalized psychiatric and medical patients and the clergy. *Journal of Religion and Health,* 35, 11–19.

Skog, O. J., Teixeira, Z., Barrias, J., & Moreira, R. (1995). Alcohol and suicide: The Portuguese experience. *Addiction,* 90(8), 1053–1061.

Skolnick, A. (1990). Religious exemptions to child neglect laws still being passed despite convictions of parents. *Journal of the American Medical Association,* 264, 1226, 1229,1233.

Skolnick, J. H. (1958). Religious affiliation and drinking behavior. *Quarterly Journal of Studies on Alcohol,* 19, 452–470.

Skyring, A., Modan, B., Crocetti, A., & Hammerstrom, C. (1963). Some epidemiological and familial aspects of coronary heart disease: Report of a pilot study. *Journal of Chronic Disease,* 16, 1267–1279.

Sloan, R. P., Baglella, E., & Powell, T. (1999). Religion, spirituality, and medicine. *Lancet,* 353, 664–667.

Sloane, D. M., & Potvin, R. H. (1986). Religion and delinquency: Cutting through the maze. *Social Forces,* 65, 87–105.

Smedstad, L. M., Vaglum, P., Kvien, T. K., & Moum, T. (1995). The relationship between self-reported pain and sociodemographic variables, anxiety, and depressive symptoms in rheumatoid arthritis. *Journal of Rheumatology,* 22, 514–520.

Smith, A. C. (1982). *Schizophrenia and Madness.* London: Allen & Unwin.

Smith, A. H., Pool, D. I., Pearce, N. E., Lyon, J. L., Lilley, B. M., Davis, P. B., & Prior, I. A. M. (1985). Mortality among New Zealand Maori and non-Maori Mormons. *International Journal of Epidemiology,* 14, 265–271.

Smith, B. W. (1996). Coping as a predictor of outcomes following the 1993 Midwest flood. *Journal of Social Behavior and Personality,* 11, 225–239.

Smith, C. B., Weigert, A. J., & Thomas, D. L. (1979). Self-esteem and religiosity: An analysis of Catholic adolescents from five cultures. *Journal for the Scientific Study of Religion,* 18, 51–60.

Smith, D. K., Nehemkis, A. M., & Charter, R. A. (1983–1984). Fear of death, death attitude, and religious conviction in the terminally ill. *International Journal of Psychiatry in Medicine,* 13, 221–232.

Smith, D. M. (1986). Safety of faith healing. *Lancet,* March 15, 621.

Smith, E. D. (1992). Hypertension management with church-based education: A pilot study. *Journal of the National Black Nurses Association,* 6(1),19–28.

Smith, E. D., Merritt, S. L., & Patel, M. K. (1997). Church-based education: An outreach program for African Americans with hypertension. *Ethnic Health,* 2(3), 243–253.

Smith, P. M. (1956). Prisoners' attitudes toward organized religion. *Religious Education,* 51, 462–464.

Smith, R. E., Wheeler, G., & Diener, E. (1975). Faith without works: Jesus people, resistance to temptation, and altruism. *Journal of Applied Social Psychology,* 5, 320–330.

Smith, S., Freeland, M., Heffler, S., McKusick, D., & the Health Expenditures Projection Team (1998). The next ten years of health spending: What does the future hold? *Health Affairs,* 17, 128–140.

Smith, T. W. (1998). A review of church attendance measures. *American Sociological Review,* 63, 131–136.

Smith, T. W., Allred, K. D., Morrison, C. A., & Carlson, S. D. (1989). Cardiovascular reactivity and interpersonal influence: Active coping in a social context. *Journal of Personality and Social Psychology,* 56, 209–218.

Snow, L. F. (1978). Sorcerers, saints, and charlatans: Black folk healers in urban America. *Culture, Medicine and Psychiatry,* 2, 69–72.

Snowdon, D. A., Phillips, R. L., & Frazer, G. E. (1984). Meat consumption and fatal ischemic heart disease. *Preventive Medicine,* 13, 490–500.

Snyder, C. R., Harris, C., Anderson, J. R., Holleran, S. A., Irving, L. M., Sigmon, S. T., Yoshinobu, L., Gibb, J., Langelle, C., & Harney, P. (1991). The will and the ways: Development and validation of an individual differences measure of hope. *Journal of Personality and Social Psychology,* 60, 570–585.

Snyder, C. R., Sympson, S. C., Michael, S. T., & Cheavens, J. (in press). The optimism and hope constructs: Variants on a positive expectancy theme. In E. Chang (ed.), *Optimism and Pessimism.* Washington, D.C.: American Psychological Association.

Snyder, C. R., Sympson, S. C., Ybasco, F. C., Borders, T. F., Babyak, M. A., & Higgins, R. L. (1996). Development and validation of the State Hope Scale. *Journal of Personality and Social Psychology,* 70, 321–335.

Snyder, D. K., Klein, M. A., Gdowski, C. L., Faulstich, C., & LaCombe, J. (1988). Generalized dysfunction in clinic and nonclinic families: A comparative analysis. *Journal of Abnormal Child Psychology,* 16, 97–109.

Snyder, H., & Sickmund, M. (1995). *Juvenile Offenders and Victims: A National Report.* Washington, D.C.: U.S. Department of Justice, Office of Juvenile Justice and Delinquency Prevention.

Snyder, H. N. (1997). *Juvenile Arrests 1996.* Washington, D.C.: U.S. Department of Justice, Office of Juvenile Justice and Delinquency Prevention.

Sobel, D. S. (1995). Rethinking medicine: Improving health outcomes with cost-effective psychosocial interventions. *Psychosomatic Medicine,* 57, 234–244.

Sodestrom, K. E., & Martinson, I. M. (1987). Patients' spiritual coping strategies: A study of nurse and patient perspectives. *Oncology Nursing Forum,* 14, 41–46.

Solomon, Z., Mikulincer, M., & Avitzur, E. (1988). Coping, locus of control, social support, and combat-related posttraumatic stress disorder: A prospective study. *Journal of Personality and Social Psychology,* 55, 279–285.

Sonnenblick, M., Friedlander, Y., & Steinberg, A. (1993). Association between wishes of terminally ill parents and decisions by their offspring. *Journal of the American Geriatric Society,* 41, 599–604.

Sorenson, A. M., Grindstaff, C. F., & Turner, R. J. (1995). Religious involvement among unmarried adolescent mothers: A source of emotional support? *Sociology of Religion,* 56, 71–81.

Souetre, E., Lozet, H., Cimarosti, I., & Martin, P. (1994). Cost of anxiety disorders: Impact of comorbidity. *Journal of Psychosomatic Research,* 38, 151–160.

Spangler, J. G., Bell, R. A., Knick, S., Michielutte, R., Dignan, M. B., & Summerson, J. H. (1998). Church-related correlates of tobacco use among Lumbee Indians in North Carolina. *Ethnicity and Disease,* 8, 73–80.

Spect, C. E., Kudull, W. A., & Brenner, D. E. (1995). History of depression as a risk factor for Alzheimer's disease. *Epidemiology,* 6, 366–369.

Spellman, C. M., Baskett, G. D., & Byrne, D. (1971). Manifest anxiety as a contributing factor in religious conversion. *Journal of Consulting and Clinical Psychology,* 35, 245–247.

Spence, C., & Danielson, T. S. (1987). The Faith Assembly: A follow-up study of faith healing and mortality. *Indiana Medicine,* March, 238–240.

Spence, C., Danielson, T. S., & Kaunitz, W. M. (1984). The Faith Assembly: A study of perinatal and maternal mortality. *Indiana Medicine*, March, 180–183.

Spencer, J. (1975). The mental health of Jehovah's witnesses. *British Journal of Psychiatry*, 126, 556–559.

Spendlove, D. C., West, D. W., & Stanish, W. M. (1984). Risk factors and the prevalence of depression in Mormon women. *Social Science and Medicine*, 18, 491–495.

Spero, M. H. (1983). Religious patients in psychotherapy. *British Journal of Medical Psychology*, 56, 287–291.

Sperry, L., & Giblin, P. (1996). Marital and family therapy with religious persons. In E. P. Shafranske (ed.), *Religion and the Clinical Practice of Psychology* (pp. 511–533). Washington, D.C.: American Psychological Association.

Spiegel, D., & Kato, P. M. (1996). Psychosocial influences on cancer incidence and progression. *Harvard Review of Psychiatry*, 4(1), 10–26.

Spiegel, D., Bloom, J. R., & Gottheil, E. (1983). Family environment as a predictor of adjustment to metastatic breast carcinoma. *Journal of Psychosocial Oncology*, 1, 33–44.

Spiegel, D., Bloom, J. R., Kraemer, H. C., & Gottheil, E. (1989). Effect of psychosocial treatment on survival of patients with metastatic breast cancer. *Lancet*, 2(8668), 888–891.

Spilka, B., Spangler, J. D., & Nelson, C. B. (1983). Spiritual support in life threatening illness. *Journal of Religion and Health*, 22, 98–104.

Spilka, B., Stout, L., Minton, B., & Sizemore, D. (1977). Death and personal faith: A psychometric investigation. *Journal for the Scientific Study of Religion*, 16, 169–178.

Spilka, B., Zwartjes, W. J., & Zwartjes, G. M. (1991). The role of religion in coping with childhood cancer. *Pastoral Psychology*, 39, 295–304.

Sporakowski, M. J., & Hughston, G. A. (1978). Prescriptions for happy marriage: Adjustments and satisfactions of couples married for 50 or more years. *Family Coordinator*, 321–327.

Spreitzer, E., & Snyder, E. E. (1974). Correlates of life satisfaction among the aged. *Journal of Gerontology*, 29, 454–458.

Srole, L., Langner, T., Michael, S. T., Opler, M. K., & Rennie, T. A. C. (1962). *Mental Health in the Metropolis: Midtown Manhattan Study*, Vol. 1. New York: McGraw-Hill.

St. George, A., & McNamara, P. H. (1984). Religion, race and psychological well-being. *Journal for the Scientific Study of Religion*, 23, 351–363.

Stack, S. (1980a). The effect of marital dissolution on suicide. *Journal of Marriage and the Family*, 42, 83–92.

Stack, S. (1980b). Religion and suicide: A reanalysis. *Social Psychiatry*, 15(2), 65–70.

Stack, S. (1981). Suicide and religion: A comparative analysis. *Sociological Focus*, 14, 207–220.

Stack, S. (1982). Suicide: A decade review of the sociological literature. *Deviant Behavior*, 4, 41–66.

Stack, S. (1983a). A comparative analysis of suicide and religiosity. *Journal of Social Psychology*, 119(2), 285–286.

Stack, S. (1983b). The effect of the decline in institutionalized religion on suicide, 1954–1978. *Journal for the Scientific Study of Religion*, 22(3), 239–252.

Stack, S. (1983c). The effect of religious commitment on suicide: A cross-national analysis. *Journal of Health and Social Behavior*, 24(4), 362–374.

Stack, S. (1985). The effect of domestic/religious individualism on suicide, 1954–1978. *Journal of Marriage and the Family*, 47, 431–447.

Stack, S. (1987). The sociological study of suicide: Methodological issues. *Suicide and Life-Threatening Behavior*, 17, 133–150.

Stack, S. (1991). The effect of religiosity on suicide in Sweden: A time-series analysis. *Journal for the Scientific Study of Religion*, 30, 462–468.

Stack, S. (1992a). The effect of divorce on suicide in Finland: A time-series analysis. *Journal of Marriage and the Family*, 54(3), 636–642.

Stack, S. (1992b). Religiosity, depression, and suicide. In J. F. Schumaker (ed.), *Religion and Mental Health* (pp. 87–97). New York: Oxford University Press.

Stack, S. (1998). Heavy metal, religiosity, and suicide acceptability. *Suicide and Life-Threatening Behavior*, 28, 388–394.

Stack, S., & Lester, D. (1991). The effect of religion on suicidal ideation. *Social Psychiatry and Psychiatric Epidemiology*, 26(4), 168–170.

Stack, S., & Wasserman, I. (1992). The effect of religion on suicide ideology: An analysis of the networks perspective. *Journal for the Scientific Study of Religion*, 31(4), 457–466.

Stack, S., & Wasserman, I. (1993). Marital status, alcohol consumption, and suicide: An analysis of national data. *Journal of Marriage and the Family*, 55, 1018–1024.

Stack, S., & Wasserman, I. (1995). The effect of marriage, family, and religious ties on African American suicide ideology. *Journal of Marriage and the Family*, 57(1), 215–222.

Stack, S., Wasserman, I. M., & Kposowa, A. (1994). The effects of religion and feminism on suicide ideology: An analysis of national survey data.

Journal for the Scientific Study of Religion, 33(2), 110–121.

Stamler, J., Wentworth, D., & Neaton, J. D. (1986). Is relationship between serum cholesterol and risk of premature death from coronary heart disease continuous and graded? Findings in 356,222 primary screenees of the Multiple Risk Factor Intervention Trial (MRFIT). *Journal of the American Medical Association*, 256, 2823–2828.

Starbuck, E. D. (1899). *The Psychology of Religion.* New York: Scribner.

Stark, R. (1968). Age and faith. *Sociological Analysis*, 29, 1–10.

Stark, R. (1971). Psychopathology and religious commitment. *Review of Religious Research*, 12, 165–176.

Stark, R. (1996). Religion as context: Hellfire and delinquency one more time. *Sociology of Religion*, 57, 163–173.

Stark, R., & Glock, C. Y. (1968). *American Piety: The Nature of Religious Commitment.* Berkeley: University of California Press.

Stark, R., Doyle, D., & Rushing, J. (1983). Beyond Durkheim: Religion and suicide. *Journal for the Scientific Study of Religion*, 22, 120–131.

Stark, R., Kent, L., & Doyle, D. P. (1982). Religion and delinquency: The ecology of a "lost" relationship. *Journal of Research in Crime and Delinquency*, 19(10), 4–24.

Stavig, G. R., Igra, A., & Leonard, A. R. (1984). Hypertension among Asians and Pacific Islanders in California. *American Journal of Epidemiology*, 119, 677–691.

Steenland, K., Johnson, J., & Nowlin, S. (1997). A follow-up study of job strain and heart disease among males in the NHANES1 population. *American Journal of Industrial Medicine*, 31, 256–260.

Steffen, P. R., Blumenthal, J., & Sherwood, A. (2000). Religious coping and blood pressure. Paper presented at the annual meeting of the American Psychosomatic Society, Savanna, Ga., March.

Stein, D., Witztum, E., Brom, D., & DeNour, A. K. (1992). The association between adolescents' attitudes toward suicide and their psychosocial background and suicidal tendencies. *Adolescence*, 27, 949–959.

Stein, D., Witztum, E., & DeNour, A. K. (1989). Adolescent attitudes toward suicide. *Israel Journal of Psychiatry and Related Sciences*, 26(1–2), 58–68.

Stein, M., Miller, A. H., & Trestmen, R. L. (1991). Depression, the immune system, and health and illness. *Archives of General Psychiatry*, 8, 171–177.

Steinbaum, Ellen. (1996). Acting on faith. *Arthritis Today* (March–April), 35–39.

Steinberg, K. K., Pernarelli, J. M., Marcus, M., Khoury, M. J., Schildraut, J. M., & Marchbanks, P. A. (1998). Increased risk for familial ovarian cancer among Jewish women. *Genetic Epidemiology*, 15, 51–59.

Steininger, M., & Colsher, S. (1978–1979). Correlates of attitudes about "the right to die" among 1973 and 1976 high school and college students. *Omega*, 9(4), 355–368.

Steinitz, L. Y. (1980). Religiosity, well-being, and weltanschauung among the elderly. *Journal for the Scientific Study of Religion*, 19, 60–67.

Steinitz, L. Y. (1981). The local church as support for the elderly. *Journal of Gerontological Social Work*, 4, 43–53.

Steketee, G., Quay, S., & White, K. (1991). Religion and guilt in OCD patients. *Journal of Anxiety Disorders*, 4, 359–367.

Steptoe, A., Wardle, J., Pollard, T. M., Canaan, L., & Davies, G. J. (1996). Stress, social support and health-related behavior: A study of smoking, alcohol consumption and physical exercise. *Journal of Psychosomatic Research*, 41, 171–180.

Stern, M. J., & Pascale, L. (1979). Life adjustment post-myocardial infarction: Determining predictive variables. *Archives of Internal Medicine*, 137, 1680–1685.

Stern, R. C., Canda, E. R., & Doershuk, C. F. (1992). Use of nonmedical treatment by cystic fibrosis patients. *Journal of Adolescent Health*, 13, 612–615.

Stevens, R. (1989). *In Sickness and in Wealth: American Hospitals in the 20th Century.* New York: Basic Books.

Stewart, R. B., & Caranosos, G. J. (1989). Medical compliance in the elderly. *Medical Clinics of North America*, 73, 1551–1563.

Stewart, S. P., & Gale, J. E. (1994). On hallowed ground: Marital therapy with couples on the religious right. *Journal of Systemic Therapies*, 13(3), 16–25.

Stewin, L., & Anderson, C. C. (1974). Cognitive complexity as a determinant of information processing. *Alberta Journal of Educational Research*, 20, 233–243.

Stillion, J. M., McDowell, E., & Shamblin, J. B. (1984). The suicide attitude vignette experience: A method of measuring adolescent attitudes toward suicide. *Death Education*, 8, 65–79.

Stolley, J. M., & Koenig, H. G. (1995). Religion, aging, and dementia. *Alzheimer Actualites* (Fondation IPSEN), 104, 6–10.

Stolley, J. M., Buckwalter, K. C., & Koenig, H. G. (1999). Prayer and religious coping for caregivers of persons with Alzheimer's disease and related disorders. *American Journal of Alzheimer's Disease and Related Disorders and Research*, 14, 181–191.

Straus, R., & Bacon, S. D. (1953). *Drinking in College*. New Haven: Yale University Press.

Strausbaugh, H., & Irwin, M. (1992). Central corticotropin-releasing hormone reduces cellular immunity. *Brain, Behavior, and Immunity*, 6, 11–17.

Strawbridge, W. J., Cohen, R. D., Shema, S. J., & Kaplan, G. A. (1997). Frequent attendance at religious services and mortality over 28 years. *American Journal of Public Health*, 87, 957–961.

Strawbridge, W. J., Shema, S. J., Cohen, R. D., Roberts, R. E., & Kaplan, G. A. (1998). Religiosity buffers effects of some stressors on depression but exacerbates others. *Journal of Gerontology* (social sciences), 53, S118–S126.

Strayhorn, J. M., Weidman, C. S., & Larson, D. B. (1990). A measure of religiousness, and its relation to parent and child mental health variables. *Journal of Community Psychology*, 18, 34–43.

Strickland, B. R., & Schaffer, S. (1971). I-E, I-E, & F. *Journal for the Scientific Study of Religion*, 10, 366–369.

Strickland, B. R., & Weddell, S. C. (1971). Religious orientation, racial prejudice, and dogmatism: A study of Baptists and Unitarians. *Journal for the Scientific Study of Religion*, 11, 395–399.

Stroebe, W., & Stroebe, M. S. (1995). *Social Psychology and Health*. Pacific Grove, Calif.: Brooks/Cole.

Strogatz, D. S., Croft, J. B., James, S. A., Keenan, N. L., Browning, S. R., Garrett, J. M., & Curtis, A. B. (1997). Social support, stress, and blood pressure in black adults. *Epidemiology*, 8, 482–487.

Strunk, O. (1959). Interest and personality patterns of pre-ministerial students. *Psychological Reports*, 5, 740.

Studer, M., & Thornton, A. (1987). Adolescent religiosity and contraceptive usage. *Journal of Marriage and the Family*, 49, 117–128.

Sturgeon, R. S., & Hamley, R. W. (1979). Religion and anxiety. *Journal of Social Psychology*, 108, 137–138.

Suarez, L., Lloyd, L., Weiss, N., Rainbolt, T., & Pulley, L. (1994). Effect of social networks on cancer-screening behavior of older Mexican-American women. *Journal of the National Cancer Institute*, 86, 775–779.

Sudsuang, R., Chentanez, V., & Veluvan, K. (1991). Effect of Buddhist meditation on serum cortisol and total protein levels, blood pressure, pulse rate, lung volume and reaction time. *Physiology and Behavior*, 50, 543–548.

Sullivan, L. E. (1989). *Healing and Restoring: Health and Medicine in the World's Religious Traditions*. New York: Macmillan.

Sullivan, R., & Wilson, M. F. (1995). New directions for research in prevention and treatment of delinquency: A review and proposal. *Adolescence*, 30(117), 1–17.

Sullivan, W. P. (1993). "It helps me to be a whole person": The role of spirituality among the mentally challenged. *Psychosocial Rehabilitation Journal*, 16, 125–134.

Sumi, K. (1997). Optimism, social support, stress, and physical and psychological well-being in Japanese women. *Psychological Reports*, 81, 299–306.

Sundar, S., Agrawal, S. K., Singh, V. P., Bhattacharya, S. K., Udupa, K. N., & Vaish, S. K. (1984). Role of yoga in management of essential hypertension. *Acta Cardiology*, 39(3), 203–208.

Sundre, D. L. (1978). The relationship between happiness and internal/external locus of control. Unpublished masters thesis, California State University, Chico.

Surwillo, W. W., & Hobson, D. P. (1978). Brain electrical activity during prayer. *Psychological Reports*, 43, 135–143.

Surwit, R. S., Schneider, M. S., & Feinglos, M. N. (1992). Stress and diabetes mellitus. *Diabetes Care*, 15, 1413–1422.

Sussman, S., Brannon, B. R., Dent, C. W., Hansen, W. B., Johnson, C. A., & Flay, B. R. (1993). Relations of coping effort, coping strategies, perceived stress, and cigarette smoking among adolescents. *International Journal of the Addictions*, 28, 599–612.

Swan, N. (1998). Drug abuse cost to society set at $97.7 billion, continuing steady increase since 1975. *NIDA Notes*. Bethesda, Md.: National Institute for Drug Abuse.

Swan, R. (1983). Faith healing, Christian science, and the medical care of children. *New England Journal of Medicine*, 302, 1639–1641.

Swan, R. (1997). Children, medicine, religion, and the law. In L. A. Barness (ed.), *Advances in Pediatrics* (chap. 15). St. Louis: Mosby.

Swanson, W. C., & Harter, C. L. (1971). How do elderly blacks cope in New Orleans? *Aging and Human Development*, 2, 210–216.

Swindell, D. H., & L'Abate, L. (1970). Religiosity, dogmatism, and repression sensitization. *Journal for the Scientific Study of Religion*, 9, 249–251.

Szasz, T. (1978). *The Myth of Psychotherapy*. Garden City, N.Y.: Doubleday/Anchor Press.

Takahasi, Y. (1989). Mass suicide by members of the Japanese Friend of the Truth Church. *Suicide and Life-Threatening Behavior*, 19, 289–296.

Talbot, N. A. (1983). The position of the Christian Science Church. *New England Journal of Medicine*, 309, 1639–1644.

Tamburrino, M. B., Franco, K. N., Campbell, N. B., Pentz, J. E., Evans, C. L., & Jurs, S. G. (1990). Postabortion dysphoria and religion. *Southern Medical Journal*, 83, 736–738.

Tapanya, S., Nicki, R., & Jarusawad, O. (1997). Worry and intrinsic/extrinsic religious orientation among Buddhist (Thai) and Christian (Canadian) elderly persons. *International Journal of Aging and Human Development*, 44, 73–83.

Targ, E. (1997). Evaluating distant healing: A research review. *Alternative Therapies in Health and Medicine*, 3(6), 74–78.

Tate, J. L. (1998). The observant Jewish physician. *Journal of the Medical Association of Georgia*, 87, 309–310.

Taub, E., Steiner, S. S., Weingarten, E., & Walton, K. G. (1994). Effectiveness of broad specturm approaches to relapse prevention in severe alcoholism: A long-term randomized controlled-trial of transcendental meditation, EMG biofeedback, and electronic neurotherapy. *Alcoholism Treatment Quarterly*, 11(1/2), 187–220.

Taubes, T. (1998). "Healthy avenues of the mind": Psychological theory building and the influence of religion during the era of moral treatment. *American Journal of Psychiatry*, 155, 1001–1008.

Tauxe, R. V. (1998). The evolution of an epidemiologist: A Unitarian-Universalist in public health. *Journal of the Medical Association of Georgia*, 87, 305–308.

Taylor, C. B., & Fortman, S. P. (1983). Psychosomatic illness review: Hypertension. *Psychosomatics*, 24, 433–448.

Taylor, C. B., Houston-Miller, N., Killen, J. D., & DeBusk, R. F. (1990). Smoking cessation after acute myocardial infarction: Effects of a nurse-managed intervention. *Annals of Internal Medicine*, 113, 118–123.

Taylor, J., & Jackson, B. B. (1990). Factors affecting alcohol consumption in Black women: Part II. *International Journal of the Addictions*, 25, 1287–1300.

Taylor, R. J. (1986). Religious participation among elderly blacks. *Gerontologist*, 26, 630–635.

Taylor, R. J., & Chatters, L. M. (1988). Church members as a source of informal social support. *Review of Religious Research*, 30, 193–203.

Taylor, R. J., & Chatters, L. M. (1991). Nonorganizational religious participation among elderly black adults. *Journal of Gerontology* (social sciences), 46, S103–111.

Taylor, R. S., Carroll, B. E., & Lloyd, J. W. (1959). Mortality among women in 3 Catholic religious orders with special reference to cancer. *Cancer*, 12, 1207–1225.

Tebbi, C. K., Mallon, J. C., Richards, M. E., & Bigler, L. R. (1987). Religiosity and locus of control of adolescent cancer patients. *Psychological Reports*, 61, 683–696.

Tellis-Nayak, V. (1982). The transcendent standard: The religious ethos of the rural elderly. *Gerontologist*, 22, 359–363.

Templer, D. I. (1972). Death anxiety in religiously very involved persons. *Psychological Reports*, 31, 361–362.

Templer, D. I., & Dotson, E. (1970). Religious correlates of death anxiety. *Psychological Reports*, 26, 895–897.

Templer, D. I., & Veleber, D. M. (1980). Suicide rate and religion within the United States. *Psychological Reports*, 47(3), 898.

Tenant-Clark, C. M., Fritz, J. J., & Beauvais, F. (1989). Occult participation: Its impact on adolescent development. *Adolescence*, 24 (96), 757–772.

Tennison, J. C., & Snyder, W. U. (1968). Some relationships between attitudes toward the church and certain personality characteristics. *Journal of Counseling Psychology*, 15, 187–189.

Thearle, M. J., Vance, J. C., Najman, J. M., Embelton, G., & Foster, W. J. (1995) Church attendance, religious affiliation, and parental responses to sudden infant death, neonatal death and stillbirth. *Omega Journal of Death and Dying*, 31, 51–58.

Thoits, P. A. (1986). Social support as coping assistance. *Journal of Consulting and Clinical Psychology*, 54, 416–423.

Thomas, L. (1982). On immunosurveillance in human cancer. *Yale Journal of Biology and Medicine*, 55, 329–333.

Thomas, L. E., & Cooper, P. E. (1980). Incidence and psychological correlates of intense spiritual experiences. *Journal of Transpersonal Psychology*, 12, 75–85.

Thomas, M. E., & Holmes, B. J. (1992). Determinants of satisfaction for Blacks and Whites. *Sociological Quarterly*, 33, 459–472.

Thomas, P. D., Goodwin, J. M., & Goodwin J. S. (1985). Effect of social support on stress-related changes in cholesterol level, uric acid level, and immune function in an elderly sample. *American Journal of Psychiatry*, 142, 735–737.

Thomas, S. B., Quinn, S. C., Billingsley, A., & Caldwell, C. (1994). The characteristics of northern Black churches with community health outreach programs. *American Journal of Public Health*, 84, 575–579.

Thompson, M. P., & Vardaman, P. J. (1997). The role of rleigion in coping with loss of a family member in homicide. *Journal for the Scientific Study of Religion*, 36, 44–51.

Thoresen, C. E. (1990). Long-term, 8-year followup of recurrent coronary prevention project: Invited Symposium. Uppsala, Sweden: First conference of the International Society of Behavioral Medicine, June 14.

Thoresen, C. E. (1998). Spirituality, health, and science: The coming revival? In S. Roth-Roemer, & S. R. Kurpius (eds.), *The Emerging Role of Counseling Psychology in Health Care* (pp. 409–431). New York: Norton.

Thorndike, E. L. (1939). American cities and states. *Annals of the New York Academy of Sciences*, 39, 213–298.

Thorne, C., Nickerson, D., & Gemmel, D. (1996). The relationship between religiosity and health-risk factors in geriatrics. *Journal of Religion and Health*, 35(2), 149–158.

Thorner, I. (1953). Ascetic Protestantism and alcoholism. *Psychiatry*, 16, 167–176.

Thornton, A., & Camburn, D. (1989). Religious participation and adolescent sexual behavior and attitudes. *Journal of Marriage and the Family*, 51, 641–653.

Thorson, J. A. (1991). Afterlife constructs, death anxiety, and life reviewing: The importance of religion as a moderating variable. *Journal of Psychology and Theology*, 19, 278–284.

Thorson, J. A. (1998). Religion and anxiety: Which anxiety? Which religion? In H. G. Koenig (ed.), *Handbook of Religion and Mental Health* (pp. 147–159). San Diego: Academic Press.

Thorson, J. A., & Powell, F. C. (1989). Death anxiety and religion in an older male sample. *Psychological Reports*, 64, 985–986.

Thorson, J. A., & Powell, F. C. (1990). Meanings of death and intrinsic religiosity. *Journal of Clinical Psychology*, 46, 379–391.

Thorson, J. A., & Powell, F. C. (1991). Life, death, and life after death: Meanings of the relationship between death anxiety and religion. *Journal of Religious Gerontology*, 8, 41–56.

Thouless, R. (1935). The tendency to certainty in religious beliefs. *British Journal of Psychology*, 6, 16–31.

Thurstone, L., & Chave, E. (1929). Attitude toward church scale. In *The Measurement of Attitude*. Chicago: University of Chicago Press.

Tiebout, H. M. (1944). Therapeutic mechanisms of Alcoholics Anonymous. *American Journal of Psychiatry*, 100, 468–473.

Tillman, J. G. (1998). Psychodynamic psychotherapy, religious beliefs, and self-disclosure. *American Journal of Psychotherapy*, 52, 273–286.

Timio, M., Verdecchia, P., Venanzi, S., Gentili, S., Ronconi, M., Francucci, B., Montanari, M., & Bichisao, E. (1988). Age and blood pressure changes: A 20-year follow-up study in nuns in a secluded order. *Hypertension*, 12, 457–461.

Tix, A. P., & Frazier, P. A. (1997). The use of religious coping during stressful life events: Main effects, moderation, and medication. *Journal of Consulting and Clinical Psychology*, 66, 411–422.

Tjeltveit, A. C., Fiordalisi, A. M., & Smith, C. (1996). Relationships among mental health values and various dimensions of religiousness. *Journal of Social and Clinical Psychology*, 15, 364–377.

Tobach, E., & Bloch, H. (1956). Effect of stress by crowding prior to and following tuberculosis infection. *American Journal of Physiology*, 187, 399–402.

Tobacyk, J. (1983). Death threat, death concerns, and paranormal beliefs. *Death Education*, 7, 115–124.

Toh, Y. M., & Tan, S. Y. (1997). The effectiveness of church-based lay counselors: A controlled outcome study. *Journal of Psychology and Christianity*, 16, 260–267.

Tondo, L., Baldessarini, R. J., Hennen, J., Minnai, G. P., Salis, P., Scamonatti, L., Masia, M., Ghiani, C., & Mannu, P. (1999). Suicide attempts in major affective disorder patients with comorbid substance use disorders. *Journal of Clinical Psychiatry*, 60(Suppl. 2), 63–69; discussion 75–76, 113–116.

Toniolo, P. G., & Kato, I. (1996). Jewish religion and risk of breast cancer. *Lancet*, 348, 760.

Toone, B. K., Cooke, E., & Lader, M. H. (1979). The effect of temporal lobe surgery on electrodermal activity: Implications for an organic hypothesis in the etiology of schizophrenia. *Psychological Medicine*, 9, 281–285.

Toor, M., Agmon, J., & Aallalouf, D. (1954). Changes of serum total lipids, total cholesterol and lipid-phosphorous in Jewish Yemenite immigrants after 20 years in Israel. *Bulletin of the Research Council of Israel*, 4, 202–203.

Torabi, M. R. (1990). Tobacco use by samples of American and Turkish students: A cross-cultural study. *International Quarterly of Community Health Education*, 10(3), 241–251.

Torrington, M., & Botha, J. L. (1981). Familial hyperchoesterolaemia and church affiliation. *Lancet*, November 14, 1120.

Toseland, R., & Rasch, J. (1979). Correlates of life satisfaction: An aid analysis. *International Journal of Aging and Human Development*, 10, 203–211.

Tournier, P. (1957). *The Meaning of Persons*. New York: Harper & Row.

Trappler, B., & Endicott, J. (1997). Religion and psychopathology (letter in response to Kendler study). *American Journal of Psychiatry*, 154, 1636.

Trappler, B., Endicott, J., & Friedman, S. (1995). Psychosocial adjustment among returnees to Judaism. *Journal of Psychology*, 129, 433–441.

Trenholm, T., Trent, J., & Compton, W. C. (1998). Negative religious conflict as a predictor of panic disorder. *Journal of Clinical Psychology*, 54, 59–65.

Trew, A. (1971). The religious factor in mental illness. *Pastoral Psychology*, 22, 21–28.

Trice, H. M., & Staudenmeier, W. J. (1989) A sociocultural history of Alcoholics Anonymous. In M. Galanter (ed.), *Treatment Research*, Vol. 7, *Recent Developments in Alcoholism* (pp. 11–36). *Treatment Research*. New York: Plenum.

Trier, K. K., & Shupe, A. (1991). Prayer, religiosity, and healing in the heartland, USA: A research note. *Review of Religious Research*, 32, 351–358.

Trimble, D. E. (1997). The Religious Orientation Scale: Review and meta-analysis of social desirability effects. *Educational and Psychological Measurement*, 57, 970–986.

Trimble, M. R., Mendez, M. F., & Cummings, J. L. (1997). Neuropsychiatric symptoms from the temporolimbic lobes. *Journal of Neuropsychiatry and Clinical Neurosciences*, 9, 429–438.

Trovato, F. (1986). The relationship between marital dissolution and suicide: The Canadian case. *Journal of Marriage and the Family*, 48, 341–348.

Trovato, F. (1992). A Durkheimian analysis of youth suicide: Canada, 1971 and 1981. *Suicide and Life-Threatening Behavior*, 22(4), 413–427.

Troyer, H. (1988). Review of cancer among 4 religious sects: Evidence that life-styles are distinctive sets of risk factors. *Social Science and Medicine*, 26, 1007–1017.

Truett, K. R., Eaves, L. J., Meyer, J. M., Heath, A. C., & Martin, N. G. (1992). Religion and education as mediators of attitudes: A multivariate analysis. *Behavior Genetics*, 22, 43–62.

Tschann, J. M., Adler, N. E., Irwin, C. E., Millstein, S. G., Turner, R. A., & Kegles, S. M. (1994). Initiation of substance use in early adolescence: The roles of pubertal timing and emotional distress. *Health Psychology*, 13, 326–333.

Tu, W. (1980). A religiophilosophical perspective on pain. In H. W. Koster, D. Kosterlitz, & L. Y. Terenius (eds.), *Pain and Society* (pp. 63–78). Weinheim-Deerfield Beach, Fla.: Verlag Chemie.

Tuchfeld, B. S. (1981). Spontaneous remission in alcoholics: Empirical observations and theoretical implications. *Journal of Studies on Alcohol*, 42, 626–641.

Tucker, D. M., Novelly, R. A., & Walker, P. J. (1987). Hyperreligiosity in temporal lobe epilepsy: Redefining the relationship. *Journal of Nervous and Mental Disease*, 175, 181–184.

Turbott, J. (1996). Religion, spirituality and psychiatry: Conceptual, cultural and personal challenges. *Australian and New Zealand Journal of Psychiatry*, 30, 720–727.

Turner, J. A., & Clancy, S. (1986). Strategies for coping with chronic low back pain: Relationship to pain and disability. *Pain*, 24, 355–364.

Turner, N. H., Ramirez, G. Y., Higginbotham, J. C., Markides, K., Wygant, A. C., & Black, S. (1994). Tri-ethnic alcohol use and religion, family, and gender. *Journal of Religion and Health*, 33, 341–352.

Turner, R. P., Lukoff, D., Barnhouse, R. T., & Lu, F. G. (1995). Religious or spiritual problem: A culturally sensitive diagnostic category in the DSM-IV. *Journal of Nervous and Mental Disease*, 183, 435–444.

Tuttle, D. H., Shutty, M. S., & DeGood, D. E. (1991). Empirical dimensions of coping in chronic pain patients: A factorial analysis. *Rehabilitation Psychology*, 36, 179–187.

Uchino, B. N., Cacioppo, J. R., & Kiecolt-Glaser, J. K. (1996). The relationship between social support and physiological processes: A review with emphasis on underlying mechanisms and implications for health. *Psychological Bulletin*, 119, 488–531.

Uhlman, J., & Steinke, P. D. (1984). Pastoral visitation to the institutionalized aged: Delivering more than a lick and a promise. *Pastoral Psychology*, 32, 231–238.

Ullman, C. (1988). Psychological well-being among converts in traditional and nontraditional religious groups. *Psychiatry*, 51, 312–322.

Ultmann, J. E., & Golomb, H. M. (1980). Principles of neoplasia: Approach to diagnosis and management. In K. J. Isselbacher, R. D. Adams, E. Braunwald, R. G. Petersdorf, & J. D. Wilson (eds.), *Harrison's Principles of Internal Medicine*, 9th ed. (p. 1588). New York: McGraw-Hill.

Underwood, L. (1999). Daily spiritual experiences scale. In *Multidimensional Measurement of Religiousness/Spirituality for Use in Health Research*. Kalamazoo, Mich.: John E. Fetzer Institute.

Unutzer, J., Patrick, D. L., Simon, G., Grembowski, D., Walker, E., Rutter, C., & Katon, W. (1997). Depressive symptoms and the cost of health services in HMO patients aged 65 and older: 84-year prospective study. *Journal of the American Medical Association*, 277, 1618–1623.

Ur, E., White, P. D., & Grossman, A. (1992). Hypothesis: Cytokines may be activated to cause depressive illness and chronic fatigue syndrome. *European Archives of Psychiatry and Clinical Neurosciences*, 241, 317–322.

U.S. Bureau of the Census. (1978). Marriage, divorce, widowhood, and remarriage by family characteristics. *Current Population Reports*, Series P-20, no. 312. Washington, D.C.: U.S. Government Printing Office.

U.S. Congress. (1989). House Select Committee on Children, Youth, and Families. *U.S. Children and Their Families: Current Conditions and Recent Trends*. Washington, D.C.: U.S. Government Printing Office.

Usui, W. M., Keil, T. J., & Durig, K. R. (1985). Socioeconomic comparisons and life satisfaction of elderly adults. *Journal of Gerontology*, 40, 110–114.

Uyanga, J. (1979). The characteristics of patients of spiritual healing homes and traditional doctors in southeastern Nigeria. *Social Science and Medicine*, 13A, 323–329.

Vaillant, G. E. (1983). *The Natural History of Alcoholism*. Cambridge, Mass.: Harvard University Press.

Van Egmond, M., & Diekstra, R. F. W. (1989). The predictability of suicidal behavior: The results of a meta-analysis of published studies. In R. F. W. Diekstra, R. Maris, S. Platt, A. Schmidtke, & G. Sonneck (eds.), *Suicide and Its Prevention* (pp. 37–61). New York: Brill.

Van Loon, A. (1998). The development of faith community nursing programs as a response to changing Australian health policy. *Health Education and Behavior*, 25, 790–799.

VandeCreek, L. (1991). Identifying the spiritually needy patient: The role of demographics. *Caregiver Journal*, 8(3), 38–47.

VandeCreek, L. (1997). Collaboration between nurses and chaplains for spiritual caregiving. *Seminars in Oncology Nursing*, 13, 279–280.

VandeCreek, L., & Cooke, B. (1996). Hospital pastoral care practices of parish clergy. *Research in the Social Scientific Study of Religion*, 7, 253–264.

VandeCreek, L., Pargament, K., Belavich, T., Cowell, B., & Friedel, L. (1995). The role of religious support when coping with surgical anxieties. Paper presented at the annual meeting of the American Psychological Association, New York City.

Varma, S., Zain, A., & Kerian, K. (1997). Experiences in religious psychotherapy. *Australian and New Zealand Journal of Psychiatry*, 31, 147–149.

Vaughan, P. (1998). *The Monogamy Myth: A Personal Handbook for Recovering from Affairs*. New York: Designer.

Veach, T. L., & Chappel, J. N. (1992). Measuring spiritual health: A preliminary study. *Substance Abuse*, 13, 139–147.

Vedhara, K., Cox, N. K. M., Wilcock, G. K., Perks, P., Hunt, M., Andersen, S., Lightman, S. L., & Shanks, N. M. (1999). Chronic stress in elderly caregivers of dementia patients and antibody response to influenza vaccine. *Lancet*, 353, 627–631.

Veith, R. C., Lewis, N., Linares, O. A., Barnes, R. F., Raskind, M. A., & Villacres, E. C. (1993). Sympathetic nervous system activity in major depression–basal and desipramine-induced alterations in plasma norepinephrine kinetics. *Archives of General Psychiatry*, 50, 1–12.

Velikova, G., Selby, P. J., Snaith, P. R., & Kirby, P. G. (1995). The relationship of cancer pain to anxiety. *Psychotherapy and Psychosomatics*, 63, 181–184.

Ventura, J. N. (1982). Parent coping behaviors, parent functioning, and infant temperament characteristics. *Nursing Research*, 31, 269–273.

Verbosky, L. A., Franco, K. N., & Zrull, J. P. (1993). The relationship between depression and length of stay in the general hospital patient. *Journal of Clinical Psychiatry*, 54, 177–181.

Verbrugge, L. M. (1979). Marital status and health. *Journal of Marriage and the Family*, 41, 267–285.

Verghese, A., John, J. K., Rajkumar, S., Richard, J., Sethi, B. B., & Trivedi, J. K. (1989). Factors associated with the course and outcome of schizophrenia in India: Results of a two-year multicentre follow-up study. *British Journal of Psychiatry,* 154, 499–503.

Verhaak, P. F. M., & Tijhuis, M. A. R. (1994). The somatizing patient in general practice. *International Journal of Psychiatry in Medicine,* 24, 157–177.

Veroff, J., Kulka, R. A., & Douvan, E. (1981). *Mental Health in America: Patterns of Help Seeking from 1957 to 1976.* New York: Basic Books.

Versluys, J. J. (1949). Cancer and occupation in the Netherlands. *British Journal of Cancer,* 3, 161–185.

Videka-Sherman, L. (1982). Coping with the death of a child: A study over time. *American Journal of Orthopsychiatry,* 52, 688–698.

Vinson, J. M., Rich, M. W., & Sperry, J. C. (1990). Early re-admissions of elderly patients with congestive heart failure. *Journal of the American Geriatrics Society,* 38, 1290–1295.

Vinyon, K. A. (1995). *Coping with chronic illness: Individual and marital adjustment of patients and spouses.* Ph.D. diss., University of Minnesota.

Vlietstra, R. E., Kronmal, R. A., Oberman, A., Frye, R. L., & Killip, T. (1986). Effect of cigarette smoking on survival of patients with angiographically documented coronary artery disease. Report from the CASS Registry. *Journal of the American Medical Association,* 255, 1023–1027.

Vogt, T. M., Lullooly, J. P., Ernst, D., Pope, C. R., & Hollis, J. F. (1992). Social networks as predictors of ischemic heart disease, cancer, stroke and hypertension. *Journal of Clinical Epidemiology,* 45, 659–666.

Von Korff, M., Le Resche, L., & Dworkin, S. F. (1993). First onset of common pain symptoms: A prospective steady of depression as a risk factor. *Pain,* 55, 251–258.

Waaler, H. T., & Hjort, P. F. (1981). Low mortality among Norwegian Seventh-Day Adventists, 1960–1977: A message on lifestyle and health? *Tidsskrift for Den Norske Laegeforening,* 101, 623–627.

Wagner, B. M. (1997). Family risk factors for child and adolescent suicidal behavior. *Psychological Bulletin,* 121, 246–298.

Wahass, S., & Kent, G. (1997). Coping with auditory hallucinations: A cross-cultural comparison between Western (British) and non-Western (Saudi Arabian) patients. *Journal of Nervous and Mental Disease,* 185, 664–668.

Waisberg, J. L., & Porter, J. E. (1994). Purpose in life and outcome of treatment for alcohol dependence. *British Journal of Clinical Psychology,* 33, 49–63.

Walden, R. T., Schaefer, L. E., Lemon, F. R., Sunshine, A., & Wynder, E. L. (1964). Effect of environment on the serum cholesterol-triglyceride distribution. *American Journal of Medicine,* 35, 269–276.

Waldfogel, S., & Meadows, S. (1996). Religious issues in the capacity evaluation. *General Hospital Psychiatry,* 18, 173–182.

Waldfogel, S., & Wolpe, P. R. (1993). Using awareness of religious factors to enhance interventions in consultation-liaison psychiatry. *Hospital and Community Psychiatry,* 44, 473–477.

Wales, J. K. (1995). The psychological stress cause diabetes? *Diabetic Medicine,* 12, 109–112.

Walker, L., & Walker, L. D. (1990). "Anniversary Reaction": Important events and timing of death in a group of Roman Catholic Priests. *Omega,* 21, 69–74.

Walker, S. R., Tonigan, J. S., Miller, W. R., Corner, S., & Kahlich, L. (1997). Intercessory prayer in the treatment of alcohol abuse independence: A pilot investigation. *Alternative Therapies in Health and Medicine,* 3(6), 79–86.

Wallace, J. G. (1972). Drinkers and abstainers in Norway. *Quarterly Journal of Studies on Alcohol* (Suppl 6), 129–151.

Wallace, J. M., & Forman, T. A. (1998). Religion's role in promoting health and reducing the risk among American youth. *Health Education and Behavior,* 25, 721–741.

Wallis, C. (1996). Faith and healing. *Time,* June 24, 58–68. Quoting Yankelovich Partners (1996) for Time-CNN, June 12–13.

Walls, C. T., & Zarit, S. H. (1991). Informal support from black churches and the well-being of elderly blacks. *Gerontologist,* 31, 490–495.

Wallston, K. A., Wallston, B. S., & DeVellis, R. (1978). Development of the Multidimensional Health Locus of Control Scales. *Health Education Monographs,* 6(2), 160–170.

Walsh, A. (1980). The prophylactic effect of religion on blood pressure levels among a sample of immigrants. *Social Sciences and Medicine,* 14B, 59–63.

Walsh, A. (1998). Religion and hypertension: Testing alternative explanations among immigrants. *Behavioral Medicine,* 24, 122–130.

Walter, T. (1997). The ideology and organization of spiritual care: Three approaches. *Palliative Medicine*, 11, 21–30.

Walters, O. S. (1957). The religious background of fifty alcoholics. *Quarterly Journal of Studies of Alcohol*, 18, 405–416.

Walton, C. G., Shultz, C. M., Beck, C. M., & Walls, R. C. (1991). Psychological correlates of loneliness in the older adult. *Archives of Psychiatric Nursing*, 5, 165–170.

Walton, K. G., Pugh, N. D. C., Gelderloos, P., & Macrae, P. (1995). Stress reduction in preventing hypertension: Preliminary support for a psychoneuroendocrine mechanism. *Journal of Alternative and Complementary Medicine*, 1(3), 263–283.

Wan, T. T. H., & Yates, A. S. (1975). Prediction of dental services utilization: A multivariate approach. *Inquiry*, 12, 143–156.

Wandrei, K. E. (1985). Identifying potential suicides among high-risk women. *Social Work*, 30, 511–517.

Wang, C. Y., & Fenske, M. M. (1996). Self-care of adults with non-insulin-dependent diabetes mellitus: Influence of family and friends. *Diabetes Educator*, 22, 465–470.

Ward, R. (1980). Age and acceptance of euthanasia. *Journal of Gerontology*, 35(3), 421–431.

Wardwell, W. I., & Bahnson, C. B. (1973). Behavioral variables and myocardial infarction in the Southeastern Connecticut Heart Study. *Journal of Chronic Disease*, 26, 447–461.

Wardwell, W. I., Bahnson, C. B., & Caron, H. S. (1963). Social and psychological factors in coronary heart disease. *Journal of Health and Human Behavior*, 4, 154–165.

Wardwell, W. I., Hyman, M., & Bahnson, C. B. (1964). Stress and coronary heart disease in three field studies. *Journal of Chronic Disease*, 17, 73–84.

Wardwell, W. I., Hyman, M., & Bahnson, C. B. (1968). Socio-environmental antecedents to coronary heart disease in 87 white males. *Social Science and Medicine*, 2, 165–183.

Warfield, R. D., & Golstein, M. B. (1996). Spirituality: The key to recovery from alcoholism. *Counseling and Values*, 40, 196–205.

Warren, R. (1990). God help me: I. Religious coping efforts as predictors of the outcomes to significant negative life events. *American Journal of Community Psychology*, 18, 793–824.

Wasman, M., Corradi, R. B., & Clemens, N. A. (1979). In-depth continuing education for clergy in mental health: Ten years of a large-scale program. *Pastoral Psychology*, 27, 251–259.

Wasserman, I., & Stack, S. (1993). The effect of religion on suicide: An analysis of cultural context. *Omega: Journal of Death and Dying*, 27(4), 295–305.

Wassersug, J. (1989). It's a miracle! *Postgraduate Medicine*, 86 (July), 76–77.

Watson, J. S. (1991). Religion as a cultural phenomenon, and national mortality rates from heart disease. *Psychological Reports*, 69, 439–442.

Watson, P. J., Hood, R. W., Morris, R. J., & Hall, J. R. (1984). Empathy, religious orientation and social desirability. *Journal of Psychology*, 117, 211–216.

Watson, P. J., Hood, R. W., Morris, R. J., & Hall, J. R. (1985). Religiosity, sin and self-esteem. *Journal of Psychology and Theology*, 13, 115–128.

Watson, P. J., Milliron, J. T., Morris, R. J., & Hood, R. W., Jr. (1995). Locus of control within a religious ideological surround. *Journal of Psychology and Christianity*, 14, 239–249.

Watson, P. J., Morris, R. J., & Hood, R. W. (1988). Sin and self-functioning: Part 1. Grace, guilt, and self-consciousness. *Journal of Psychology and Theology*, 16, 254–269.

Watson, P. J., Morris, R. J., & Hood, R. W. (1989). Sin and self-functioning: Part 4. Depression, assertiveness, and religious commitments. *Journal of Psychology and Theology*, 17, 44–58.

Watson, P. J., Morris, R. J., & Hood, R. W. (1990). Extrinsic scale factors: Correlations and construction of religious orientation types. *Journal of Psychology and Christianity*, 9, 35–46.

Wattenberg, W. (1950) Church attendance and juvenile misconduct. *Sociology and Social Research*, 14, 195–202.

Watters, W. (1992). *Deadly Doctrine: Health, Illness, and Christian God-Talk*. Buffalo, N.Y.: Prometheus.

Waxman, S. G., & Geshwind, N. (1975). The interictal behavior syndrome of temporal lobe epilepsy. *Archives of General Psychiatry*, 32, 1580–1586.

Weaver, A. J. (1993a). Depression: What clergy need to know. *Currents in Theology and Mission*, 20(1), 5–16.

Weaver, A. J. (1993b). Psychological trauma: What clergy need to know. *Pastoral Psychology*, 41, 385–407.

Weaver, A. J. (1995). Has there been a failure to prepare and support parish-based clergy in their role as front-lined community mental health workers? A review. *Journal of Pastoral Care*, 49, 129–149.

Weaver, A. J., Flannelly, L. T., Flannelly, K. J., Koenig, H. G., & Larson, D. B. (1998). An analysis of research on religious and spiritual variables in three major mental health nursing journals: 1991–1995. *Issues in Mental Health Nursing*, 19, 263–276.

Weaver, A. J., Koenig, H. G., & Larson, D. B. (1997). Marriage and family therapists and the clergy: A need for clinical collaboration, training, and research. *Journal of Marriage and Family Therapy*, 23(1), 13–25.

Weaver, A. J., Samford, J. A., Kline, A. E., Lucas, L. A., Larson, D. B., & Koenig, H. G. (1997). Psychologists and clergy working together? An analysis of eight APA journals: 1991–1994. *Professional Psychology: Research and Practice*, 28, 471–474.

Weaver, A. J., Samford, J. A., Larson, D. B., Lucas, L. A., Koenig, H. G., & Patrick, V. (1998). A systematic review of research on religion in four major psychiatric journals: 1991–1995. *Journal of Nervous and Mental Diseases*, 186, 187–190.

Webster, I. W., & Rawson, G. K. (1979). Health status of Seventh-Day Adventists. *Medical Journal of Australia*, 1(May 19), 417–420.

Webster's New World Dictionary of the American Language (1980). New York: Simon & Schuster.

Wechsler, H., & McFadden, M. (1979). Drinking among college students in New England: Extent, social correlates, and consequences of alcohol use. *Journal of Studies on Alcohol*, 40, 969–996.

Wechsler, H., Thum, D., Demone, H. W., & Dwinnell, J. (1972). Social characteristics and blood alcohol level. *Quarterly Journal of Studies on Alcohol*, 33, 132–147.

Weill, J., & Le Bourhis, B. (1994). Factors predictive of alcohol consumption in a representative sample of French male teenagers: A five-year prospective study. *Drug and Alcohol Dependence*, 35, 45–50.

Weima, J. (1965). Authoritarianism, religious conservatism and socio-centric attitudes in Roman Catholic groups. *Human Relations*, 18, 231–239.

Weinberg, N. Z., Rahdert, E., Colliver, J. D., & Glantz, M. D. (1998). Adolescent substance abuse: A review of the past 10 years. *Journal of the American Academy of Child and Adolescent Psychiatry*, 37(3), 252–261.

Weiner, H. (1979). *The Psychobiology of Hypertension*. New York: Elsevier.

Weinrich, S., Hardin, S. B., & Johnson, M. (1990). Nurses respond to Hurricane Hugo victims' disaster stress. *Archives of Psychiatric Nursing*, 4, 195–205.

Weinrich, S., Holdford, D., Boyd, M., Creanga, D., Cover, K., Johnson, K., Frank-Stromborg, M., & Weinrich, M. (1998). Prostate cancer education in African-American churches. *Public Health Nursing*, 15, 188–195.

Weis, D., Matheus, R., & Shank, M. J. (1997). Health care delivery in faith communities: The parish nurse model. *Public Health Nursing*, 14, 368–372.

Weisner, T. S., Belzer, L., & Stolze, L. (1991). Religion and families of children with developmental delays. *American Journal of Mental Retardation*, 95, 647–662.

Weiss, A. S., & Mendoza, R. H. (1990). Effects of acculturation into the Hare Krishna movement on mental health and personality. *Journal for the Scientific Study of Religion*, 29, 173–184.

Weissman, M. M., Prusoff, B. A., & Klerman, G. L. (1978). Personality and the prediction of long-term outcome of depression. *American Journal of Psychiatry*, 135, 797–800.

Weitzman, L. J. (1985). *The Divorce Revolution: The Unexpected Social and Economic Consequences for Women and Children in America*. New York: Free Press.

Welford, A. T. (1947). Is religious behavior dependent upon affect or frustration? *Journal of Abnormal and Social Psychology*, 42, 310–319.

Weltha, D. A. (1969). Some relationships between religious attitudes and the self-concept. *Dissertation Abstracts International*, 30, 2782-B.

Wenneberg, S. R., Schneider, R. H., Walton, K. G., MacClean, C. R., Levitsky, D. K., Mandarino, J. V., Waziri, R., & Wallace, R. K. (1997). Anger expression correlates with platelet aggregation. *Behavioral Medicine*, 22, 174–177.

Wenneberg, S. R., Schneider, R. H., Walton, K. G., MacClean, C. R., Levitsky, D. K., Salerno, J. W., Wallace, R. K., Mandarino, J. V., Rainforth, M. V., & Waziri, R. (1997). A controlled study of the effects of the Transcendental Meditation program on cardiovascular reactivity and ambulatory blood pressure. *International Journal of Neuroscience*, 89(1–2), 15–28.

Werebe, M. J. G. (1983). Attitudes of French adolescents toward sexuality. *Journal of Adolescence*, 6, 145–159.

Werman, D. (1972). The teaching of the history of psychiatry. *Archives of General Psychiatry*, 26, 287–289.

Werner, O. R., Wallace, R. K., Charles, B., Janssen, G., Stryker, T., & Chalmers, R. A. (1986). Long-term endocrinologic changes in subjects practicing the Transcendental meditation and TM-Sidhi program. *Psychosomatic Medicine*, 48(1–2), 59–66.

West, G. E., & Simons, R. L. (1983). Sex differences in stress, coping resources, and illness among the elderly. *Research on Aging*, 5, 235–268.

West, R. O., & Hayes, O. B. (1968). Diet and serum cholesterol levels: A comparison between vegetarians and nonvegetarians in Seventh-day Adventist group. *American Journal of Clinical Nutrition*, 21, 853–862.

Westberg, G. F. (1984). Churches are joining the health care team. *Urban Health* (October), 34–36.

Westman, A. S., & Canter, F. M. (1985). Fear of death and the concept of extended self. *Psychological Reports*, 56, 419–425.

Weymeyer, Peggy (1995). Religion and the power of prayer to heal the sick. *ABC World News Tonight*, December 20.

White, G. (1991). Prison ministry, Department of Human Resources chaplains face budget ax. *Atlanta Constitution* (August 24), p. E6.

Whitehead, P. C. (1970). Religious affiliation and use of drugs among adolescent students. *Journal for the Scientific Study of Religion*, 9, 152–154.

Whitlatch, A. M., Meddaugh, D. I., & Langhout, K. J. (1992). Religiosity among Alzheimer's disease caregivers. *American Journal of Alzheimer's Disease and Related Disorders and Research*, 11–20.

Whitlock, F. A., & Schapira, K. (1967). Attempted suicide in Newcastle upon Tyne. *British Journal of Psychiatry*, 113, 423–434.

Whitt, H. P., Gordon, C. C., & Hofley, J. R. (1972). Religion, economic development and lethal aggression. *American Sociological Review*, 37, 193–201.

Wickerstrom, D. L., & Fleck, J. R. (1983). Missionary children: Correlates of self-esteem and dependency. *Journal of Psychology and Theology*, 11, 226–235.

Wicks, A. C., Lowe, R. F., & Jones, J. J. (1974). Alcohol: A cause of diabetes in Rhodesia. *South African Medical Journal*, 48, 1115–1117.

Wicks, R. J., Parsons, R. D., & Capps, D. (1985). *Clinical Handbook of Pastoral Counseling*, Vol. 1. New York: Paulist Press.

Wiebe, K. F., & Fleck, J. R. (1980). Personality correlates of intrinsic, extrinsic, and non-religious orientations. *Journal of Psychology*, 105, 181–187.

Wiedman, D. (1990). Big and Little Moon Peyotism as health care delivery systems. *Medical Anthropology*, 12(4), 371–387.

Wierson, M., Forehand, R., & McCombs, A. (1988). The relationship of early adolescent functioning to parent-reported and adolescent perceived interparental conflict. *Journal of Abnormal Child Psychology*, 16, 707–718.

Wiggins, J. S. (1969). Content dimensions in the MMPI. In J. N. Butcher (ed.), *MMPI: Research Developments and Clinical Applications*. New York: McGraw-Hill.

Wikan, U. (1988). Bereavement and loss in two Muslim communities: Egypt and Bali compared. *Social Science and Medicine*, 27, 451–460.

Wilbert, J. (1991). Does pharmacology corroborate the nicotine therapy and practices of South American shamanism? *Journal of Ethnopharmacology*, 32(1–3), 179–186.

Will, G. F. (1998). The gospel from science. *Newsweek* (November 9), 88.

Willams, R. (1989). *The Trusting Heart: Great News about Type A Behavior*. New York: Times Books.

Willett, W. C., Green, A., Stampfer, M. J., Speizer, F. E., Colditz, G. A., Rosner, B., Monson, R. R., Stason, W., & Hennekens, C. H. (1987). Relative and absolute excess risks of coronary heart disease among women who smoke cigarettes. *New England Journal of Medicine*, 317, 1303–1309.

Williams, A. B., Shahryarinejad, A., Andrews, S., & Alcabes, P. (1997). Social support for HIV-infected mothers: Relation to HIV care seeking. *Journal of the Association of Nurses in AIDS Care*, 8, 91–98.

Williams, D. R., Larson, D. B., Buckler, R. E., Heckmann, R. C., Pyle, & C. M. (1991). Religion and psychological distress in a community sample. *Social Science and Medicine*, 32, 1257–1262.

Williams, G. (1998). How prayer heals: Proof of the power of faith. *McCall's* (December), 90, 92–93, 96.

Williams, J. M., Stout, J. K., & Erickson, L. (1986). Comparison of the importance of alcoholics anonymous and outpatient counseling to maintenance of sobriety among alcohol abusers. *Psychological Reports*, 58, 803–806.

Williams, R., & Dickson, R. A. (1995). Economics of schizophrenia. *Canadian Journal of Psychiatry*, 40(7, Suppl. 2), S60–S67.

Williams, R., & Hunt, K. (1997). Psychological distress among British South Asians: The contribution of stressful situations and subcultural differences in the West of Scotland Twenty-07 Study. *Psychological Medicine, 27*, 1173–1181.

Williams, R. B., Barefoot, J. C., Califf, R. M., Haney, T. L., Saunders, W. B., Pryor, D. B., Hlatky, M. A., Siegler, I. C., & Mark, D. B. (1992). Prognostic importance of social and economic resources among medically treated patients with angiographically documented coronary artery disease. *Journal of the American Medical Association, 267*, 520–524.

Williams, R. B., Haney, T. L., Lee, K. L., Kong, Y., Blumenthal, J. A., & Whalen, R. E. (1980). Type A behavior hostility and coronary artherosclerosis. *Psychosomatic Medicine, 42*, 539–549.

Williams, R. L., & Cole, S. (1968). Religiosity, generalized anxiety, and apprehension concerning death. *Journal of Social Psychology, 75*, 111–117.

Willits, F. K., & Crider, D. M. (1988). Religion and well-being: Men and women in the middle years. *Review of Religious Research, 29*, 281–294.

Wills, T. A. (1986). Stress and coping in early adolescence: Relationships to substance use in urban school samples. *Health Psychology, 5*, 503–529.

Wilson, B. F., & Schoenborn, C. A. (1989). A healthy marriage. *American Demographics* (November).

Wilson, D. R., Widmer, R. B., Cadoret, R. J., & Judiesch, K. (1983). Somatic symptoms: A major feature of depression in a family practice. *Journal of Affective Disorders, 5*, 199–207.

Wilson, G. E. (1965). Christian Science and longevity. *Journal of Forensic Science, 1*, 43–60.

Wilson, J. (1978). *Religion in American Society*. Englewood Cliffs, N.J.: Prentice Hall.

Wilson, J., & Musick, M. (1996). Religion and marital dependency. *Journal for the Scientific Study of Religion, 35*(1), 30–40.

Wilson, M. R., & Filsinger, E. E. (1986). Religiosity and marital adjustment: multidimensional interrelationships. *Journal of Marriage and the Family, 48*, 147–151.

Wilson, W. (1967). Correlates of avowed happiness. *Psychological Bulletin, 67*, 294–306.

Wilson, W., & Kawamura, W. (1967). Rigidity, adjustment, and social responsibility as possible correlates of religiousness: A test of three points of view. *Journal for the Scientific Study of Religion, 6*, 279–280.

Wilson, W., & Miller, H. L. (1968). Fear, anxiety, and religiousness. *Journal for the Scientific Study of Religion, 7*, 111.

Wilson, W. P. (1972). Mental health benefits of religious salvation. *Diseases of the Nervous System, 36*, 382–386.

Wilson, W. P. (1998). Religion and the psychoses. In H. Koenig (ed.), *Handbook of Mental Health and Religion* (pp. 161–172). San Diego: Academic Press.

Wilson, W. P., Larson, D. B., & Meier, P. D. (1983). Religious life of schizophrenics. *Southern Medical Journal, 76*, 1096–1100.

Windle, R. C., & Windle, M. (1997). An investigation of adolescents' substance use behaviors, depressed affect, and suicidal behaviors. *Journal of Child Psychology and Psychiatry, 38*(8), 921–929.

Wineberg, H. (1994). Marital reconciliation in the United States: Which couples are successful? *Journal of Marriage and the Family, 56*, 80–88.

Wingard, E. B. (1982). The sex differential in mortality rates. *American Journal of Epidemiology, 115*, 205–216.

Winkelstein, W., & Rekate, A. C. (1969). Age trend of mortality from coronary artery disease in women and observations on the reproductive patterns of those affected. *American Heart Journal, 67*, 481–488.

Winkelstein, W., Stenchever, M. A., & Lilienfeld, A. M. (1958). Occurrence of pregnancy, abortion, and artificial menopause among women with coronary artery disease: A preliminary study. *Journal of Chronic Diseases, 7*, 273–286.

Wirth, D. P. (1995). The significance of belief and expectancy within the spiritual healing encounter. *Social Science and Medicine, 41*, 249–260.

Wittchen, H. U., & Essau, C. A. (1993). Epidemiology of panic disorder: progress and unresolved issues. *Journal of Psychiatric Research, 27*(Suppl. 1): 47–68.

Witter, R. A., Stock, W. A., Okum, M. A., & Haring, M. J. (1985). Religion and subjective well-being in adulthood: A quantitative synthesis. *Review of Religious Research, 26*, 332–342.

Wittkowski, J., & Baumgartner, I. (1977). Religiosität und Einstellung zu Tod und Sterben bei alten Menschen (Religiosity and attitude toward death and dying in elderly persons). *Zeitschrift für Gerontologie, 10*, 61–68.

Witztum, E., Greenberg, D., & Basberg, H. (1990). Mental illness and religious change. *British Journal of Medical Psychology, 63*, 33–41.

Wolbarst, A. L. (1932). Circumcision and penile cancer in men. *Lancet*, January 16, 150–153.

Wolf, A. M., & Colditz G. A. (1998). Current estimates of the economic cost of obesity in the United States. *Obesity Research, 6*, 97–106.

Wolff, G. (1939). Cancer and race with special reference to the Jews. *American Journal of Hygiene, 29*, 121–137.

Wolinsky, F. D., & Stump, T. E. (1996). Age and the sense of control among older adults. *Journal of Gerontology*, 51B, S217–S220.

Woloshin, S., Schwartz, L. M., Tosteson, A. N., Chang, C. H., Wright, B., Plohman, J., & Fisher, E. S. (1997). Perceived adequacy of tangible social support and health outcomes in patients with coronary artery disease. *Journal of General Internal Medicine*, 12, 613–618.

Wood, J. B., & Parham, I. A. (1990). Coping with perceived burden: Ethnic and cultural issues in Alzheimer's family caregiving. *Journal of Applied Gerontology*, 9, 325–339.

Woodruff, J. T. (1985). Premarital sexual behavior and religious adolescents. *Journal for the Scientific Study of Religion*, 24, 343–366.

Woods, T. E., Antoni, M. H., Ironson, G. H., & Kling, D. W. (1999). Religiosity is associated with affective and immune status in symptomatic HIV-infected gay men. *Journal of Psychosomatic Research*, 46,165–176.

Woodward, K. (1997). Is God listening? *Newsweek* (March 31), 56–65.

Wootton, R. J., & Allen, D. F. (1983). Dramatic religious conversion and schizophrenic decompensation. *Journal of Religion and Health*, 22, 212–220.

World Almanac (1997). *World Almanac and Book of Facts.* New York: World Almanac Books.

Worthington, E. L. (1986). Religious counseling: A review of published empirical research. *Journal of Counseling and Development*, 64, 421–431.

Worthington, E. L. (1989). Religious faith across the life span: Implications for counseling and research. *Counseling Psychologist*, 17, 555–612.

Worthington, E. L. (1991). Psychotherapy and religious values: An update. *Journal of Psychology and Christianity*, 10, 211–223.

Worthington, E. L., Kurusu, T. A., McCullough, M. E., & Sandage, S. J. (1996). Empirical research on religion and psychotherapeutic processes and outcomes: A 10-year review and research prospectus. *Psychological Bulletin*, 119, 448–487.

Wright, D., & Cox, E. (1971). Changes in moral belief among sixth-form boys and girls (ages 16–20) over a seven-year period in relation to religious belief, age, and sex difference. *British Journal of Social and Clinical Psychology*, 10, 332–341.

Wright, J. C. (1959). Personal adjustment and its relationship to religious attitude and certainty. *Religious Education*, 54, 521–523.

Wright, K. (1998). Professional, ethical, and legal implications for spiritual care in nursing. *Image: Journal of Nursing Scholarship*, 30, 81–83.

Wright, L. S., Frost, C. J., & Wisecarver, S. J. (1993). Church attendance, meaningfulness of religion, and depressive symptomatology among adolescents. *Journal of Youth and Adolescence*, 22, 559–568.

Wright, S. D., Pratt, C. C., & Schmall, V. L. (1985). Spiritual support for caregivers of dementia patients. *Journal of Religion and Health*, 24, 31–38.

Wynder, E. L., Lemon, F. R., & Bross, I. J. (1959). Cancer and coronary artery disease among Seventh-Day Adventists. *Cancer*, 12, 1016–1028.

Xiao, S., Young, D., & Zhang, H. (1998). Taoistic cognitive psychotherapy for neurotic patients: A preliminary clinical trial. *Psychiatry and Clinical Neurosciences*, 52(suppl.), S238–241.

Yang, B. (1992). The economy and suicide: A time-series study of the U.S.A. *American Journal of Economics and Sociology*, 51(1), 87–99.

Yang, B., & Lester, D. (1991). Correlates of state-wide divorce rates. *Journal of Divorce and Remarriage*, 15(3–4), 219–223.

Yang, M. S., Yang, M. J., Liu, Y. H., & Ko, Y. C. (1998). Prevalence and related risk factors of licit and illicit substances use by adolescent students in southern Taiwan. *Public Health*, 112(5), 347–352.

Yates, J. W., Chalmer, B. J., St. James, P., Follansbee, M., & McKegney, F. P. (1981). Religion in patients with advanced cancer. *Medical and Pediatric Oncology*, 9, 121–128.

Yelsma, P., & Montambo, L. (1990). Patients' and spouses' religious problem-solving styles and their physiological health. *Psychological Reports*, 66, 857–858.

Yesavage, J. A., Brink, T. L., & Rose, T. L. (1983). Development and validation of a geriatric depression screening scale. *Journal of Psychiatric Research*, 17, 37–52.

Yeung, P. P., & Greenwald, S. (1992). Jewish Americans and mental health: Results of the NIMH Epidemiologic Catchment Area study. *Social Psychiatry and Psychiatric Epidemiology*, 27, 292–297.

Young, G., & Dowling, W. (1987). Dimensions of religiosity in old age: Accounting for variation in types of participation. *Journal of Gerontology*, 42, 376–380.

Young, M., & Daniels, S. (1980). Born-again status as a factor in death anxiety. *Psychological Reports*, 47, 367–370.

Young, M., & Daniels, S. (1981). Religious correlates of death anxiety among high school students in the rural south. *Death Education*, 4, 223–233.

Young, N. K. (1997). The effects of alcohol and other drugs on children. *Journal of Psychoactive Drugs*, 29(1), 23–42.

Youth Risk Behavior Survey (1995). *Youth Risk Behavior Surveillance–United States, 1993*. Washington, D.C.: U.S. Department of Health and Human Services.

Zaldivar, A., & Smolowitz, J. (1994). Perceptions of the importance placed on religion and folk medicine by non-Mexican-American Hispanic adults with diabetes. *Diabetes Educator*, 20, 303–306.

Zamarra, J. W., Schneider, R. H., Besseghini, I., Robinson, D. K., & Salerno, J. W. (1996). Usefulness of the transcendental meditation program in the treatment of patients with coronary artery disease. *American Journal of Cardiology*, 77, 867–870.

Zautra, A., Beier, E., & Cappel, L. (1977). The dimensions of life quality in a community. *American Journal of Community Psychology*, 5(1), 85–97.

Zborowski, M. (1952). Cultural components in responses to pain. *Journal of Social Issues*, 8, 16–30.

Zeidner, M., & Hammer, A. L. (1992). Coping with missile attack: Resources, strategies, and outcomes. *Journal of Personality*, 60, 709–746.

Zhang, J., & Jin, S. (1996). Determinants of suicide ideation: A comparison of Chinese and American college students. *Adolescence*, 31(122), 451–467.

Zhang, J., & Thomas, D. L. (1991). Familial and religious influences on suicidal ideation. *Family Perspective*, 25, 301–321.

Zhang, J., & Thomas, D. L. (1994). Modernization theory revisited a cross-cultural study of adolescent conformity to significant others in mainland China, Taiwan, and the U.S.A. *Adolescence*, 29, 885–903.

Zhou, Y. F., Leon, M. B., Waclawiw, M. A., Popma, J. J., Yu, Z. X., Finkel, T., & Epstein, S. E. (1996). Association between prior cytomegalovirus infection and the risk of restenosis after coronary atherectomy. *New England Journal of Medicine*, 1335, 624–630.

Zilboorg, G., & Henry, G. W. (1941). *A History of Medical Psychology*. New York: Norton.

Zill, N., & Schoenborn, C. A. (1990). Developmental, learning, and emotional problems: Health of our nation's children, United States, 1988. *Advance Data*. National Center for Health Statistics, No. 190, November 16, 1990 (pp. 1–18).

Zill, N., Morrison, D. R., & Coiro, M. J. (1993). Long-term effects of parental divorce on parent-child relationships, adjustment, and achievement in young adulthood. *Journal of Family Psychology*, 7(1), 91–103.

Zinnbauer, B. J., Pargament, K. I., Cole, B., Rye, M. S., Butter, E. M., Belavich, T. G., Hipp, K. M., Scott, A. B., & Kadar, J. L. (1998). Religion and spirituality: Unfuzzying the fuzzy. *Journal for the Scientific Study of Religion*, 36, 549–564.

Zollinger, T. W., Phillips, R. L., & Kuzman, J. W. (1984). Breast cancer survival rates among Seventh-Day Adventists and non-Seventh-Day Adventists. *American Journal of Epidemiology*, 119, 503–509.

Zorn, C. R. (1997). Factors contributing to hope among noninstitutionalized elderly. *Applied Nursing Research*, 10(2), 94–100.

Zorn, C. R., & Johnson, M. T. (1997). Religious well-being in noninstitutionalized elderly women. *Health Care for Women International*, 18 (3), 209–219.

Zucker, D. K., Austin, F., Fair, A., & Branchey, L. (1987). Associations between patient religiosity and alcohol attitudes and knowledge in an alcohol treatment program. *International Journal of the Addications*, 22, 47–53.

Zuckerman, D. M., Kasl, S. V., & Ostfeld, A. M. (1984). Psychosocial predictors of mortality among the elderly poor: The role of religion, well-being, and social contacts. *American Journal of Epidemiology*, 119, 410–423.

Zuckerman, M., & Lubin, B. (1965). *Manual for the Multiple Affect Adjective Check List*. San Diego: Educational and Industrial Testing Service.

INDEX

Baptists
  health behaviors of, 76, 365, 367, 457
  health services usage and, 415–416, 425, 451
  historical perspectives of, 20, 45, 48
  measures of, 496–498, 500
  mental health of, 104, 138, 157, 171, 199
  religious coping by, 84, 131, 152, 451–452
  sexual permissiveness and, 373–374, 376–379
benefits from health services, perception of,
    430–433
Benson, Herbert, 21, 58
benzenes, immune function and, 279–280
bereavement. *See also* coping
  mental heath impact of, 92, 121, 209, 215
  physical health impact of, 192–193, 296
  as process, 310, 342
bias, in publications, 71–74, 493
Bible. *See also* scripture reading
  beliefs about, measures of, 4, 20, 23, 496–
    497, 499, 504
  health effects of: as negative, 227; as positive,
    27, 29, 53–54
  in historical timeline, 27, 29, 31–32, 37, 40, 47
  marital satisfaction and, 196–197, 199–200
biofeedback, 261, 348
biological theories
  of mental health, 147–148, 204, 220, 222–223
  of religious experiences, 264, 272–275,
    470–472
biomedical factors, of medical service usage,
    410–411
blood-letting, historical use of, 39, 42
blood pressure, pathologic. *See* hypertension
blood pressure programs, church-based, 262–
    263, 365, 401
blood transfusions, refusal of, 66
born-again experience, 8, 22, 28, 105, 129, 173
brain function
  cerebrovascular disease and, 264–265,
    271–275
  historical studies of, 9, 34, 39, 43, 45, 49
  in religious experiences, 264, 271–275,
    470–472
brain imaging studies, 156–157, 271
breast cancer
  ethnicity and, 312, 315, 400–401
  genetic factors of, 293–294, 301
  immune dysfunction with, 282–285, 288,
    290
  mortality with, 314, 321
  per religious affiliation, 301–303, 305
  religious coping with, 65, 88–89
  screening programs for, 65, 293–294, 306,
    316, 399–401

Buddhists and Buddhism
  dimensions of, 7, 18–23, 468, 498, 504
  health effects of, 149, 287, 305–306, 352; as
    positive, 56, 362
  historical perspectives of, 28, 30, 56

Calvin, John, 38–39, 42, 496
Canada
  mental health and, 101–113, 168, 170, 196
  religious coping trends, 92–93, 149, 311
cancer
  diagnosis timing, 315–316
  natural history of, 293–294, 316, 345, 352–353
  prevalence of, 292–293
  psychosocial influences on, 296–298, 307
  religion's effect on, 10, 305, 309, 385: adapta-
    tion to, 307, 309–314; course of, 307, 314–
    316; development of, 307–309; as negative,
    64–65, 400
  religious affiliation and, 298–307
  religious coping with, 80, 85, 307, 309–314:
    by caregivers, 82, 87–90, 313
  screening programs for, 294–295, 315,
    399–402
  well-being in, 103, 106, 150, 209–210
cancer adaptation
  by caregivers, 88–89, 313
  grieving stages in, 309–310
  religious coping for, 80, 85, 307, 309–314
  spiritual caregivers for, 313–314
  of survivors, 314–315
cancer course
  psychosocial factors of, 296–298, 307
  religiousness and, 307, 314–316
cancer development
  immune function and, 282–285, 288, 290,
    295–296
  religious influences on, 307–309
cancer mortality, 293, 299–300, 302–305,
    321–322
cancer screening, 294–295, 315
cancer survival, religion's effect on, 314–315
cancer treatments, 316
caregivers. *See* health professionals; religious pro-
    fessionals
catastrophizing, 208
catecholamines, immune function and, 281–283
Catholic clergy, health factors of, 157–158,
    319–320
Catholics and Catholicism
  cancer and, 299–300, 400
  cardiovascular disease and, 241–243, 246, 258
  cerebrovascular disease and, 269–270, 273
  depression and, 120–121, 127